THIS BOOK BELONGS TO
PICU SJUH.
PLEASE TREAT ME
WITH RESPECT.
I AM TO REMAIN ON
PICU.
THANKYOU.
X.

Paediatric Oncology

Paediatric Oncology

Third Edition

Edited by

Ross Pinkerton MD FRCPI FRCPCH
Professor of Oncology, University of Queensland
and Director of Cancer Services, Mater Hospitals,
Brisbane, Australia

Piers N. Plowman
Senior Consultant Clinical Oncologist, Hospital for
Sick Children, Great Ormond Street, London; and
The Royal Hospital of St Bartholomew, London, UK

and

Rob Pieters MD MSc PhD
Professor of Pediatric Oncology/Hematology
Erasmus University Medical Center &
Sophia Children's Hospital
Rotterdam, The Netherlands

ARNOLD

A member of the Hodder Headline Group
LONDON

First published in Great Britain in 2004 by
Arnold, a member of the Hodder Headline Group,
338 Euston Road, London NW1 3BH

http://www.arnoldpublishers.com

Distributed in the United States of America by
Oxford University Press Inc.,
198 Madison Avenue, New York, NY 10016
Oxford is a registered trademark of Oxford University Press

British Library Cataloguing in Publication Data
A catalogue record for this book is available from the British Library

Library of Congress Cataloging-in-Publication Data
A catalog record for this book is available from the Library of Congress

ISBN 0 340 80775 X

1 2 3 4 5 6 7 8 9 10

Commissioning Editor: Joanna Koster
Development Editor: Sarah Burrows
Project Editor: Anke Ueberberg
Production Controller: Lindsay Smith
Cover Design: Stewart Larking
Index: Indexing Specialists (UK) Ltd

Typeset in 10/12 pt Minion by Charon Tec Pvt. Ltd, Chennai, India
Printed and bound in UK by Butler & Tanner Ltd.

What do you think about this book? Or any other Arnold title?
Please send your comments to **feedback.arnold@hodder.co.uk**

Contents

Contributors

B. Abdulkarim
Paediatric Unit
Department of Radiation Oncology
Institut Gustave-Roussy
Villejuif, France

Rita Alaggio MD
Consultant Peadiatric Pathologist
Department of Oncological Science
University Hospital of Padova
Padova, Italy

John Anderson BA(Oxon) MBBS MRCP PhD
CRUK Clinical Lecturer in Paediatric Oncology
Unit of Molecular Haematology and Cancer Biology
Institute of Child Health and Great Ormond Street Hospital
London, UK

A. Bernard
Paediatric Unit
Department of Radiation Oncology
Institut Gustave-Roussy
Villejuif, France

Alan V. Boddy BSc(Hons) PhD
Senior Lecturer
Northern Institute for Cancer Research
University of Newcastle
Newcastle upon Tyne, UK

H. Brisse MD
Service de Radiodiagnostic,
Institut Curie
Paris, France

Mark F. H. Brougham BSc MRCP
Department of Paediatric Haematology and Oncology
Royal Hospital for Sick Children
Edinburgh, UK

Gabriele Calaminus MD
Consultant Paediatric Oncologist
Department of Paediatric Haematology and Oncology
University of Düsseldorf

Children's Hospital
Düsseldorf, Germany

Modesto Carli MD
Professor of Paediatrics
Division of Haematology/Oncology
Department of Paediatrics
University Hospital of Padova
Padova, Italy

Giovanni Cecchetto MD
Associate Professor of Paediatric Surgery
Division of Paediatric Surgery
Department of Paediatrics
University Hospital of Padova
Padova, Italy

L. Desjardins MD
Service d'Ophthalmologie
Institut Curie
Paris, France

François Doz
Département d'Oncologie Pédiatrique
Institut Curie
Paris, France

Jackie Edwards
Clinical Nurse Specialist
Paediatric Oncology Outreach Nursing Team
Royal Marsden NHS Trust
Sutton, Surrey, UK

Helmut Gadner MD FRCP(G)
St Anna's Children's Hospital and Children's
Research Cancer Institute
Vienna, Austria

Anthony Gordon PhD
Microarray Business Unit Manager
MWG-Biotech (UK & Ireland) Ltd
Wolverton Mill South
Milton Keynes, UK

Nicholas Goulden
Royal Children's Hospital
Bristol, UK

Nicole Grois MD
Children's Research Cancer Institute
Vienna, Austria

R. G. Grundy
Clinical Senior Lecturer in Paediatric Oncology
Birmingham Children's Hospital
Birmingham, UK

Jyoti Gupta BSc(Hons) MB BS
Specialist Registrar
Gloucestershire Hospitals NHS Trust
Cheltenham General Hospital
Cheltenham, Gloucestershire, UK

Jean-Louis Habrand
Paediatric Unit
Department of Radiation Oncology
Institut Gustave-Roussy
Villejuif, France

Richard D. W. Hain MBBS MSc MD MRCP(UK) FRCPCH Dip Pal Med
LATCH Senior Lecturer in Paediatric Palliative Medicine
Department of Child Health
University of Wales College of Medicine
Llandough Hospital, Cardiff
Vale of Glamorgan
Wales, UK

Ian Malcolm Hann MD FRCPath FRCP FRCPCH
Consultant in Paediatric Haematology
Professor of Haematology
Great Ormond Street Hospital for Children NHS Trust
London, UK

Janet Hardy BSc FRACP MD
Director of Palliative Care
Mater Hospital
Brisbane, Australia

Darren R. Hargrave MBChB MRCP(UK) FRCPCH
Consultant Paediatric Oncologist
Royal Marsden Hospital
Sutton, Surrey, UK

Olivier Hartmann MD
Director of Paediatric Unit
Institute Gustave Roussy
Villejuif, Paris

Louise Hooker RGN RSCN MSc
Lead Cancer Nurse
Southampton General Hospital
Southampton, UK

Stewart J. Kellie MBBS FRACP
Consultant Paediatric Oncologist and Neuro-Oncologist
Department of Oncology
The Children's Hospital at Westmead
Sydney; and

Clinical Associate Professor
University of Sydney
Sydney, Australia

Ewa Koscielnak MD
Paediatric Oncology Unit
Olga Hospital
Stuttgart, Germany

Ruth Ladenstein MD
Paediatric Oncologist/Haematologist
St Anna's Children's Hospital
Vienna, Austria

Linda S. Lashford PhD FRCP MRCPCH
Director of Translational Research
Cancer Research Campaign
London, UK

Stephen P. Lowis BA(Hons) BM BCh PhD MRCP MRCPCH
MacMillan Consultant in Paediatric and Adolescent Oncology
Bristol Royal Hospital for Sick Children
Bristol, UK

Jillian R. Mann MBBS FRCP FRCPCH DCH
Emeritus Professor of Paediatric Oncology
University of Birmingham
Emeritus Consultant Paediatric Oncologist
Birmingham Children's Hospital
Birmingham, UK

Keith P. McCarthy MB BS FRCPath
Consultant Histopathologist
Gloucestershire Hospitals NHS Trust
Department of Histopathology
Cheltenham General Hospital
Cheltenham, Gloucestershire, UK

Heather P. McDowell MBBS PhD FRCPCH FRCP
Consultant Paediatric Oncologist
Royal Liverpool Children's NHS Trust
Alder Hey, Liverpool, UK

Boo Messahel MBCHB MRCPCH
Department of Paediatrics
Royal Marsden Hospital
Sutton, Surrey, UK

Christopher D. Mitchell MB PhD FRCP
Consultant Paediatric Oncologist
John Radcliffe Hospital
Headington, Oxford, UK

Bruce Morland MBChB MRCP(UK) DM FRCPCH
Consultant Paediatric Oncologist
Department of Oncology
Birmingham Children's Hospital NHS Trust
Birmingham, UK

David Newell
Northern Institute For Cancer Research
The Medical School
University of Newcastle upon Tyne
Newcastle Upon Tyne, UK

Anthony Oakhill MBChB DCH MRCP FRCP
Professor of Childhood Leukaemia and Transplantation
Bristol Royal Hospital for Children
Bristol, UK

Odile Oberlin MD
Paediatric Oncologist
Paediatric Department,
Institut Gustave-Roussy
Villejuif, France

Joseph A. O'Donoghue PhD
Associate Attending Physicist
Department of Medical Physics
Memorial Sloan-Kettering Cancer Center
New York, NY, USA

Catherine Patte MD
Institut Gustave-Roussy
Villejuif, France

Andrew D. J. Pearson MD FRCP FRCPCH
Professor of Paediatric Oncology
Department of Child Health
Royal Victoria Infirmary
Newcastle upon Tyne, UK

Thierry Philip MD
Director of Centre Leon Berard
Lyon, France

Rob Pieters MD MSc PhD
Head of Paediatric Oncology/Haematology
Erasmus MC
University Medical Center Rotterdam
Sophia Children's Hospital
Rotterdam, The Netherlands

Ross Pinkerton MD FRCPI FRCPCH
Director of Cancer Services
Mater Hospital
Brisbane, Australia

Piers N. Plowman
Senior Consultant Clinical Oncologist
Hospital for Sick Children
Great Ormond Street, London; and
St Bartholomew's Hospital
West Smithfield
London, UK

Jon Pritchard FRCPH FRCP(Ed) MRCP Hon FAAP
Consultant Paediatric Oncologist
Royal Hospital for Sick Children
Edinburgh, UK

Kathy Pritchard-Jones PhD FRCPE FRCPCH
CRC Senior Lecturer in Paediatric Oncology
The Royal Marsden NHS Trust
Sutton, Surrey, UK

Pramila Ramani MBBS PhD FRCPath
Consultant Paediatric Pathologist
Department of Histopathology
Bristol Royal Infirmary
Bristol, UK

Kanchan Rao MBBS MNAMS MRCP
Fellow in Blood and Marrow Transplantation
Great Ormond Street Hospital for Children NHS Trust
London, UK

Frank Saran MD FRCR
Department of Radiotherapy and
Department of Paediatric Oncology
Royal Marsden NHS Trust
Sutton, Surrey, UK

X. Sastre MD
Laboratoire d'Anatomie Pathologie
Institut Curie
Paris, France

Martin Schrappe MD PhD
Chairman
ALL-BFM Study Group
Department of Paediatric Haematology and Oncology
Hannover Medical School, Hannover, Germany

Elizabeth A. Shafford MBBS DCH MRCP
Clinical Research Fellow & Honorary Clinical Assistant
Paediatric Haematology and Oncology
Royal London Hospital
Whitechapel, London, UK

Janet Shipley PhD
Molecular Cytogenetics
Institute of Cancer Research
Sutton, Surrey, UK

Owen P. Smith MA MB BA Mod FRCPath FRCPCH, FRCP
Consultant Paediatric Haematologist
Our Lady's Hospital for Sick Children, and
St James's Hospital Dublin; and
Professor of Haematology
Trinity College Dublin
Dublin, Ireland

Rubin Soomal BSc MRCP FRCR
Department of Radiotherapy and
Department of Paediatric Oncology
Royal Marsden NHS Trust
Sutton, Surrey, UK

Guido Sotti MD
Chief Division of Radiotherapy
University Hospital of Padova
Padova, Italy

Richard Sposto PhD
Group Statistician
Children's Oncology Group; and
Associate Professor of Research
Department of Preventive Medicine
University of Southern California
Arcadia, CA, USA

Helen A. Spoudeas DROG MD FRCPCH FRCP
University College London
The London Centre for Paediatric Endocrinology
Middlesex Hospital
London, UK

Michael C. G. Stevens MD FRCP FRCPCH
CLIC Professor of Paediatric Oncology
Institute of Child Health
Royal Hospital for Children
Bristol, UK

Charles A. Stiller MA MSc
Childhood Cancer Research Group
Department of Paediatrics
University of Oxford
Oxford, UK

D. Stoppa-Lyonnet MD PhD
Unité de Génétique Oncologique
Institut Curie
Paris, France

Marry van den Heuvel-Eibrink MD PhD
Erasmus MC,
University Medical Center Rotterdam
Sophia Children's Hospital
Rotterdam, The Netherlands

Gareth J. Veal BSc(Hons) PhD
Northern Institute For Cancer Research
The Medical School
University of Newcastle upon Tyne
Newcastle upon Tyne, UK

Paul Veys MBBS MRCP FRCPath FRCPCH
Director of Blood and Marrow Transplantation
Great Ormond Street Hospital for Children NHS Trust
London, UK

W. Hamish B. Wallace MD FRCP FRCPCH
Consultant Paediatric Oncologist
Department of Paediatric Haematology and Oncology
Royal Hospital for Sick Children
Edinburgh, UK

Jeremy Whelan MD FRCP MBBS
Consultant Medical Oncologist, The Middlesex Hospital
University College Hospitals NHS Trust
London, UK

Jean-Michel Zucker MD
Département d'Oncologie Pédiatrique
Institut Curie
Paris, France

Preface

This book aims to present a succinct, but detailed, contemporary overview of the most important aspects of managing children with cancer. The choice of authors is intended to give the book a European flavour with emphasis on the treatment philosophies of SIOP and the larger European collaborative groups in contrast to that of most American texts.

The chapters on individual diseases contain details of clinical presentation, diagnostic work up, new imaging techniques and current treatments with chemotherapy, radiotherapy and surgery. Treatments are not presented in a didactic fashion but rather as discussions of the pros and cons of different strategies.

Since the last edition the sections on the molecular basis of childhood cancers and molecular pathology have been expanded to incorporate the rapid progress in these areas. Similarly, there are completely revised chapters on novel therapeutic approaches to both chemotherapy and radiotherapy. A number of new authors have been brought in to strengthen the chapters on haematogical malignancies and haematopoetic stem cell transplantation. There remains an emphasis on avoiding, detecting and managing late sequelae and the chapters on community and palliative care have been expanded.

The book is aimed at all members of the multidiscplinary team involved in tertiary care and also at general paediatricians concerned with shared care. It is hoped that it will meet the needs of anyone who requires an accessible summary of clinical features and modern management of children with cancer.

List of abbreviations

5-FU	5-fluorouracil	COMT	catechol-O-methyltransferase
5-HIAA	5-hydroxyindolacetic acid	CP	cyclophosphamide
6-MP	6-mercaptopurine	CPDN	cystic partly differentiated nephroblastoma
6-TGN	6-thioguanine nucleotide	CR	complete remission
ABMT	autologous bone marrow transplantation	CRT	conformal radiotherapy
ACTH	adrenocorticotrophic hormone	CSF	cerebrospinal fluid
AFP	alpha-fetoprotein	CT	computed tomography
aGvHD	acute graft-versus-host disease	CTL	cytotoxic T lymphocytes
ALCL	anaplastic large-cell lymphoma	CTV	clinical target volume
ALDH	aldehyde dehydrogenase	Cy	cyclophosphamide
ALL	acute lymphoblastic leukaemia	CYC	cyclophosphamide
ALT	alanine aminotransaminase	Cyclo	cyclophosphamide
ALP	alkaline phosphatase	DAH	diffuse alveolar haemorrhage
AML	acute myeloid leukaemia	DFS	disease-free survival
APC	adenomatous polyposis coli	DHFR	dihydrofolate reductase
APL	acute promyelocytic leukaemia	DI	diabetes insipidus
Ara-C	cytosine arabinoside	DIC	disseminated intravascular coagulation
AST	aspartate aminotransferase	DLBCL	diffuse large B-cell lymphoma
ATG	antithymocyte globulin	DL_{CO}	carbon monoxide diffusion capacity
ATRA	all-*trans*-retinoic acid	DLI	donor lymphocyte infusion
AUC	area under the curve	DLT	dose-limiting toxicity
β-hCG	beta-human chorionic gonadotrophin	DNA	deoxyribonucleic acid
BAL	bronchoalveolar lavage	DPD	dihydropyrimidine dehydrogenase
BED	biologically effective dose	DS	Down's syndrome
BFM	Berlin–Frankfurt–Munster	DTC	differentiated thyroid cancer
BMD	bone mineral density	EBV	Epstein–Barr virus
BMT	bone marrow transplantation	EDTA	ethylenediamine tetra-acetate
Bu	busulphan	EFS	event-free survival
CAE	chloroacetate esterase	EFT	Ewing's family of tumours
CAH	congenital adrenal hyperplasia	EM	electron microscopy
CBF	core binding factor	EOE	extraosseous Ewing's sarcoma
CCG	Children's Cancer Group	ESR	erythrocyte sedimentation rate
CDK	cyclin-dependent kinase	FAP	familial adenomatous polyposis
CEA	carcinoembryonic antigen	FDG-PET	fluorodeoxyglucose positron emission tomography
CFS	congenital fibrosarcoma		
CFU-GM	colony-forming unit-granulocyte macrophage	FdUMP	5-fluorodeoxyuridine monophosphate
CGH	comparative genomic hybridization	FEV_1	forced expiratory volume in 1 second
cGvHD	chronic graft-versus-host disease	FFS	failure-free survival
cGy	centigrays	FGF	fibroblast growth factor
CML	chronic myeloid leukaemia	FISH	fluorescence *in situ* hybridization
CMN	congenital mesoblastic nephroma	FLU	fludarabine
CMV	cytomegalovirus	FPGS	folylpolyglutamate synthetase
		FSH	follicle-stimulating hormone

FTC	follicular thyroid cancer		MRI	magnetic resonance imaging
FTI	farnesyl transferase inhibitor		MSD	matched sibling donor
G-CSF	granulocyte colony-stimulating factor		MTC	medullary carcinoma of the thyroid
GCT	germ cell tumour		MTD	maximum tolerated dose
GFR	glomerular filtration rate		MTX	methotrexate
GGTI	geranylgeranyl transferase inhibitor		MUD	matched unrelated donor
GHRH	growth hormone-releasing hormone		NF (-1, -2)	neurofibromatosis (type 1, type 2)
GIST	gastrointestinal stromal tumours		NHL	non-Hodgkin's lymphoma
GM-CSF	granulocyte/monocyte colony-stimulating factor		NPC	nasopharyngeal cancer
			NRSTSs	non-rhabdo soft tissue sarcomas
GnRH	gonadotrophin-releasing hormone		NSE	neuron-specific enolase
GTV	gross tumour volume		NSpE	non-specific esterase
GvHD	graft-versus-host disease		NK	natural killer
GvL	graft versus leukaemia		NPA	nasopharyngeal aspirate
GvT	graft versus tumour		OER	oxygen enhancement ratio
HBsAg	hepatitis B surface antigen		OS	overall survival
HDR	high-dose rate		PAS	periodic acid–Schiff
HEPA	high-efficiency particulate air filtration		PBPC	peripheral blood progenitor cell
HHV6	human herpesvirus type 6		PBSC	peripheral blood stem cell
HLA	human leucocyte antigen		PCA	patient controlled analgesia
HLH	haemophagocytic lymphohistiocytosis		PCR	polymerase chain reaction
HPLC	high-performance liquid chromatography		PDGF	platelet-derived growth factor
HSCR	haemopoietic stem cell rescue		PEM	protein energy malnutrition
HUS	haemolytic uraemic syndrome		PET	positron emission tomography
HVA	homovanillic acid		PFS	progression-free survival
ICCC	International Classification of Childhood Cancer		Ph+	Philadelphia chromosome positive
			PNET	primitive neuroectodermal tumour
ICP	intracranial pressure		POG	Pediatric Oncology Group
IFO	ifosfamide		PPB	pleuropulmonary blastoma
IGF	insulin-like growth factor		pPNET	peripheral primitive neuroectodermal tumour
IMRT	intensity-modulated radiotherapy			
IPA	invasive pulmonary aspergillosis		PR	partial remission
IPS	idiopathic pneumonia syndrome		PTC	papillary thyroid cancer
ITP	idiopathic thrombocytopenic purpura		PTV	planning target volume
JMML	juvenile myelomonocytic leukaemia		RAEB	refractory anaemia with excess blasts
JSC	juvenile secreting carcinoma		RB	retinoblastoma
KIR	killer inhibitory receptor		RBE	relative biological effectiveness
LC	Langerhans cell		RE	relative effectiveness
LCL	large-cell lymphoma		RFR	relative failure rate
LCH	Langerhans cell histiocytosis		RIC	reduced-intensity conditioning
LDH	lactate dehydrogenase		RMS	rhabdomyosarcoma
LDR	low-dose rate		RR	relapse rate
LET	linear energy transfer		RSV	respiratory syncytial virus
LFS	leukaemia-free survival		RTK	receptor tyrosine kinase
LH	luteinizing hormone		SBB	Sudan black B
LOH	loss of heterozygosity		SCT	stem cell transplantation
MAO	monoamine oxidase		SLD	sum of the largest diameter
MDR-AML	myelodysplastic syndrome-related AML		SMN	second malignant neoplasm
MDS	myelodysplastic syndrome		SPECT	single photon emission computed tomography
MHMA	3-methoxy-4-hydroxymandelic acid			
MHPG	3-methoxy-4-hydroxy-phenylglycol		SRS	stereotactic radiosurgery
MPNST	malignant peripheral nerve sheath tumour		SS	synovial sarcoma
MPO	myeloperoxidase		STI	signal transduction inhibitor
MRC	Medical Research Council		STS	soft tissue sarcoma
MRD	minimal residual disease		TBI	total body irradiation

TdT	terminal deoxynucleotidyl transferase	UD	unrelated donor
TMA	thrombotic microangiopathy	UKCCSG	United Kingdom Children's Cancer Study Group
TMD	transient myeloproliferative disorder		
TNF	tumour necrosis factor	VCA	viral capsid antigen
TPA	tissue plasminogen activator	VEGF	vascular endothelial growth factor
TPMT	thiopurine methyltransferase	VMA	vanillylmandelic acid
TS	thymidylate synthase	VOD	veno-occlusive disease
TSH	thyroid-stimulating hormone	VP-16	etoposide
TTP	thrombotic thrombocytopenic purpura	WT	Wilms' tumour
UCB	umbilical cord blood		

Reference annotation

The reference lists are annotated, where appropriate, to guide readers to key primary papers and major review articles, as follows:

♦ key review papers
• papers that discuss the results of a major clinical trial.

We hope that this feature will render extensive lists of references more useful to the reader and will help to encourage self-directed learning among both trainees and practising physicians.

PART 1

Scientific and diagnostic principles

Aetiology and epidemiology

CHARLES A. STILLER

INCIDENCE

Cancer is predominantly a disease of ageing and is very rare in childhood. In western populations, only around 0.5 per cent of all cancers occur in children aged under 15 years. The incidence rate is typically in the range 110–150 per million children per year;[1] this translates into a risk of 1 in 600 to 1 in 450 that a child will be affected during the first 15 years of life.

Childhood cancers exhibit a great diversity of histological type and anatomical site but the carcinomas most frequently seen in western adults – those of lung, female breast, stomach and large bowel – are all extremely rare among children. Cancer incidence data for adults are nearly always grouped according to the International Classification of Diseases (ICD). In the ICD, however, cancers other than leukaemias, lymphomas, Kaposi's sarcoma, mesothelioma and cutaneous melanomas are classified by site of origin. While this is satisfactory for the great majority of neoplasms in adults, it is more appropriate for childhood tumours to be classified according to their histology. In the International Classification of Childhood Cancer (ICCC),[2] the groups are defined according to codes for morphology as well as topography from the second edition of the International Classification of Diseases for Oncology (ICD-O). The 12 major diagnostic groups are as follows: leukaemias; lymphomas; brain and spinal tumours; sympathetic nervous system tumours; retinoblastoma; kidney tumours; liver tumours; bone tumours; soft tissue sarcomas; gonadal and germ cell tumours; epithelial tumours; other and unspecified malignant neoplasms.

The largest population-based series of childhood cancers in the world is the National Registry of Childhood Tumours, which includes virtually all children in England, Scotland and Wales with cancer diagnosed since 1962. Table 1.1 shows the incidence rates for Great Britain during 1986–95, a period when the average child population was 10.6 million.

About one-third of all childhood cancers are leukaemias, and, of these, about 80 per cent are of the acute lymphoblastic type (ALL). Between a quarter and a fifth are brain and spinal tumours, of which astrocytoma is the most common histological type. Neuroblastoma, retinoblastoma, Wilms' tumour and hepatoblastoma – the distinctive embryonal tumours of childhood – account for 16 per cent of all registrations. Lymphomas account for a further 9 per cent, with non-Hodgkin's lymphoma (NHL) somewhat more common than Hodgkin's disease. Langerhans cell histiocytosis has been omitted from Table 1.1 as registration of this group of disorders is thought to be incomplete and their status as neoplasms has been controversial; they are all included in the third edition of ICD-O, but with many subtypes coded as non-malignant. In the German Childhood Cancer Registry the annual incidence is 5 per million;[3] incidence is highest in the first year of life, and boys are affected one and a half times as often as girls. Myelodysplastic syndrome other than juvenile or chronic myelomonocytic leukaemia, which is included in the ICCC subgroup for chronic myeloid leukaemia, was also not coded as malignant until the third edition of ICD-O and registration has been incomplete. Many cases may also have been initially diagnosed as acute myeloid leukaemia. Total incidence is probably 3–4 per million children per year.[4]

Different diagnostic groups have distinctive age distributions. The incidence of ALL is highest among children

Table 1.1 *Registration rates for childhood cancers in England, Scotland and Wales, 1986–95 (National Registry of Childhood Tumours data). Total rates are standardized to world population*

Diagnostic group/ subgroup (ICCC)	Total registrations	Annual rates per million for age group (years)				Total (age-standardized)	Sex ratio (M/F)
		0	1–4	5–9	10–14		
I Leukaemia	4454	33.4	73.5	32.3	26.4	43.4	1.3
(a) ALL	3611	18.1	63.7	27.1	18.9	35.3	1.3
(b) ANLL	676	12.0	7.8	4.2	6.1	6.5	1.2
(c) CML	96	0.9	1.4	0.6	0.7	0.9	1.7
(d, e) Other and unspecified	71	2.3	0.6	0.4	0.7	0.7	1.1
II Lymphomas	1305	1.1	7.6	12.4	18.6	11.8	2.3
(a) Hodgkin's disease	514	–	1.2	4.3	9.5	4.5	2.1
(b, c) NHL	757	0.7	6.1	7.7	8.8	7.0	2.4
(d, e) Other and unspecified	34	0.4	0.3	0.3	0.3	0.3	2.8
III Brain and spinal	3242	29.7	33.2	32.6	26.1	30.7	1.1
(a) Ependymoma and choroid plexus	314	5.1	4.8	2.0	1.9	3.1	1.2
(b) Astrocytoma	1352	8.5	14.2	13.8	11.2	12.8	1.0
(c) PNET	652	6.2	7.6	6.9	4.0	6.2	1.5
(d) Other glioma	414	2.6	3.1	5.2	3.5	3.9	1.0
(e) Other specified	319	3.1	1.9	3.2	3.7	2.9	1.2
(f) Unspecified	191	4.2	1.6	1.6	1.7	1.8	1.0
IV Sympathetic nervous	918	34.3	17.8	3.2	0.7	9.4	1.2
(a) Neuroblastoma	904	34.2	17.6	3.2	0.6	9.3	1.2
(b) Other	14	0.1	0.3	0.1	0.1	0.1	0.3
V Retinoblastoma	439	23.6	8.2	0.6	0.0	4.6	1.1
VI Renal tumours	772	14.7	16.6	4.0	0.9	7.9	1.0
(a) Wilms' tumour etc.	754	14.5	16.6	3.9	0.6	7.7	1.0
(b) Renal carcinoma	16	–	–	0.1	0.4	0.1	1.3
(c) Other and unspecified	2	0.3	–	–	–	0.0	–
VII Hepatic tumours	125	5.0	1.7	0.5	0.6	1.2	1.9
(a) Hepatoblastoma	96	4.7	1.6	0.2	0.2	1.0	2.0
(b) Hepatic carcinoma	29	0.3	0.1	0.3	0.4	0.3	1.6
VIII Bone tumours	567	0.8	0.9	4.3	11.2	5.0	1.1
(a) Osteosarcoma	296	–	0.2	2.3	6.1	2.6	1.0
(c) Ewing's sarcoma	229	0.1	0.6	1.7	4.3	2.0	1.2
(b, d, e) Other and unspecified	42	0.7	0.0	0.2	0.8	0.4	1.0
IX Soft tissue sarcoma	988	13.9	11.7	7.1	8.4	9.5	1.2
(a) Rhabdomyosarcoma	564	5.7	9.1	4.4	2.9	5.5	1.3
(b) Fibrosarcoma	113	2.3	0.5	0.8	1.5	1.0	1.1
(c, d) Other specified	244	4.1	1.7	1.6	3.2	2.3	1.1
(e) Unspecified	67	1.9	0.5	0.4	0.8	0.6	1.2
X Gonadal and germ cell	445	10.3	4.7	1.8	4.9	4.3	0.9
(a) Intracranial/intraspinal germ cell	131	2.0	0.6	0.9	2.0	1.2	1.6
(b) Other extragonadal germ cell	105	4.9	1.9	0.1	0.2	1.1	0.3
(c) Gonadal germ cell	188	3.2	2.1	0.7	2.3	1.8	1.2
(d, e) Other and unspecified	21	0.1	0.1	0.1	0.4	0.2	0.2
XI Carcinoma and melanoma	456	0.5	1.4	2.8	9.2	4.0	0.8
(a) Adrenocortical carcinoma	15	–	0.2	0.1	0.1	0.1	0.3
(b) Thyroid carcinoma	54	–	0.1	0.3	1.2	0.5	0.5
(c) Nasopharyngeal carcinoma	25	–	–	0.1	0.6	0.2	3.2
(d) Malignant melanoma	160	0.4	0.7	1.2	2.8	1.4	0.8
(e) Skin carcinoma	83	0.1	0.2	0.5	1.7	0.7	1.1
(f) Other carcinoma	119	–	0.2	0.5	2.8	1.0	0.9
XII Other and unspecified	90	1.8	0.9	0.6	0.8	0.9	0.7
Total	13 801	169.1	178.3	102.1	108.0	132.6	1.2

ALL, acute lymphoblastic leukaemia; ANLL, acute non-lymphocytic leukaemia; CML, chronic myeloid leukaemia; ICCC, International Classification of Childhood Cancer; NHL, non-Hodgkin's lymphoma; PNET, primitive neuroectodermal tumour; –, no registrations in this age group.

aged 2–3 years. Early age peaks in incidence are also found for the embryonal tumours; indeed, for neuroblastoma, retinoblastoma and hepatoblastoma, the highest incidence is found in the first year of life. By contrast, Hodgkin's disease, osteosarcoma, Ewing's sarcoma and malignant melanoma show a marked increase in incidence with age that continues into early adulthood. A third pattern of incidence related to age is seen in fibrosarcoma, where a peak in infancy is followed by a very low incidence, which then increases in the 10–14 year age group. The apparently similar pattern for gonadal germ cell tumours is in fact a combination of different age distributions for the two sexes. In boys the incidence is highest in early childhood and then falls sharply; the start of the postpubertal rise through adolescence is barely discernible before the age of 15 years. In girls, incidence is lower in early childhood, but the increase in the years following puberty takes place at an earlier age than in boys.

Overall, childhood cancer is about one-fifth more common among boys than among girls. The male predominance is greatest for lymphomas, liver tumours and nasopharyngeal carcinoma, and less marked for leukaemia, brain tumours, neuroblastoma and soft tissue sarcomas. The two sexes have similar incidences of retinoblastoma and Wilms' tumour. Only for extragonadal, non-intracranial germ cell tumours, malignant melanoma and some carcinomas, notably those of the adrenal cortex and thyroid, is there an excess of girls. The markedly different age distribution of gonadal germ cell tumours in the two sexes has been mentioned previously. For the other main diagnostic groups the sex ratio varies relatively little with age.

The patterns of incidence described above are typical of those found in mainly white populations throughout Europe, North America and Oceania. The principal systematic exceptions occur in eastern Europe, where the incidence of ALL is somewhat lower than in the West and the peak at age 2–3 years is less marked,[5] whereas Hodgkin's disease has a rather higher incidence, particularly before the age of 10 years.[1] Published data on variations in incidence with ethnic group in western countries largely concern comparisons between blacks and whites in the USA. Overall, the incidence of childhood cancer in blacks is lower than in whites, mainly because incidence of ALL in blacks is only half that in whites.[1] Several other diagnostic groups have a slightly lower incidence in American blacks, and Ewing's sarcoma is hardly ever seen. Children of Asian ethnic origin in Britain appear to have a higher incidence of Hodgkin's disease, particularly in early childhood, and of germ cell tumours, but a lower incidence of rhabdomyosarcoma.[6,7]

Greater variations in incidence are found between other regions of the world. The most striking long-standing example is the extremely high incidence of Burkitt's lymphoma in some parts of tropical Africa and in Papua New Guinea where it is by far the commonest cancer among children.

In Britain, ALL has a higher incidence in areas of higher socioeconomic status, particularly in early childhood.[8] The lower incidence in American and African blacks may be at least partly an effect of social class. A higher incidence of Hodgkin's disease, predominantly of the nodular sclerosing subtype, among older children and young adults has been associated with higher socioeconomic status in several studies.[9] In many developing countries, Hodgkin's disease has a higher incidence among young children, and the mixed cellularity subtype is more common, a pattern which seems to be linked to poor socioeconomic conditions.[10] Neuroblastoma may be slightly more common in children of lower socioeconomic status.[11,12]

There is no evidence of any major change in the incidence of childhood cancer during recent years in most regions of the world. In the United States, for example, there have been only small changes in overall incidence since the mid-1970s.[13] There was a rather sudden increase in the incidence of central nervous system (CNS) tumours in the mid-1980s, largely accounted for by low-grade gliomas and consistent with improved detection following the widespread introduction of nuclear magnetic resonance scanning.[14] In Sweden, also, there was an increase in incidence of CNS tumours which was most marked for low-grade astrocytoma,[15] and it has been suggested that this could again be an artefact of improved detection.[16] In north-west England, incidence rates for both pilocytic astrocytoma and primitive neuroectodermal tumours increased by 1 per cent per year between 1954 and 1998, and these increases could not be accounted for by changes in reporting or diagnostic practice.[17] Recent results from the Czech Republic indicate that the incidence of ALL in eastern European children aged 1–4 years has been increasing with improved socioeconomic conditions, resulting in a more marked early childhood peak, similar to that found in western industrialized counties.[18] Population screening of infants for neuroblastoma in Japan led to the diagnosis of large numbers of cases that would never have presented clinically, giving rise to a dramatic increase in recorded incidence.[19] There are two other exceptions to the pattern of, at most, moderate increases in incidence, namely AIDS-related cancers in sub-Saharan Africa and thyroid carcinoma in the region around Chernobyl. Both of these topics are discussed in the following section.

AETIOLOGY

Very little is known about the aetiology of most childhood cancers. For many diagnostic groups, the occurrence of the highest incidence at an early age and the cell type of origin strongly suggest that causative factors operate before birth and possibly even before conception.

The *MLL-AF4* and *TEL-AML1* fusion genes, which are characteristic, respectively, of infant null cell ALL and many cases of childhood common ALL, have been detected in neonatal blood spots of children with these diseases, providing confirmation that leukaemia can be initiated by chromosome translocation events *in utero*.[20,21] Many aetiological studies of childhood tumours have been concerned largely with exposures occurring during the mother's pregnancy, although postnatal factors have also been investigated. Most of the relevant studies published up to 1997 were included in Little's comprehensive review of childhood cancer epidemiology.[22]

This section will concentrate on putative risk factors that have been most frequently investigated or that have been the subject of more recent publications. They have been somewhat arbitrarily divided into environmental risk factors, genetic factors and other birth characteristics which could be markers for environmental or genetic risk. Some predisposing genetic abnormalities may have environmental origins and gene–environment interactions could well be important in the induction of malignant disease.

Environmental risk factors

The only environmental factor well established as the cause of more than a handful of cases in most regions of the world is ionizing radiation. The relationship between antenatal obstetric irradiation and subsequent cancer in the child was established more than 40 years ago through the pioneering work of Stewart *et al.*[23] At that time, exposure to diagnostic X-rays in pregnancy may have caused as many as 5 per cent of all childhood malignant neoplasms, but reductions in both the frequency of X-ray examination and the dose of radiation used at each examination will have reduced the proportion substantially in later years. No overall excess of childhood cancer was found among persons exposed *in utero* to radiation from the atomic bombs in Japan, but among those with adequate dosimetry there was an excess relative risk of two per gray between 1950 and 1984.[24] Ultrasound has now largely superseded obstetric X-ray examination in pregnancy, and there is no evidence for any increased risk of childhood cancer associated with obstetric ultrasound.[25]

In the past, the use of X-rays to treat benign childhood conditions, such as 'enlarged thymus' and tinea capitis also caused subsequent malignant neoplasms.[26,27] The groups of persons thus irradiated represented a small proportion of the total childhood population of the countries concerned, and the great majority of the resulting cancers occurred during adulthood. Radiotherapy for cancer can also give rise to second primary neoplasms. Although the cumulative risk can be high, many of the second primaries occur in later life[28] and so the number of childhood tumours caused by radiotherapy for a previous cancer is very small. Follow-up studies of children exposed to much lower doses of radiation from diagnostic cardiac catheterization have shown no evidence of an overall increased risk of cancer or leukaemia.[29,30]

Environmental radiation could also be a cause of childhood cancer, especially leukaemia. Among children who survived the atomic bombs there was an increased risk of leukaemia which reached a peak at 6–7 years after exposure.[31] There was also an excess of leukaemia among children in the area of Utah, in the United States, that received the highest doses of fallout from nuclear weapons tests, although this was based on very few cases.[32] In the Nordic countries there was a slightly higher risk of leukaemia in children who would have received higher doses of radiation to their bone marrow as a result of fallout from atmospheric nuclear weapons testing, but otherwise it was not possible to detect any dose–response relationship.[33]

The European Childhood Leukaemia/Lymphoma Incidence Study (ECLIS) has shown little evidence of any increase in leukaemia incidence attributable to fallout from the Chernobyl nuclear power plant accident in 1986.[5] ECLIS did not include the most heavily exposed areas of Belarus and Ukraine that were closest to Chernobyl. In Belarus the incidence of leukaemia remained fairly constant.[34] In a cohort study in Ukraine, the risk of leukaemia in the first 10 years of life among children born in 1986 in Zhitomir, one of the most heavily contaminated regions, was over three times that among children born in a control region that received little or no fallout from Chernobyl.[35] The numbers of cases were rather small, however, and while the cumulative incidence in Zhitomir was somewhat higher than in other populations, the control region had an unusually low incidence and the scale of any excess was almost certainly overstated.

Within 4 years of the accident, the numbers of cases of thyroid cancer diagnosed in children and adolescents in the most heavily contaminated areas rose dramatically. Some of the increase undoubtedly resulted from intensive screening for what is often a fairly indolent disease. Even if it is assumed, however, that all thyroid tumours diagnosed before 1991 were unrelated to Chernobyl, a large part of the subsequent rise in incidence can be attributed to radiation exposure, mainly radioactive iodine. Between 1986–90 and 1991–95, incidence in the most severely affected areas of Belarus, Ukraine and Russia rose by a factor of 7–9.[36–38] Further evidence for a genuine, Chernobyl-related increase is provided by the more aggressive histology and greater frequency of extrathyroidal extension of these tumours compared with thyroid carcinomas in western European children that were presumably not radiation-induced.[39] The association with short-lived radioactive fallout is strengthened by the fact that no thyroid cancers were seen among 9472 children from areas of Belarus within 150 km of Chernobyl who were born between 1987 and 1989 and would thus have been conceived after the accident.[40]

It has been suggested that inhalation of radon, a natural radioactive gas that is present everywhere but in varying concentrations, may result in irradiation of the bone marrow and thereby increase the risk of leukaemia. Ecological studies indicate that the incidence of childhood leukaemia may be related to radon exposure, but case–control studies have not shown any significant association and the number of attributable cases, if any, is likely to be small.[41]

Excessive exposure to the ultraviolet component of sunlight is known to increase the risk of skin cancer (predominantly in adults). An association in international data between ultraviolet radiation and retinoblastoma incidence[42] was not present within the United States, and at an international level was non-significant after adjusting for ethnic group and tropical climate.[43] There is no conclusive evidence that other non-ionizing radiations can cause cancer. There has been public concern for 20 years about the possible health effects of extremely low-frequency magnetic fields (EMF) emitted by electrical sources such as power transmission lines and domestic wiring. By far the largest number of epidemiological studies of EMF have concerned the possible association of childhood leukaemia with exposure to power frequency (50–60 Hz) fields. Most studies found a raised risk for the highest exposure level, although this was often not statistically significant. Two pooled analyses of data from case–control studies have yielded similar results.[44,45] There was no evidence of an effect from the lower exposure levels that are experienced by the overwhelming majority of children. There was, however, a relative risk of around 2 with exposure levels above $0.3\,\mu T$[45] or above $0.4\,\mu T$.[44]

On the basis of control data from studies that were not restricted to children living in the vicinity of high-voltage transmission lines, fewer than 2 per cent of children in western European countries and fewer than 5 per cent in North America are exposed to levels above $0.3\,\mu T$. A more recent study from Germany was similar to many previous ones in that it produced a non-significant raised risk for the highest exposure level, in this instance above $0.2\,\mu T$;[46] inclusion of this study in a pooled analysis would probably not materially alter the results. Allowance for known confounding factors in both pooled analyses made little difference to the results. The explanation for the consistently elevated risk at higher exposure levels is unknown, but it may be partly accounted for by selection bias. Central nervous system tumours are the only other group of childhood cancers to have been studied in sufficient numbers in relation to EMF; there is no evidence

of an association with EMF comparable with that for leukaemia.[47]

Cancer incidence among workers exposed to magnetic fields at 16.7 Hz has been investigated in several European countries where this is the operating frequency for electric railways, but there has been only one study of the effects in children.[48] The results, while non-significant, did not exclude a small excess risk, but the attributable risk must be very low as so few children live close enough to electrified lines to receive substantial exposure. In another study, there was little evidence that exposure to magnetic fields inside infant incubators increased the risk of childhood leukaemia.[49]

There have been reports of the possible carcinogenic effects of many different drugs taken by mothers during pregnancy. The only one of these agents firmly established as a transplacental carcinogen is diethylstilboestrol (DES), a hormone which was given to pregnant women with threatened abortion in some countries until the early 1970s. Exposure to this drug in utero caused clear cell adenocarcinoma of the vagina or cervix mostly in young women, although a few cases were observed in girls aged under 15 years. The cumulative risk of clear cell adenocarcinoma during the first 35 years of life among DES-exposed females is between 1 in 1000 and 1 in 10 000.[50] DES-exposed offspring have not so far been found to have an increased risk for other cancers.[50,51] As the use of DES was discontinued about 30 years ago, and there is no direct evidence for a transgenerational effect, it is unlikely that further childhood cancers attributable to DES will be seen in the future.

Several case–control studies of neuroblastoma have found a raised risk associated with maternal use of sex hormones during pregnancy.[52–54] Interpretation is difficult because of inconsistency between studies in the specific hormones for which data were collected and raised risks were found.

There have been several case reports of neuroblastoma in the offspring of mothers who took the antiepileptic drug phenytoin during pregnancy, but case–control studies have failed to find any consistent association between use of phenytoin or other anticonvulsant drugs in pregnancy and childhood cancer.[22] In a cohort study of over 2500 children whose mothers had previously been hospitalized for epilepsy and who were thus presumably exposed to anticonvulsants in utero, there was no excess of cancer overall or of any specific diagnostic group.[55] Various other drugs taken during pregnancy have been associated with a raised risk of particular childhood cancers in individual case–control studies, but hardly any of these findings have been replicated.[22]

Drugs given to children themselves have occasionally been reported as conferring an increased risk of malignant disease. In Shanghai, an association was found between use of the antibiotic chloramphenicol by children and subsequent risk of acute leukaemia of both lymphoblastic and non-lymphocytic types.[56] Chloramphenicol is less widely used in western countries and this finding has not been repeated.

Early suggestions of an association between human growth hormone treatment and leukaemia were not confirmed in an analysis of more than 24 000 North American patients in the National Cooperative Growth Study, among whom three cases of leukaemia were observed compared with 3.42 expected.[57]

Among 40 children with juvenile rheumatoid arthritis who were given the alkylating agent chlorambucil, three (7.5 per cent) developed acute non-lymphocytic leukaemia (ANLL),[58] and there have been several later reports of leukaemia following chlorambucil treatment.[59] Several agents used in the chemotherapy of cancer are also themselves carcinogenic but, as with radiotherapy, the number of childhood cancers caused by these drugs must be very low.

A case–control study that found that intramuscular vitamin K given to infants to prevent vitamin K deficiency bleeding was associated with a threefold risk of childhood leukaemia[60] caused much controversy and public concern. A pooled analysis of six case–control studies from Britain and Germany, including the one which gave rise to the controversy, found little evidence for a raised risk of leukaemia or other cancer among children recorded as having received intramuscular vitamin K.[61] For many study subjects, however, there was no record of whether or not vitamin K had been given. When vitamin K status was imputed for individual children in this category on the basis of hospital policy and perinatal morbidity, the odds ratio for leukaemia rose to 1.21 and was statistically significant, but when the earliest, hypothesis-generating study was excluded, it fell to 1.06 and was non-significant. Interpretation is rendered difficult by the poor quality of much of the vitamin K data. Overall, and in several individual studies, the odds ratio for no record of vitamin K status compared with a definite record that no vitamin K had been given was higher than that for intramuscular vitamin K.

Numerous domestic and other environmental exposures have been linked with childhood cancers. The most frequently investigated substances have included pesticides, and many epidemiological studies have yielded some positive results.[62] Interpretation is limited by the wide range of cancers studied, variation in the timing of exposure, ranging from before conception to during the child's lifetime, the small number of exposed subjects in many studies and the lack of information on specific pesticides. Nevertheless, the number of positive results and the fact that exposure to pesticides has been associated with related cancers in adults, notably acute leukaemias, lymphomas, CNS tumours and soft tissue sarcomas, suggest that this would be a fruitful area for further research. The most recent studies have followed the existing pattern of finding positive results for a variety of childhood cancers, namely leukaemia,[63] NHL[63,64] and neuroblastoma[65] but with diverse timing of exposure and little information on the types of chemicals involved. Domestic exposure to solvents other than pesticides has been much less often investigated. A recent American case–control study provided some evidence that frequent exposure to model-building or artwork using solvents is a risk factor for childhood ALL,[66] but the numbers of children in the high-exposure categories were very small.

Exposure to benzene is an established risk factor for acute myeloid leukaemia (AML) in adults, but investigations in relation to leukaemia and other cancers in children have been generally inconclusive, and many studies have used a diversity of proxies for benzene exposure. Of the three most recent studies that included substantial numbers of cases, one from Sweden that also included adolescents and young adults found an increased risk of AML with car density in the patient's area of residence at diagnosis,[67] but this measure is heavily confounded with population density and socioeconomic status. In Greater London children with leukaemia were more likely to live in areas with higher benzene levels, estimated largely from traffic flow data.[68] The remaining study, in Denmark, included leukaemia, lymphomas and CNS tumours and used calculated levels of benzene and nitrogen dioxide at all addresses from pregnancy to diagnosis;[69] there was no link between air pollution and leukaemia and the only positive finding, an increased risk for Hodgkin's disease with exposure to pollutants during pregnancy, may well have been due to chance.

Following experimental evidence that transplacental exposure to certain N-nitroso compounds can induce nervous system tumours, several epidemiological studies of childhood brain tumours, leukaemia and other cancers have investigated a possible association with exposure to sources of these compounds, most frequently cured meats and tobacco smoke. Most studies have found an association with high maternal consumption of cured meats in pregnancy, but there was limited consistency of results between studies, numbers of cases in some studies were small, and recall and selection biases could not be ruled out; moreover, childhood brain tumour incidence rose at a time when residual nitrite levels in cured meats fell sharply.[70]

In a study of drinking water contaminants as possible risk factors for childhood leukaemia, there was no association with nitrate levels during pregnancy or postnatally;[71] raised risks were found for a few other contaminants but these were not statistically significant and have yet to be confirmed in other studies.

Tobacco smoke is a potent source of N-nitroso compounds although it also contains other carcinogens. The offspring of mothers who smoke during pregnancy have an increased risk of adverse effects, including low birth weight and perinatal mortality, but the evidence on parental smoking and cancer in children has been somewhat inconclusive. In a meta-analysis of more than 30 studies,[72] there was a 10 per cent increase in risk of all neoplasms with maternal smoking during pregnancy but no evidence for an increased risk of any specific cancer. Paternal smoking was associated with a significantly raised risk of brain tumours and lymphomas, but the latter result was based on rather small numbers; recent large studies were compatible with a weak effect of paternal smoke on the risk of other neoplasms.

There is little consistent evidence to link maternal alcohol consumption during pregnancy with most childhood cancers, but three studies have found a positive association for ANLL.[22]

Several studies, including a large, international case–control study,[73] have indicated a protective effect against childhood CNS tumours of maternal consumption of vitamin supplements during pregnancy. Maternal folate supplements taken in pregnancy, which are protective against neural tube defects, were found in a recent Australian study to be associated with a significant reduction in the risk of common ALL.[74] This finding should be treated with caution, however, as it was based on fewer than 100 cases and has yet to be replicated, and a substantial increase in the use of folate by pregnant women was not accompanied by a commensurate reduction in the incidence of ALL.

When 48 studies on parental occupations and cancer were reviewed,[75] the most consistent associations were for leukaemia with paternal exposure to solvents, paints and motor vehicle-related employment, and for CNS tumours with paternal exposure to paints. A wide range of other occupational exposures were found on occasion to be associated with a raised risk of certain childhood cancers but with little consistency between studies. Subsequent studies have tended to follow a similar pattern.

The possible role of parental exposure to ionizing radiation in the causation of childhood cancer, especially leukaemia, aroused considerable interest in the context of excesses of leukaemia in the vicinity of certain nuclear installations in Britain. A case–control study in west Cumbria, which includes the Sellafield reprocessing plant, found an association of recorded paternal preconceptual external dose with risk of leukaemia and NHL,[76] but it has since been shown that radiation to the fathers could not account for the striking and persistent excess among young people in the village of Seascale near the plant.[77] In a national registry-based study which excluded the west Cumbria cases that were the subject of the earlier study, fathers of children with leukaemia or NHL were significantly more likely than fathers of controls to have been radiation workers.[78] No dose–response relation

could be detected based on individual exposure records, however, and the highest risk was for the lowest dose range, making it likely that this was a chance finding or that the raised risk resulted from exposure to infective or other agents. In a cohort study, the incidence of cancer and leukaemia among children of nuclear industry employees was similar to that in the general population.[79] In the case–control study, there was a significant association of childhood cancer with mother's radiation work but this was based on only 15 cases and three controls, and only four of the case children had mothers who were radiation workers during pregnancy.[78] An increased risk of leukaemia for children of female radiation workers was also found in a case–control study in Moscow, but the numbers of exposed subjects were again small.[80] In England and Wales and in Germany, as in other countries, there is no evidence of a general increase in the incidence of childhood leukaemia around nuclear power stations.[81,82] No consistent associations have been found with employment of either parent in occupations that tend to involve relatively high exposure to electromagnetic fields.[22]

Exposure to infections certainly plays a part in the aetiology of some childhood cancers. The classic example is that of Burkitt lymphoma in the tropics, where its incidence is very high. Children with Burkitt lymphoma in these regions generally have raised antibody titres for Epstein–Barr virus (EBV), whereas in temperate regions, where Burkitt lymphoma has a much lower incidence, few patients have raised EBV titres.[83] In the high-incidence regions, malaria is endemic and this is believed to cause a continuous, intense, antigenic stimulus, which alters response to EBV infection so that the latter gives rise to Burkitt lymphoma. A malaria suppression programme in part of Tanzania apparently contributed to, but was not wholly responsible for, a temporary reduction in the incidence of Burkitt lymphoma.[84] Three-quarters of childhood Hodgkin's disease may be a rare response to EBV infection together with an as yet unidentified cofactor.[85] EBV positivity has been found more frequently in cases occurring below the age of 10 years or of mixed cellularity subtype, and this may entirely account for the higher proportion of EBV-associated cases in developing countries.[86] The great majority of cases of nasopharyngeal carcinoma, especially in countries of medium to high incidence, are probably EBV-related.[85]

In a large cohort study of patients of all ages undergoing cardiothoracic transplantation, the risk of EBV-associated lymphoproliferative disease was 40 per 1000 person-years among the 66 children aged under 5 years at transplantation, and 19 per 1000 person-years among the 123 children aged 5–14 years.[87] The risk was particularly high during the year immediately following transplantation and among patients who were EBV seronegative before transplantation.

Infection with human immunodeficiency virus (HIV), whether by direct maternal transmission or through external sources such as contaminated blood products, carries an enormously increased risk of Kaposi's sarcoma and certain types of lymphoma. The regions of Africa most severely affected by the AIDS epidemic have seen a marked increase in the incidence of Kaposi's sarcoma in childhood. In Kyadondo County, Uganda, the age-standardized rate of Kaposi's sarcoma rose from 2.5 per million in the period 1960–71 to 55.8 per million in the period 1991–97, when it accounted for a third of all childhood cancers;[88] the incidence of Burkitt lymphoma also increased, although less dramatically, from 9.5 to 34.3 per million. Among children in a case–control study in the same area, HIV infection was associated with significantly increased risks of Kaposi's sarcoma [odds ratio (OR) = 94.9] and Burkitt lymphoma (OR = 7.5) but not with other cancers.[89] In western populations, by contrast, Kaposi's sarcoma remains rare even among HIV-infected children, but the risk of NHL, especially Burkitt lymphoma, is increased among children with HIV by a factor of 500 to 2000 depending on age and length of time since infection.[90–92] Leiomyosarcoma, which is exceptionally rare in childhood, also has an unusually high incidence among HIV-infected children and this may be a result of frequent EBV infection of smooth-muscle cells in patients with immune deficiency.[93] With current and anticipated levels of infection, HIV-related tumour are expected to remain rare among children in developed countries, although it is possible that small aggregations will occur in localities where there is a relatively high prevalence of HIV among women of child-bearing age.

Hepatocellular carcinoma is most frequently found among children in regions where the same tumour has a high incidence in adults. The association of hepatocellular carcinoma with hepatitis B infection is well known, and in areas where hepatitis B is common a large proportion of children with hepatocellular carcinoma are chronic HBsAg carriers.[94] In Europe, where hepatocellular carcinoma is very rare in children, a large proportion of patients also appear to be HbsAg-positive.[95] Some mothers of HBsAg-positive case children are themselves infected with hepatitis B but the infection need not have been transmitted to the children antenatally. Mass immunization against hepatitis B in Taiwan has been followed by a reduction in the incidence of hepatocellular carcinoma in childhood.[96] A decline in incidence may be expected in other countries where hepatitis B is endemic if immunization is introduced.

The finding of SV40 DNA sequences in cells from ependymomas and choroid plexus tumours raised the possibility that these tumours could have been induced by polio vaccines administered between 1955 and 1963 that were contaminated with SV40, but population studies have shown no difference in incidence between exposed and unexposed cohorts.[97]

The advent of the early childhood peak of leukaemia incidence in the most affluent western populations in the mid-20th century, and the persistently lower incidence in socioeconomically disadvantaged ethnic groups and less developed countries has suggested that ALL could be associated with an infectious agent linked to public hygiene conditions; this theory is supported by the striking inverse correlation between childhood leukaemia incidence and the hepatitis A force of infection among US whites and blacks and in Japan in the 20th century,[98] although this should not be taken to imply that hepatitis A itself is implicated in the aetiology of leukaemia. The JC polyomavirus has been suggested as a candidate agent but this seems unlikely since two studies failed to find genomic sequences of JC virus in leukaemic blast cells from children with this disease.[99,100] Similarly, no trace was found of sequences from the other polyomaviruses that can infect humans, BK virus[99,100] and SV40.[100] The absence in one study of any excess of herpesvirus genome in blood samples from children with common ALL compared with those from children with a diversity of other tumours suggests that herpesviruses, including EBV, HHV-6 and HHV-8, are also unlikely to be aetiologically involved as transforming agents.[101]

Although viruses are known to cause leukaemia in certain other species, notably cats, the absence in a large case–control study of any association between childhood leukaemia and pet ownership or exposure to an ill pet suggests that infectious agents of domestic animals are unlikely to have a role in its aetiology.[102]

Possible relationships between maternal infections during pregnancy and childhood cancer have been investigated in a large number of epidemiological studies. The two viral infections most frequently studied in this context have been influenza and varicella; as with several of the other putative risk factors considered above, there has been a variety of positive and negative findings and no clearly unequivocal associations have emerged.[22]

Greaves[103] proposed a hypothesis linking the 'common' immunophenotype of ALL, the commonest childhood cancer, with exposure to infection during infancy. Under this hypothesis, common ALL is the result of a sequence of two spontaneous mutations. The first would be associated with proliferation of B-cell precursors in utero and associated random mistakes in their replication. If immune stimulation of mature lymphoid tissue generates a positive feedback proliferation signal to the B-cell precursors, whose turnover in bone marrow is highest in early infancy, then the greater immunological challenge resulting from delayed exposure to infection may produce a less regulated proliferative stress. This in turn would bring about the second mutation in a cell belonging to a clone which had already expanded after the first mutation, and it is that second mutation that would precipitate clinically overt leukaemia. If this model is correct, then children with common ALL might be expected to have relatively few infections in the first months of life and correspondingly more shortly before the onset of leukaemia; the risk of ALL could also vary with the number of immunizations in infancy and the duration of breast-feeding.

Epidemiological evidence on specific infections in early childhood and subsequent leukaemia has so far been equivocal.[22] Children who attended day care outside the home from an early age would be expected to have earlier exposure to common infections but in two studies this was not found to be protective against leukaemia.[104,105] Differences between children with ALL and healthy control infants in HLA haplotypes related to susceptibility to infection, however, support an infectious aetiology.[106]

Several case–control studies[107–109] have found a significantly raised risk of leukaemia among children who had fewer immunizations, although in some of them this obtained for all childhood cancers and not just for leukaemia. An American case–control study found that conjugate Hib vaccination in infancy, introduced in the late 1980s, had a significant protective effect against childhood ALL.[110] A cohort study based on a trial in Finland comparing conjugate Hib vaccination at the ages of 3 months and 2 years found a 28 per cent lower incidence of leukaemia in the early vaccination arm, although this was not statistically significant.[111]

In a national case–control study in the UK, there was a borderline statistically significant 11 per cent reduction in risk of leukaemia for children who were ever breast-fed compared with those who were never breast-fed, and the effect was slightly more marked for breast-feeding of more than 6 months' duration.[112] When the results were combined with those of other studies, the results for leukaemia were broadly similar, and there was also some evidence of a reduction in risk of both Hodgkin's disease and NHL with breast-feeding for longer than 6 months. For all cancers combined, other than leukaemia and lymphomas, there was also a small protective effect, but this was unrelated to duration of feeding.

Seasonality in the occurrence of childhood cancer by date of birth or date of diagnosis would point strongly to an aetiological role for infection. The latest studies of seasonality in relation to childhood leukaemia in Britain, the United States and Denmark have, however, produced little convincing evidence. The range of variation between low and high rates has been fairly small and there has been only limited consistency in the timing of peaks in incidence between countries, regions or periods.[113–116]

There is a well established trend of lower risk of ALL with increasing birth order;[117] the highest risk is among first-born and only children, who of course could not be exposed to infection from older siblings. Children born more than 5 years after their last preceding sibling might have less opportunity to be infected by older siblings at an early age and they were also found to have a higher risk of ALL in one American study,[118] although no such effect was found in a more recent study by the same group.[104] The finding of a higher incidence of childhood ALL in isolated areas is also consistent with reduced exposure to infections in early childhood being a risk factor.

Kinlen[119] suggested that leukaemia might be a rare response to some unidentified, possibly subclinical, infection and that variations in incidence are related to variations in the level of herd immunity. Outbreaks of the infection would be most likely to occur in situations where susceptible and infected persons are brought together by high levels of population mixing, often as a result of migration. Support has been given to this hypothesis by the finding of an increased incidence of childhood leukaemia in several types of communities experiencing a high degree of population mixing, including rural new towns, areas receiving large numbers of servicemen, migrant construction workers or wartime evacuees, and towns with large increases in the level of commuting.[120] Increased incidence in areas of England and Wales with relatively modest levels of population mixing suggests that a substantial proportion of childhood leukaemia could be attributable to below-average herd immunity to an infectious agent.[121,122] There is also evidence of a role for population mixing from studies in Hong Kong[123] and in rural areas of Canada,[124] Greece and Italy.[125] Findings of increased risk of leukaemia among young children of fathers in occupations with high contact levels in rural Scotland and Sweden, even in the absence of population mixing, lend further support to the hypothesis, and particularly to the role of adults in transmitting the infection.[126–128]

Spatial and space-time clustering of cases of childhood leukaemia have been found in large series in several countries, including an international study covering 16 European countries and Australia,[123,129,130] although some other studies have failed to detect clustering.[131,132] A tendency for childhood leukaemia cases to cluster is consistent with an infectious aetiology and has often been interpreted as supporting the hypotheses of Kinlen[119] or Greaves,[103] although of course in some instances an excess of cases of leukaemia could be linked to some other environmental exposure or have arisen by chance.

The role of most environmental exposures in the aetiology of childhood cancer is far from clear. Obstetric X-ray examination is certainly carcinogenic, but accounts for well under 5 per cent of all current cases of childhood cancer. The only well established environmental causes in Western populations, other than ionizing radiation, are intrauterine DES exposure and infection with hepatitis B and HIV, which together can account for only a tiny fraction of all cases. Large numbers of other risk factors for childhood cancer have been reported, each one yielding a positive finding in at most a handful of studies, with negative findings for the same factor in other studies. It is impossible to tell from published reports how much of this inconsistency is due to causal factors being missed because of the small numbers of cases in many of these studies, how much to other variations in study design or in the population prevalence of risk factors, and how much to chance in the absence of causation. It seems very likely, however, that for most of the factors studied, either the associated excess risk is small or exposure is rare, and consequently studies of very large numbers of cases would be required to establish them conclusively as agents in the causation of childhood cancer.

Some recent case–control studies have been based on unusually large numbers of cases.[73,104,133] For some specific putative risk factors, notably parental smoking,[72] electromagnetic fields[44,45] and vitamin K,[61] previous studies have been aggregated in order to produce results based on larger numbers of subjects, either by calculating weighted averages of risk estimates or by combining individual records. While systematic reviews of clinical trials are well established, the use of similar techniques in epidemiology is still in its infancy.[134] This approach is perhaps particularly attractive and appropriate for childhood cancer epidemiology, where there is a real need for a systematic evaluation of the very large number of existing studies, often of large numbers of possible risk factors and involving fairly small numbers of cases of any particular diagnostic subgroup. It would have the additional advantage that, as new studies are reported, existing reviews can relatively easily be updated to incorporate their findings, and their conclusions can be modified accordingly.

Genetic epidemiology

Epidemiologically, genetic factors in the aetiology of childhood cancer may be detected in two ways: namely, through familial aggregations of childhood cancers with other diseases and through the presence of some constitutional genetic abnormality which may be manifested in distinctive associations of cancer with other conditions such as congenital abnormalities in the affected child.

The clearest example of a childhood cancer due to an inherited genetic condition is retinoblastoma. The genetics of this tumour are reviewed in Chapter 2. Many families have been identified with retinoblastoma in several members, and often in more than one generation. In a large proportion of these familial cases both eyes are affected. An unusually early age of onset can often distinguish heritable from non-heritable forms of a cancer, and the median age at diagnosis for bilateral

retinoblastoma is under a year, compared with over 2 years for unilateral tumours.[135] The usual definition of heritable retinoblastoma is any case in which there are bilateral tumours or a positive family history. By these criteria around 45 per cent of cases in western populations are heritable, although two-thirds of children with this form have no previous family history.[135] The frequent bilateral involvement and early age of onset accord well with the 'two-hit' mutational model of Knudson,[136] whereby retinoblastoma can be explained as the result of two mutations in what is now known to be the retinoblastoma suppressor gene *RB1* on chromosome 13q14. In sporadic cases the first mutation is postzygotic, whereas in heritable cases it is prezygotic, being either inherited itself or as a rare germ cell mutation which can then be inherited by future generations. The pattern of inheritance is essentially Mendelian autosomal dominant with a penetrance of about 90 per cent, although this is probably reduced in the rare unilateral heritable cases, and so the offspring of survivors of heritable retinoblastoma have a risk of nearly 50 per cent that they will themselves develop retinoblastoma. Survivors also have an extremely high risk of developing a second primary tumour, which in many cases cannot be ascribed to the treatment given for retinoblastoma. The relative risk is highest of all for osteosarcoma, for which the incidence among survivors of heritable retinoblastoma is hundreds of times that in the general population.[137] Many other types of second primary have also been observed, including malignant melanoma and carcinomas of the lung and bladder, and the risk of a second malignant neoplasm persists well into adulthood.[138]

In comparison with retinoblastoma, familial aggregations of other embryonal tumours are rare and a correspondingly much smaller proportion of cases can be regarded as genetic on the basis of family history. In the National Wilms' Tumor Study in the USA, a family history of Wilms' tumour was found in only 37 out of 3442 cases (1.1 per cent).[139] As survival rates are substantially higher than they were a generation ago, the proportion of Wilms' tumour cases with family history will presumably rise, but will nevertheless fall well short of the proportion of retinoblastoma patients with other family members affected.[140] Also in contrast to retinoblastoma, there are at least three, and possibly four or more, familial Wilms' tumour susceptibility genes, all presumably rare or of low penetrance.[141]

Familial aggregations of neuroblastoma and hepatoblastoma are even rarer, and there is little published information other than case reports. There is, however, a well documented association between hepatoblastoma and familial adenomatous polyposis coli.[142]

In the Li–Fraumeni syndrome, unusually large numbers of several types of cancer occur among members of the same family. The cancers involved include soft tissue sarcoma, adrenocortical carcinoma (ACC), premenopausal breast carcinoma, brain and spinal cord tumours and osteosarcoma, and there is a roughly 20-fold relative risk of childhood cancer.[143] Germ line mutations have been detected in the TP53 tumour suppressor gene on chromosome 17p13 in many affected families. Among 28 families with germ line TP53 mutations, there were significantly raised risks for each of the cancers listed above, and also for Wilms' tumour.[144] Other Li–Fraumeni families do not appear to have any germ line TP53 mutation and this could be due to chance, failure to detect TP53 mutations, or some other abnormality.[145] For example, germ line mutations of hSNF5[146] or hCHK2[147] can give risk to aggregations of cancers similar to those in some Li–Fraumeni families. Germ line mutations of TP53 have been detected in a high proportion of cases in two series of children with ACC but no family history of cancer.[148,149] In southern Brazil, the incidence of childhood ACC is around 10 times as high as in the rest of the world. A specific, inherited TP53 mutation was found in 35 of 36 affected children from that region, nearly all of whom had no immediate family history of other tumours characteristic of Li–Fraumeni syndrome.[150] The causes of this mutation are unknown but seem likely to be environmental.

Several other familial neoplastic syndromes can give rise to cancer in childhood.[151] The most numerous group of cases consists of those associated with neurofibromatosis type 1 (NF-1), which appears to account for 0.6 per cent of all childhood cancers. NF-1 is inherited as an autosomal dominant, but many cases are the result of new mutations. The most frequent cancers among children with NF-1 are tumours of the CNS. Overall, the risk of brain and spinal tumours is over 40 times that in the general population; the risk of optic nerve glioma is increased about 1000-fold. Malignant peripheral nerve sheath tumours can develop at the site of a neurofibroma, and many of these tumours in childhood are associated with NF-1. There is also an increased risk of rhabdomyosarcoma, and the relative risk for all types of soft tissue sarcoma combined is over 50. Various other cancers can occur in children with NF-1, and of these the commonest are the leukaemias: the risk of juvenile myelomonocytic leukaemia is about 200 times that in the rest of the population and ALL has a relative risk of about 5.[152]

Other familial syndromes characterized by the occurrence of tumours in affected members of a kindred account for considerably fewer cases of cancer in childhood.[153] They include multiple endocrine neoplasia type 2, associated with medullary carcinoma of the thyroid; dysplastic naevus syndrome (malignant melanoma); basal cell naevus syndrome or Gorlin's syndrome (medulloblastoma and basal cell carcinoma); and Turcot's syndrome (brain tumours and carcinoma of the colon).

If a child has cancer without known family history, then the risk of childhood cancer also developing in a sibling of that child is approximately doubled.[154] In a population-based study in the Nordic countries, the relative risk of cancer before the age of 20 years in siblings of children and adolescents who themselves had cancer before the age of 20 was 1.7, but after exclusion of families with known hereditary cancer syndromes the relative risk fell to 1.0.[155]

Familial aggregations of childhood cancer are largely explained by known genetic conditions and the contributions of as yet undefined hereditary syndromes and common environmental exposures are likely to be very small. Twins are a particularly interesting, although very small, subgroup of childhood cancer sib pairs. The concordance rate is especially high for leukaemia occurring in monozygotic twins during infancy. In most of these cases, the leukaemia arises in a single cell clone in utero in one twin and is then spread to the other by their shared placental circulation.[156]

Among genetic conditions which are not themselves neoplastic, the one most frequently associated with childhood cancer is Down's syndrome. The risk of leukaemia is increased about 50-fold in the first 5 years of life, and 10-fold in older Down's syndrome children.[157] Of this total, around 60 per cent are ALL and 40 per cent are ANLL. Thus, although a majority of children with Down's syndrome and leukaemia have ALL, the relative risk of ANLL is higher. Within the broad category of ANLL, the relative risk is highest for the megakaryoblastic subtype. The incidence of most solid tumours among children and adults with Down's syndrome tends to be lower than expected.[157,158] A complete absence of neuroblastoma in Down's syndrome has been tentatively ascribed to overproduction of the chromosome 21 coded S-100b protein, which inhibits the development of neuroblastoma.[159] There is evidence, however, of an increased risk of germ cell tumours.[158] Overall, 0.8 per cent of children with cancer and 2–2.5 per cent of children with leukaemia have Down's syndrome.

Tuberous sclerosis affects an estimated 1 in 15 000 children. These children have a relative risk of 75 for brain tumours and 50 for rhabdomyosarcoma, resulting in an 18-fold increased risk for all cancers combined.[151] About 0.1 per cent of childhood cancers are associated with tuberous sclerosis.

Certain genetically determined immune deficiency syndromes carry an increased risk of cancer, although as these syndromes are themselves very rare they account for less than 0.1 per cent of all cases of childhood cancer. Most of these cancers are lymphomas occurring in children with ataxia telangiectasia, and more than one-tenth of all children with this condition develop lymphoma or leukaemia before the age of 15.[160] Non-Hodgkin's lymphoma occurs at a similarly increased rate among children with Wiskott–Aldrich syndrome.[161] There is also an increased risk of non-Hodgkin's lymphoma and leukaemia among children with other rare, congenital immunodeficiency disorders, including Bloom's syndrome, common variable immunodeficiency syndrome, X-linked agammaglobulinaemia, IgA deficiency, severe combined immunodeficiency and Duncan's disease.[162] Among children with Fanconi's anaemia reported to the international register for that disease, 14 per cent had developed ANLL or myelodysplasia by the age of 15.[163] The risk for children with Shwachman–Diamond syndrome could be even higher.[164]

Wilms' tumour can occur in association with several malformation syndromes.[165] The complex of abnormalities including aniridia, genitourinary defects and mental retardation is associated with a chromosomal deletion at 11p13, which includes the Wilms' tumour suppressor gene *WT1*, and about 30 per cent of affected children develop Wilms' tumour. In a population-based record linkage study in Denmark, children with sporadic aniridia had a relative risk of 67 for developing Wilms' tumour.[166] Denys–Drash syndrome, whose characteristics include nephropathy and intersex disorders, is also associated with mutations of *WT1*; the incidence of Wilms' tumour is around 90 per cent.[165] Children with Beckwith–Wiedemann syndrome, which is associated with abnormalities at 11p15, have a cumulative risk of cancer of around 10 per cent in the first 4 years of life.[167] The most frequent cancer is Wilms' tumour, indicating the existence of a second Wilms' tumour suppressor gene, *WT2*, at this locus; the risk of neuroblastoma and hepatoblastoma is also significantly raised. Hemihypertrophy, either alone or as part of the Beckwith–Wiedemann syndrome, is associated with hepatoblastoma and ACC as well as Wilms' tumour.[168] A wide range of cancers has been described in children with Sotos syndrome.[169] Children with Costello syndrome appear to be particularly susceptible to rhabdomyosarcoma, although the risk has yet to be formally estimated.[170]

A higher than expected number of children of Pakistani ancestry with cancer in the West Midlands of England had autosomal recessive disorders, suggesting that parental consanguinity increases the risk of cancer.[171] In the United Arab Emirates, where half of all families are consanguineous, there was a higher than expected rate of consanguinity in the families of children with ALL.[172] For Hodgkin's disease and NHL, however, both of which have raised incidence in Middle Eastern countries, the proportions of children from consanguineous families were significantly low.

In a population-based study of over 20 000 childhood cancers of all types, 4.4 per cent of children with solid tumours had a congenital anomaly, significantly higher than the 2.6 per cent of those with leukaemia or lymphoma.[173] Congenital anomalies were found in over 6 per cent of children with Wilms' tumour, Ewing's sarcoma, hepatoblastoma or germ cell tumours. Neural tube defects and anomalies of the eye, ribs and spine were more common than in population controls but without being restricted to any particular type of cancer.

At present, under 5 per cent of childhood cancers can be directly attributed to genetic conditions. Variations in incidence between ethnic groups, however, as discussed in the first section of this chapter, have long suggested that hereditary factors govern susceptibility to a much larger proportion of childhood cancers. There is also a growing body of evidence that genetic variation influences the susceptibility of individuals to the development of malignant disease, especially leukaemia, following environmental exposures. For example, as mentioned above, specific HLA haplotypes may increase the risk of leukaemia following infection. Particular polymorphisms of several other genes have been found with increased frequency among children with leukaemia and these may heighten susceptibility to a range of putative carcinogens.[174–178]

Other birth characteristics

Several possible risk factors for childhood cancer are considered here which cannot with confidence be classified exclusively as either environmental or genetic in origin.

Overall there has been little consistent evidence to associate most childhood cancers with fetal loss or other maternal fertility problems.[22] Following several anecdotal reports of cancer in children conceived with assisted reproduction technology (ART), cancer incidence has been studied in three cohorts of children born following ART. Among 2507 live-born children in Britain, two cancers were observed compared with 3.5 expected;[179] among 5856 born in Sweden there were four cancers compared with 3.6 expected;[180] and among 5249 born in Victoria, Australia, there were six cancers compared with 4.3 expected.[181] The statistical power of these studies was low, however, and while there is little sign of a marked increase in cancer risk following ART, studies of larger data sets will be required for the risk to be reliably calculated.

Early studies found that the numbers of deaths from childhood cancer among twins were only 80 per cent of expected, and it was suggested that this might be due to prenatal selection against embryos with a disposition to develop cancer during childhood.[182] In pooled analyses of childhood cancer occurrence in twins from six studies, the standardized incidence ratio for all cancers of 81 [95% confidence interval (CI) = 67–96] and the standardized mortality ratio of 85 (95% CI = 74–95) were both significantly low and confirmed that the risk in twins is reduced by 15–20 per cent compared with singleton births.[183]

A national case–control study based on birth records and including over 3000 children with ALL who were born in England and Wales was consistent with previous smaller studies in finding significant increasing trends in risk of ALL with increasing maternal and paternal age despite the countervailing decrease in risk with higher birth order.[117] The relationship still obtained after the exclusion of children with Down's syndrome, for which high maternal age is a strong risk factor. There has been little consistency between studies in relation to parental age for other childhood cancers.

For most types of childhood cancer the results from studies of length of gestation, birth weight and stature at birth are inconclusive and positive associations have not in general been confirmed in later studies. While several studies have found a raised relative risk for birth weight above thresholds ranging from 3.5 to 4.5 kg in children with ALL, several others have not.[22] Notably, a recent population-based study in California which obtained data from birth certificates, and was thus not subject to selection or recall biases that tend to affect interview-based studies, found only a modest, non-significant increase in risk with birth weight above 4 kg.[184] If there is a real association, then it seems likely that high birth weight is a marker for some other risk factor rather than affecting the risk of leukaemia in its own right. A raised risk of hepatoblastoma among children of low birth weight has been noted in Japan, with a particularly marked excess for those weighing less than 1 kg at birth.[185] An investigation of 15 hepatoblastoma patients weighing under 1.5 kg at birth was inconclusive, but it seems likely that the association is due to some as yet unidentified environmental factor, possibly relating to medical treatment in the neonatal period.[186]

SURVIVAL RATES

In 1960, the age-standardized annual mortality rate from neoplasms among children aged 1–14 years in England and Wales was 86 per million. Neoplasms accounted for 16 per cent of all deaths in this age group and were the second most important cause after accidents. By 1999, mortality from neoplasms had more than halved to 34 per million, although, as mortality from all causes had decreased by two-thirds, they accounted for 21 per cent of deaths and still ranked second after accidents. This dramatic reduction in mortality reflects an equally dramatic improvement in survival rates for children with cancer.

In the 1960s, survival rates were generally low. Retinoblastoma, Hodgkin's disease, astrocytoma, craniopharyngioma and fibrosarcoma were the only major diagnostic subgroups with a 5-year survival rate of over 50 per cent. Towards the end of the 1960s the 5-year survival rate for childhood leukaemia was still only around 10 per cent. Since then, there have been great advances in the treatment of most childhood cancers, and these have resulted in markedly higher survival rates. Figures 1.1–1.3 show the 5-year survival rates for children in the principal diagnostic subgroups in the National Registry of Childhood Tumours who were diagnosed in successive

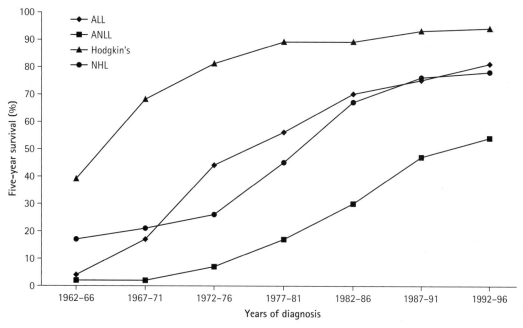

Figure 1.1 *Trends in 5-year survival rates for children with acute lymphoblastic leukaemia (ALL), acute non-lymphocytic leukaemia (ANLL), Hodgkin's disease and non-Hodgkin's lymphoma (NHL) diagnosed between 1962 and 1996 in Great Britain. (Source: National Registry of Childhood Tumours.)*

5-year periods from 1962 to 1996. There have been substantial improvements for almost every diagnostic group. During the 1960s, the main beneficiaries were children with Hodgkin's disease and Wilms' tumour. In the 1970s, there were further improvements for both these diagnostic groups but the increases in survival rates also occurred over a much wider range of childhood cancers; the most spectacular improvements were in ALL and NHL. In the 1980s, survival improved substantially for children with ANLL, osteosarcoma, Ewing's sarcoma and gonadal germ cell tumours. By the mid-1990s, 5-year survival exceeded 50 per cent for every diagnostic group shown in Figures 1.1–1.3. The EUROCARE collaboration has revealed considerable variation in survival between European

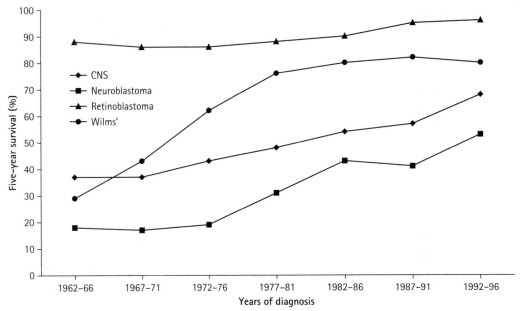

Figure 1.2 *Trends in 5-year survival rates for children with central nervous system (CNS) tumours, neuroblastoma, retinoblastoma and Wilms' tumour diagnosed between 1962 and 1996 in Great Britain. (Source: National Registry of Childhood Tumours.)*

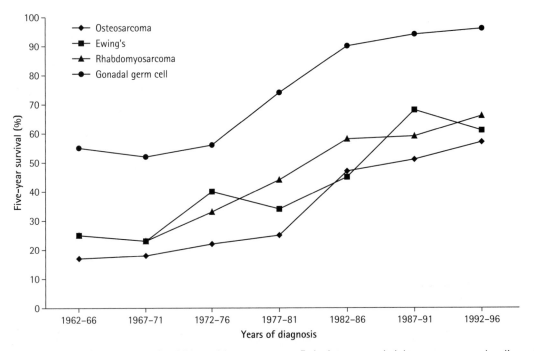

Figure 1.3 *Trends in 5-year survival rates for children with osteosarcoma, Ewing's sarcoma, rhabdomyosarcoma and malignant gonadal germ cell tumours diagnosed between 1962 and 1996 in Great Britain. (Source: National Registry of Childhood Tumours.)*

countries,[187] and comparative studies between Europe and the USA are in progress.

Undoubtedly these increases in survival rates are directly related to advances in treatment, as described in detail in other chapters. During this period of great technical developments in childhood cancer treatment, there were also major changes in patterns of referral. At one time most children with cancer were treated at local hospitals, there were few clinicians specializing in paediatric oncology, and opportunities for participation in collaborative studies of treatment were limited. Treatment has gradually become more centralized and larger numbers of children have been entered in national and international clinical trials and studies. For several types of cancer, survival has been found to be higher among children who were treated at specialist centres or who were entered in national or international clinical trials.[188,189]

STUDIES OF LONG-TERM SURVIVORS

As a consequence of the improved survival rates described above, the number of adult survivors of childhood cancer has greatly increased. Figure 1.4 shows the numbers of persons in Britain who were aged 18 and over at the end of successive calendar years and were known to have had cancer in childhood. By 1971 there were already over 1000 such survivors. Since then, the numbers have increased steadily and at the end of 2000 there were almost 15 000 adult survivors. At that point, about 1 in 1000 young adults aged 18–24 years, 1 in 1400 of those aged 25–29 years, and 1 in 2200 of those aged 30–39 years were survivors of cancer diagnosed before the age of 15 years; 17 per cent of adult survivors were aged at least 40 years, and the proportion in older age groups will continue to increase. Eventually, more than 1 in 1000 adults of all ages will be survivors of childhood cancer.

As the number of long-term survivors has risen, there has been a correspondingly increased interest in their subsequent health, and several studies of large series of survivors of childhood cancer are in progress. These studies focus on several questions: whether the patients are really cured, their quality of life, their risk of developing a second malignant neoplasm, the likelihood of their having children of their own, and the health of those children. Late effects and long-term follow-up are discussed in detail in other chapters. The following is a brief review of the epidemiological data.

Although there is a small risk of very late relapse, the great majority of 5-year survivors do appear to be cured, with only a 10 per cent risk of death from recurrent tumour or a treatment-related effect during the next

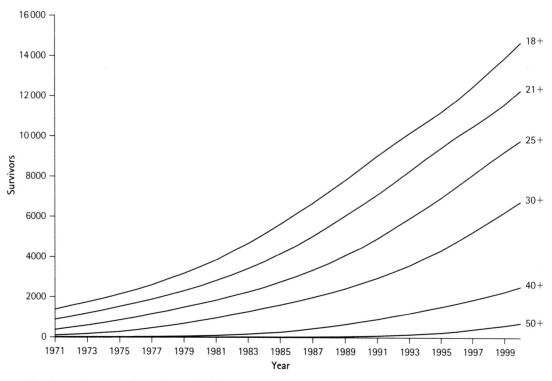

Figure 1.4 *Numbers of known adult survivors of childhood cancer in Great Britain at the end of successive calendar years, 1971–2000. Each curve shows the numbers of survivors who had attained at least the specified age in years. (Source: National Registry of Childhood Tumours.)*

10 years.[190–192] A recent population-based study from the Nordic countries found that subsequent mortality among 5-year survivors diagnosed in the 1980s was 39 per cent less than for those diagnosed between 1960 and 1979;[192] moreover, substantial reduction in mortality from the original cancer was not offset by any increase in treatment-related mortality.

Current indications are that the risk of developing a second primary neoplasm within 25 years following treatment for childhood cancer is about 4 per cent.[193–195] The risk depends partly upon the treatment given for the original tumour; some second tumours are radiation-induced,[28] and there is an increased risk of leukaemia among survivors who were treated with alkylating agents or epipodophyllotoxins.[196,197] There is also a genetic element in the aetiology of some second tumours, exemplified by the enormously increased risk of osteosarcoma and high risk of various other cancers among survivors of heritable retinoblastoma. The incidence of second tumours among survivors of childhood cancer may alter in the future. This may result partly from the changing distribution of original tumour types among survivors, as improvements in survival rates have not been uniform across all diagnostic groups, and partly from alterations in methods of treatment for most childhood cancers. Little is known about the risk among very long-term survivors, as they reach ages of 40 and above, the period of life during which the incidence of many of the common cancers rises markedly in the general population. These questions will be investigated through continuing follow-up studies of large series of childhood cancer survivors in the USA,[198] the UK and elsewhere.

Some survivors are rendered infertile by their treatment but many others will have children. Among about 900 female survivors treated mainly before 1970, there were 57 per cent of the expected number of live births.[199] Many of the children born to survivors are as yet very young and few have been followed up for a long period, and at present only tentative conclusions can be drawn regarding their health. Women given abdominal radiotherapy have an increased risk of low-birth-weight babies, apparently because of a direct effect of radiation on the uterus rather than a genetic effect.[200] There is little evidence of a substantially increased risk of cancer in the offspring of survivors after hereditary cancer syndromes have been taken into account.[201,202] The only group known to have a markedly higher risk consists of the children born to survivors of heritable retinoblastoma, as described above. The incidence of congenital malformations in the offspring of childhood cancer survivors appears to be little different from that observed in the population.[203,204] The longer-term health of the offspring of survivors and the health of children born to survivors who received more modern treatment for their cancers are currently under investigation.

KEY POINTS

- The risk that a child will develop cancer during the first 15 years of life is between 1 in 600 and 1 in 450.
- Well established environmental risk factors account for a very small proportion of cases.
- Obstetric irradiation may have caused 5 per cent of childhood cancers in the past but probably accounts for hardly any nowadays.
- Infection with Epstein–Barr virus, hepatitis B or HIV is definitely a cause of substantial numbers of cases in some tropical populations but accounts for far fewer in industrialized countries.
- Infection is probably involved in the aetiology of childhood leukaemia but its precise role remains to be elucidated.
- Certain rare genetic conditions are associated with childhood cancer but account for under 5 per cent of cases.
- If a child has cancer without family history then the risk of childhood cancer in a sibling is doubled, but virtually all the excess risk can be accounted for by known hereditary syndromes.
- Survival continues to increase and eventually 1 in 1000 adults will be survivors of childhood cancer.
- The risk of a second malignant neoplasm within 25 years of diagnosis of childhood cancer is about 4 per cent, but this may change and very little is known about the risk among very long-term survivors.
- The long-term health of survivors and the children born to them is under investigation.

REFERENCES

♦1. Parkin DM, Kramarova E, Draper GJ et al., eds. International Incidence of Childhood Cancer, Vol II. IARC Scientific Publications No. 144. Lyon: IARC, 1998.

2. Kramarova E, Stiller CA. The international classification of childhood cancer. Int J Cancer 1996; **68**: 759–65.

3. Kaatsch P, Spix C, Michaelis J. Annnual Report 2000. German Childhood Cancer Registry. Mainz: Deutsches Kinderkrebsregister, 2002.

4. Hasle H, Wadsworth LD, Massing BG et al. A population-based study of childhood myelodysplastic syndrome in British Columbia, Canada. Br J Haematol 1999; **106**: 1027–32.

5. Parkin DM, Clayton D, Black RJ et al. Childhood leukaemia in Europe after Chernobyl: 5-year follow-up. Br J Cancer 1996; **73**: 1006–12.

6. Stiller CA, McKinney PA, Bunch KJ *et al.* Childhood cancer and ethnic group in Britain: a United Kingdom Children's Cancer Study Group (UKCCSG) study. *Br J Cancer* 1991; **64**: 543–8.

7. Powell JE, Parkes SE, Cameron AH, Mann JR. Is the risk of cancer increased in Asians living in the UK? *Arch Dis Child* 1994; **71**: 398–403.

8. Draper GJ, Vincent TJ, O'Connor CM, Stiller CA. Socio-economic factors and variations in incidence rates between County Districts. In: Draper GJ, ed. *The Geographical Epidemiology of Childhood Leukaemia and Non-Hodgkin Lymphoma in Great Britain 1966–83. Studies on Medical and Population Subjects No. 53.* London: HMSO, 1991; 37–45.

9. Alexander FE, Ricketts TJ, McKinney PA, Cartwright RA. Community lifestyle characteristics and incidence of Hodgkin's disease in young people. *Int J Cancer* 1991; **48**: 10–14.

10. Stiller CA, Parkin DM. International variations in the incidence of childhood lymphomas. *Paediatr Perinat Epidemiol* 1990; **4**: 302–23.

11. Carlsen NLT. Epidemiological investigations on neuroblastomas in Denmark 1943–1980. *Br J Cancer* 1986; **54**: 977–88.

12. Davis S, Rogers MAM, Pendergrass TW. The incidence and epidemiologic characteristics of neuroblastoma in the United States. *Am J Epidemiol* 1987; **126**: 1063–74.

13. Linet MS, Ries LAG, Smith MA, *et al.* Cancer surveillance series: recent trends in childhood cancer incidence and mortality in the United States. *J Natl Cancer Inst* 1999; **91**: 1051–8.

14. Smith MA, Freidlin B, Ries LAG, Simon R. Trends in reported incidence of primary malignant brain tumors in children in the United States. *J Natl Cancer Inst* 1998; **90**: 1269–77.

15. Hjalmars U, Kulldoorff M, Wahlquist Y, Lannering B. Increased incidence rates but no space-time clustering of childhood astrocytoma in Sweden, 1973–1992. *Cancer* 1999; **85**: 2077–90.

16. Smith MA, Freidlin B, Ries LAG, Simon R. Increased incidence rates but no space-time clustering of childhood astrocytoma in Sweden, 1973–1992. *Cancer* 2000; **88**: 1492–3.

17. McNally RJ, Kelsey AM, Cairns DP *et al.* Temporal increases in the incidence of childhood solid tumors seen in northwest England (1954–1998) are likely to be real. *Cancer* 2001; **92**: 1967–76.

18. Hrusák O, Trka J, Zuna J *et al.* Acute lymphoblastic leukemia incidence during socioeconomic transition: selective increase in children from 1 to 4 years. *Leukemia* 2002; **16**: 720–5.

19. Ajiki W, Tsukuma H, Oshima A, Kawa K. Effects of mass screening for neuroblastoma on incidence, mortality, and survival rates in Osaka, Japan. *Cancer Causes Control* 1998; **9**: 631–6.

20. Gale KB, Ford AM, Repp R, *et al.* Backtracking leukemia to birth: identification of clonotypic gene fusion sequences in neonatal blood spots. *Proc Natl Acad Sci USA* 1997; **94**: 13950–4.

21. Wiemels JL, Cazzaniga G, Daniotti M *et al.* Prenatal origin of acute lymphoblastic leukaemia in children. *Lancet* 1999; **354**: 1499–503.

♦22. Little J. *Epidemiology of Childhood Cancer.* IARC Scientific Publications No. 149. Lyon: IARC, 1999.

23. Stewart A, Webb J, Hewitt D. A survey of childhood malignancies. *Br Med J* 1958; **1**: 1495–508.

24. Yoshimoto Y, Delongchamp R, Mabuchi K. *In-utero* exposed atomic bomb survivors: cancer risk update. *Lancet* 1994; **344**: 345–6.

25. Salvesen KA, Eik-Nes SH. Ultrasound during pregnancy and birthweight, childhood malignancies and neurological development. *Ultrasound Med Biol* 1999; **25**: 1025–31.

26. Ron E, Modan B, Boice JD *et al.* Tumors of the brain and nervous system after radiotherapy in childhood. *N Engl J Med* 1988; **319**: 1033–9.

♦27. Ron E, Lubin JH, Shore RE *et al.* Thyroid cancer after exposure to external radiation: a pooled analysis of seven studies. *Radiat Res* 1995; **141**: 259–77.

28. Garwicz S, Anderson H, Olsen JH *et al.* Second malignant neoplasms after cancer in childhood and adolescence: a population-based case-control study in the 5 Nordic countries. *Int J Cancer* 2000; **88**: 672–8.

29. McLaughlin JR, Kreiger N, Sloan MP *et al.* An historical cohort study of cardiac catheterization during childhood and the risk of cancer. *Int J Epidemiol* 1993; **22**: 584–91.

30. Modan B, Keinan L, Blumstein T, Sadetzki S. Cancer following cardiac catheterization in childhood. *Int J Epidemiol* 2000; **29**: 424–8.

31. Shimizu Y, Schull WJ, Kato H. Cancer risk among atomic bomb survivors: the RERF Life Span Study. *J Am Med Assoc* 1990; **264**: 601–4.

32. Stevens W, Thomas DC, Lyon JL *et al.* Leukemia in Utah and radioactive fallout from the Nevada test site. *J Am Med Assoc* 1990; **264**: 585–91.

33. Darby SC, Olsen SH, Doll R *et al.* Trends in childhood leukaemia in the Nordic countries in relation to fallout from atmospheric nuclear weapons testing. *Br Med J* 1992; **304**: 1005–9.

34. Gapanovich VN, Iaroshevich RF, Shuvaeva LP *et al.* Childhood leukemia in Belarus before and after the Chernobyl accident: continued follow-up. *Radiat Environ Biophys* 2001; **40**: 259–67.

35. Noshchenko AG, Moysich KB, Bondar A *et al.* Patterns of acute leukaemia occurrence among children in the Chernobyl region. *Int J Epidemiol* 2001; **30**: 125–9.

36. Antonelli A, Miccoli P, Derzhitski VE *et al.* Epidemiologic and clinical evaluation of thyroid cancer in children from the Gomel region (Belarus). *World J Surg* 1996; **20**: 867–71.

37. Tronko MD, Bogdanova TI, Komissarenko IV *et al.* Thyroid carcinoma in children and adolescents in Ukraine after the Chernobyl nuclear accident: statistical data and clinicomorphologic characteristics. *Cancer* 1999; **86**: 149–56.

38. Ivanov VK, Gorsky AI, Tsyb AF *et al.* Dynamics of thyroid cancer incidence in Russia following the Chernobyl accident. *J Radiol Prot* 1999; **19**: 305–18.

39. Pacini F, Vorontsova T, Demidchik EP *et al.* Post-Chernobyl thyroid carcinoma in Belarus children and adolescents: comparisons with naturally occurring thyroid carcinoma in Italy and France. *J Clin Endocrinol Metab* 1997; **82**: 3563–9.

40. Shibata Y, Yamashita S, Masayakin VB *et al.* 15 years after Chernobyl: new evidence of thyroid cancer. *Lancet* 2001; **358**: 1965–6.

♦41. Laurier D, Valenty M, Tirmarche M. Radon exposure and the risk of leukemia: a review of epidemiological studies. *Health Phys* 2001; **81**: 272–88.

42. Hooper ML. Is sunlight an aetiological agent in the genesis of retinoblastoma? *Br J Cancer* 1999; **79**: 1273–6.

43. Jemal A, Devesa SS, Fears TR, Fraumeni JF. Retinoblastoma incidence and sunlight exposure. *Br J Cancer* 2000; **82**: 1875–8.

♦44. Ahlbom A, Day N, Feychting M *et al.* A pooled analysis of magnetic fields and childhood leukaemia. *Br J Cancer* 2000; **83**: 692–8.

♦45. Greenland S, Sheppard AR, Kaune WT *et al.* A pooled analysis of magnetic fields, wire codes and childhood leukaemia. *Epidemiology* 2000; **11**: 624–34.

46. Schüz J, Grigat J-P, Brinkmann K, Michaelis J. Residential magnetic fields as a risk factor for childhood acute leukaemia: results from a German population-based case-control study. *Int J Cancer* 2001; **91**: 728–35.

♦47. Advisory Group on Non-ionising Radiation (chairman Sir Richard Doll). *ELF Electromagnetic Fields and the Risk of Cancer. Report of an Advisory Group on Non-ionising Radiation. Documents of the NRPB, vol 12, no. 1.* Chilton: National Radiological Protection Board, 2001.

48. Schüz J, Grigat JP, Brinkmann K, Michaelis J. Childhood acute leukaemia and residential 16.7 Hz magnetic fields in Germany. *Br J Cancer* 2001; **84**: 697–9.

49. Söderberg KC, Naumburg E, Anger G *et al.* Childhood leukemia and magnetic fields in infant incubators. *Epidemiology* 2002; **13**: 45–9.

♦50. Giusti RM, Iwamoto K, Hatch EE. Diethylstilbestrol revisited: a review of the long-term health effects. *Ann Intern Med* 1995; **122**: 778–88.

51. Hatch EE, Palmer JR, Titus-Ernstoff L *et al.* Cancer risk in women exposed to diethylstilbestrol *in utero. J Am Med Assoc* 1998; **280**: 630–4.

52. Michalek AM, Buck GM, Nasca PC *et al.* Gravid health status, medication use, and risk of neuroblastoma. *Am J Epidemiol* 1996; **143**: 996–1001.

53. Olshan AF, Smith J, Cook MN *et al.* Hormone and fertility drug use and the risk of neuroblastoma: a report from the Children's Cancer Group and the Pediatric Oncology Group. *Am J Epidemiol* 1999; **150**: 930–8.

54. Schüz J, Kaletsch U, Meinert R *et al.* Risk factors for neuroblastoma at different stages of disease. Results from a population-based case-control study in Germany. *J Clin Epidemiol* 2001; **54**: 702–9.

55. Olsen JH, Boice JD, Fraumeni JF. Cancer in children of epileptic mothers and the possible relation to maternal anticonvulsant therapy. *Br J Cancer* 1990; **62**: 996–9.

56. Shu XO, Gao YT, Brinton LA *et al.* A population-based case-control study of childhood leukemia in Shanghai. *Cancer* 1988; **62**: 635–44.

♦57. Allen DB, Rundle AC, Graves DA, Blethen SL. Risk of leukemia in children treated with human growth hormone: review and reanalysis. *J Pediatr* 1997; **131**: S32–6.

58. Buriot D, Prieur A-M, Lebranchu Y *et al.* Leucémie aigue chez trois enfants atteints d'arthrite chronique juvénile traités par le Chlorambucil. *Arch Franc Pediat* 1979; **36**: 592–8.

59. Kauppi MJ, Savolainen HA, Anttila V-J, Isomaki HA. Increased risk of leukaemia in patients with juvenile chronic arthritis treated with chlorambucil. *Acta Paediatr* 1996; **85**: 248–50.

60. Golding J, Greenwood R, Birmingham K, Mott M. Childhood cancer, intramuscular vitamin K, and pethidine given during labour. *Br Med J* 1992; **305**: 341–6.

♦61. Roman E, Fear NT, Ansell P *et al.* Vitamin K and childhood cancer: analysis of individual patient data from six case-control studies. *Br J Cancer* 2002; **86**: 63–9.

♦62. Zahm SH, Ward MH. Pesticides and childhood cancer. *Environ Health Perspect* 1998; **106**: 893–908.

63. Meinert R, Schüz J, Kaletsch U *et al.* Leukemia and non-Hodgkin's lymphoma in childhood and exposure to pesticides: results of a register-based case-control study in Germany. *Am J Epidemiol* 2000; **151**: 639–46.

64. Buckley JD, Meadows AT, Kadin ME *et al.* Pesticide exposures in children with non-Hodgkin lymphoma. *Cancer* 2000; **89**: 2315–21.

65. Daniels JL, Olshan AF, Teschke K *et al.* Residential pesticide exposure and neuroblastoma. *Epidemiology* 2001; **12**: 20–7.

66. Freedman DM, Stewart P, Kleinerman RA *et al.* Household solvent exposures and childhood acute lymphoblastic leukemia. *Am J Public Health* 2001; **91**: 564–7.

67. Nordlinder R, Järvholm B. Environmental exposure to gasoline and leukemia in children and young adults – an ecology study. *Int Arch Occup Environ Health* 1997; **70**: 57–60.

68. Best N, Cockings S, Bennett J *et al.* Ecological regression analysis of environmental benzene exposure and childhood leukaemia: sensitivity to data inaccuracies, geographical scale and ecological bias. *J R Stat Soc A* 2001; **164**: 155–74.

69. Raaschou-Nielsen O, Hertel O, Thomsen BL, Olsen JH. Air pollution from traffic at the residence of children with cancer. *Am J Epidemiol* 2001; **153**: 433–43.

♦70. Blot WJ, Henderson BE, Boice JD. Childhood cancer in relation to cured meat intake: review of the epidemiological evidence. *Nutr Cancer* 1999; **34**: 111–18.

71. Infante-Rivard C, Olson E, Jacques L, Ayotte P. Drinking water contaminants and childhood leukemia. *Epidemiology* 2001; **12**: 13–19.

♦72. Boffetta P, Trédaniel J, Greco A. Risk of childhood cancer and adult lung cancer after childhood exposure to passive smoking: a meta-analysis. *Environ Health Perspect* 2000; **108**: 73–82.

73. Preston-Martin S, Pogoda JM, Mueller BA *et al.* Prenatal vitamin supplementation and risk of childhood brain tumors. *Int J Cancer* 1998; Suppl. 11: 17–22.

74. Thompson JR, FitzGerald P, Willoughby MLN, Armstrong BK. Maternal folate supplementation in pregnancy and protection against acute lymphoblastic leukaemia in childhood: a case-control study. *Lancet* 2001; **358**: 1935–40.

♦75. Colt JS, Blair A. Parental occupational exposures and risk of childhood cancer. *Environ Health Perspect* 1998; **106**: 909–25.

76. Gardner MJ, Snee MP, Hall AJ *et al.* Results of case-control study of leukaemia and lymphoma among young people near Sellafield nuclear plant in West Cumbria. *Br Med J* 1990; **300**: 423–9.

77. Kinlen LJ. Can paternal preconceptional radiation account for the increase of leukaemia and non-Hodgkin's lymphoma in Seascale? *Br Med J* 1993; **306**: 1718–21.

78. Draper GJ, Little MP, Sorahan T *et al.* Cancer in the offspring of radiation workers: a record linkage study. *Br Med J* 1997; **315**: 1181–8.

79. Roman E, Doyle P, Maconochie N *et al.* Cancer in children of nuclear industry employees: report on children aged under 25 years from nuclear industry family study. *Br Med J* 1999; **318**: 1443–50.

80. Smulevich VB, Solionova LG, Belyakova SV. Parental occupation and other factors and cancer risk in children: II Occupational factors. *Int J Cancer* 1999; **83**: 718–22.

81. Bithell JF, Dutton SJ, Draper GJ, Neary NM. Distribution of childhood laukaemias and non-Hodgkin lymphomas near nuclear installations in England and Wales. *Br Med J* 1994; **309**: 501–5.

82. Kaatsch P, Kaletsch U, Meinert R, Michaelis J. An extended study on childhood malignancies in the vicinity of German nuclear power plants. *Cancer Causes Control* 1998; **9**: 529–33.

83. Gutierrez MI, Bhatia K, Barriga F *et al.* Molecular epidemiology of Burkitt's lymphoma from South America: differences in breakpoint location and Epstein–Barr virus association from tumors in other world regions. *Blood* 1992; **79**: 3261–6.

84. Geser A, Brubaker G, Draper CC. Effect of a malaria suppression program on the incidence of African Burkitt's lymphoma. *Am J Epidemiol* 1989; **129**: 740–52.

♦85. Parkin DM, Pisani P, Munoz N, Ferlay J. The global health burden of infection associated cancers. *Cancer Surv* 1999; **33**: 5–33.

86. Glaser SL, Lin RJ, Stewart SL *et al.* Epstein–Barr virus-associated Hodgkin's disease: epidemiologic characteristics in international data. *Int J Cancer* 1997; **70**: 375–82.

87. Swerdlow AJ, Higgins CD, Hunt BJ *et al.* Risk of lymphoid neoplasia after cardiothoracic transplantation. A cohort study of the relation to Epstein–Barr virus. *Transplantation* 2000; **69**: 897–904.

88. Wabinga HR, Parkin DM, Wabwire-Mangen F, Nambooze S. Trends in cancer incidence in Kyadondo County, Uganda, 1960–1997. *Br J Cancer* 2000; **82**: 1585–92.

89. Newton R, Ziegler J, Beral V *et al.* A case-control study of human immunodeficiency virus infection and cancer in adults and children residing in Kampala, Uganda. *Int J Cancer* 2001; **92**: 622–7.

90. Evans JA, Gibb DM, Holland FJ *et al.* Malignancies in UK children with HIV infection acquired from mother to child transmission. *Arch Dis Child* 1997; **76**: 330–3.

91. Biggar RJ, Frisch M, Goedert JJ for the AIDS-Cancer Match Registry Study Group. Risk of cancer in children with AIDS. *J Am Med Assoc* 2000; **284**: 205–9.

92. Caselli D, Klersy C, de Martino M *et al.* for the Italian Register for HIV Infection in Children. Human immunodeficiency virus-related cancer in children: incidence and treatment outcome – report of the Italian register. *J Clin Oncol* 2000; **18**: 3854–61.

93. McClain KL, Leach CT, Jenson HB *et al.* Association of Epstein–Barr virus with leiomyosarcomas in young people with AIDS. *N Engl J Med* 1995; **332**: 12–18.

94. Hsu H-C, Wu M-Z, Chang M-H *et al.* Childhood hepatocellular carcinoma develops exclusively in hepatitis B surface antigen carriers in three decades in Taiwan. *J Hepatol* 1987; **5**: 260–7.

95. Leuschner I, Harms D, Schmidt D. The association of hepatocellular carcinoma in childhood with hepatitis B virus infection. *Cancer* 1988; **62**: 2363–9.

96. Chang M-H, Chen C-J, Lai MS *et al.* Universal hepatitis B vaccination in Taiwan and the incidence of hepatocellular carcinoma in children. *N Engl J Med* 1997, **336**: 1855–9.

♦97. Strickler HD, Goedert JJ. Exposure to SV40-contaminated poliovirus vaccine and the risk of cancer: a review of the epidemiological evidence. *Dev Biol Stand* 1998; **94**: 235–44.

98. Smith MA, Simon R, Strickler HD *et al.* Evidence that childhood acute lymphoblastic leukemia is associated with an infectious agent linked to hygiene conditions. *Cancer Causes Control* 1998; **9**: 285–98.

99. MacKenzie J, Perry J, Ford AM *et al.* JC and BK virus sequences are not detectable in leukaemic samples from children with common acute lymphoblastic leukaemia. *Br J Cancer* 1999; **81**: 898–9.

100. Smith MA, Strickler HD, Granovsky M *et al.* Investigation of leukemia cells from children with common acute lymphoblastic leukemia for genomic sequences of the primate polyomaviruses JC virus, BK virus, and Simian virus 40. *Med Pediatr Oncol* 1999; **33**: 441–3.

101. MacKenzie J, Gallagher A, Clayton RA *et al.* Screening for herpesvirus genomes in common acute lymphoblastic leukemia. *Leukemia* 2001; **15**: 414–21.

102. Swensen AR, Ross JA, Shu XO *et al.* Pet ownership and childhood acute leukemia (USA and Canada). *Cancer Causes Control* 2001; **12**: 301–3.

103. Greaves MF. Speculations on the cause of childhood acute lymphoblastic leukemia. *Leukemia* 1988; **2**: 120–5.

104. Neglia JP, Linet MS, Shu XO *et al.* Patterns of infection and day care utilization and risk of childhood acute lymphoblastic leukaemia. *Br J Cancer* 2000; **82**: 234–40.

105. Rosenbaum PF, Buck GM, Brecher ML. Early child-care and preschool experiences and the risk of childhood acute lymphoblastic leukemia. *Am J Epidemiol* 2000; **152**: 1136–44.

106. Taylor GM, Dearden S, Payne N *et al.* Evidence that an *HLA-DQA1-DQB1* haplotype influences susceptibility to childhood common acute lymphoblastic leukaemia in boys provides further support for an infection-related aetiology. *Br J Cancer* 1998; **78**: 561–5.

107. Kneale GW, Stewart AM, Kinnier Wilson LM. Immunizations against infectious diseases and childhood cancers. *Cancer Immunol Imunother* 1986; **21**: 129–32.

108. Hartley AL, Birch JM, McKinney PA *et al.* The Inter-Regional Epidemiological Study of Childhood Cancer (IRESCC): past medical history in children with cancer. *J Epidemiol Comm Health* 1988; **42**: 235–42.

109. Schüz J, Kaletsch U, Meinert R *et al.* Association of childhood leukaemia with factors related to the immune system. *Br J Cancer* 1999; **80**: 585–90.

110. Groves FD, Gridley G, Wacholder S *et al.* Infant vaccinations and risk of childhood acute lymphoblastic leukaemia in the USA. *Br J Cancer* 1999; **81**: 175–8.

111. Auvinen A, Hakulinen T, Groves F. Haemophilus influenzae type B vaccination and risk of childhood leukaemia in a vaccine trial in Finland. *Br J Cancer* 2000; **83**: 956–8.

112. UK Childhood Cancer Study Investigators. Breastfeeding and childhood cancer. *Br J Cancer* 2001; **85**: 1685–94.

113. Ross JA, Severson RK, Swensen AR *et al.* Seasonal variations in the diagnosis of childhood cancer in the United States. *Br J Cancer* 1999; **81**: 549–53.

114. Higgins CD, dos-Santos-Silva I, Stiller CA, Swerdlow AJ. Season of birth and diagnosis of children with leukaemia: an analysis of over 15 000 UK cases occurring from 1953–95. *Br J Cancer* 2001; **84**: 406–12.

115. Feltbower RG, Pearce MS, Dickinson HO *et al.* Seasonality of birth for cancer in Northern England, UK. *Paediatr Perinat Epidemiol* 2001; **15**: 338–45.

116. Sorensen HT, Pedersen L, Olsen JH, Rothman KJ. Seasonal variation in month of birth and diagnosis of early childhood acute lymphoblastic leukemia (letter). *J Am Med Assoc* 2001; **285**: 168–9.

117. Dockerty JD, Draper GJ, Vincent TJ *et al.* Case-control study of parental age, parity and socioeconomic level in relation to childhood cancers. *Int J Epidemiol* 2001; **30**: 1428–37.

118. Kaye SA, Robison LL, Smithson WA *et al.* Maternal reproductive history and birth characteristics in childhood acute lymphoblastic leukemia. *Cancer* 1991; **68**: 1351–5.

119. Kinlen L. Evidence for an infective cause of childhood leukaemia: comparison of a Scottish new town with nuclear reprocessing sites in Britain. *Lancet* 1988; **2**: 1323–7.

♦120. Kinlen LJ. Epidemiological evidence for an infective basis in childhood leukaemia. *Br J Cancer* 1995; **71**: 1–5.

121. Stiller CA, Boyle PJ. Effect of population mixing and socioeconomic status in England and Wales, 1979–85, on lymphoblastic leukaemia in children. *Br Med J* 1996; **313**: 1297–300.

122. Dickinson HO, Parker L. Quantifying the effect of population mixing on childhood leukaemia risk: the Seascale cluster. *Br J Cancer* 1999; **81**: 144–51.

123. Alexander FE, Chan LC, Lam TH *et al.* Clustering of childhood leukaemia in Hong Kong: association with the childhood peak and common acute lymphoblastic leukaemia and with population mixing. *Br J Cancer* 1997; **75**: 457–63.

124. Koushik A, King WD, McLaughlin JR. An ecologic study of childhood leukemia and population mixing in Ontario, Canada. *Cancer Causes Control* 2001; **12**: 483–90.

125. Kinlen LJ, Petridou E. Childhood leukemia and rural population movements: Greece, Italy, and other countries. *Cancer Causes Control* 1995; **6**: 445–50.

126. Kinlen LJ. High-contact paternal occupations, infection and childhood leukaemia: five studies of unusual population-mixing of adults. *Br J Cancer* 1997; **76**: 1539–45.

127. Kinlen LJ, Bramald S. Paternal occupational contact level and childhood leukaemia in rural Scotland: a case-control study. *Br J Cancer* 2001; **84**: 1002–7.

128. Kinlen L, Jiang J, Hemminki K. A case-control study of childhood leukaemia and paternal occupational contact level in Sweden. *Br J Cancer* 2002; **86**: 732–7.

129. Alexander FE, Boyle P, Carli PM *et al.* Spatial clustering of childhood leukaemia: summary results from the EUROCLUS project. *Br J Cancer* 1997; **77**: 818–24.

130. Birch JM, Alexander FE, Blair V *et al.* Space-time clustering patterns in childhood leukaemia support a role for infection. *Br J Cancer* 2000; **82**: 1571–6.

131. Muirhead CR. Childhood leukemia in metropolitan regions in the United States: a possible relation to population density? *Cancer Causes Control* 1995; **6**: 383–8.

132. Dockerty JD, Sharples KJ, Borman B. An assessment of spatial clustering of leukaemias and lymphomas among young people in New Zealand. *J Epidemiol Community Health* 1999; **53**: 154–8.

133. UK Childhood Cancer Study Investigators. The United Kingdom childhood cancer study: objectives, materials and methods. *Br J Cancer* 2000; **82**: 1073–102.

134. Dickersin K. Systematic reviews in epidemiology: why are we so far behind? *Int J Epidemiol* 2002; **31**: 6–12.

135. Draper GJ, Sanders BM, Brownbill PA, Hawkins MM. Patterns of risk of hereditary retinoblastoma and applications to genetic counselling. *Br J Cancer* 1992; **66**: 211–19.

136. Knudson AG. Mutation and cancer: statistical study of retinoblastoma. *Proc Natl Acad Sci USA* 1971; **68**: 820–3.

137. Draper GJ, Sanders BM, Kingston JE. Second primary neoplasms in patients with retinoblastoma. *Br J Cancer* 1986; **53**: 661–71.

138. Sanders BM, Jay M, Draper GJ, Roberts EM. Non-ocular cancer in relatives of retinoblastoma patients. *Br J Cancer* 1989; **60**: 358–65.

139. Breslow NE, Beckwith JB. Epidemiological features of Wilms' tumor: results of the National Wilms' Tumor Study. *J Natl Cancer Inst* 1982; **68**: 429–36.

140. Li FP, Williams WR, Gimbrere K *et al.* Heritable fraction of unilateral Wilms' tumor. *Pediatrics* 1988; **81**: 147–9.

141. Rapley EA, Barfoot R, Bonaïti-Pellié C *et al.* Evidence for susceptibility genes to familial Wilms tumour in addition to *WT1*, *FWT1* and *FWT2*. *Br J Cancer* 2000; **83**: 177–83.

142. Kingston JE, Herbert A, Draper GJ, Mann JR. Association between hepatoblastoma and polyposis coli. *Arch Dis Child* 1983; **58**: 959–62.

♦143. Varley JM, Evans DGR, Birch JM. Li-Fraumeni syndrome – a molecular and clinical review. *Br J Cancer* 1997; **76**: 1–14.

144. Birch JM, Alston RD, McNally RJQ *et al.* Relative frequency and morphology of cancers in carriers of germline TP53 mutations. *Oncogene* 2001; **20**: 4621–8.

♦145. Li FP. Molecular epidemiology studies of cancer in families. *Br J Cancer* 1993; **68**: 217–19.

146. Sévenet N, Sheridan E, Amram D *et al.* Constitutional mutations of the *hSNF5/INI1* gene predispose to a variety of cancers. *Am J Hum Genet* 1999; **65**: 1342–8.

147. Bell DW, Varley JM, Szydlo TE *et al.* Heterozygous germ line *hCHK2* mutations in Li–Fraumeni syndrome. *Science* 1999; **286**: 2528–31.

148. Wagner J, Portwine C, Rabin K *et al.* High frequency of germline p53 mutations in childhood adrenocortical cancer. *J Natl Cancer Inst* 1994; **86**: 1707–10.

149. Varley JM, McGown G, Thorncroft M *et al.* Are there low-penetrance TP53 alleles? Evidence from childhood adrenocortical tumors. *Am J Hum Genet* 1999; **65**: 995–1006.

150. Ribeiro RC, Sandrini F, Figueiredo B *et al.* An inherited p53 mutation that contributes in a tissue-specific manner to pediatric adrenal cortical carcinoma. *Proc Natl Acad Sci USA* 2001; **98**: 9330–5.

151. Narod SA, Stiller C, Lenoir GM. An estimate of the heritable fraction of childhood cancer. *Br J Cancer* 1991; **63**: 993–9.

152. Stiller CA, Chessells JM, Fitchett M. Neurofibromatosis and childhood leukaemia/lymphoma: a population-based UKCCSG study. *Br J Cancer* 1994; **70**: 969–72.

♦153. Lindor NM, Greene MH, Mayo Familial Cancer Program. The concise handbook of family cancer syndromes. *J Natl Cancer Inst* 1998; **90**: 1039–71.

154. Draper GJ, Heaf MM, Kinnier Wilson LM. Occurrence of childhood cancers among sibs and estimation of familial risks. *J Med Genet* 1977; **14**: 81–90.

155. Winther JF, Sankila R, Boice JD *et al*. Cancer in siblings of children with cancer in the Nordic countries: a population-based cohort study. *Lancet* 2001; **358**: 711–17.

156. Ford AM, Ridge SA, Cabrera ME *et al*. In utero rearrangements in the trithorax-related oncogene in infant leukaemias. *Nature* 1993; **363**: 358–60.

157. Hasle H, Clemmensen IH, Mikkelsen M. Risks of leukaemia and solid tumours in individuals with Down's syndrome. *Lancet* 2000; **355**: 165–9.

♦158. Hasle H. Pattern of malignant disorders in individuals with Down's syndrome. *Lancet Oncol* 2001; **2**: 429–36.

159. Satgé D, Sasco AJ, Carlsen NLT *et al*. A lack of neuroblastoma in Down syndrome: a study from 11 European countries. *Cancer Res* 1998; **58**: 448–52.

160. Morrell D, Cromartie E, Swift M. Mortality and cancer incidence in 163 patients with ataxia-telangiectasia. *J Natl Cancer Inst* 1986; **77**: 89–92.

161. Sullivan KE, Mullen CA, Blaese RM, Winkelstein JA. A multi-institutional survey of the Wiskott-Aldrich syndrome. *J Pediatr* 1994; **125**: 876–85.

♦162. Mueller BU, Pizzo PA. Cancer in children with primary or secondary immunodeficiencies. *J Pediatr* 1995; **126**: 1–10.

163. Butturini A, Gale RP, Verlander PC *et al*. Hematologic abnormalities in Fanconi anemia: an International Fanconi Anemia Registry study. *Blood* 1994; **84**: 1650–5.

164. Smith OP, Hann IM, Chessells JM *et al*. Haematological abnormalities in Shwachman–Diamond syndrome. *Br J Haematol* 1996; **94**: 279–84.

165. Coppes MJ, Haber DA, Grundy PE. Genetic events in the development of Wilms' tumor. *N Engl J Med* 1994; **331**: 586–90.

166. Grønskov K, Olsen JH, Sand A *et al*. Population-based risk estimates of Wilms tumor in sporadic aniridia: A comprehensive mutation screening procedure of PAX6 identifies 80% of mutations in aniridia. *Hum Genet* 2001; **109**: 11–19.

167. DeBaun MR, Tucker MA. Risk of cancer during the first four years of life in children from The Beckwith–Wiedemann Syndrome Registry. *J Pediatr* 1998; **132**: 398–400.

168. Sotelo-Avila C, Gonzalez-Crussi F, Fowler JW. Complete and incomplete forms of Beckwith–Wiedemann syndrome: Their oncogenic potential. *J Pediatr* 1980; **96**: 47–50.

169. Hersh JH, Cole TR, Bloom AS *et al*. Risk of malignancy in Sotos syndrome. *J Pediatr* 1992; **120**: 572–4.

170. Gripp KW, Scott CI, Nicholson L *et al*. Five additional Costello syndrome patients with rhabdomyosarcoma: proposal for a tumor screening protocol. *Am J Med Genet* 2002; **108**: 80–7.

171. Powell JE, Kelly AM, Parkes SE *et al*. Cancer and congenital abnormalities in Asian children: a population-based study from the West Midlands. *Br J Cancer* 1995; **72**: 1563–9.

172. Bener A, Denic S, Al-Mazrouei M. Consanguinity and family history of cancer in children with leukemia and lymphomas. *Cancer* 2001; **92**: 1–6.

173. Narod SA, Hawkins MM, Robertson CM, Stiller CA. Congenital anomalies and childhood cancer in Great Britain. *Am J Hum Genet* 1997; **60**: 474–85.

174. Larson RA, Wang Y, Banerjee M *et al*. Prevalence of the inactivating ^{690}C-T polymorphism in the NAD(P)H: quinone oxidoreductase (NQO1) gene in patients with primary and therapy-related myeloid leukemia. *Blood* 1999; **94**: 803–7.

175. Wiemels JL, Pagnamenta A, Taylor GM *et al*. A lack of a functional NAD(P)H: quinone oxidoreductase allele is selectively associated with pediatric leukemias that have *MLL* fusions. *Cancer Res* 1999; **59**: 4095–9.

176. Sinnett D, Krajinovic M, Labuda D. Genetic susceptibility to childhood acute lymphoblastic leukemia. *Leuk Lymphoma* 2000; **38**: 447–62.

177. Davies SM, Robison LL, Buckley JD *et al*. Glutathione s-transferase polymorphisms in children with myeloid leukemia: a children's cancer group study. *Cancer Epidemiol Biomarkers Prev* 2000; **9**: 563–6.

178. Krajinovic M, Sinnett H, Richer C *et al*. Role of *NQO1*, *MPO* and *CYP2E1* genetic polymorphisms in the susceptibility to childhood acute lymphoblastic leukemia. *Int J Cancer* 2002; **97**: 230–6.

179. Doyle P, Bunch KJ, Beral V, Draper GJ. Cancer incidence in children conceived with assisted reproduction technology. *Lancet* 1996; **352**: 452–3.

180. Bergh T, Ericson A, Hillensjo T *et al*. Deliveries and children born after in-vitro fertilisation in Sweden 1982–95: a retrospective cohort study. *Lancet* 1999; **354**: 1579–85.

181. Bruinsma F, Venn A, Lancaster P *et al*. Incidence of cancer in children born after in-vitro fertilization. *Hum Reprod* 2000; **15**: 604–7.

182. Hewitt D, Lashof JC, Stewart AM. Childhood cancer in twins. *Cancer* 1966; **19**: 157–61.

183. Murphy MFG, Whiteman D, Hey K *et al*. Childhood cancer incidence in a cohort of twin babies. *Br J Cancer* 2001; **84**: 1460–2.

184. Reynolds P, Von Behren J, Elkin EP. Birth characteristics and leukemia in young children. *Am J Epidemiol* 2002; **155**: 603–13.

185. Tanimura M, Matsui I, Abe J *et al*. Increased risk of hepatoblastoma among immature children with a lower birth weight. *Cancer Res* 1998; **58**: 3032–5.

186. Maruyama K, Ikeda H, Koizumi T, Tsuchida Y. Prenatal and postnatal histories of very low birthweight infants who developed hepatoblastoma. *Pediatr Int* 1999; **41**: 82–9.

♦187. Terracini B, Coebergh J-W, Gatta G *et al*. Childhood cancer survival in Europe: an overview. *Eur J Cancer* 2001; **37**: 810–16.

♦188. Stiller CA. Centralised treatment, entry to trials and survival. *Br J Cancer* 1994; **70**: 352–62.

189. Stiller CA, Eatock EM. Patterns of care and survival for children with acute lymphoblastic leukaemia diagnosed between 1980–94. *Arch Dis Child* 1999; **81**: 202–8.

190. Robertson CM, Hawkins MM, Kingston JE. Late deaths and survival after childhood cancer; implications for cure. *Br Med J* 1994; **309**: 162–6.

191. Mertens AC, Yasui Y, Neglia JP *et al.* Late mortality experience in five-year survivors of childhood and adolescent cancer: the Childhood Cancer Survivor Study. *J Clin Oncol* 2001; **19**: 3163–72.

192. Möller TR, Garwicz S, Barlow L *et al.* Decreasing late mortality among five-year survivors of cancer in childhood and adolescence: a population-based study in the Nordic countries. *J Clin Oncol* 2001; **19**: 3173–81.

193. Hawkins MM, Draper GJ, Kingston JE. Incidence of second primary tumours among childhood cancer survivors. *Br J Cancer* 1987; **56**: 339–47.

194. Olsen JH, Garwicz S, Hertz H *et al.* Second malignant neoplasms after cancer in childhood or adolescence. *Br Med J* 1993; **307**: 1030–6.

195. Neglia JP, Friedman DL, Yasui Y *et al.* Second malignant neoplasms in five-year survivors of childhood cancer: childhood cancer survivor study. *J Natl Cancer Inst* 2001; **93**: 618–29.

196. Hawkins MM, Kinnier Wilson LM, Stovall MA *et al.* Epipodophyllotoxins, alkylating agents and radiation and risk of secondary leukaemia after childhood cancers. *Br Med J* 1992; **304**: 951–8.

197. Smith MA, Rubinstein L, Anderson JR *et al.* Secondary leukemia or myelodysplastic syndrome after treatment with epipodophyllotoxins. *J Clin Oncol* 1999; **17**: 569–77.

198. Robison LL, Mertens AC, Boice JD *et al.* Study design and cohort characteristics of the Childhood Cancer Survivor Study: a multi-institutional collaborative project. *Med Pediatr Oncol* 2002; **38**: 229–39.

199. Hawkins MM, Smith RA, Curtice LJ. Childhood cancer survivors and their offspring studied through a postal survey of general practitioners: preliminary results. *J R Coll Gen Pract* 1988; **38**: 102–5.

200. Li F, Gimbere K, Gelber RD *et al.* Outcome of pregnancy in survivors of Wilms' tumor. *J Am Med Assoc* 1987; **257**: 216–19.

201. Hawkins MM, Draper GJ, Winter DL. Cancer in the offspring of survivors of childhood leukaemia and non-Hodgkin lymphoma. *Br J Cancer* 1995; **71**: 1335–9.

202. Sankila R, Olsen JH, Anderson H *et al.* Risk of cancer among offspring of childhood-cancer survivors. *N Engl J Med* 1998; **338**: 1339–44.

203. Hawkins MM. Is there evidence of a therapy-related increase in germ-cell mutation among childhood cancer survivors? *J Natl Cancer Inst* 1991; **83**: 1643–50.

204. Meistrich ML, Byrne J. Genetic disease in offspring of long-term survivors of childhood and adolescent cancer treated with potentially mutagenic therapies. *Am J Hum Genet* 2002; **70**: 1069–71.

2

The molecular basis of children's cancers

JOHN ANDERSON & KATHY PRITCHARD-JONES

INTRODUCTION

Cancer develops as a result of changes in the structure and function of genes. Since the identification of the first viral proto-oncogenes in the 1980s, there has been an exponential increase in the number of known genes involved in cancer development, and a gradually evolving picture of the complex network of pathways typically disturbed in cancer cells. Moreover, it has become apparent that individual cancers may undergo a lengthy evolutionary process involving multiple genes, and that there may be genetic heterogeneity within individual tumours. This chapter will give an overview of the molecular processes at play in cancer development, and then illustrate these principles with reference to individual paediatric cancer types.

THE CONCEPTS OF ONCOGENES AND TUMOUR SUPPRESSOR GENES

Oncogenes and tumour suppressor genes are normal genes that perform important regulatory functions in normal cells, but which have become aberrantly activated or repressed in cancer cells. It is this process of genetic change in oncogenes and tumour suppressor genes that results ultimately in the malignant transformation of cells.

Oncogenes and mechanisms of activation

Oncogenes are, literally, cancer-causing genes. Under normal physiological conditions, oncogenes perform important functions often related to control of cell division. However, deregulated expression of oncogenes disrupts the normal constraints on cellular growth and division, resulting in tumour formation.

The first oncogenes were discovered following analysis of retroviruses that were capable of infecting cells and transforming them into malignant cells.[1] In some cases, genes isolated from acute transforming retroviruses were themselves capable of causing malignant transformation when transfected into mammalian cells.[2,3] Human and other mammalian homologues of the viral genes were found. The RAS family of genes were amongst the first to be discovered in this way. N-RAS, K-RAS and H-RAS are closely related proteins of about 21 kDa. H-RAS and K-RAS have viral oncogene counterparts carried by the Harvey and Kirsten strains of murine sarcoma virus. Each of the wild-type cellular genes can give rise to a transforming oncogene by single amino acid substitution. The mutated forms are oncogenes and the wild-type forms are referred to as proto-oncogenes. Subsequently, other oncogenes have been similarly discovered and confirmed, because of evidence of activation in tumours and the capacity of the activated form to transform cells, such as fibroblasts, in culture.

Over 100 oncogenes are now known and the number is still growing. In cancer, deregulation of oncogenes can occur by a variety of mechanisms. Viral infection has been found to be a relatively uncommon pathway of oncogene activation. Most oncogenes are native genes activated as a result of somatic rearrangements of the genome resulting from random mutation associated with failure of repair of DNA damage following, for example, exposure to carcinogens or radiation. For example, oncogenes can become overexpressed following their translocation to a new genetic locus where they come under the influence of new genetic regulatory elements in the form of promoters and enhancers. By these means, the c-*myc* gene becomes activated following its juxtaposition to the immunoglobulin heavy chain enhancer as a result of a t(8;14)(q24;q32) reciprocal translocation in Burkitt lymphoma (see below and Figure 2.1a). The consequence is high levels of expression (greater than physiological) of c-*myc* protein in tumour cells.[4] An alternative mechanism of deregulation of c-*myc* is genomic amplification. Typically, this involves the generation of tandem repeats of a large genetic element

containing several contiguous genes, referred to as an amplicon. A homologue of c-*myc* with expression limited to cells of neural crest origin is *MYCN*. In common with c-*myc*, it can become activated as a result of chromosomal translocation (rare) or genomic amplification (common). Both amplification and juxtaposition of novel genetic elements may result in overexpression of proteins that are otherwise present in their wild-type form.[5,6] The overexpression might simply reflect levels of expression, or alternatively there may be a failure of down-regulation in response to normal cellular homeostatic mechanisms.

Alternatively, new oncogenes can sometimes be generated as a result of chromosomal translocations in cancer cells involving breakpoints within genes, typically occurring within intronic (non-coding) sequences. An example of this is the PAX3-FKHR fusion protein formed by the translocation t(2;13)(q35;q14) in alveolar rhabdomyosarcoma (Figure 2.1b).[7,8] The PAX3-FKHR fusion is oncogenic, whereas PAX3 and FKHR themselves are not (see below).

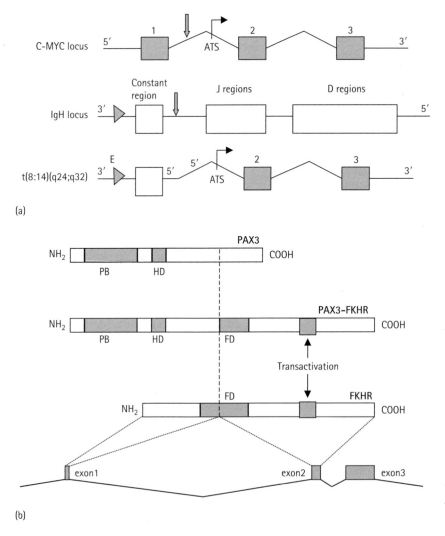

(a)

(b)

Figure 2.1 *Examples of two different mechanisms of oncogene activation by chromosomal translocation. (a) The translocation t(8;14)(q24;q32) in Burkitt lymphoma and mature B-cell leukaemia fuses the C-MYC oncogene with the immunoglobulin heavy chain enhancer (E). Respective chromosomal breakpoints are shown as filled arrows. Note fusion of the 5′ ends of the genes. Although exon 1 of C-MYC is missing, a functional reading frame is generated because there is an alternative transcription start site (ATS) within intron 1.(b) The translocation t(2;13)(q35;q14) of alveolar rhabdomyosarcoma causes the generation of a fusion gene encoding a single open reading frame for a chimeric protein PAX3-FKHR in which the paired domain (PD) and homeodomain (HD) DNA binding elements of PAX3 are coupled with a strong transcription activation domain from FKHR protein.*

In contrast, oncogenic RAS proteins are present at physiological levels and are activated by point mutation rather than chromosomal rearrangement. Early transformation assays using mutated RAS revealed the phenomenon of oncogene complementation, whereby mutant *RAS* and deregulated c-*myc* could cooperate in some cell lines to initiate transformation but neither oncogene alone was sufficient.[9,10] Like MYC, normal RAS is a component of a complex signalling pathway that instructs cells to progress through the cell cycle. However, MYC is a transcription factor that is thought to regulate expression of target genes that result in cell cycle progression and inhibition of differentiation, whereas RAS proteins are located at the cell surface and transduce signals from extracellular signals such as growth factors, through complex pathways of intracellular signalling, the end results of which include mitogenesis. Mutations in RAS result in proteins that are constitutively active and provide mitogenic signals in the absence of extraneous growth factors. Individual genetic events may be responsible for one or more of these changes, but typically several different genetic hits are required to initiate the process of full tumorigenesis.

Tumour suppressor genes and mechanisms of their inactivation

Tumour suppressor genes typically code for proteins that play important negative regulatory roles in control of cell growth and division. Hence, loss of this negative regulation may cause uncontrolled growth. Because loss of protein function is required, both genomic copies of a tumour suppressor are usually lost in the tumorigenic process through processes such as mutation or deletion. There are two common exceptions to this maxim. Firstly, in some cases of inherited cancer, the loss of the first copy of the tumour suppressor is inherited whilst the second is an acquired second hit. An example is inherited mutations of the tumour suppressor genes *p53* or *pRB* in the clinical syndromes of Li–Fraumeni and familial retinoblastoma respectively (see below). Here there is a constitutional mutation of one allele, which places somatic cells at increased risk of malignancy. Tumorigenesis is initiated once function of the wild-type allele is lost following a spontaneous mutating event. A second theoretical exception is where a tumour suppressor gene is imprinted, i.e. it is normally expressed from one allele only (Figure 2.2).

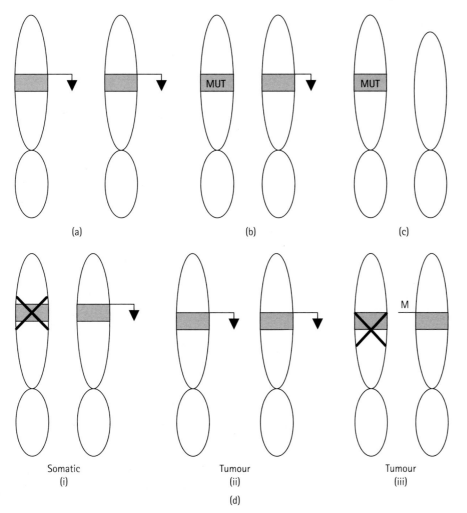

(a)   (b)   (c)

Somatic   Tumour   Tumour
(i)   (ii)   (iii)
(d)

Figure 2.2 *Mechanisms of disruption of normal and imprinted genes. (a) A normal cell showing biallelic expression. (b) Mutation of a single copy of a tumour suppressor gene predisposes to, but is insufficient for, tumorigenesis. (c) Acquired mutation or 'second hit' results in tumorigenesis. (d) (i) An imprinted allele is expressed from one chromosome only; (ii) loss of imprinting results in biallelic expression; (iii) mutation of the non-imprinted allele results in complete loss of expression following a single hit.*

In this situation, a single genetic hit (of the allele that is normally expressed) is sufficient for loss of function. A cluster of imprinted genes at chromosome region 11p15.5 may contain several tumour suppressors that are deleted from the active (non-imprinted) allele in a number of cancers (see section on 'Wilms' tumour'). Loss of function mutations of tumour suppressor genes can occur by a variety of mechanisms. For example, genes can be completely deleted (often in large regions involving several contiguous genetic elements), individually mutated to generate a non-functional gene, or their expression can be silenced, e.g. by altered methylation of their promoter region(s).

Although many oncogenes are capable by themselves, or in combination with one other gene, of promoting tumorigenesis in experimental cell line transformation assays, studies of patterns of deregulation of oncogenes and mutation of tumour suppressors in actual cancers have revealed a more complex picture. Typically there are multiple pathways contributing to tumorigenesis involving several different classes of oncogenes and tumour suppressor genes.[11]

THE COMPONENTS OF MALIGNANT TRANSFORMATION

In-built into normal tissues are multiple homeostatic pathways that regulate the processes of cell growth and division and thereby function as checkpoints against the development of tumours. To form a malignancy, cells need to undergo a series of phenotypic changes allowing them to escape from normal growth regulation. Alterations in a number of oncogenes and/or tumour suppressor genes are needed to drive these phenotypic changes.

Immortalization

Normal cells stimulated to grow in culture have a finite replicative potential; after a finite number of cell divisions, cells are unable to divide further, at which point replicative senescence is said to have occurred. Typically, cells undergo 60 or more doublings before senescence. Under normal circumstances, senescent cells in culture remain viable. However, further replication can occur in senescent cells through disruption of the tumour suppressor genes *pRB* or *p53*, and these cells will eventually undergo cell death (crisis). Out of a population of cells in crisis, an occasional immortalized cell may emerge. Unlike the situation with normal cells, tumour cells, once established as a cell line in culture, do not usually undergo crisis, indicating that prior immortalization has occurred during the process of tumorigenesis. The molecular processes defining senescence are becoming more clearly defined.[12]

One component of the process leading towards crisis is the shortening of the non-coding ends of chromosomes, or telomeres, that occurs at each cell division. Telomeres are composed of thousands of copies of a 6 bp repeat sequence. Approximately 50–100 bp of telomere DNA is lost during each cell division. After 50 or so divisions, telomeres have virtually disappeared. Exposure of non-telomere DNA at the ends of chromosomes will result in end-to-end chromosome fusions that are characteristic of cells in crisis and lead to cell death by apoptosis. Cancer cells become immortal by preventing telomere shortening during cycling. The most commonly observed mechanism of telomere protection is upregulation in cancer of cells of the enzyme telomerase, which adds DNA to the chromosome ends at each round of DNA replication.[13,14] Telomere shortening appears to be a natural defence mechanism against deregulated cell growth, and telomere protection is the tumour cell's response to allow limitless replicative potential.

Growth factor autonomy

The decision of a normal cell to divide is controlled largely by factors in the extracellular environment. Hence, normal cells divide in accordance with physiological need. Conversely, cell division is inhibited in the absence of physiological requirement. This constraint on cell division functions as a check against the uncontrolled proliferation that is a feature of oncogenesis. Cells receive growth cues from their environment in the form of signalling molecules and extracellular matrix.

The most common mechanism of growth signalling is via diffusible molecules, or growth factors, produced by one cell type in order to stimulate a second (heterotypic signalling). Alternatively, the ligands for growth factor receptors may be membrane-bound themselves, such that ligand/receptor interaction can occur during cell–cell interaction. Growth factor receptors on the target cell transduce the signal from the growth factor ligand through complex intracellular pathways. Frequently the end result of signal transduction is transcriptional activation of genes that are important in cell cycle progression and cell death decisions. Growth factor receptors transduce the signals from their cognate ligands via a variety of different molecular pathways, the control and interactions of which are gradually being elucidated. A second mechanism of growth signalling is through interaction with extracellular matrix (ECM). Extracellular matrix is a macromolecular meshwork of proteins that can anchor cells in position within a tissue. Extracellular matrix receptors, or integrins, both attach a cell to its ECM and signal that the cell is attached. The result of signalling depends on the type of integrin, and different integrin combinations variously result in quiescence, division or migration.[15]

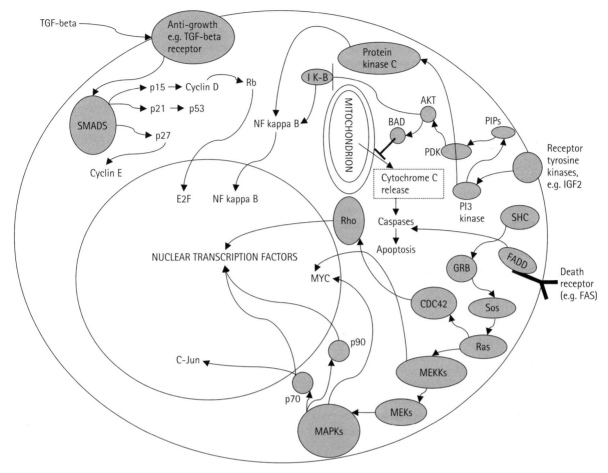

Figure 2.3 *Overview of some signalling pathways commonly disrupted in human cancers.*

Figure 2.3 demonstrates some signal transduction pathways, including many that are altered in cancer cells. Many pathways are cell type-specific. As a clearer picture is emerging of the huge repertoire of genetic alterations that can contribute to malignant transformation, it is becoming apparent that virtually all parts of signal transduction pathways can be oncogenic. Many oncogenic changes may function by disrupting the balance of the homeostatic network of signal transduction pathways.

EXAMPLES OF SIGNAL-TRANSDUCING ONCOGENES

Many cancer cells upregulate production of soluble mitogenic ligands for their own growth factor receptors, thereby creating autologous signalling loops. For example, tumour growth factor-α (TGFα) is often secreted by human sarcomas, and signals their own proliferation. Pro-growth combinations of integrins, which are heterodimeric receptors, may be preferentially expressed in cancer cells. For example, the particular combinations αvβ3 and α6β4 have known roles in cellular mobility and ability to invade ECM, and are associated with more highly metastatic tumours. Cell surface receptor tyrosine kinases (RTKs)

may be upregulated through different mechanisms, overexpression or mutation. For example, overexpression of epidermal growth factor receptor erbB is described in brain and breast cancer and high circulating levels of the receptor may prove to be an important prognostic factor for stratifying patients with breast cancer[16] or nephroblastoma.[17] Mutation and/or overexpression can both result in ligand-independent signalling of RTKs. In this way, missense mutation of the c-*met*, c-*kit* and *RET RTK* proto-oncogenes results in constitutive activation of the tyrosine kinase domain,[18] whereas truncation of the epidermal growth factor receptor lacking most of the cytoplasmic domain is constitutively activated. One of the most commonly mutated genes in cancer is *RAS*, which is a cell membrane molecule that interacts with RTKs and transduces signals following its coupling with guanosine triphosphate (GTP). Mutations of *RAS* that maintain it in its activated RAS-GTP form result in its constitutive activation and signalling in the absence of exogenous growth factor. RAS activation results in activation of the RAS–Raf–MAP kinase signalling pathway, which in turn interacts with a number of oncogenic transcription factors to elicit generally pro-growth signals. In about

25 per cent of human cancers, RAS proteins are mutated and give mitogenic signals in the absence of their normal upstream regulators.[19]

Inhibition of cell death

Programmed cell death (apoptosis) plays a critical role in normal development. Early insights came from the nematode worm *Caenorhabditis elegans*, an organism in which developmental cell divisions and the cell fate of all progeny cells have been painstakingly mapped. Of interest is the number of cells whose programmed fate is to die by the process of apoptosis, thereby allowing room for other cells to migrate or providing shape to the organism in a highly regulated manner. The limited number of genes that regulate apoptosis in *C. elegans* have mammalian homologues which form families of apoptosis-regulating proteins. These include the Bcl2 family of apoptosis-regulating molecules and the downstream effector caspases that initiate the proteolytic cleavage cascade resulting in apoptosis.[20] Many of the Bcl2 family members are involved in the regulation of release of cytochrome C from the inner mitochondrial membrane. Cytoplasmic cytochrome C is thought to trigger subsequent apoptosis through activation of caspase 9 and effector caspases. Pathways of apoptosis that are independent of cytochrome C release but culminate in caspase activation have also been discovered, e.g. pathways downstream from the tumour necrosis factor (TNF) family of death receptors which activate caspase 8 via FADD (FAS-associated death domain).[21]

Apoptosis is a protective mechanism against propagation of damage for cells with deregulated growth. DNA damage resulting from an insult such as ultraviolet (UV) irradiation results in induction of the *p53* tumour suppressor gene, and *p53* protects the cell through stimulating either growth arrest or apoptosis. It is therefore of great interest that *p53* itself is the single most commonly mutated gene in human cancer. The implication is that defects in the cell damage response pathways allow defects to go unchecked and result in the propagation of those defects in a tumour.[21]

Perhaps not surprisingly, many pro- and anti-apoptotic agents have been found to be over- or under-expressed in cancer cells. The anti-apoptotic *BCL2*, which inhibits cytochrome C release, is overexpressed in B-cell follicular non-Hodgkin's lymphoma as a result of a chromosomal translocation that juxtaposes the *BCL2* gene to the immunoglobulin heavy chain enhancer element.[22] In neuroblastoma, inactivation of caspase 8 appears to be essential for inhibition of apoptosis and this may reflect the capacity of *MYCN* oncogene to induce apoptosis in a number of cell types.[23] Anti-apoptotic survival signals downstream from the PI3 kinase-AKT/PKB pathway mitigate apoptosis in a large proportion of human tumours. In many paediatric cancers, this pathway is activated through deregulated expression of insulin-like growth factor 2 (IGF2), which occurs via transcriptional and epigenetic mechanisms.[24]

Angiogenesis and metastasis

Malignant cells divide frequently and have high metabolic activity. They therefore have a relatively high requirement for nutrients and oxygen, which necessitates the formation of a tumour vasculature. Failure of the blood supply will result in death of the tumour. During development, blood supply develops concomitant with tissue growth. Tumorigenesis involves the recapitulation of many aspects of normal development, including angiogenesis. However, tumour growth is often much faster than developmental growth, implying that vascular invasion into the tumour must also proceed at a high rate to maintain tumour viability.

In order for cancer cells to disseminate and form metastatic disease, they need the ability to migrate into adjacent and distant tissues. Typically, distant metastases result from dissemination through blood or lymphatic vessels, resulting in micro-deposits in distant organs or lymph nodes. This multistep process requires invasion into the vessel, adhesion to vessel endothelium at distant sites, and invasion out of the vessel and into surrounding tissues. This process may require production of proteins that break down ECM, whereas expression of adhesion molecules may be required for tumour cells to attach to microvessel endothelium.[25,26]

There are numerous examples of genes that are specifically upregulated in cancer to confer a more metastatic phenotype or allow tumour angiogenesis to proceed. For both angiogenic and metastatic genes, there is evidence that their deregulation can be an important aspect of tumour progression but not part of the initial process of malignant transformation. In a recent study of tumour progression of human melanoma in a mouse xenograft model, only a subpopulation of cells had the capacity to metastasize to distant organs, and metastatic capacity was associated with overexpression of a number of genes such as *rhoC* and *thymosin β4*.[27] Large numbers of gene products have now been linked with enhanced metastatic capacity. These genes may be secreted factors such as matrix metalloproteinases, involved in the disruption of extracellular structures, or cell surface molecules such as αvβ3 integrin and cell–cell adhesion molecules (CAMs), involved in cell–cell interaction and responses. Similarly, there is evidence that rudimentary tumours lack angiogenic factors, and therefore their growth is curtailed.[25,26] However, secondary genetic changes, perhaps made more likely because of an inherent genomic instability that also predisposes to the malignant transformation, result in the evolution of a tumour with the capacity to stimulate blood vessel invasion. Studies in several animal tumour models suggest that induction of angiogenic factors is a mid-stage process allowing development of tumours to diameters greater than 100 μm, but further changes are then required for tumours to invade into neighbouring structures.

As with growth factor signalling there are angiogenesis and invasion inducers and countervailing inhibitors.[28] A prototypic secreted angiogenic factor is vascular endothelial growth factor, a secreted cytokine produced by many tumour types, which is a ligand for vascular endothelial cell receptor tyrosine kinases.[29] Other angiogenic factors in tumour cells include basic and acidic fibroblast growth factors.

Following the discovery of genes that are upregulated to allow tumour angiogenesis, there is great interest in the potential therapeutic use of small molecule inhibitors of these factors. It is apparent that different tumour types employ distinct mechanisms of angiogenesis, so it might be that anti-angiogenic therapy will need to be directed to a particular tumour's pathway. Similarly, local growth of many tumours can be managed with surgery and radiotherapy, but the tumours are incurable because of their capacity to metastasize to multiple sites. Agents to prevent growth of metastatic deposits may become another novel therapeutic approach.

METHODS IN GENE DISCOVERY AND ANALYSIS

There has been an exponential increase in knowledge about gene function that has come about following the development of technologies such as microarray analysis, rapid-throughput DNA sequencing, culminating in the publication of the major component of the human genome sequence, and gene targeting in animal models, including transgenics, 'knock-ins', and 'knock-outs'.

Clues from cytogenetics

Historically, a first step towards delineation of genes critical in specific tumour types has come from analysis of gross chromosomal rearrangements characteristic of at least a proportion of cases of that tumour type. Tumour-specific karyotypic abnormalities have been seen in a wide range of tumours, both solid and haematological. Typically, chromosomal translocations provide more information on the site of involved genes than do deletions, as even the smallest microscopically visible deletion can still encompass many genes. Moreover, the size of a characteristic deleted region may vary considerably between tumours of different types. Defining common regions of overlap

between tumours carrying cytogenetically identical deletions goes some way to identifying putative tumour suppressor genes within deletions. The deletion at 11p15.5 is common to Wilms' tumour, rhabdomyosarcoma and hepatoblastoma. Common region of overlap analysis has defined a smaller region that still contains many sequences (see section on 'Wilms' tumour').

In contrast, the cloning of genes disrupted at the breakpoints of invariant translocations has resulted in the discovery of new oncogenes or confirmed the role of known oncogenes in particular forms of cancer.

The human genome

The availability of the majority of the sequence of the genomes of human beings and other organisms has revolutionized genetic analysis. The human genome is now thought to consist of approximately 40 000 coding sequences, which are available to researchers through online databases.[30,31] This has been possible through the use of automated sequence technology and data analysis. Powerful computer technology means that researchers can search databases of sequences to perform alignments of putative novel genes.

More recent still is the availability of microarrays of genes, which allow functional characterization of samples in terms of expression of more than 20 000 sequences at a time. The challenge for the future is the interpretation of data. Patterns of expression need to be related to function and networks of activated genes need to be discovered. However, powerful bioinformatic tools such as clustering algorithms are already having an impact on clinical thinking, e.g. in paediatric brain tumours and leukaemia.[32,33] Adaptations of oligonucleotide arrays permit rapid-throughput screening for mutations in known genes.

Gene targeting

Gene targeting technology allows the determination of roles of individual genes *in vivo* by analysing the phenotypic or developmental effects of overexpression or loss of expression. Mice are particularly useful for gene targeting of cancer-associated genes as they are relatively easy to breed and the phenotype can be more easily extrapolated to the human situation than is possible with alternative organisms such as *Drosophila* or *Xenopus*.

TRANSGENIC ORGANISMS

These organisms result from the insertion of a gene of interest into an organism by micro-injection of naked DNA (the transgene) into the pro-nucleus of a fertilized egg. Eggs are then surgically implanted into the uterus of a pseudo-pregnant mother. Integration of the transgene is random and expression is dependent on site (or sites) of insertion. Typically, multiple tandem repeats of a transgene are inserted. As well as the coding sequence, the transgene contains regulatory elements that direct gene expression to a cell lineage and/or a developmental stage of choice. For example, the *MYCN* oncogene, which is frequently deregulated in neuroblastoma, has been overexpressed in neural crest cells of transgenic mice through the insertion of the *MYCN* coding sequence, under the regulation of a tyrosine hydroxylase promoter. Transgenic mice develop a disease that closely resembles human neuroblastoma.[34] However, many other experiments that have targeted oncogenes to appropriate promoters, in an attempt to recapitulate oncogene activation in tumorigenesis, have resulted in mice with severe developmental defects or viable mice that fail to develop malignancies.[35,36] These results suggest that oncogene activation occurs in complex sequential pathways that are not amenable to simple manipulation.

KNOCK-OUTS

Generation of knock-out mice has become a classical method of determining gene function. The principle is that a gene is functionally removed (either one copy or both) from the germ line of an organism and the normal physiological or developmental role is deduced from the phenotype. A proliferation of a specific cell type in a knock-out organism is consistent with a normal physiological role for that gene in apoptosis of those cells. Generation of 'knock-outs' makes use of embryonic stem (ES) cells and exploits the process of homologous recombination. In the cancer field, the technique has been most fruitfully applied in the mouse. ES cells are derived from blastocysts and are cell lines that are capable, in a physiological environment, of pluripotential differentiation. As with all cell lines, targeting vectors can be used to introduce genes into cells. To generate knock-outs, a gene of interest is replaced with a selection marker such as a neomycin resistance gene and neomycin-resistant cell clones are screened by Southern blot for replacement of the wild-type allele. Genetically manipulated ES cells, if physically inserted into a blastocyst, are capable of transmitting their genome into multiple lineages to generate chimeric mice. If germ-line transmission follows, the resulting generation will be fully heterozygous for the inserted genetic element. Breeding of heterozygotes to make homozygotes is sometimes required to disclose the full phenotype.

KNOCK-INS

As with knock-outs, knock-in technology has been most successfully applied in mice. Here the concept is the replacement of a wild-type allele by a functional but altered allele. For example, a mutation of a gene that results in a dominant phenotype could replace the wild-type allele.

Alternatively, a fusion gene resulting from a chromosomal translocation could be inserted into the locus of the wild-type undisrupted allele.[37,38] The advantage of knock-ins over transgenic approaches is that the gene is regulated by the physiologically relevant genetic elements.

Knock-out strategies have been informative in delineating both similarities and differences of gene function between murine and human backgrounds. Numerous examples exist of knock-out organisms that have revealed the key roles genes play in development and cancer. Knock-outs of tumour suppressor genes might be expected to result in tumours. Knock-ins of dominant oncogenes, such as translocation-associated fusion genes, have disclosed interesting and often severe phenotypes. However, mice bearing identical germ-line mutations to human genetic predisposition syndromes often have strikingly different phenotypes, thereby demonstrating the limitations of this approach and possible different roles and interactions of homologous proteins between species.[39,40] Increasing use is being made of conditional transgenes and gene targeting to elucidate roles of oncogenes *in vivo*. This technology exploits genetic elements, the expression of which is conditional on the administration of exogenous ligands such as tetracycline or tamoxifen.[41,42] The ligands can be administered to live-born animals or pregnant mothers carrying transgenic offspring to delineate the roles of genes in adult tissues or during development, respectively. Conditional gene targeting is also possible and this technology has exploited genetic elements from other species to control rearrangement of genes during development or in adult tissues. For example, genes encoding Cre recombinase from *Drosophila melanogaster* can be introduced as transgenes and used to insert or excise targeted elements in a tissue-specific manner. *In vivo* activation of transgenes, knock-ins and knock-outs is possible.[38]

LEUKAEMIA AND LYMPHOMA

Leukaemia and non-Hodgkin's lymphoma are described and distinguished in terms of cellular morphology, cell surface markers and propensity to aggregate in marrow or organs of the reticuloendothelial system. Although there is some overlap between clinical entities, molecular cytogenetics has tended to confirm classical morphology by identifying molecular rearrangements that are characteristic of a disease type (Table 2.1). Transcriptional profiling of leukaemic cells by microarray analysis has promise for both contribution to differential diagnosis and understanding of critical genes.[43] The increase in understanding of leukaemogenesis in recent years has been paralleled by increased understanding of normal haemopoiesis. Many genes that are critical in leukaemogenesis have important roles in specification of haemopoietic differentiation.

Table 2.1 *Reciprocal chromosomal translocations in solid tumours*

Tumour histology	Fusion gene	Chromosomal rearrangement
Alveolar rhabdomyosarcoma	PAX3-FKHR	t(2;13)(q35;q14)
	PAX7-FKHR	t(1;13)(p36;q14)
Ewing's family of tumours	EWS-FLI1	t(11;22)(q24;q12)
	EWS-ERG	t(21;22)(q22;q12)
	EWS-ETV1	t(7;22)(p22;q12)
	EWS-FEV	t(2;22)(q33;q12)
	EWS-E1AF	t(17;22)(q12;q12)
Alveolar soft part sarcoma, renal cell carcinoma (rare)	ASPL-TFE3	t(X;17)(p11.2;q25)
Synovial sarcoma	SYT-SSX1	t(X;18)(p11;q11)
	SYT-SSX2	t(X;18)(p11;q11)
	SYT-SSX4	t(X;18)(p11;q11)
Desmoplastic small round-cell tumour	EWS-WT1	t(11;22)(p13;q12)
Congenital fibrosarcoma, cellular mesoblastic nephroma	ETV6-NTRK3	t(12;15)(p13;q25)
Clear cell sarcoma of soft parts	EWS-ATF1	t(12;22)(q13;q12)
Myxoid liposarcoma	FUS-CHOP	t(12;16)(q13;p11)
	EWS-CHOP	t(12;22)(q13;q12)
Extraskeletal myxoid chondrosarcoma	EWS-TEC	t(9;22)(q22;q12)
	TAF2N-TEC	t(9;17)(q22;q12)
Myxoid chondrosarcoma	EWS-CHN	t(9;22)(q22;q13)
Dermatofibrosarcoma protuberans	COL1A1-PDG	t(17;22)(q22;q13)

More than 100 genetic changes or chromosomal rearrangements involved in leukaemia have now been defined. Some are leukaemia subtype-specific, such as most gene fusions caused by chromosomal translocation, and some are generic, such as *p53* or *RAS* mutations or deletion of CDK4 inhibitors. Most genetic changes in leukaemia are acquired DNA alterations in haemopoietic stem cells. More rarely, inherited mutations, such as in *p53* or *NF1*, can predispose to leukaemia.

Burkitt lymphoma

In Burkitt lymphoma and mature B-cell acute lymphoblastic leukaemia (ALL), there is activation of the c-*myc* oncogene as a result of chromosomal translocations, which juxtaposes the full-length c-*myc* proto-oncogene with an immunoglobulin gene enhancer element (Figure 2.1). In most cases this is caused by translocation t(8;14)(q24;q32) in which an immunoglobulin heavy chain enhancer is juxtaposed to the c-*myc* locus. Rarer, but functionally analogous, translocations involve chromosomes 2 and 22, sites of the kappa and lambda light chains, respectively.[5]

C-MYC is a transcription factor that is deregulated by overexpression, usually as a result of genomic amplification, in many cancer types. Like *MYCN*, which can be amplified in neuroblastoma, rhabdomyosarcoma, retinoblastoma and small cell lung cancer, it is a transcription factor containing a basic helix-loop-helix (bHLH) DNA binding domain that forms heterodimers with another bHLH family member, MAX, to form a transcription activation complex. A complex network of interacting related bHLH family members regulate MYC/MAX transcription. Overexpression of MYC results in preferential formation of transcriptionally active MYC/MAX heterodimers.[44] In cell transfection experiments, MYC overexpression results in enhanced proliferation, inhibition of differentiation, and apoptosis, suggesting that additional survival factors are required *in vivo* to offset MYC-induced apoptosis.[45] In transgenic mice containing a c-*myc* expression cassette conditionally overexpressed under the regulation of the immunoglobulin heavy chain enhancer, and only in the absence of doxycycline, lymphomas and leukaemias developed at high frequency and osteosarcomas at low frequency. Interestingly, inactivation of the *MYC* oncogene, through addition of doxycycline, resulted in tumour regression associated with differentiation and apoptosis of tumour cells. This suggests that *myc* can initiate tumorigenesis and that its continued overexpression is required for continued tumour growth.[42,46]

T–lineage leukaemia

Several genes have been discovered through their involvement in translocations involving the T-cell receptor loci, resulting in T-cell leukaemias (Table 2.2). Typically this results in an expression in T-lineage cells of transcription factors that are normally not expressed in T cells. LMO1, LMO2 and TAL1 have been elucidated in this way. Interestingly, LMO and TAL1 proteins are thought to be part of a DNA binding transcription complex and their activation through translocation is probably responsible for directing T-cell differentiation in leukaemia.

Table 2.2 *Major translocations in leukaemia and lymphoma of childhood*

Translocation	Genes	Disease
t(8;14)(q24;q32)	*C-MYC* and *IgH*	Burkitt lymphoma, mature B-cell leukaemia
t(2;8)(p12;q24)	*IgK* and *C-MYC*	Burkitt lymphoma, mature B-cell leukaemia
t(8;22)(q24;q11)	*C-MYC* and *IgK*	Burkitt lymphoma, mature B-cell leukaemia
t(4;11)(q21;q23)	*AF4* and *MLL*	ALL
t(6;11)(q21;q23)	*AF6q21* and *MLL*	AML
t(9;11)(p22;q23)	*AF9* and *MLL*	AML, ALL
t(11;19)(q23;p13)	*MLL* and *ELL*	AML
t(11;19)(q23;p13)	*MLL* and *ENL*	AML, ALL
t(12;21)(p13;q22)	*AML1* and *TEL (ETV6)*	Pre-B ALL
t(8;21)(q22;q22)	*ETO* and *AML1*	AML (M2)
Inv(16)(p13;q22)	*MYH11* and *CBFβ*	AML
t(15;17)(q22;q21)	*PML* and *RARα*	AML (M3)
t(11;17)(q23;q21)	*PLZF* and *RARα*	AML (M3)
t(5;17)(q32;q21)	*NPM* and *RARα*	AML (M3)
t(1;19)(q23;p13)	*PBX1* and *E2A*	Pre-B ALL
t(17;19)(q23;p13)	*HLF* and *E2A*	Pre-B ALL
t(9;22)(q34;q11)	*BCR* and *ABL*	Adult type CML/pre-B ALL
t(10;14)(q24;q11)	*HOX11* and *TCRα/δ*	T-cell ALL
t(11;14)(p13;q11)	*RBTN-2* and *TCRα/δ*	T-cell ALL
t(11;14)(p15;q11)	*RBTN-1* and *TCRα/δ*	T-cell ALL
t(8;14)(q24;q11)	*C-MYC* and *TCRα/δ*	T-cell ALL
t(7;9)(q34;q32)	*TCRβ* and *TAL*	T-cell ALL
t(2;5)(p23;q35)	*ALK* and *NPM*	Anaplastic large-cell lymphoma

ALL, acute lymphoblastic leukaemia; AML, acute myeloid leukaemia.

INFANT LEUKAEMIA AND *MLL* GENE REARRANGEMENTS

Although the outcome for children with ALL has improved significantly, a subgroup of patients who have cytogenetic rearrangements disrupting the *MLL* gene on chromosome region 11q23 have very poor prognosis. Most of these children are infants, and indeed the prognostic significance of *MLL* gene rearrangement in children older than 1 year old is not so clear as in the infant group.[47,48] The majority of leukaemias associated with *MLL* rearrangement express predominantly lymphoid markers but their immunophenotype differs from the majority of cases of pre-B ALL. For example, they are generally CD10-negative and often co-express the myeloid antigens CD15 and CD65.

MLL is a large protein with sequence homology to the *Drosophila* gene *trithorax*. Gene targeting experiments in mice indicate that *MLL*, like *trithorax*, is a positive regulator of expression of important developmental patterning genes known as hox genes. Its presence is required for maintenance, although not initiation, of expression of hox genes and, as a result, homozygous deletion of *MLL* is embryo lethal with multiple defects in neural crest-derived structures.[49] Three altered forms of MLL protein have been described in leukaemias with 11q23 disruption. Most commonly there is fusion to one of about 30 partner genes. In all cases, the fusion involves the N terminus of *MLL* fused in-frame with the C terminus of the partner gene. More rarely there can be a partial tandem duplication

of *MLL* or an internal deletion of exon 8. In all the fusion proteins, as well as proteins derived from deletion and duplication, there is conservation of the three AT hooks and the CxxC domain, and the rearranged gene is always in frame such that a chimeric protein of altered size is generated. This indicates that there is a necessary gain of function contributed by the partner or the rearrangement. This is borne out by the observation that expression of *MLL* N terminus alone is insufficient to immortalize cells in transformation assays.[50] It is thought that the AT hooks are involved in binding to DNA whereas the CxxC domain is involved in protein–protein interaction and transcriptional repression.[51] Partner genes of *MLL* fall into two functional categories, either cytoplasmic signalling molecules or nuclear transcription factors. The AT hooks and CxxC domains are required for transformation, consistent with a role for the N terminus region of *MLL* in binding specific DNA target sequences.[50] However, the contribution of the C terminus fusion partners is less apparent. One mechanism seems to be the gain of transcriptional function. For example, with the fusion partners *ENL* and *ELL*, ability to immortalize myeloid progenitors correlates with ability to transactivate reporter genes in transient assays, and the transactivation domains are both necessary and sufficient for immortalization when fused to *MLL*. However, in the *MLL-CBP* fusion, a HAT domain of CBP has transcription activation properties and is necessary but not sufficient for immortalization. A further domain of *CBP*, the bromodomain, is also required. This domain may play a role in chromatin remodelling of DNA at regions of *MLL* target genes.[52]

The two other types of *MLL* rearrangement seen in leukaemia, deletion of exon 8 and tandem duplication of the N terminus, both result in the formation of new *MLL* derivatives, one smaller and the other larger. The mechanism of how the rearranged elements of *MLL* function in these proteins is not well understood.

Experiments to study the mechanism of *MLL*-associated leukaemogenesis through knock-in of the fusion gene are likely to yield interesting results. Chimeric animals generated from *MLL-AF9* ES cells develop acute myeloid and lymphoid leukaemia at around 6 months of age, indicating that the fusion protein can initiate leukaemogenesis *in vivo* in more than one lineage.[37,53] Interestingly, knock-in of a MLL-lacZ into the MLL locus is also leukaemogenic (although at lower frequency), suggesting that haploinsufficiency of MLL may also predispose to malignant transformation.[54] However, many attempts to obtain stable expression of MLL fusion proteins in cell lines or transgenic mice have failed. This may be because of an apoptotic response to very high-level expression of the fusion genes.[55]

Identification of target genes of rearranged *MLL* molecules may disclose pathways, the disruption of which could be exploited therapeutically. It is known, for example, that many hox genes regulated by *MLL* in normal development are also targets of the rearranged *MLL* molecules in leukaemia. A recent comprehensive analysis of gene expression in cases of leukaemia with *MLL* rearrangement, and cases of *MLL*-negative acute pre-B lymphoblastic leukaemia, revealed numerous genes specifically associated with *MLL* rearrangement and allowed the description of a gene expression profile that was markedly different from *MLL*-negative ALL.[33] Further work is needed to use this information to determine important genes for therapeutic targeting and identify possible important new prognostic indicators.

AML1 and its roles in acute myeloid leukaemia (AML) and ALL

The *AML1* gene, also known as *Runx1* or *CBFA2*, is the most common target for chromosomal translocations in human leukaemia. Although originally described as being disrupted in AML, it has since been found to be involved in a high proportion of cases of ALL as well.

AML1 is a transcription factor that binds DNA as a heterodimer with core binding factor β (CBFβ). AML1-CBFβ binding sites are defined by a core motif TGTGGT and are frequently adjacent to binding sites for other transcription factors, and AML1-CBFβ is known to cooperate in transcription activation. AML1 also interacts with factors such as p300, ALY and YAP, which stimulate transcription

indirectly by recruitment of RNA polymerase II or histone acetylation. AML1-CBFβ target genes have been well characterized and include *GM-CSF*, *IL3*, myeloperoxidase and *CD11a*, as well as non-haemopoietic targets such as c-*fos*. Gene targeting experiments show that AML1 null mice have impaired differentiation of haemopoietic stem cells in the fetal liver[56] suggesting that disruption of AML1 function, as a result of gene rearrangement, may contribute to leukaemogenesis by inhibiting differentiation.

AML1 IN MYELOID LEUKAEMIA

AML1 is disrupted in a translocation t(8;21)(q22;q22) associated with AML, in which it is fused with the *ETO* gene on chromosome 8 to form the chimeric product *AML-ETO*. *AML-ETO* is thought to contribute to malignant transformation in a number of ways. Firstly, it blocks AML1-CBFβ-induced transactivation of target genes such as *GM-CSF* and *IL3* through the association of *ETO* with *NcoR*, and histone deacetylases which function as transcriptional repressors.[57] Secondly, other genes, such as the anti-apoptotic gene *Bcl2*, are transcriptionally activated by *AML-ETO* despite not being normal transcriptional targets of AML1-CBFβ.[58] Attempts to delineate the function of *AML-ETO* by gene targeting have been disappointing. *AML-ETO* knock-in mice are embryo lethal and have a phenotype that resembles *AML1* null mice. Conditional transgenic *AML-ETO* mice with transgene expression restricted to adult mice do not develop leukaemia despite successful expression of the transgene in haemopoietic cells, suggesting that further genetic events are required for leukaemia development.[41] Recently, similar results have been obtained with a conditional knock-in *AML1-ETO* strain.[59] These interesting findings are consistent with the finding that *AML-ETO* mRNA can still be detected in blood samples of patients in remission who do not subsequently relapse.[60,61]

AML1 IN ALL

The translocation t(12;21)(p13;q22) is found in about 25 per cent of children with pre-B ALL, although in many cases it is not apparent with conventional cytogenetics, and its presence is revealed only by molecular diagnostic techniques.[62] The translocation results in the fusion gene *TEL-AML1*. TEL is a member of the ETS family of transcription factors (see section on 'Ewing's family tumours', and, in the fusion, the 5′ helix-loop-helix DNA binding portion of TEL is fused in-frame with both DNA binding and transactivation domains of AML1.[63]TEL-AML associates with CBFβ and competes with AML1-CBFβ for binding to the AML1-CBFβ core motif. However, TEL-AML functions as a transcription repressor of AML1 targets that are normally transcriptionally activated by AML1-CBFβ.[64,65] Interestingly, the normal *TEL* allele is deleted in many but not all ALL patients with t(12;21), suggesting that *TEL* itself has tumour suppressor properties that are partially abrogated as a result of fusion with *AML1*.[66]

Chronic myeloid leukaemia (CML) and Philadelphia chromosome

Adult-type CML is rare in childhood and is characterized by a reciprocal chromosomal translocation t(9;22)(q34;q11) known as the Philadelphia chromosome. This was the first consistent cytogenetic abnormality to be described in human malignancy. It involves the in-frame fusion of the c-*ABL* oncogene on chromosome 9 with *BCR* gene on chromosome 22 to generate a chimeric protein. Like all fusion genes generated by reciprocal translocations in human cancer, the two components of the fusion are in an open reading frame one with another. In adult-type CML, a fusion protein of about 210 kDa, known as p210, is generated. The c-*ABL* proto-oncogene is a cytoplasmic tyrosine kinase with poorly understood roles in directing cellular life/death decisions. The p210 protein has greater tyrosine kinase activity than ABL and demonstrates transforming potential when introduced into primary cells and cell lines.[67,68] More common within paediatric practice is the occurrence of the Philadelphia chromosome in cases of ALL. This is seen in only about 5 per cent or fewer of cases of paediatric ALL but in about 20 per cent of cases of adult ALL. The fusion protein is generated as a result of a different intronic breakpoint in BCR, resulting in a smaller protein called p190, which has greater tyrosine kinase and transforming activity than p210. The presence of p190 in children with ALL confers a very poor prognosis, and bone marrow transplantation in first remission is needed to cure the disease. Glivec, which targets the receptor tyrosine kinases c-kit, abl, and PDGFRβ, has an emerging role in the targeted therapy against BCR-ABL in CML.

Large-cell anaplastic lymphoma

Understanding of Ki-l-positive anaplastic large-cell lymphoma moved from a first description in the mid-1980s to characterization of genes involved in a specific translocation some 10 years later. This condition is characterized by large pleomorphic tumour cells, expression of lymphocyte activation antigens CD30, CD25, CD71 and HLA-DR,[69,70] and a non-random chromosome translocation t(2;5)(p23;q35).[71] Positional cloning using fluorescence *in situ* hybridization (FISH) to order cosmid clones led to the identification of the genes involved as nucleophosmin (NPM) on chromosome 5q35, and a previously undescribed protein tyrosine kinase, ALK, on chromosome 2p23.[72] The rearrangement results in the amino terminus of NPM being linked to the catalytic domain of ALK. ALK is normally expressed in small intestine, testis and brain, but is not expressed in lymphoid cells. The normal NPM protein is a non-ribosomal protein involved in the assembly of preribosomal particles to form large and small ribosomal subunits. The transcription and translation of NPM are cell cycle-regulated, peaking just before the S-phase and declining to baseline levels just before the onset of G2. Thus, one would predict that the translocation leads to dysregulation of the ALK kinase activity.

RETINOBLASTOMA AS A PARADIGM OF THE TWO-HIT HYPOTHESIS OF TUMOUR SUPPRESSOR GENES

Approximately 25–30 per cent of cases of retinoblastoma (RB) have a family history, making it the prototype of cancer predisposition syndromes and a paradigm for the two-hit hypothesis of inherited mutated tumour suppressor genes. In a mathematical analysis based on observed incidence and age of onset of RB in familial and sporadic forms, Knudson formulated a hypothesis that contended that only two genetic events were required for tumour initiation. In hereditary cases, the first event (or 'hit') is inherited and only a single additional random event is required. Therefore familial tumours are usually multifocal, frequently bilateral and tend to have an earlier age of onset than sporadic forms, which are typically unifocal.

Analysis of the genetics of RB led to the discovery of the predisposition gene, termed *RB*, on chromosome region 13q14. The gene has been shown to encode a key regulator of the cell cycle, which transduces growth signals via binding and inhibiting of the transcripion factor E2F1. Hence, the normal effect of *RB* is inhibitory. If *RB* is phosphorylated following activation of D-type cyclins, it releases its inhibition of E2F1 which permits transition from G1 to S-phase of the cell cycle. Hence loss of *RB* function results in uncontrolled, or unchecked, proliferation. *RB* function can also be lost through overactivity of cyclins (e.g. cyclin D or CDK4 and CDK6) or through loss of cyclin-dependent kinase inhibitors (CDKI). The CDKIs are themselves tumour suppressor genes, whose expression is lost by mutation of genes or their promoters in many cancer types. Indeed, it seems likely that loss of normal G1-S checkpoint regulation is a feature of most, if not all, cancers, although different mechanisms exist, e.g. mutation of *RB*, loss of CDKIs (such as p16INK4A) or expression of adenovirus protein E1A, which interacts with *RB*.

RB is now known to be one of a family of proteins, the other family members being p107 and p130. Together with pRB, p107 and p130 represent a family of closely related proteins that play critical roles in the regulation of cell proliferation. A degree of redundancy might help explain the specificity and limited repertoire of tumour types in patients with familial RB mutation. These patients are prone to RB only in early life, and in adolescence are at increased risk of osteosarcoma. However, large numbers of sporadic tumour types, especially in adults, have high incidences of acquired RB mutations. It is possible that mutated RB has a limited role in initiating tumorigenesis, except in the retina, but its loss is essential in many cell types for tumour progression. The situation is more confused by the study of RB knock-out mice which develop pituitary tumours but not RB.[73] This suggests differences between species in the relative importance of RB in regulating the cell cycle in different cell types.

WILMS' TUMOUR

Wilms' tumour (nephroblastoma) is an embryonal kidney cancer that affects 1 in 10 000 children worldwide each year and accounts for around 6 per cent of childhood cancers in the UK. Knudson and Strong[74] proposed that his two-hit model could also apply to Wilms' tumour (WT), even though the genetic component is not as obvious as in RB, with fewer than 1 per cent having a family history. A small number of children with WT have specific congenital malformation syndromes, suggesting that they, too, may be carriers of mutations in a WT-predisposition gene. The first association to be recognized was that of WT with sporadic aniridia, congenital absence of the irises. This was termed the WAGR syndrome, due to the frequent occurrence of other characteristic abnormalities (WT, aniridia, genitourinary malformation and mental retardation). These patients have a constitutional deletion encompassing chromosome 11p13, although aniridia is fully penetrant, and hence a marker for the syndrome, WT develops in only 30–50 per cent. Gonadal tumours are also occasionally seen in this syndrome. The 11p13 deletion can rarely be inherited, either by carriers of balanced translocations who transmit an unbalanced form, or by carriers of submicroscopic deletions who have escaped the abnormal genital phenotype. By deletion mapping of individuals with varying phenotypes, the aniridia locus can be

separated from the WT locus within 11p13, whereas the WT locus cannot be separated from that for genitourinary malformation, suggesting that tumorigenesis and malformation can be pleiotropic effects of mutation in the same gene.[75] This led to the isolation of PAX6 as the aniridia gene and WT1 as the gene predisposing to both WT and genitourinary malformation.

Several other recognized syndromes carry an increased risk of WT (Table 2.3). They can be grouped into the overgrowth syndromes, of which the commonest is Beckwith–Wiedemann syndrome (BWS) but includes the X-linked Simpson–Golabi–Behmel syndrome, and syndromes associated with nephrotic syndrome, including Denys–Drash syndrome (DDS) and Perlman syndrome.[76–80] Although rare, they have proved important in localizing WT-predisposition genes. It is now clear that there are several WT genes that may be responsible for both genetic and sporadic forms of WT.

The *WT1* gene at 11p13

The aforementioned chromosome 11p13 deletions both localized a WT-predisposition gene and provided evidence that WT, like RB, could be due to loss of function of a gene. By positional cloning, a WT-predisposition gene within chromosome 11p13 was isolated.[81,82] The gene, designated WT1, encodes a protein with four zinc fingers, a structural motif of transcription factors. The gene is the subject of both alternate splicing and RNA editing, to produce eight potential isoforms of the WT1 protein, which differ in their DNA binding specificity and effects on transcription.[75] WT1 is expressed only in certain tissues, particularly the developing kidney and gonad, in keeping with its having a role in malformation and tumorigenesis of these organs.[83] Children with the WAGR syndrome carry a germ line complete deletion of one WT1 allele. In the majority of tumours that develop in these children, a second hit in the remaining WT1 allele can be found, in accordance with Knudson's model.[84,85] Some cases of children with bilateral WT have similarly been shown to follow germ line WT1 mutation.[86] In several large studies of sporadic WTs, it is now clear that homozygous WT1 gene mutations are

Table 2.3 *Congenital malformation syndromes predisposing to Wilms' tumour (WT)*

Syndrome	Locus	Gene(s)	Mutation type	Risk of WT
WAGR	11p13	WT1	Complete deletion of WT1	30–50%
Denys–Drash/Frasier	11p13	WT1	Missense mutation/aberrant splicing of WT1	30–50%
Overgrowth syndromes				
Beckwith–Wiedemann	11p15.5	p57/IGF2/H19	Abnormal imprinting	<10%
Hemihypertrophy	?	?		<1%
Simpson–Golabi–Behmel	Xq26	GPC3	Loss of function	~1%
Perlman	?	?		?

WAGR, Wilms' tumour, aniridia, genitourinary malformation and mental retardation.

present in only 5–15 per cent of tumours.[87] The majority of these *WT1* mutations produce a truncated protein. However, many cases have now been described where the *WT1* mutation produces an altered protein that may have gained new properties or may interfere with the action of the remaining normal WT1 protein (a so-called 'dominant-negative' effect).[88,89] Therefore, although homozygous inactivating mutations of *WT1* may be sufficient for the development of WT, this is not the only genetic pathway that results in this tumour phenotype.

Denys–Drash and Frasier syndromes

In a rather pleasing confirmation of a biological prediction, the *WT1* gene was shown to underlie the Denys–Drash syndrome (DDS).[90] Disruption of this single gene was predicted to account for the triad of pseudohermaphroditism, WT and nephrotic syndrome based on specific expression of *WT1* in the three cell types that are defective (i.e. developing gonad, metanephric blastema and podocyte layer of the renal glomerulus, respectively). The germ-line mutations found in this syndrome mainly affect DNA binding. These *WT1* mutations have a dominant effect on gonadal development and podocyte function, whereas they are recessive for tumorigenesis. The related Frasier syndrome (genital malformation combined with a later-onset nephrotic syndrome and predisposition to gonadal tumours) has been shown to be due also to constitutional *WT1* mutation. Characterization of constitutional *WT1* mutations in these patients shows that these syndromes probably represent part of a spectrum of *WT1*-associated disorders that includes rare cases of isolated nephrotic syndrome.[91] Finally, a comparison of DDS with the WAGR syndrome emphasizes that complete absence of one allele of the *WT1* gene has less severe effects on development of the gonad and podocytes than does the presence of a mutated protein. Rapid genetic screening for *WT1* mutations in patients with features of DDS is now possible, as 50 per cent of the mutations are identical and the majority are confined to the zinc finger region of the gene.

Since the cloning of the *WT1* gene, much work has been done towards understanding its biological activity. In *in vitro* experiments, it has been shown to function as a transcriptional regulator of many different genes, either increasing or decreasing their expression depending on the target gene and on the WT1 isoform.[92] A more powerful approach to understanding a gene's biology can be gene 'knock-out' experiments. Homozygous null mice are not viable and die at midgestation. There is no induction of metanephric kidney formation, with massive apoptosis of the metanephric blastema and failure of gonadal development. Subsequently, 'knock-in' technology has created a mouse strain lacking the ability to produce +KTS isoforms on one *WT1* allele. Heterozygous mice develop glomerulosclerosis and represent a murine model of Frasier syndrome.[93] These experiments show that WT1 is essential for genitourinary development in the mouse and therefore probably also in humans.

Precursor lesions for WT

In a comprehensive study of WT specimens submitted to the National Wilms' Tumour Study (NWTS) pathology review panel, Beckwith *et al.*[94] found that nearly all cases of bilateral WT and 40 per cent of unilateral WT are associated with nephrogenic rests in the adjacent normal kidney. These rests consist of areas of persistent but disorganized fetal renal tissue and are categorized into 'intralobar' and 'perilobar' depending on whether their morphology reflects early or late stages of nephrogenesis, respectively. Do these nephrogenic rests result from the first 'hit' in the *WT1* gene, representing true precursors, with the development of WT resulting from loss of the remaining *WT1* allele? Observations on the tumours of patients with the WAGR syndrome would suggest that this is the case, as nearly all of them have associated rests of the intralobar variety. Two small studies of allele loss and/or *WT1* mutation in nephrogenic rests show that *WT1* may already be homozygously mutated in intralobar and occasional perilobar nephrogenic rests, suggesting that further genetic events are necessary for tumour development.[95]

Several genes for WT

Originally, allele loss or loss of heterozygosity (LOH) was used as a marker for the location of tumour suppressor genes involved in WT. Consistent allele loss had been found in WT only for chromosome 11p (in approximately one-third) and for 16q (in approximately 20 per cent).[96,97] In the case of 11p, fine mapping studies have shown that in one-third of tumours with allele loss, this is confined to the most telomeric part of the short arm (11p15) and does not include the *WT1* locus at 11p13.[96,98] This suggested that there might be a second WT locus on chromosome 11, located at 11p15. This idea was supported by the mapping of the locus for Beckwith–Wiedemann syndrome to 11p15.5 (see below). This locus is known to contain several genes implicated in BWS, some of which may contribute to sporadic forms of WT. Linkage studies on pedigrees of familial WT have provided evidence for the existence of at least three familial WT genes on 17q, 19q and elsewhere in the genome.[99–101] Thus, there are several genes that can predispose to WT. It is possible that somatic mutations in these genes also cause sporadic WT and that they act in synergy or in sequence to produce a similar phenotype.

Beckwith–Wiedemann syndrome

In the 1960s, Wiedemann and Beckwith described a syndrome of fetal overgrowth with macroglossia, generalized organomegaly and omphalos, together with characteristic facial features. A proportion of children with this syndrome have hemihypertrophy, which may be limited to only one part of the body. As part of the original description, it was recognized that these children had an increased risk of childhood tumours, particularly the embryonal type (WT, rhabdomyosarcoma, hepatoblastoma), as well as adrenocortical carcinoma. Only 10 per cent of children with BWS develop tumours and the commonest type is WT, which accounts for about half of all tumours.[78] Of interest is the fact that the children with hemihypertrophy or early nephromegaly seem to be at higher risk, but the tumour does not necessarily develop on the hypertrophied side.[102]

BWS usually occurs sporadically but rarely may be familial, being inherited as an autosomal dominant. In the sporadic form, occasional patients have been found to have constitutional karyotypic abnormalities that involve duplication of part of the short arm of chromosome 11p15.[103–105] Familial cases have also been mapped to this same region by linkage analysis.[106,107] However, elucidating the 'BWS gene' has not proved straightforward and has led to the recognition that an epigenetic phenomenon known as imprinting may play an important role in several childhood embryonal tumours. The 11p15 region is very well mapped and contains many genes, several of which have been implicated in the development of BWS. To understand how these genetic changes interact and the possible genotype–phenotype correlations seen in BWS, it is necessary to first review the phenomenon of imprinting and how it affects the BWS gene cluster at 11p15.5.

Imprinting in WT

Imprinting is defined as when the expression of each allele of a gene depends on the parental origin of that allele. The imprinting pattern must therefore be erased and re-established in the germ cell of each individual. The molecular mechanism may involve methylation of the promoter of a gene. A minority of genes, which seem to be mainly active during embryogenesis, are imprinted and may be transcribed exclusively from either paternal or maternal alleles. In the mouse, over 50 genes are known to be imprinted in a restricted number of chromosomal regions (see www.mgu.har.mrc.ac.uk/imprinting/imprinting.html). The syntenic region of human chromosome 11p15.5 is the distal region of mouse chromosome 7, which contains a large cluster of imprinted genes. Their human counterparts are also imprinted and include five genes implicated in BWS (see Figure 2.4). Although they lie very close to each other, these genes are differentially imprinted, with $H19$, $KVLQT1$ and $CDKN1C/p^{57KIP2}$ being expressed from the maternal allele, and $IGF2$ and $LIT1$ from the paternal allele. $IGF2$ encodes a fetal mitogen and $CDKN1C/p^{57KIP2}$ encodes an inhibitor of the cell cycle. Overexpression of the former and mutation or loss of the latter could be expected to contribute to overgrowth and tumorigenesis. The causative role of the other genes in BWS and WT is less clear. $KVLQT1$ encodes a voltage-gated potassium channel defective in the long QT syndrome. Both $H19$ and $LIT1$ (long QT intronic transcript 1) encode only RNAs, with the latter being transcribed in the antisense orientation to $KVLQT1$. A model has been proposed whereby these genes lie within two imprinted subdomains: the more telomeric contains the $IGF2$ and $H19$ genes and the more centromeric domain includes $CDKN1C/p^{57KIP2}$, $LIT1$ and $KVLQT1$ (see Figure 2.4). Disturbances of methylation in either domain could affect

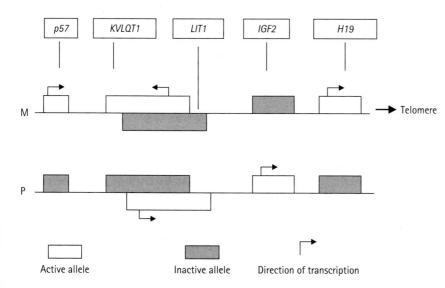

Figure 2.4 *Locus of imprinted alleles at human chromosome region 11p15.5. M and P, maternally and paternally inherited chromosomes, respectively.*

imprinting and cause the BWS phenotype through bial-lelic expression of the growth-promoting *IGF2* or silencing of the growth suppressing *CDKN1C/p57KIP2*.

So, which gene is the BWS gene? In those few cases who are constitutionally trisomic for 11p15, there is duplication of the paternal allele, giving two active copies of the *IGF2* gene. Many other cases, with trisomy 11p15, have achieved the same gene dosage by loss of imprinting of the maternal *IGF2* allele so that it has become abnormally active.[108] Thus, although *IGF2* is not 'the BWS gene' in the conventional sense of encoding a mutant protein in affected individuals, its level of expression is certainly disregulated and is likely to be causative for the syndrome in at least some cases. Constitutional mutations of *CDKN1C/p57KIP2* occur in a small fraction of patients with BWS.[109,110] Another way of inactivating this gene may be through altered methylation of *LIT1*. The interactions of alterations in *CDKN1C/p57KIP2* and *IGF2* have been investigated in mouse models. The *CDKN1C/p57KIP2* knock-out mouse has overlapping phenotypic features with BWS.[111] By crossing these animals onto a strain with loss of imprinting of *IGF2*, some features are shown to be *IGF2*-independent, which may explain how BWS can arise from mutations in either gene.[112] In the future, it may be possible to predict the tumour risk in individuals with BWS by detailed molecular analysis of these two imprinted domains, but it is premature on the current evidence base to remove patients from screening programmes.[113,114]

Imprinting may explain the observation that in most of the cases of sporadic WT that show LOH, the allele that is lost is the maternal one.[115] Since the *WT1* gene at 11p13 is not imprinted in either fetal kidney or in WTs, and since the allele loss may be confined to 11p15, this may mean that for most WTs with 11p LOH, this reflects abnormalities at 11p15 rather than involvement of the *WT1* gene. Allele loss (LOH), usually by mitotic recombination, is the commonest method by which a mutant gene becomes homozygous in the tumour, as seen in retinoblastoma.[116] However, loss of imprinting (LOI) is an alternative mechanism to achieve the same functional results if tumorigenesis is dependent on gene dosage. Loss of imprinting occurs somatically in sporadic WTs.[108] This results in two active copies of the *IGF2* gene, and the double dose of *IGF2* may promote tumour growth. Tumours with LOI of *IGF2* also show aberrant imprinting of the *H19* gene with hypermethylation of its promoter and lack of expression,[117] and this may be functionally important as *H19* has tumour suppressor activity.[118] Disregulation of both *IGF2* and *H19* has been found in 28 out of 37 WTs analysed.[117,119] Thus, this may be an important defect in the majority of WTs, which can be achieved through several different genetic pathways. Neither somatic mutation nor altered imprinting of the *p57* gene seem to be important in sporadic WT.[120]

Simpson–Golabi–Behmel syndrome

This X-linked overgrowth syndrome has several phenotypic features in common with BWS, but is distinguished by hypertelorism, polydactyly and supernumerary nipples.[80,121] The risk of WT is probably lower than in BWS, but many fewer cases have been described worldwide. The gene underlying this syndrome was identified as *glypican 3* through analysis of constitutional translocations.[122] Glypicans are cell surface heparan sulphate proteoglycans that play essential roles in development by modulating cellular responses to growth factors and morphogens. It is uncertain at present whether they act through or independently of the IGF2 pathway.[123] Somatic mutation of *GPC3* is not common in sporadic WT.[124]

Perlman syndrome

Perlman described a much rarer autosomal recessive syndrome with some phenotypic overlap with BWS but a high perinatal mortality and much greater risk of WT in survivors. Virtually all the affected individuals have genitourinary abnormalities, with hypospadias (in males) and nephroblastomatosis. Although fewer than 10 affected families have been described worldwide, this syndrome is important from a genetic point of view as it probably involves yet another WT gene.[79]

Other known genes associated with WT

WT occurs occasionally in families with a pattern of familial cancer consistent with the Li–Fraumeni syndrome.[125] However, germ-line *p53* gene mutations do not seem to confer a particularly high risk of WT, whereas they do for sarcomas and adrenocortical carcinoma, although a few cases of WT in Li–Fraumeni syndrome families have been described.[126] Somatic *p53* mutation in sporadic WT is uncommon (5 per cent) and is associated with anaplastic histology and a poor outcome.[127]

Heritability of WT

In large studies in both Europe and the USA, the incidence of familial WT is 1–2 per cent.[128,129] Most pedigrees are small with only two or three affected members. However, linkage studies in the few large pedigrees have provided evidence for the existence of two familial WT genes, designated *FWT1* and *FWT2* at 17q12–21 and 19q12, respectively.[99,100] Analysis of collected smaller pedigrees show that further *FWT* genes must exist.[101] However, none has yet been identified. What is the risk for the offspring of the ever increasing number of survivors of both unilateral and bilateral WT? So far, four studies, which together cover 462 survivors of unilateral WT, have revealed only four cases among 362 offspring with a calculated maximum 3 per cent lifetime risk of any such offspring.[130] However, it is the bilateral cases that are expected to be germ-line carriers of mutation in a WT predisposition gene; what is the risk to their offspring? There are now epidemiological data that suggest that a proportion of bilateral and multicentric cases may be due to somatic mutation occurring postzygotically.[131] They may therefore be at low risk of transmitting the gene. The true proportion of bilateral cases with germ-line mutations will await a survey of their offspring, of which none has yet been reported.

SMALL ROUND–CELL TUMOURS OF CHILDHOOD

Non-Hodgkin's lymphoma, neuroblastoma, Ewing's sarcoma, rhabdomyosarcoma, retinoblastoma, desmoplastic small round-cell tumour and WT are sometimes collectively referred to as the small round-cell tumours of childhood. Distinguishing between these tumour types is usually easily accomplished by conventional morphology and immunohistochemistry. In a few instances, however, tumours are relatively undifferentiated and it is in these cases that molecular genetic analysis can be contributory.

In paediatric practice, diagnostic molecular cytogenetics is becoming established as an important adjunct to conventional histological analysis in rhabdomyosarcoma and Ewing's family of tumours, which both have typical chromosomal translocations. This has been made possible by the introduction of new molecular techniques, to complement conventional cytogenetics. Using the technique of interphase FISH, cells can be analysed directly without any need for tissue culture; furthermore, retrospective analysis is also possible if snap-frozen samples are available, although FISH analysis of formalin-fixed tissue is problematic and not yet a part of diagnostic work-up. A further means of detecting translocations is by analysis of tumour RNA by reverse transcriptase polymerase chain reaction (RT-PCR) for the presence of chimeric transcripts. Success of RT-PCR is critically dependent on the quality of extracted RNA, which in turn is dependent on tumour being transported fresh to the laboratory and snap-frozen or extracted immediately. The recent introduction of solutions to protect RNA in samples through inhibition of ribonucleases is likely to improve the percentage of informative cases. However, a critical feature of all diagnostic work will be controls for the expression of housekeeping genes in the tumour samples, as a guard against false-negative results.

Alveolar rhabdomyosarcoma

In rhabdomyosarcoma, a consistent chromosomal abnormality – a translocation t(2;13)(q35;q14) – was first noted in 1987 by Douglass et al.[132] This is very strongly associated with alveolar histology. Using the candidate gene approach, Barr et al.[133] were able to demonstrate that the relevant gene on chromosome 2 was the human homologue of the mouse PAX3 gene. Subsequent work identified the involved gene on chromosome 13 as a novel human homologue of the Drosophila forkhead gene, now termed FKHR. A smaller proportion of alveolar rhabdomyosarcoma cases are associated with a variant translocation, t(1;13)(p36;q14), which causes a fusion between the FKHR gene on chromosome 13 and the PAX7 gene on chromosome 1.[134] PAX3, PAX7 and FKHR are all transcription factors that bind specific target genes through interaction with target DNA sequences in the promoters, and then stimulate transcription through interaction of transactivation domains with the basal transcriptional proteins.

In tumours with the t(2;13)(q35;q14) translocation, the chimeric fusion gene on the derivative chromosome 13 contains the PAX3 DNA binding elements known as paired box, homeodomain and octapeptide, and a small part of the forkhead DNA binding domain.[8,135] However, FKHR contributes a transcription activation domain and it is likely that the gain of function associated with expression of PAX3-FKHR fusion in rhabdomyosarcoma is derived, at least in part, from enhanced transcription of PAX3 target genes.[136] Introduction of PAX3-FKHR expressing vectors into a variety of cell types has resulted in tumorigenesis or enhanced malignancy, whereas downregulation of PAX3-FKHR expression using antisense or competitor transcription factors has inhibited cell growth or resulted in apoptosis.[137,138]

More recent work has focused on the mechanism by which PAX3-FKHR transforms cells and the genes that are critically regulated by it. The likely role of PAX3 in tumorigenesis can be summarized from its important developmental role, the study of which has been greatly aided by the existence of naturally occurring mutants. Mutations of PAX3 were first described in mice with the splotch (Sp) phenotype. Mice that are heterozygous for a splotch mutation have white belly spots (the 'splotches'), whereas homozygotes have a severe phenotype involving neural tube defects and a severe muscle phenotype. In the human, mutations within PAX3 similar to those seen in splotch mice lead to Waardenburg syndrome (WS) type 1 and type 3. Type 1 WS consists of deafness, heterochromic irides and a prominent white forelock. In addition to these abnormalities, limb defects are seen in type 3 WS. Very rare individuals homozygous for PAX3 mutations have major limb abnormalities with complete absence of muscles.

An explanation for the phenotypes of Splotch and Waardenberg follows from a close examination of normal expression patterns of PAX3 in development. In normal mouse embryos, *PAX3* expression can be first seen at day 8.5 in the dorsal neural tube, in the region that gives rise to the neural crest, and in the lateral dermatome of the condensing somites. At days 9.5–10.5, *PAX3*-expressing cells can be seen in the limb premuscle masses, suggesting that these cells have de-epithelialized from the lateral dermomyotome to form a migratory population destined to become the muscles of the limbs, diaphragm and tip of the tongue. Moreover, mesenchymal cells migrating into limb buds in the 9-day mouse embryo continue to express *PAX3* mRNA. *PAX3* expression is also seen, although this is at lower levels in the myotome cells derived from the somite that give rise to the non-migrating muscles of the trunk. In splotch mutants, migration from the dermomyotome is absent, suggesting that *PAX3*, or genes it regulates, is critical for this developmental migration.[139] More recently, an important anti-apoptotic cell survival role for *PAX3* and *PAX7* in early development has been described.[140]

Hence *PAX3-FKHR* expression in clinical tumours is associated with alveolar histology, which itself is associated with increased rate of distant metastases. Results from cell biology experiments indicate it to be critical for cell transformation and survival, and to confer new invasive properties to cells that recapitulate some features of the developmental role of *PAX3*. Several attempts have been made to correlate expression of the fusion genes with clinical behaviour and histological appearances of patient samples. Such studies are difficult because of the problems of obtaining adequate samples from patients treated uniformly and with centralized review of histology. However, several conclusions are apparent: firstly, a proportion of alveolar tumours (approximately 10–20 per cent) lack either *PAX3-FKHR* or *PAX7-FKHR* expression but might be associated with alternate mechanisms of activation of these *PAX* genes; secondly, alveolar histology is sometimes not seen in a sample expressing *PAX3-FKHR* or *PAX7-FKHR*, and this may be because of minimal sample size, another possible source of confusion being the existence of solid variant alveolar histology which lacks the clefts and alveolar spaces but is associated with the characteristic fusions; finally, whereas the outcome for patients with *PAX3-FKHR* is poor (overall survival 20–40 per cent), patients with *PAX7-FKHR* are less likely to have metastatic disease despite alveolar histology, have metastases limited to lymph nodes and bone, and have a better overall survival.[141,142] The question remains as to whether it is histology or molecular genetics that correlates best with response to treatment and outcome. Current protocols stratify patients based on the presence of alveolar histology (classical or solid variant) and molecular genetics is likely to contribute to the histological diagnosis in a proportion of cases. To determine the relative prognostic significance of fusion genes and histology will require multivariate survival analysis of very large prospective studies of uniformly treated patients. It is important that the significance of the fusion genes is critically assessed and that they do not become accepted as adverse features without firm evidence.

OTHER GENES INVOLVED IN RHABDOMYOSARCOMA

Like many embryonal tumours, *IGF2* is expressed at high levels in rhabdomyosarcoma and this is associated with epigenetic changes at chromosome region 11p15.5, a region that includes a number of imprinted genes, some of which are potential tumour suppressors or oncogenes. *IGF2* is mitogenic and may provide an important anti-apoptotic survival role. Cell culture evidence suggests that *PAX3-FKHR* and *IGF2* may cooperate in transformation of myoblasts. The genes that regulate *PAX3* and/or *PAX3-FKHR* expression in rhabdomyosarcoma are becoming better defined.[143,144] In normal development, combinatorial signalling from notocord and neural tube, including SHH signalling, is important. *PTCH* knock-out mice, which effectively have unopposed SHH signalling, develop medulloblastomas and rhabdomyosarcomas, the latter associated with high expression of the transcription factor GLI-1, which is also observed in human rhabdomyosarcoma.[145] However, *PAX3* expression in these tumours has not been demonstrated and it is uncertain how far they resemble the human counterpart.

Ewing's family of tumours and other gene fusions involving *EWS*

In 1984, a number of groups described a chromosomal translocation, t(II;22)(q24;qI2), in Ewing's sarcoma, peripheral neuroepithelioma and Askin tumour. The presence of this characteristic chromosomal translocation now effectively defines Ewing's family of tumours, comprising Ewing's sarcoma, extraosseous Ewing's and peripheral primitive neuroectodermal tumour (pPNET). Using a reverse genetics approach, the breakpoints in the two chromosomes were cloned. Phylogenetically conserved DNA fragments adjacent to the breakpoints were then used to identify transcribed sequences, including a hybrid transcript. Subsequent screening of complementary DNA libraries using these conserved sequences led to the identification of the *EWS* gene on chromosome 22 and the human homologue of the murine *FLI-l* gene on chromosome 11. The breakpoints in the two genes are very consistent, so that the translocation results in the substitution of the *EWS* RNA-binding domain by the DNA-binding domain of *FLI-1*, which thereby comes under the control of the *EWS* promoter.[146] As one might expect, both *FLI-1* and *EWS/FLI-1* are able to bind the same nucleotide target sequences in a specific manner, but the *EWS* sequences present in the *EWS/FLI-1* chimera act as potent activators of transcription and have a different tissue specificity to the human *FLI-1* promoter.[147] *EWS/FLI-1* causes a phenotype distinct from that caused by wild-type *FLI-1* as the chimeric protein possesses a transforming ability that *FLI-1* lacks, when expressed at comparable levels. Therefore, the oncogenic effect is not simply a result of deregulated expression of the *FLI-1* DNA-binding domain. Overall about 90 per cent of tumours within Ewing's family have *EWS-FLI-1*, and other family members have one of a number of variant translocations still involving the N terminus of *EWS*. Alternate intronic breakpoints in both *EWS* and *FLI-1* result in a number of different isoforms of *EWS-FLI-1*. Type 1 transcripts (*EWS* exon 7 fused with *FLI-1* exon 6) account for 60 per cent of all cases, whilst type 2 transcripts (*EWS* exon 7 to *FLI-1* exon 5) are seen in about 25 per cent. There is some evidence that type 1 transcript is a positive predictor of outcome in multivariate analysis compared with the other isoforms or translocations.[148] This finding is borne out at the cellular level, as tumours with type 1 transcripts have also been shown to have a lower proliferation rate.[149] Moreover, in transient transfection experiments, there is lower transactivation of reporters with *FLI-1*-sensitive promoter sequences following co-transfection with type 1 *EWS-FLI-1* compared with type 2 transcript. This suggests a simple model of type 1 *EWS-FLI-1* being a weaker transcription factor and resulting in a less malignant phenotype due to factors such as reduced cellular proliferation.

A further translocation found in Ewing's sarcoma is between *EWS* and *ERG*, lying on chromosome 21, which also encodes an ETS-like DNA-binding protein related to FLI-1.[150,151] The *EWS* gene, rather like the *MLL* and *AML1* genes in leukaemia, has been shown to be highly promiscuous and to be fused to a number of different partners in a number of different malignancies. In each case, the paradigm of *EWS-FLI-1* holds with *EWS* providing transcriptional activation and the partner gene providing DNA-binding elements and thereby conferring the specificity of the ensuing malignant transformation. Little is known about other genetic changes in Ewing's family tumours. However, recent evidence suggest that *p53* mutation is seen in a subset of tumours with typical histology but is associated with worse prognosis.[152]

A particularly illuminating and intriguing example relevant to paediatric oncology is the *EWS-WT1* fusion seen in desmoplastic small round-cell tumours. The fusion protein in this malignancy involves three of the four zinc fingers (DNA-binding elements) of *WT1* fused to the N terminus of *EWS* containing its transactivation domain. Like all other fusion genes involving *EWS*, fusion gene expression is driven by the normally ubiquitously expressed *EWS* promoter. *EWS-WT1* is capable of transforming cells. It is therefore thought that the *WT1* zinc fingers confer the specificity of transformation by binding to some normal *WT1* targets, whilst *EWS* regulates transcriptional activation. Despite the ubiquitous activity of *EWS*

promoter in somatic cells, there is a strong tissue specificity of desmoplastic small round-cell tumours (80 per cent abdominal primaries). This suggests either limitation in the cells in which the chromosomal translocation is able to occur, or that the fusion protein itself is limited in the cell types it is capable of transforming.

Several other *EWS* fusions are characteristic of other tumour types (see Table 2.1). It is probably simplistic to assume that the *EWS* part of the fusion provides the same function in each tumour type. However, it is the other fusion partner that is typically associated with tumour specificity, e.g. ETS-type transcription factors in Ewing's family tumours, WT1 for desmoplastic small round-cell tumour (DSRCT), and CHOP in myxoid liposarcoma.

Neuroblastoma

Neuroblastoma (NB) arises from primitive neural crest cells and is the most common solid tumour outside the central nervous system (CNS) and the most common neoplasm diagnosed in infancy. There have been a few reported cases of familial NB, although, as for WT, they are rare. As with many other tumour types, clues to the aetiology of neuroblastoma have emerged as a result of molecular cytogenetic studies. The constitutional cytogenetic abnormalities in a few familial cases have been useful in indicating regions (1p36 and 17q23) that are important in sporadic neuroblastoma.[153,154] In sporadic tumours, cytological evidence for gene amplification in the form of double minutes (DM) and homogeneously staining regions (HSR) represent amplification of a region containing (amongst several other potentially important genes) the *MYCN* oncogene, which occurs in 20–25 per cent of cases and is a proven independently adverse prognostic factor. It is usually associated with metastatic disease but when it occurs in localized neuroblastoma or in infant neuroblastoma, treatment is upgraded to equivalent intensity to that used for metastatic disease. More recently, gain of chromosome region 17q23-qter and loss of 1p36, which occur in about 50 and 35 per cent, respectively, and are also known to be adverse prognostic factors, have been compared with *MYCN* amplification in a large multivariate survival analysis.[155] Two interesting findings emerge: that 17q gain is an independent adverse prognostic factor, and that *MYCN* amplification never occurs in the absence of one of the other two changes.

Cell transfection experiments have revealed the apparently conflicting roles of MYC proteins of enhancement of proliferation, inhibition of differentiation and increased sensitivity to apoptosis. One resolution of this conflict is that *MYCN* deregulation requires anti-apoptotic survival signals for its proliferative effect to outweigh the cell death pathways. It is possible that 17q gain and/or 1p36 loss contribute to such survival signalling. More direct evidence comes from the discovery of inactivation of the key pro-apoptotic caspase 8 in neuroblastomas with *MYCN* amplification.[23] In tumour samples, the inactivation occurs as a result of methylation of the promoter region of the caspase 8 gene. Other investigators have, however, failed to repeat these obervations.[156,157] Interestingly, in a transgenic mouse model of neuroblastoma in which a *MYCN* transgene is overexpressed in neural crest cells through placement downstream of a tyrosine hydroxylase promoter, the tumours derived occurred at a very high frequency and were histologically and cytogenetically similar to human neuroblastoma with a similar pattern of whole or partial chromosome gains and losses.[34] The implication from this experiment is that *MYCN* deregulation can be an initiating event in neuroblastoma but several secondary changes are needed for tumour progression. Other regions of cytogenetic alteration in neuroblastoma include 11q23 with LOH in 44 per cent of cases, and 14q23-qter with LOH in 22 per cent of cases. Genes responsible for neuroblastoma at these regions have not been identified.

Of special interest are infant neuroblastomas, especially those that fall into the category of stage 4S disease. Here the natural history of the disease is for spontaneous regression to occur, although there may be a significant delay between presentation and regression so that treatment is often necessary. Regression usually occurs without residual tumour or scarring, suggesting that apoptosis might be an important factor in initiating it. However, the molecular basis underlying stage 4S regression is not known. A molecular understanding of why stage 4S regresses might ultimately be applicable to other cases of infant neuroblastoma where the clinical likelihood of spontaneous regression is not clear-cut.

OSTEOSARCOMAS

Compared with most of the other paediatric malignancies, the molecular pathology of osteosarcomas is relatively poorly understood. This may be accounted for in part by the relative rarity of the tumours and the need for decalcification of specimens. Cytogenetic analysis has revealed that the tumours tend to be aneuploid but that many samples show multiple clones with different degrees of ploidy.[158] Comparative genomic hybridization (CGH) analysis has revealed many non-random regions of gain or loss, and 8q or 1q21 gains have been linked with shorter overall survival.[159]

Patients affected with hereditary retinoblastoma have a 1000 times increased risk of osteosarcoma, and the important role for *RB* mutation has been confirmed in sporadic osteosarcoma tumour samples where the loss of heterozygosity for the *RB* gene locus (and presumed point mutations of non-deleted allele) have been described in about 60 per cent of cases.[160] Retinoblastoma pathway inactivation may also occur through an alternate mechanism such as loss of *p16* expression[161] and/or CDK4/cyclin D1 amplification.[162] *p53* is mutated in about 50 per cent of cases of osteosarcoma.[163,164] Additionally, the *p53* pathway may be disrupted through *MDM2* overexpression.[165]

PAEDIATRIC CENTRAL NERVOUS SYSTEM TUMOURS

The role of the sonic hedgehog (SHH) signalling pathway in medulloblastoma has been known for several years following the discovery that medulloblastoma (as well as basal cell carcinomas) is seen in patients with Gorlin syndrome and its mouse model, which constitutes germ-line mutations in the SHH receptor PTCH.[145,166] About 10–20 per cent of sporadic medulloblastoma tumours harbour PTCH mutation, suggesting an essential role for this pathway in the disease.[167] More recently, the relationship between SHH signalling, histogenesis and pathological classification has been elucidated following gene expression profiling of embryonal brain tumours using DNA gene arrays.[32] Using a variety of computational approaches to data analysis, it has been possible to identify distinct expression patterns of highly discriminatory genes that are highly predictive of pathological type. Interestingly, the same data set has identified differences between desmoplastic and classical medulloblastoma. Desmoplastic tumours specifically had high expression of *PTCH*, *GLI*, *MYCN* and *IGF2*, indicative of activation of the SHH pathway. In contrast, activation of genes of the SHH pathway is not seen in classical medulloblastoma, which is not associated with inherited mutations resulting in aberrant sonic signalling. SHH signalling is essential for mammalian CNS development and causes proliferation of cerebellar granule cells. *ZIC* and *NSCL1* are genes that are expressed exclusively in these cells. The finding of high-level expression of *ZIC* and *NSCL1* in medulloblastoma, but lack of expression in other embryonal tumours, adds weight to the embryological origin of medulloblastoma being the cerebellar granule cells.[32] One target of SHH signalling is the GLI transcription factors. The recent description of mutations in SUFU in a small percentage of medulloblastomas lacking PTCH mutations suggests that GLI is the key downstream oncogenic target because SUFU's role is to sequester GLI proteins and target them for degradation.[168] However, in a mouse model of medulloblastoma, injection of SHH into the cerebellum causes tumours to form even in a GLI-1 null background.[169] The role of other GLI proteins and other SHH targets needs to be defined in these cell types. The elucidation of the importance of the SHH pathway in medulloblastoma suggests novel approaches for directed therapy. In this regard it is interesting that the oncogenic mutations in *Smo* and *Ptch* can be reversed with cyclopamine.[170]

There are several putative molecular prognostic factors in medulloblastoma, a disease for which risk group stratification and targeted therapy of aggressive cases is a priority. High *TrkC* expression, in particular, has been linked to improved survival,[171] although gene expression profiling is still capable of predicting more favourable outcomes within the *TrkC*-low category.[32] The ErbB receptors homo- and heterodimerize to form functional receptors and are expressed in medulloblastoma. Both high expression of ErbB2 and co-expression of ErbB2/ErbB4 dimers are adverse prognostic indicators.[172]

Rhabdoid tumours developing in the brain have been termed atypical teratoid/rhabdoid tumours. A number of different cytogenetic or molecular genetic mechanisms result in biallelic hSNF5/INI1 inactivation, which is characteristic of this tumour type. Point mutations rather than deletions appear to be the most common genetic change in brain rhabdoids, although the functional significance of this is unknown.[173]

The extreme heterogeneity of clinical grade within gliomas suggests that they constitute many different diseases and that elucidation of molecular genetics will be important for developing rational approaches to therapy, especially for high-grade tumours. Malignant gliomas arise in association with neurofibromatosis type 1, Li–Fraumeni and Turcot syndromes. For example, within high-grade glioblastomas, presence of *p53* mutation or epidermal growth factor receptor (EGFR) amplification appear to define two mutually exclusive groups. Activation of EGFR, platelet-derived growth factor (PDGF) and RAS signalling are described in high-grade astrocytomas. Like medulloblastoma and the embryonal tumours, it is possible that gene expression profiling might be of value in determining key genes and identifying new prognostic groups.[174]

Gliomas are largely adult tumours and it is important to distinguish to what extent paediatric gliomas can be considered a separate entity. However, within the glioma family, paediatric ependymomas appear to be a distinct clinical entity. There is currently little molecular genetic information on these tumours. CGH indicates regions prone to gain of chromosomal material, the most common of which is 1q.[175] Lack of chromosomal rearrangement correlates with younger age at presentation, suggesting a distinct histogenesis.[176]

CANCER PREDISPOSITION SYNDROMES

The familial Wilms' predisposition syndromes and the importance of the retinoblastoma protein as a cell cycle regulator and as a paradigm for the tumour suppressor gene and the two-hit hypothesis have already been discussed.

The Li–Fraumeni syndrome (LFS)

This is a familial association of early-onset soft tissue sarcomas with breast cancer and was first described in the 1960s.[177] The LFS gene was mapped by linkage analysis to chromosome 17p and found to be the *p53* gene (now termed *TP53*), one of the most mutated genes in cancer. The sequence of the gene was analysed in affected members of LFS families and found to be mutated in the germ line.[178] The mutations were all missense ones and tended to affect only a few residues. Subsequently, larger analyses have confirmed *TP53* to underlie virtually all cases of classic Li–Fraumeni families and also about 10 per cent of LFS-like families, in which there is clustering of the same spectrum of tumours but in insufficient numbers to meet the strict criteria for LFS.[179] These larger analyses have shown that the mutational spectrum in the *TP53* gene in LFS is wider than was first thought, but they still cluster within exons 5–8, which encode the domains critical for DNA binding and protein–protein interactions.

TP53 was initially thought to be an oncogene until it was realized that early experiments were performed with a mutated form of the protein that had acquired transforming properties. It is a multifunctional protein with roles in cell cycle control and apoptosis. It is loss of normal *TP53* function that is important in tumour progression. This can be achieved either by gene deletion/nonsense mutations or by sequestration of *TP53* by binding to other abnormal cellular proteins. Somatic *TP53* mutations are common in many adult cancers but relatively rare in most childhood cancers. Exceptions are soft tissue sarcomas and WT with anaplastic morphology. Analyses for germ-line *TP53* gene mutations in children with apparently sporadic forms of tumours falling within the LFS spectrum have shown that approximately 5 per cent of osteosarcomas, 5 per cent of rhabdomyosarcomas and virtually all cases of adrenocortical carcinoma are due to such a predisposing mutation.[180,181] Children and young adults who develop second primary tumours are also more likely to have a germ-line *TP53* mutation, which is found in 7 per cent of such cases.[182]

Neurofibromatosis type 1 (NF-1)

This is known to be associated with an increased risk of a few specific childhood cancers, such as juvenile myelomonocytic leukaemia and brain tumours. Following the cloning of the *NF-1* gene in 1990, it has become apparent that *NF-1* mutations are also found in cancers not normally associated with neurofibromatosis type 1.[183] The *NF-1* gene encodes a GTPase-activating protein, termed neurofibromin, that is involved in negative regulation of RAS signal transduction pathways and is highly expressed in brain. RAS proteins are known to be important in regulating cell growth and transformation and in transmitting differentiation signals. When *NF-1* is mutant, certain RAS pathways may be constitutively active, and therefore *NF-1* has been termed a tumour suppressor. Due to its high molecular weight, it is difficult to exclude *NF-1* mutation as being the cause of tumours. Whereas it has been shown to be homozygously mutated in tumours that develop in patients with NF-1, the incidence of *NF-1* mutation in sporadic brain tumours in children seems to be low.[184] However, the increasing understanding of the RAS signalling pathway may yet lead to treatments designed to block the effects of constitutively active RAS.[185]

Immunodeficiency syndromes

Enormous progress has been made recently in isolating genes that underlie the many rare immunodeficiency syndromes of childhood. These mostly predispose to leukaemias and lymphomas and it has been unclear how much of the increased risk of cancer development is due either to defective immune destruction of a postulated background level of nascent tumour cells or to the underlying genetic defect promoting accumulation of mutations and increasing the number of tumour progenitors. Now that the genes for ataxia-telangiectasia[186] and Bloom's syndrome[187] have been isolated, it is clear that defects in DNA replication and/or repair control genes are responsible for many of these syndromes. It is therefore possible that they predispose to cancer by allowing a rapid accumulation of mutations in other cancer-causing genes. Defective immunosurveillance may also play a role but apart from Epstein–Barr virus-associated lymphoproliferative disease and Hodgkin's disease, there is little association between immunodeficiency and cancer.

KEY POINTS

- Cancer arises following activating mutations of oncogenes and/or inactivating mutations of tumour suppressor genes.
- Oncogenesis is a multistep process involving immortalization, growth factor autonomy, inhibition of cell death pathways and the capacity to invade local tissues and/or promote blood vessel growth.
- Understanding of mechanisms of tumorigenesis has been greatly facilitated by technological advances, including sequence databases, microarray analysis and gene targeting in animal models.
- Cytogenetic analysis has identified many oncogenes and tumour suppressors deregulated as a result of chromosomal rearrangement.
- Many cytogenetic rearrangements help define tumour subtypes as well as providing mechanistic insight and diagnostic tools.
- Future therapies for difficult tumours may be increasingly directed towards 'molecular signatures'.

REFERENCES

1. Temin HM. Origin of retroviruses from cellular moveable genetic elements. *Cell* 1980; **21**(3): 599–600.
2. Blair DG, Cooper CS, Oskarsson MK *et al.* New method for detecting cellular transforming genes. *Science* 1982; **218**(4577): 1122–5.
3. Fasano O, Birnbaum D, Edlund L *et al.* New human transforming genes detected by a tumorigenicity assay. *Mol Cell Biol* 1984; **4**(9): 1695–705.
4. Hecht JL, Aster JC. Molecular biology of Burkitt's lymphoma. *J Clin Oncol* 2000; **18**(21): 3707–21.
5. Boxer LM, Dang CV. Translocations involving c-myc and c-myc function. *Oncogene* 2001; **20**(40): 5595–610.
6. Zimmerman K, Alt FW. Expression and function of myc family genes. *Crit Rev Oncog* 1990; **2**(1): 75–95.
7. Turc-Carel C, Lizard-Nacol S, Justrabo E *et al.* Consistent chromosomal translocation in alveolar rhabdomyosarcoma. *Cancer Genet Cytogenet* 1986; **19**(3–4): 361–2.
8. Galili N, Davis RJ, Fredericks WJ *et al.* Fusion of a fork head domain gene to PAX3 in the solid tumour alveolar rhabdomyosarcoma. *Nat Genet* 1993; **5**(3): 230–5.
9. Birrer MJ, Segal S, DeGreve JS *et al.* L-myc cooperates with ras to transform primary rat embryo fibroblasts. *Mol Cell Biol* 1988; **8**(6): 2668–73.
10. Ralston R. Complementation of transforming domains in E1a/myc chimaeras. *Nature* 1991; **353**(6347): 866–8.
11. Hanahan D, Weinberg RA. The hallmarks of cancer. *Cell* 2000; **100**(1): 57–70.
12. Hayflick L. Mortality and immortality at the cellular level. A review. *Biochemistry (Mosc)* 1997; **62**(11): 1180–90.
13. Counter CM, Avilion AA, LeFeuvre CE *et al.* Telomere shortening associated with chromosome instability is arrested in immortal cells which express telomerase activity. *EMBO J* 1992; **11**(5): 1921–9.
14. Greenberg RA, Chin L, Femino A *et al.* Short dysfunctional telomeres impair tumorigenesis in the INK4a(delta2/3) cancer-prone mouse. *Cell* 1999; **97**(4): 515–25.
15. Giancotti FG, Ruoslahti E. Integrin signaling. *Science* 1999; **285**(5430): 1028–32.
16. Slamon DJ, Godolphin W, Jones LA *et al.* Studies of the HER-2/neu proto-oncogene in human breast and ovarian cancer. *Science* 1989; **244**(4905): 707–12.
17. Ghanem MA, Van Der Kwast TH, Den Hollander JC *et al.* Expression and prognostic value of epidermal growth factor receptor, transforming growth factor-alpha, and c-erb B-2 in nephroblastoma. *Cancer* 2001; **92**(12): 3120–9.
18. Schmidt L, Duh FM, Chen F *et al.* Germline and somatic mutations in the tyrosine kinase domain of the MET

proto-oncogene in papillary renal carcinomas. *Nat Genet* 1997; **16**(1): 68–73.

19. Medema RH, Bos JL. The role of p21ras in receptor tyrosine kinase signaling. *Crit Rev Oncog* 1993; **4**(6): 615–61.

20. Evan G, Littlewood T. A matter of life and cell death. *Science* 1998; **281**(5381): 1317–22.

21. Evan GI, Vousden KH. Proliferation, cell cycle and apoptosis in cancer. *Nature* 2001; **411**(6835): 342–8.

22. Gauwerky CE, Haluska FG, Tsujimoto Y *et al.* Evolution of B-cell malignancy: pre-B-cell leukemia resulting from MYC activation in a B-cell neoplasm with a rearranged BCL2 gene. *Proc Natl Acad Sci USA* 1988; **85**(22): 8548–52.

23. Teitz T, Wei T, Valentine MB *et al.* Caspase 8 is deleted or silenced preferentially in childhood neuroblastomas with amplification of MYCN. *Nat Med* 2000; **6**(5): 529–35.

24. Rainier S, Johnson LA, Dobry CJ *et al.* Relaxation of imprinted genes in human cancer. *Nature* 1993; **362**(6422): 747–9.

25. Carmeliet P, Jain RK. Angiogenesis in cancer and other diseases. *Nature* 2000; **407**(6801): 249–57.

26. Hanahan D, Folkman J. Patterns and emerging mechanisms of the angiogenic switch during tumorigenesis. *Cell* 1996; **86**(3): 353–64.

27. Clark EA, Golub TR, Lander ES, Hynes RO. Genomic analysis of metastasis reveals an essential role for RhoC. *Nature* 2000; **406**(6795): 532–5.

28. Bergers G, Javaherian K, Lo KM *et al.* Effects of angiogenesis inhibitors on multistage carcinogenesis in mice. *Science* 1999; **284**(5415): 808–12.

29. Yancopoulos GD, Davis S, Gale NW *et al.* Vascular-specific growth factors and blood vessel formation. *Nature* 2000; **407**(6801): 242–8.

30. McPherson JD, Marra M, Hillier L *et al.* A physical map of the human genome. *Nature* 2001; **409**(6822): 934–41.

31. Sachidanandam R, Weissman D, Schmidt SC *et al.* A map of human genome sequence variation containing 1.42 million single nucleotide polymorphisms. *Nature* 2001; **409**(6822): 928–33.

32. Pomeroy SL, Tamayo P, Gaasenbeek M *et al.* Prediction of central nervous system embryonal tumour outcome based on gene expression. *Nature* 2002; **415**(6870): 436–42.

33. Armstrong SA, Staunton JE, Silverman LB *et al.* MLL translocations specify a distinct gene expression profile that distinguishes a unique leukemia. *Nat Genet* 2002; **30**(1): 41–7.

34. Weiss WA, Aldape K, Mohapatra G *et al.* Targeted expression of MYCN causes neuroblastoma in transgenic mice. *EMBO J* 1997; **16**(11): 2985–95.

35. Anderson MJ, Shelton GD, Cavenee WK, Arden KC. Embryonic expression of the tumor-associated PAX3-FKHR fusion protein interferes with the developmental functions of Pax3. *Proc Natl Acad Sci USA* 2001; **98**(4): 1589–94.

36. Okuda T, Cai Z, Yang S *et al.* Expression of a knocked-in AML1-ETO leukemia gene inhibits the establishment of normal definitive hematopoiesis and directly generates dysplastic hematopoietic progenitors. *Blood* 1998; **91**(9): 3134–43.

37. Dobson CL, Warren AJ, Pannell R *et al.* The mll-AF9 gene fusion in mice controls myeloproliferation and specifies acute myeloid leukaemogenesis. *EMBO J* 1999; **18**(13): 3564–74.

38. Collins EC, Pannell R, Simpson EM *et al.* Inter-chromosomal recombination of Mll and Af9 genes mediated by cre-loxP in mouse development. *EMBO Rep* 2000; **1**(2): 127–32.

39. Zhang Z, Liu Q, Lantry LE *et al.* A germ-line p53 mutation accelerates pulmonary tumorigenesis: p53-independent efficacy of chemopreventive agents green tea or dexamethasone/myo-inositol and chemotherapeutic agents taxol or adriamycin. *Cancer Res* 2000; **60**(4): 901–7.

40. Clarke AR. Murine models of neoplasia: functional analysis of the tumour suppressor genes Rb-1 and p53. *Cancer Metastasis Rev* 1995; **14**(2): 125–48.

41. Rhoades KL, Hetherington CJ, Harakawa N *et al.* Analysis of the role of AML1-ETO in leukemogenesis, using an inducible transgenic mouse model. *Blood* 2000; **96**(6): 2108–15.

42. Jain M, Arvanitis C, Chu K *et al.* Sustained loss of a neoplastic phenotype by brief inactivation of MYC. *Science* 2002; **297**(5578): 102–4.

43. Yeoh EJ, Ross ME, Shurtleff SA *et al.* Classification, subtype discovery, and prediction of outcome in pediatric acute lymphoblastic leukemia by gene expression profiling. *Cancer Cell* 2002; **1**(2): 133–43.

44. Cole MD, McMahon SB. The Myc oncoprotein: a critical evaluation of transactivation and target gene regulation. *Oncogene* 1999; **18**(19): 2916–24.

45. Pelengaris S, Khan M, Evan G. c-MYC: more than just a matter of life and death. *Nat Rev Cancer* 2002; **2**(10): 764–76.

46. Felsher DW, Bishop JM. Reversible tumorigenesis by MYC in hematopoietic lineages. *Mol Cell* 1999; **4**(2): 199–207.

47. Heerema NA, Sather HN, Ge J *et al.* Cytogenetic studies of infant acute lymphoblastic leukemia: poor prognosis of infants with t(4;11) – a report of the Children's Cancer Group. *Leukemia* 1999; **13**(5): 679–86.

48. Behm FG, Raimondi SC, Frestedt JL *et al.* Rearrangement of the MLL gene confers a poor prognosis in childhood acute lymphoblastic leukemia, regardless of presenting age. *Blood* 1996; **87**(7): 2870–7.

49. Yagi H, Deguchi K, Aono A *et al.* Growth disturbance in fetal liver hematopoiesis of Mll-mutant mice. *Blood* 1998; **92**(1): 108–17.

50. Lavau C, Szilvassy SJ, Slany R, Cleary ML. Immortalization and leukemic transformation of a myelomonocytic precursor by retrovirally transduced HRX-ENL. *EMBO J* 1997; **16**(14): 4226–37.

51. Zeleznik-Le NJ, Harden AM, Rowley JD. 11q23 translocations split the 'AT-hook' cruciform DNA-binding region and the transcriptional repression domain from the activation domain of the mixed-lineage leukemia (MLL) gene. *Proc Natl Acad Sci USA* 1994; **91**(22): 10610–14.

52. Ayton PM, Cleary ML. Molecular mechanisms of leukemogenesis mediated by MLL fusion proteins. *Oncogene* 2001; **20**(40): 5695–707.

53. Corral J, Lavenir I, Impey H *et al.* An Mll-AF9 fusion gene made by homologous recombination causes acute leukemia in chimeric mice: a method to create fusion oncogenes. *Cell* 1996; **85**(6): 853–61.

54. Dobson CL, Warren AJ, Pannell R et al. Tumorigenesis in mice with a fusion of the leukaemia oncogene Mll and the bacterial lacZ gene. EMBO J 2000; 19(5): 843–51.

55. Caslini C, Shilatifard A, Yang L, Hess JL. The amino terminus of the mixed lineage leukemia protein (MLL) promotes cell cycle arrest and monocytic differentiation. Proc Natl Acad Sci USA 2000; 97(6): 2797–802.

56. Okuda T, van Deursen J, Hiebert SW et al. AML1, the target of multiple chromosomal translocations in human leukemia, is essential for normal fetal liver hematopoiesis. Cell 1996; 84(2): 321–30.

57. Meyers S, Lenny N, Hiebert SW. The t(8;21) fusion protein interferes with AML-1B-dependent transcriptional activation. Mol Cell Biol 1995; 15(4): 1974–82.

58. Klampfer L, Zhang J, Zelenetz AO et al. The AML1/ETO fusion protein activates transcription of BCL-2. Proc Natl Acad Sci USA 1996; 93(24): 14059–64.

59. Higuchi M, O'Brien D, Kumaravelu P et al. Expression of a conditional AML1-ETO oncogene bypasses embryonic lethality and establishes a murine model of human t(8;21) acute myeloid leukemia. Cancer Cell 2002; 1(1): 63–74.

60. Nucifora G, Larson RA, Rowley JD. Persistence of the 8;21 translocation in patients with acute myeloid leukemia type M2 in long-term remission. Blood 1993; 82(3): 712–15.

61. Saunders MJ, Brereton ML, Adams JA et al. Expression of AML1/MTG8 transcripts in clonogenic cells grown from bone marrow of patients in remission of acute myeloid leukaemia with t(8;21). Br J Haematol 1997; 99(4): 921–4.

62. Romana SP, Poirel H, Leconiat M et al. High frequency of t(12;21) in childhood B-lineage acute lymphoblastic leukemia. Blood 1995; 86(11): 4263–9.

63. Golub TR, Barker GF, Bohlander SK et al. Fusion of the TEL gene on 12p13 to the AML1 gene on 21q22 in acute lymphoblastic leukemia. Proc Natl Acad Sci USA 1995; 92(11): 4917–21.

64. Hiebert SW, Sun W, Davis JN et al. The t(12;21) translocation converts AML-1B from an activator to a repressor of transcription. Mol Cell Biol 1996; 16(4): 1349–55.

65. Uchida H, Downing JR, Miyazaki Y et al. Three distinct domains in TEL-AML1 are required for transcriptional repression of the IL-3 promoter. Oncogene 1999; 18(4): 1015–22.

66. Stegmaier K, Pendse S, Barker GF et al. Frequent loss of heterozygosity at the TEL gene locus in acute lymphoblastic leukemia of childhood. Blood 1995; 86(1): 38–44.

67. Daley GQ, Van Etten RA, Baltimore D. Induction of chronic myelogenous leukemia in mice by the P210bcr/abl gene of the Philadelphia chromosome. Science 1990; 247(4944): 824–30.

68. Kabarowski JH, Allen PB, Wiedemann LM. A temperature sensitive p210 BCR-ABL mutant defines the primary consequences of BCR-ABL tyrosine kinase expression in growth factor dependent cells. EMBO J 1994; 13(24): 5887–95.

69. Agnarsson BA, Kadin ME. Ki-1 positive large cell lymphoma. A morphologic and immunologic study of 19 cases. Am J Surg Pathol 1988; 12(4): 264–74.

70. Kadin ME, Sako D, Berliner N et al. Childhood Ki-1 lymphoma presenting with skin lesions and peripheral lymphadenopathy. Blood 1986; 68(5): 1042–9.

71. Mason DY, Bastard C, Rimokh R et al. CD30-positive large cell lymphomas ('Ki-1 lymphoma') are associated with a chromosomal translocation involving 5q35. Br J Haematol 1990; 74(2): 161–8.

72. Morris SW, Kirstein MN, Valentine MB et al. Fusion of a kinase gene, ALK, to a nucleolar protein gene, NPM, in non-Hodgkin's lymphoma. Science 1994; 263(5151): 1281–4.

73. Williams BO, Schmitt EM, Remington L et al. Extensive contribution of Rb-deficient cells to adult chimeric mice with limited histopathological consequences. EMBO J 1994; 13(18): 4251–9.

74. Knudson AG Jr, Strong LC. Mutation and cancer: a model for Wilms' tumor of the kidney. J Natl Cancer Inst 1972; 48(2): 313–24.

75. Hastie ND. The genetics of Wilms' tumor – a case of disrupted development. Annu Rev Genet 1994; 28: 523–58.

76. Denys P, Malvaux P, Van Den Berghe H et al. [Association of an anatomo-pathological syndrome of male pseudohermaphroditism, Wilms' tumor, parenchymatous nephropathy and XX/XY mosaicism]. Arch Fr Pediatr 1967; 24(7): 729–39.

77. Drash A, Sherman F, Hartmann WH, Blizzard RM. A syndrome of pseudohermaphroditism, Wilms' tumor, hypertension, and degenerative renal disease. J Pediatr 1970; 76(4): 585–93.

78. Sotelo-Avila C, Gonzalez-Crussi F, Fowler JW. Complete and incomplete forms of Beckwith–Wiedemann syndrome: their oncogenic potential. J Pediatr 1980; 96(1): 47–50.

79. Greenberg F, Copeland K, Gresik MV. Expanding the spectrum of the Perlman syndrome. Am J Med Genet 1988; 29(4): 773–6.

80. Neri G, Gurrieri F, Zanni G, Lin A. Clinical and molecular aspects of the Simpson–Golabi–Behmel syndrome. Am J Med Genet 1998; 79(4): 279–83.

81. Call KM, Glaser T, Ito CY et al. Isolation and characterization of a zinc finger polypeptide gene at the human chromosome 11 Wilms' tumor locus. Cell 1990; 60(3): 509–20.

82. Gessler M, Poustka A, Cavenee W et al. Homozygous deletion in Wilms tumours of a zinc-finger gene identified by chromosome jumping. Nature 1990; 343(6260): 774–8.

83. Pritchard-Jones K, Fleming S, Davidson D et al. The candidate Wilms' tumour gene is involved in genitourinary development. Nature 1990; 346(6280): 194–7.

84. Baird PN, Groves N, Haber DA et al. Identification of mutations in the WT1 gene in tumours from patients with the WAGR syndrome. Oncogene 1992; 7(11): 2141–9.

85. Brown KW, Wilmore HP, Watson JE et al. Low frequency of mutations in the WT1 coding region in Wilms' tumor. Genes Chromosomes Cancer 1993; 8(2): 74–9.

86. Huff V, Miwa H, Haber DA et al. Evidence for WT1 as a Wilms tumor (WT) gene: intragenic germinal deletion in bilateral WT. Am J Hum Genet 1991; 48(5): 997–1003.

87. Little M, Wells C. A clinical overview of WT1 gene mutations. Hum Mutat 1997; 9(3): 209–25.

88. Haber DA, Timmers HT, Pelletier J et al. A dominant mutation in the Wilms tumor gene WT1 cooperates with the viral oncogene E1A in transformation of primary kidney cells. Proc Natl Acad Sci USA 1992; 89(13): 6010–14.

89. Little MH, Williamson KA, Mannens M *et al.* Evidence that WT1 mutations in Denys–Drash syndrome patients may act in a dominant-negative fashion. *Hum Mol Genet* 1993; **2**(3): 259–64.

90. Pelletier J, Bruening W, Kashtan CE *et al.* Germline mutations in the Wilms' tumor suppressor gene are associated with abnormal urogenital development in Denys–Drash syndrome. *Cell* 1991; **67**(2): 437–47.

91. Koziell A, Charmandari E, Hindmarsh PC *et al.* Frasier syndrome, part of the Denys Drash continuum or simply a WT1 gene associated disorder of intersex and nephropathy? *Clin Endocrinol (Oxf)* 2000; **52**(4): 519–24.

92. Reddy JC, Hosono S, Licht JD. The transcriptional effect of WT1 is modulated by choice of expression vector. *J Biol Chem* 1995; **270**(50): 29976–82.

93. Hammes A, Guo JK, Lutsch G *et al.* Two splice variants of the Wilms' tumor 1 gene have distinct functions during sex determination and nephron formation. *Cell* 2001; **106**(3): 319–29.

94. Beckwith JB, Kiviat NB, Bonadio JF. Nephrogenic rests, nephroblastomatosis, and the pathogenesis of Wilms' tumor. *Pediatr Pathol* 1990; **10**(1–2): 1–36.

95. Park S, Bernard A, Bove KE *et al.* Inactivation of WT1 in nephrogenic rests, genetic precursors to Wilms' tumour. *Nat Genet* 1993; **5**(4): 363–7.

96. Wadey RB, Pal N, Buckle B *et al.* Loss of heterozygosity in Wilms' tumour involves two distinct regions of chromosome 11. *Oncogene* 1990; **5**(6): 901–7.

97. Maw MA, Grundy PE, Millow LJ *et al.* A third Wilms' tumor locus on chromosome 16q. *Cancer Res* 1992; **52**(11): 3094–8.

98. Mannens M, Slater RM, Heyting C *et al.* Molecular nature of genetic changes resulting in loss of heterozygosity of chromosome 11 in Wilms' tumours. *Hum Genet* 1988; **81**(1): 41–8.

99. Rahman N, Arbour L, Tonin P *et al.* Evidence for a familial Wilms' tumour gene (FWT1) on chromosome 17q12-q21. *Nat Genet* 1996; **13**(4): 461–3.

100. McDonald JM, Douglass EC, Fisher R *et al.* Linkage of familial Wilms' tumor predisposition to chromosome 19 and a two-locus model for the etiology of familial tumors. *Cancer Res* 1998; **58**(7): 1387–90.

101. Rapley EA, Barfoot R, Bonaiti-Pellie C *et al.* Evidence for susceptibility genes to familial Wilms tumour in addition to WT1, FWT1 and FWT2. *Br J Cancer* 2000; **83**(2): 177–83.

102. DeBaun MR, Siegel MJ, Choyke PL. Nephromegaly in infancy and early childhood: a risk factor for Wilms tumor in Beckwith–Wiedemann syndrome. *J Pediatr* 1998; **132**(3 Pt 1): 401–4.

103. Henry I, Bonaiti-Pellie C, Chehensse V *et al.* Uniparental paternal disomy in a genetic cancer-predisposing syndrome. *Nature* 1991; **351**(6328): 665–7.

104. Weksberg R, Shen DR, Fei YL *et al.* Disruption of insulin-like growth factor 2 imprinting in Beckwith–Wiedemann syndrome. *Nat Genet* 1993; **5**(2): 143–50.

105. Mannens M, Hoovers JM, Redeker E *et al.* Parental imprinting of human chromosome region 11p15.3-pter involved in the Beckwith–Wiedemann syndrome and various human neoplasia. *Eur J Hum Genet* 1994; **2**(1): 3–23.

106. Koufos A, Grundy P, *et al.* Familial Wiedemann–Beckwith syndrome and a second Wilms tumor locus both map to 11p15.5. *Am J Hum Genet* 1989; **44**(5): 711–19.

107. Ping AJ, Reeve AE, Law DJ *et al.* Genetic linkage of Beckwith–Wiedemann syndrome to 11p15. *Am J Hum Genet* 1989; **44**(5): 720–3.

108. Ogawa O, Eccles MR, Szeto J *et al.* Relaxation of insulin-like growth factor II gene imprinting implicated in Wilms' tumour. *Nature* 1993; **362**(6422): 749–51.

109. Hatada I, Ohashi H, Fukushima Y *et al.* An imprinted gene p57KIP2 is mutated in Beckwith–Wiedemann syndrome. *Nat Genet* 1996; **14**(2): 171–3.

110. Lee MP, DeBaun M, Randhawa G *et al.* Low frequency of p57KIP2 mutation in Beckwith–Wiedemann syndrome. *Am J Hum Genet* 1997; **61**(2): 304–9.

111. Zhang P, Liegeois NJ, Wong C *et al.* Altered cell differentiation and proliferation in mice lacking p57KIP2 indicates a role in Beckwith–Wiedemann syndrome. *Nature* 1997; **387**(6629): 151–8.

112. Caspary T, Cleary MA, Perlman EJ *et al.* Oppositely imprinted genes p57(Kip2) and igf2 interact in a mouse model for Beckwith–Wiedemann syndrome. *Genes Dev* 1999; **13**(23): 3115–24.

113. DeBaun MR, Niemitz EL, McNeil DE *et al.* Epigenetic alterations of H19 and LIT1 distinguish patients with Beckwith–Wiedemann syndrome with cancer and birth defects. *Am J Hum Genet* 2002; **70**(3): 604–11.

114. Bliek J, Maas SM, Ruijter JM *et al.* Increased tumour risk for BWS patients correlates with aberrant H19 and not KCNQ1OT1 methylation: occurrence of KCNQ1OT1 hypomethylation in familial cases of BWS. *Hum Mol Genet* 2001; **10**(5): 467–76.

115. Wilkins RJ. Genomic imprinting and carcinogenesis. *Lancet* 1988; **1**(8581): 329–31.

116. Cavenee WK, Dryja TP, *et al.* Expression of recessive alleles by chromosomal mechanisms in retinoblastoma. *Nature* 1983; **305**(5937): 779–84.

117. Steenman MJ, Rainier S, Dobry CJ *et al.* Loss of imprinting of IGF2 is linked to reduced expression and abnormal methylation of H19 in Wilms' tumour. *Nat Genet* 1994; **7**(3): 433–9.

118. Hao Y, Crenshaw T, Moulton T *et al.* Tumour-suppressor activity of H19 RNA. *Nature* 1993; **365**(6448): 764–7.

119. Moulton T, Crenshaw T, Hao Y *et al.* Epigenetic lesions at the H19 locus in Wilms' tumour patients. *Nat Genet* 1994; **7**(3): 440–7.

120. Okamoto K, Morison IM, Taniguchi T, Reeve AE. Epigenetic changes at the insulin-like growth factor II/H19 locus in developing kidney is an early event in Wilms tumorigenesis. *Proc Natl Acad Sci USA* 1997; **94**(10): 5367–71.

121. Li M, Shuman C, Fei YL *et al.* GPC3 mutation analysis in a spectrum of patients with overgrowth expands the phenotype of Simpson–Golabi–Behmel syndrome. *Am J Med Genet* 2001; **102**(2): 161–8.

122. Pilia G, Hughes-Benzie RM, MacKenzie A *et al.* Mutations in GPC3, a glypican gene, cause the Simpson–Golabi–Behmel overgrowth syndrome. *Nat Genet* 1996; **12**(3): 241–7.

123. Chiao E, Fisher P, Crisponi L *et al.* Overgrowth of a mouse model of the Simpson–Golabi–Behmel syndrome is

independent of IGF signaling. *Dev Biol* 2002; **243**(1): 185–206.

124. White GR, Kelsey AM, Varley JM, Birch JM. Somatic glypican 3 (GPC3) mutations in Wilms' tumour. *Br J Cancer* 2002; **86**(12): 1920–2.

125. Hartley AL, Birch JM, Tricker K *et al.* Wilms' tumor in the Li–Fraumeni cancer family syndrome. *Cancer Genet Cytogenet* 1993; **67**(2): 133–5.

126. Birch JM, Alston RD, McNally RJ *et al.* Relative frequency and morphology of cancers in carriers of germline TP53 mutations. *Oncogene* 2001; **20**(34): 4621–8.

127. Bardeesy N, Falkoff D, Petruzzi MJ *et al.* Anaplastic Wilms' tumour, a subtype displaying poor prognosis, harbours p53 gene mutations. *Nat Genet* 1994; **7**(1): 91–7.

128. Breslow N, Beckwith JB, Ciol M, Sharples K. Age distribution of Wilms' tumor: report from the National Wilms' Tumor Study. *Cancer Res* 1988; **48**(6): 1653–7.

129. Pastore G, Carli M, Lemerle J *et al.* Epidemiological features of Wilms' tumor: results of studies by the International Society of Paediatric Oncology (SIOP). *Med Pediatr Oncol* 1988; **16**(1): 7–11.

130. Hawkins MM, Winter DL, Burton HS, Potok MH. Heritability of Wilms' tumour. *J Natl Cancer Inst* 1995; **87**(17): 1323–4.

131. Breslow N, A Olshan, Beckwith JB, Green DM. Epidemiology of Wilms tumor. *Med Pediatr Oncol* 1993; **21**(3): 172–81.

132. Douglass EC, Valentine M, Etcubanas E *et al.* A specific chromosomal abnormality in rhabdomyosarcoma. *Cytogenet Cell Genet* 1987; **45**(3–4): 148–55.

133. Barr FG, Galili N, Holick J *et al.* Rearrangement of the PAX3 paired box gene in the paediatric solid tumour alveolar rhabdomyosarcoma. *Nat Genet* 1993; **3**(2): 113–17.

134. Davis RJ, D'Cruz CM, Lovell MA *et al.* Fusion of PAX7 to FKHR by the variant t(1;13)(p36;q14) translocation in alveolar rhabdomyosarcoma. *Cancer Res* 1994; **54**(11): 2869–72.

135. Shapiro DN, Sublett JE, Li B *et al.* Fusion of PAX3 to a member of the forkhead family of transcription factors in human alveolar rhabdomyosarcoma. *Cancer Res* 1993; **53**(21): 5108–12.

136. Bennicelli JL, Edwards RH, Barr FG. Mechanism for transcriptional gain of function resulting from chromosomal translocation in alveolar rhabdomyosarcoma. *Proc Natl Acad Sci USA* 1996; **93**(11): 5455–9.

137. Bernasconi M, Remppis A, Fredericks WJ *et al.* Induction of apoptosis in rhabdomyosarcoma cells through down-regulation of PAX proteins. *Proc Natl Acad Sci USA* 1996; **93**(23): 13164–9.

138. Ayyanathan K, Fredericks WJ, Berking C *et al.* Hormone-dependent tumor regression in vivo by an inducible transcriptional repressor directed at the PAX3-FKHR oncogene. *Cancer Res* 2000; **60**(20): 5803–14.

139. Bober E, Franz T, Arnold HH *et al.* Pax-3 is required for the development of limb muscles: a possible role for the migration of dermomyotomal muscle progenitor cells. *Development* 1994; **120**(3): 603–12.

140. Borycki AG, Li J, Jin F *et al.* Pax3 functions in cell survival and in pax7 regulation. *Development* 1999; **126**(8): 1665–74.

141. Kelly KM, Womer RB, Sorensen PH *et al.* Common and variant gene fusions predict distinct clinical phenotypes in rhabdomyosarcoma. *J Clin Oncol* 1997; **15**(5): 1831–6.

142. Anderson J, Gordon T, McManus A *et al.* Detection of the PAX3-FKHR fusion gene in paediatric rhabdomyosarcoma: a reproducible predictor of outcome? *Br J Cancer* 2001; **85**(6): 831–5.

143. Khan J, Bittner ML, Saal LH *et al.* cDNA microarrays detect activation of a myogenic transcription program by the PAX3-FKHR fusion oncogene. *Proc Natl Acad Sci USA* 1999; **96**(23): 13264–9.

144. Khan J, Wei JS, Ringner M *et al.* Classification and diagnostic prediction of cancers using gene expression profiling and artificial neural networks. *Nat Med* 2001; **7**(6): 673–9.

145. Hahn H, Wojnowski L, Zimmer AM *et al.* Rhabdomyosarcomas and radiation hypersensitivity in a mouse model of Gorlin syndrome. *Nat Med* 1998; **4**(5): 619–22.

146. Delattre O, Zucman J, Plougastel B *et al.* Gene fusion with an ETS DNA-binding domain caused by chromosome translocation in human tumours. *Nature* 1992; **359**(6391): 162–5.

147. May WA, Lessnick SL, Braun BS *et al.* The Ewing's sarcoma EWS/FLI-1 fusion gene encodes a more potent transcriptional activator and is a more powerful transforming gene than FLI-1. *Mol Cell Biol* 1993; **13**(12): 7393–8.

148. de Alava E, Kawai A, Healey JH *et al.* EWS-FLI1 fusion transcript structure is an independent determinant of prognosis in Ewing's sarcoma. *J Clin Oncol* 1998; **16**(4): 1248–55.

149. de Alava E, Panizo A, Antonescu CR *et al.* Association of EWS-FLI1 type 1 fusion with lower proliferative rate in Ewing's sarcoma. *Am J Pathol* 2000; **156**(3): 849–55.

150. Zucman J, Melot T, Desmaze C *et al.* Combinatorial generation of variable fusion proteins in the Ewing family of tumours. *EMBO J* 1993; **12**(12): 4481–7.

151. Sorensen PH, Lessnick SL, Lopez-Terrada D *et al.* A second Ewing's sarcoma translocation, t(21;22), fuses the EWS gene to another ETS-family transcription factor, ERG. *Nat Genet* 1994; **6**(2): 146–51.

152. de Alava E, Antonescu CR, Panizo A *et al.* Prognostic impact of P53 status in Ewing sarcoma. *Cancer* 2000; **89**(4): 783–92.

153. Laureys G, Speleman F, Opdenakker G *et al.* Constitutional translocation t(1;17)(p36;q12–21) in a patient with neuroblastoma. *Genes Chromosomes Cancer* 1990; **2**(3): 252–4.

154. Biegel JA, White PS, Marshall HN *et al.* Constitutional 1p36 deletion in a child with neuroblastoma. *Am J Hum Genet* 1993; **52**(1): 176–82.

155. Bown N, Cotterill S, Lastowska M *et al.* Gain of chromosome arm 17q and adverse outcome in patients with neuroblastoma [see comments]. *N Engl J Med* 1999; **340**(25): 1954–61.

156. Banelli B, Casciano I, Croce M *et al.* Expression and methylation of CASP8 in neuroblastoma: Identification of a promoter region. *Nat Med* 2002; **8**(12): 1333–5.

157. Teitz T, Lahti JM, Kidd VJ. Reply to 'Expression and methylation of CASP8 in neuroblastoma: identification of a promoter region'. *Nat Med* 2002; **8**(12): 1335.

158. Bridge JA, Nelson M, McComb E et al. Cytogenetic findings in 73 osteosarcoma specimens and a review of the literature. Cancer Genet Cytogenet 1997; **95**(1): 74–87.

159. Tarkkanen M, Elomaa I, Blomqvist C et al. DNA sequence copy number increase at 8q: a potential new prognostic marker in high-grade osteosarcoma. Int J Cancer 1999; **84**(2): 114–21.

160. Belchis DA, Meece CA, Benko FA et al. Loss of heterozygosity and microsatellite instability at the retinoblastoma locus in osteosarcomas. Diagn Mol Pathol 1996; **5**(3): 214–19.

161. Maitra A, Roberts H, Weinberg AG, Geradts J. Loss of p16(INK4a) expression correlates with decreased survival in pediatric osteosarcomas. Int J Cancer 2001; **95**(1): 34–8.

162. Tarkkanen M, Karhu R, Kallioniemi A et al. Gains and losses of DNA sequences in osteosarcomas by comparative genomic hybridization. Cancer Res 1995; **55**(6): 1334–8.

163. Lonardo F, Ueda T, Huvos AG et al. p53 and MDM2 alterations in osteosarcomas: correlation with clinicopathologic features and proliferative rate. Cancer 1997; **79**(8): 1541–7.

164. Masuda H, Miller C, Koeffler HP et al. Rearrangement of the p53 gene in human osteogenic sarcomas. Proc Natl Acad Sci USA 1987; **84**(21): 7716–19.

165. Ladanyi M, Park CK, Lewis R et al. Sporadic amplification of the MYC gene in human osteosarcomas. Diagn Mol Pathol 1993; **2**(3): 163–7.

166. Hahn H, Wicking C, Zaphiropoulous PG et al. Mutations of the human homolog of Drosophila patched in the nevoid basal cell carcinoma syndrome. Cell 1996; **85**(6): 841–51.

167. Raffel C, Jenkins RB, Frederick L et al. Sporadic medulloblastomas contain PTCH mutations. Cancer Res 1997; **57**(5): 842–5.

168. Taylor MD, Liu L, Raffel C et al. Mutations in SUFU predispose to medulloblastoma. Nat Genet 2002; **31**(3): 306–10.

169. Weiner HL, Bakst R, Hurlbert MS et al. Induction of medulloblastomas in mice by sonic hedgehog, independent of Gli1. Cancer Res 2002; **62**(22): 6385–9.

170. Taipale J, Chen JK, Cooper MK et al. Effects of oncogenic mutations in Smoothened and Patched can be reversed by cyclopamine. Nature 2000; **406**(6799): 1005–9.

171. Grotzer MA, Janss AJ, Fung K et al. TrkC expression predicts good clinical outcome in primitive neuroectodermal brain tumors. J Clin Oncol 2000; **18**(5): 1027–35.

172. Gilbertson RJ, Perry RH, Kelly PJ et al. Prognostic significance of HER2 and HER4 coexpression in childhood medulloblastoma. Cancer Res 1997; **57**(15): 3272–80.

173. Sevenet N, Lellouch-Tubiana A, Schofield D et al. Spectrum of hSNF5/INI1 somatic mutations in human cancer and genotype–phenotype correlations. Hum Mol Genet 1999; **8**(13): 2359–68.

174. Nutt CL, Mani DR, Betensky RA et al. Gene expression-based classification of malignant gliomas correlates better with survival than histological classification. Cancer Res 2003; **63**(7): 1602–7.

175. Ward S, Harding B, Wilkins P et al. Gain of 1q and loss of 22 are the most common changes detected by comparative genomic hybridisation in paediatric ependymoma. Genes Chromosomes Cancer 2001; **32**(1): 59–66.

176. Dyer S, Prebble E, Davison V et al. Genomic imbalances in pediatric intracranial ependymomas define clinically relevant groups. Am J Pathol 2002; **161**(6): 2133–41.

177. Li FP, Fraumeni JF Jr. Soft-tissue sarcomas, breast cancer, and other neoplasms. A familial syndrome? Ann Intern Med 1969; **71**(4): 747–52.

178. Malkin D, Li FP, Strong LC et al. Germ line p53 mutations in a familial syndrome of breast cancer, sarcomas, and other neoplasms. Science 1990; **250**(4985): 1233–8.

179. Eeles RA. Germline mutations in the TP53 gene. Cancer Surv 1995; **25**: 101–24.

180. Sameshima Y, Tsunematsu Y, Watanabe S et al. Detection of novel germ-line p53 mutations in diverse-cancer-prone families identified by selecting patients with childhood adrenocortical carcinoma. J Natl Cancer Inst 1992; **84**(9): 703–7.

181. Toguchida J, Yamaguchi T, Dayton SH et al. Prevalence and spectrum of germline mutations of the p53 gene among patients with sarcoma. N Engl J Med 1992; **326**(20): 1301–8.

182. Malkin D, Jolly KW, Barbier N et al. Germline mutations of the p53 tumor-suppressor gene in children and young adults with second malignant neoplasms. N Engl J Med 1992; **326**(20): 1309–15.

183. Seizinger BR. NF1: a prevalent cause of tumorigenesis in human cancers? Nat Genet 1993; **3**(2): 97–9.

184. Scheurlen WG, Senf L. Analysis of the GAP-related domain of the neurofibromatosis type 1 (NF1) gene in childhood brain tumors. Int J Cancer 1995; **64**(4): 234–8.

185. Yan N, Ricca C, Fletcher J et al. Farnesyltransferase inhibitors block the neurofibromatosis type I (NF1) malignant phenotype. Cancer Res 1995; **55**(16): 3569–75.

186. Savitsky K, Bar-Shira A, Gilad S et al. A single ataxia telangiectasia gene with a product similar to PI-3 kinase. Science 1995; **268**(5218): 1749–53.

187. Ellis NA, Groden J, Ye TZ et al. The Bloom's syndrome gene product is homologous to RecQ helicases. Cell 1995; **83**(4): 655–66.

3

Solid tumour pathology and molecular diagnostics

PRAMILA RAMANI, ANTHONY GORDON & JANET SHIPLEY

Childhood tumours are a large and varied group. They can be confusing to the novice and can pose significant diagnostic challenges to even the most experienced pathologist.

Pathologists are usually faced with the question: 'Is the lump benign or malignant, and what is the precise diagnosis?' Despite the development of new techniques, the conventional histological (morphological) examination remains the gold standard in diagnostic pathology.[1] A step-by-step investigative approach is necessary, carefully analysing the results generated by the available methodology. All the results are integrated and interpreted in the context of the clinical and radiological features before a final diagnosis is rendered.

METHODOLOGY

The techniques available to the pathologist are as follows:
- light microscopy
- electron microscopy
- chromosomal and molecular analysis.

Light microscopy

This involves the utilization of three histological staining methods: routine, histochemistry and immunohisto-chemistry.

ROUTINE

The traditional, simple haematoxylin and eosin (H&E) stain helps the pathologist answer four crucial questions:

Is the lesion really a neoplasm?
As an example, nodular fasciitis often presents as a rapidly enlarging lump and shows mitotic figures. It thus mimics a sarcoma but is a reactive process. A well-prepared section stained with H&E will show the characteristic zonal pattern of nodular fasciitis and confirm the diagnosis.[2]

Is it malignant?
The features that usually indicate malignancy are mitotic activity, necrosis and pleomorphism (variability in the size and shape of the cells). However, certain malignant tumours display a deceptively benign appearance by the absence of these features. An example is alveolar soft part sarcoma, a high-grade sarcoma which lacks mitotic figures.[3]

If so, what is the precise diagnosis?
The H&E stain is useful for placing tumours in broad diagnostic categories such as small round-cell tumour (SRCT), spindle-shaped or epithelioid sarcoma, and carcinoma or melanoma. If a SRCT displays overt differentiation, e.g. strap cells indicating myogenic differentiation, a prompt diagnosis of rhabdomyosarcoma (RMS) can be made.

However, in the case of an undifferentiated or poorly differentiated tumour, the precise identification of the histogenesis (proper histological type or kind of differentiation) often requires the aid of ancillary techniques.

Is it useful for prognostication?

The H&E stain is utilized for categorizing neuroblastic tumours into favourable versus unfavourable prognostic groups. The typing of alveolar versus embryonal RMS can also be done in the majority of cases using this basic stain.

HISTOCHEMISTRY

The commonly used stain is the reticulin stain, which is particularly helpful in identifying the septa in alveolar-type RMS. In limited situations, periodic acid–Schiff (PAS) stain (with and without diastase digestion) for glycogen versus mucin can also be helpful.

IMMUNOHISTOCHEMISTRY

Immunohistochemistry (IHC) is a technique that identifies cellular constituents (antigens) by means of antigen–antibody interactions. The expression of certain antigens or cluster of antigens is characteristic of some tumours. The antigens may be proteins, polypeptides, carbohydrates or lipid molecules that bear one or more antibody-binding sites. The site of the antibody binding is visualized under the light microscope.

IHC plays an important role in establishing histogenesis at the light microscopic level. Its main advantage lies in the precise identification of cell type. It can be utilized to locate gene products in tissue sections as well as cytospin, imprint or touch preparations. The development of IHC has resulted in refinements to diagnosis and prognosis over the past few decades, and it is now the most widely available ancillary technique.[4] A large number of antibodies are commercially available for the diagnostic work-up. Several technological procedures for enhancing the sensitivity of the technique and the detection of previously undetectable antigens are also used.[5]

This technique produces a series of positive and negative stains, which are then matched with the appearances seen on the H&E. The correct interpretation of a positive immunoreaction first requires its confirmation in the tumour cells. Next, its precise cellular location (membrane, nuclear or cytoplasmic) and its character (diffuse or perinuclear cytoplasmic) are verified against the expected reaction.[6]

After making the initial histological evaluation on a routine H&E stain, the pathologist selects a screening panel of antibodies to analyse the tumour. Tables 3.1 and 3.2 summarize the immunocytochemical findings that are seen in the usual childhood tumours. For example, a basic set of antibodies for the initial work-up of a SRCT may employ the use of NB84 or synaptophysin for neuroblastoma,

myogenin or desmin for RMS, CD99 for primitive neuroectodermal tumour (PNET)/Ewing's sarcoma (ES), and CD45 (leucocyte common antigen) for lymphoma (Table 3.1). The results of the preliminary panel dictate what additional immunostains are necessary to confirm a diagnosis.

Limitations of IHC

While IHC removes the degree of subjectivity inherent in H&E staining, potential pitfalls exist in the interpretation, as none of the antibodies is either sensitive or specific.[7] In addition, some antibodies display aberrant activity. The pathologist has to be aware of the false-positive and false-negative reactions and assess each case in a thoughtful manner. A confirmatory panel is important for a confident diagnosis.

Neuroblastoma PNET/ES also show a variable degree of neural differentiation including the expression of NB84[8] and synaptophysin.[9] In this scenario, CD99 serves as a reliable marker to distinguish the two neural tumours.[9,10]

PNET/ES More than 95 per cent of these tumours are positive for CD99.[7,9] However, it is not a specific marker as it also marks the vast majority of lymphoblastic lymphoma and acute lymphoblastic leukaemias (ALLs),[11,12] which may be negative for CD45 and other lymphoid markers. If the clinical and histological features are suggestive of PNET/ES, positivity of the tumour cells with various neural marker(s) assists the diagnosis.[9] In this setting, it is also important to see a negative reaction for lymphoid markers such as TdT, CD34 and CD43 to confidently exclude lymphoblastic lymphoma/leukaemia.[7,12,13]

Rhabdomyosarcoma Desmin is not a specific marker of RMS.[14] The picture is complicated by the fact that various lymphoid,[15] neural[16,17] and epithelial markers[16,17] may be immunopositive in RMS. Therefore it is important to confirm the diagnosis of RMS by staining for highly specific and sensitive indicators of myogenic differentiation such as myogenin and myoD1.[18]

Non-Hodgkin's lymphoma Anaplastic large-cell lymphoma (ALCL), which has a small-cell variant, may be negative for CD45. In these cases, the diagnosis can be confirmed using antibodies against CD30 and ALK1 protein.

Desmoplastic small-cell tumour This can be confirmed with antibodies to WT1.[19]

Electron microscopy

Like light microscopy, electron microscopy (EM) provides another direct morphologic approach to establish the diagnosis. It uses a beam of electrons rather than a beam of light as used by the light microscope, enabling examination at a very high magnification. It helps the

Table 3.1 *Immunohistochemical panel used to distinguish undifferentiated, small round-cell tumours[a]*

Antibody to	NB	PNET/ES	RMS	NHL	DSCRT
Neural/neuroendocrine markers					
NB 84	++	+	+/−	−	+
Synaptophysin	+	+/−	−	−	+
Neurofilament	+	+	+/−	−	−
NSE	+	++	+/−	−	++
PGP 9.5	+	+	+/−	−	+
S-100	−	+	+/−	−	−
Myogenic group					
Desmin	−	+/−	++	−	++
MyoD1	−	−	+	−	−
Myogenin	−	−	++	−	−
Muscle-specific actin	−	−	++	−	+
Lymphoid/myeloid group					
CD45 (LCA)	−	−	−	+	−
Tdt	−	−	−	+	−
CD34	−	−	−	+	−
CD43	−	−	−	+	−
CD30	−	−	−	+	−
Misc					
CD99	−	+	+/−	+	+
WT1	−	−	−	−	++
FLI1	−	+	−	+	+
Epithelial markers					
Pan-cytokeratin	−	+	+/−	−	++
EMA	−	−	−	+ in ALCL	++

[a] A critical assessment involving correlation with the H&E and judicious interpretation of immunohistochemistry is essential.

ALCL, anaplastic large-cell lymphoma; DSCRT, desmoplastic small round-cell tumour; EMA, epithelial membrane antigen; FLI1, *FLI1* gene product; LCA, leucocyte common antigen; NB, neuroblastoma; NHL, non-Hodgkin's lymphoma; NK, not known; NSE, neuron-specific enolase; PGP 9.5, protein gene product 9.5; PNET/ES, primitive neuroectodermal tumour/Ewing's sarcoma; RMS, rhabdomyosarcoma; Tdt, terminal deoxynucleotidyl transferase; WT1, Wilms' tumour 1 gene product.
++, strong reaction in most cases; +, positive reaction; +/−, occasional, usually focal reaction; −, negative reaction.

Table 3.2 *Immunohistochemical panel used to distinguish monomorphic spindle cell tumours in childhood (other than rhabdomyosarcoma)*

Antibody to	MPNST	SS	AS	AFH	FS	LMS
S-100	++	+/−	−	−	−	+/−
Cytokeratin	−[a]	++	+/−	−	−	+
EMA	+/−	++		−	−	+/−
CD34	−[a]	−[a]	++	−	−	−
Desmin	+/−	−	+/−	+	−	++
Myogenin	−	+/−	NK	−	+/−	−
Caldesmon	−	−	NK	+	NK	+

AFH, angiomatoid fibrous histiocytoma; AS, angiosarcoma; EMA, epithelial membrane antigen; FS, fibrosarcoma; LMS, leiomyosarcoma; MPNST, malignant peripheral nerve sheath tumour; NK, not known; SS, synovial sarcoma.
++, strong reaction in most cases; +, positive reaction; +/−, occasional, usually focal reaction; −, negative reaction;
[a], typically negative but rare positive results reported.

pathologist to study the components of individual cells rather than the architectural patterns or a group of cells.[20] EM has the advantage of detecting cellular organelles that were not suspected, whereas IHC involves hypothesis testing. Its main drawback is that the area examined is small, this being an inherent sampling limitation. The other disadvantage in comparison to IHC is that it cannot be used for phenotyping of lymphomas. The two should be regarded as complementary and not as competitive techniques.[21,22]

As IHC has become firmly established as the most convenient and widely available ancillary technique, the role of EM has diminished. The main arguments against its frequent use are the purchase and maintenance costs of the necessary equipment and technical support.[23] It is also often considered (incorrectly) as a slow process. Consequently, it is now used sparingly and selectively in difficult cases by pathologists.[22,24]

However, EM still remains a valuable tool in the hands of a pathologist experienced in operating and evaluating the fine structure.[25] It is also re-emerging in importance as it is becoming increasingly apparent that IHC can lead to incorrect diagnosis.[1,26,27] Thus a pathologist should save a small portion of the tumour in glutaraldehyde fixative for processing. Sections can be viewed and a definitive diagnosis made available within 36 hours of receipt of the specimen.[23]

Selected indications for EM

- Small round-cell tumours (SRCTs) – EM can confidently establish the diagnosis of a difficult SCRT, where the IHC is inconclusive, non-contributory or the tissue sample is too small for a firm conclusion.[25] In addition, it can be pivotal in diagnosing a SCRT in an unusual location or clinical context, such as the presence of blastema only in the lung or liver metastasis from Wilms' tumour. Box 3.1 summarizes the diagnostic EM findings seen in the common SCRTs.
- Spindle-cell sarcomas (non-RMS)[22]
- Epithelioid tumours, including various sarcomas, carcinoma and melanoma[22]
- Brain tumours, e.g. ependymoma[22]
- Bone tumours – small-cell osteosarcoma vs. PNET/ES vs. mesenchymal chondrosaroma[24]
- Renal tumours – identification of rhabdoid tumour and PNET
- Intra-abdominal – mesothelioma vs. intra-abdominal desmoplastic round-cell tumour
- Langerhans cell histiocytosis.

Chromosomal and molecular analyses

Four main approaches are available to aid the pathologist in the diagnosis of paediatric solid tumours: conventional cytogenetics, fluorescence *in situ* hybridization (FISH), microarray analyses and reverse transcription polymerase chain reaction (RT-PCR).

CONVENTIONAL CYTOGENETICS

Conventional cytogenetics can give large amounts of information about chromosome gains, losses and

Box 3.1 *The diagnostic ultrastructural features of four small round-cell tumours of childhood*[24]

Neuroblastoma
Neural differentiation demonstrated by cytoplasmic membrane-bound dense-core secretory granules. Cell processes containing numerous microtubules and neurosecretory granules. Cell junctions are common

Rhabdomyosarcoma
Myogenic differentiation characterized by alternating arrays of cytoplasmic thin actin and thick myosin filaments; Z-band-like material. 'Indian-file' alignment of ribosomes along thick filaments, intermediate filaments and occasionally glycogen are other features

Primitive neuroectodermal tumour/Ewing's sarcoma
No specific features but large amounts of cytoplasmic and extracellular glycogen, variable number of cell junctions and occasional intermediate filaments are usually seen; cells closely apposed but no matrix

Non–Hodgkin's lymphoma
No diagnostic features. Cell–cell attachments almost always absent between the lymphoma cells, abundant polyribosomes and occasional intermediate filaments

---

rearrangements, particularly various translocations that are diagnostic in some types of paediatric solid tumours. In order to obtain chromosome spreads from a tumour sample, a number of processes have to be undertaken and fresh tumour material has to be available. Tumour material has to be disaggregated, either mechanically or enzymatically, then placed in cell culture conditions which allow rapid growth of tumour cells, preferably without the growth of any normal cells that may be present in the sample. Rapidly growing cell cultures are then harvested in the presence of a metaphase inhibitor such as colcemid to ensure the highest possible number of cells in mitosis. Harvested cells are then swollen in a hypotonic solution and fixed before being dropped onto slides to produce the chromosome spreads.

However, two major factors have limited the use of conventional cytogenetics in paediatric solid tumour diagnostics. First, it is difficult to grow paediatric solid tumour cells to produce metaphase chromosome spreads representative of the tumour and free from normal cell metaphases. Secondly, solid tumour chromosome rearrangements are frequently very complex, making identification of these rearrangements very difficult, if not impossible, by standard Giemsa banding techniques. Conventional paediatric cytogenetics is also time-consuming and cytogeneticists require extensive training before they are able to assess chromosome rearrangements accurately. Not all tumours have characteristic chromosome changes associated with them, which may be useful in diagnosis and prognostication. A highly informative database of published cytogenetic cases, collated by Felix Mitelman – the 'Mitelman Database of Chromosome Aberrations in Cancer' – is available on the internet (http://cgap.nci. nih.gov/chromosomes/Mitelman) (Mitelman online). This database also gives details of any cytogenetic-molecular biological and clinical correlations for each tumour type.

FLUORESCENCE *IN SITU* HYBRIDIZATION TECHNIQUES

Fluorescence *in situ* hybridization involves labelling nucleic acids with fluorochromes, their hybridization to material *in situ*, followed by the visualization of specifically bound label under an epifluorescence microscope. FISH has certain advantages over conventional cytogenetics, being able to be undertaken on very small amounts of material (including frozen and formalin-fixed paraffin-embedded material), not necessarily requiring metaphase chromosome spreads (interphase FISH), and being able to give accurate information about specific chromosome rearrangements and copy number changes. Two main forms of FISH can be undertaken for diagnostic cytogenetics, using either whole chromosome paints (WCPs) onto chromosome spreads or locus-specific probes onto chromosome spreads or interphase nuclei.

WCP FISH is often used in conjunction with conventional cytogenetics, particularly in situations where chromosomal rearrangements are complex or the morphology of chromosome banding is poor. Recent developments in FISH now allow WCP FISH to be undertaken using single chromosome paints or multiple chromosome paint sets. In multiple paint sets, combinations of various fluorochromes can be used to give up to 24 or more separate colours, one for each chromosome. Twenty-four colour karyotyping techniques, called multifluor-FISH (M-FISH) or spectral karyotyping (SKY), thus allow rearrangements of each individual chromosome to be assessed. Twenty-four colour karyotyping has enabled the classification of chromosome arrangements that would have been impossible with conventional cytogenetics.

Locus-specific FISH is routinely used for assessing the presence of diagnostic chromosomal translocations in paediatric solid tumours where chromosomal breakpoints have been defined or gain/loss of chromosomal material is important in the biology of the tumour (Plate 1). In the identification of chromosomal breakpoints, two forms of locus-specific FISH probes, translocation flanking or translocation conjoining, can be used, depending on which particular translocations are to be investigated.

Translocation flanking probes co-localize in normal cells but produce split signals on derivative chromosomes and interphase cells. Markers flanking a gene are of particular use where multiple different translocation partner genes are fused to a consistent gene. Thus, probes flanking the consistent partner gene can be used to identify the presence of a number of variant translocations. Conjoining probes are located on each of the normal chromosomes that come together on a consistent derivative. Thus, they are split in a normal interphase cell and come together in an interphase cell containing the specific translocation. For optimal diagnosis, use of both conjoining and flanking probes should be as close as possible to translocation breakpoints to eliminate the presence of false-positive/false-negative results.

Comparative genomic hybridization (CGH) is another derivation of FISH technology. It is carried out by differential fluorescence labelling of tumour and normal DNA samples, which are then co-hybridized onto normal metaphase chromosomes. The ratio of tumour to normal fluorescence intensity along the length of each chromosome is determined and plotted. Gains and losses in tumour material can then be seen across the genome. CGH can be used for molecular cytogenetic prognosis in paediatric solid tumours where gains, amplifications and losses have been shown to be predictors of outcome. CGH has the advantages of requiring only very small amounts of genomic DNA, being able to use microdissected and paraffin-embedded, formalin-fixed material. However, the resolution of changes seen by CGH is approximately 10 Mbp and hence small deletions can be missed. Rarely a chromosomal gain/loss/amplification can be of diagnostic value (e.g. co-amplification in the 1p36 region of the *PAX7* locus and 13q14 region of the *FOX1A10* locus indicates amplification of the *PAX7-FOX1A10* fusion gene in alveolar rhabdomyosarcoma). Online databases of CGH studies and publications are available on the internet for further information (www.ncbi.nlm.nih.gov/sky/) (see also Struski et al.[28]).

A recent variation of the CGH technique has been the development of differentially labelling and co-hybridizing control and test probes derived from the RNA in tissues. This profiles differential patterns of expression across the genome and has been termed comparative expressed sequence hybridization (CESH).[29] The CESH profiles and regions of differential expression identified may be useful in classifying tumours and in predicting tumour behaviour.[29,30]

MICROARRAY ANALYSES

Another recent advance in fluorescence hybridization technology applicable to molecular diagnosis has been the development of microarray technology. Of interest is their use in expression profiling for the classification of tumours.[31–33] Microarray technology involves the fluorescence labelling of RNA samples that are then hybridized onto arrays of gene sequences consisting of a large number of cDNA clones or oligonucleotide spots attached to a glass slide surface, or a silicon chip onto which oligonucleotides have been synthesized at particular positions. Following hybridization, washing, scanning and image analysis, the relative level of expression of each gene represented on the array can be determined. Present technology allows the large-scale parallel analysis of gene expression of up to 30 000–40 000 individual human genes to be used for expression profiling. Very large amounts of data are produced from microarray expression experiments, and to find expression patterns that represent specific tumour types in this data requires sophisticated statistical methods to be applied to data sets. These methods include clustering analysis where no prior information about the data set is used (K-means, hierarchical clustering, self-organizing maps) and molecular classifier analysis using training sets of known cancer samples (support vector machines, neural networks)[34,35] (for review, see Knudsen[36]). Expression profiles from a number of different tumour types have been studied with the aim of using them to identify small numbers of genes whose expression pattern can subsequently be used to classify unknown tumour samples. Small classifier sets of genes have already been reported in certain cancer types, such as B-cell lymphoma,[37] although they have not yet been widely used to classify paediatric solid tumours (RMS;[38] for review, see Triche et al.[39]). Expression profiling has also been used to investigate the current classification of adult soft tissue sarcomas, which can be problematic.[40]

REVERSE TRANSCRIPTION POLYMERASE CHAIN REACTION

Reverse transcription polymerase chain reaction (RT-PCR) is a method that can be used diagnostically to detect the presence of fusion gene transcripts associated with specific chromosome translocations (Plate 1). In order to perform a diagnostic RT-PCR, the genes involved in the translocation breakpoint need to be known and PCR primers corresponding to the gene sequences optimized. Tumour RNA must first be extracted, cDNA produced from the RNA and then a PCR reaction performed. The presence or absence of a band on a gel then indicates the presence or absence of a fusion gene transcript. RT-PCR can be highly sensitive, is inherently translocation-specific, is less labour-intensive than conventional cytogenetics or FISH, can be performed on formalin-fixed, paraffin-embedded material and can be adapted to high throughput.[41,42] However, RT-PCR has some disadvantages compared with conventional cytogenetics and FISH. It can only be used where the sequence

of chromosome translocation breakpoint fusion genes has been identified and it does not detect variant products unless these are specifically tested for, intact RNA is required and the method can be prone to artifacts and contamination.

A recent development of RT-PCR has been the introduction of real-time PCR, which uses smaller amounts of material and is more sensitive than normal RT-PCR. It is quantitative, can be multiplexed to investigate multiple fusion gene products at the same time and is capable of being adapted to high throughput using 384-well formats.[43,44] Real-time PCR is also sensitive enough to detect cells containing translocations in peripheral blood samples.

For all molecular cytogenetic diagnostics, best practice should involve, where possible, more than one test (conventional cytogenetics or FISH or RT-PCR) to fully confirm a diagnosis. Tests should also be carried out with the investigator blinded to the sample details and with positive and negative controls. It should be noted that, although of great diagnostic value in paediatric cancer due to their absence in normal tissue, pathognomonic chromosomal translocations and their resultant fusion genes only have positive diagnostic value (summarized in Table 3.3). Studies looking into the presence of translocations in paediatric solid tumours (RMS, Ewing's sarcoma and synovial sarcoma) have not identified a 100 per cent correlation between pathology and the presence of a pathognomonic translocation.[45–47] For example, Anderson et al.[45] and Sorensen et al.[48] found only 70–75 per cent of alveolar RMS examined to contain a PAX3-FOX1A10 or PAX7-FOX1A10 fusion gene product. The reason why there has not been 100 per cent correlation between pathology and detection of a specific translocation is not known, but it may be due to factors such as the variable biology found within tumour groups, the presence of as yet unidentified chromosomal translocations, variable fusion gene products, alternative mechanisms affecting pathways within cells or technical considerations.[49]

TUMOURS OF THE CENTRAL NERVOUS SYSTEM

Although neuroimaging has improved dramatically over the past few years, tissue diagnosis remains essential.[50] The WHO classification[51] provides an excellent framework for recognition of paediatric central nervous system (CNS) tumours. Approximately 88 per cent fall into four main histological types (Table 3.4)[52] Germ cell tumours comprise 2 per cent and choroid plexus tumours 1 per cent of the primary brain tumours. Uncommon tumours include neuronal and mixed neuronal-glial tumours (ganglioglioma, desmoplastic infantile astrocytoma and ganglioglioma, dysembryoplastic neuroepithelial tumour

Table 3.3 *Summary of molecular cytogenetic rearrangements used in the diagnosis of paediatric solid tumours*

Tumour	Cytogenetic rearrangement	Molecular rearrangement
Neuroblastoma	dms/hsr 2p24	*MYCN* amplification?
	gain 17q21-qter	
Alveolar RMS	t(2;13)(q35;q14)	*PAX3-FOX1A10*
	t(1;13)(p36;q14)	*PAX7-FOX1A10*
Embryonal RMS		LOH 11p
Ewing's family of tumours and pPNET	t(11;22)(q24;q12)	*EWS-FLI1*
	t(21;22)(q22;q12)	*EWS-ERG*
	t(7;22)(p22;q12)	*EWS-ETV1*
	t(17;22)(q12;q12)	*EWS-E1AF*
	t(2;22)	*EWS-FEV*
MEM and DSRCT	t(11;22)(p13;q12)	*EWS-WT1*
CCS (MMSP)	(12;22)(q13;q12)	*EWS-ATF1*
Myxoid chondrosarcoma	t(9;22)(q22;q12)	*EWS-CHN*
	t(9;17)(q22;q11)	*TAF2N-CHN*
	t(9;15)(q22;q21)	*TCF12-TEC*
PNET	i(17q)	Loss *TP53*
Synovial sarcoma	t(X;18)(p11;q11)	*SYT-SSX1 or SSX2 or SSX4*
Germ cell tumour	i(12p)	?
ASPS	t(X;17)(p11.2;q25)	*ASPL-TFES*
CFS and CMN	t(12;15)(p13q25)	*ETV6-NTRK3*
Myxoid liposarcoma	t(12;16)(q13;p11)	*CHOP-FUS*

ASPS, alveolar soft part sarcoma; CCS, clear cell sarcoma (or malignant melanoma of the soft parts); CFS, congenital fibrosarcoma; CMN, congenital mesoblastic nephroma.; DSRCT, desmoplastic small round-cell tumour; MEM, malignant ectomesenchymoma; PNET, primitive neuroectodermal tumour; pPNET, peripheral primitive neuroectodermal tumour; RMS, rhabdomyosarcoma.

Table 3.4 *The main histological types of central nervous system tumours*

Primary brain tumours	Percentage frequency
Low-grade astrocytoma – pilocytic and diffuse	37
High-grade astrocytoma – anaplastic and glioblastoma multiforme	8
Embryonal tumour (PNET) including medulloblastoma	20
Ependymoma	13
Craniopharyngioma	10

PNET, primitive neuroectodermal tumour.

and central neurocytoma), astrocytic tumours such as pleomorphic xanthoastrocytoma,[53] and embryonal tumours including atypical teratoid/rhabdoid tumours.[54] Meningioma, oligodendroglioma, Schwannoma and haemangioblastoma are rare. The clinical, neuroimaging, pathological and molecular genetic features of all these tumours are described in the *WHO Classification of Tumours*.[51]

The distribution of the CNS tumours and the differential diagnosis according to location are given in Table 3.5. The Childhood Brain Tumour Consortium study[55] has highlighted the limitations of the WHO classification of supratentorial astrocytic tumours. The proposed refined

criteria are reproducible and reliably divide these tumours into three distinct prognostic groups. Brainstem gliomas comprise up to 20 per cent of childhood brain tumours, and can be classified into two distinct clinicopathological and biological entities.[56]

Astrocytomas

These occur throughout the CNS, including the spinal cord. About 50 per cent of astrocytomas are supratentorial; the other 50 per cent are infratentorial, of which 35 per cent are located in the cerebellum and 15 per cent in the brain stem.[52] All astrocytomas express the cytoplasmic intermediate filament, glial fibrillary acidic protein (GFAP), to a variable degree.[57]

PILOCYTIC ASTROCYTOMA (WHO GRADE I)[51]

Pilocytic astrocytomas are the most common gliomas in children. Their characteristic location is the cerebellum, hypothalamus or optic nerve rather than the cerebral hemisphere. These are stable or slow-growing masses; rare examples undergo malignant transformation.[58]

Macroscopic features

These are discrete, soft tumours which show a marked tendency to undergo cystic degeneration. Other regressive changes such as calcification and haemorrhage are also seen.

Table 3.5 *Distribution and differential diagnosis of childhood central nervous system tumours*[52]

Location	%	Region	%	Histological type	%
Supratentorial	40	Cerebral hemisphere	35	Astrocytoma	65
				PNET	15
				Ependymoma	15
				Other	5
		Parasellar	40	Craniopharyngioma/GCT	
		Thalamus and basal ganglia	10	Astrocytoma	
		Pineal	10	Pineal/GCT	
		Intraventricular	3	Choroid plexus tumours,	
		Meninges	2	ependymoma	
Infratentorial	52	Cerebellar	75	Pilocytic astrocytoma	
				Medulloblastoma	
		Brainstem	25	Low-grade astrocytoma	33
				High-grade astrocytoma	66
Spinal cord	8	Intramedullary		Astrocytoma	32
				Ependymoma	17
		Extramedullary		Developmental	47
				Schwannoma	
				Meningioma	

PNET, primitive neuroectodermal tumour; GCT, germ cell tumour.

Pilocytic astrocytomas of the optic nerve and chiasm are less well circumscribed than those located in the cerebellum. In the brainstem, these are usually dorsal and exophytic.[56]

Microscopic features

Typically, pilocytic astrocytomas show a biphasic appearance composed of loose, spongy areas alternating with compact cellular areas (Plate 2a). The spongy areas contain microcysts and astrocytes with oval to round nuclei. In the more compact areas, the astrocytes have thin nuclei and bipolar cytoplasmic processes. Rosenthal fibres and eosinophilic bodies are characteristic features. The contrast enhancement, seen on imaging, is due to vascular proliferation.

The growth fraction, as determined by Ki67/MIB-1 labelling index (LI), is usually in the region of 1 per cent.[59] The suprasellar pilocytic astrocytoma of infants does not show the classic histological features.[60] The mitotic activity is usually increased in contrast to the classic variety. This subtype usually displays aggressive behaviour.

DIFFUSE ASTROCYTOMA (WHO GRADE II)[61]

Diffuse astrocytomas invade the adjacent brain structures and have an intrinsic tendency to progress to a more malignant phenotype. Approximately 10 per cent occur in children. These are usually located supratentorially and are uncommon in the cerebellum.

Macroscopic features

As this is an infiltrating tumour, the boundaries between the tumour and normal parenchyma are indistinct. These may show cystic change.

Microscopic features

This is a moderately cellular tumour composed of well-differentiated astrocytes set in a loosely woven matrix. There is no necrosis or microvascular proliferation. Mitotic activity is generally absent. Depending on the predominant astrocytic component, three histological variants are recognized: protoplasmic, fibrillary and gemistocytic. The growth fraction of these astrocytomas ranges from 1 to 4 per cent.

Prognostic features

The gemistocytic variant undergoes malignant progression more rapidly than the fibrillary type.[62] A growth fraction with a LI >5 per cent predicts a shorter survival.[63]

ANAPLASTIC ASTROCYTOMA (WHO GRADE III)[64]

This is also a diffusely infiltrating astrocytoma with a tendency for malignant progression to glioblastoma. The time interval for progression to glioblastoma is an average of 2 years.[65]

Macroscopic features

This has a similar infiltrative pattern to that of diffuse astrocytoma, but cysts are less common.

Microscopic features

In comparison to low-grade astrocytomas, these display increased cellularity, nuclear atypia and marked mitotic activity. There is no microvascular proliferation or necrosis. The growth fraction is 5–10 per cent.

Prognostic features

The presence of an oligodendroglial component is associated with a significant increase in survival.[64]

GLIOBLASTOMA MULTIFORME (WHO GRADE IV)[66]

This is the most malignant astrocytic tumour; 9 per cent occur in children, in whom it is usually located in the brainstem. Unlike pilocytic astrocytomas, this is rare in the cerebellum and spinal cord.

Macroscopic features

These are poorly delineated masses with a variegated appearance due to necrosis, haemorrhage and cystic changes.

Microscopic features

The size and appearance of the malignant astrocytes are variable and this inherent heterogeneity may lead to undergrading in stereotactic biopsies.[67] Generally, these are highly cellular, pleomorphic and mitotic tumours. Necrosis (Plate 2b) and/or microvascular proliferation are essential diagnostic features. The latter usually palisades around the necrotic foci. A variable number of the tumour cells express GFAP (Plate 2c).

The growth fraction is a mean of 15–20 per cent,[63] and higher proliferation is seen in the small undifferentiated cells, in contrast to the gemistocytes.

Genetics

No pathognomonic chromosomal aberrations have yet been found for astrocytoma.[68] Relatively few juvenile astrocytoma karyotypes have been reported (31 cases; see http://cgap.nci.nih.gov/chromosomes/Mitelman). It has been found that they exhibit complex chromosomal rearrangements, although less frequently than adult forms. The molecular cytogenetic prognosis of paediatric astrocytomas, like adult forms, seems to be generally related to the frequency of aberrations, with grade I and grade II astrocytomas showing fewer aberrations than grade III and IV forms, or (one-third) showing no aberrations at all.[68]

Embryonal tumours

These are undifferentiated round-cell tumours which can show divergent patterns of differentiation. This group of tumours encompasses distinct clinicopathological entities. The infratentorial embryonal tumour is medulloblastoma, while supratentorial embryonal tumours include PNETs and ependymoblastomas. Medulloepitheliomas and atypical teratoid/rhabdoid tumours are distinct entities.

MEDULLOBLASTOMAS

Seventy per cent of medulloblastomas arise in the vermis and the peak age of occurrence is 7 years.

Macroscopic features

The consistency and the boundaries are variable.

Microscopic features

Four histopathological variants are recognized:

- *Classic medulloblastoma* – this is composed of embryonal undifferentiated cells. Neuroblastic rosettes, ganglion cells and apoptosis are other features.
- *Desmoplastic variant* – this is composed of reticulin-free nodules of low cellularity (Plate 3a). The tumour cells within these nodules show neuronal differentiation.[69] Between the nodules are densely packed, proliferating cells set in a reticulin-rich stroma.
- *Medulloblastomas with extensive nodularity and advanced neuronal differentiation* – these show intranodular nuclear uniformity and cell streaming in a fine fibrillary background and occur predominantly in children younger than 3 years of age.
- *Large-cell variant* – this medulloblastoma is rare and resembles the rhabdoid/atypical teratoid tumours of the cerebellar region.[70]

Immunohistochemically, the tumour cells are positive for synaptophysin (Plate 3b). In addition, a variety of other markers, such as nestin, GFAP, neurofilament and vimentin, may be seen in the tumour cells.

Prognosis

Desmoplastic medulloblastomas and medulloblastomas with extensive nodularity are associated with a better outcome.[71] The large-cell variant is biologically more aggressive and the survival of children with this type is significantly shorter.[70] Glial differentiation is associated with a worse prognosis.[72] TrkC expression[73] and low MYC mRNA[74] are associated with a good clinical outcome.

Genetics

Mitelman online reports 181 PNET cases showing clonal chromosomal aberrations. Deletions of 10q, 11 and 17p [often through associated i(17q)] are the most frequently seen cytogenetics changes, although none of these is pathognomonic. However, the presence of i(17q) can offer limited aid to the diagnosis of these tumours.[75] Loss of 17p11.2-p13 has also been seen by CGH studies of PNETs and, at the molecular level, is associated with loss of *TP53*, although again this is not diagnostic for PNET.[76]

Ependymomas

These can occur at any site along the ventricular system and in the spinal canal. They develop in the posterior fossa (65 per cent) and in the spinal cord (10 per cent),[52] followed by the lateral ventricles and the third ventricle

(25 per cent). Supratentorial tumours can occur outside the ventricular system, originating from the embryonic ependymal remnants in the brain parenchyma.

Macroscopic features

These are soft, greyish-red tumours and may show haemorrhage, necrosis and cysts.

Microscopic features

Ependymomas are well circumscribed, moderately cellular tumours. Mitoses are rare or absent. Rosettes are a helpful diagnostic feature. True rosettes have columnar cells around a central lumen. However, these are rarely seen. The majority of ependymomas show perivascular rosettes which are composed of tumour cells arranged radially around the blood vessels (Plate 4).

The histopathological variants are cellular ependymoma, papillary ependymoma, clear cell ependymoma and tancytic ependymoma, but these have no bearing on prognosis.

Ependymomas display GFAP, predominantly around the blood vessels. S100, vimentin and epithelial membrane antigen (EMA) positivity is also seen. The LI has been correlated with a poor prognosis.[77,78]

ANAPLASTIC EPENDYMOMA

Anaplastic ependymoma is malignant and corresponds to WHO grade III.

Microscopic features

Perivascular rosettes are seen but true rosettes are absent. It shows high cell density and increased mitotic activity and often microvascular proliferation and pseudopalisading necrosis, of which the former two have been correlated to poor outcome. However, as precise criteria for the grading of classic versus anaplastic ependymomas have not been defined, the results of various studies show conflicting data regarding the survival of patients with classic and anaplastic ependymomas.

Genetics

A relatively large number of clonal chromosomal aberrations have been reported for ependymoma, although no pathognomonic chromosomal aberrations have been described. Gain of 1q and loss of 22 are the most common changes detected by comparative genomic hybridization in paediatric ependymoma.[79,80] Children with structural (mainly partial) genomic imbalances show a significantly worse outcome than those with tumours with a numerical or balanced genomic profile.[81]

Craniopharyngioma

These are the most common non-neuroepithelial tumours occurring in children aged 5–14 years. They are slow-growing and correspond to WHO grade I.[82] The majority

are intrasellar and suprasellar in location. The papillary variant is located in the ventricle and is rare in children.

Macroscopic features

Craniopharyngiomas have solid and cystic components.

Microscopic features

These tumours are composed of broad bands, strands and trabeculae of squamous cells with peripheral palisading. Keratinous nodules and dystrophic calcification are diagnostically helpful characteristics. A LI >7 per cent is a useful indicator of recurrence.[83]

Genetics

Very few molecular cytogenetic data have been published for craniopharyngiomas and no diagnostic information has been discerned.

Germ cell tumours (GCTs)[84]

Sixty-eight per cent of germ cell tumours occur in the second decade, although congenital examples are well recognized. The majority of the GCTs in the pineal gland are seen in boys, while those in the suprasellar region are generally seen in girls. The male:female ratio for germinomas is 1.5:2.1; for non-germinomatous tumours the ratio is 1:3. As with their extragonadal counterparts, CNS GCTs occur in the midline and the histology is also identical to that seen in the extracranial sites.

Choroid plexus tumours[85]

These are intraventricular tumours which arise from the choroid plexus epithelium. They typically manifest in children and are the most frequently occurring tumours during the first year of life.

Choroid plexus papilloma (CPP) is a benign, slow-growing tumour. Histologically it closely resembles the non-neoplastic choroid plexus.

Choroid plexus carcinoma (CPC) shows cellular atypia, necrosis, mitosis[86] and cellular stratification with invasion of the brain and CSF metastases.

The mean LI for CPP is 1.9 per cent, while that for CPC is 13.8 per cent.

Atypical teratoid and rhabdoid tumours

Typically, these tumours occur in boys younger than 2 years of age and are associated with poor prognosis.[54] Some infants with malignant rhabdoid tumour of the kidney also have a CNS embryonal tumour. These tumours may cause diagnostic confusion with medulloblastoma.[87]

Microscopic features

The characteristic feature of this group of tumours is the rhabdoid cell. It is present in addition to primitive neuroectodermal, mesenchymal and epithelial cells. Immunohistochemically, the rhabdoid cells are consistently reactive to epithelial membrane antigen and vimentin. Electron microscopy shows intermediate filaments arranged in whorls.

Genetics

Thirty-four karyotypes of rhabdoid tumours (both CNS and renal) have been reported with one overall consistent chromosomal aberration, (del)(22q11.12), having been noted. The deletion is thought to involve loss of the *INF1* gene region and is also seen in teratoid tumours.[88] Loss of 22q11.2 can hence be used to aid diagnosis of atypical teratoid and rhabdoid tumours.[75,87]

NEUROBLASTIC TUMOURS

Neuroblastic tumours are the most common extracranial malignant solid tumours of childhood, and account for 6–10 per cent of all childhood cancers.

These are tumours of the autonomic nervous system that may arise in any site of autonomic ganglia or paraganglia. These tumours are distinct entities from the central PNETs (e.g. medulloblastoma) and peripheral PNETs/Ewing's sarcoma group of tumours. According to the conventional terminology, neuroblastic tumours are classified into three main categories: neuroblastoma (NB), ganglioneuroblastoma (GNB) and ganglioneuroma (GN).[89]

The first priority of the pathologist is to secure enough viable tissue for confirmation of the diagnosis.

Tissue is then taken for biological studies following the recommended guidelines.[90]

The pre-chemotherapy tumour specimens, from either the primary or metastatic sites (Plate 5a), are optimal material for establishing the histopathological diagnosis and evaluating the prognosis. While a diagnosis can be established by fine-needle aspiration biopsy of the primary and metastatic sites, it is unsuitable for the histopathological classification that is required for the risk assessment.[91,92]

DIAGNOSTIC FEATURES

Depending on the proportion of the two main cell components, neuroblastic/ganglionic and Schwann cells, neuroblastic tumours are typed into four main categories,[92] as shown in the Table 3.6. Consonant with the variable maturation that neuroblastic tumours display, a wide range of gross and microscopic appearances are seen.

Macroscopic features

Neuroblastomas are encapsulated masses of variable colour and consistency. Usually they are soft, red-brown (Plate 5b), and typically contain flecks of calcification. Haemorrhage and necrosis are other features. On the other hand, GNs are firm, grey-white, solid tumours without haemorrhage and necrosis. The nodular type of ganglioneuroblastoma (GNB, n) shows haemorrhagic nodules in a tumour which is otherwise like a GN.

Microscopic features

The undifferentiated NB is rare, but carries a very poor prognosis. It is the archetypal malignant small round-cell

Table 3.6 *Histopathological classification of the neuroblastic tumours (NT)*[91,92]

Type	Definition	Subtype	Criteria
NB	<50% of the tumour tissue is composed of Schwannian stroma or Schwannian stroma-poor NT	1. Undifferentiated	No discernible differentiation on H&E; IHC and EM are essential for diagnosis
		2. Poorly differentiated	Less than 5% ganglionic differentiation
		3. Differentiating	5–50% ganglionic differentiation
GNB intermixed	>50% of the NT is composed of Schwannian stroma		The neuroblastic foci in the stroma are not visible grossly; and are composed of differentiating neuroblasts
GNB neuroblastic nodular or composite			Abrupt demarcation between nodules and GNB or GN
GN	Schwannian stroma predominant NT	1. Maturing	Predominantly composed of Schwannian stroma with randomly scattered mature ganglion cells and immature neuroblasts
		2. Mature	Fully mature ganglion cells embedded in the Schwannian stroma

EM, electron microscopy; GNB, ganglioneuroblastoma; GN, ganglioneuroma; IHC, immunohistochemistry; NB, neuroblastoma.

tumour (Plate 5c) that requires ancillary techniques for diagnosis (Table 3.1 and Box 3.1).

As the primitive neuroblasts differentiate into ganglion cells, the cell size progressively enlarges and the nucleus and cytoplasm show maturation (Plates 5d–f). The Schwannian stroma is composed of Schwann cells, perineural cells, neuritic processes and fibrous tissue. A semiquantitative method of assessment is utilized to define and subtype neuroblastic tumours (Table 3.6).

PROGNOSTIC FEATURES

Histological criteria

These were set out in the International Classification, which is based on the Shimada system,[91,92] and its prognostic significance has been confirmed recently.[93] It is based on a conceptual framework of age-linked maturation, which starts with NB, proceeds to GNB (intermixed) and reaches the final stage of GN. It divides neuroblastic tumours into two prognostic groups – favourable histology (FH) and unfavourable histology (UH) – taking three variables into consideration: degree of differentiation, mitosis-karyorrhexis index (MKI) and age (see Box 3.2).

The MKI represents cellular turnover. The average number of proliferating (mitotic) and apoptotic (karyorrhectic) cells, obtained by counting 5000 cells, is enumerated and NB is categorized as showing low (<2 per cent), intermediate (2–4 per cent) or high (>4 per cent) MKI.

The behaviour of nodular GNB is not always unfavourable. Histopathological assessment of the nodule, as assessed by the age-linked classification, determines the prognosis.[94] A recent study combining histology with *MYCN* status identified four subsets of patients.[95] Of the patients with FH, the majority were non-*MYCN*-amplified and had an excellent prognosis regardless of age. The majority of the *MYCN*-amplified tumours almost always fell into the UH category and had the worst prognosis regardless of age. More importantly, the histology was predictive of poor outcome in patients (>1.5 years) with UH non-amplified tumours.[95]

Expression of neurotrophin receptors

High levels of tyrosine kinase receptor *TrkA* expression are seen in low-stage tumours without *MYCN* amplification and correlate strongly with survival.[96] Similarly, expression of *TrkC* is predominantly found in lower stage tumours, and like *TrkA*, it is not detected in *MYCN*-amplified tumours.[97] However, expression of full-length *TrkB* is strongly associated with *MYCN*-amplified tumours.[98]

CD44 Expression

The standard molecule of CD44, a transmembrane glycoprotein, can be detected in neuroblastoma samples employing immunohistochemistry. CD44 expression has been associated with a favourable outcome.[99] There is

Box 3.2 *Prognostic classification of neuroblastic tumours*[93]

Favourable histology

Neuroblastoma, <1.5 years
Poorly differentiated, low MKI
Poorly differentiated, intermediate MKI
Differentiating, low MKI
Differentiating, intermediate MKI

Neuroblastoma, 1.5–5 years
Differentiating, low MKI

Neuroblastoma, ≥5 years
GNB – intermixed
GN – mature and maturing

Unfavourable histology

Neuroblastoma, <1.5 years
Undifferentiated
Poorly differentiated, high MKI
Differentiating, high MKI

Neuroblastoma, 1.5–5 years
Undifferentiated
Poorly differentiated, high MKI
Poorly differentiated, intermediate MKI
Differentiating, high MKI
Differentiating, intermediate MKI

Neuroblastoma, ≥5 years
GNB – nodular (composite)

GN, ganglioneuroma; GNB, ganglioneuroblastoma; MKI, mitosis-karyorrhexis index; NB, neuroblastoma.

also a strong correlation between the absence of CD44 and *MYCN* amplification[100] and the absence of *TrkA* expression.[101]

Genetics

Although not pathognomonic, a number of consistent molecular cytogenetic aberrations have been found through study of the more than 200 reported neuroblastoma karyotypes (Mitelman online) and the many neuroblastoma CGH studies (http://www.helsinki.fi/~lgl_www/CMG.html) (for review, see Bown[102]). Although not strictly of diagnostic value, these chromosomal changes are very useful as markers of poor prognosis. The markers include 1p36 loss, ploidy, *MYCN* amplification and gain of 17q.[70] 80 per cent of cases show evidence of 1p36 loss and 25–30 per cent show amplification of the *MYCN* gene, which is associated with poorer prognosis. However, recently, gain of 17q (specifically 17q21-qter), the most common cytogenetic change in neuroblastoma, has been shown to be the most important cytogenetic marker of prognosis, with greater power than loss of 1p36, ploidy or *MYCN* amplification.[103,104] The underlying molecular events of 1p36 loss and 17q gain are as yet unknown, although much attention has been paid to this area of research. Chromosome 11q loss without *MYCN* amplification is not only associated with advanced stage disease but is also suggestive of relapse in low stage disease.[105]

RENAL TUMOURS

Renal tumours in childhood comprise about 7 per cent of all tumours in children up to 15 years of age. The relative incidence of renal tumours of childhood is shown in the Table 3.7.[106]

Clear cell sarcoma of the kidney (CCSK) and rhabdoid tumour of kidney (RTK) are biological entities distinct from Wilms' tumour (WT). CCSK, RTK and WT, anaplastic type, are classed as unfavourable histology in the National Wilms' Tumour Study (NWTS) and the second UKCCSG Wilms' Tumour Study. The 4-year event-free survival seen in the second UK Wilms' Tumour Study was 36 per cent for RTK; for WT, anaplastic type, the figure was 29 per cent, as compared with 82 per cent for WT, favourable histology.[107]

In the current International Society of Paediatric Oncology (SIOP) and UKCCSG protocols,[108] these three renal tumours are placed in the high-risk treatment category (Box 3.3). A preoperative biopsy is performed to provide the diagnosis in the UKCCSG protocol.[109] Monophasic and biphasic WT, CCSK, tumours in the older age group and rarer tumours can be difficult to interpret. Provided the biopsy is adequate, a diagnosis can usually be reached with the aid of ancillary techniques.

The SIOP approach is to give preoperative chemotherapy first, the diagnosis being based on imaging studies. The nephrectomy specimen provides confirmation of the diagnosis, staging of the tumour and categorization of risk.

UKCCSG protocols follow the NWTS staging criteria (Box 3.4). Unlike the SIOP protocol, pre-treatment biopsy does not upstage the tumour. The local staging for this protocol is also done following chemotherapy and is important for stages IV and V. The pathologist should be provided with the information relevant to the staging, including the pre- or intraoperative tumour rupture and metastases.

Table 3.7 *The incidence of renal tumours*

Renal tumour	Relative percentage
Wilms' tumour, favourable histology	80
Wilms' tumour, anaplastic	4
Mesoblastic nephroma	5
Clear cell sarcoma	4
Rhabdoid tumour	2
Miscellaneous	5

Wilms' tumour (nephroblastoma)

The peak incidence of WT is between 2 and 6 years; it is uncommon in neonates. Cases of adult WT often prove to be other neoplastic entities, including PNETs. WT has been described in the extrarenal sites. It may be sporadic or familial. Unlike other renal tumours, WT may be associated with several syndromes, such as WAGR (WT, aniridia, genitourinary anomalies, and mental retardation) and Denys–Drash syndrome.

Macroscopic features

Wilms' tumours show a lobulated, soft, grey appearance with areas of haemorrhage, necrosis and cystic degeneration (Plate 6a). Ten per cent are multifocal, a feature that is associated with an increased likelihood of tumour formation in the remaining kidney. Bilateral tumours are present in 5–6 per cent of cases.

Box 3.3 *Renal tumours: the revised SIOP (International Society of Paediatric Oncology) working classification*[108]

For pre-treated cases

Low-risk tumours
- Mesoblastic nephroma
- Cystic partially differentiated nephroblastoma
- Completely necrotic nephroblastoma

Intermediate-risk tumours
- Nephroblastoma – epithelial type
- Nephroblastoma – stromal type
- Nephroblastoma – mixed type
- Nephroblastoma – regressive type
- Nephroblastoma – focal anaplasia

High-risk tumours
- Nephroblastoma – blastemal type
- Nephroblastoma – diffuse anaplasia
- Clear cell sarcoma of the kidney
- Rhabdoid tumour of the kidney

For primary nephrectomy cases

Low-risk tumours
- Mesoblastic nephroma
- Cystic partially differentiated nephroblastoma

Intermediate-risk tumours
- Non-anaplastic nephroblastoma and its variants
- Nephroblastoma – focal anaplasia

High-risk tumours
- Nephroblastoma – diffuse anaplasia
- Clear cell sarcoma of the kidney
- Rhabdoid tumour of the kidney

Microscopic features

The classic triphasic variety shows the blastemal, stromal and epithelial components (Plate 6b). The blastema is the undifferentiated element. The epithelial component comprises tubular and glomeruloid structures. The stromal elements are undifferentiated mesenchymal cells, muscle, fat, cartilage and bone. If one element comprises more than two-thirds of the total, the tumour is categorized accordingly.

Box 3.4 *Pathological staging of renal tumours*[108]

Stage I

(a) The tumour is confined to the kidney or surrounded by a fibrous capsule if outside the normal contours of the kidney. The renal capsule or pseudocapsule may be infiltrated with the tumour but it does not reach the outer surface. It is completely resected.

(b) The tumour may be protruding (bulging) into the pelvis system and dipping into the ureter (but it is not infiltrating the walls).

(c) The vessels of the renal sinus are not involved.

(d) Intrarenal vessel involvement may be present.

Fine-needle aspiration or percutaneous core needle biopsy (Tru-Cut) does not upstage the tumour.

Stage II

(a) The tumour extends beyond the kidney or penetrates the capsule and/or the fibrous pseudocapsule into the perirenal fat but is completely resected.

(b) The tumour infiltrates the renal sinus and/or invades blood and lymphatic vessels outside the renal parenchyma but is completely resected.

(c) The tumour infiltrates the adjacent organs or vena cava but is completely resected.

Stage III

(a) The tumour has been incompletely excised.

(b) The abdominal lymph nodes are involved.

(c) The tumour has ruptured pre- or intraoperatively.

(d) Tumour implants are present on the peritoneal surface.

(e) Tumour thrombi are present at the resection margins of the vessels or the ureter.

(f) A wedge biopsy prior to the nephrectomy or surgery.

Stage IV

The presence of metastases: haematogenous (lung, liver, bone, brain) or lymph node metastases beyond the abdominopelvic region (e.g. mediastinal nodes).

Stage V

Bilateral renal tumours at diagnosis; each tumour should be substaged separately.

Anaplasia The only histological feature of adverse prognostic significance is anaplasia, as it is resistant to chemotherapy.[110] It is encountered in 4–5 per cent of WT specimens and is recognized by the presence of nuclear enlargement (threefold) or one multipolar mitotic figure (Plate 6c). Depending on the distribution and location, it may be may be focal or diffuse, the prognosis being worse for diffuse anaplasia. Focal anaplasia is confined to one or more clearly defined loci within the primary tumour, without evidence of anaplasia or prominent nuclear atypia in extratumoral or extrarenal sites. Intrarenal multiple foci are acceptable when each is small enough to be contained on a single microscope section. Diffuse anaplasia is diagnosed when a WT fulfils any one of the following four criteria:

- anaplastic changes in the primary tumour are more extensive than those defined for focal anaplasia
- tumour cells with anaplastic changes are present in the intrarenal or extrarenal vessels, renal sinus, extracapsular or metastatic sites
- anaplasia is focal but there is nuclear atypia elsewhere in the tumour
- anaplasia is present in a biopsy sample.

Chemotherapy response Chemotherapy usually results in massive necrosis of the immature and actively proliferating cell types.[111,112] For example, the blastemal component is aggressive but chemosensitive at all stages. The mature components such as skeletal muscle are resistant to chemotherapy, as are the anaplastic cells.

Nephrogenic rests (NRs) These are abnormally persistent foci of embryonal cells that are capable of developing into WTs.[113] NRs are found adjacent to 30–40 per cent of WTs and may be perilobar (Plate 6d) or intralobar. Both types may be dormant, hyperplastic or sclerosing. They may develop into WTs or regress.

Intralobar NRs can be located anywhere in the renal lobe, and these foci merge imperceptibly with the renal tissue. They are composed of stroma and are usually associated with WAGR and Denys–Drash syndromes. The perilobar NRs, on the other hand, are confined to the periphery of the renal lobe, are sharply demarcated from the normal renal tissue and are usually triphasic. These are associated with overgrowth syndromes and have a low malignant potential.

Both cystic nephromas and cystic partially differentiated nephroblastomas are thought to represent relatively mature variants of WT. Both are encapsulated and consist of multiple cystic spaces separated by delicate septa with no significant solid component. Cystic nephromas have no embryonal elements. Simple surgical removal is usually the only therapy required for both entities.[114] An intrafamilial aggregation of cases of cystic nephromas and pleuropulmonary blastomas has been reported.[115]

Genetics

Although over 200 karyotypes and a number of CGH studies have been published on WT, no translocations of consistent chromosomal aberrations have been identified that would aid its diagnosis. The *WT1* gene has been implicated in some cases and there are several candidate genes for a second WT locus also on 11p. It is suggested that *WT1* and *WT2* are important tumour suppressor genes in the disease. Two familial WT loci, FWT1 and FWT2, involved in around 5 per cent of cases, have also been described, although the genes involved remain to be identified.[116] Loss of 1p and 16q material has been noted in allelic imbalance studies and formation of der(16)(q10-21;q10-13) is associated with these and other tumours, including those in Ewing's family. This chromosome rearrangement and an isochromosome for 1q which is also found in a small proportion of WTs result in gain of 1q material. Loss of heterozygosity on 1p and 16q may serve to stratify WT patients into biologically favourable and unfavourable subgroups.[117] Gain of 1q material and overexpression of genes from this chromosome arm have recently been associated with subsequent relapse in WTs with favourable histology.[118,119]

Mesoblastic nephroma

Mesoblastic nephroma is the commonest congenital renal tumour and virtually never occurs after 3 years of age.

Macroscopic features

This tumour usually arises centrally within the kidney, and nearly all cases extensively involve the renal sinus. Therefore the surgeon and the pathologist should take particular care to establish that the medial aspect of the nephrectomy specimen is free of tumour.

Microscopic features

There are two histological types: classical and cellular. The cellular type has infiltrative margins. Most cases of recurrent type are cellular. Even non-stage 1 mesoblastic nephroma is treated with surgery alone. Rare instances of local recurrences and metastases have been reported. They develop within the first 12 months after nephrectomy, grow rapidly and are resistant to chemotherapy.

Genetics

Sixteen published case karyotypes are present in the Mitelman online database for both mesoblastic and cystic nephroma. As yet there have been no chromosomal aberrations identified for cystic nephroma; however, congenital mesoblastic nephroma has been shown to contain the same t(12;15)(p13;q25) translocation as is found in congenital fibrosarcoma, which results in the fusion of the *ETV6-NTRK3* genes.

Clear cell sarcoma of the kidney (CCSK)[120]

This is also known as bone-metastasizing renal tumour. The peak incidence is 2–4 years of age. Unlike WT, CCSKs are unilateral and solitary tumours.

Microscopic features

Clear cell sarcoma of the kidney is the most commonly misdiagnosed renal tumour of childhood as it can display a variety of histological patterns. Cytologically, the tumour cells look bland and mitoses are rare (Plate 7). An arborizing vascular pattern is a characteristic and diagnostically helpful feature.

Immunohistochemistry The tumour cells are positive only for vimentin, and usually negative for epithelial, myogenic and neural markers.

Rhabdoid tumour of the kidney (RTK)

This tumour occurs in the first 3 years of life. It may be associated with hypercalcaemia and synchronous or metachronous brain tumours.

Microscopic features

Rhabdoid tumour of the kidney is composed of sheets of large cells with abundant cytoplasm and eccentric large nuclei with very prominent eosinophilic central nucleoli (Plate 8a). The cytoplasm may contain intracytoplasmic inclusions. Histologically, it can mimic several other neoplasms.[121]

Immunohistochemistry reveals non-specific staining with a variety of markers. A characteristic feature that is invaluable in making the diagnosis is the presence of large oval or round cytoplasmic inclusions composed of 8- to 10-nm filaments by electron microscopy (Plate 8b).

SOFT TISSUE SARCOMAS

Sarcomas are malignant tumours that show differentiation along mesenchymal lineages such as skeletal muscle, adipose tissue, fibrous tissue, vascular tissue and peripheral nerves. Rhabdomyosarcoma (RMS) is thought to arise from immature mesenchymal cells that are committed to skeletal muscle lineage. Undifferentiated sarcomas, on the other hand, cannot be ascribed to any specific lineage. Some tumours may also display multilineage markers. One example is ectomesenchymoma, which shows evidence of skeletal muscle and neuronal lineage.

The distribution of the soft tissue sarcomas (STSs), as seen in the Kiel Paediatric Tumour Registry,[122] is presented in Table 3.8.

Rhabdomyosarcomas

In addition to the known prognostic factors of primary site, clinical group and tumour size, Newton *et al.*[123] found that the histological type was strongly predictive of survival by multivariate analysis. The International Classification of Rhabdomyosarcomas,[123] with its addition,[124] recognizes three prognostic groups (Table 3.9) and three histological types (embryonal, alveolar and anaplastic).

Table 3.8 *Soft tissue tumours in childhood*

Tumour type	Percentage
Rhabdomyosarcoma	45
PNET/ES	23
MPNST	7
Synovial sarcoma	6
Leiomyosarcoma	4
Fibrosarcoma	2
Others[a]	13

[a] Others – malignant fibrous histiocytoma, liposarcoma, rhabdoid tumour of soft parts, angiosarcoma, epithelioid sarcoma and clear cell sarcoma.
PNET/ES, primitive neuroectodermal tumour/extraosseous Ewing's sarcoma; MPNST, malignant peripheral nerve sheath tumour.

EMBRYONAL RMS (ERMS)

These show a variable differentiation ranging from blastemal mesenchymal cells to those resembling the mature cross-striated muscle cells. The majority of the tumour cells are elongated or spindle-shaped. They may be closely packed or set in a loose myxoid stroma (Plate 9a).

Botryoid subtype of ERMS
Macroscopic features This shows grape-like masses protruding into a cavity or lumen (Plate 9b).

Microscopic features The diagnosis requires the demon-stration of the cambium layer (Plate 9c). This is a subepithelial layer condensation of tumour cells, often several layers thick. It is separated from the epithelium by a loose stroma. The tumour cells may show evidence of myogenesis.

Spindle cell subtype of ERMS[125]
Microscopic features This shows cigar-shaped or spindle cells arranged in fascicles in a collagen-rich or collagen-poor stroma.

ALVEOLAR RMS (ARMS)

Alveolar RMS occurs in two forms: the classical or the solid alveolar. Tumour cells line connective tissue septa forming a pattern reminiscent of lung alveoli. These spaces may be packed solid with tumour cells (Plate 10a). Reticulin stain delineates the septa (Plate 10b).

In the solid alveolar pattern, the reticulin is absent. RMSs displaying both an embryonal and an alveolar pattern are classified as alveolar. An alveolar pattern, of course, may not be evident in a small sample.

Immunohistochemically, the tumour cells display nuclear myogenin (Plate 10c) and myoD1 positivity.

Table 3.9 *Prognostic groups of rhabdomyosarcoma*

Prognostic group	5-year survival (%)	Subtype	Incidence (%)	Location
Favourable	95	Embryonal, botryoid	6	Nasal cavity, nasopharynx, bile duct, urinary bladder, vagina
	88	Embryonal, spindle cell	3	Paratesticular, head and neck, extremities, orbit
Intermediate	66	Embryonal, NOS	49	Head and neck including orbit, genitourinary tract, extremities, pelvis and retroperitoneum
Poor	53	Alveolar, NOS or solid variant	31	Extremities, head and neck, trunk and perineum
	45	Anaplasia, diffuse	2	Lower extremities, retroperitoneum, head and neck
	44	Undifferentiated sarcoma	3	Extremities

NOS, not otherwise specified.

Undifferentiated sarcoma[124,125] is diagnosed by excluding specific sarcomas using IHC and EM. These are negative for all markers, except vimentin.

ANAPLASTIC (DIFFUSE) SUBTYPE[124]

The anaplastic tumour cells contain nuclei which are hyperchromatic, large (at least three times the size of the neighbouring nuclei), and with atypical mitotic figures. This can be seen in both the embryonal and the alveolar subtypes. It is classified as diffuse when large groups or sheets of anaplastic cells are present in the tumour.

Ectomesenchymomas are rare neoplasms usually consisting of RMSs (embryonal or alveolar type) with neoplastic, neuroblastic or neuroectodermal elements.[126] The primary sites include external genitalia, pelvis/abdomen, head and neck and extremities.

Post-chemotherapy differentiation of tumour cells into mature skeletal muscle cells is seen in botryoid and embryonal subtypes.[127] Decreased proliferative activity and cytodifferentiation are associated with a favourable outcome in patients with botryoid RMS[127] and those located in the pelvic region.[128]

Genetics

Two pathognomonic translocations have been identified in RMS which occur specifically in the alveolar subtype (ARMS) and which are of high diagnostic value. The first translocation to be identified was the t(2;13)(q35;q14), which results in the fusion of the *PAX3* gene at 2q35 and the *FOX1A10* (FKHR) gene at 13q14. Subsequently, a variant translocation was identified, t(1;13)(p36;q14), which was shown to result in the fusion of the *PAX7* gene at 1p36 and the *FOX1A10* gene at 13q14 (for review, see Anderson *et al.*[45]). RT-PCR, FISH and real-time RT-PCR have all been used to identify translocation-positive ARMS by a number of workers.[43] Cytogenetics, FISH and RT-PCR studies of ARMS have shown, using these techniques individually and combined, that only 70–75 per cent are positive for the *PAX-FOX1A10* translocations.[45,129] Recent data have also shown that a prognostic difference exists between translocation-positive ARMS cases, with the *PAX3-FOX1A10* fusion cases showing a significantly worse prognosis than the *PAX7-FOX1A10* fusion cases.[45,48,130] Microarray gene expression profiling has also been applied to ARMS in order to try and separate ARMS from the ERMS subtype at the molecular level.[38] At present, no classifier set of expressed genes have been identified that have sufficient power to be used in clinical diagnosis. The molecular cytogenetics of the ERMS subtype are not well understood (66 ERMS karyotypes reported, compared with 110 ARMS) and no ERMS translocations or specific chromosomal aberrations have been identified to aid in their molecular diagnosis.[129,131]

Non–RMS sarcomas

MALIGNANT PERIPHERAL NERVE SHEATH TUMOUR

In the largest paediatric series, 20 per cent of the malignant peripheral nerve sheath tumours (MPNSTs) were found to occur in the setting of neurofibromatosis NF1.[132] The tumour is usually axial, central or situated proximally in the extremities.

In its classic form, an MPNST arises as a fusiform mass in a major nerve, and in NF1 patients it may arise in a pre-existing neurofibroma. It is a non-encapsulated mass with a glistening, fleshy, grey-white cut surface with areas of necrosis.

Microscopic features

These show a range of appearances from tumours resembling a neurofibroma to those indistinguishable from a fibrosarcoma. Typically, they are composed of tapered spindle cells with buckled nuclei compactly arranged in fascicles. An epithelioid, glandular or round-cell component may be seen.

Tumour necrosis involving more than 25 per cent, larger tumour size, age more than 7 years and NF1 was associated with adverse prognosis.[132]

Genetics

Over 80 MPNST karyotypes have been reported (Mitelman online) and as yet no consistent chromosomal aberrations have been identified that are of diagnostic value. It has been reported that the t(X;18)(p11;q11) associated with synovial sarcomas (resulting in the *SYT-SSX1*, *SYT-SSX2* or *SYT-SSX4* fusion genes) is also found in MPNST,[133–135] although other reports have recently suggested otherwise.[136–138]

SYNOVIAL SARCOMA

This occurs in adolescence and in young adults. It is usually located in the soft tissue on the extremities, most often in the vicinity of the large joints. Head and neck and viscera are other sites.[139]

Macroscopic features

The para-articular tumours are generally attached to the joint capsules, tendon sheaths and bursae.

Microscopic features

The characteristic pattern is biphasic, composed of varying proportions of epithelial cells, resembling those of a carcinoma, and a fibrosarcoma-like area composed of spindle cells. The monophasic spindle cell (or rarely epithelial) and poorly differentiated round-cell types are rare.

Immunohistochemically, 90 per cent are positive for cytokeratin and/or epithelial membrane antigen in both cell types.[139,140]

Genetics

Synovial sarcomas are characterized by a pathognomonic translocation, the t(X;18)(p11;q11), which is found in over 95 per cent of cases.[44,47,133] At the molecular level, this translocation results in fusion gene products combining the 18q11 SYT gene and one of the Xp11 SSX1, SSX2 or SSX4 genes, creating SYT-SSX1, SYT-SSX2 or SYT-SSX4 fusion genes, respectively.[141] As well as being of strong diagnostic value (82 papers reported cytogenetic-molecular biological and clinical correlations; Mitelman online), studies have also noted prognostic differences between the different fusion genes. Patients found to have a SYT-SSX1 fusion gene display a shorter survival than patients with SYT-SSX2.[142] There is also a strong relationship between tumour subtype and translocation, with biphasic synovial sarcomas being found to contain the SYT-SSX1 fusion and monophasic tumours found to contain the SYT-SSX2 fusion.[141,143–145]

LEIOMYOSARCOMA

These are rare in children, occurring in the subcutaneous and deep locations of the trunk, head and neck, lower and upper limbs.[146]

Microscopic features

The tumour is typically composed of fascicles of eosinophilic spindle cells with cigar-shaped nuclei. These are low-grade lesions and behave in a relatively indolent fashion. These are positive for desmin, actin,[146] and caldesmon,[147] but negative for myogenin.[18]

FIBROSARCOMA

Fibrosarcomas show a biphasic age distribution, with one peak in infancy and children less than 2 years of age and the second in adolescence. In the former group, the prognosis is excellent, while in the latter, fibrosarcoma behaves as an aggressive tumour.[148]

Macroscopic features

These show a firm, fleshy cut surface with focal haemorrhage and necrosis.

Microscopic features

Both the types show similar features, being composed of uniform, spindle-shaped tumour cells arranged in a herring-bone pattern.

Immunohistochemically, spindle cells stain for vimentin and variably for muscle markers including muscle-specific and smooth muscle actin.[148]

Genetics

An almost cytogenetically cryptic, yet consistent, chromosomal translocation, the t(12;15)(p13;q25), has recently been identified in congenital fibrosarcoma. This translocation had not been previously noted in any of the 40 published karyotypes. Molecular cloning of the breakpoint determined the translocation to result in an ETV6-NTRK3 gene fusion. Further RT-PCR studies of congenital fibrosarcoma have shown the ETV6-NTRK3 fusion gene product to be in all the small number of cases studied, indicating that this is a very valuable diagnostic marker.[149] Interestingly this fusion gene product has also been found in congenital mesoblastic nephroma, indicating a basic molecular biological link between these two previously unrelated tumour types.

RARE STSs

These include angiomatoid fibrous histiocytoma, alveolar soft part sarcoma, epithelioid sarcoma, clear cell sarcoma, epithelioid haemangioendothelioma and angiosarcoma.

Genetics

Only 10 karyotypes of alveolar soft part sarcomas (ASPSs) have been reported, although a recurrent chromosomal aberration, der(17), has been shown to result from a non-reciprocal t(X;17)(p11.2;q25). Molecular cloning of this translocation breakpoint has shown it to result in the fusion of the Xp11.2 TFE3 gene with a novel gene on 17q25, designated APSL. RT-PCR analyses of cases so far studied have shown this to be a pathognomonic translocation and hence another valuable diagnostic marker.[150]

Clear cell sarcomas or malignant melanoma of the soft parts display a well characterized diagnostic pathognomonic translocation, the t(12;22)(q13;12), resulting in the fusion of the EWS-AFT1 genes.[151] Similar to the related Ewing's sarcoma EWS translocations, the precise position of breakpoints within the EWS gene can vary, making FISH a particularly useful diagnostic method in these tumours.[152]

For epithelioid sarcoma, haemangioendothelioma and angiosarcoma little molecular cytogenetics is known with only 10, 1 and 12 karyotypes having been published for epithelioid sarcoma, haemangioendothelioma and angiosarcoma respectively. As yet there have been no specific molecular cytogenetic markers identified in these tumours to aid diagnosis.

MYOFIBROMATOSIS[153]

This may present as a solitary, multiple or generalized form. The prognostic implications are worst for the generalized forms, due to visceral involvement.

Macroscopic features

These are firm discrete or infiltrating nodules with a solid, grey-white cut surface.

Microscopic features

This shows a zonal pattern comprising bundles and fascicles of spindle-shaped cells at the periphery, which blend with round cells arranged in a haemangiopericytoma-like pattern centrally.

Immunohistochemically, the lesional cells show staining with vimentin and smooth muscle actin, while desmin staining is variable.

PERIPHERAL PRIMITIVE NEUROECTODERMAL TUMOUR/EWING'S SARCOMA

These tumours have been described by a multitude of names, such as malignant small cell tumour of the thoracopulmonary region (Askin tumour), skeletal and extraskeletal Ewing's sarcoma (ES), malignant peripheral neuroepithelioma and paravertebral small cell tumour.

All these tumours are considered to belong to Ewing's family of tumours on the basis of similar tissue culture studies, pathological findings, proto-oncogene expression and cytogenetic features.[154] ES and peripheral primitive neuroectodermal tumour (pPNET) are currently viewed as the ends of a spectrum, with ES at the undifferentiated end and pPNET with neural differentiation at the other. Eighty per cent of these tumours present before 20 years of age, and only 14 per cent occur below 5 years of age. The distribution between the sexes is approximately equal.

The common sites of involvement are the soft tissues of the trunk, chest wall, paraspinal region, extremities and head and neck. They are increasingly being recognized in the viscera and various solid organs as reviewed by Ladanyi and Bridge.[155]

Macroscopic features

These tumours are either well defined masses with a fibrous capsule or infiltrative in nature. The cut surface displays a fleshy and grey-white appearance. Haemorrhage and necrosis are more marked in post-chemotherapy specimens.

Microscopic features

This group of tumours is usually composed of small, round cells. ES is usually composed of sheets of cells with uniform cytology and minimal mitoses. pPNETs display a lobular arrangement with pleomorphism and mitoses. Rosettes are uncommon, and ganglion cells are seen rarely in pPNETs. The significance of neural differentiation in relation to prognosis is debatable.[156,157]

Histochemical stains show the presence of glycogen in 30 per cent of the cases. The most sensitive marker is CD99; its expression (assessed using various antibodies) is seen in more 95 per cent of cases.[7,9] A membranous pattern of staining is seen in the majority of the tumour cells. Other markers, including neural/neuroendocrine and vimentin, are less sensitive.[9] However, CD99 suffers from the drawback that it is not specific for pPNET/ES. It can be seen in other round-cell tumours of childhood such as rhabdomyosarcoma,[9] lymphoblastic leukaemia/lymphoma,[12] as well as extramedullary myeloid-cell tumours.[158] Therefore, it is used as part of a panel of antibodies to diagnose pPNET/ES.

Recently, immunostaining of tumour cells with the *FLI* fusion gene product has been reported; however, like CD99, it marks a high proportion of lymphoblastic lymphomas.[159]

TUMOURS OF BONE AND CARTILAGE

In the first two decades of life, most bone tumours are primary. Secondary tumours include neuroblastoma and rhabdomyosarcoma, particularly of the alveolar subtype.

The two main primary malignant bone tumours are osteosarcoma and primitive neuroectodermal tumour/Ewing's sarcoma (pPNET/ES). In aggregate, these two tumours account for approximately 5 per cent of all cancers in children. Osteosarcomas account for about 60 per cent of the malignant neoplasms of bone, while pPNET/ES account for 20–30 per cent;[160] lymphomas comprise 6 per cent and chondrosarcomas 4 per cent; fibrosarcomas and malignant fibrous histiocytomas make up the remainder.

Radiological-pathological correlation is essential for an accurate evaluation of a bone biopsy specimen.[161] The potential pitfalls encountered along the way to the correct diagnosis include a diminutive biopsy, where the diagnostic features of a specific entity are entirely absent. For example, a biopsy which reveals a 'high-grade sarcoma' without the accompanying malignant osteoid might not permit the definitive diagnosis of osteosarcoma. The radiological findings are then critical. On the other hand, a highly destructive osteolyic tumour may have the imaging features of pPNET/ES yet be an osteosarcoma on biopsy.

Osteosarcoma

The majority of cases of osteosarcoma occur in males, with a peak incidence in the second decade of life. There is a propensity for osteosarcomas to occur in the metaphyseal region of the long tubular bones (distal femur, proximal tibia, proximal humerus). Osteosarcoma of the axial skeleton and hands and feet is rare.

Macroscopic features

The marrow cavity is often involved and there may be 'skip' lesions composed of tumour nodules separated by apparently normal marrow cavity. The consistency varies from firm to rock hard and gritty. The colour is white-tan or red-yellow depending on the amount of viable tumour. Secondary changes such as necrosis, haemorrhage and cyst formation are frequent, particularly in the post-chemotherapy specimens (Plate 11a). Conventional osteosarcoma usually breaches the bone and periosteum and extends into the surrounding soft tissues. Both the proximal and distal margins are generally well defined. The epiphyseal plate acts as a barrier to tumour spread.

Microscopic features

The histopathology of osteosarcoma is very diverse[162] and almost a dozen subtypes have been described which may have prognostic significance. Five to 10 per cent of the osteosarcomas in children fulfil the criteria for one of the distinct variants. Certain subtypes of osteosarcoma, such as postirradiation or that associated with Paget's disease, do not occur in children.

By definition, osteosarcoma is a high-grade spindle cell neoplasm that produces osteoid. The osteoid has a fine, lace-like pink appearance (Plate 11b). The tumour cells display pleomorphism, hyperchromasia and increased mitotic rate with abnormal mitotic figures. There may be predominantly fibroblastic, osteoblastic or chondroblastic differentiation.

Most osteosarcomas are resected after preoperative chemotherapy. Most studies show that if the tumour is more than 90 per cent necrotic, the prognosis is excellent.[162]

Immunohistochemistry is of little value in diagnosis.

TELANGIECTATIC OSTEOSARCOMA

Radiologically and pathologically, this may be mistaken for a benign lesion such as an aneurysmal bone cyst. The criterion used to make the diagnosis of this subtype is an X-ray showing a purely lytic lesion simulating the appearance of an aneurysmal bone cyst.

Macroscopic features

This shows a large cavity or cystic spaces separated by septa containing blood.

Microscopic features

Tissue is often arranged in small strands as in aneurysmal bone cysts and giant cell tumours of bone. Unlike conventional osteosarcoma, tumour osteoid is hard to recognize and a diligent search has been made for malignant cells which are admixed with benign giant cells in the septal wall or floating free in the blood.

SMALL-CELL OSTEOSARCOMA

This may resemble PNET/ES. The diagnosis can only be made if tumour cells show osteoid production.[163] This is a round-cell tumour of bone, which may be difficult to distinguish from PNET/ES lymphoma and mesenchymal chondrosarcoma.

PERIOSTEAL OSTEOSARCOMA

Patients tend to be in the same age group as those with conventional osteosarcoma. Typically, it involves the diaphysis of the femur or the tibia. The radiological appearance is that of a flat-based lesion extending off the periosteum, with spicules of bone extending into the soft tissues. By definition, there should be no medullary involvement.

Microscopic features

Lobules of cartilage show central bone formation and spindle cells peripherally. The prognosis for this subtype appears to be excellent.

Genetics

Over 100 osteosarcoma karyotypes have been published (Mitelman online) (for review[164]), however they are frequently very complex and no tumour specific chromosomal aberrations have been so far identified. Many CGH studies have also been undertaken and again no tumour specific chromosomal changes have been found (www.helsinki.fi/~lgl_www/CMG.html).

Peripheral PNET/ES

As mentioned previously, these tumours belong to the same family because of similar morphological and molecular cytogenetic features. Typically, ES occurs in males. Any portion of the skeleton may be involved, but the diaphysis of the long bones is the commonest site.

Macroscopic features

This is a destructive and permeative tumour. Periosteal reactive new bone formation gives rise to an onion-skin appearance on X-ray.

Microscopic features

These are similar to the features seen in the soft tissue and viscera (Plate 12a). In addition to the small-cell variant of osteosarcoma and mesenchymal chondrosarcoma, both of which are rare, an important differential diagnosis is precursor B-lymphoblastic lymphoma. Like pPNET/ES, it also displays CD99 positivity (Plate12b) and other immunocytochemical stains may be necessary to establish the diagnosis.

Genetics

Ewing's sarcoma is the best-studied paediatric solid tumour from a cytogenetic point of view, with 306 published karyotypes and over 200 papers detailing cytogenetic-molecular biological and clinical correlations (see Mitelman online). It was the first sarcoma to be identified with a pathognomonic translocation, the t(11;22)(q24;q12). This translocation results in the fusion of the EWS and FLI1 genes, and subsequently a number of other derivative translocations involving the EWS gene have been identified[165–167] (Table 3.10). These translocations are highly useful in the diagnosis of

Table 3.10 *The frequency of variant EWS translocations and subsequent fusion genes in Ewing's sarcoma and pPNET*

Chromosomal translocation	Fusion gene	Percentage occurrence in Ewing's sarcoma and pPNET
t(11;22)(q24;q12)	EWS-FLI1	90–95%
t(21;22)(q22;q12)	EWS-ERG	5–10%
t(7;22)(p22;q12)	EWS-ETV1	~1%
t(17;22)(q12;q12)	EWS-EIAF	<1
t(2;22)(q33;q12)	EWS-FEV	<1

pPNET/ES, peripheral primitive neuroectodermal tumour.

Ewing's tumours. Along with ESs, pPNETs also display the same *EWS* variant translocation and fusion genes, suggesting a basic biological link between these two tumour types and enabling detection of these translocations to aid in the diagnosis of both tumour types. It should be noted that not all cases of pPNET/ES studied show evidence of the known variant *EWS* translocations and that other tumour types have been described with this fusion gene (e.g. Dagher *et al.*[46]). The translocation breakpoints of the *EWS* gene are variable, being seen in introns 7–10 and there are five common *EWS* fusion gene partners (Table 3.10).

Frequently, complex chromosomal rearrangements can mask these translocations; neither single RT-PCR reactions nor conventional cytogenetics are ideally suited to the simultaneous identification of all possible *EWS* variant translocations. In this instance, diagnostic FISH using *EWS* flanking probes should be used to screen all possible breakpoints, in conjunction with a range of variant translocation-specific RT-PCRs or consensus primer RT-PCR to allow multiple method confirmation of *EWS* variant translocations.[168] The cytogenetics of ES and pPNET are often complex, and no diagnostic cytogenetic abnormalities, other than *EWS* variant translocations, have been identified. Numerous CGH studies of ES have found that many changes occur in this tumour type, the most frequent being gain of chromosome 8, 12 and 1q21-22 (www.helsinki.fi/~lgl_www/CMG.html). Gain of chromosome 12 and 1q predicts a worse outcome.[169] Prognostic significance is attributed to the different *EWS-FLI* fusion gene subtypes. In patients with localized disease, type I fusions (*EWS* exon 7 fused to *FLI-1* exon 6) are associated with a better prognosis than fusion subtypes including additional exons from either *EWS* or *FLI-1*.

DESMOPLASTIC SMALL ROUND-CELL TUMOUR

Desmoplastic small round-cell tumour (DSRCT) is a rare tumour with unique clinicopathological and genetic features.[170] It affects young adults, predominantly males, and the patients typically present with abdominal pain, distension and occasionally ascites. Large tumour masses typically involve the mesentery and pelvis with multiple peritoneal implants. This tumour has now been reported in several other sites, including the mediastinum, CNS, paratesticular region, parotid and bone.[171]

Macroscopic features
Desmoplastic small round-cell tumour is a grey-white tumour with myxoid areas and necrotic foci.

Microscopic features
It has a characteristic pattern composed of variably sized nests of tumour embedded in a fibrous stroma (Plate 13). The tumour cells resemble a small round-cell tumour with epithelial or neuroendocrine features, and a wide range of histological features including a spindle cell type have now been described.[170]

Immunohistochemistry demonstrates a combination of epithelial (cytokeratin and EMA), neural (e.g. neuron-specific enolase) and muscle markers (desmin, rarely actin).[172] The cytoplasmic, dot-like positivity seen with desmin is characteristic, but myogenic markers such as myogenin and MyoD1 are negative.[173] WT1 immunostaining appears to be a very sensitive test[19] and is also reliable in distinguishing DSRCT from PNET/ES[174] and other small round-cell tumours.[19]

Under electron microscopy the majority of the neoplastic cells within the nests are closely apposed and surrounded by a basal lamina. Small, well-formed junctions are seen in a small proportion of cases. Juxtanuclear intermediate filaments are usually seen in the cytoplasm. There is no evidence of myogenic differentiation, and rarely dense-core neurosecretory granules are seen.[173]

Genetics
Although little cytogenetics has been published for DSRCT, a pathognomonic and hence diagnostically valuable translocation, t(11;22)(p13;q12), has been characterized. This results in fusion of the *EWS* gene on chromosome 22 and the Wilms' tumour gene *WT1* on chromosome 11.[175] Additional PCR studies have shown the presence of the *EWS-WT1* fusion in a number of further DSRCT cases.[176,177]

RETINOBLASTOMA

This is the most common intraocular tumour in childhood.

Macroscopic features
Five different patterns may be seen: endophytic, exophytic, mixed endophytic and exophytic, diffuse infiltrating type and complete spontaneous regression. The endophytic

retinoblastoma grows towards the vitreous (Plate 14), while the exophytic type grows towards the subretinal space and may cause retinal detachment.[178]

Microscopic features

This is a SRCT in which the well differentiated examples show rosettes and fleurettes indicating photoreceptor differentiation. Characteristically it displays numerous mitotic figures, apoptosis, necrosis and calcification. A differentiated tumour composed entirely of fleurettes has a much better prognosis.[179] A high mitotic index does not imply a poor outcome.[180] The most important prognostic factors are invasion of the lamina cribrosa, full thickness of the choroid and the cut end of the optic nerve.[178]

Genetics

Around 90 per cent of retinoblastoma cases are sporadic, whereas the remainder occur in a familial setting. The *RB1* gene has been implicated in both settings and the patterns of genetic change led to the 'two hit' hypothesis of losing function of both alleles in the development of the tumour.[181] This may occur through a combination of mutation and loss of the wild-type allele. Although loss of *RB1* gene function is critical, other changes are also associated with the development of the tumour.

GERM CELL TUMOURS

Germ cell tumours (GCTs) are biphasic with regard to age and biology, with one peak occurring before 3 years and the second at 15–20 years of age.[182]

The histological classification used by the UKCCSG[183] is modified from Dehner[184] and is shown in Box 3.5. The British Testicular Tumour Panel classification[185] is also shown in the box for comparison. Both the classifications can be applied to GCT occurring at the gonadal and all the extragonadal sites (sacrococcygeal, intracranial, mediastinal and vulva/vagina), as shown in Table 3.11.

MATURE TERATOMAS

These are composed of one or more mature tissue types, derived from the three embryonic layers and arranged in a haphazard fashion. They are grossly heterogeneous solid and cystic neoplasms.

IMMATURE TERATOMAS

These contain immature tissues, the predominant being neural tissue (Plate 15), and can be graded according to the quantity of the immature neural components into three grades.[186,187] These usually have mature teratomatous elements as well. Small foci of yolk sac tumour may also be present,[188] which may not be detected if the tumour has not been adequately sampled. The presence

Box 3.5 *Comparison of nomenclature between Dehner and the British Testicular Tumour Panel Terminology (BTTP) classification*[185]

Dehner classification	BTTP classification
I. Germinoma	Seminoma
A. ITGCN	Spermatocytic seminoma
B. Invasive (seminoma/ dysgerminoma)	
II. Teratoma	Teratoma
A. Mature	Mature = TD
B. Immature	Immature = TD
C. Malignant	TD with malignant GCT component(s) = (MTI)
III. Embryonal carcinoma (adult type)	MTU
IV. Endodermal sinus or YST	YST
V. Choriocarcinoma	MTT
VI. Gonadoblastoma (pure or invasive)	Gonadoblastoma
VII. Malignant GCT of mixed histological pattern	Mixed malignant GCT

ITGCN, intratubular germ cell neoplasia (extremely rare in childhood); GCT, germ cell tumour; MTI, malignant teratoma intermediate; MTT, malignant teratoma trophoblastic; MTU, malignant teratoma undifferentiated (no mature or organoid tissues); TD, teratoma differentiated; YST, yolksac tumour.

of yolk sac tumour is correlated to the behaviour rather than to the age or the grade of the immature neural component,[187] and surgery alone is effective in the majority of the cases.[189,190]

YOLK SAC TUMOUR (ENDODERMAL SINUS TUMOUR)

Macroscopic features

These tumours are solid, soft, friable, grey and mucoid in appearance. They may show areas of haemorrhage and necrosis (Plate 16a).

Microscopic features

The histology and cytology vary widely.[188] About 50 per cent show glomeruloid structures such as Schiller–Duval bodies (Plate 16b). IHC shows alpha-fetoprotein (AFP) and cytokeratin in the tumour cells.

DYSGERMINOMAS/SEMINOMAS

These are composed of uniform cells with a clear cytoplasm and the cells are arranged in sheets or nests. IHC

Table 3.11 *Features of germ cell tumours (GCTs) at specific sites*[191]

Site	Age (%)[a]	Relative incidence (%)[191]	Features
Ovary	>10 years (46)	39	Mature teratomas (76%),[191] immature teratomas, malignant GCTs (dysgerminoma, YST) and those occurring in the dysgenetic testis (gonadoblastoma and dysgerminoma)[188]
Testis	<2 years (46)	7	Malignant (70%, YST is the most common)[191] followed by mature teratomas. Immature elements are not commonly seen. The biology of mature and immature teratomas is similar[200] In adolescents and young adults – adult-type tumours such as seminoma and non-seminomatous GCT
Sacrococcygeal	<2 years (82) typically neonates	36	Female predominance (64%), majority (65%) are mature teratomas, 14% recur as YSTs. In children, more than 1 year, the majority are malignant
Mediastinal	>10 years	4	In males, 20% are associated with Klinefelter's syndrome. Mediastinal GCTs in males may be associated with haematological malignancies[201]
Intracranial	>10 years (50)	5	Generally in males as pineal or suprasellar masses Germinomas, teratomas, YSTs[84]
Other	<2 years (70)	9	Mature teratomas

YST, yolk sac tumour.
[a] The percentage in brackets refers to the incidence of cases that occur in that age group.

shows a positive reaction of the tumour cells for placental alkaline phosphatase.

While an intratubular germ cell neoplasia lesion is seen in the seminiferous tubules of GCTs in postpubertal patients, similar lesions are not present in the vast majority of children with normal gonads. The key clinicopathological features of GCTs at gonadal and extragonadal sites are given in Table 3.11.[182,191]

Genetics

Loss of 1p36, similar to that found in neuroblastoma, is a recurrent feature in paediatric GCTs, although it is not a diagnostic marker.[192] Gain of 12p material, frequently through the presence of an i(12p), is associated with adolescent/adult testicular GCT. Identifying this change may be useful in confirming the non-paediatric nature of a tumour.[193]

HEPATIC TUMOURS

In children, as in adults, the most common malignant hepatic tumours are metastatic, usually neuroblastoma, lymphoma, rhabdomyosarcoma and Wilms' tumour.[194]

Malignant tumours comprise 55–68 per cent of the primary hepatic tumours in children; the remainder are

Table 3.12 *Incidence of malignant hepatic tumours*

Tumour type	Percentage
Hepatoblastoma	26–36
Hepatocellular carcinoma	19–20
Undifferentiated sarcoma	7–9
Angiosarcoma	<2
Other malignant tumours	<1

benign. The relative frequency of these malignant tumours in paediatric patients (birth to 20 years) is shown in Table 3.12.

Hepatoblastoma

Hepatoblastomas almost always arise in an otherwise normal liver. Ninety per cent of patients have elevated serum AFP levels. The majority of hepatoblastomas occur in children under the age of 5 years.

Macroscopic features

Seventy to 80 per cent of hepatoblastomas are solitary, and these develop most often in the right lobe. It is usually a partially encapsulated, solid and/or cystic mass. The solid areas are lobulated and tan-green in colour.

Table 3.13 *Microscopic patterns of hepatoblastomas*

Histological pattern (%)	Architectural patterns	Cytology	Comments
Epithelial type			
Fetal (31)	Trabeculae two to three cells thick	Resemble normal hepatocytes low N/C	Best prognosis of all in early studies[202] but related to other factors[197]
Embryonal (19)	A variety such as acini, rosettes and trabeculae	Higher N/C, mitotic figures >2/10 hpf	
Macrotrabecular (3)	Trabeculae (>10 cells thick)	Variable N/C	Difficult to distinguish from HCC
Small-cell, undifferentiated (3)	Sheets of small round cells	Highest N/C, mitotic figures >2/10 hpf	Uniformly poor outcome,[203] other patterns necessary for the diagnosis, AFP-negative, cytokeratin +
Mixed type	Spindle cells with osteoid and other sarcomatoid elements		
Teratoid features (10)			Ectodermal, mesodermal, endodermal derivatives
Non-teratoid (34)			

AFP, alpha-fetoprotein; HCC, hepatocellular carcinoma; hpf, high-power field; N/C, nuclear cytoplasmic ratio.

The average diameter of a hepatoblastoma is 10–12 cm. Changes such as necrosis, haemorrhage and calcification are more common in post-chemotherapy tumours.[195,196]

Microscopic features

These are classified into two main types: epithelial (56 per cent) (Plate 17a) or mixed epithelial-mesenchymal (44 per cent). They are further subclassified into six histological patterns, as shown in the Table 3.13.[197]

The fetal and embryonal epithelial cells are usually positive for AFP (Plate 17b) while all the epithelial types are positive for cytokeratins.

Hepatocellular carcinoma

Hepatocellular carcinoma (HCC) is a tumour of older children with a peak incidence between 10 and 14 years. The majority of these tumours are either multifocal or involve both lobes at the time of diagnosis. Microscopically these resemble HCC in adults.

FIBROLAMELLAR HCC

This is a distinctive variant which arises in the non-cirrhotic liver (90 per cent) in young patients. Serum AFP levels are elevated in only about 10–15 per cent of the cases. It has a more favourable prognosis than ordinary HCC.[198,199]

Macroscopic features

The majority of cases involve the left lobe, but both the lobes may be affected. The tumours are solitary, well circumscribed, tan-white, grey or brown in colour. They show a central, stellate scar.

Microscopic features

Fibrolamellar HCC shows large, polygonal cells with abundant pink cytoplasm. These cells are divided into cords by fibrous tissue.

Undifferentiated (embryonal) sarcoma

This is also known as malignant mesenchymoma or mesenchymal sarcoma. More than 50 per cent of the cases occur in children between the age of 6 and 10 years.

Macroscopic features

The tumour presents as a well demarcated, solitary mass, usually >10 cm in diameter. It is soft and myxoid with necrosis, haemorrhage and cystic degeneration.

Microscopic features

This tumour is composed of spindle, oval or stellate cells set in a myxoid stroma. Multinucleated and cytologically bizarre cells with numerous mitotic cells and PAS-positive hyaline globules may be seen in the tumour cells or in the stroma. IHC reveals variable reactivity to desmin, muscle-specific actin and cytokeratin, but not myoglobin.

Genetics

Forty-six hepatoblastoma and 12 angiosarcoma karyotypes have been published. Little is known about the molecular cytogenetics of these tumour types.

KEY POINTS

- Good communication between the paediatric oncologist and the pathologist is essential at all stages.
  - The oncologist and the surgeon must provide the pathologist with the full clinical information available as well as the operative findings. They influence tumour handling and are relevant to the final diagnosis, which is always made in the context of the clinico-radiological features.
  - Tumour samples must arrive fresh in the laboratory for appropriate triaging. It is therefore important to let the pathologist know when the sample will be available.
  - Multidisciplinary meetings are vital for discussing individual cases. They also promote mutual understanding and broaden perspectives generally.
- The clinician cannot usually expect an instant diagnosis.
  - In all but the most straightforward cases, to make a confident diagnosis, it is necessary for the pathologist to employ a combination of different techniques, which may take hours or days to complete.
  - It takes time for the pathologist to analyse and interpret the results. Sometimes it is necessary to consult the relevant trial protocols, the literature or take a second opinion.
  - Molecular changes associated with paediatric tumours may have a diagnostic and/or prognostic value.
- Fusion genes are associated with particular types of paediatric tumours such as Ewing's sarcoma or alveolar rhabdomyosarcoma.
- Reverse-transcriptase PCR and fluorescence *in situ* hybridization, used for the detection of aberrations, have become important tools in the evaluation of certain types of paediatric tumour.
- Tissue handling and technical considerations can optimize the information available for patient management.

REFERENCES

♦1. Pfeifer JD, Hill DA, O'Sullivan MJ, Dehner LP. Diagnostic gold standard for soft tissue tumours: morphology or molecular genetics? *Histopathology* 2000; **37**: 485–500.

2. Benign fibrous tissue tumours. In: Weiss SW, Goldblum JR, eds. *Enzinger's and Weiss' Soft Tissue Tumours.* St Louis: Mosby, 2001; 247–307.

3. Coffin CM, Dehner LP. Soft tissue tumours of nosologic uncertainty. In: Coffin CM, Dehner LP, O'Shea PA, eds. *Pediatric Soft Tissue Tumours: A Clinical, Pathological, and Therapeutic Approach.* Baltimore: Williams & Wilkins, 1997; 311–41.

4. Parham DM, Holt H. Immunodiagnosis of childhood malignancies. *Mol Biotechnol* 1999; **12**: 207–16.

5. Chan JKC. Advances in immunohistochemical techniques: toward making things simpler, cheaper, more sensitive, and more reproducible. *Adv Anat Pathol* 1998; **5**: 314–25.

6. Siedal T, Balaton AJ, Battifora H. Interpretation and quantification of immunostains. *Am J Surg Pathol* 2001; **25**: 1204–7.

♦7. Devoe K, Weidner N. Immunohistochemistry of small round-cell tumors. *Semin Diagn Pathol* 2000; **17**: 216–24.

8. Miettinen M, Chatten J, Paetau A, Stevenson A. Monoclonal antibody NB84 in the differential diagnosis of neuroblastoma and other small round cell tumors. *Am J Surg Pathol* 1998; **22**: 327–32.

9. Ramani P, Rampling D, Link M. Immunocytochemical study of 12E7 in small round-cell tumours of childhood: an assessment of its sensitivity and specificity. *Histopathology* 1993; **23**: 557–61.

10. Pappo AS, Douglass EC, Meyer WH *et al.* Use of HBA 71 and anti-beta 2-microglobulin to distinguish peripheral neuroepithelioma from neuroblastoma. *Hum Pathol* 1993; **24**: 880–5.

11. Riopel M, Dickman PS, Link MP, Perlman EJ. MIC2 analysis in pediatric lymphomas and leukemias. *Hum Pathol* 1994; **25**: 396–9.

12. Soslow RA, Bhargava V, Warnke RA. MIC2, TdT, bcl-2, and CD34 expression in paraffin-embedded high-grade lymphoma/acute lymphoblastic leukemia distinguishes between distinct clinicopathologic entities. *Hum Pathol* 1997; **28**: 1158–65.

13. Lucas DR, Bentley G, Dan ME *et al.* Ewing sarcoma vs lymphoblastic lymphoma. A comparative immunohisto-chemical study. *Am J Clin Pathol* 2001; **115**: 11–17.

14. Parham DM, Dias P, Kelly DR *et al.* Desmin positivity in primitive neuroectodermal tumors of childhood. *Am J Surg Pathol* 1992; **16**: 483–92.

15. Pinto A, Tallini G, Novak RW *et al.* Undifferentiated rhabdomyosarcoma with lymphoid phenotype expression. *Med Pediatr Oncol* 1997; **28**: 165–70.

16. Coindre J-M, DeMescarel A, Trojani M. Immunohistochemical study of rhabdomyosarcoma. Unexpected staining with S100 protein and cytokeratin. *J Pathol* 1988; **155**: 127–32.

17. Miettinen M, Rapola J. Immunohistochemical spectrum of rhabdomyosarcoma and rhabdomyosarcoma-like tumors. Expression of cytokeratin and the 68-kD neurofilament protein. *Am J Surg Pathol* 1989; **13**: 120–32.

18. Cessna MH, Zhou H, Perkins SLTSR *et al.* Are myogenin and MyoD1 expression specific for rhabdomyosarcoma? A study of 150 cases, with emphasis on spindle cell mimics. *Am J Surg Pathol* 2001; **25**: 1150–7.

19. Barnoud R, Sabourin JC, Pasquier D *et al.* Immunohisto-chemical expression of WT1 by desmoplastic small round cell tumor: a comparative study with other small round cell tumors. *Am J Surg Pathol* 2000; **24**: 830–6.

20. Mierau GW. Techniques in paediatric pathology. In: Stocker JT, Dehner LP, eds. *Pediatric Pathology.* Philadelphia: Lippincott Williams & Wilkins, 2001; 45–53.

21. Mierau GW, Berry PJ, Malott RL, Weeks DA. Appraisal of the comparative utility of immunohistochemistry and electron microscopy in the diagnosis of childhood round cell tumors. *Ultrastruct Pathol* 1996; **20**: 507–17.

22. Ordonez NG, Mackay B. Electron microscopy in tumor diagnosis: indications for its use in the immunohistochemical era. *Hum Pathol* 1998; **29**: 1403–11.

23. Erlandson RA, Rosai J. A realistic approach to the use of electron microscopy and other ancillary diagnostic techniques in surgical pathology. *Am J Surg Pathol* 1995; **19**: 247–50.

24. Mawad JK, Mackay B, Raymond AK, Ayala AG. Electron microscopy in the diagnosis of small round cell tumors of bone. *Ultrastruct Pathol* 1994; **18**: 263–8.

25. Mierau GW, Weeks DA, Hicks MJ. Role of electron microscopy and other special techniques in the diagnosis of childhood round cell tumors. *Hum Pathol* 1998; **29**: 1347–55.

26. Dehner LP. On trial: a malignant small cell tumor in a child: four wrongs do not make a right. *Am J Clin Pathol* 1998; **109**: 662–8.

♦27. Mierau GW. Electron microscopy for tumour diagnosis: is it redundant? *Histopathology* 1999; **35**: 99–101.

28. Struski S, Doco-Fenzy M, Cornillet-Lefebvre P. Compilation of published comparative genomic hybridization studies. *Cancer Genet Cytogenet* 2002; **135**: 63–90.

29. Lu YJ, Williamson D, Clark J *et al.* Comparative expressed sequence hybridization to chromosomes for tumor classification and identification of genomic regions of differential gene expression. *Proc Natl Acad Sci USA* 2001; **98**: 9197–202.

30. Lu Y, Williamson D, Wang R *et al.* New approach to expression profiling for classification and prediction of clinical behavior. *Gene Chromosome Cancer* 2003; **38**: 207–14.

♦31. Alizadeh AA, Ross DT, Perou CM, van de RM. Towards a novel classification of human malignancies based on gene expression patterns. *J Pathol* 2001; **195**: 41–52.

♦32. Bertucci F, Houlgatte R, Nguyen C *et al.* Gene expression profiling of cancer by use of DNA arrays: how far from the clinic? *Lancet Oncol* 2001; **2**: 674–82.

♦33. Lakhani SR, Ashworth A. Microarray and histopathological analysis of tumours: the future and the past? *Nat Rev Cancer* 2001; **1**: 151–7.

34. Ramaswamy S, Tamayo P, Rifkin R *et al.* Multiclass cancer diagnosis using tumor gene expression signatures. *Proc Natl Acad Sci USA* 2001; **98**: 15149–54.

35. Khan J, Wei JS, Ringner M *et al.* Classification and diagnostic prediction of cancers using gene expression profiling and artificial neural networks. *Nat Med* 2001; **7**: 673–9.

♦36. Knudsen S. *A Biologist's Guide to Analysis of DNA Microarray Data.* New York: Wiley-Interscience, 2002.

37. Alizadeh AA, Eisen MB, Davis RE *et al.* Distinct types of diffuse large B-cell lymphoma identified by gene expression profiling. *Nature* 2000; **403**: 503–11.

38. Khan J, Simon R, Bittner M *et al.* Gene expression profiling of alveolar rhabdomyosarcoma with cDNA microarrays. *Cancer Res* 1998; **58**: 5009–13.

♦39. Triche TJ, Schofield D, Buckley J. DNA microarrays in pediatric cancer. *Cancer J* 2001; **7**: 2–15.

40. Nielsen TO, West RB, Linn SC *et al.* Molecular characterisation of soft tissue tumours: a gene expression study. *Lancet* 2002; **359**: 1301–7.

41. Kushner BH, LaQuaglia MP, Cheung NK *et al.* Clinically critical impact of molecular genetic studies in pediatric solid tumors. *Med Pediatr Oncol* 1999; **33**: 530–5.

42. Athale UH, Shurtleff SA, Jenkins JJ *et al.* Use of reverse transcriptase polymerase chain reaction for diagnosis and staging of alveolar rhabdomyosarcoma, Ewing sarcoma family of tumors, and desmoplastic small round cell tumor. *J Pediatr Hematol Oncol* 2001; **23**: 99–104.

43. Peter M, Gilbert E, Delattre O. A multiplex real-time pcr assay for the detection of gene fusions observed in solid tumors. *Lab Invest* 2001; **81**: 905–12.

44. Bijwaard KE, Fetsch JF, Przygodzki R *et al.* Detection of SYT-SSX fusion transcripts in archival synovial sarcomas by real-time reverse transcriptase-polymerase chain reaction. *J Mol Diagn* 2002; **4**: 59–64.

♦45. Anderson J, Gordon A, Pritchard-Jones K, Shipley J. Genes, chromosomes, and rhabdomyosarcoma. *Genes Chromosomes Cancer* 1999; **26**: 275–85.

46. Dagher R, Pham TA, Sorbara L *et al.* Molecular confirmation of Ewing sarcoma. *J Pediatr Hematol Oncol* 2001; **23**: 221–4.

47. Guillou L, Coindre J, Gallagher G *et al.* Detection of the synovial sarcoma translocation t(X; 18) (SYT; SSX) in paraffin-embedded tissues using reverse transcriptase-polymerase chain reaction: a reliable and powerful diagnostic tool for pathologists. A molecular analysis of 221 mesenchymal tumors fixed in different fixatives. *Hum Pathol* 2001; **32**: 105–12.

48. Sorensen PH, Lynch JC, Qualman SJ *et al.* PAX3-FKHR and PAX7-FKHR gene fusions are prognostic indicators in alveolar rhabdomyosarcoma: a report from the children's oncology group. *J Clin Oncol* 2002; **20**: 2672–9.

49. Barr FG. Translocations, cancer and the puzzle of specificity. *Nat Genet* 1998; **19**: 121–4.

50. Rorke LB. Pathologic diagnosis as the gold standard. *Cancer* 1997; **79**: 665–7.

51. International Agency for Research on Cancer. *WHO Classification of Tumours: Pathology and Genetics of Tumours of the Nervous System.* Lyon: IARC, 2000.

52. Becker LE, Halliday WC. Central nervous system tumours of childhood. *Perspect Pediatr Pathol* 1987; **10**: 86–134.

53. Giannini C, Scheithauer BW, Burger PC *et al.* Pleomorphic xanthoastrocytoma: what do we really know about it? *Cancer* 1999; **85**: 2033–45.

54. Rorke LB, Packer RJ, Biegel JA. Central nervous system atypical teratoid/rhabdoid tumors of infancy and childhood: definition of an entity. *J Neurosurg* 1996; **85**: 56–65.

55. Gilles FH, Brown WD, Leviton A *et al.* Limitations of the World Health Organization classification of childhood supratentorial astrocytic tumors. Childhood Brain Tumour Consortium. *Cancer* 2000; **88**: 1477–83.

56. Fisher PG, Breiter SN, Carson BS *et al.* A clinicopathologic reappraisal of brain stem tumor classification. Identification of pilocytic astrocytoma and fibrillary astrocytoma as distinct entities. *Cancer* 2000; **89**: 1569–76.

57. Becker LE. The nervous system. In: Stocker JT, Dehner LP, eds. *Pediatric Pathology.* Philadelphia: Lippincott, Williams & Wilkins, 2000; 385–97.

58. Tomlinson FH, Scheithauer BW, Hayostek CJ *et al.* The significance of atypia and histologic malignancy in pilocytic astrocytoma of the cerebellum: a clinicopathologic and flow cytometric study. *J Child Neurol* 1994; **9**: 301–10.

59. Giannini C, Scheithauer BW, Burger PC *et al.* Cellular proliferation in pilocytic and diffuse astrocytomas. *J Neuropathol Exp Neurol* 1999; **58**: 46–53.

60. Tihan T, Fisher PG, Kepner JL *et al.* Pediatric astrocytomas with monomorphous pilomyxoid features and a less favorable outcome. *J Neuropathol Exp Neurol* 1999; **58**: 1061–8.

61. Kleihues P, Davis RL, Ohgaki H *et al.* Diffuse astrocytoma. In: Kleihues P, Cavanee WK, eds. *Tumours of the Nervous System.* Lyon: IARC, 2000; 22–6.

62. Peraud A, Ansari H, Bise K, Reulen HJ. Clinical outcome of supratentorial astrocytoma WHO grade II. *Acta Neurochir (Wien)* 1998; **140**: 1213–22.

63. Jaros E, Perry RH, Adam L *et al.* Prognostic implications of p53 protein, epidermal growth factor receptor, and Ki-67 labelling in brain tumours. *Br J Cancer* 1992; **66**: 373–85.

64. Kleihues P, Davis RL, Coons SW, Burger PC. Anaplastic astrocytoma. In: Kleihues P, Cavanee WK, eds. *Tumours of the Nervous Sytem.* Lyon: IARC, 2000; 27–8.

65. Watanabe K, Sato K, Biernat W *et al.* Incidence and timing of p53 mutations during astrocytoma progression in patients with multiple biopsies. *Clin Cancer Res* 1997; **3**: 523–30.

66. Kleihues P, Burger PC, Collins VP *et al.* Glioblastoma. In: Kleihues P, Cavanee WK, eds. *Tumours of the Nervous System.* Lyon: IARC, 2000; 29–39.

67. Burger PC, Kleihues P. Cytologic composition of the untreated glioblastoma with implications for evaluation of needle biopsies. *Cancer* 1989; **63**: 2014–23.

♦68. Hiem S, Mitelman F. *Cancer Cytogenetics: Chromosomal and Molecular Genetic Aberrations of Tumour Cells.* New York: Wiley-Liss, 1995.

69. Eberhart CG, Kaufman WE, Tihan T, Burger PC. Apoptosis, neuronal maturation, and neurotrophin expression within medulloblastoma nodules. *J Neuropathol Exp Neurol* 2001; **60**: 462–9.

70. Brown HG, Kepner JL, Perlman EJ *et al.* 'Large cell/anaplastic' medulloblastomas: a Pediatric Oncology Group Study. *J Neuropathol Exp Neurol* 2000; **59**: 857–65.

71. Giangaspero F, Perilongo G, Fondelli MP *et al.* Medulloblastoma with extensive nodularity: a variant with favorable prognosis. *J Neurosurg* 1999; **91**: 971–7.

72. Janss AJ, Yachnis AT, Silber JH *et al.* Glial differentiation predicts poor clinical outcome in primitive neuroectodermal brain tumors. *Ann Neurol* 1996; **39**: 481–9.

73. Grotzer MA, Janss AJ, Fung K *et al.* TrkC expression predicts good clinical outcome in primitive neuroectodermal brain tumors. *J Clin Oncol* 2000; **18**: 1027–35.

74. Grotzer MA, Hogarty MD, Janss AJ *et al.* MYC messenger RNA expression predicts survival outcome in childhood primitive neuroectodermal tumor/medulloblastoma. *Clin Cancer Res* 2001; **7**: 2425–33.

♦75. Biegel JA. Cytogenetics and molecular genetics of childhood brain tumors. *Neurooncology* 1999; **1**: 139–51.

76. Koga T, Iwasaki H, Ishiguro M *et al.* Frequent genomic imbalances in chromosomes 17,19 and 22q in peripheral nerve sheath tumours detected by comparative genomic hybridization analysis. *J Pathol* 2002; **197**: 98–107.

77. Rushing EJ, Brown DF, Hladik CL *et al.* Correlation of bcl-2, p53, and MIB-1 expression with ependymoma grade and subtype. *Mod Pathol* 1998; **11**: 464–70.

78. Prayson RA. Clinicopathologic study of 61 patients with ependymoma including MIB-1 immunohistochemistry. *Ann Diagn Pathol* 1999; **3**: 11–18.

79. Carter M, Nicholson J, Ross F *et al.* Genetic abnormalities detected in ependymomas by comparative genomic hybridisation. *Br J Cancer* 2002; **86**: 929–39.

80. Ward S, Harding B, Wilkins P *et al.* Gain of 1q and loss of 22 are the most common changes detected by comparative genomic hybridisation in paediatric ependymoma. *Genes Chromosomes Cancer* 2001; **32**: 59–66.

81. Dyer S, Prebble E, Davison V *et al.* Genomic imbalances in pediatric intracranial ependymomas define clinically relevant groups. *Am J Pathol* 2002; **161**: 2133–41.

82. Fisher PG, Jenab J, Goldthwaite PT *et al.* Outcomes and failure patterns in childhood craniopharyngiomas. *Childs Nerv Syst* 1998; **14**: 558–63.

83. Nishi T, Kuratsu J, Takeshima H *et al.* Prognostic significance of the MIB-1 labeling index for patient with craniopharyn-gioma. *Int J Mol Med* 1999; **3**: 157–61.

84. Rosenblum MK, Matsutani M, Van Meir EG. Germ cell tumours. In: Kleihues P, Cavenee WK, eds. *Tumours of the Nervous System.* Lyon: IARC, 2000; 207–14.

85. Aguzzi A, Brandner S, Paulus W. Choroid plexus tumours. In: Kleihues P, Cavenee WK, eds. *Tumours of the Nervous System.* Lyon: IARC, 2000; 83–6.

86. Chow E, Jenkins JJ, Burger PC *et al.* Malignant evolution of choroid plexus papilloma. *Pediatr Neurosurg* 1999; **31**: 127–30.

87. Burger PC, Yu IT, Tihan T *et al.* Atypical teratoid/rhabdoid tumor of the central nervous system: a highly malignant tumor of infancy and childhood frequently mistaken for medulloblastoma: a Pediatric Oncology Group study. *Am J Surg Pathol* 1998; **22**: 1083–92.

88. Versteege I, Sevenet N, Lange J *et al.* Truncating mutations of hSNF5/INI1 in aggressive paediatric cancer. *Nature* 1998; **394**: 203–6.

89. Joshi VV, Cantor AB, Altshuler G *et al.* Recommendations for modification of terminology of neuroblastic tumors and prognostic significance of Shimada classification. A clinicopathologic study of 213 cases from the Pediatric Oncology Group. *Cancer* 1992; **69**: 2183–96.

90. Ambros PF, Ambros IM. Pathology and biology guidelines for resectable and unresectable neuroblastic tumors and bone marrow examination guidelines. *Med Pediatr Oncol* 2001; **37**: 492–504.

91. Shimada H, Ambros IM, Dehner LP *et al.* The International Neuroblastoma Pathology Classification (the Shimada system). *Cancer* 1999; **86**: 364–72.

92. Shimada H, Ambros IM, Dehner LP *et al.* Terminology and morphologic criteria of neuroblastic tumors: recommendations by the International Neuroblastoma Pathology Committee. *Cancer* 1999; **86**: 349–63.

93. Shimada H, Umehara S, Monobe Y *et al.* International neuroblastoma pathology classification for prognostic evaluation of patients with peripheral neuroblastic tumors. *Cancer* 2001; **92**: 2451–61.

94. Umehara S, Nakagawa A, Matthay KK *et al.* Histopathology defines prognostic subsets of ganglioneuroblastoma, nodular. *Cancer* 2000; **89**: 1150–61.

95. Goto S, Umehara S, Gerbing RB *et al.* Histopathology (International Neuroblastoma Pathology Classification) and

MYCN status in patients with peripheral neuroblastic tumors. *Cancer* 2001; **92**: 2699–708.

96. Nakagawara A, Arima N, Scavarda NJ *et al.* Association between high levels of expression of the TRK gene and favourable outcome in human neuroblastoma. *N Engl J Med* 1993; **328**: 847–54.

97. Yamashiro DJ, Nakagawara A, Ikegaki N *et al.* Expression of TrkC in favourable human neuroblastomas. *Oncogene* 1996; **12**: 37–41.

98. Brodeur GM, Nakagawara A, Yamashiro DJ *et al.* Expression of TrkA, TrkB and TrkC in human neuroblastomas. *J Neurooncol* 1997; **31**: 49–55.

99. Combaret V, Gross N, Lasset C *et al.* Clinical relevance of TRKA expression on neuroblastoma: comparison with N-MYC amplification and CD44 expression. *Br J Cancer* 1997; **75**: 1151–5.

100. Lastowska M, Cullinane C, Variend S *et al.* Comprehensive genetic and histopathologic study reveals three types of neuroblastoma tumors. *J Clin Oncol* 2001; **19**: 3080–90.

101. Kramer K, Cheung NK, Gerald WL *et al.* Correlation of MYCN amplification, Trk-A and CD44 expression with clinical stage in 250 patients with neuroblastoma. *Eur J Cancer* 1997; **33**: 2098–100.

♦102. Bown N. Neuroblastoma tumour genetics: clinical and biological aspects. *J Clin Pathol* 2001; **54**: 897–910.

103. Bown N, Cotterill S, Lastowska M *et al.* Gain of chromosome arm 17q and adverse outcome in patients with neuroblastoma. *N Engl J Med* 1999; **340**: 1954–61.

104. Bown N, Lastowska M, Cotterill S *et al.* 17q gain in neuroblastoma predicts adverse clinical outcome. UK Cancer Cytogenetics Group and the UK Children's Cancer Study Group. *Med Pediatr Oncol* 2001; **36**: 14–19.

105. Luttikhuis ME, Powell JE, Rees SA *et al.* Neuroblastomas with chromosome 11q loss and single copy MYCN comprise a biologically distinct group of tumours with adverse prognosis. *Br J Cancer* 2001; **85**: 531–7.

106. Beckwith JB. Renal tumors. In: Stocker JT, Askin FB, eds. *Pathology of Solid Tumours in Children*. London: Chapman & Hall Medical, 1998; 1–23.

●107. Mitchell C, Jones PM, Kelsey A *et al.* The treatment of Wilms' tumour: results of the United Kingdom Children's Cancer Study Group (UKCCSG) second Wilms' tumour study. *Br J Cancer* 2000; **83**: 602–8.

108. Vujanic GM, Sandstedt B, Harms D *et al.* Revised International Society of Paediatric Oncology (SIOP) working classification of renal tumors of childhood. *Med Pediatr Oncol* 2002; **38**: 79–82.

109. Vujanic GM, Kelsey A, Mitchell C *et al.* The role of biopsy in the diagnosis of renal tumors of childhood: results of the UKCCSG Wilms' Tumor Study 3. *Med Pediatr Oncol* 2003; **40**: 18–22.

110. Faria P, Beckwith JB, Mishra K *et al.* Focal versus diffuse anaplasia in Wilms' tumor – new dimensions with prognostic significance – a report from the National Wilms' Tumour Study Group. *Am J Surg Pathol* 1996; **20**: 909–20.

111. Beckwith JB, Zuppan C, Browning NG. Histological analysis of aggressiveness and responsiveness in Wilms' tumour. *Med Pediatr Oncol* 1996; **27**: 422–8.

112. Zuppan C, Beckwith JB, Weeks DA. The effect of pre-operative chemotherapy on the histologic features of

Wilms' tumour. An analysis of the cases from the Third National Wilms' Tumour Study. *Cancer* 1991; **68**: 385–94.

♦113. Beckwith JB. Precursor lesions of Wilms' tumour: clinical and biological implications. *Med Pediatr Oncol* 1993; **21**: 158–68.

♦114. Eble JN, Bonsib SM. Extensively cystic renal neoplasms: cystic nephroma, cystic partially differentiated nephroblastoma, multilocular cystic renal cell carcinoma, and cystic hamartoma of renal pelvis. *Semin Diagn Pathol* 1998; **15**: 2–20.

115. Priest JR, Watterson J, Strong L. Pleuropulmonary blastoma: a marker for familial disease. *J Pediatr* 1996; **128**: 220–4.

♦116. Dome JS, Cooper MJ. Recent advances in Wilms' tumor genetics. *Curr Opin Pediatr* 2002; **14**: 5–11.

117. Grundy PE, Telzerow PE, Breslow N *et al.* Loss of heterozygosity for chromosome 16q and 1p in Wilms' tumours predicts an adverse outcome. *Cancer Res* 2002; **54**: 2331–3.

118. Lu YJ, Hing S, Williams R *et al.* Chromosome 1q expression profiling and relapse in Wilms' tumour. *Lancet* 2002; **360**: 385–6.

119. Hing S, Lu YJ, Summersgill B *et al.* Gain of 1q is associated with adverse outcome in favorable histology Wilms' tumors. *Am J Pathol* 2001; **158**: 393–8.

120. Argani P, Perlman EJ, Breslow NE *et al.* Clear cell sarcoma of the kidney: a review of 351 cases from the National Wilms' Tumor Study Group Pathology Center. *Am J Surg Pathol* 2000; **24**: 4–18.

121. Weeks DA, Beckwith JB, Mierau GW, Zuppan CW. Renal neoplasms mimicking rhabdoid tumor of kidney. A report from the National Wilms' Tumor Study Pathology Center. *Am J Surg Pathol* 1991; **15**: 1042–54.

♦122. Harms D. Soft tissue sarcomas in the Kiel Paediatric Tumour Registry. *Curr Top Pathol* 1995; **89**: 31–45.

123. Newton WA Jr, Gehan EA, Webber BL *et al.* Classification of rhabdomyosarcomas and related sarcomas. Pathologic aspects and proposal for a new classification – an Intergroup Rhabdomyosarcoma Study. *Cancer* 1995; **76**: 1073–85.

♦124. Qualman SJ, Coffin CM, Newton WA *et al.* Intergroup Rhabdomyosarcoma Study: update for pathologists. *Pediatr Dev Pathol* 1998; **1**: 550–61.

♦125. Leuschner I. Spindle cell rhabdomyosarcoma: histologic variant of embryonal rhabdomyosarcoma with association to favorable prognosis. *Curr Top Pathol* 1995; **89**: 261–72.

126. Boue DR, Parham DM, Webber B *et al.* Clinicopathologic study of ectomesenchymomas from Intergroup Rhabdomyosarcoma Study Groups III and IV. *Pediatr Dev Pathol* 2000; **3**: 290–300.

127. Coffin CM, Rulon J, Smith L *et al.* Pathologic features of rhabdomyosarcoma before and after treatment: a clinico-pathologic and immunohistochemical analysis. *Mod Pathol* 1997; **10**: 1175–87.

128. Ortega JA, Rowland J, Monforte H *et al.* Presence of well-differentiated rhabdomyoblasts at the end of therapy for pelvic rhabdomyosarcoma: implications for the outcome. *J Pediatr Hematol Oncol* 2000; **22**: 106–11.

129. Gordon T, McManus A, Anderson J *et al.* Cytogenetic abnormalities in 42 rhabdomyosarcoma: a United Kingdom Cancer Cytogenetics Group Study. *Med Pediatr Oncol* 2001; **36**: 259–67.

130. Anderson J, Gordon T, McManus A et al. Detection of the PAX3-FKHR fusion gene in paediatric rhabdomyosarcoma: a reproducible predictor of outcome? Br J Cancer 2001; **85**: 831–5.

131. Kelly KM, Womer RB, Sorensen PH et al. Common and variant fusions predict distinct clinical phenotypes in rhabdomyosarcoma. J Clin Oncol 1997; **15**: 1831–6.

132. Meis JM, Enzinger FM, Martz KL, Neal JA. Malignant peripheral nerve sheath tumors (malignant schwannomas) in children. Am J Surg Pathol 1992; **16**: 694–707.

133. Hiraga H, Nojima T, Abe S et al. Diagnosis of synovial sarcoma with the reverse transcriptase-polymerase chain reaction: analyses of 84 soft tissue and bone tumors. Diagn Mol Pathol 1998; **7**: 102–10.

134. Vang R, Biddle DA, Harrison WR et al. Malignant peripheral nerve sheath tumor with a t(X; 18). Arch Pathol Lab Med 2000; **124**: 864–7.

135. O'Sullivan MJ, Kyriakos M, Zhu X et al. Malignant peripheral nerve sheath tumors with t(X; 18). A pathologic and molecular genetic study. Mod Pathol 2000; **13**: 1336–46.

136. Coindre J-M, Hostein I, Benhattar J et al. Malignant peripheral nerve sheath tumors are t(X; 18) negative sarcomas. Molecular analysis of 25 cases occurring in neurofibromatosis type 1 patients, using two different RT-PCR based methods of detection. Mod Pathol 2002; **15**: 589–92.

137. Liew MA, Coffin CM, Fletcher JA et al. Peripheral nerve sheath tumors from patients with neurofibromatosis type 1 do not have the chromosomal translocation t(X; 18). Pediatr Dev Pathol 2002; **5**: 165–9.

138. Tamborini E, Agus V, Perrone F et al. Lack of SYT-SSX fusion transcripts in malignant peripheral nerve sheath tumors on RT-PCR analysis of 34 archival cases. Lab Invest 2002; **82**: 609–18.

♦139. Fisher C. Synovial sarcoma. Ann Diagn Pathol 1998; **2**: 401–21.

140. Pelmus M, Guillou L, Hostein I et al. Monophasic fibrous and poorly differentiated synovial sarcoma: immunohistochemical reassessment of 60 t(X; 18)(SYT-SSX)-positive cases. Am J Surg Pathol 2002; **26**: 1434–40.

♦141. Ladanyi M. Fusions of the SYT and SSX genes in synovial sarcoma. Oncogene 2001; **20**: 5755–62.

142. Ladanyi M, Antonescu CR, Leung DH et al. Impact of SYT-SSX fusion type on the clinical behavior of synovial sarcoma: a multi-institutional retrospective study of 243 patients. Cancer Res 2002; **62**: 135–40.

143. Birdsall S, Osin P, Lu YJ et al. Synovial sarcoma specific translocation associated with both epithelial and spindle cell components. Int J Cancer 1999; **82**: 605–8.

144. Antonescu CR, Kawai A, Leung DH et al. Strong association of SYT-SSX fusion type and morphologic epithelial differentiation in synovial sarcoma. Diagn Mol Pathol 2000; **9**: 1–8.

145. Panagopoulos I, Mertens F, Isaksson M et al. Clinical impact of molecular and cytogenetic findings in synovial sarcoma. Genes Chromosomes Cancer 2001; **31**: 362–72.

146. Saint Aubain SN, Fletcher CD. Leiomyosarcoma of soft tissue in children: clinicopathologic analysis of 20 cases. Am J Surg Pathol 1999; **23**: 755–63.

147. Ceballos KM, Nielsen GP, Selig MK, O'Connell JX. Is anti-h-caldesmon useful for distinguishing smooth muscle and myofibroblastic tumors? An immunohistochemical study. Am J Clin Pathol 2000; **114**: 746–53.

148. Coffin CM, Jaszcz W, O'Shea PA, Dehner LP. So-called congenital-infantile fibrosarcoma: does it exist and what is it? Pediatr Pathol 1994; **14**: 133–50.

149. Bourgeois JM, Knezevich SR, Mathers JA, Sorensen PH. Molecular detection of the ETV6-NTRK3 gene fusion differentiates congenital fibrosarcoma from other childhood spindle cell tumors. Am J Surg Pathol 2000; **24**: 937–46.

150. Ladanyi M, Lui MY, Antonescu CR et al. The der(17)t(X; 17) (p11; q25) of human alveolar soft part sarcoma fuses the TFE3 transcription factor gene to ASPL, a novel gene at 17q25. Oncogene 2001; **20**: 48–57.

151. Zucman J, Delattre O, Desmaze C et al. EWS and ATF-1 gene fusion induced by t(12; 22) translocation in malignant melanoma of soft parts. Nat Genet 1993; **4**: 341–5.

152. Speleman F, Delattre O, Peter M et al. Malignant melanoma of the soft parts (clear-cell sarcoma): confirmation of EWS and ATF-1 gene fusion caused by a t(12; 22) translocation. Mod Pathol 1997; **10**: 496–9.

153. Weiss SW, Goldblum JR. Fibrous tissue tumours of infancy and childhood. In: Weiss SW, Goldblum JR, eds. Enzinger's and Weiss' Soft Tissue Tumours. St Louis: Mosby, 2001; 347–408.

♦154. Dehner LP. The evolution of the diagnosis and understanding of primitive and embryonic neoplasms in children: living through an epoch. Mod Pathol 1998; **11**: 669–85.

♦155. Ladanyi M, Bridge JA. Contribution of molecular genetic data to the classification of sarcomas. Hum Pathol 2000; **31**: 532–8.

♦156. Terrier P, Llombart-Bosch A, Contesso G. Small round blue cell tumors in bone: prognostic factors correlated to Ewing's sarcoma and neuroectodermal tumors. Semin Diagn Pathol 1996; **13**: 250–7.

157. Parham DM, Hijazi Y, Steinberg SM et al. Neuroectodermal differentiation in Ewing's sarcoma family of tumors does not predict tumor behavior. Hum Pathol 1999; **30**: 911–18.

158. Menasce LP, Banerjee SS, Beckett E, Harris M. Extra-medullary myeloid tumour (granulocytic sarcoma) is often misdiagnosed: a study of 26 cases. Histopathology 1999; **34**: 391–8.

159. Folpe AL, Hill CE, Parham DM et al. Immunohistochemical detection of FLI-1 protein expression: a study of 132 round cell tumors with emphasis on CD99-positive mimics of Ewing's sarcoma/primitive neuroecto-dermal tumor. Am J Surg Pathol 2000; **24**: 1657–62.

160. Unni KK. Dahlin's Bone Tumours: General Aspects and Data on 11,087 Cases. Philadelphia: Lippincott-Raven, 1996.

♦161. Patterson K. The pathologic handling of skeletal tumors. Am J Clin Pathol 1998; **109**: S53–S66.

162. Raymond AK, Chawla SP, Carrasco CH et al. Osteosarcoma chemotherapy effect: a prognostic factor. Semin Diagn Pathol 1987; **4**: 212–36.

163. Inwards CY, Unni KK. Bone tumors. In: Sternberg SS, ed. Diagnostic Surgical Pathology. Philadelphia: Lippincott Williams & Wilkins, 1999; 263–315.

♦164. Ragland BD, Bell WC, Lopez RR, Siegal GP. Cytogenetics and molecular biology of osteosarcoma. Lab Invest 2002; **82**: 365–73.

♦165. Kim J, Pelletier J. Molecular genetics of chromosome translocations involving EWS and related family members. Physiol Genomics 1999; **1**: 127–38.

Colour plates

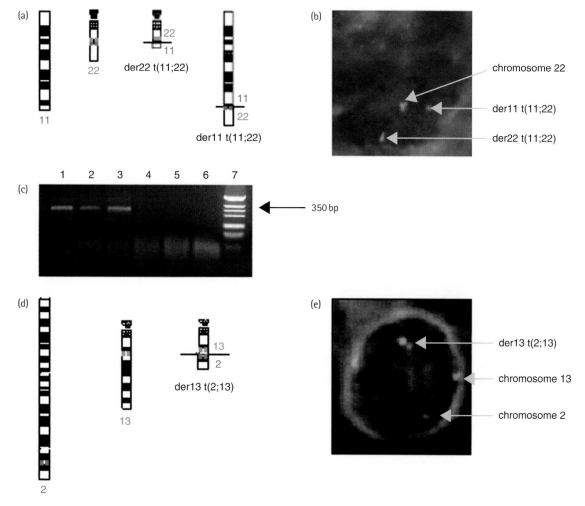

Plate 1 *Examples of molecular diagnoses of paediatric solid tumours. (a) An ideogram of chromosomes 11 and 22 and the derivative chromosomes that result from the translocation t(11;22)(q23;q12) associated with Ewing's family of tumours. The green and red spots on chromosome 22 represent the probes flanking the breakpoint region at the EWS gene. If the translocation is present these markers are no longer juxtaposed. (b) An interphase nucleus showing separate red and green signals consistent with disruption of the EWS gene. As there are two copies of each chromosome in normal cells, the juxtaposed red and green signals indicate a normal copy chromosome 22 in addition to the rearranged chromosomes. (c) Gel showing the products of reverse transcription PCR (RT-PCR) analysis for the EWS–FLI1 fusion gene product associated with Ewing's tumours. Lane 1: Ewing's tumour; lane 2: Ewing's tumour; lane 3: cell line known to be positive for the type I fusion gene and which gives a 350-bp product with the primers used (exon 7 of the EWS gene fuses with exon 6 of FLI1); lane 4: cell line negative for this fusion gene product; lanes 5, 6: negative PCR controls; lane 7: size marker, a 1-kb ladder. (d) An ideogram of chromosomes 2 and 13 and the derivative 13 chromosome that results from the t(2;13)(q35;q14) associated with alveolar rhabdomyosarcomas. The red spots represent the position of the probe used distal to the PAX3 gene on chromosome 2, and the green spots represent a marker centromeric to the FKHR (FOX1A10) on chromosome 13. (e) If the translocation is present, these probes become juxtaposed as shown in the interphase nuclei from an alveolar rhabdomyosarcoma.*

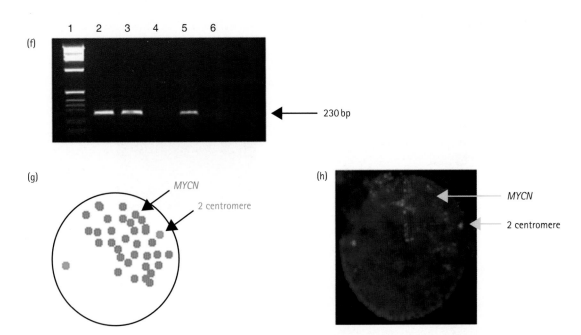

Plate 1 *(Continued) (f) Gel showing the products of RT-PCR analysis for the PAX3-FKHR fusion gene product associated with alveolar rhabdomyosarcomas. Lane 1: size marker, a 1-kb ladder; lane 2: alveolar rhabdomyosarcoma; lane 3: alveolar rhabdomyosarcoma; lane 3: cell line negative for this fusion gene product; lane 5: cell line positive for this 230-bp fusion gene product. (g) Diagram of an interphase nucleus representing multiple copies of the* MYCN *gene relative to a marker for the centromere of chromosome 2. (h) An interphase nucleus from a neuroblastoma where amplification of the* MYCN *gene has prognostic value. (The authors thank Sandra Hing for images of the RT-PCR analyses.)*

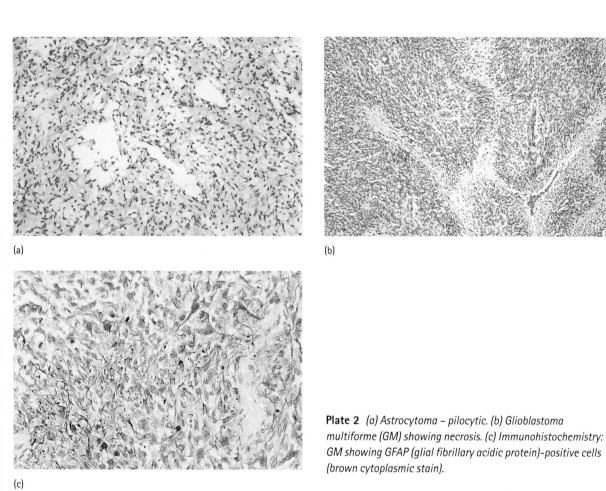

Plate 2 *(a) Astrocytoma – pilocytic. (b) Glioblastoma multiforme (GM) showing necrosis. (c) Immunohistochemistry: GM showing GFAP (glial fibrillary acidic protein)-positive cells (brown cytoplasmic stain).*

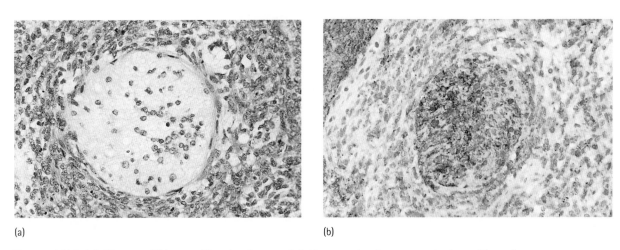

(a)

(b)

Plate 3 *(a) Medulloblastoma. (b) Immunohistochemistry: medulloblastoma showing synaptophysin-positive cells (brown cytoplasmic stain).*

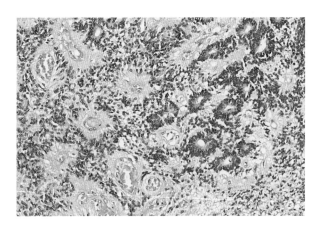

Plate 4 *Ependymoma showing pseudorosettes.*

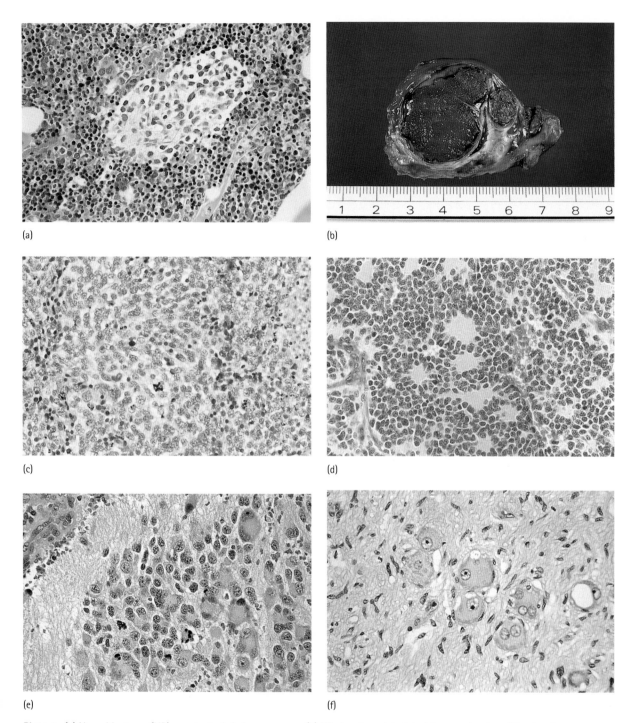

Plate 5 *(a) Neuroblastoma (NB) – metastasis in bone marrow. (b) NB showing a lobulated, haemorrhagic, solid cut surface. (c) NB, undifferentiated showing high mitosis-karyorrhexis index. (d) NB, poorly differentiated forming rosettes. (e) NB, differentiating. (f) Ganglioneuroma – Schwann cell stroma containing mature ganglion cells.*

(a)

(b)

(c)

(d)

(e)

(f)

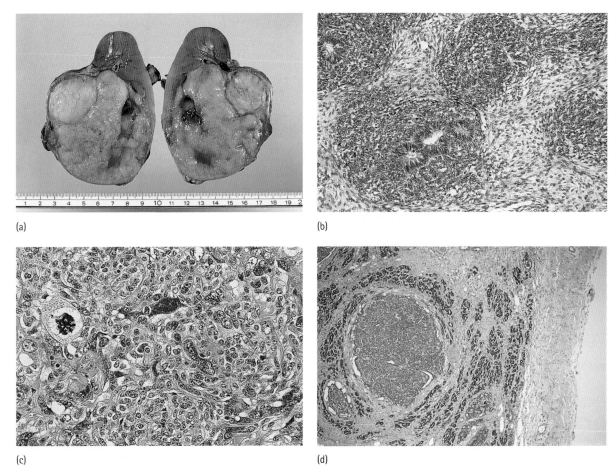

(a)

(b)

(c)

(d)

Plate 6 *(a) Bisected kidney showing Wilms' tumour (WT). (b) WT showing blastema, tubules and mesenchyme. (c) WT – anaplastic showing abnormal mitotic figures and nuclear gigantism. (d) Subcapsular nephrogenic rests.*

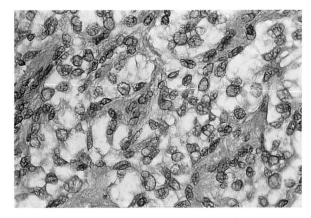

Plate 7 *Clear cell sarcoma of the kidney.*

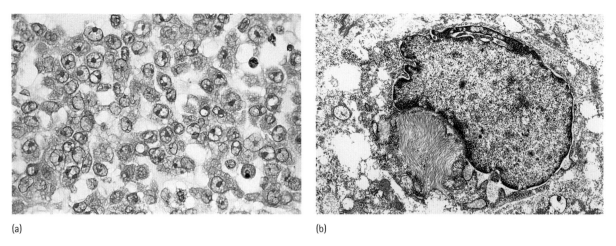

Plate 8 *(a) Malignant rhabdoid tumour of the kidney (MRTK). (b) Electron microscopy: MRTK showing cytoplasmic paranuclear whorls.*

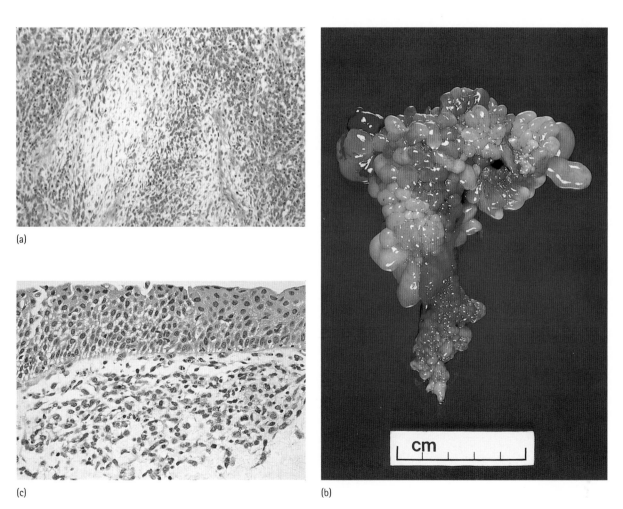

Plate 9 *(a) Embryonal rhabdomyosarcoma (ERMS) showing hypo- and hypercellular areas. (b) ERMS: botryoid type. (c) ERMS: botryoid type showing the cambium layer.*

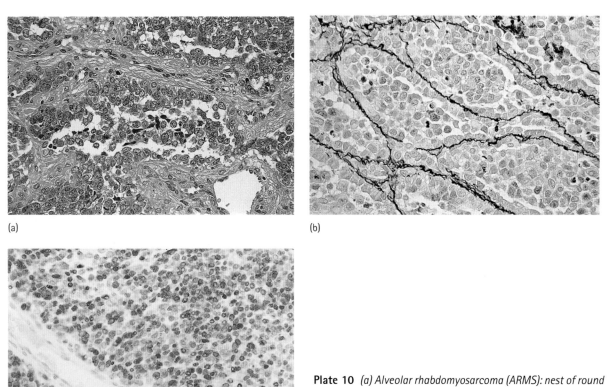

(a)

(b)

(c)

Plate 10 *(a) Alveolar rhabdomyosarcoma (ARMS): nest of round cells separated by fibrous band (pink). (b) ARMS: reticulin stain (black) surrounding nests of cells. (c) Immunohistochemistry: rhabdomyosarcoma showing nuclear myogenin positivity (brown).*

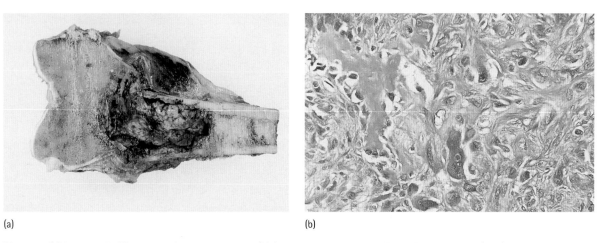

(a)

(b)

Plate 11 *(a) Lower end of femur showing osteosarcoma. (b) Osteosarcoma tumour cells producing osteoid (pink).*

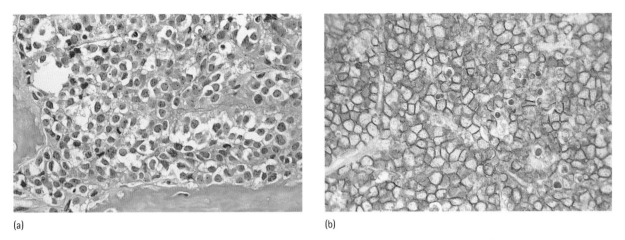

(a)   (b)

Plate 12 *(a) Ewing's sarcoma (ES) composed of undifferentiated small cells. (b) Immunohistochemistry: membranous CD99 positivity of ES tumour cells.*

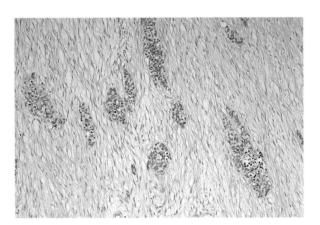

Plate 13 *Desmoplastic small round-cell tumour showing the nests of tumour cells in a fibrous stroma.*

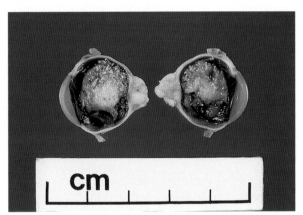

Plate 14 *Retinoblastoma.*

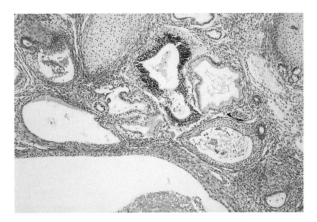

Plate 15 *Immature teratoma.*

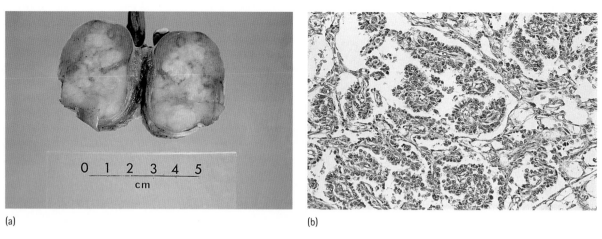

(a)

(b)

Plate 16 *(a) Testis showing solid, grey tumour. (b) Yolk sac tumour showing a papillary pattern.*

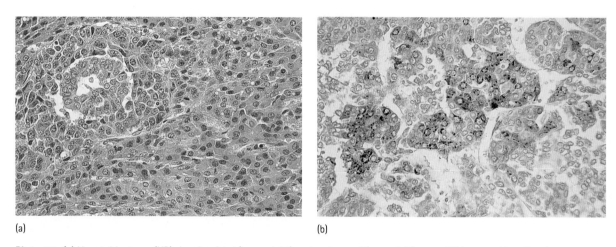

(a)

(b)

Plate 17 *(a) Hepatoblastoma (HB) showing fetal (lower right) and embryonal (upper left) areas. (b) Immunohistochemistry: HB showing alpha-fetoprotein-positive epithelial cells (stained brown).*

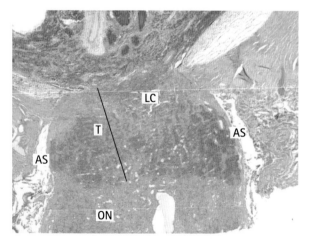

Plate 18 *Unilateral retinoblastoma: retrolaminar optic nerve involvement. AS: arachnoïdal space, ON: optic nerve, T: tumour involvement and LC: lamina cribrosa.*

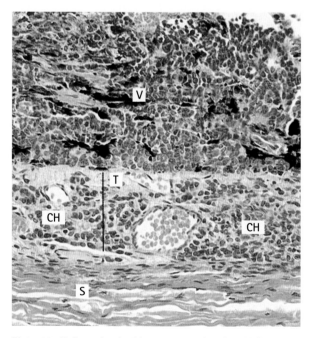

Plate 19 *Unilateral retinoblastoma: massive choroidal involvement. V: vitreous, T: deep choroïdal tumour involvement, S: sclera, and CH: choroïd.*

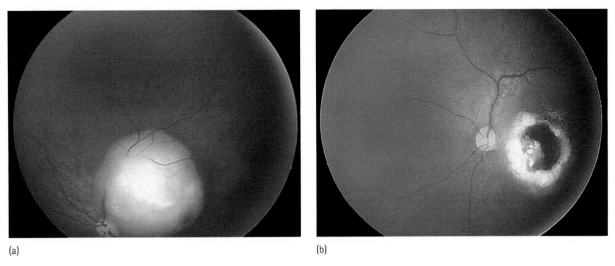

(a)

(b)

Plate 20 *Bilateral retinoblastoma: treatment of a posterior pole tumour using the combination of intravenous carboplatin and tumour local hyperthermia through a transpupillary irradiation using a diode laser.*

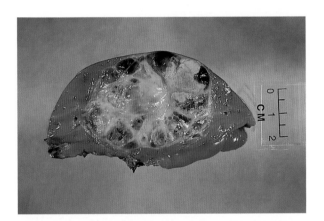

Plate 21 *Hepatoblastoma: cut surface of resected tumour.*

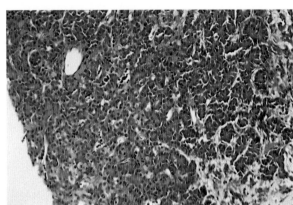

Plate 23 *Hepatoblastoma: embryonal subtype.*

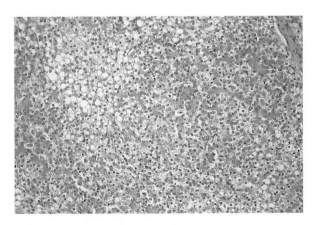

Plate 22 *Hepatoblastoma: fetal subtype.*

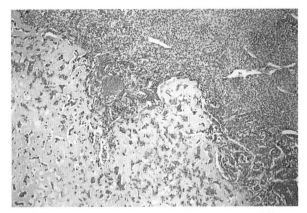

Plate 24 *Hepatoblastoma: anaplastic, fetal/embryonal and osteoid areas.*

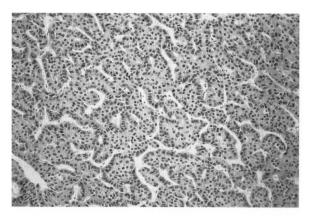

Plate 25 *Hepatoblastoma: macrotrabecular subtype.*

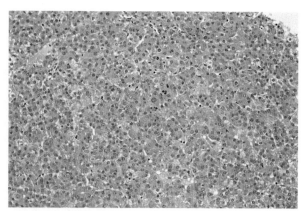

Plate 26 *Hepatocellular carcinoma.*

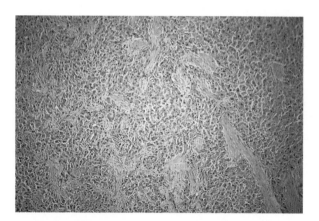

Plate 27 *Fibrolamellar hepatocellular carcinoma.*

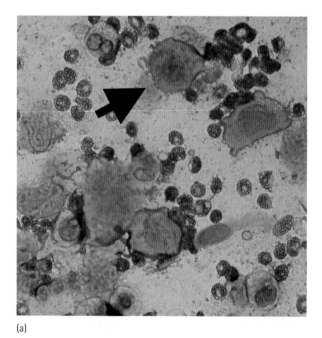

(a)

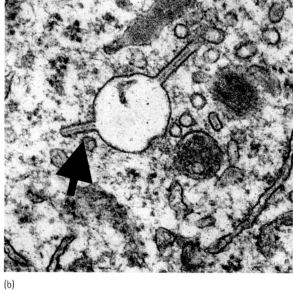

(b)

Plate 28 *(a) Langerhans cells stain intensely for CD1a; (b) Birbeck granules appearing in the shape of a tennis racket.*

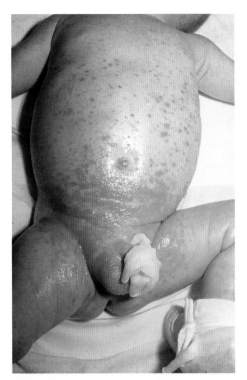
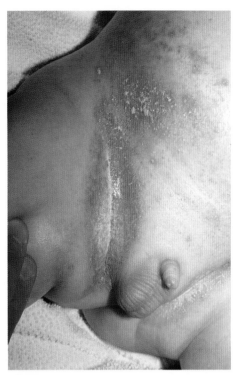

(a)　　　　　　　　　　　　　　(b)
Plate 29 *(a) Widespread macular papular eruption with marked involvement of the diaper area; (b) scaling eruptions in the groin with tendency to form scars.*

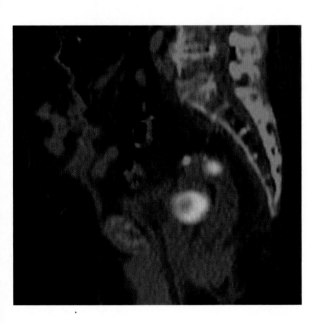

Plate 30 *A fused CT and PET image that localizes the presacral uptake from the PET scan onto the CT scan indicating metastatic spread to a regional lymph node. Such methods of combining anatomical details with biological tumour information are likely to improve staging accuracy and aid target definition for radiotherapy planning in the future. (Reproduced with the kind permission of CTI Molecular Imaging.)*

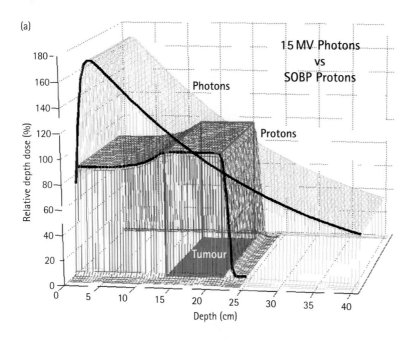

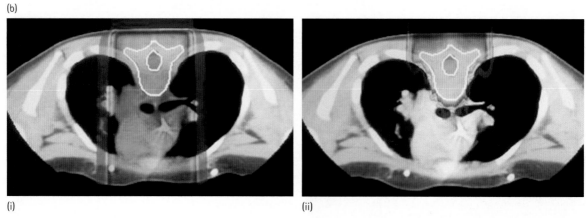

(i) (ii)

Plate 31 *Comparison of the depth–dose characteristics of photons and protons. (a) The graph demonstrates the differences of dose distribution with increasing depth of tissue for a photon and a proton beam. For this deep-seated tumour, there is minimal radiation dose deposited beyond the defined planning target volume compared with a single photon beam. (b) Dose distribution for a spinal field for a child lying in a prone position such as is required for the treatment of patients with primitive neuroectodermal tumours of the central nervous system. Compared with a conventional photon beam (i), a proton beam (ii) significantly reduces the dose outside the planning target volume, particularly to the heart, thus potentially reducing radiotherapy-associated late sequelae. (Reproduced with the kind permission of Nancy Tarbell, MGH, Boston, Massachusetts, USA.)*

♦166. de Alava E, Gerald WL. Molecular biology of the Ewing's sarcoma/primitive neuroectodermal tumor family. *J Clin Oncol* 2000; **18**: 204–13.

♦167. Sandberg AA, Bridge JA. Updates on cytogenetics and molecular genetics of bone and soft tissue tumors: Ewing sarcoma and peripheral primitive neuroectodermal tumors. *Cancer Genet Cytogenet* 2000; **123**: 1–26.

168. Morishita T, Bolander ME, Zhang K *et al.* A method for accurate detection of translocation junctions in Ewing family of tumors. *Mol Biotechnol* 2001; **18**: 97–104.

169. Hattinger CM, Potschger U, Tarkkanen M *et al.* Prognostic impact of chromosomal aberrations in Ewing tumours. *Br J Cancer* 2002; **86**: 1763–9.

170. Ordonez NG. Desmoplastic small round cell tumor: I: a histopathologic study of 39 cases with emphasis on unusual histological patterns. *Am J Surg Pathol* 1998; **22**: 1303–13.

171. Lae ME, Roche PC, Jin L *et al.* Desmoplastic small round cell tumor: a clinicopathologic, immunohistochemical, and molecular study of 32 tumors. *Am J Surg Pathol* 2002; **26**: 823–35.

172. Gerald W, Ladanyi M, de Alava E *et al.* Clinical, pathologic, and molecular spectrum of tumors associated with t(11; 22) (p13; q12): desmoplastic small-round cell tumor and its variants. *J Clin Oncol* 1998; **16**: 3028–36.

173. Ordonez NG. Desmoplastic small round cell tumor: II: an ultrastructural and immunohistochemical study with emphasis on new immunohistochemical markers. *Am J Surg Pathol* 1998; **22**: 1314–27.

174. Hill DA, Pfeifer JD, Marley EF *et al.* WT1 staining reliably differentiates desmoplastic small round cell tumor from Ewing sarcoma/primitive neuroectodermal tumor. An immunohistochemical and molecular diagnostic study. *Am J Clin Pathol* 2000; **114**: 345–53.

175. Ladanyi M, Gerald W. Fusion of the EWS and WT1 genes in the desmoplastic small round cell tumor. *Cancer Res* 1994; **54**: 2837–40.

176. Barnoud R, Delattre O, Peoc'h M *et al.* Desmoplastic small round cell tumour: RT-PCR analysis and immunohisto-chemical detection of Wilms' tumor gene WT1. *Pathol Res Pract* 1998; **194**: 693–700.

177. Hill DA, O'Sullivan MJ, Zhu X *et al.* Practical Application of molecular genetic testing as an aid to the surgical pathologic diagnosis of sarcomas: a prospective study. *Am J Surg Pathol* 2002; **26**: 965–77.

178. McLean IW. Retinoblastomas, retinocytomas, and pseudoretinoblastomas. In: Spencer W, ed. *Ophthalmic Pathology*. Philadelphia: WB Saunders, 1996; 1332–438.

179. Margo C, Hidayat A, Kopelman J, Zimmerman LE. Retinocytoma. A benign variant of retinoblastoma. *Arch Ophthalmol* 1983; **101**: 1519–31.

180. Schwimer CJ, Prayson RA. Clinicopathologic study of retinoblastoma including MIB-1, p53, and CD99 immunohistochemistry. *Ann Diagn Pathol* 2001; **5**: 148–54.

181. Knudson A. Statistical study of retinoblastoma. *Proc Natl Acad Sci USA* 1971; **68**: 820–3.

♦182. Perlman EJ, Hawkins EP. Pediatric germ cell tumors: protocol update for pathologists. *Pediatr Dev Pathol* 1998; **1**: 328–35.

●183. Mann JR, Raafat F, Robinson K *et al.* The UKCCSG second Germ Cell Tumour Study: carboplatin, etoposide, and bleomycin are effective treatment for children with malignant extracranial germ cell tumours, with acceptable toxicity. *J Clin Oncol* 2000; **18**: 3809–18.

184. Dehner LP. Gonadal and extragonadal germ cell neoplasms-teratomas in childhood. In: Finegold MJ, ed. *Pathology of Neoplasia in Children and Adolescents*. Philadelphia: WB Saunders, 1986; 282–312.

185. Ulbright TM, Roth LM. Testicular and paratesticular tumours. In: Sternberg SS, ed. *Diagnostic Surgical Pathology*. Philadelphia: Lippincott Williams and Wilkins, 1999; 1973–2033.

186. Norris HJ, Zirkin HJ, Benson WL. Immature (malignant) teratoma of the ovary: a clinical and pathologic study of 58 cases. *Cancer* 1976; **37**: 2359–72.

187. Heifetz SA, Cushing B, Giller R *et al.* Immature teratomas in children: pathologic considerations: a report from the combined Pediatric Oncology Group/Children's Cancer Group. *Am J Surg Pathol* 1998; **22**: 1115–24.

188. Perlman EJ. Germ cell tumours. In: Stocker JT, Askin FB, eds. *Pathology of Solid Tumours in Children*. London: Chapman & Hall Medical, 1998; 213–34.

189. Marina NM, Cushing B, Giller R *et al.* Complete surgical excision is effective treatment for children with immature teratomas with or without malignant elements: A Pediatric Oncology Group/Children's Cancer Group Intergroup Study. *J Clin Oncol* 1999; **17**: 2137–43.

190. Cushing B, Giller R, Ablin A *et al.* Surgical resection alone is effective treatment for ovarian immature teratoma in children and adolescents: a report of the pediatric oncology group and the children's cancer group. *Am J Obstet Gynecol* 1999; **181**: 353–8.

191. Malogolowkin MH, Mahour GH, Krailo M, Ortega JA. Germ cell tumors in infancy and childhood: a 45-year experience. *Pediatr Pathol* 1990; **10**: 231–41.

192. Bussey KJ, Lawce HJ, Himoe E *et al.* Chromosomes 1 and 12 abnormalities in pediatric germ cell tumors by interphase fluorescence in situ hybridization. *Cancer Genet Cytogenet* 2001; **125**: 112–18.

193. Rodriguez E, Houldsworth J, Reuter VE *et al.* Molecular cytogenetic analysis of i(12p)-negative human male germ cell tumors. *Genes Chromosomes Cancer* 1993; **8**: 230–6.

♦194. Stocker JT. Hepatic tumors in children. *Clin Liver Dis* 2001; **5**: 259–81.

195. Heifetz SA, French M, Correa M, Grosfeld JL. Hepatoblastoma: the Indiana experience with preoperative chemotherapy for inoperable tumors; clinicopathological considerations. *Pediatr Pathol Lab Med* 1997; **17**: 857–74.

196. Saxena R, Leake JL, Shafford EA *et al.* Chemotherapy effects on hepatoblastoma. A histological study. *Am J Surg Pathol* 1993; **17**: 1266–71.

197. Conran RM, Hitchcock CL, Waclawiw MA *et al.* Hepatoblastoma: the prognostic significance of histologic type. *Pediatr Pathol* 1992; **12**: 167–83.

198. Berman MA, Burnham JA, Sheahan DG. Fibrolamellar carcinoma of the liver: an immunohistochemical study of nineteen cases and a review of the literature. *Hum Pathol* 1988; **19**: 784–94.

199. Craig JR, Peters RL, Edmondson HA, Omata M. Fibrolamellar carcinoma of the liver: a tumor of adolescents and young

adults with distinctive clinico-pathologic features. *Cancer* 1980; **46**: 372–9.

200. Silver SA, Wiley JM, Perlman EJ. DNA ploidy analysis of pediatric germ cell tumors. *Mod Pathol* 1994; **7**: 951–6.

♦201. deMent SH. Association between mediastinal germ cell tumors and hematologic malignancies: an update. *Hum Pathol* 1990; **21**: 699–703.

202. Haas JE, Muczynski KA, Krailo M *et al.* Histopathology and prognosis in childhood hepatoblastoma and hepatocarcinoma. *Cancer* 1989; **64**: 1082–95.

203. Haas JE, Feusner JH, Finegold MJ. Small cell undifferentiated histology in hepatoblastoma may be unfavorable. *Cancer* 2001; **92**: 3130–4.

4

Pathology of leukaemia

OWEN P. SMITH & IAN HANN

INTRODUCTION

Leukaemia is the most common form of childhood cancer, representing approximately 30 per cent of all cancers in children. Acute lymphoblastic leukaemia (ALL) is the dominant type, accounting for approximately 80–85 per cent of childhood leukaemia, with acute myeloblastic leukaemia (AML) representing approximately 15–20 per cent and juvenile myelomonocytic leukaemia (JMML) 2–3 per cent. There is a significant peak in incidence between 3 and 5 years of age but this peak is noticeably absent in many developing countries, leading to theories that exposures, e.g. to infections associated with modernization, may lead to leukaemia. Males are about 1.5 times more commonly affected than females, except in T-cell ALL where the male/female ratio is 4:1 and in infant leukaemia where there is a female preponderance.

Childhood leukaemia represents a very heterogeneous group of malignancies characterized by the accumulation of immature lymphocytes and phagocytes in the bone marrow and blood. These transformed haemopoietic stem cells exhibit aberrant differentiation patterns with increased self-renewal capability, and ultimately they inhibit the growth of normal lymphoid, erythroid, granulocytic and megakaryocytic precursors in the bone marrow by direct and indirect mechanisms. Recent advances in the molecular biology, cytogenetics and immunology of childhood leukaemias, together with improvements in intensive chemotherapy and supportive care regimens, bone marrow transplantation and the realization of therapies targeted to oncogenic transcription factors, regulators of apoptosis, and other biological response modifiers will hopefully improve the current impressive cure rates, considered by many to be the success story of cancer treatment during the 20th century.

HISTORICAL PERSPECTIVE

While it is generally agreed that leukaemia was first described independently by Bennett, Craigie and Virchow in 1845,[1–3] clinical and microscopic descriptions were reported earlier, by Alfred Velpeau in 1827[4] and Alfred Francois Donne in 1844.[5] The recognition of leukaemia as a distinct pathological entity and not a 'symptomatic suppuration of the blood' as it was felt to be until 1847, is credited to Virchow,[6] who was also the first to give this condition its rightful name, *Weisses Blut* (white blood or leukaemia).[3] In 1857, Friedreich[7] described the first case of acute leukaemia, thus allowing a classification into acute and chronic forms. The staining methods developed by Ehrlich at the end of the 19th century enabled accurate cytological descriptions of these disorders. The concept of a myelogenous form was put forward as early as 1878 by Neumann;[8] however, it took a further 25 years for this to be realized when Naegeli[9] discovered that the myeloblast was the precursor of neutrophilic granulocytes. Subtypes of AML were recognized in 1913 by Reschad and Schilling-Torgau[10] with their description of monocytic leukaemia, which was subsequently reclassified by Watkins and Hall[11] in 1940 into myelomonocytic and the true monocytic varieties. Further subtypes were subsequently described: erythroleukaemia by Di Guglielmo[12] in 1946; promyelocytic leukaemia by Hillestad[13] in 1957; megakaryoblastic leukaemia by Lewis and Szur[14] in 1963; and the hypogranular variant of promyelocytic leukaemia by Golomb et al.[15] in 1980.

The first great breakthrough in the treatment of acute leukaemia came in 1948, when Farber et al.[16] in Boston reported that remissions, albeit short-lived, could be readily achieved with the folic acid antagonist aminopterin. Within 5 years of their discovery, the purine antagonists (mercaptopurine) and corticosteroids had become available for therapeutic usage, and hence the era of 'modern' chemotherapy was born.

EPIDEMIOLOGY

The incidence of ALL varies significantly throughout the world, with rates ranging from nine to 47 per million for male children, and from seven to 43 per million for females. Incidence rates are highest in the USA among whites and in Australia, Costa Rica and Germany.[17] Most European countries have intermediate rates, while the lowest quoted rates are found among American blacks, Indians and Kuwaitis. There is a significant peak in incidence between 3 and 5 years of age, but this peak is noticeably absent in many developing countries, leading to theories that certain exposures, e.g. to infections associated with modern lifestyles, may lead to leukaemia.[17] Boys are about 1.5 times more commonly affected than girls except in T-cell ALL, where the male:female ratio is 4:1, and in infant leukaemia, where there is a female preponderance.

AML constitutes a minority of cases of leukaemia in childhood, with a relative incidence of 10–12 per cent in the first decade of life, rising to approximately double that by the age of 15 years. In the first 4 weeks of life, by contrast, AML does predominate over ALL. In the UK there are approximately 50–60 new childhood AML cases every year. There is considerable worldwide variation in relative incidence but some of the comparative data, not being population-based, must be treated with caution. In Japan and some parts of Africa, AML appears to be more common than ALL throughout childhood, and in northern Turkey there is a reported high incidence of monocytic leukaemia.[17]

The most striking genetic association is with Down's syndrome, in which there is a 20-fold increased risk of leukaemia. Other chromosomal disorders associated with an increased risk of childhood leukaemia include Klinefelter's syndrome, Turner's syndrome, those with XYY and XYY mosaic karyotypes, and those with trisomy 13. Genetic instability syndromes (Fanconi's anaemia, ataxia telangiectasia, Bloom's syndrome)[18] and most of the inherited bone marrow failure syndromes (Fanconi's anaemia, Shwachman–Diamond syndrome, Kostman's syndrome, dyskeratosis congenita, amegakaryocytic thrombocytopenia, Diamond–Blackfan anaemia and thrombocytopenia with absent radii) have an increased risk of developing leukaemia. Also, host genomic polymorphisms in genes such as NQ01 and MTHFR, as well as HLA class II alleles and inflammatory response genes, probably play a role in leukaemia susceptibility.[19]

Familial leukaemia cases have been described over many decades, and can cluster in families that experience a high risk of cancers, including brain tumours, colon and stomach cancer. This could suggest a genetic component to the aetiology but may also reflect a shared environmental exposure, e.g. ionizing radiation, chemicals such as benzene, viruses (human T-cell leukaemia/lymphoma virus type II, Epstein–Barr virus) and bacteria (Helicobacter pylori). However, the precise role, if any, that these exposures play in the development of childhood leukaemia remains to be determined.[19]

A variety of consistent structural chromosomal translocations have been described in childhood leukaemia. Besides being an aid to classification and diagnosis, these translocations appear to initiate disease and often arise prenatally, as has been demonstrated from twin studies.[20] Although the occurrence of acute leukaemia in identical (monozygotic) infant twins is rare, molecular studies on such children in the recent past have shown a very high degree of concordance for ALL; in other words, the risk of developing a genetically identical (usually MLL gene fusion positive) leukaemia rises to 100 per cent for the unaffected identical twin sibling. This suggests that the development of MLL rearrangements in utero is pivotal in subsequent leukaemia development, but it also justifies continued efforts to evaluate prenatal exposure to environmental agents such as DNA topoisomerase II inhibitors. If a twin develops ALL with TEL-AML1 fusion gene at age 2–6 years, then the concordance rate for leukaemia development for the identical twin sibling drops to 5 per cent.[20] It should be remembered that this still represents a huge increased risk (100-fold) of developing leukaemia and is highly suggestive that some other molecular/cellular event has occurred, e.g. an aberrant systemic inflammatory response to infection. Put another way, early exposure to infection may be protective against the disease and delayed exposure (due to fewer siblings or delayed entry into day care) in susceptible individuals may predispose to ALL.[19,20]

Treatment with alkylating agents is also associated with an increased incidence, and these leukaemias may present with a myelodysplastic (MDS) prodrome. Typically, these cases present within 4–6 years of initial therapy, with a much lower risk after 10 years, and commonly the associated cytogenetic abnormalities involve deletions of the long arms of chromosomes 5 and 7.[21] The development of AML after prolonged exposure to an epipodophyllotoxin is now well established, but the quantity of the risk is controversial. Within the Medical Research Council (MRC) (United Kingdom) studies, the incidence in children treated primarily for ALL is 0.3 per cent and has not increased overall since the introduction of two short intensive blocks of epipodophyllotoxin chemotherapy. Much higher incidences reported from the USA have been associated with different epipodophyllotoxin drug scheduling, usually given once or twice weekly for longer periods, and this information must not be allowed to cloud the real issue, which is that cure of leukaemia is paramount and the risk of secondary AML is very small if appropriate scheduling of epipodophyllotoxins is followed. Those exposed to the epipodophyllotoxins have a leukaemia with a short latency period and are most frequently of monocytic or myelomonocytic subtype with characteristic involvement of the *ALL-1* gene on chromosome 11 (q2,3).[21]

PATHOGENESIS

Acute leukaemias are acquired genetic disorders, as somatic mutations can be detected in the bone marrow or peripheral blood. They usually arise when the normal haemopoietic stem cell undergoes dysregulated proliferation and clonal expansion, following a structural and/or numerical change in its genetic material. The change usually results in qualitative and/or quantitative alterations in the proteins (growth factors, growth factor receptors, cytoplasmic signal transducers, nuclear transcription factors) that regulate cell cycle control, apoptosis, cell proliferation and differentiation, and thus turn housekeeping genes into 'tumour' genes.

The majority of these genetic changes involve translocation events leading to activation of an oncogene or anti-apoptotic gene. The breakpoints involved in some of these translocations have identified new cellular proto-oncogenes that contribute to the leukaemic process. These novel fusion products, usually acting as *trans*-activating proteins (transcription factors), ultimately lead to block(s) in cellular differentiation and aberrant cell proliferation. For example, a cellular differentiation blockade event is seen in acute promyelocytic leukaemia where the t(15;17) translocation involving the retinoic acid receptor is implicated, whereas the expression of a leukaemia-specific anti-apoptotic gene, e.g. *bcr-abl*, is observed in chronic myeloid leukaemia (CML) and Philadelphia chromosome positive ALL.

As stated above, many of the genes that are involved in translocation events are transcription factors and a small number of these genes may have different translocation partners (translocational promiscuity), leading to the concept of master genes – genes whose products regulate many different processes in normal haemopoiesis which, when mutated, can give rise to different forms of leukaemia depending on their promiscuous partner. The most common structural genetic abnormality in childhood leukaemia is a fusion of two genes, *TEL* (chromosome 12) and *AML1* (chromosome 21). Several different translocation events have been shown to target the 21q22 region of chromosome 21 and disrupt the *AML1* gene. *AML1* encodes a DNA binding protein that is part of a core binding protein factor complex (CBF) implicated in the transcriptional regulation of a variety of genes involved in haemopoiesis, including GM-CSF and myeloperoxidase. In the normal situation, *AML1* interacts with a transactivator (TA) and core binding factor β (CBFβ). In t(3;21) and t(8;21) translocations, the TA portion is replaced by *EAP*, *MDS-1* or *EVI-1* genes (chromosome 3) or *ETO* (chromosome 8). Replacement of the TA domain means that, although *AML1/ETO* or *AML1/EVI-1* can bind to target genes, they cannot activate them. In addition, inv 16 generates a core binding factor β/smooth muscle myosin heavy chain (CBFβ/SMMHC) fusion which similarly cannot activate target genes. Other mechanisms may also perturb *AML1*, as the t(12;21) generating a TEL/AML1 fusion protein involves a virtually intact AML1 protein, complete with its transactivating domain. Other genes also function as 'master genes', the most prominent being the mixed lineage leukaemia gene (*MLL*) which shares homology to the *Drosophila* gene *trithorax* and which, when mutated by translocation, can lead to a variety of acute leukaemias – the 11q23 abnormalities.[21]

Other genetic alterations that lead, directly or indirectly, to defective clonal haemopoiesis with the potential to evolve into leukaemia include chromosome number and, at a more subtle level, there may also be gene deletions, especially involving chromosomes 5 and 7,[22] or single nucleotide base changes in genes such as *Flt3* and *p53*,[23–26] or overexpression of anti-apoptotic proteins such as Bcl-2[27–29] or the *ras* family.[30,31] Unfortunately, a comprehensive account of what is currently known about the pathobiological basis of leukaemogenesis is far beyond the scope of this chapter, but molecular insights into specific leukaemia subgroups are outlined below.

CLINICAL MANIFESTATIONS

The clinical features seen in childhood leukaemia are related to inhibition of normal haemopoiesis by leukaemic replacement of the bone marrow and also by extramedullary involvement. Any combination of cytopenias may be seen at presentation and these are usually reflected in the patients' symptoms and signs, i.e. fever and granulocytopenia, bruising/bleeding and thrombocytopenia, fatigue/pallor and anaemia. Whilst bone and joint pain is less frequently seen at presentation, neurological manifestations, such as impaired vision and headache, are more common in AML than in ALL.

More specific clinical features are seen in association with certain subtypes of leukaemia. Infants with ALL, as well as AML, present with a relatively unique constellation of features, including a high circulating blast count, massive organomegaly and central nervous system (CNS) involvement. Whilst the majority of these cases will have the translocation t(4;11), it should be remembered that a similar presentation is seen in infants with the translocation t(1;22)/AML megakaryoblastic subtype (M7), although the circulating blast count is usually much lower and there is usually leucoerythroblastosis obvious on the blood smear. Children with T-cell ALL may present with signs associated with the presence of a mediastinal mass and a high white cell count (usually $>100 \times 10^9$/L) and there is a male predominance. In children with Burkitt-like pathology (mature B-cell ALL), a leukaemic presentation is almost specific for the sporadic type. The sporadic form also frequently involves the testis, ovary, pleura, cerebrospinal fluid, peripheral lymph nodes and the pharynx in approximately 15 per cent of cases. Coagulopathy was frequently a problem in AML-acute promyelocytic leukaemia (M3) prior to the use of all-*trans* retinoic acid (ATRA) and was felt to be multifactorial in origin, but disturbances in the primary fibrinolytic pathway are at the forefront of its pathogenesis. Gum hypertrophy, CNS and skin infiltration (leukaemia cutis) are not uncommon in the monocytoid varieties, AML-M4 and AML-M5. The majority of cases of congenital/infant leukaemia are AML-M5, and more than 50 per cent of these have skin infiltration, the so-called 'blueberry muffin'. Isolated extramedullary collections of AML, more commonly known as 'granulocytic sarcoma' or 'chloroma', occur in less than 2 per cent of childhood AML cases. These tumours can occur anywhere but have a predilection for the paranasal sinuses, orbit, skin, CNS, respiratory and gastrointestinal tracts, and lymph node regions. Difficulty with marrow aspiration 'dry tap' and pancytopenia are usually seen in association with marrow fibrosis in megakaryoblastic leukaemia, AML-M7.

CLASSIFICATION AND DIAGNOSIS

The first internationally accepted classification of acute leukaemia was proposed in 1975 by a group of French, American and British (FAB) haematologists.[32] The classification was subsequently revised and expanded on two further occasions and is considered by many the gold standard for subclassifying AML on the basis of lineage commitment and degree of blast differentiation.[33] The same pattern did not apply to ALL as there was no clear association between morphological, immunophenotypic and genetic correlates with the exception of the distinctive L3 and its variants. The major problem with the FAB classification was that it failed to incorporate evolving new immunological and cytogenetic data that were shedding light onto the pathobiological basis of leukaemogenesis. The classification also failed to contribute to better treatment designs in acute leukaemia. In 1988, the Morphologic Immunological and Cytogenetic (MIC) Group recognized for the first time the importance of subgrouping leukaemia by cytogenetics,[34] and in 2001 the World Health Organization (WHO) published its classification that incorporated not only morphological, immunological and cytogenetic data but also molecular genetic studies that have a direct correlation to laboratory and clinical features of acute leukaemia (Table 4.1).[35] Numerous differences between the WHO and FAB classifications exist, but a detailed discussion goes beyond the scope of this chapter.

Morphology

According to FAB criteria, ALL can be subdivided into three groups, L1, L2 and L3, from the morphological appearance of lymphoblasts in the blood and marrow (Table 4.2). With L1 disease, the lymphoblasts usually have uniformly inconspicuous nucleoli. L2 blasts consist of large heterogeneous cells with more cytoplasm, irregular nuclei and prominent nucleoli, and L3 blasts are characterized by large size with abundant, deeply basophilic cytoplasm, round nuclei, prominent nucleoli and cytoplasmic vacuoles. Rarely, ALL may present with an associated hypereosinophilia. This may precede the diagnosis of ALL and is usually seen when the translocation t(5;14)(q31.1;q32.3) is present.

In AML, the morphological basis of the FAB system relies on identifying the lineage (myeloblast, monoblast, erythroblast and megakaryoblast) and degree of differentiation of the leukaemic cells. The FAB classification for AML is divided into eight groups (M0–M7) with a number of subgroups (Table 4.3). The diagnosis of AML is made when 30 per cent or more of the nucleated cells in the marrow are blasts of non-lymphoid origin. Whilst good morphology and cytochemistry remain the gold standard for diagnosing AML, a number of morphological problems still exist with the present FAB criteria. Approximately 15 per cent of AML samples are difficult to classify using the present nomenclature. This is best illustrated in leukaemias evolving from a myelodysplastic

Table 4.1 *World Health Organization (WHO) classification of acute leukaemia with corresponding FAB classification subtypes*

WHO classification[a] subtypes[b]	Corresponding FAB
Precursor lymphoblastic leukaemia/lymphoblastic lymphoma	
Precursor B-cell acute lymphoblastic leukaemia/lymphoma	L1, L2
Precursor T-lymphoblastic leukaemia/lymphoblastic lymphoma	L1, L2
Burkitt lymphoma/leukaemia	
Endemic Burkitt lymphoma/leukaemia	L3
Sporadic Burkitt lymphoma/leukaemia	L3
Immunodeficiency-associated Burkitt lymphoma/leukaemia	L3
AML with recurrent genetic abnormalities	
AML with (t8;21)(q22;q22); *AMLI-ETO*	M2 > M1 > M4 > M0
AML with abnormal marrow eosinophilia and inv(16)(p13q22) or t(16:16)(p13;q22): *CBFβ-MYH11*	M4Eo > M4 > M2 > M1
Acute promyelocytic leukaemia with t(15:17)(q22;q12); *PML-RARα*	M3 > M2 > M1
AML with 11q23 abnormalities; *MLL* rearrangements	M5M4 > M2 > M1 > M0
AML with multilineage dysplasia	
Following a myelodysplastic syndrome or myeloproliferative disorder or without antecedent myelodysplastic syndrome	M2 > M4 > M6
AML and myelodysplastic syndrome, therapy-related	
Alkylating agent-related	M2 > M4 > M6
Topoisomerase type II inhibitor-related	M5 > M4 > M2 > M1
Other types	
AML not otherwise categorized	
Acute myeloid leukaemia minimally differentiated	M0
Acute myeloid leukaemia without maturation	M1
Acute myeloid leukaemia with maturation	M2
Acute myelomonocytic leukaemia	M4
Acute monoblastic leukaemia	M5
Acute erythroid leukaemia	M6
Acute megakaryoblastic leukaemia	M7
Acute basophilic leukaemia	–
Acute panmyelosis with myelofibrosis	M7; ?M1; ?MDS
Myeloid sarcoma	–

FAB, French-American-British; MDS, myelodysplastic syndrome.
[a] For details, see Second MIC Cooperative Study Group.[34]
[b] For details, see Bennett *et al*.[32,33]

Table 4.2 *FAB morphologic classification for acute lymphoblastic leukaemia*

	L1	L2	L3
Size of blast	Small, uniform	Large, variable	Medium to huge, uniform
Amount of cytoplasm	Scanty	Variable	Molecule
Cytoplasmic basophilia	Slight	Variable	Intense
Cytoplasmic vacuoles	Variable	Variable	Prominent
Nucleus	Regular, occasional clefting, homogenous chromatin	Irregular, clefting, common heterogenous chromatin	Regular, non-cleft, finely stripped chromatin
Nucleolus	0–1, inconspicuous	1 or more, prominent	2–5 prominent
Nuclear/cytoplasmic ratio	High	Low	Low

FAB, French-American-British.

or pre-leukaemic disorder, in some AML-M3 and AML-M5b types that contain less than 30 per cent blasts in the bone marrow and the stipulation that 50 per cent or more erythroblasts should be present before making the diagnosis of AML-M6 and -M7. Furthermore, the FAB classification lacks a category for hybrid and biphenotypic leukaemias, eosinophilic, basophilic and mast cell and primitive erythroblastic leukaemias.

Table 4.3 *FAB classification of acute myeloid leukaemia (AML) divided into eight groups*

FAB category	Criteria for FAB typing	Cytochemistry
M0 (AML with minimal evidence of myeloid maturation)	Morphologically undifferentiated blasts Myeloid phenotype Lymphoid markers negative	<3% blasts positive for SBB or MPO No Auer rods present on SBB or MPO Esterases negative in the blast cells
M1 (AML without maturation)	Blasts >90% of BM NEC Maturing monocytic cells <10% Maturing granulocytes <10%	3–100% blasts positive for SBB or MPO Usually localized pattern of positivity SBB- or MPO-positive Auer rods frequently present Chloroacetate-positive cells <10% NSE- or BE-positive cells scanty or absent
M2 (AML with maturation)	Blasts 30–89% of NEC Maturing granulocytes >10% of NEC Monocytic component <20%	3–100% blasts positive for SBB or MPO Usually localized pattern of positivity SBB- or MPO-positive Auer rods frequently present SBB- or MPO-negative neutrophils may be present if dysplastic Chloroacetate-positive cells >10% (maturing granulocytes) NSE- or BE-positive cells scanty or absent
M3 (hypergranular promyelocytic leukaemia) M3 variant (hypogranular promyelocytic leukaemia)	M3 shows marrow replacement by granular and hypergranular promyelocytes M3 variant shows mainly agranular basophilic cells, bilobed nuclei	SBB and MPO show characteristic heavy staining filling the cytoplasm Multiple SBB- or MPO-positive Auer rods present, often obscured by heavy cytoplasmic staining Majority of cells are chloroacetate esterase-positive Auer rods are chloroacetate-positive Leukaemic promyelocytes show a deep pink cytoplasmic blush with PAS stain t(15;17) demonstrable by cytogenetics, RT-PCR or FISH Microparticulate nuclear PML protein pattern
M4 (acute myelomonocytic leukaemia)	Blasts >30% of NEC Granulocyte component >20% of BM NEC	Esterase stains show a mixture of chloroacetate and NSE- or BE-positive cells, usually >20% of each Some cells may show both types of esterase 3–100% blasts positive for SBB or MPO, localized

	Monocytic component >20% of BM NEC	pattern in the myeloblasts, scattered pattern in monoblasts/monocytes SBB- or MPO-positive Auer rods common SBB- or MPO-negative neutrophils if dysplasia present
M4EO	Typical large 'eosinophils' present which define presence of inv/del/t(16)	Usually conforms to M4 by conventional criteria, but may occasionally be M2 by FAB criteria Inv/del/t(16) demonstrable by cytogenetics, RT-PCR or FISH
M5a and M5b [acute monoblastic leukaemia without maturation (M5a) and with maturation (M5b)]	Blasts >30% of BM NEC >80% monocytic component of BM NEC M5a when monoblasts >80% of BM NEC M5b when monoblasts <80% of BM NEC	Usually >80% of BM cells show NSE or BE positivity Chloroacetate-positive cells usually rare, but always <20% SBB and MPO may be negative in the blasts/monocytes SBB- or MPO-positive Auer rods rare
M6 (erythroleukaemia)	Erythroid cells (all stages) >50% of BM Cells Myeloid blasts >30% of BM NEC	Some/many erythroid precursors positive on PAS stain. Rarely all negative Some myeloid blasts SBB- or MPO-positive SBB- or MPO-positive Auer rods occasionally present
M7 (acute megakaryoblastic leukaemia)	Blasts mainly megakaryoblasts shown by immunological methods	Immunological confirmation of megakaryocytic blasts required (>30%) Trephine biopsy may be helpful Megakaryoblasts may show platelet-like granules on PAS stain Focal NSE (but not BE) positivity may be present Myeloid blasts may show SBB or MPO positivity and rarely Auer rods

BE, butyrate esterase; BM, bone marrow; FAB, French American British; FISH, fluorescence *in situ* hybridization; MPO, myeloperoxidase; NEC, non-erythroid compartment; NSE, non-specific esterase; PAS, periodic acid–Schiff; SBB, Sudan black B.

Cytochemistry

There are no positive diagnostic cytochemical stains that distinguish ALL. Lymphoblasts are negative for myeloperoxidase (MPO), chloroacetate esterase (CAE) and non-specific esterase (NSpE), but very fine positive cytoplasmic granules may rarely be present with Sudan black B (SBB). Characteristic block positivity (rosary bead pattern), usually on a clear background (in contrast to AML, especially M1, M4, M5 and M6) with periodic acid–Schiff (PAS) staining, may corroborate a diagnosis of ALL; however, it should be remembered that similar reactivity can be seen in some cases of AML-M6 and -M7 (Table 4.3). Terminal deoxynucleotidyl transferase (TdT) is positive in >90 per cent of ALL cases, but it can also be positive in up to 10 per cent of AML cases. T-cell ALL cases usually show block positivity with acid phosphatase stain predominantly in the area of the Golgi apparatus, which shows up as a strong, focal 'red dot like' structure. ALL L3 blasts often stain with oil red O due to the presence of neutral lipids within the cytoplasmic vacuoles.

Cytochemical staining is usually required for the initial categorization of AML and the most widely used stains include MPO, SBB, NSpE, CAE and PAS. The relationship between cytochemical staining, morphology and immunophenotype of AML blasts is shown in Table 4.4.

Immunophenotype

Immunophenotyping of blast cells by flow cytometric analysis (FCM) in suspected cases of ALL is essential in making the correct diagnosis. The ability to detect intracellular antigens by FCM has considerably improved the diagnostic accuracy of immunophenotyping. Nuclear TdT, cytoplasmic CD79a (B-lineage), CD3 (T-lineage) and MPO (myeloid lineage) are reliably detectable.

Simultaneous assessment of the three cytoplasmic antigens with multicolour FCM, together with membrane markers such as CD34 and CD45 to identify the blast cells, is a powerful technique which virtually eliminates the possibility of misdiagnosis.

In B-cell ALL, immunological classification includes four subgroups (Table 4.5): early B precursor or Pro-B ALL, B-precursor ALL, pre-B ALL and mature B-ALL.[36] Pro-B ALL, thought to be derived from a very immature B-cell precursor, is characterized by a CD10-negative immunophenotype and the absence of cytoplasmic μ (cy-μ). It is most often observed in infants with ALL, especially those with abnormalities involving chromosome 11q23 (*MLL* gene locus). The other three subgroups can be distinguished by using CD19, cy-μ and surface immunoglobulin (smIg). B-precursor ALL only shows CD19, pre-B ALL expresses CD19 and cy-μ, and B-ALL shows CD19 and smIg. The malignant nature of the ALL cells is determined by TdT, CD10 and CD34. As stated above, TdT is present in the vast majority of cases of ALL (except B-ALL). CD10 (common ALL antigen), in association with CD19, CD22, TdT, cytoplasmic CD79a and CD34, and lack of cy-μ, and smIg expression are seen in most cases of B-lineage ALL, so-called 'common precursor-B' ALL or 'early precursor-B' ALL. CD34 positivity is usually not present in pre-B ALL and may be positive in some cases of B-cell ALL. Other antibodies that may help in defining ALL include HLA-DR, CD20 and CD22 (Table 4.5). Cytoplasmic CD22 appears early in the B-cell development and is consistently positive in B-ALL, and CD79a, a relatively new marker developed by the St Judes' Children's Research Hospital to identify B cells in ALL cases, is highly sensitive for B cells.[37–39]

Expression of a myeloid antigen can be seen in some ALLs, especially those of precursor-B lineage. Conversely, some AMLs may express a lymphoid-associated marker. These leukaemias, which are very rare in children, may

Table 4.4 *Cytochemical and immunophenotyping of acute leukaemias*

FAB	Cytochemical	Markers
M0	MPO−, SB−, CAE−, NSE−	CD13, CD33, CD34, TdT+/−, HLA-DR, cyMPO
M1	MPO+, SB+, CAE+, NSE−	CD13, CD33, HLA-DR, cyMPO
M2	MPO+, SB+, CAE+, NSE−	CD13, CD33, HLA-DR, cyMPO
M3	MPO+, SB+, CAE+, NSE−	CD13, CD33, cyMPO
M4	MPO+, SB+, CAE+, NSE+	CD13, CD33, HLA-DR, cyMPO, CD14
M5	MPO+, SB+, CAE−, NSE+	CD13, CD33, HLA-DR, cyMPO, CD14
M6	MPO+, SB+, PAS+	CD13+/−, CD33+/−, cyMPO, glycophorin A
M7	MPO−, SB+/−, PAS+	CD33, CD41, CD61, cyMPO
ALL (L1)	MPO−, SB−, PAS+	CD19, CD10+/−, sIg−
ALL (L3)	MPO−, SB−, PAS+	CD19, sIg+, kappa or lambda light chain
T-ALL	MPO−, SB−, PAS+	CD3, cyCD3+

CAE, chloroacetate esterase; cy, cytoplasmic; MPO, myeloperoxidase; NSE, non-specific esterase; PAS, periodic acid–Schiff; SB, Sudan black; sIg, surface immunoglobulin.

represent the neoplastic transformation of a stem cell at a stage prior to lineage commitment and they should not be confused with biclonal (or multiclonal) acute leukaemias defined as the coexistence of two or more distinct leukaemia populations with different phenotypes. Much controversy has surrounded the criteria for identifying such leukaemias and a variety of terms have been used, such as hybrid, biphenotypic, mixed-lineage, My+ ALL and Ly+ AML, thus creating a great deal of confusion. More recently, strict and well defined criteria have been proposed, incorporating criteria and scoring systems to define biphenotypic leukaemia (Table 4.6) by multiparameter FCM using lineage-specific (MPO, CD22, CD79a, CD3) and/or lineage-associated antigens.[40] It should be remembered that at the time of writing no clinical studies have been published showing any significant prognostic implication for these leukaemias.

Whilst the immunophenotypic classification of T-cell ALL is more controversial, a general consensus is beginning to emerge (Table 4.7).[41] The coexpression of cytoplasmic CD3 and TdT/CD34 alone is diagnostic of T-ALL.[41] A more comprehensive classification dividing T-ALL into four subgroups has been proposed (Table 4.7), but given the fact that therapeutic response and prognosis have little, if any, correlation with such subgrouping, the general consensus that is emerging is either to divide it into pre-T-cell and T-cell ALL or not to divide T-ALL into any subtype.[42,43] However, the one immunophenotypic marker that continues to have prognostic implications in T-ALL in terms of disease-free survival is CD10. Two studies found that T-ALL cases that expressed CD10 had a better prognosis than those without CD10 expression in terms of remission rate and event-free survival.[44,45]

Monoclonal antibodies directed against 'specific' myeloid antigens may be of value in separating those 10–20 per cent of cases of acute leukaemia where it is difficult to differentiate AML from ALL on morphological and cytochemical grounds. Antibodies commonly used in cataloguing AML include the panmyelomonocytic markers CD13 and CD33, which are positive in over 90 per cent of cases of AML (and are positive in 20 per cent of precursor B-ALL). CD41 (platelet glycoprotein IIb/IIIa) and CD42 (platelet glycoprotein Ib) are frequently positive in megakaryoblastic leukaemia; CD15 and CD11b, which are present on immature and mature myeloid cells as well as immature monocytic precursors, and CD14, with its more monocytic specificity, are of particular help in diagnosing AML-M4 and AML-M5 varieties. Interestingly, CD19, usually found on B cells, and stem cell antigen CD34, are frequently seen in AML-M2 with the t(8;21) translocation.[46,47] The prognostic implications of these various antigen associations in AML remain to be determined.

Table 4.5 *Immunophenotypic classification of B-lineage acute lymphoblastic leukaemia (ALL)*

Marker	Pro-B ALL	B-precursor ALL	Pre-B ALL	B-ALL
CD10	−	+	+/−	+/−
CD19	+	+	+	+
CD20	+/−	+/−	+/−	+
CD22	+	−	−	+
CD34	+	+	−	−
cyCD79a	+	+	+	+
HLA-DR	+	+	+	+
Cy-μ	−	−	+	−
Surface Ig	−	−	−	+
TdT	+	+	+/−	−

ALL, acute lymphoblastic leukaemia; cy, cytoplasmic; Ig, immunoglobulin; TdT, terminal deoxynucleotidyl transferase.

Table 4.6 *Scoring system for biphenotypic acute leukaemias (BALs)[a]*

Points	B-lineage	T-lineage	Myeloid lineage
2	CD79α cy IgM (cy) CD22	CD3 (cy/m) Anti-TCRα/β Anti-TCRγ/δ	MPO
1	CD19 CD10 CD20	CD2 CD5 CD8 CD10	CD13 CD33 CD65s CD117
0.5	TdT CD24	TdT CD7 CD1a	CD14 CD15 CD64

cy, cytoplasmic; m, membrane; MPO, myeloperoxidase; TCR, T-cell receptor; TdT, terminal deoxynucleotidyl transferase.
[a] Total scores must exceed 2 for the myeloid lineage and 1 for the lymphoid lineages. The value of each marker is given in the first column.

Table 4.7 *Immunophenotypic classification of T-cell acute lymphoblastic leukaemia (ALL)*

	CD1	CD2	CD3	SCD3	SCD3	CD4	CD5	CD7	CD8	TdT
Pre-T cell	−	−	+	−	−	−	−	+	−	+
Early cortical	−	+(75%)	+	−	−	−	+(90%)	+	−	+
Late cortical	+	+	+	+	+(25%)	+(90%)	+	+	+(90%)	+
Medullary	−	+	+	+	+	+/−	+	+	+/−	+/−

ALL, acute lymphoblastic leukaemia; CD3, cytoplasmic CD3; SCD3, surface CD3; TdT, terminal deoxynucleotidyl transferase.

Box 4.1 *Cytogenetic abnormalities in acute lymphoblastic leukaemia (ALL)*

Structural chromosomal changes in B-ALL
- t(9;22)(934;911)
- Cryptic t(12;21)(p13;q22)
- t(1;19)(q23;p13)
- t(8;14)(924;932) and variants
- MLL rearrangements (11q23)
  - → t(4;11)(q21;q23)
  - → t(6;11)(q27,Q23)
  - → t(9;11)(p12;q23)
  - → t(10;11)(p12;q23)
  - → t(11;19)(q23;p13.3)

Structural chromosomal changes in T-ALL
- t(10;14)(q24;q11)
- t(7;10)(q35;Q24)
- t(1;14)(p15;q11)
- t(7;9)(q34;q32)
- t(11;14)(p15;q11)
- t(11;14)(p13;q1)
- t(7;11)(q35;p13)
- t(8;14)(q24;q11)
Others

Numerical chromosomal abnormalities
- Hypodiploid
- Hyperdiploid (47–49 chromosomes)
- Hyperdiploid (>50 chromosomes)
- Near triploidy
- Near tetraploidy

Cytomolecular genetics

Cytogenetic analysis of leukaemic blasts provides important information in up to 90 per cent of cases of ALL that is clinically relevant for diagnosis and prognosis of childhood leukaemia (Box 4.1).[48] There are two major classes of cytogenetic aberrations: those that result in the visible loss or gain of chromosomal material and those that result in a balanced exchange without apparent loss or gain of DNA.[49] Loss may be characterized as partial (deletion, del) or complete loss of a chromosome (monosomy). Gains may refer to portions of chromosomes (e.g. duplications) or whole chromosomes (trisomy, tetrasomy). Unidentified abnormal chromosomes are labelled as markers (mar). Balanced alterations involve the reciprocal exchange of genetic material either between two or more chromosomes (translocations, t) or between various portions of one chromosome (inversions, inv).

Whilst this type of conventional cytogenetic data (karyotypic analysis) has provided information that led to identification and localization of genes involved in leukaemogenesis, there are a number of limitations. Firstly, only a few cells in metaphase are analysed. Secondly, analysis is entirely dependent upon the production of high-quality metaphase preparations and is significantly restricted for cells that have low mitotic rates or cannot easily be grown in culture. It is also very labour-intensive. For these reasons, and because conventional karyotypic analysis may not reveal all cytogenetic abnormalities and gene alterations, molecular cytogenetics in the form of fluorescent *in situ* hybridization (FISH) and polymerase chain reaction (PCR) has been employed to increase the sensitivity level for detection of genetic defects.[50–53]

Although specific cytogenetic abnormalities in ALL can be related to immunophenotype, with the exception of t(8;14)(q24;q32) and its FAB L3 variants, they do not show a close relationship to the FAB subtype. On the other hand, in AML, chromosomal abnormalities, including t(8;21)(q22;q22) FAB M2, t(15;17)(q22;q21) FAB M3, inv(16)(p13;q22) FAB M4 E0 and t(9;11)(q2;q23) FAB M5, have been associated with specific morphological features (Table 4.8).

In terms of numeric changes, hyperdiploidy, which is the most frequent chromosomal abnormality in ALL, has been identified in over 40 per cent of cases of precursor-B-cell disease (Box 4.1). High hyperdiploidy (51–65 chromosomes), which occurs in approximately 27 per cent of ALL cases, is associated with a particularly favourable response to anti-metabolite blood therapy, which translates into an event-free survival in excess of 85 per cent.[54–56] This karyotype is usually associated with other good risk features of age ≥1 and <10 years, a low white cell count and pre-B immunophenotype.[57] Within the high hyperdiploid group, children with chromosomal numbers between 56 and 67 do better than the subgroup with 51–55, translating into event-free survivals of 86 and 72 per cent at 5 years, respectively. These chromosomal genes normally involve chromosomes 4, 6, 10, 14, 17, 18, 21 and the X chromosome. Trisomies involving chromosomes 4, 6, 10 and 17 are associated with a good prognosis, whilst trisomy 5, a rare abnormality in childhood ALL, is associated with a poor prognosis.[58–60]

Gene expression profiles

Recent advances in DNA microarray assay technology in association with bioinformatics has enabled gene expression profiles to be produced that categorize specific leukaemias. For example, Golub *et al.*[61] analysed 27 patients with ALL and 11 with AML and were able to define 50 of 1100 genes that allow ALL to be distinguished from AML, but also B-lineage ALL from T-lineage ALL, with approximately 100 per cent accuracy. Further studies on bigger ALL samples have been able to identify several prognostic cytogenetic subgroups of B-lineage

Table 4.8 *Morphological, immunological and cytogenetic (MIC) classification of acute leukaemia*

MIC group	FAB	Immunological markers							Karyotype
		CD2	CD7	CD10	CD19	TdT	cIg	cIg	
ALL									
Early B-precursor ALL	L1, L2		−	−/+	+	+	−	−	t(4;11); t(9;22)[a]
Common ALL	L1, L2		−	+	+	+	−	−	6q−; near-haploid; del(12), or t(9;22)
Pre-B ALL	L1		−	+	+	+	+	−	t(1;19); t(9;22)
B-cell ALL	L3		−	+/−	+	−	−	−	t(8;14); t(2;8); t(8;22)
Early T-precursor ALL	L1, L2	+	+		−	+			t/del(9p)
T-cell ALL	L1, L2	+	+		−	+			6q−

MIC group	FAB	Immunological markers						Karyotype
		CD7	CD19	CD13	CD33	GPA	CD41	
AML								
M2/t(8;21)	M2	−	−	+	+	−	−	t(8;21)(q22;q22)
M3/t(15;17)	M3, M3v	−	−	+	+	−	−	t(15;17)(q22;q12)
M5a/del(11q23)	M5a (M5b, M4)	−	−	+	+	−	−	t/del(11)(q23)
M4Eo/inv(16)	M4Eo	−	−	+	+	−	−	del/inv(16)(q23)
M1/t(9;22)	M1 (M2)	−	−	+	+	−	−	t(9;22)(q34;q11)
M2/t(6;9)	M2 or M4 with basophilia	−	−	+	+	−	−	
M1/inv(3)	M1m (M2, M4, M7) with thrombocytosis	−	−	+	+	−	−	Inv(3)(q21; q26)
M5b/t(8;16)	M5b with phagocytosis	−	−	+	+	−	−	T(8;16)(p11;p13)
M2	M2 with basophilia	−	−	+	+	−	−	t/del(12)(p11–13)
Bason/t(12p) M4/+4	M4 (M2)	−	−	+	+	−	−	+4

+, positive; −, negative; no symbol, not specified by MIC workshop.

FAB, French–American–British Classification; GPA, glycophorin A; TdT, terminal deoxynucleotidyl transferase.

[a] CD10 is usually negative in case of t(4;11) and positive in case of t(9;22).

ALL – hyperdiploid >50, t(12;21), t(1;19) and MLL – with 95–100 per cent accuracy.[62] This technique may also be able to predict those patients who will do less well with combination chemotherapy regimens and who will therefore be candidates for more intense/experimental therapies. This molecular genetic strategy may also be powerful enough to shed further light onto the genetic drivers of leukaemogenesis, and in addition may generate a patient leukaemic-specific gene fingerprint that will warrant individualized treatment approaches.

BIOLOGICAL SUBSETS

Infant leukaemias

11q23

As stated above, infant leukaemias tend to have a unique clinical presentation with high circulating blast counts, massive organomegaly and CNS involvement. After neuroblastoma these are the commonest malignancies

seen in infancy and they account for approximately 4 per cent of childhood ALL and 10 per cent of childhood AML. Unlike in older children, in whom ALL is the predominant leukaemia, in infants it is only marginally more common. The majority of infant leukaemias, both AML and ALL, are associated with a translocation involving 11q23 and its various partners in 50 and 80 per cent of cases, respectively. The commonest translocations involving 11q23 in ALL are t(4;11) and t(11;19), and in approximately two-thirds of cases involve the CD10-negative B-lineage precursor cell (also called Pro-B ALL), with the rest consisting of common/pre-B types. The single most common translocation in AML involving this region occurs at t(9;11)(p22;q2,3) and is associated with monocytic morphology (AML-M5).[63] 11q23 translocations of differing types are seen in children with ALL who have been treated with the epipodophyllotoxins, etoposide (VP16) and teniposide (VM26), and have developed secondary AML.[64–66]

The gene involved in these chromosomal translocations that maps to 11q23 was cloned by a number of groups; hence the many abbreviations ascribed to it

(*HRX*, *ALL-1* and *MLL*).[67-69] A 15-kb mRNA is transcribed from 11q23 and translated into a 430-kDa protein. This protein shares sequence homology with the *Drosophila trithorax* regulator, which plays a key role in the embryonic development of the fruit fly. The precise leukaemogenic events that result from the expression of this protein have not been fully elucidated, but probably involve impairment of the transcription factor function of *MLL*, as a result of which the translocation breaks the gene between the two DNA binding regions.

t(1;22)(p13;q13)

This subtype of AML, megakaryoblastic leukaemia (M7), has been predominantly described in very young non-Down's syndrome children who do not have a preceding transient abnormal myelopoiesis or evidence of myelodysplasia.[70,71] The translocation involves two oncogenes, N-*ras* located in the breakpoint 1p13, and c-*sis* located at chromosome 22p13.[72] N-*ras* is felt to be activated due to its translocation and this in turn leads to the malignant phenotype, whilst the c-*sis* gene encodes for platelet-derived growth factor β (PDGFβ) and its dysregulation gives rise to marked increases in c-*sis* m-RNA in megakaryoblasts.[73,74] The increase in PDGFβ protein in the marrow microenvironment is felt to play an important role in the genesis of the widespread bone marrow fibrosis that is usually seen in these infants. The marrow fibrosis ultimately leads to extramedullary haemopoiesis which presents as massive hepatosplenomegaly and paraspinal haemopoietic outgrowths. Children with t(1;22)(p13;q13)/M7 are said to respond less well to chemotherapy and stem cell replacement therapies than do children with M7 without the translocation.

DOWN'S SYNDROME

Trisomy 21 Down's syndrome results in an approximately 20-fold increased risk of developing leukaemia when compared with constitutionally normal children.[75] Other unique haematological associations with this syndrome include:[76]

- transient abnormal myelopoiesis (TAM) – a spontaneously regressing clonal myeloproliferation that can mimic AML and occurs almost exclusively in children in the first few weeks of life
- a peak incidence of AML occurring under 4 years of age
- the association of MDS with the development of AML
- the propensity of megakaryoblastic subtype with or without marrow and hepatic fibrosis.

Down's syndrome children who develop TAM require close follow-up over the first 4 years of life, as approximately 20 per cent will develop AML.[77] The pathobiological basis by which constitutional trisomy 21 produces myeloproliferation and leukaemia development is not known.

Although the acute leukaemias seen in children with Down's syndrome are similar morphologically to the corresponding leukaemias in constitutionally normal children, their response to chemotherapy is better and this favourable response to treatment may in part be due to enhanced intracellular metabolism by cytarabine to cytarabine triphosphate by the Down's syndrome blast cells.[78] Given this increased AML blast sensitivity to cytarabine, those children with Down's syndrome and those with the t(9:11) represent a unique subgroup that will most likely benefit from high-dose cytarabine-based regimens. As a rule, stem cell transplantation is not considered in first complete remission in this group of children.

AML

t(8;21)(q22;q22)

The commonest cytogenetic abnormality seen in paediatric AML is the t(8;21)(q22;q22) translocation, occurring in approximately 20 per cent of AML-M2 cases. This reciprocal translocation involving the *ETO* gene on chromosome 8 and the *AML1* gene on chromosome 21 results in a fusion gene whose product is most likely to behave as an aberrant transcription factor. It is usually associated with Auer rods, bone marrow eosinophilia and sex chromosome loss (−Y in males and −X in females), and has a relatively good prognosis, despite its detection in bone marrow remission samples many years after completion of therapy.[79]

t(15;17)(q22;q11–21)

This translocation has been documented in 80–90 per cent of patients with AML-M3 and AML-3 variant (M3v). It occurs almost exclusively in these two FAB types and is invariably associated with coagulopathy. The gene involved on chromosome 17 is the retinoic acid receptor alpha gene (*RARα*), a member of the steroid/thyroid superfamily of nuclear transcription factors.[80] The *RARα* gene is fused to the *PML* gene, another putative transcription factor on chromosome 15. The *PML-RARα* fusion transcript is only present in the leukaemic clone and encodes for a protein that probably inhibits promyelocytic differentiation via the *RARα* receptor. The explanation for ATRA responsiveness in AML-M3 has not been fully elucidated, but is most likely to result from the retinoid altering the function of the PML-RARα fusion protein or disinhibiting the effect of the fusion protein on normal *RARα* activity. It is interesting that the rare subtype of AML-M3 harbouring the t(11;17)-(q23;q21) translocation, and hence involving the *RARα* receptor, is primarily refractory to ATRA therapy.[81,82]

inv(16)(p13;q22)

The subtype acute myelomonocytic leukaemia with eosinophils (AML-M4Eφ) is characterized by atypical eosinophils and abnormalities of chromosome 16(q22). The commonest cytogenetic defects are inv(16)(p13;q22) and del(16)(q22). The inversion involves the *CBFβ* gene, a transcription factor, and the myosin heavy-chain gene (*MYH11*) creating a fusion protein. Similar to the t(15;17) and t(8;21) chromosomal translocations, abnormalities involving 16(q22) have a higher complete remission rate, but unlike these, patients with the 16(q22) abnormality have a higher rate of CNS relapse.[83]

t(9;11)(9p21;q23)

Acute myeloid leukaemia with 11q23 abnormalities is usually associated with monocytic features. As stated above, although more than 30 chromosomal loci can participate in the 11q23 translocation, most involve 9q22, 6q27, 10p12, 27q21, or 19p13.1.[84] Until relatively recently, it was felt that all children with AML 5a or 5b with associated 11q23 abnormality had a poor prognosis with generally high remission rates but short survival times. Recent data from several groups have shown a clear survival advantage in children with the t(9;11), with event-free survival as high as 86 per cent.[85–87] It may be that monoblastic leukaemias with this translocation are highly sensitive to cytotoxic kill by etoposide and cytarabine as *in vitro* studies have indicated.[78]

t(6;9)(p23;q34)

The t(6;9)(p23;q34) is a rare translocation, usually seen in AML-M2 and AML-M4, and is associated with a poor prognosis. The function of the fusion protein resulting from the juxtaposition of the *DEK* gene on chromosome 6 and the *CAN* gene on chromosome 9 has yet to be determined. Bone marrow basophilia is commonly seen with this translocation.

3q ABNORMALITIES

Although rare in children, abnormalities involving breakpoints at 3q21 and 3q26 have been described in the majority of AML subtypes and are associated with poor clinical outcome.

MONOSOMIES 7, 5/DELETIONS 7q, 5q

Cytogenetic abnormalities involving chromosome 7 (loss of chromosome 7 or deletions of the long arm) are detected in childhood MDS, and AML in particular, with therapy-related MDS/AML following exposure to alkylating agents. In addition, monosomy 7 or 7q- occurs in MDS/AMLs that develop in children with constitutional disorders such as Fanconi's anaemia, Shwachman–Diamond syndrome, Kostman's syndrome, neurofibromatosis type 1 and familial monosomy.[88] Whether the MDS/AML with associate chromosome 7 abnormality occurs in a constitutionally normal or abnormal individual, the prognosis is extremely poor, with stem cell replacement therapy offering a better chance of cure. Two critical regions have been identified, one in band 7q22 and another in bands 7q32-q35, suggesting that these regions contain novel tumour suppressor gene(s), whose loss of function contributes to leukaemic transformation or tumour progression.[88]

Unlike monosomy 7, which is associated with approximately 7 per cent of *de novo* cases of paediatric AML, abnormalities involving the 5q chromosome are rarely seen. When present they are usually, similar to chromosome 7 abnormalities, seen in association with secondary AML (therapy-related) and AML evolving from MDS. The amount of chromosome deleted varies from patient to patient, but the most commonly deleted region involves 5q31.1.[89,90] This region encodes for the putative tumour suppressor gene, interferon regulatory factor-1 (*IFR-1*),[90] and is juxtaposed to a region encoding for many cytokine genes that display haemopoietic activity.

B–ALL

CRYPTIC t(12;21)(p13;q22)

A translocation between the short arm of chromosome 12 and the long arm of chromosome 21 was first reported in 1994 and subsequently shown to be the commonest genetic translocation in childhood ALL,[50] occurring in approximately 25 per cent of patients.[49–51] The cryptic translocation results in the *TEL/AML1* fusion gene. The TEL protein is a member of the ETS family of transcription factors.[49] The other target in this translocation is the *AML1* (*CBFA2*) gene, a member of the family of core binding factor (CBF) genes. AML1 represents one of three CBFα subunits that, together with a common CBFβ subunit, comprise functional transcription factors. Both *AML1* and *CBFβ* are involved in the translocation of several translocations in AML. CBF onco-proteins, such as the TEL/AML1 fusion product, modulate endogenous CBF activities, which is probably relevant in leukaemia transformation.

The presence of this fusion gene defines a subgroup of children with a better-than-average prognosis and interestingly this may be related to sensitivity to L-asparaginase therapy. Due to the prognostic significance of this cryptic translocation, it is essential that molecular screening for the translocation should be standard practice for improving the management of such patients.

t(8;14)(q24;q32) AND VARIANTS (L3)

The translocation t(8;14)(q24;q11) and variant forms, t(2;8)(p13;q24) and t(8;22)(q24;q32), are found in

Burkitt lymphoma and also occur in mature B-cell or Burkitt-type ALL (FAB L3). The translocation results in the activation of the c-*myc* oncogene through juxtaposition with Ig heavy-[t(8;14)] or light-chain loci [t(2;8) or t(8;22)], the former occurring more commonly. These cases constitute about 2 per cent of childhood ALL.

The breakpoint on chromosome 8 corresponds to the c-*myc* oncogene, and those on chromosome 14, 2 and 22 correspond to heavy chain, kappa and lambda light chains, respectively. Therefore, the translocations are always between the c-*myc* oncogene and an immunoglobulin gene. This translocation results in dysregulation of the c-*myc* gene and this is considered the mechanism for the mature B-cell clonal proliferation.[91] These cytogenetic abnormalities can now be detected not only by karyotyping but also by Southern blotting, PCR and FISH.[92]

Leukaemia of mature B cells more frequently involves the testis, ovary, pleura, cerebrospinal fluid, peripheral nodes and pharynx, factors that in the past probably contributed to a poorer outcome.[93] However, more recently, these patients were found to respond very well to short-term intensive chemotherapy as compared with typical ALL therapeutic regimens, and hence urgent cytogenetic or molecular confirmation of these genetic lesions is essential to treatment planning.

t(1;19)(q23;p13)

First described in 1984, this translocation is seen in approximately 5 per cent of childhood ALL cases.[94,95] It is associated with a pre-B immunophenotype and the blasts express cytoplasmic immunoglobulin (cy-μ) in a high percentage (>90 per cent) of cases.[95] Outcomes for children with ALL harbouring the t(1;19)(q23;p13) translocation treated with contemporary therapeutic protocols are comparable to those children without the translocation. RT-PCR looking for the cryptic t(1;19) is the preferred investigational tool,[96] as identification of the translocation can be missed in up to 50 per cent of cases when conventional cytogenetic analysis is used. Although this translocation is an independent prognostic factor for poor outcome, these children do usually present with high risk factors, such as high white cell counts and CNS disease.[96] Furthermore, the presence of this genotype, found in one-quarter of pre-B ALL (cy-μ-positive) cases, explains the poor prognosis previously reported with this phenotype.[96]

This translocation juxtaposes the *E2A* gene with the *PBX1* gene. E2A proteins function as transcriptional activators, which are essential for normal B-cell development.[96] The translocation creates an *E2A/ PBX1* fusion gene on the der(19) chromosome. Cases of t(1;19) ALL without detection of *E2A/PBX1* fusion transcripts have been described, suggesting that this translocation is molecularly heterogenous.

T-ALL

T-ALL accounts for approximately 10–15 per cent of cases of childhood ALL and usually presents with a high white cell count in males aged between 6 and 8 years.[97] These children usually have bulky extramedullary disease (hepatosplenomegaly with peripheral lymphadenopathy and overt CNS leukaemia), some having an anterior mediastinal mass, and white cell counts in excess of $100 \times 10^9/L$ are not unusual.[97] Historically, children with T-ALL had a worse outcome than those with B-ALL. However, with the use of more intensive chemotherapeutic protocols, this prognostic difference has been eliminated. Those children with T-cell ALL who relapse tend to do so earlier following cessation of thiopurine continuation therapy.

Although, T-cell ALL and B-cell ALL share some cytogenetic abnormalities, there are some characteristic changes that are specific to T-cell ALL. Numerical abnormalities such as hyperdiploidy are more frequently demonstrated in B-cell ALL, whereas pseudodiploidy (normal chromosomal number with structural abnormality) and near tetraploidy (chromosome >65) are more frequently seen in T-cell ALL. These cytogenetic changes translate into prognostic outcomes, i.e. cases of B-cell (hyperdiploid/near-tetraploid) ALL do better in terms of event-free survival.[97]

Genetic changes in T-ALL involve the T-cell receptor genes (TCR), *TCR-alpha* and *TCR-delta*. Rearrangements involving the TCR loci occur in up to 30 per cent of cases.[98] Several different proto-oncogenes are activated by translocations in T-ALL, the commonest being stem cell leukaemia (SCL) on the *TAL-1* gene, which is aberrantly expressed after translocation from 1p32-33 into the *TCR-alpha/delta* or *TCR-beta* locus. Most patients with *SCL/TAL-1* dysregulation have one or both *TCR-delta* genes deleted and express a CD3-positive *TCR-alpha/ beta*-positive phenotype. The important translocations involve the *TCR-alpha/delta* locus at 14q11 and are t(1;14), t(8;14), t(10;14) and t(11;14). Those involving the *TCR-beta* locus at 7q32-36 include t(1;7), t(7;9), t(7;11) and t(7;19). The prognosis of patients with *SCC/ TAL-1* expression is indistinguishable from that of patients without it. Space does not allow further exploration of the molecular genetic basis of T-ALL and readers are referred to the references cited above.

Miscellanea

ALL WITH EOSINOPHILIA AND t(5;14)(q31;q32)

Eosinophil proliferation is associated with immature B-lineage ALL with the translocation t(5;14)(q31;q32).[99] This translocation joins the interleukin-3 (IL-3) gene to the Ig heavy chain gene. The eosinophilia is probably reactive, i.e. through IL-3 gene activation, as the clonal cytogenetic lesion is not seen in the eosinophils themselves and serum IL-3 levels have been found to correlate with disease activity.[99]

Eosinophilia has been demonstrated in L1 and L2 blasts. The eosinophils demonstrate strong reactivity with MPO and SBB, moderate activity with NSpE, and are negative for CAE, AP, PAS and toluidine blue. Not all cases of ALL with eosinophilia manifest the t(5;14) chromosome rearrangement. The eosinophils may demonstrate myelodysplastic change. This type of ALL is usually more difficult to manage because of cardiac and pulmonary infiltration of eosinophils, and this tends to occur more frequently in males and in older children.[99]

APLASTIC/HYPOPLASTIC ALL

Transient pancytopenia and hypoplastic/aplastic bone marrow occur in a small number of children prior to the onset of ALL. A transient recovery of normal blood counts is followed by overt leukaemia in weeks to months. Dysplastic change is not seen in the blood or marrow and the blasts are usually of L1 FAB subtype and CD10-positive.[100] There is usually an association with a history of fever and an infectious disease prodrome; a preponderance of girls has also been noted.[100] Immunophenotype and cytogenetic analysis are not usually helpful and differentiating the marrow findings from bone marrow necrosis can be extremely difficult. It is recommended that the bone marrow should be repeated at a different site or at a later date, but in fact it usually becomes obvious with time.

DETECTION AND MONITORING OF RESIDUAL DISEASE

Molecular and cellular biological assays have defined the concept of minimal residual disease (MRD) where detection of 'leukaemia specific' DNA or RNA or 'leukaemia associated' antigens is achievable at levels of sensitivity that are much greater than morphological or karyotypic analysis.[101] The two most common methods used for MRD assessment are the detection of cells expressing abnormal immunophenotypes by FCM, and of leukaemia-associated molecular targets, e.g. fusion transcripts, such as the *BCR-ABL*, *TEL-AML1* and clone-specific immunoglobulin and T-cell receptor gene rearrangement.[102,103] Sensitivities of these two methods differ; namely, FCM can routinely detect as few as 0.01 per cent leukaemia cells in the blood or marrow, whilst PCR-based assays usually detect one leukaemia cell in 10^4–10^6 normal cells, and hence most investigators to date have used the latter technique.[98,104,105]

The majority of clinical MRD studies to date have been in childhood ALL, both during and after treatment.

Low levels or absence of MRD after completion of induction therapy appear to predict good outcome by both immunophenotyping and PCR clonality studies. However, it is important to note that quantitation of levels of MRD can be relevant in particular types of leukaemia. A steady decrease of MRD levels during treatment is associated with a good prognosis, whereas persistent high levels or increases in MRD positivity generally lead to clinical relapse. Several prospective studies have indicated that sequential sampling, preferably using a quantitative approach, allows stratification of patient risk of relapse. However, it is important to note that although this technique is a powerful and independent prognostic indicator in certain types of childhood leukaemia, it has not been proven that planning treatment according to MRD results will improve outcome or decrease toxicity.

KEY POINTS

- Childhood leukaemia comprises a very heterogenous group of malignancies.
- Diagnosis relies on morphological, immunophenotypic and cytomolecular genetic evaluation as defined by the French-American-British (FAB) and World Health Organization classifications.
- Similar to its epidemiology, the pathobiological basis of childhood leukaemia is complex, involving gene–enviroment interactions.
- Biological subsets based on clinical and molecular genetic characteristics allow specific treatment regimens to be given.
- Quantitative PCR-based MRD analysis has changed our definition of remission and thus has allowed us to identify very high-risk and very low-risk patients in terms of relapse. However, this approach requires further evaluation in a prospective manner.
- Gene expression microarray has not only identified biologicallly relevant subgroups of ALL based on distinctive gene expression profiles but may also have the ability to identify subgroups of patients who are most likely to relapse on a given therapeutic protocol or develop myelodysplasia following cure of their leukaemia.

REFERENCES

1. Bennett JH. Case of hypertrophy of the spleen and liver, in which death took place from suppuration of the blood. *Edinb Med Surg J* 1845; **64**: 413–23.

2. Craigie D. Case of disease of the spleen, in which death took place in consequence of the presence of purulent matter in the blood. *Edinb Med Surg J* 1845; **64**: 400–13.

3. Virchow R. Weisses Blut. *Froriep's Notizen* 1845; **36**: 151–7.

4. Velpeau A. Sur la resorption du pus et sur l'alteration du sang dans les maladies *Rev Med* 1827; **2**: 218–34 (as quoted by R. Virchow in *Virchows Arch Path Anat Physiol* 1853; **5**: 56–65).

5. Donne A. *Cours de Microscopie Complementaire des Etudes Medicales, Anatomie Microscopique et Physiologie des Fluides.* Paris: Baillière, 1844; 132–6.

6. Virchow R. 'Zur pathologischen Physiologie des Blutes. II Weisses Blut. *Virchows Arch Path Anat Physiol* 1847; **1**: 563–72.

7. Friedreich N. Ein neuer Fall von Leukaemie. *Arch Pathol Anat* 1857; **12**: 37–68.

8. Neumann E. Ueber myelogene Leukamie. *Berl Klin Wochenschr* 1878; **15**: 131–43.

9. Naegeli O. Ueber rotes Knochenmark und myeloblasten. *Dtsch Med Wochenschr* 1900; 26: 287–90.

10. Reschad H, Schilling-Torgau V. Ueber eine neue Leukaemie durch echte uebergangsforfen (Splenocytenleukamie) und ihre Bedeutung fur die Selbstandigkeit dieser Zellen. *Munchen Med Wochenschr* 1913; **60**: 1981–4.

11. Watkins CH, Hall BE. Monocytic leukaemia of the Naegeli and Schilling types. *Am J Clin Pathol* 1940; **10**: 387–96.

12. Di Guglielmo G. Les maladies erythremisques. *Rev Hematol* 1946; **1**: 355–9.

13. Hillestad LK. Acute promyelocytic leukaemia. *Acta Med Scand* 1957; **159**: 189–94.

14. Lewis SM, Szur L. Malignant myelosclerosis. *Br Med J* 1963; **2**: 472–5.

15. Golomb HM, Rowley JD, Vardiman J *et al.* 'Microgranular' acute promyelocytic leukaemia: a distinct clinical entity. *Blood* 1980; **55**: 253–9.

16. Farber S, Diamond LK, Mercer RD *et al.* Temporary remissions in acute leukaemia in children produced by folic antagonist, 4 aminopteroylglutamic acid (aminopterin). *N Engl J Med* 1948; **238**: 787–93.

17. Linet MS. The leukaemias: epidemiological aspects. In: Likenfield AM, ed. *Monographs in Epidemiology and Biostatistics.* Oxford: Oxford University Press, 1985.

18. Stivrins TJ, Davis R, Sanger W *et al.* Transformation of Fanconi's anaemia to acute non lymphocytic leukaemia associated with emergence of monosomy 7. *Blood* 1984; **64**: 173–6.

19. Greaves M. Clinical review: science, medicine and the future *Br Med J* 2002; **324**: 283–7.

20. Greaves M. A natural history of paediatric acute leukaemia. *Blood* 1993; **82**: 1043–51.

21. Pui CH, Ribeiro R, Hancock M *et al.* Acute myeloid leukaemia in children treated with epipodophyllotoxins for acute lymphoblastic leukaemia. *N Engl J Med* 1991; **325**: 1682–7.

22. Martinez-Climent JA, Lane NJ, Rubin CM *et al.* Clinical and prognostic signficance of chromosomal abnormalities in childhood acute myeloid leukaemia de novo. *Leukemia* 1995; **9**: 95–101.

23. Kastan MB, Radin AI, Kuerbits SJ *et al.* Levels of p53 protein increase with maturation in human haemopoietic cells. *Cancer Res* 1991; **51**: 4279–86.

24. Slingerland J, Minden M, Benchimol S. Mutations of the p53 gene in human acute myelogenous leukaemia. *Blood* 1991; **77**: 1500–7.

25. Fenaux P, Preudhomme C, Quiquandon I *et al.* Mutations of the p53 gene in acute myeloid leukaemia. *Br J Haematol* 1992; **80**: 178–83.

26. Fenaux P, Jonveaux P, Quiquandon I *et al.* p53 mutations in acute myeloid leukaemia with 17p monosomy. *Blood* 1991; **78**: 1652–7.

27. Sachs L, Lotem J. Control of programmed cell death in normal and leukaemic cells: new implications for therapy. *Blood* 1993; **82**: 15–21.

28. Campos L, Rouault JP, Sabido O *et al.* High expression of bcl-2 protein in acute myeloid leukaemia cells is associated with poor response to chemotherapy. *Blood* 1993; **81**: 3091–6.

29. Lowenberg B, van Putten WLJ, Touw IP *et al.* Autonomous proliferation of leukaemic cells in vitro as a determinant of prognosis in adult acute myeloid leukaemia. *N Engl J Med* 1993; **328**: 614–19.

30. Cline MJ. Mechanisms of disease: the molecular basis of leukaemia. *N Engl J Med* 1994; **330**: 328–36.

31. Yunis J, Boot AJM, Mayer MG *et al.* Mechanisms of ras mutation in myelodysplastic syndrome. *Oncogene* 1989; **4**: 609–14.

●32. Bennett JM, Catovsky D, Daniel MT *et al.* Proposals for the classification of the acute leukaemias. French-American-British Cooperative Group. *Br J Haematol* 1976; **33**: 451–8.

●33. Bennett JM, Catovsky D, Daniel MT *et al.* Proposed revised criteria for the classification of acute myeloid leukaemia. *Ann Intern Med* 1985; **103**: 620–5.

●34. Second MIC Cooperative Study Group. Morphologic, immunologic and cytogenetic (MIC) working classification of the acute leukaemias. *Br J Haematol* 1988; **68**: 487–94.

●35. Jaffe ES, Harris NL, Stein H, Vardiman JW, eds. *World Health Organization Classification of Tumours. Pathology and Genetics of Tumours of Haematopoietic and Lymphoid Tissues.* Lyon: IARC, 2001.

36. Jennings CD, Foon KA. Recent advances in flow cytometry. Application to the diagnosis of haematologic malignancy. *Blood* 1997; **90**: 2863–92.

37. Borowitz MJ, Di Giuseppe JA. Acute lymphoblastic leukaemia. In: Knowles DM, ed. *Neoplastic Hematology*, 2nd edn. Philadelphia: Lippincott Williams & Wilkins, 2001; 1643–65.

●38. Pui C-H, Evans WE. Acute lymphoblastic leukaemia *N Engl J Med* 1998; **339**: 605–15.

39. Astsaturov IA, Matutes E, Moritla R *et al.* Differential expression of B29 (CD79b) and MB-1 (CD79a) proteins in acute lymphoblastic leukaemia. *Leukemia* 1996; **10**; 769–73.

●40. Bene MC, Castoldi G, Knapp W *et al.* Proposals for the immunological classification of acute leukaemias. European Group for the Immunological Characterisation of Leukaemias (EGIL). *Leukemia* 1995; **9**: 1783–6.

41. Borowitz MJ, Bray R, Gascoyne R et al. US Canadian Census recommendations on the immunophenotypic analysis of haematologic neoplasma by cytometry. Data analysis and interpretation. Cytometry 1997; 30: 236–44.

42. Copeland EA, McGuire EA. The biology and treatment of acute lymphoblastic leukaemia in adults. Blood 1995; 85: 1151–68.

43. Head DR, Behm FG. Acute lymphoblastic leukaemia and the lymphoblastic lymphomas of Childhood. Semin Diagn Pathol 1995; 12: 325–34.

44. Shuster JJ, Falletta JM, Pullen DJ et al. Prognostic factors in childhood T-cell acute lymphoblastic leukaemia. A Pediatric Oncology Group Study. Blood 1990; 75: 166–73.

45. Dowell BL, Borowitz MJ, Boyell JM et al. Immunologic and clinico-pathologic features of common acute lymphoblastic leukaemia. A Pediatric Oncology Group Study. Cancer 1987; 59: 2020–6.

46. Kita K, Nakase K, Miwa H. Phenotypical characteristics of acute myelocytic leukaemia associated with the t(8;21) (q22'2) chromosomal abnormality: frequent expression of immature B-cell antigen CD19 together with stem cell antigen. Blood 1992; 80: 470–7.

47. Smith FO, Lampkin BC, Versteeg C et al. Expression of lymphoid-associated cell surface antigens by childhood acute myeloid leukaemia cells lack prognostic significance. Blood 1992; 79: 2415–22.

48. Raimondi SC, Mathew S. Conventional cytogenetic techniques in the diagnosis of childhood acute lymphoblastic leukemia. Methods Mol Biol 2003; 220: 73–82.

49. Rubnitz JE, Look AT. Molecular genetics of childhood leukaemias. J Pediatr Hematol Oncol 1998; 20: 1–7.

●50. Romain SP, Le Coriat M, Berger R. E(12; 21): a new recurrent translocation in acute lymphoblastic leukaemia. Genes Chromosomes Cancer 1994; 9: 184–91.

51. Rubnitz JE, Pui CH, Downing JR. The role of TEL fusion genes in paediatric leukaemia. Leukemia 1999; 13: 6–13.

52. Ramakers-Van Waerden NL, Pieters R, Loonen AH et al. Tel/AML1 gene fusion is related to in vitro drug sensitivity for L-asparaginase in childhood acute lymphoblastic leukaemia. Blood 2002; 96: 1094–9.

53. Pui CHH, Raimondi SC, Dodge RK et al. Prognostic importance of structural chromosomal abnormalities in children with hyperdiploid (>50 chromosomes) acute lymphoblastic leukaemia. Blood 1989; 73: 1989–95.

54. Trueworthy R, Shuster J, Look T et al. Ploidy of lymphoblasts is the strongest predictor of treatment outcome in B-progenitor cell acute lymphoblastic leukaemia of childhood: a Pediatric Oncology Group study. J Clin Oncol 1992; 10: 606–11.

55. Raimondi SC, Pui C, Hancock ML et al. Heterogeneity of hyperdiploid (51–67) childhood acute lymphoblastic leukaemia. Leukemia 1996; 10: 213–24.

●56. Harris MB, Schuster JJ, Carroll A et al. Trisomy of leukaemia cell chromosomes 4 and 10 identifies children with B-progenitor cell acute lymphoblastic leukaemia with a very low risk of treatment failure: a Pediatric Oncology Group Study. Blood 1992; 79: 3316–24.

●57. Jackson JF, Boyett J, Pallen J et al. Favourable prognosis associated with hyperdiploidity in children with acute lymphoblastic leukaemia correlates with extra chromosome 6. Cancer 1990; 66: 1184–9.

●58. Heerema NA, Sather NH, Sensel MG et al. Prognostic impact of trisomies 10, 17 and 5 among children with acute lymphoblastic leukaemia and high hyperdiploidy (>50 chromosomes). J Clin Oncol 2000; 18: 1876–87.

59. Sandoval C, Mayer SP, Oxkaynak MF et al. Trisomy 5 as a sole cytogenetic abnormality in pediatric acute lymphoblastic leukemia. Cancer Genet Cytogenet 2000; 118: 69–71.

60. Pui CH, Crist WM. Biology and treatment of acute lymphoblastic leukaemia. J Pediatr 1994; 124: 491–6.

61. Golub TR, Slonim DK, Tamayo P et al. Molecular classification of cancer: Class discovery and class prediction by gene expression monitoring. Science 1999; 286: 531–7.

●62. Yeoh EJ, Williams K, Patel D et al. Expression profiling of paediatric acute lymphoblastic leukaemia (ALL) blasts at diagnosis accurately predicts both risk of relapse and of developing therapy induced acute myeloid leukaemia. Blood 2001; Suppl. 1.

63. Fourth International Workshop on Chromosomes in Leukaemia. A prospective study of acute non-lymphocytic leukaemia. Cancer Genet Cytogenet 1984; 11: 249.

64. Abe R, Sandberg AA. Significance of abnormalities involving chromosomal segment 11q22-25 in acute leukaemia. Cancer Genet Cytogenet 1984; 13: 121–7.

65. Pui C-H, Raimondi SC, Murphy SB et al. An analysis of leukaemic cell chromosomal features in infants. Blood 1987; 69: 1289–93.

66. Pui C-H, Behm FG, Raimondi SC et al. Secondary acute myeloid leukaemia in children treated for acute lymphoid leukaemia. N Engl J Med 1989; 321: 136–42.

67. Tkachuk D, Kohler S, Cleary M. Involvement of a homologue of Drosophila trithorax by 11q23 chromosomal translocations in acute leukaemia. Cell 1992; 71: 691–700.

●68. Gu Y, Nakamura T, Alder H et al. The t(4: 11) chromosome translocation of human acute leukaemias fuses the ALL-1 gene, related to Drosophilia trithorax to the AF-4 gene. Cell 1992; 71: 701–8.

●69. Zieman-van der Poel S, McCabe NR, Gill HJ et al. Identification of a gene, MLL, that spans the breakpoint in 11q23 translocations associated with human leukaemias. Proc Natl Acad Sci USA 1991; 88: 10735–9.

70. Zipursky A, Brown EJ, Chistensen H et al. Transient myeloproliferative disorder (transient leukaemia) and haematologic manifestations of Down syndrome. Clin Lab Med 1999; 19: 157–67.

71. Lu G, Altman AJ, Benn PA. Review of cytogenetic changes in acute megakaryoblastic leukaemia: one disease or several? Cancer Genet Cytogenet 1993; 67: 81–9.

72. Lion T, Haas OA, Harbott J et al. The translocation t(1;22)(p13;q13) is a non-random marker specifically associated with acute megakaryoblastic leukaemia in young children. Blood 1992; 79: 3325–30.

73. Sunami S, Fuse A, Simizu A et al. The c-sis gene expression in cells from a patient with acute megakaryoblastic leukaemia with Down's syndrome. Blood 1987; 70: 368–71.

74. Marcus RE, Hibbin JA, Matutes S et al. Megakaryoblastic transformation of myelofibrosis with expression of c-cis oncogene. Scand J Haematol 1986; **36**: 186–93.

75. Robinson IL, Nesbitt ME Jr, Salter HN et al. Down syndrome and acute leukaemia in children: a ten year retrospective study from Children's Cancer Study Group. J Pediatr 1984; **105**: 235–42.

76. Creutzig U. Treatment of acute myeloid leukaemia in children. In: Pui Ching-Hon, ed. Treatment of Acute Leukemias: New Directions for Clinical Research. Totowa NJ: Humana Press, 2002; 237–54.

●77. Taub JW, Huang X, Matherly LH et al. Expression of chromosome 21-localised genes in acute leukaemia: differences between Down syndrome and non-Down syndrome blast cells and relationship to in vitro sensitivity to cytosine arabinoside and daunorubicin. Blood 1999; **94**: 1393–400.

●78. Zwann CM, Kaspers GJ, Pieters R et al. Cellular drug resistance in childhood acute myeloid leukaemia is related to chromosomal abnormalities. Blood 2002; **100**: 3352–60.

79. Nucifora G, Larson RA, Rowley JD et al. Persistence of the 8: 21 translocation in patients with acute myeloid leukaemia type M2 in long term remission. Blood 1993; **82**: 712–15.

80. Evans R. The steroid and thyroid hormone receptor superfamily. Science 1988; **240**: 889–94.

81. Warrell RP, Maslak P, Eardley A et al. Treatment of acute promyelocytic leukaemia with ATRA: an update of the New York experience. Leukemia 1994; **8**: 929–33.

●82. Biondi A, Rovelli A, Cantu-Rajnoldi A et al. Acute promyelocytic leukaemia in children: experience of AIEOP. Leukemia 1994; **8**: 1264–8.

83. Holmes R, Keating MJ, Cork A et al. A unique pattern of central nervous system leukaemia in acute myelomonocytic leukaemia associated with inv(16)(p13q22). Blood 1985; **65**: 1071–8.

84. Moorman AV, Hagemeijer A, Charrin C et al. The translocation t(9; 11)(q23; p13.1) and t(11; 19)(q23; p13.13.3): a cytogenetic and clinical profile of 53 patients. Leukemia 1998; **12**: 788–91.

●85. Lie SO, Abrahamsson J, Clausen N et al. Treatment stratification based on initial in vivo response in acute myeloid leukaemia in children without Down syndrome: results of NOPHO-AML. Br J Haematol 2003; **122**: 217–25.

●86. Pui CH, Raimondi SC, Srivastava DK et al. Prognostic factors in infants with acute myeloid leukaemia. Leukemia 2000; **14**: 684–6.

●87. Pui CH, Raimondi SC, Tong X. Favourable impact of the t(9; 11) in childhood acute myeloid leukaemia. J Clin Oncol 2002; **20**: 2303–9.

88. Fischer K, Frohling S, Scherer, SW et al. Molecular cytogenetic delineation of deletions and translocations involving chromosome band 7q22 in myeloid leukaemia. Blood 1997; **80**: 2036–41.

89. Le Beau M, Lemons R, Espinosa R et al. IL4 and IL5 map to human chromosome 5 in a region encoding growth factors and receptors and are deleted in myeloid leukaemias with the del(5q). Blood 1989; **73**: 647–53.

90. Miyamoto M, Fujita T, Kimura Y et al. Regulated expression of a gene encoding a nuclear factor, IRF-1, that specifically binds to INF-beta gene regulatory elements. Cell 1988; **54**: 903–6.

91. Siebert R, Mathiesen P, Harder S et al. Application of interphase fluorescence in situ hybridization for the detection of the Burkitt translocation t(8; 14)(q24; q32) in B-cell lymphoma. Blood 1998; **91**: 984–90.

92. Mederos LJ. Intermediate and high-grade diffuse non-Hodgkins' lymphoma in the working formulation. In: Jaffe ES, ed. Surgical Pathology of the Lymph Nodes and Related Organs, 2nd edn. Philadelphia: WB Saunders, 1995; 283–343.

93. Hoelzer D, Ludwig W, Eckhard E et al. Improved outcome to adult B-cell acute lymphoblastic leukaemia. Blood 1996; **87**: 495–508.

94. Carroll AJ, Crist WM, Parmley RT et al. Pre-B cell leukaemia associated with chromosome translocations 1:19. Blood 1994; **63**: 721–4.

95. Crist WM, Carroll AJ, Schuster JJ et al. Poor prognosis of children with pre-B lymphoblastic leukaemia is associated with the t(1; 19)(q23; p13): a Pediatric Oncology Group study. Blood 1990; **76**: 117–24.

96. Hungar SP. Chromosomal translocations involving the E2A gene in acute lymphoblastic leukaemia: clinical features and molecular pathogenesis. Blood 1996; **87**: 1211–16.

●97. Uckum FM, Sensel MG, Sun L et al. Biology and treatment of childhood T-Lineage acute lymphoblastic leukaemia, Blood 1998; **91**: 735–46.

98. Campana D, Coustan-Smith E. Detection of minimal residual disease in acute leukemia by flow cytometry. Cytometry 1999; **38**: 139–52.

99. Meekev TC, Haroy D, William C et al. Activation of the interleukin-3 gene by chromosomal translocation in acute lymphocytic leukaemia with eosinophilia. Blood 1990; **76**: 285–8.

100. Matloub YH, Brunning RD, Arthur DC et al. Severe aplastic anaemia preceding acute lymphoblastic leukaemia. Cancer 1993; **71**: 234–68.

●101. Pui CH, Campana D, Evans WE. Childhood acute lymphoblastic leukaemia: current status and future perspectives. Lancet Oncol 2001; **2**: 597–607.

●102. Campana D, Pui CH. Detection of minimal residual disease in acute leukaemia methodological advances and clinical significance. Blood 1995; **85**: 1416–34.

103. Pui CH Campana D. New definition of remission in childhood acute lymphoblastic leukemia. Leukemia 2000; **14**: 783–5.

104. Szczepanski T, Orfao A, van der Velden V et al. Minimal residual disease in leukaemia patients. Lancet Oncol 2001; **2**: 409–17.

●105. Coustan-Smith E, Behm FG, Sanchez J et al. Immunological detection of minimal residual disease in children with acute lymphoblastic leukaemia. Lancet 1998; **351**: 550–4.

5

Pathology of lymphoma

JYOTI GUPTA & KEITH P. McCARTHY

INTRODUCTION

Lymphomas can be classified into Hodgkin's lymphoma (HL) and non-Hodgkin's lymphoma (NHL). The classification system of choice worldwide is the World Health Organization (WHO) classification, which was an update and expansion of the Revised European-American Lymphoma (REAL) classification[1,2] (see Boxes 5.1 and 5.2).

In developed countries NHLs represent 60–70 per cent of all childhood lymphomas,[3] affecting children mainly between 7 and 10 years of age. In a Dutch study the male:female ratio recorded was 2.5.[4] There is, however, an increased incidence in children with inherited or acquired immunodeficiencies.[5,6] The remaining 30–40 per cent of childhood lymphomas are HLs, the incidence of which increases steadily throughout life and with a male:female ratio of 2.7.

In contradistinction to adult NHLs, which are often low to intermediate grade, paediatric NHLs are frequently high-grade lymphomas and are clinically aggressive.[7] Low-grade tumours of both B and T cells do occur rarely in children.[8] Extranodal disease is also the more common one, as is a leukaemic phase, particularly in lymphoblastic lymphoma.

There are three main types of paediatric NHL:

- Burkitt and atypical Burkitt lymphomas (35–50 per cent of cases)
- lymphoblastic lymphoma (30–40 per cent)
- large-cell lymphomas (15–25 per cent).

Box 5.1 *WHO classification of lymphoid neoplasms. Tumours occurring in childhood*

B-cell neoplasms
- → Precursor B-cell neoplasm
  - • Precursor B-lymphoblastic leukaemia/lymphoma
    - → Mature (peripheral) B-cell neoplasm
      - – Diffuse large B-cell lymphoma
      - – Follicular lymphoma
      - – Burkitt lymphoma
      - – [Mantle cell]

T-cell and natural killer neoplasms
- → Precursor T-cell neoplasm
  - • Precursor T-lymphoblastic leukaemia/lymphoma
    - → Mature (peripheral) T-cell neoplasm
      - • Anaplastic large-cell lymphoma
        - – T-NHL cell, primary systemic type
          - – [Anaplastic large cell lymphoma
        - – T-NHL cell, primary cutaneous type]
  - • [*Mycosis fungoides*]
  - • [Peripheral T-cell, not otherwise characterized]

[] = very rare.
T-NHL, T-cell non-Hodgkin's lymphoma.

Box 5.2 *Hodgkin's lymphoma (WHO classification 1999)*

- Nodular lymphocyte-predominant Hodgkin's lymphoma
- Classical Hodgkin's lymphoma
  - Nodular sclerosis Hodgkin's lymphoma (grades 1 and 2)
  - Lymphocyte-rich Hodgkin's lymphoma
  - Mixed cellularity Hodgkin's lymphoma
  - Lymphocyte depletion Hodgkin's lymphoma

Anaplastic large-cell lymphomas (ALCLs) are an increasingly identified subgroup, in some studies accounting for even 25 per cent of paediatric lymphomas.[9] All other subtypes of NHL, including follicular lymphoma, are rare.[10,11]

Burkitt lymphoma is of B-cell phenotype, and in the WHO classification there are three subtypes: endemic, non-endemic (sporadic) and immunodeficiency-associated.[2] In the REAL classification, Burkitt-like lymphoma was defined as a variant of diffuse large B-cell lymphoma (DLBCL) with features resembling Burkitt lymphoma.[1] The new WHO classification has replaced this term with atypical Burkitt lymphoma, which is defined as a variant of Burkitt lymphoma.[2] The distinction between Burkitt and atypical Burkitt is based on subtle morphological differences, and their diagnostic reproducibility is open to serious contention. They do not appear to have different aetiology or clinical behaviour. It must therefore be debatable whether atypical Burkitt lymphoma is in fact a real entity.

Lymphoblastic lymphomas are tumours that are histologically indistinguishable from acute lymphoblastic leukaemia (ALL), as all are derived from precursor B or T cells. The number of blasts in the bone marrow is used to distinguish lymphoblastic lymphoma from ALL, i.e. if more than 25 per cent of blasts are in the bone marrow it is ALL. Eighty per cent of lymphoblastic lymphomas are of T-cell origin and the remainder are of B-cell origin.[12]

The majority of paediatric large-cell lymphomas (LCLs) are DLBCLs. In general, B-cell lineage LCLs have centroblastic or immunoblastic morphological features, lack CD30 expression, affect older patients and demonstrate less advanced disease. Peripheral T-cell lymphomas do rarely occur, and by convention ALCL is considered separately. Follicular lymphoma, one of the commonest lymphomas in adults, is rarely found in children and tends to present extranodally.[13]

Hodgkin's lymphoma represents 30–40 per cent of childhood lymphomas. As with adult HL, paediatric HL can be divided into nodular lymphocyte-predominant HL and classic HL (nodular sclerosis, mixed cellularity, lymphocyte depletion, lymphocyte-rich). The histological subtype is not an independent prognostic factor for survival except where irradiation alone is used for localized disease, when mixed cellularity HL fares less well.[14]

The mechanism by which oncogenes are activated in paediatric NHL usually involves genetic alterations that correlate with cell lineage (i.e. B-cell immunoglobulin and T-cell receptor genes). The loss or inactivation of the multitumour suppressor (*MTS1*) gene, which has a role in the regulation of tumour suppression genes, may be important in certain lymphoblastic lymphomas.[15] In paediatric Hodgkin's disease, deregulated cytokine production may be important.[15,16]

BURKITT LYMPHOMA

In the Working Formulation and Kiel classifications, Burkitt lymphoma was previously referred to as small, non-cleaved cell, Burkitt lymphoma.

CLINICAL FEATURES

Burkitt lymphoma occurs endemically in Africa and parts of New Guinea and is seen sporadically elsewhere in the world. The sporadic form is the predominant type in Europe and the USA and affects older children and young adults, whereas the endemic form affects children ranging in age from 3 to 15 years.[9]

The endemic form is strongly associated with the Epstein–Barr virus (EBV), which can be found in up to 95 per cent of cases. The association with sporadic and HIV-associated cases is less clear; EBV is seen in only 20 per cent of sporadic cases and 30–40 per cent of HIV-positive cases. High antibody titre to EBV antigen may be associated with a better prognosis.[17] The precise role of EBV in the pathogenesis of Burkitt lymphoma is still unclear. Burkitt lymphoma usually shows a dramatic response to chemotherapy, but spontaneous remission occurs only rarely,[18] although it may involve viral-induced immortalization of B cells in which the translocation involving C-*MYC* and light- or heavy-chain genes becomes transposed.

PATHOLOGICAL FEATURES

Usually the normal intestinal wall or lymph node architecture is completely effaced by a monomorphic population of cohesive medium-sized lymphoid cells. These are admixed with macrophages containing apoptotic debris, which give the characteristic 'starry sky' appearance (Figure 5.1). The growth pattern is usually diffuse but occasionally an apparently follicular pattern is present due to follicular colonization.

The neoplastic cells have nuclei that are large and rounded or oval. Chromatin is dense and clumped and tends to obscure the nucleoli (classically two to five in

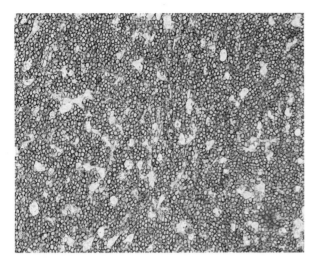

Figure 5.1 *Burkitt lymphoma showing 'starry sky' appearance.* (CD20 magnification × 20.)

number). The abundant basophilic cytoplasm contains characteristic vacuoles which may not be easily seen in histological sections. It is important to remember that these may also be seen in other lymphoma subtypes, particularly when cells are degenerate. Characteristically, the proliferation fraction approaches 100 per cent, which, with the possible exception of atypical Burkitt lymphoma, is unique and is an extremely useful diagnostic feature. The neoplastic cells often infiltrate around nerves, muscles and other normal structures, compressing rather than destroying them.[19] The histological features of sporadic and endemic types of Burkitt lymphoma are identical.

DIFFERENTIAL DIAGNOSIS

The differential diagnosis includes other types of high-grade lymphomas such as B- and T-lymphoblastic lymphoma and the small-cell variant of DLBCL. If fixation is poor, Burkitt lymphoma may lose its characteristic cytological and morphological features (such as the monotonous appearance and the 'starry sky' pattern). The high proliferation index may help to distinguish Burkitt lymphoma from DLBCL and true lymphoblastic lymphoma, which generally have a lower proliferation rate. Although cytoplasmic vacuoles are best demonstrated in cytological preparations, they may be seen at the edge of sections, where cells are tending to separate, provided that the area chosen retains relatively good preservation.

In the unusual case where Burkitt lymphoma grows in a follicular or nodular pattern, there may be superficial resemblance to follicle centre cell lymphomas, and this impression may be further strengthened by the positivity for CD10. High-power examination should clarify the cytology of the Burkitt lymphoma cells, which is quite different from centrocytes or centroblasts.

True lymphoblastic lymphomas are terminal deoxynucleotide transferase (TdT)-positive, whereas Burkitt lymphoma is always negative. However, TdT may be technically difficult to interpret and care should be taken when there is a negative result. If the lymph node is well fixed, then the morphological characteristics remain an essential part of distinguishing these tumours from Burkitt lymphoma.

IMMUNOPHENOTYPICAL CONSIDERATIONS

Immunophenotypically, the Burkitt lymphoma cell is indistinguishable from a peripheral B cell, although the positivity for CD10 suggests derivation from germinal centre cells. Neoplastic cells express monoclonal pan B-cell markers (CD19, 20, 22 and 79a) and CD10, and are sIgM-positive. They are always negative for CD5 and CD23. Ki67 is a useful marker in the differentiation of Burkitt lymphoma from other high-grade lymphoma subtypes and TdT is always negative. The tumour cells may be positive for EBV-associated antigens such as LMP-1 and may, similarly, be positive on *in situ* hybridization for EBERs (small RNA molecules found in the latent state).

GENETIC AND CYTOGENETIC CONSIDERATIONS

The vast majority of cases, whatever the subtype, show a chromosomal translocation involving the C-*MYC* gene (chromosome 8).[15] The commonest abnormality is t(8:14)(q24;q32), which results in the translocation of C-*MYC* into the heavy-chain (IgH) gene locus. This locus is actively transcribing in B cells and the translocation results in C-*MYC* being influenced by the IgH gene promoter, producing constitutive expression of C-MYC protein, which is a powerful cell-proliferation protein. Variant chromosome translocations include t(2;8)(p11;q24) and t(8;22)(p24;q11), in which the C-*MYC* gene is translocated into the actively transcribing immunoglobulin kappa light-chain gene and the immunoglobulin lambda light-chain gene, respectively.

Burkitt lymphoma may also show promiscuous rearrangements of T-cell receptor genes, especially of the T-cell receptor gamma chain genes. Such rearrangements are usually only partial and appear to be secondary events.

ATYPICAL BURKITT LYMPHOMA/ BURKITT–LIKE LYMPHOMA

GENERAL CONSIDERATIONS

There is considerable controversy concerning this entity, not least because published studies show that its diagnosis has extremely poor reproducibility.[20] Both the REAL classification and the new WHO classification consider there to be a subtype of high-grade lymphoma with features intermediate between DLBCL and Burkitt lymphoma. The REAL system implies that this should be considered a variant of DLBCL, whereas the WHO defines it as an entity similar to Burkitt lymphoma. It is the opinion of the authors that atypical Burkitt lymphoma and Burkitt-like lymphoma may actually be the same entity – poorly fixed or poorly processed Burkitt lymphoma. It is well recognized that the conditions of fixation and processing may significantly alter several aspects of cytomorphology, including cell size and nuclear appearance. Reports in which atypical/Burkitt-like NHL is regarded as a separate entity have suggested a number of characteristic features. The tumour is said to occur slightly more commonly in adults than in children, and may also be seen in patients with immunosuppression. It more frequently presents primarily as a nodal rather than an extranodal disease,[21] and there may be a shorter long-term survival in Burkitt-like lymphoma, compared with Burkitt, particularly in adults.[22,23]

PATHOLOGICAL FEATURES

Atypical Burkitt lymphoma is said to show subtle morphological differences from Burkitt lymphoma, the main one being greater cellular pleomorphism. The cells are of intermediate size (possibly slightly larger than typical Burkitt lymphoma cells) and have round to oval nuclei that show more nuclear irregularity than in Burkitt lymphoma. The chromatin is more clumped and nucleoli more prominent, but fewer in number, compared with Burkitt lymphoma. The 'starry sky' appearance is less often seen than in Burkitt lymphoma. Cases have a high proliferation index, as judged by MIB-1 or Ki67 staining, approaching that of Burkitt lymphoma.

DIFFERENTIAL DIAGNOSIS

The main differential diagnoses are Burkitt lymphoma and DLBCL. Lymphoblastic lymphoma, especially in small or poorly fixed samples, may also pose a diagnostic difficulty, but staining for TdT (only positive in true lymphoblastic lymphomas) should be decisive.

IMMUNOPHENOTYPICAL CONSIDERATIONS

Like Burkitt lymphoma and DLBCL, this entity possesses a mature B-cell phenotype, showing positivity for pan B markers (e.g. CD19, CD20, CD22, CD79a). It is CD5– and usually CD10+. It may have surface immunoglobulin (IgM or IgG), but is always negative for TdT. There are no published data concerning the percentage of cases showing bcl-2 positivity.

Accurate estimation of the percentage of cells in cycle may allow a pragmatic distinction between DLBCL and atypical Burkitt lymphoma/Burkitt-like lymphoma. The diagnosis of atypical Burkitt lymphoma/Burkitt-like lymphoma should not be made if the proliferation index falls below 98 per cent.

GENETIC AND CYTOGENETIC CONSIDERATIONS

As a mature B-cell lymphoma, this entity shows both IgH and IgL gene rearrangements, detectable by both restriction enzyme analysis and polymerase chain reaction. C-*MYC* rearrangements are reportedly less common than in Burkitt lymphoma, but this can be attributed to the heterogeneity of lymphoma subtypes included under this heading. *Bcl-2* gene rearrangements have been reported in 30 per cent of patients,[1] in contrast to Burkitt lymphoma where no such rearrangements occur, but again this may represent cases of DLBCL included erroneously.

DIFFUSE LARGE B–CELL LYMPHOMA

In the Kiel classification, this entity is divided into various subsets – centroblastic, B-immunoblastic and B-large cell anaplastic. There is no convincing evidence for a distinction between centroblastic and immunoblastic lymphomas and these groups were therefore combined in subsequent classification systems under the term diffuse large B-cell lymphoma (DLBCL). In the REAL classification, all high-grade B-cell lymphomas other than distinct clinicopathological entities such as Burkitt lymphoma are included under this heading. The new WHO classification similarly recognizes that there is no prognostic difference between large B-cell lymphomas containing centroblasts only, immunoblasts only, or a combination thereof, although because of its distinctive clinicopathological features, primary mediastinal large B-cell lymphoma is considered separately.

In adults, a proportion of cases of DLBCL represent transformation of pre-existing low-grade B-cell lymphoma or even transformation of nodular lymphocyte-predominant Hodgkin's disease; in childhood, in contrast, almost all cases represent *de novo* high-grade disease.

PATHOLOGICAL FEATURES

Diffuse large B-cell lymphoma grows in a diffuse pattern, effacing the lymph node or normal tissue architecture, perhaps with extensive necrosis. There may be a high mitotic count, even a 'starry sky' appearance similar to Burkitt lymphoma, representing a high mitotic and apoptotic rate. The constituent cells are intermediate to large in size with nuclei greater in diameter than tissue macrophage nuclei; a feature of use in distinguishing it from Burkitt lymphoma, where the nuclei are never larger than those of the interspersed macrophages. Nucleoli are usually prominent and the cells have a moderate amount of variably basophilic cytoplasm.

DLBCL can exhibit marked cytological and morphological variation, depending only in part on the relative proportions of centroblasts and immunoblasts. Centroblasts are intermediate to large cells that may contain the classical rounded or ovoid nucleus shape or cerebriform or polylobated nucleus. Several relatively inconspicuous nucleoli are distributed around the nuclear membrane. Immunoblasts are usually larger cells whose nuclei have a prominent nuclear membrane, open chromatin and a single, large central eosinophilic nucleolus and they have variable amounts of cytoplasm. There may be marked plasmacytoid differentiation, with eccentrically placed nuclei in which there is peripherally condensed chromatin.

Occasionally, one cell type is in excess, but this does not alter the diagnosis of DLBCL. For example, 'T-cell-rich B-cell lymphoma' is a histological pattern of DLBCL in which there is a marked predominance of mature or activated T cells, but this is not a distinct subtype. If there is an excess of other non-neoplastic cells, such as reactive plasma cells, mature B-cells, macrophages and eosinophils, the tumour may resemble a peripheral T-cell lymphoma. The malignant cells must, therefore, be carefully identified.

In some cases, bizarre tumour giant cells may be seen which have a superficial resemblance to Reed–Sternberg cells. If an anaplastic morphology is prominent, the tumour may be mistaken for ALCL.

Mediastinal B-cell lymphoma is characterized by its 'compartmentalizing' pattern of fibrosis, producing small packets of tumour cells surrounded by strands of sclerosis.

DIFFERENTIAL DIAGNOSIS

On H&E staining there may be some similarity with a number of different tumours such as poorly differentiated carcinoma, plasmablastic myeloma and malignant melanoma. These can be excluded by appropriate immunohistochemical staining. ALCL is also easily excluded by immunohistochemistry.

Where accompanying inflammatory cells mimic the appearance of peripheral T-cell lymphoma, careful examination of immunohistochemistry should reveal the B-cell phenotype of the cytologically atypical cells.

The distinction of DLBCL from Burkitt lymphoma and atypical Burkitt lymphoma/Burkitt-like lymphoma is the main problem. This topic has already been addressed but points that should be emphasized are the presence of intracytoplasmic vacuoles, the proliferation index, the presence of bcl-2 positivity and CD10 positivity (although DLBCL may be positive, Burkitt lymphoma is always positive).

IMMUNOPHENOTYPICAL CONSIDERATIONS

As a neoplasm of mature B cells, DLBCL shows positivity for pan B-cell markers (CD19, 20, 22 and 79a). Most are CD45+ (leucocyte common antigen), although immunoblastic lymphomas may occasionally be negative. CD44 expression may be a prognostic indicator in localized large B-cell lymphoma.[24] TdT is always negative, and cells show variable expression of CD5, CD10 and cytoplasmic and surface immunoglobulin. A small percentage of cases express CD30, which does not mean that they should be regarded as ALCLs, and they are rarely CD15-positive.

Thymic B-cell lymphoma also has a mature B-cell phenotype and is more likely to express CD30 than other types of DLBCL. It is usually immunoglobulin-negative.

GENETIC AND CYTOGENETIC CONSIDERATIONS

Twenty-five per cent of cases have the t(14;18)(q32;q23) chromosomal translocation, characteristic of follicle centre cell lesions,[9] which inserts the entire BCL-2 gene on chromosome 18 into the actively transcribing IgH locus on chromosome 14. This results in the constitutive expression of the anti-apoptotic gene BCL-2 and may indicate transformation from a pre-existing low-grade lymphoma. The presence of the translocation may also indicate poorer response to therapy.[25]

In 30–40 per cent of cases there is some form of cytogenetic abnormality involving the BCL-6/LAZ3 gene on chromosome 3q27.[1] Rearrangement of the C-MYC gene is uncommon, but can occur in association with other genetic rearrangements.[25] The commonest variant is the t(8;14)(q23;q35) translocation, demonstrating that the presence of this abnormality is not pathognomonic for Burkitt lymphoma.

PRECURSOR B-LYMPHOBLASTIC LEUKAEMIA/LYMPHOMA

In the Kiel classification these were referred to as malignant lymphoma, lymphoblastic B-cell type, and in the Working Formulation as malignant lymphoma lymphoblastic (convoluted cell, non-convoluted cell). Lymphoblastic lymphomas showing B-lineage differentiation are less common than their T-cell counterparts. Like the latter, a high proportion involve bone marrow and central nervous system.

PATHOLOGICAL FEATURES

There is usually diffuse replacement of normal nodal architecture by a monotonous infiltrate of non-cohesive, but closely packed, uniform, medium-sized lymphoblasts. These characteristically grow in an interfollicular pattern, which is a useful feature in establishing the diagnosis. The neoplastic cells contain large round or convoluted nuclei with a fine chromatin pattern and inconspicuous nucleoli. The cytoplasm is scanty, varying from pale to slightly basophilic in colour. Morphologically, the neoplastic cells are identical to those seen in ALL,[26] and in well-preserved tissues the distinction from Burkitt lymphoma should be easy.

Mitotic figures are frequent, although less so than in Burkitt lymphoma. Necrosis may be extensive, which may hamper the tissue diagnosis.

DIFFERENTIAL DIAGNOSIS

B- and T-lymphoblastic lymphomas may resemble each other, especially if the fixation is suboptimal. In T-lymphoblastic lymphoma the cells are more heterogeneous and the nuclei usually show some convolution. Immunohistochemistry should clarify the phenotype. Chloroma (a soft tissue deposit of primitive myeloid cells) can resemble a wide variety of tumour types, including lymphoblastic lymphoma, but the presence of maturing myeloid cells and scattered immature eosinophils should arouse suspicion regarding this possibility. Immunohistochemistry should allow a definite diagnosis, with choroma being positive for MT1, CD11c and negative for TdT.

Small round-cell tumours of childhood, such as Ewing's sarcoma, peripheral neuroectodermal tumours and neuroblastoma, may closely resemble lymphoblastic lymphoma but these can also usually be excluded by immunohistochemistry.

IMMUNOPHENOTYPICAL CONSIDERATIONS

B-lymphoblastic lymphoma expresses early B-cell markers (CD19, CD22, CD79a) with variable CD20 expression. There is also variable positivity for CD10, CD13, CD33 and CD34. Surface immunoglobulin is negative although cytoplasmic immunoglobulin may be expressed. TdT is usually positive, although it is lost in the more differentiated tumours. The lymphomas may be subclassified, as for acute lymphoblastic leukaemia, as common, pre-B and pre-pre-B.[9,27]

GENETIC AND CYTOGENETIC CONSIDERATIONS

There are no consistent characteristic cytogenetic abnormalities, although, as in leukaemia, various broad groupings of abnormality are recognized, including hypodiploid, pseudodiploid and hyperdiploid (whether there are less than 51 chromosomes, or 51 or more). The prognostic significance of cytogenetic changes in NHL is unclear.

T–CELL LYMPHOMAS

T-cell phenotype NHLs occurring in children are almost always of lymphoblastic subtype.[28] However, peripheral T-cell lymphoma, although rare, does occur.[29] ALCL frequently marks with CD3 and other T-cell markers,[30] although for the purposes of classification and treatment, it is regarded as a separate entity. It is thus important to exclude a diagnosis of ALCL by staining for CD30, ALK-1 and epithelial membrane antigen (EMA), especially since the 'small-cell' variant may morphologically resemble T-cell lymphoma.[30]

T–cell lymphoblastic lymphoma (TLL)

PATHOLOGICAL FEATURES

At the lowest power, TLL has a relatively uniform appearance with a diffuse, monotonous growth pattern. Although a 'starry sky' appearance may be present, this is less prominent than in Burkitt lymphoma. There is frequently extracapsular extension in the nodes and the infiltrate is usually paracortical, possibly sparing the germinal centres.[31] Most cells are 1.5–2 times the diameter of a small lymphocyte and have a high nucleocytoplasmic ratio, with only a thin rim of cytoplasm. Cytoplasmic vacuolation is less conspicuous than that seen in Burkitt lymphoma.[32] The nuclear chromatin may be either dispersed or very finely condensed. Nucleoli are of variable number and are usually inconspicuous.[31] There may be subpopulations of cells, including larger, more obviously blastic cells with larger nucleoli, and cells similar to mature small lymphocytes. The mitotic rate and apoptotic rate are high, but less than in Burkitt lymphoma. 'Convoluted' and 'non-convoluted' subtypes are described, although this distinction has no clinical significance.[33]

IMMUNOPHENOTYPICAL CONSIDERATIONS

Terminal deoxynucleotide transferase positivity is extremely useful in confirming the diagnosis.[34] TLL also expresses pan-T markers (CD2, CD3, CD5 and CD7) and there may be coexpression of CD4, CD8 and CD1a. Fifty to 60 per cent of cases express CD10[35] and tumours may occasionally be positive for CD79a. It is important to realize that this does not signify bi-lineage differentiation.[2] Positivity for CD1a, CD4 and CD8 appears to correlate with stage of differentiation, although it is unclear whether this relates to clinical behaviour.[28,36]

Rarely, cases show true bi-lineage differentiation with expression of myeloid markers such as CD13 and CD33, although myeloblastic lesions may themselves express T-cell antigens.[28] A case of TLL arising 9 months after the diagnosis of acute myeloblastic leukaemia has been reported.[37] Both cytomegalovirus and EBV have been associated with TLL,[38,39] although the biological relevance of this is unclear.

GENETIC AND CYTOGENETIC CONSIDERATIONS

Although TLL is not defined by a specific cytogenetic abnormality,[40] in approximately 30 per cent of cases there are cytogenetic abnormalities involving either the T-cell receptor beta chain locus (7q35), the T-cell receptor gamma chain locus (7p14) or the T-cell receptor alpha/ delta receptor loci (14q11).[41] These aberrations may result in the inappropriate activation of cellular oncogenes, a situation that parallels the activation of *BCL-2* in follicle centre cell lymphoma.[42] In TLL, the precise nature of the oncogenes being activated is not known. *MYC*, *RBTN-1*, *RBTN-2* and *HOX-11* have been described.[43]

Deletion of 9p occurs in about one-third of cases of TLL, resulting in loss of the tumour suppressor gene *CDKN2a*, the gene product of which inhibits cyclin-dependent kinase-4. In 25 per cent of cases, a deletion of the locus 1p32 is present (although it is karyotypically visible in only 5 per cent of cases).[44] This is the site of the *TAL-1* gene (also known as *SCL* or *TCL-5*) which encodes a transcription factor containing a basic helix-loop-helix motif fundamental in haemopoietic stem cell development.[45] It binds as a heterodimer to the *E2A* and *HEB/HTF4* gene products, but the *TAL-1* gene product can act as both an activator and a repressor of transcription.[46] Overexpression of *TAL-1* is the commonest molecular abnormality found in T-cell leukaemia.[47]

Although rearrangement of the T-cell receptor chain loci can be used as a diagnostic tool, it should be remembered that such rearrangements, especially of the gamma chain, are promiscuous and are also found in myeloid lesions as well as in B-lineage lesions.[48–51]

ANAPLASTIC LARGE-CELL LYMPHOMA

There are several subtypes of ALCL. The 'classical' or 'common' subtype is seen most frequently and was the first variant to be recognized.[52] The 'small cell' and the 'lymphohistiocytic' subtypes are of importance since these may easily be mistaken for peripheral T-cell lymphoma.[53]

Amongst other subtypes are the 'sarcomatoid' variant (possessing a spindle cell morphology which may lead to a misdiagnosis of a soft tissue tumour), the 'giant cell' variant and the 'Hodgkin-like' variant.[53,54]

It is now recognized that ALCL is a disease entity distinct from Hodgkin's disease.[55] The view that truly intermediate forms exist is now discounted.[56] 'Hodgkin-like' cases (possibly with classical Hodgkin and Reed–Sternberg cells, a nodular growth pattern and capsular thickening) should be considered to be Hodgkin-like ALCL only if they express ALK-1 protein, and as HL if this is negative.[57] Mixed forms of ALCL (in which two or more subtypes can be identified) are common and one pattern may predominate at relapse.[58]

ALCL was originally defined by its positivity for CD30, a cell surface protein that is a part of the tumour necrosis factor–nerve growth factor receptor family.[59] CD30 is normally found on activated B and T cells and sometimes on activated macrophages.[55] The function of CD30 remains unknown.[60] Overexpression may also be seen in germ cell tumours, and this must be remembered if the presentation or morphology is unusual.[61]

Although the main differential diagnosis of ALCL is HL (CD30 expression is also a feature of classical HL), other lymphomas and lymphoproliferative disorders can be CD30-positive.[55] DLBCL (especially mediastinal B-cell lymphoma) may be CD30-positive, and some lesions show extreme cellular pleomorphism. Although it is now known that B-cell NHL may express a fusion protein involving the protein encoded by the *ALK* gene, this is probably best regarded as a separate entity to ALCL.[62–64]

In certain lymphohistiocytic proliferations of the skin, including regressing atypical histiocytosis and lymphomatoid papulosis,[65] CD30 positivity may occur in cells that morphologically resemble ALCL cells. These are usually negative both for ALK-1 and EMA and should not therefore be considered as isolated skin deposits of ALCL,[53] unless there is obvious lymph node or other site involvement. Isolated lymphohistiocytic proliferations of the skin are self-limiting and may be cured by local surgery, whereas skin and lymph node involvement by ALCL requires chemotherapy.[65]

PATHOLOGICAL FEATURES

The 'hallmark cell' characterizes ALCL. This is approximately equivalent in size to a macrophage, is mononuclear and has a characteristic 'reniform', 'horseshoe' or 'grooved' nuclear shape. These are seen in all variants of ALCL and should be identified in order for the diagnosis to be made. ALCL may show great nuclear pleomorphism and may even contain cells that are morphologically and immunophenotypically indistinguishable from Hodgkin and Reed–Sternberg cells. Paradoxically, ALCL may also show little or no nuclear pleomorphism and may even, in the small-cell variant, consist predominantly of cells that are relatively small in size.

The chromatin is usually coarsely clumped and may be condensed on the nuclear membrane. Nucleoli are usually prominent and may be multiple. There is generally a moderate amount of eosinophilic cytoplasm. Intensification of eosinophilia within the region of the Golgi complex may be apparent if fixation and staining conditions are optimal.

Tumour cells may be seen growing in cohesive sheets within paracortical areas (hence the confusion with metastatic carcinoma), but a characteristic feature is an intrasinusoidal growth pattern, as distinct from HL. A tendency for perivascular growth is associated with the small-cell and lymphohistiocytic variants.

In the small-cell variant, the characteristic hallmark cells may be sparse, most of the atypical cells being small to intermediate in size, with insignificant nucleoli and markedly irregular, possibly cerebriform, nuclear outline.[66] The cytoplasm is scanty. In the lymphohistiocytic variant there is predominance of epithelioid and non-epithelioid histiocytes, and atypical cells are rare.[67,68] As in the small-cell variant, these tend to be smaller, although hallmark cells may be found. It is often difficult to distinguish between the lymphohistiocytic and small-cell variants and these may in fact be biologically related.

In the giant-cell type, the majority of cells are extremely large and multinucleate, often with bizarre morphological features.[52,69] In the sarcomatoid variant, the atypical cells have a spindle cell morphology and there may be a myxoid stroma.[54] Other variants include the neutrophil-rich variant[70] and the Hodgkin-like variant (in which there may be capsular thickening and banded sclerosis).[53] This last variant not only leads to diagnostic difficulties, but also suggests a possible relationship between the two entities.[57] It is now generally accepted that, morphologically at least, there are cases of overlap between the two diseases, although use of immunohistochemistry for ALK-1 and PAX-5 (the former characteristic of ALCL, the latter of HL) usually allows distinction to be made.[53] Some authorities believe that this subtype does not exist as a separate entity and that most such cases are, in reality, HL.[71]

IMMUNOPHENOTYPICAL CONSIDERATIONS

The staining pattern of CD30 is usually accentuated on the cell membrane, although positive staining of the Golgi complex may impart a 'dot-like' positivity.[53] EMA is positive in approximately 50 per cent of cases, also staining the cell membrane and Golgi complex.[72] CD45 is positive in only 50 per cent of cases, which also leads to early confusion with metastatic carcinoma.

ALK-1 and ALK-C are monoclonal antibodies against ALK protein and are most commonly used.[7] Polyclonal ALK antibodies may give false-positive results and are best avoided. ALK-1 stains not only the NPM-ALK fusion protein that results from the commonest cytogenetic marker of ALCL, the t(2;5)(p23;p35), but also its variants.[53] The staining pattern varies depending on the cytogenetic abnormality. The commonest pattern (associated with t(2;5)(p23;p35)) is cytoplasmic, nuclear and nucleolar. The second commonest pattern is predominantly cytoplasmic and cytoplasmic membrane staining and is associated with the t(1;2)(q25;p23) abnormality.

In the small-cell variant, the more characteristic cytoplasmic and nuclear staining may be seen in the scattered hallmark cells, whereas in the small atypical cells there may be predominant nuclear staining.[74]

In children, ALK-positive ALCL is the norm and, unlike in adults, ALK positivity has no prognostic significance.[75] Rare cases of ALK-negative ALCL do, however, occur in children.

Childhood ALCL is a proliferation of cytotoxic T-cells and, as such, exhibits either a T-cell phenotype or a null cell phenotype. Tumour cells may express any or all of a variety of T-cell markers, but the variability means that it is not recommended to attempt to assign phenotype using only one or two antibodies. Even in those cases that are consistently negative, it may prove possible to assign a T-cell phenotype by finding positivity for either granzyme B, perforin or TIA-1 (although this last is not particularly specific). These are characteristic markers of cytotoxic T-cells.[76,77] Rare cases may express CD56, suggesting a natural killer cell phenotype.[76]

Stains for EBV (such as LMP-1) are almost always negative.[77]

CYTOGENETIC AND GENETIC CONSIDERATIONS

The t(2;5)(p23;q35) translocation is found in approximately 75 per cent of cases,[67] although incidence depends on method of deletion. The *ALK* gene on chromosome 2p23 fuses with the *NPM* (nucleophosmin) gene on chromosome 5q35.[7] NPM codes for an ubiquitously expressed intranuclear phosphoprotein that binds RNA and transports ribonucleoproteins between the nucleolus and the cytoplasm and is normally located in the nucleolus. ALK, a member of the insulin receptor family that is normally located in the cell membrane, is a tyrosine kinase.[79] Its normal role appears to be in nervous system development, and it is not normally expressed in haemopoietic cells.[80] The expression of the fusion protein is both in frame and functional,[63] and retains the cytoplasmic kinase domain of *ALK* fused to the 5′ end of the *NPM* gene.[81] It is a constitutively active kinase under the action of the strong NPM promoter.[82] The fusion protein loses the nuclear localization signal of wild-type NPM but it is still capable of dimerization.[64] Homodimerization results in cytoplasmic localization, heterodimerization (with wild-type ALK) in nuclear and nucleolar localization; it is the homodimers that are thought to be oncogenic.[83]

There are several variants of this cytogenetic abnormality, all involving the *ALK* gene on chromosome 2p23. The second commonest, found in approximately 15 per cent of cases, is the t(1;2)(q25;p23), which produces a fusion protein of ALK and tropomysin 3.[84] This fusion protein has no nuclear localization signal and staining is therefore exclusively cytoplasmic.

Five per cent of cases have an inversion of chromosome 2, inv(2)(p23;q35), which results in a fusion protein of *ALK* and *ATIC-2*, a gene that codes for an enzyme involved in purine nucleotide synthesis.[84] This is also restricted to the cytoplasm. Several other cytogenetic abnormalities, all involving 2p23, have been described in cases of ALCL.

T-cell receptor gene rearrangements can be found in 90 per cent of cases using either polymerase chain reaction (PCR) or Southern blotting techniques. Immunoglobulin genes are not found rearranged.

HODGKIN'S LYMPHOMA

The currently accepted classifications for HL are the REAL and the revised WHO systems.[43] In recent years it has been recognized that there are two distinct disease entities encompassed by the term Hodgkin's lymphoma – namely, classical Hodgkin's lymphoma (CHL) and nodular lymphocyte-predominant Hodgkin's lymphoma (NLPHL).[85–87]

Classical Hodgkin's lymphoma

In CHL, the Hodgkin and Reed–Sternberg cells are derived from follicle centre cells that have participated in the primary immune response but have not completed the normal process of somatic hypermutation in the germinal centre that is part of the primary immune response.[88] Somatic hypermutation is the mechanism whereby the specificity and strength of binding of B cells to antigen are increased, thus allowing a more targeted secondary immune response.[89] In CHL, an abnormally high number of somatic hypermutations occur, many leading to non-functional rearranged immunoglobulin heavy-chain genes. It is in the environs of the germinal centre itself that the transforming event seems to arise.[90,91] There may also be mutations in the *IκBα* gene, suggesting that an abnormality of the nuclear factor κB signalling pathway is a fundamental pathogenetic mechanism.[92] This is consistent with the characteristic inflammatory response of HL.[88]

PATHOLOGICAL FEATURES

The Reed–Sternberg (RS) cell has traditionally been described as binucleate or multinucleate, but in fact has a single bilobed or multilobed nucleus. The cell is usually 10–15 times larger than a small lymphocyte with a single, centrally placed and prominent nucleolus and a small to moderate amount of amphophilic cytoplasm. The Hodgkin cell is the 'mononuclear' variant which, although highly suggestive of HL, is not diagnostic of the condition.[93] The presence of so-called 'mummified' cells, which are degenerate variants of Hodgkin and RS cells,[43] may aid diagnosis. These are smaller than Hodgkin or RS cells with hyperchromatic nuclei, smudged chromatin, insignificant nucleoli and eosinophilic cytoplasm. At low power they may be prominent.

HL tends to have a paracortical growth pattern around follicles which may show quite marked hyperplasia. In contradistinction to ALCL,[43] the cellular background to the Hodgkin and RS cells does not usually involve the sinuses. In lymphocyte-rich HL there are few atypical cells in a large number of small lymphocytes and histiocytes. The presence of numerous, often highly atypical and pleomorphic, Hodgkin and RS cells with relatively few surrounding reactive cells is the characteristic appearance of lymphocyte-depleted HL. Mixed cellularity HL contains atypical cells in moderate numbers set in a background of small lymphocytes, eosinophils, histiocytes and plasma cells.[93]

In all the preceding subtypes, features of nodular sclerosis are absent. Nodular sclerosing HL is defined by the presence of two out of three of the following: banded sclerosis, capsular thickening or lacunar cells.[93] The latter are another variant of Hodgkin and RS cells in which the atypical cell appears to be placed within a 'lacuna' or clear space. They may not have all of the usual morphological characteristics of RS cells, although it has been suggested that they are artefactual; due to tissue retraction associated with fibrosis, they can be seen in the 'cellular phase' of nodular sclerosing HL where there is no established banded sclerosis.[94] It should also be noted that sclerosis must be as thick, acellular and eosinophilic bands; diffuse, ill-defined sclerosis should not be regarded as indicating nodular sclerosing HL.[28]

If the features of nodular sclerosis are present, the cellularity of the residual lymphoid tissue is not relevant in subcategorization, although an attempt has been made to grade the disease.[95] Grade 1 disease has fewer and/or less pleomorphic atypical cells than grade 2 disease. One study has suggested that cellular-phase nodular sclerosing HD may have a worse prognosis,[96] but the clinical usefulness of grading is still contentious.[97–99]

IMMUNOPHENOTYPICAL CONSIDERATIONS

Hodgkin and RS cells are almost invariably positive for CD30 and a negative result should throw doubt on the diagnosis. Conversely, a number of other tumours, such as ALCLs, some high-grade B-NHLs and germ cell tumours, may also be CD30-positive.[43,100] The function of CD30 is largely unknown, although its activation, by binding with its ligand, is thought to result in cell proliferation and apoptosis.[62,101]

Despite its lymphoid origin, CHL is consistently negative for CD45. CD15 positivity is found in approximately 80 per cent of HL, which can be useful since NHL is rarely positive.[102] Approximately 40 per cent of HL cases are positive with the pan B-cell marker, CD20, but HL is usually negative with CD79a. Rarely, T-cell markers such as CD3 may be positive, but in this case it is important to exclude ALCL.

ALK-1 is never positive and EMA very rarely in CHL,[43] in contrast to ALCL. Variable expression of T-cell markers, such as CD2 and granzyme B, may occur.[88] Overall, approximately 50 per cent of CHLs in Europe and the United States are EBV-positive depending on subtype.[102,103] The pattern of protein expression, with positivity for antibodies against latent membrane protein 1 and EBNA1, indicates type 2 latent infection.[103] The most appropriate method of detecting EBV infection is *in situ* hybridization for EBERs (small RNA molecules found in the latent state).[103]

GENETIC AND CYTOGENETIC CONSIDERATIONS

There are no consistent karyotypic abnormalities in CHL, although the absence of the typical translocations seen in B-NHL and ALCL may help the diagnosis.[104] Frequent, apparently random, abnormalities involving 14q may occur and the marked variability of karyotypes between cells from the same case indicates that genomic instability is a characteristic of HL. There is a relatively high frequency of amplification and gain of chromosomal material in various distinct regions.[105]

In most cases of HL, aneuploidy and hypertetraploidy are seen in both Hodgkin and RS cells.[43]

It is now recognized that the majority of cases of HL have rearranged immunoglobulin genes.[102,106,107] Those cases expressing B-cell antigens are reported to be more likely to have such rearrangments.[107] The use of single-cell amplification techniques has allowed the separation of Hodgkin and RS cells from the surrounding reactive infiltrate. These findings are consistent with the postulated B-cell origin, although rearranged T-cell receptor chain genes in the absence of rearranged immunoglobulin genes have been described.[108]

Nodular lymphocyte–predominant Hodgkin's lymphoma (NLPHL)

CLINICAL CONSIDERATIONS

In children this is a relatively uncommon tumour type. It is considered to be a relatively indolent lesion, often presenting as localized disease, characteristically as an enlarged node or nodal mass high in the neck or axilla. There is a small risk of transformation to high-grade B-cell NHL, occurring in about 5 per cent of cases.[109] Case reports of transformation to T-cell lymphoma presumably represent instances of coincidental second malignancy.[110]

The original Lukes and Butler classification of HL recognized two variants of lymphocyte-predominant Hodgkin's lymphoma – a nodular form (also called 'nodular paragranuloma') and a diffuse form.[94] It is now generally agreed that cases of the diffuse variant are either NHL (T-cell rich B-cell lymphoma) or lymphocyte-rich CHL.[43]

NLPHL has an ill-defined relationship with progressive transformation of germinal centres (PTGC). In this condition, there is lymph node enlargement without systemic symptoms. Histologically, there is follicular enlargement, with germinal centres appearing disrupted, expanded and infiltrated by small B lymphocytes[28] which are CD5+ and derived from the mantle zone. PTGC may present as an independent entity or precede, occur synchronously with or occur subsequently to NLPHL.[111,112]

NLPHL is derived from follicle centre cells, but there is more B-cell differentiation than in CHL.[43]

PATHOLOGICAL FEATURES

Nodal architecture is completely or partly effaced by a vaguely nodular lymphoid proliferation. This does not resemble normal follicular architecture and the nodularity may be exceedingly difficult to discern, in contrast to follicle centre cell lymphoma often accentuated by immunohistochemistry with pan B- and pan T-cell markers.[45,102]

The proliferation consists of mature and polyclonal small lymphocytes, together with a variable number of histiocytes, possibly forming small granulomata and a small number of lymphocytic and histiocytic (L&H) or 'popcorn' cells. These cells have nuclei, often bilobated or multilobated,[28] that are three to four times the size of a small lymphocyte and in which the chromatin is condensed on the nuclear membrane. They characteristically have small nucleoli that are less prominent than those seen in CHL. In contrast, RS cells are often multiple and less eosinophilic. The other components of CHL – eosinophils, plasma cells and neutrophils – are absent in NLPHL.

IMMUNOPHENOTYPICAL CONSIDERATIONS

'Popcorn' cells are CD15- or CD30-negative, in contrast to classical Hodgkin's lymphoma.[43] Moreover, L&H cells characteristically express CD45 and CD79a, unlike CHL. They are also more frequently positive with other B-cell markers, such as CD19, CD20 and CD22,[102] and stain with BCL-6. Between 40 and 50 per cent are EMA-positive.[102,113]

The surrounding small lymphocytes are a mixture of CD20+ B cells and CD3+ T cells, with B cells being predominant in the nodular areas. The L&H cells within the nodules may be surrounded by a ring of CD3+, CD57+ T cells, a phenomenon not seen in CHL.[114,115] Staining for follicular dendritic cells (e.g. CD21) highlights large networks within the nodules and demonstrates that the nodules are expanded and broken-up follicles.[102]

CYTOGENETIC AND GENETIC CONSIDERATIONS

There are no known recurrent cytogenetic abnormalities occurring in NLPHL.[102] Single-cell PCR demonstrates that L&H cells show rearrangement of the immunoglobulin heavy- and light-chain genes.[116] Sequencing of rearranged immunoglobulin heavy-chain genes has shown that, as in CHL, the cells are undergoing excessive somatic hypermutation.[117] The resulting genes which appear to have been positively selected by an antigen[88] are functional, thus explaining the evidence of B-cell differentiation, but in contrast to CHL, hypermutation continues after the transforming event.

KEY POINTS

- Atypical Burkitt lymphoma is an entity of dubious reality that is poorly reproducible.
- Peripheral T-cell lymphoma does (rarely) occur in childhood and should not be overlooked as a possible diagnosis.
- Anaplastic large-cell lymphoma is a tumour of cytotoxic T cells and usually contains the t(2;5) translocation.
- Nodular lymphocyte-predominant Hodgkin's lymphoma is an entity separate from classical Hodgkin's lymphoma; it is more closely related to B-cell non-Hodgkin's lymphoma.

REFERENCES

1. Chan JKC, Banks PM, Clearly ML et al. A revised European-American classification of lymphoid neoplasms proposed by the international lymphoma study group. A summary version. Am J Clin Pathol 1995; 103(5): 543–60.
2. Harris NL, Jaffe ES, Diebold J et al. World Health Organization classification of neoplastic disease of the haematopoietic and lymphoid tissues: report of the clinical advisory committee meeting – Airlie House, Virginia, November 1997. J Clin Oncol 1999; 17(12): 3835–49.
3. Carter RL, McCarthy KP. Features of specific tumours, section 2. In: Pinkerton CR, Plowman PN, eds. Paediatric Oncology, 2nd edn. London: Chapman & Hall Medical, 1997.
4. Coeberg JW, Van der Does-Van den Berg A, Kamps WA et al. Malignant lymphomas in children in The Netherlands in the period 1973–1985: incidence in relation to leukaemia: a report from the Dutch Childhood Leukaemia Study Group. Med Pediatr Oncol 1991; 19(3): 169–74.
5. Filipovich AH, Mathur A, Kamat D et al. Primary immunodeficiencies: genetic risk factors for lymphoma. Cancer Res 1992; 52(suppl): 5465s–7s.
6. Filipovich AH, Mathur A, Kamat D et al. Lymphoproliferative disorders and other tumours complicating immunodeficiencies. Immunodeficiency 1994; 5(2): 91–112.
7. Wright D, McKeever P, Carter R. Childhood non-Hodgkin's lymphomas in the United Kingdom: findings from the UK Children's Cancer Study Group. J Clin Pathol 1997; 50(2): 128–34.
8. Bucsky P, Feller AC, Reiter A et al. Low grade malignant non-Hodgkin's lymphomas and peripheral pleomorphic T-cell lymphomas in childhood – a BFM group report. Klin Pediatr 1990; 202(4): 258–61.
9. Ramsay A. High grade lymphomas in lymph nodes (including paediatric cases). CPD Cell Pathol 2002; 4(1): 13–17.
10. Sandlund JT, Downing JR, Crist WM. Non-Hodgkin's lymphoma in childhood. N Engl J Med 1996; 334(19): 1238–48.
11. Kjeldsberg CR, Wilson JF, Berard C. Non-Hodgkin's lymphoma in children. Hum Pathol 1983; 14: 612–27.
12. Head D, Behm F. Acute lymphoblastic leukaemia and the lymphoblastic lymphomas of childhood. Semin Diagn Pathol 1995; 12: 325–34.
13. Pinto A, Hutchison RE, Grant LH et al. Follicular lymphomas in paediatric patients. Mod Pathol 1990; 3(3): 308–13.
14. Shankar AG, Ashley S, Radford M et al. Does histology influence outcome in childhood Hodgkin's disease? Results from the United Kingdom Children's Cancer Study Group. J Clin Oncol 1997; 15(7): 2622–30.
15. Goldsby RE, Carroll WL. The molecular biology of paediatric lymphomas. J Pediatr Hematol Oncol 1998; 20(4): 282–96.
16. Gruss HJ, Herrmann F, Drexler HG. Hodgkin's disease: A cytokine-producing tumour – a review. Crit Rev Oncog 1994; 5(5): 473–538.
17. Levine PH, Kamaraju LS, Connelly RR. The American Burkitt Lymphoma Registry: eight years' experience. Cancer 1982; 49(5): 1016–22.
18. Magrath IT. Management of high-grade lymphomas. Oncology 1998; 12(10): 40–8.
19. Perkin SL. Work-up and diagnosis of paediatric non-Hodgkin's lymphoma. Pediatr Dev Pathol 2000; 3(4): 374–90.
20. Lones MA, Auperin A, Raphael M et al. Mature B-cell lymphoma/leukaemia in children and adolescent: intergoup pathologist consensus with the revised European-American Lymphoma Classification. Ann Oncol 2000; 11(1): 47–51.
21. Perkins SL, Segal GH, Kjeldsberg CR. Classification of non-Hodgkin's lymphomas in children. Semin Diagn Pathol 1995; 12: 303–13.
22. Pavlova Z, Parker JW, Taylor CR et al. Small noncleaved follicular center cell lymphoma: Burkitt and non-Burkitt variants in the U.S. Cancer 1987; 59: 1892–902.

23. Miliaukas JR, Berard CW, Young RC *et al.* Undifferentiated non-Hodgkin's lymphoma (Burkitt and non-Burkitt types). The relevance of making this histologic distinction. *Cancer* 1982; **50**(10): 2115–21.

24. Drillenburg P, Wielenga VJ, Kramer MH *et al.* CD 44 expression predicts disease outcome in localized large B cell lymphoma. *Leukemia* 1999; **13**(9): 1448–55.

25. Kramer MH, Hermans J, Wijburg E *et al.* Clinical relevance of BCL2, BCL6, and MYC rearrangements in diffuse large B-cell lymphoma. *Blood* 1998; **92**(9): 3152–62.

26. Berry CL. *Paediatric Pathology*, 3rd edn. London: Springer-Verlag, 1996.

27. Mirro J Jr. Pathology and immunology of acute leukaemia. *Leukemia* 1992; **6**(suppl 4): 13–15.

28. Warnke RA, Weiss LM, Chan JKC *et al.* Tumors of the lymph nodes and spleen. *Atlas of Tumor Pathology.* Washington, DC: Armed Forces Institute of Pathology, 1995.

29. Gordon BG, Weisenburger DD, Warkentin PI *et al.* Peripheral T-cell lymphoma in childhood and adolescence. A clinicopathological study of 22 patients. *Cancer* 1993; **71**(1): 257–63.

30. Benharroch D, Meguerian-Bedovan Z, Lamant L *et al.* ALK-positive lymphoma: a single disease with a broad spectrum of morphology. *Blood* 1998; **91**: 2076–84.

31. Nathwani BN, Kim H, Rappaport H. Malignant lymphoma, lymphoblastic. *Cancer* 1976; **38**: 964–83.

32. Koo CH, Rappaport H, Sheibani K *et al.* Imprint cytology of non-Hodgkin's lymphomas. Based on a study of 212 immunologically characterised cases; correlation of touch imprints with tissue sections. *Hum Pathol* 1989; **20**: 1–137.

33. The Non-Hodgkin's Lymphoma Pathologic Classification Project. National Cancer Institute sponsored study of classifications of non-Hodgkin's lymphomas: summary and description of a working formulation for clinical usage. *Cancer* 1982; **49**: 2112–35.

34. Orazi A, Cattoretti G, Joh K, Neiman RS. Terminal deoxynucleotidyl transferase staining of malignant lymphomas in paraffin sections. *Mod Pathol* 1994; **7**: 582–6.

35. Conde-Sterling DA, Aguilera NS, Nandedkar MA, Abbondanzo SL. Immunoperoxidase detection of CD10 in precursor T-lymphoblastic lymphoma/leukemia: a clinico-pathologic study of 24 cases. *Arch Pathol Lab Med* 2000; **124**: 704–8.

36. Czuczman MS, Dodge RK, Stewart CC *et al.* Value of immunophenotype in intensively treated adult acute lymphoblastic leukemia: cancer and leukemia Group B study 8364. *Blood* 1999; **93**: 3931–9.

37. Thomas X, Anglaret B, Treille-Ritouet D *et al.* Occurrence of T-cell lymphoma in a patient with acute myelogenous leukemia. *Ann Hematol* 1996; **73**: 95–8.

38. Hirose Y, Takeshita S, Konda S, Takiguchi T. Detection of human cytomegalovirus in pleural fluid of lymphoblastic lymphoma T-cell type. *Int J Hematol* 1994; **59**: 81–9.

39. Su I, Hsieh HC, Lin KH *et al.* Aggressive peripheral T-cell lymphomas containing Epstein-Barr viral DNA: a clinicopathologic and molecular analysis. *Blood* 1991; **77**: 799–808.

40. Glassman AB, Hopwood V, Hayes KJ. Cytogenetics as an aid in the diagnosis of lymphomas. *Ann Clin Lab Sci* 2000; **30**(1): 72–4.

41. Rabbitts TH, Boehm T, Mengle-Gaw L. Chromosomal abnormalities in lymphoid tumours: mechanism and role in tumour pathogenesis. *Trends Genet* 1988; **4**: 300–4.

42. McCarthy KP. Molecular diagnosis of lymphomas and associated diseases. *Cancer Metast Rev* 1997; **16**: 109–25.

43. Jaffe ES, Harris NL, Stein H, Vardiman JW, eds. *Pathology and Genetics of Tumours of Haematopoietic and Lymphoid Tissues.* Lyon: IARC Press, 2001.

44. Brown L, Cheng J-T, Chen Q *et al.* Site-specific recombination of the *tal-1* gene is a common occurrence in human T-cell leukaemia. *EMBO J* 1990; **9**: 3343–51.

45. Sanchez MJ, Bockamp EO, Miller J *et al.* Selective rescue of early haematopoietic progenitors in Scl(−/−) mice by expressing Scl under the control of a stem cell enhancer. *Development* 2001; **128**: 4815–27.

46. Haung S, Brandt SJ. mSin3A regulates murine erythroleukemia cell differentiation through association with the TAL1 (or SCL) transcription factor. *Mol Cell Biol* 2000; **20**: 2248–59.

47. Robb L, Begley CG. The SCL/TAL1 gene: roles in normal and malignant haematopoiesis. *Bioessays* 1997; **19**: 607–13.

48. Davey MP, Bongiovanni KF, Kaulfersch W *et al.* Immunoglobululin and T-cell receptor gene re-arrangement and expression in human lymphoid leukemia cells at different stages of maturation. *Proc Natl Acad Sci USA* 1986; **83**: 8759–63.

49. Greaves MF, Furley AJW, Chan LC *et al.* Inappropriate rearrangement of immunoglobulin and T-cell receptor genes. *Immunol Today* 1987; **8**: 115–16.

50. Pelicci P-G, Knowles DM, Dall-Favera R. Lymphoid tumors displaying rearrangements of both immunoglobin and T-cell receptor genes. *J Exp Med* 1985; **162**: 1015–24.

51. Cheng GY, Minden MD, Toyonaga B *et al.* T cell receptor and immunoglobulin gene rearrangement in acute myeloblastic leukemia. *J Exp Med* 1986; **163**: 414–24.

52. Kadin ME. Anaplastic large cell lymphoma and its morphological variants. *Cancer Surv* 1997; **30**: 77–86.

53. Stein H, Foss H, Dürktop H *et al.* CD30$^+$ anaplastic large cell lymphoma: a review of its histopathologic, genetic, and clinical features. *Blood* 2000; **96**: 3681–95.

54. Chan JKC, Buchanan R, Fletcher CDM. Sarcomatoid variant of anaplastic large cell lymphoma. *Am J Surg Pathol* 1990; **14**: 383–90.

55. Frizzera G. The distinction of Hodgkin's disease from anaplastic large cell lymphoma. *Semin Diagn Pathol* 1992; **9**: 291–6.

56. Stein H. Ki-1-anaplastic large cell lymphoma: is it a discrete entity? *Leuk Lymphoma* 1993; **10**: 81–4.

57. Foss HD, Reusch R, Demael G *et al.* Frequent expression of the B-cell-specific activator protein in Reed–Sternberg cell of classical Hodgkin's disease provides further evidence for its B-cell origin. *Blood* 1999; **94**: 3108–13.

58. Benharroch D, Megueerian-Bedoyan Z, Lamant L *et al.* ALK-positive lymhoma: a single disease with a broad spectrum of morphology. *Blood* 1998; **91**: 2076–84.

59. Smith CA, Farrah T, Goodwin RG. The TNF receptor superfamily of cellular and viral proteins: Activation, co-stimulation, and death. *Cell* 1994; **76**: 759–62.

60. Chiarle R, Podda A, Prolla G *et al.* CD30 in normal and neoplastic cells. *Clin Immunol* 1999; **90**: 157–64.

61. Hittmair A, Rogatsch H, Mikuz A, Feichtinger H. CD30 expression in seminoma. *Hum Pathol* 1992; **27**: 1166–71.

62. Haralambieva E, Pulford K, Lamant L *et al.* Anaplastic large cell lymphomas of B-cell phenotype are anaplastic lymphoma kinase (ALK) negative and belong to the spectrum of diffuse large B-cell lymphomas. *Br J Haematol* 2000; **109**: 584–91.

63. Drexler HG, Gignac SM, von Wasielewski R *et al.* Pathobiology of *NPM-ALK* and variant fusion genes in anaplastic large cell lymphoma and other lymphomas. *Leukemia* 2000; **14**: 1533–59.

64. Falini B, Pulford K, Pucciarini K *et al.* Lymphomas expressing ALK fusion protein(s) other than NPM-ALK. *Blood* 1999; **94**(10): 3509–15.

65. Paulli M, Berti E, Rosso R *et al.* CD30/Ki-1-positive lymphoproliferative disorders of the skin–clinicopathologic correlation and statistical analysis of 86 cases: a multicentric study from the European Organization for Research and Treatment of Cancer Cutaneous Lymphoma Project Group. *J Clin Oncol* 1995; **13**: 1343–54.

66. Kinney MC, Collins RD, Greer JP *et al.* Small-cell-predominant variant of primary Ki-1 (CD30)+ T-cell lymphoma. *Am J Pathol* 1993; **17**: 859–68.

67. Stein H, Mason DY, Gerdes J *et al.* The expression of the Hodgkin disease associated antigen Ki-1 in reactive and neoplastic lymphoid tissue: evidence that Reed–Sternberg cells and histiocytic malignancies are derived from activated lymphoid cells. *Blood* 1985; **66**: 848–58.

68. Pileri S, Falini B, Delsol G *et al.* Lymphohistiocytic T-cell lymphoma (anaplastic large cell lymphoma CD30+ /Ki-1+ with a high content of reactive histiocytes). *Histopathology* 1990; **16**: 383–91.

69. Harris NL, Jaffe ES, Stein H *et al.* A revised European-American classification of lymphoid neoplasms: a proposal from the International Lymphoma Study Group. *Blood* 1994; **84**: 1361–92.

70. McCluggage WG, Walsh MY, Bhuracha H. Anaplastic large cell malignant lymphoma with extensive eosinophilic or neutrophilic infiltration. *Histopathology* 1998; **32**: 110–15.

71. Jaffe ES. Anaplastic large cell lymphoma: the shifting sands of diagnostic hematopathology. *Mod Pathol* 2001; **14**: 219–28.

72. Agnarsson BA, Kadin ME. Ki-1 positive large cell lymphoma: a morphologic and immunologic study of 19 cases. *Am J Surg Pathol* 1988; **12**: 264–74.

73. Ten Berghe RL, Oudejans JJ, Pulford K *et al.* NPM-ALK expression as a diagnostic marker in cutaneous CD30-positive T-cell lymphoproliferative disorders. *J Invest Dermatol* 1998; **110**: 578.

74. Falini B, Bigerna B, Fizzotti M *et al.* ALK expression defines a distinct group of T/null lymphomas ('ALK lymphomas') with a wide morphological spectrum. *Am J Pathol* 1998; **153**: 875–86.

75. Falini B, Pileri S, Zinzani PL *et al.* ALK+ lymphoma: clinico-pathological findings and outcome. *Blood* 1999; **93**: 2697–706.

76. Felgar RE, Salhany KE, Macon WR *et al.* The expression of TIA-1+ cytolytic-type granules and other cytolytic lymphocyte-associated markers in CD30+ anaplastic large cell lymphomas (ALCL): correlation with morphology, immunophenotype, ultrastructure, and clinical features. *Hum Pathol* 1999; **30**: 228–36.

77. Krenacs L, Wellmann A, Sorbara L *et al.* Cytotoxic cell antigen expression in anaplastic large cell lymphomas of T- and null-cell type and Hodgkin's disease: evidence for distinct cellular origin. *Blood* 1997; **89**: 980–9.

78. Morris SW, Kirstein MN, Valentine MB *et al.* Fusion of a kinase gene, *ALK*, to a nucleolar protein gene, *NPM*, in non-Hodgkin's lymphoma. *Science* 1994; **263**: 1281–4.

79. Morris SW, Naeve C, Mathew P *et al.* ALK, the chromosome 2 gene locus altered by the t(2;5) in non-Hodgkin's lymhoma, encodes a novel neural receptor tyrosine kinase that is highly related to leukocyte tyrosine kinase (LTK). *Oncogene* 1997; **14**: 2175–88.

80. Iwahar T, Fujimoto J, Wen DZ *et al.* Molecular characterization of ALK, a receptor tyrosine kinase expressed specifically in the nervous system. *Oncogene* 1997; **14**: 439–49.

81. Kadin ME, Morris SW. The t(2;5) in human lymphomas. *Leuk Lymphoma* 1998; **29**: 249–56.

82. Bischof D, Pulford K, Mason DY, Morris SW. Role of the nucleophosmin (NPM) portion of the non-Hodgkin's lymphoma-associated NPM-anaplastic lymphoma kinase fusion protein in oncogenesis. *Mol Cell Biol* 1997; **17**: 2312–25.

83. Mason DY, Pulford KAF, Bischof D *et al.* Nucleolar localization of the nucleophosmin anaplastic lymphoma kinase is not required for malignant transformation. *Cancer Res* 1998; **58**: 1057–62.

84. Duyster J, Bai R, Morris SW. Translocations involving anaplastic lymphoma kinase (ALK). *Oncogene* 2001; **20**: 5623–37.

85. Uherova P, Valdez R, Ross CW *et al.* Nodular lymphocyte predominant Hodgkin lymphoma. An immunophenotypic reappraisal based on a single-institutional experience. *Am J Clin Pathol* 2003; **119**(2): 192–8.

86. Lukes R, Butler J, Hicks E. Natural history of Hodgkin's disease as related to its pathological picture. *Cancer* 1966; **19**: 317–44.

87. Lukes R, Butler J. The pathology and nomenclature of Hodgkin's disease. *Cancer Res* 1966; **26**: 1063–83.

88. Staudt LM. The molecular and cellular origins of Hodgkin's disease. *J Exp Med* 2000; **191**: 207–12.

89. Jacob J, Kelsoe G, Rajewsky K, Weiss U. Intraclonal generation of antibody mutants in germinal centers. *Nature* 1991; **354**: 389–92.

90. Kanzler H, Küppers R, Hansmann ML, Rajewsky. Hodgkin and Reed–Sternberg cells in Hodgkin's disease represent the outgrowth of a dominant tumor clone derived from (crippled) germinal centre B cells. *J Exp Med* 1986; **184**: 389–92.

91. Bräuninger A, Hansmann ML, Strickler JG *et al.* Identification of common germinal-center B-cell precursors in two patients with both Hodgkin's disease and non-Hodgkin's lymphoma. *N Engl J Med* 1999; **340**: 1239–47.

92. Emmerich F, Meiser M, Hummel M *et al.* Overexpression of I kappa B alpha without inhibition of NF-kappaB activity and mutations in the I kappaB alpha gene in Reed–Sternberg cells. *Blood* 1999; **94**: 3129–34.

93. Marafiotic T, Hummel M, Anagnostopoulos I *et al.* Classical Hodgkin's disease and follicular lymphoma originating from the same germinal center B cell. *J Clin Oncol* 1999; **17**: 3804–9.

94. Lukes RJ, Craver LF, Hall TC *et al.* Report of the nomenclature committee. *Cancer Res* 1966; **26**: 1063–83.

95. MacLennan K, Bennett M, Tu A *et al.* Relationship of histopathologic features to survival and relapse in nodular sclerosing Hodgkin's disease. *Cancer* 1989; **64**: 1686–93.

96. Colby T, Hoppe R, Warnke R. Hodgkin's disease: a clinico-pathologic study of 659 cases. *Cancer* 1981; **49**: 1848–58.

97. Wijlhulzen T, Vrints L, Jairam R *et al.* Grades of nodular sclerosis (NSI–NSII) in Hodgkin's disease: are they of independent prognostic value? *Cancer* 1989; **63**: 1150–3.

98. Ferry J, Linggood R, Convery K *et al.* Hodgkin's disease, nodular sclerosis type: implications of histologic subclassification. *Cancer* 1993; **71**: 457–63.

99. Georgii A, Hasenclever D, Fischer R *et al.* Histopathological grading of nodular sclerosing Hodgkin's reveals significant differences in survival and relapse. *Proceedings of the Third International Workshop on Hodgkin's Lymphoma 1995, Kolne, Germany;* 1995.

100. Ferreriro JA. Ber-H2 expression in testicular germ cell tumors. *Hum Pathol* 1994; **25**: 522–4.

101. Gruss HJ, Boiani N, Williams DE *et al.* Pleiotropic effects of the CD30 ligand on CD30-expressing cells and lymphoma cell lines. *Blood* 1994; **83**: 2045–56.

102. Harris NL. Hodgkin's disease: classification and differential diagnosis. *Mod Pathol* 1999; **12**: 159–76.

103. Weiss L, Chen Y, Liu X, Shibata D. Epstein–Barr virus and Hodgkin's disease: a correlative *in situ* hybridization and polymerase chain reaction study. *Am J Pathol* 1991; **139**: 1259–65.

104. Schlegelberger B, Weber-Matthiesen K, Himmler A *et al.* Cytogenetic findings and results of combined immunophenotyping and karyotyping in Hodgkin's disease. *Leukemia* 1994; **8**: 72–80.

105. Joos S, Kupper M, Ohl S *et al.* Genomic imbalances including amplification of the tyrosine kinase gene JAK2 in CD30+ Hodgkin cells. *Cancer Res* 2000; **60**: 549–52.

106. Kamel O, Chang P, Hsu F *et al.* Clonal VDJ recombination of the immunoglobulin heavy chain gene by PCR in classical Hodgkin's disease. *Am J Clin Pathol* 1995; **104**: 419–23.

107. Tamaru J, Hummel M, Zemlin M *et al.* Hodgkin's disease with a B-cell phenotype often shows a *VDJ* rearrangement and somatic mutations in the *VH* genes. *Blood* 1994; **84**: 708–15.

108. Seitz V, Hummel M, Marafioti T *et al.* Detection of clonal T-cell recepta gamma-chain gene rearrangements in Reed–Sternberg cells of classic Hodgkin disease. *Blood* 2000; **95**: 3020–4.

109. Hansmann ML, Stein H, Fellbaum C *et al.* Nodular paragranuloma can transform into high-grade malignant lymphoma of B type. *Hum Pathol* 1989; **20**: 1169–75.

110. Miettinen M, Franssila KO, Saxén E. Hodgkin disease, lymphocytic predominance nodular. Increased risk for subsequent non-Hodgkin's lymphomas. *Cancer* 1983; **51**: 2293–300.

111. Ferry JA, Zukerberg LR, Harris NL. Florid progressive transformation of germinal centers. A syndrome affecting young men, without early progression to nodular lymphocyte predominance Hodgkin's disease. *Am J Surg Pathol* 1992; **16**: 252–8.

112. Osborne BM, Butler JJ, Gresik MV. Progressive transformation of germinal centers: comparison of 23 pediatric patients to the adult population. *Mod Pathol* 1992; **5**: 135–40.

113. Falini B, Dalla Favara R, Pileri S *et al.* bcl6 gene rearrangement and expression in Hodgkin's disease. *Proceedings of the Third International Workshop on Hodgkin's Lymphoma 1995, Kolne, Germany;* 1995.

114. Poppema S. The nature of the lymphocytes surrounding Reed–Sternberg cells in nodular lymphocyte-predominance and in other types of Hodgkin's disease. *Am J Pathol* 1989; **135**: 351–7.

115. Kamel O, Gelb A, Shibuha, Warnke RA. Leu-7 (CD57) reactivity distinguishes nodular lymphocyte-predominance Hodgkin's disease from nodular sclerosing Hodgkin's disease, T-cell-rich B-cell lymphoma, and follicular lymphoma. *Am J Pathol* 1993; **142**: 541–6.

116. Delabie J, Tierens A, Wu G *et al.* Lymphocyte-predominance Hodgkin's disease: lineage and clonality determination using a single cell assay. *Blood* 1994; **84**: 3291–8.

117. Marafioti TM, Hummel I, Anagnostopoulos HD *et al.* Origin of nodular lymphocyte-predominant Hodgkin's disease from a clonal expansion of highly mutated germinal-centre B cells. *N Engl J Med* 1997; **337**: 453–8.

Radiation biology

JOSEPH A. O'DONOGHUE

Radiation biology deals with the interaction of radiation, primarily ionizing radiation, with biological systems. The effects of ionizing radiation extend over a vast range of timescales, from 10^{-15} seconds, which is the time over which a primary ionization event occurs, to many years after the initial exposure, when consequences of that exposure may still arise. Radiation biology includes aspects of many disciplines such as physics, chemistry, biology and clinical oncology.

Ionizing radiation is a very biologically effective form of energy. For example, a dose of 10 Gy (gray) will kill almost all mammalian cells present, i.e. generally less than 1 per cent of cells that experience a dose of this magnitude will survive. However, if the same amount of energy that is represented by 10 Gy were deposited in the form of heat, it would only raise the temperature by 0.002°C and produce negligible biological consequences. Partly as a consequence of its extreme potency, ionizing radiation can be measured very precisely. Moreover, there are well defined quantitative relationships between the measurable characteristics of ionizing radiation, in particular the absorbed dose, and the biological effects produced. These factors combine to make radiation biology a quantitative discipline.

The biological effects of ionizing radiation fall into two general categories: non-stochastic and stochastic. Non-stochastic refers to the deterministic effects of radiation and generally relates to situations where the severity of the effect is proportional to the dose. A typical question would be how much damage is caused by radiation, e.g. the toxicity produced by some therapeutic procedure. These are the sorts of biological effects discussed in this chapter. Stochastic refers to the probabilistic effects of radiation, where the severity of the effect is not related to dose but the incidence of that effect is related to dose. A typical question in this context would be what is the risk of some event occurring, e.g. the cancer risk from a diagnostic procedure.

IONIZING RADIATION

By definition, ionizing radiation is radiation that produces ionization events, i.e. the ejection of one or more electrons from atoms or molecules. Ionizing radiation is conventionally classified as either directly or indirectly ionizing. Directly ionizing radiation consists of charged particles such as electrons, protons, alpha particles and heavy ions. Indirectly ionizing radiation consists of uncharged particles such as photons and neutrons. Even for indirectly ionizing radiation, the vast majority of ionizations are actually produced by charged particles, such as electrons or protons, that have been knocked out of their atoms by primary interactions with the uncharged particles.

For biological purposes the fundamental unit of ionizing radiation is the absorbed dose. This is the energy absorbed per unit mass in material. The SI unit of absorbed dose is the gray (Gy), defined as 1 joule per kilogram (J/kg). In water, which is the main component of biological materials, the mean energy deposited per ionization is 32 eV [1 eV (electron volt) = 1.6×10^{-19} J]; 1 Gy is therefore approximately equivalent to 2×10^{17} ionizations/kg, or 2×10^5 ionizations for a cell of mass 10^{-9} g.

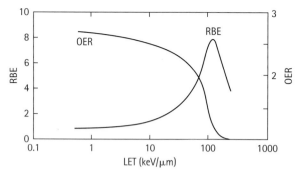

Figure 6.1 *Schematic representation of the relationship between relative biological effect (RBE) and oxygen enhancement ratio (OER) with linear energy transfer (LET). RBE has a maximum around 100 keV/μm. The oxygen effect is maximum for low-LET radiation and becomes smaller as the LET increases. (After Barendsen et al.[1])*

As a charged particle passes through material, it loses its energy by a series of interactions. The linear energy transfer (LET) is defined as the energy deposited per unit length of particle trajectory. This is an important determinant of the biological effectiveness of radiation and ranges from ~0.2 keV/μm for the electrons and X- or gamma-ray photons typically encountered in radiation therapy, to >100 keV/μm for alpha particles and heavy ions. High-LET radiation (e.g. alpha particles) produces more biological damage per unit dose than low-LET radiation (e.g. electrons). This is a direct consequence of the much denser distribution of ionizations along the particle track. Differences in the effectiveness of ionizing radiation may be expressed in terms of the relative biological effectiveness (RBE). The RBE is defined as the ratio of doses of 'standard' to 'test' radiation that is required to produce some specified biological effect. The standard radiation is generally taken to be 250 kVp X-rays or ^{60}Co gamma rays. A typical curve of RBE as a function of LET is shown in Figure 6.1.[1] It should be noted that the numerical value of the RBE for a given LET is not fixed but may depend on the nature and severity of the biological effect under observation. Most radiation used in clinical radiotherapy, including that produced by linear accelerators, brachytherapy sources and beta-emitting radionuclides, is of a low-LET nature and it is reasonable to assume that the RBE is close to 1.0. Only in unusual cases (e.g. proton or neutron irradiation, alpha-particle radioimmunotherapy) would significant changes in RBE become a major consideration.

Chemical effects of ionizing radiation

Ionizing radiation can directly produce chemical damage in critical biological molecules such as DNA. This is the primary cause of biological damage produced by high-LET radiation where the distribution of ionization events is very dense. In contrast, for low-LET radiation, a greater amount of biological damage is produced by an indirect route. The major component of biological systems is water. Ionizing radiation can cause the breakdown of water into OH. and H. radicals in a process termed radiolysis. These are reactive chemical species which can go on to cause chemical damage in addition to that produced by direct ionization. The amount and types of reactive species produced by ionizing radiation are dependent on the presence or absence of molecular oxygen. When oxygen is present, chemical damage that might otherwise repair spontaneously is 'fixed' due to electron capture by oxygen. In addition, an increased number of reactive species are generated in the presence of oxygen. Oxygen is thus a powerful radiosensitizer. For low-LET radiation, an approximately threefold higher dose is required in the absence of oxygen than in its presence to produce the same radiochemical or radiobiological effects. This ratio is called the oxygen enhancement ratio (OER). The OER is dependent on the LET, as illustrated in Figure 6.1.[1]

Damage to DNA

The primary molecular target that determines the cellular effects of ionizing radiation is DNA. The evidence for this consists of a number of observations, including the following:

- Large quantities of radiation delivered to the cytoplasm by short-range alpha particles do not result in significant cell death, whereas relatively small amounts delivered to the nucleus do.[2]
- Auger electron emitters directly incorporated into the DNA of mammalian cells via nucleosides such as (^{125}I) iodo- or (^{77}Br) bromo-deoxyuridine give rise to high-LET-type survival curves.[3,4] In contrast, when the Auger emitters are located extracellularly, bound to the plasma membrane or distributed within the cytoplasm, cell survival curves are of low-LET type, with initial shoulders and much shallower slopes.[5,6]
- Non-radioactive halogenated pyrimidines incorporated into DNA dramatically increase the radiosensitivity of mammalian cells.[7]
- Cells with defects in DNA repair are much more sensitive to the effects of ionizing radiation.[8,9]

Many distinct lesions in DNA have been identified, including single- and double-strand breaks, chemical changes in nucleotide bases, fragmentation of sugar moieties and DNA–protein cross-linkages.[10] Almost all of these molecular lesions are efficiently repaired by a variety of mechanisms.[11,12] The most biologically significant damage to DNA seems to consist of complex double-strand breaks with local multiply damaged sites.[13]

Radiation–induced cell death

Ionizing radiation causes cell death. This can be manifest through mitotic or apoptotic pathways. The process of mitotic cell death is characterized by the loss of reproductive integrity, although sterilized cells may go through several divisions before the progeny die. Actual cell death occurs at mitosis accompanied by cellular swelling, nuclear and cytoplasmic disorganization, and loss of membrane integrity. Apoptosis refers to a 'programmed' form of cell death and dismantlement that has a number of characteristic features,[14,15] such as the appearance of phosphatidylserine on the outer cell membrane, so-called 'blebbing' of the plasma membrane, leading to cellular dissolution into numerous membrane-bound fragments and a regular pattern of DNA fragmentation. The effects of ionizing radiation in terms of cell death can be studied *in vitro* by cell survival assays and analysed in terms of cell survival curves.

CELL SURVIVAL CURVES

The relationship between clonogenic survival and radiation dose is approximately exponential, which means that a given dose increment sterilizes a constant proportion of cells. For example if a dose x reduces survival to 10 per cent then $2x$ would reduce survival to 1 per cent, $3x$ to 0.1 per cent, and so on. Expressed as a semi-logarithmic plot, a pure exponential survival curve would be a straight line. However, rather than a straight line, the vast majority of survival curves for single doses delivered at high dose rates have a distinct concave-down curvature. This means that radiation becomes more effective per unit dose as the dose increases. This is illustrated in Figure 6.2.

There are a number of 'models' of radiation response that make predictions about the shapes of survival curves. The target model predicts that survival curves should have a 'shoulder' region of relatively low effectiveness and become straight lines thereafter. The theory of 'dual radiation action'[16] predicts curves that are linear-quadratic in shape, i.e. they start off linear but continuously bend downwards as the dose increases. Various hypotheses based on assumptions about the repair of radiation damage predict survival curves that have intermediate shapes.[17,18] It is unlikely that the correct model of the underlying process can be chosen simply based on the fitting of survival curves to experimental data as all the models can usually fit the data adequately. Partly because of its simplicity, the linear-quadratic (LQ) fit is the most commonly used in practice.

The LQ survival curve

The general features of the LQ survival curve are illustrated in Figure 6.3. The surviving fraction (SF) as a function of dose (d) is given by the following equation:

$$SF = \exp(-\alpha d - \beta d^2) \quad (6.1)$$

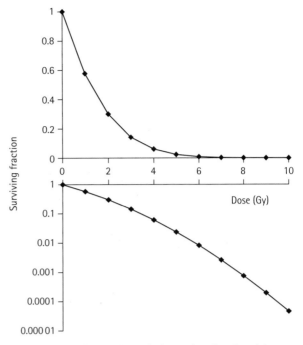

Figure 6.2 *The clonogenic survival curve is a plot of surviving fraction of irradiated cells as a function of dose. It is usually depicted on a semi-logarithmic scale as shown in the lower panel. On this scale most survival curves have downward curvature.*

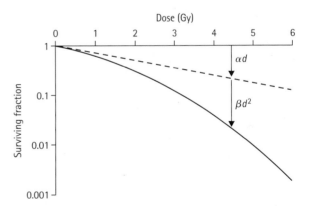

Figure 6.3 *The linear-quadratic (LQ) survival curve is the one that is most commonly used. On a semi-logarithmic scale the initial slope is given by the α parameter. As the dose (d) increases, the quadratic component of cell kill (βd^2) becomes more important. The ratio α/β describes the curvature of the survival curve.*

The parameters α and β are constants that describe the shape of the curve. One possible biophysical interpretation of these parameters is that α equals the rate of cell kill by a single-hit mechanism and β equals the rate of cell kill caused by the interaction of two sublethal hits, but this is probably an oversimplification. On a semi-logarithmic plot, the LQ curve is continuously bending with an initial slope, α. At low doses the αd term is the main determinant of survival, but as the dose increases, the βd^2 term becomes more important. The ratio α/β describes the curvature of the survival curve. Lower values of α/β have greater curvature than higher values.

THE 5 Rs

Some of the key features that govern the response of cell populations to ionizing radiation have been systematized as the '5 Rs' of radiobiology,[19] which refer to radiosensitivity, repair, redistribution, repopulation and reoxygenation.

RADIOSENSITIVITY

Clinically, tumours vary in their response to radiation therapy.[20] At one end of the scale are tumours such as the lymphomas, neuroblastomas or small-cell lung cancers, which are clinically responsive and for which local control can be achieved with relatively low doses of radiation. At the other end of the scale are tumours such as glioblastoma multiforme or renal cell carcinoma for which local control by radiation is unlikely with currently achievable doses. These variations in clinical responsiveness are reflected to some extent in the radiosensitivity of cell lines grown *in vitro*.[21,22]

REPAIR

When tumour cells grown in culture are irradiated by low-LET radiation, given a period of 'rest' and then irradiated again, the initial low portion of the survival curve reappears (Figure 6.4). This is usually interpreted as being due to repair of radiation damage. The process of repair has approximately exponential kinetics, with the amount of repairable damage decreasing by half every 1–2 hours.[23,24] This has implications for fractionated radiotherapy where treatment is usually delivered by a series of relatively low individual doses of approximately 2 Gy separated by significant periods of time. In such circumstances, the overall level of cell kill is determined by the initial low effectiveness part of the survival curve, as illustrated by Figure 6.5. Another manifestation of repair is seen in the dose-rate dependency of response (Figure 6.6).[25] For low-LET dose rates in the approximate range 0.01–1.0 Gy/min, higher dose rates are more effective than lower dose rates per unit dose. This is usually interpreted to reflect repair that takes place during irradiation. However, the biological effectiveness is relatively constant for dose rates >1 Gy/min.

REDISTRIBUTION

It is well known that there is differential radiosensitivity throughout the cell cycle.[26] Cells in S-phase are generally

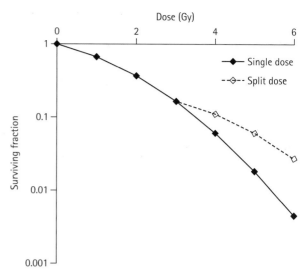

Figure 6.4 *Schematic representation of a split-dose survival curve. When cells are allowed several hours to recover from a first dose, the survival curve for a second dose retraces the initial low effectiveness component.*

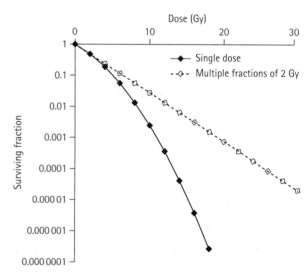

Figure 6.5 *Illustration of fractionated irradiation with individual doses of 2 Gy. The resultant survival curve represents a continuous re-expression of the initial low effectiveness part of the single-dose survival curve.*

the most resistant to radiation, while those at G2/M are most sensitive (Figure 6.7). Cells that are in the most sensitive phase when irradiation occurs will be preferentially killed. For acute radiation exposures, this produces a partial cell synchrony and a change in the overall sensitivity of the population. However, this synchrony is rapidly lost, because of natural variation in the rates at which cells pass through the cycle, in a process called redistribution. As a consequence of redistribution, it is usually assumed that the radiosensitivity of the cell population

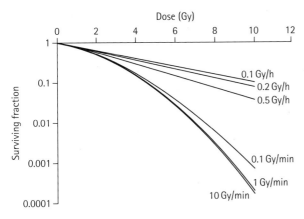

Figure 6.6 *Within the range of dose rates from approximately 0.01 to 1.0 Gy/min, higher dose rates are more biologically effective per unit dose than low dose rates. (After Hall.[25])*

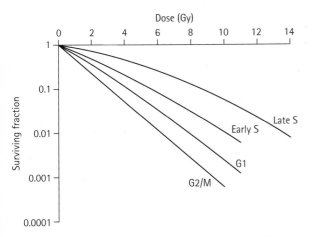

Figure 6.7 *There is differential sensitivity to ionizing radiation throughout the cell cycle. S-phase is the most resistant while G2/M is the most sensitive. (After Sinclair.[26])*

does not change with time due to cell cycle effects for standard fractionated radiotherapy.

REPOPULATION

Tumour cells in culture are capable of very rapid proliferation, with doubling times as short as 1–2 days. However, doubling times for the growth of visible tumours in patients are much longer.[27,28] The reasons for this discrepancy are twofold. Firstly, not all tumour cells may be actively proliferating in measurable clinical disease, and secondly, there is a high rate of cell loss.[27] When tumours are treated by radiotherapy, prolongation of or insertion of time gaps into treatment reduces the tumour control rate unless total doses are increased to compensate. This is usually attributed to allowing more time for tumour cell proliferation.[29–31] For treatments of head and neck cancer that are longer than 3–4 weeks, it has been estimated that around 0.5–1.0 Gy per additional day must be delivered to

maintain a similar level of tumour response.[32–35] By making some assumptions about the radiosensitivity of tumour cells *in vivo*, this would imply clonogenic cell doubling times of 2–3 days.[34,36]

REOXYGENATION

The oxygenation status of cells is a major determinant of their radiosensitivity. The oxygen effect is greatest for sparsely ionizing radiation (e.g. X-rays or beta particles) and is absent for densely ionizing radiation (e.g. alpha particles). Regions of local hypoxia are a common feature of many human cancers as evidenced by histological studies, P_{O_2} probe measurements and scintigraphic imaging.[37–40] Hypoxic cells can be as much as three times more radio-resistant to radiation than well oxygenated cells. Experiments in animal tumours have shown that the proportion of hypoxic cells remains approximately constant during fractionated radiation treatment.[41] This implies that some of the tumour cells that were previously hypoxic become aerobic. The process of reoxygenation appears to be essentially complete within 24 hours.

The existence of reoxygenation does not mean that hypoxia is not an important factor in tumour response. In fact, the pre-treatment tumour hypoxia status is emerging as an important determinant of relapse-free survival and overall clinical outcome.[38,42,43] This appears to be largely independent of the treatment modality used and implies that hypoxia is associated with a more aggressive tumour phenotype. In particular, hypoxia is associated with tumours that are more likely to metastasize.[44–46]

EFFECT OF RADIATION ON NORMAL TISSUES

The severity of non-stochastic responses in normal tissues following radiation increases with dose, when the dose is above a certain threshold. To generate detectable responses, many cells must be killed, as the death of only a few cells will not have a significant effect on physiological function. However, when a tissue is irradiated, its response involves more than just the death of the individual cells from which it is composed. It is also important to consider the effect produced in the tissue as a whole. Some of the biological factors that influence normal tissue response are described below.

FUNCTIONAL RESERVE

Some organs can tolerate higher radiation doses than others and still remain capable of function. Systemic irradiation of bone marrow with doses of around 2 Gy can cause potentially life-threatening complications. For the intestine, kidney, lung, liver and heart, local tolerance doses are higher (20–45 Gy), and for mature bone and cartilage, bladder and the central nervous system (CNS), they are higher still (50–70 Gy).[47,48] Tolerance doses for organs may also vary from patient to patient, depending on the nature and quantity of their previous treatments.

TISSUE ORGANIZATION

In broad terms, normal tissues may be organized in a serial or parallel manner. In a serial structure, damage to part of an organ can cause major functional impairment (e.g. spinal cord). In a parallel structure, function may be maintained even when a large part of the organ is damaged (e.g. liver). Purely serial or parallel structures are at opposite ends of a spectrum and tissues may have aspects of both types of organization. This is particularly important in relation to the spatial distribution of radiation dose throughout the tissue.

KINETICS OF CELLULAR DEPLETION AND REPOPULATION

Normal tissues are composed of complex systems of cells where the equilibrium between birth and death is kept in balance by regulatory mechanisms. The manner in which cell populations regenerate may also have an impact on radiation response. Organ systems such as the gastro-intestinal epithelium or the haemopoietic system have a 'hierarchical' or H-type organization.[49] This refers to the situation where there is a distinct population of clonogenic but functionally incompetent stem cells which feed into a maturing compartment with limited functional capacity and proliferative potential. This finally supplies a fully functional compartment with no ability for division. Ionizing radiation sterilizes the sensitive stem cells but physiological damage is not observed until replacements for the lost functional cells fail to arrive. The response of an H-type system is characterized by a progressive diminution of functional cell number until a nadir is reached followed by compensatory accelerated proliferation. The time to expression of radiation damage is primarily determined by the lifetime of functional cells and is relatively insensitive to dose.

Other organ systems may be different. Michalowski[49] described a 'flexible' or F-type organization that seemed to better explain the kinetic organization of some organs than the classical H-type organization. The F-type system consists of a cell population that is not only functionally competent but also capable of proliferation. Routine cellular turnover involves the loss of cells, capable of both division and function, at the end of their natural lifetime. In an unirradiated tissue, the demand for compensatory proliferation is relatively weak and replacement cells are produced by a steady-state but indolent turnover. Exposure to ionizing radiation renders a dose-dependent proportion of the cell population

non-viable. As cells attempt to divide in order to restore tissue function, latent radiation damage is expressed as abortive mitoses. Depending on the amount of latent radiation damage present, this may lead to a potentially catastrophic 'avalanche' of cell death as more and more cells are recruited to divide. For an F-type organization, the time to expression of radiation damage will be inversely dose-dependent.

Pure H- or F-type organizations are at opposite ends of a spectrum and tissues may have aspects of both.[50]

Acute and late effects

Normal tissue responses to radiation are conventionally categorized as acute or late effects. Acute effects develop relatively quickly over a period of days to weeks and are characterized by cellular depletion followed by proliferative recovery. The period over which these symptoms occur is related to the turnover times of the cell populations in the organ systems involved. This behaviour corresponds to the H-type proliferative structure described above. So long as the organ system is not irretrievably compromised and the temporary reduction of tissue function is survivable, there will be a nadir where the tissue effect is at its most severe followed by a recovery to something resembling normality. Examples include radiation damage in various epithelia and the haemopoietic system. Acute responses generally occur over similar times to the duration of treatment. This means they can be assessed as they develop and treatments can, in principle, be adjusted to alleviate symptoms, such as by introducing time gaps. Dose–response relationships for acute effects are relatively insensitive to changes in fraction size.

Late responses in normal tissues develop over a longer time than acute effects, typically months to years, and are again related to the relevant cellular turnover times of the organ systems involved. Late responses are usually characterized by progressive atrophy and fibrosis. Examples include fibrotic reactions in endothelial tissue, atrophic damage to kidney and liver, and delayed damage to the CNS including the spinal cord. Late responses occur over times longer than treatment durations, cannot be seen developing during treatment and their severity is not predictable on the basis of acute effects. Unlike the case for acute effects, inserting a break in treatment will not spare late occurring damage. For these reasons, late effects in normal tissues are usually dose-limiting for clinical radiotherapy. Dose–response relationships for late effects are highly sensitive to changes in fraction size.

A distinction must be made between the classic late effect syndrome described above and so-called consequential late effects.[51] These represent a continuation and development of acute effects that do not properly heal and may eventually lead to symptoms such as necrosis and chronic ulceration. Although these develop over protracted timescales, their origin suggests that methods of alleviating acute effects, including the use of time gaps in treatment, may reduce the incidence of consequential late effects.

Data from tumours grown in experimental animals and from the analysis of clinical dose–response relationships indicate that, in most cases, the behaviour of tumours is closer to that of acute-responding rather than late-responding normal tissues. In particular, the therapeutic effects of radiation on tumours may be significantly reduced by prolongation of treatment unless doses are increased to compensate.

THE LQ MODEL FOR FRACTIONATED RADIOTHERAPY

Quantitative differences in the fractionation sensitivity of acute, late and tumour effects may be usefully described using the LQ model. The use of the LQ survival curve as the basis for a model of normal tissue and tumour responses to radiation was first advanced in the early 1980s.[52,53] Since then it has been of great value in the analysis of clinical data and in the design of altered fractionation schemes. It is based on the assumption that not just cell survival but also dose–response relationships in general can be decomposed into linear and quadratic components.

As described previously (equation 6.1), the clonogenic survival of mammalian cells in culture following single acute doses of radiation can generally be described by the following:

$$SF = \exp(-\alpha d - \beta d^2)$$

Assuming that each fraction has an identical effect, the surviving fraction after n fractions of size d will be given by

$$SF_n = [\exp(-\alpha d - \beta d^2)]^n = \exp(-\alpha D - \beta Dd) \quad (6.2)$$

where $D = nd$ is the total dose. If we use the quantity $E = -\ln(SF_n)$ as a metric for biological effect, we can write

$$E = \alpha D[1 + d/(\alpha/\beta)] \quad (6.3)$$

In this notation, the quantity $[1 + d/(\alpha/\beta)]$ represents the relative effectiveness (RE)[52,54] of the total dose, D, when delivered at a high dose rate in fractions of size d, i.e.

$$RE = 1 + d/(\alpha/\beta) \quad (6.4)$$

The quantity $D[1 + d/(\alpha/\beta)]$ has units of dose and may be thought of as the dose required to produce the biological effect E if given as a very large number of very small fractions. This quantity has been called the 'biologically effective dose' (BED):

$$BED = D[1 + d/(\alpha/\beta)] \quad (6.5)$$

The main advantage of BED for computational purposes is that there is a linear relationship between it and biological response, i.e.

$$E = \alpha \times BED \quad (6.6)$$

This formalism is not the only one possible for the LQ model but it has the advantage that for any treatment schedule the BED is given by

$$BED = RE \times D \quad (6.7)$$

By making some assumptions about the nature and kinetics of repair of radiation damage, it is possible to calculate the RE for radiation delivered in a variety of ways. In particular, this type of analysis may be extended to brachytherapy, targeted radionuclide therapy and fractionated treatment with multiple daily doses.[54–57] The BED/RE formalism thus enables a unified approach to clinical radiobiology calculations.

Although numerical values of α and β may be derived from the analysis of survival data for tumour cells grown in culture, it is usually not possible to assign meaningful values to these parameters in the context of a normal tissue dose–response relationship. However, it is possible to estimate the ratio α/β. The α/β ratio is an important concept in clinical radiobiology. It characterizes the degree of non-linearity associated with the dose–response relationship.[58–60] Acute responses are generally associated with high values of α/β (≥ 10 Gy), indicating that the dose–response relationship is relatively insensitive to changes in fraction size. Late responses are associated with low values of the α/β ratio (~ 3 Gy), indicating a pronounced dependency on fraction size. For purposes of calculation, the α/β ratio for tumours is generally taken to be around 10 Gy, similar to that for acute normal tissue responses.

The effects of repopulation can also be factored into the LQ model. The simplest assumption is that cellular proliferation is exponential with a growth constant λ. The BED can then be written as

$$BED(t) = D[1 + d/(\alpha/\beta)] - \lambda/\alpha t \quad (6.8)$$

In this equation, BED(t) is now explicitly dependent on time t and represents the effect of radiation modified by concurrent cellular proliferation. The parameter λ/α represents how much more radiation has to be given to make up for proliferation in terms of Gy/day. For head and neck cancer, this value has been estimated as around 0.5–1.0 Gy/day.[32–35]

Although certainly an oversimplification, such a model may be applied to systems where rapid cellular proliferation is an important factor, such as tumours and acute-responding normal tissues, but not late-responding tissues where proliferation over the course of treatment is unlikely. It indicates that the biological effect produced in a proliferating cell population is determined primarily by the total dose, modified by the radiobiological effectiveness of that dose and the time over which it is delivered.

Altered fractionation

Mechanistically, the major radiobiological advantage associated with fractionation of external beam radiotherapy is the differential increase in repair of radiation damage in late-responding normal tissues in comparison to tumours. In terms of the LQ model, this can be understood as a consequence of differences in the shapes of the underlying dose–response relationships.

External beam radiotherapy given with curative intent is almost always delivered as a series of relatively small fractions, each of the order of 2 Gy. These fractions are usually delivered at a rate of one per day for each weekday (Monday to Friday) with no treatment at weekends. This means treatment is actually composed of a series of biphasic blocks. Each block consists of a high-intensity phase of five fractions delivered in a total time of 4 days from beginning to end, followed by a low-intensity phase of 3 days where no treatment is given. This treatment schema evolved empirically over the course of many decades since the introduction of cancer therapy using X- and γ-rays and is obviously shaped by the conventional 'working week'.

Over the last 15 years or so, and to a significant extent driven by LQ model analyses, there has been a great deal of interest in the clinical investigation of altered fractionation patterns. These generally have one or both of the following features:

- *Reduced fraction size.* Treatment with fraction sizes significantly less than 2 Gy is generally termed hyperfractionation. The rationale is to enable higher total radiation doses to be delivered for a similar level of late complications – as these responses are very dependent on fraction size.
- *Shorter overall times.* Treatments delivered as multiple fractions per day and/or without weekend gaps are generally referred to as accelerated fractionation. The rationale here is to minimize the impact of tumour cell proliferation by reducing the time over which treatment is given.

Most experimental fractionation schemes have elements of both of these features and may be referred to as accelerated hyperfractionation. This has been taken to its logical extreme in the CHART approach.[61,62]

Iso–effect and treatment schedule calculations using the LQ model

Iso-effect curves are plots of total dose versus fraction size or fraction number for a constant biological effect and have a long history in clinical radiobiology.[63–65] These are generally derived from clinical evaluation of differing treatment schedules that are judged to produce equivalent biological effects. In the early 1980s it was recognized that there is a fundamental distinction between iso-effect curves for acute and late-responding normal tissues.[66] Late responses have consistently steeper iso-effect curves than acute responses. Theoretical iso-effect curves can also be generated by the LQ model and used as the basis for the design of altered fractionation schemes.

From equation (6.5) for BED, if the fraction size, d, is specified, the number of fractions, n, is given by

$$n = \frac{BED}{d\left(1 + \dfrac{d}{\alpha/\beta}\right)} \qquad (6.9)$$

Alternatively, if n is specified, d is given by solving the quadratic equation

$$d = \frac{\sqrt{(\alpha/\beta)^2 + 4BED\,(\alpha/\beta)/n} - (\alpha/\beta)}{2} \qquad (6.10)$$

Equations (6.9) and (6.10) can be used to generate pairs of values of d and n that produce biological effects equal to some value of BED for any specified value of α/β. Figure 6.8 shows a set of theoretical iso-effect curves of total dose versus fraction size for a range of values of the α/β ratio. These are all calculated to be equivalent to 30 fractions of 2 Gy. It can be seen that the dependency of iso-effective dose on fraction size is much greater for low values of α/β than for high values.

Equation (6.5) for the BED applies if all the fractions are the same size ($= d$). However, if the individual doses are not all the same but are given by d_i, ($i = 1$ to n) the BED is given by

$$BED = \sum_{i=1}^{n} d_i\left(1 + \frac{d_i}{\alpha/\beta}\right) \qquad (6.11)$$

This indicates that the overall BED of a series of fractions is the sum of the BEDs for each individual fraction. In the simpler case of an overall treatment consisting of two parts (a and b) the total BED is given by

$$BED_{total} = BED_a + BED_b \qquad (6.12)$$

Conversely if BED_{total} represents the intended treatment and only a part of this treatment (BED_a) has been given, the remaining treatment to be delivered (BED_b) is just

$$BED_b = BED_{total} - BED_a \qquad (6.13)$$

The set of equations (6.9)–(6.13) are the basis for much of the scheduling correction calculations of interest in clinical radiobiology.

Whenever a radiotherapeutic treatment is prescribed, a spectrum of acute and late normal tissue and tumour responses is implicitly defined. This will depend on the dose distribution and fractionation pattern specified for the treatment. If a treatment schedule is subsequently altered by design or accident, the relative responses of acute, late and tumour tissues will diverge from the original

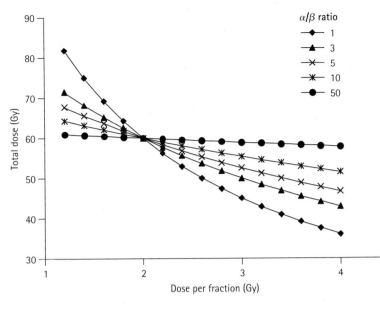

Figure 6.8 *Theoretical iso-effect curves generated using the LQ model for a variety of α/β ratios. The biological effects are calculated to be equivalent to 30 fractions of 2 Gy. The slope of the iso-effect curve is greater for lower values of the α/β ratio.*

intent. For example, an increase in fraction size from the prescribed value may necessitate a significant decrease in total dose in order to maintain an acceptable level of late normal tissue damage. However, acute effects and tumour responses will not be affected to the same extent by the change in fraction size. This means that the reduction in total dose, imposed by late-responding normal tissues, may cause a significant decrease in the effects of treatment on the tumour (and also on acute-responding normal tissues). Another example would be the insertion of a time gap into treatment. This could arise deliberately as the result of a clinical decision to alleviate acute normal tissue responses, or inadvertently due to patient absence, but it will reduce the therapeutic effect on the tumour and will not spare late effects. Situations such as the above do occur in clinical practice and when they do the LQ model can be used to provide suggestions on how to proceed.

Guidelines for schedule corrections using the LQ model

A key role of clinical radiobiology in the context of recommending 'corrections' is to ensure that the clinical significance of the unavoidable divergence in the spectrum of biological effects between intended and delivered treatments is minimized.

In order to achieve this goal, we can draw up a procedure as follows:

1 Understand the clinical priorities. Consider whether it is more important to deliver the specified level of therapy to the tumour or not to exceed the specified level of damage to normal tissues. This will set the context of the results of the model calculations.
2 Calculate the relevant BEDs for late effects and acute effects and/or tumour responses for the treatment initially prescribed and for that delivered so far. This

information enables calculation of the target BEDs that the remainder of treatment should aim to deliver.
3 Calculate how these BEDs may actually be delivered in terms of fraction sizes and numbers – bearing in mind any practical constraints.
4 Calculate the overall effects of the possible alternative treatments in terms of late and acute and/or tumour responses.
5 Decide on the most appropriate course of action.

All empirical models, including the LQ model, are more reliable when they are used in an 'interpolative' rather than an 'extrapolative' setting. For this reason it is useful to adopt some constraints or 'rules of thumb' in the context of scheduling calculations. These seek to ensure that recommendations derived from modelling do not go beyond the validity of the model. On this basis it is recommended that the upper limit of fraction sizes for schedule corrections are kept below ~3.5 Gy and certainly not more than 5 Gy, and also that the lower limit be greater than ~1.2 Gy and certainly not less than 1.0 Gy.

If a time gap in treatment has occurred, for whatever reason, the recommendations of the Working Party set up by the United Kingdom Royal College of Radiologists are to attempt to deliver the same number of fractions in the same overall time as originally intended.[67] This minimizes the impact of cellular proliferation on outcome. Although this is not always possible, especially if the problem is caused by a long time gap, it should be borne in mind that multiple fractions per day or treatment over weekends may provide an option to reduce the discrepancy in overall treatment time. If multiple fractions per day are being considered, it is best to have at least 6 hours (and preferably 8 hours) between fractions. The use of multiple fractions per day may require a dose reduction based on an incomplete repair calculation.[58]

SYSTEMIC RADIOTHERAPY WITH BIOLOGICALLY TARGETED RADIONUCLIDES

For disseminated or diffuse malignant disease, a systemic approach to treatment is required. The achievement of simultaneously selective and systemic therapy cannot be achieved by purely physical means but requires the exploitation of biological differences between cancerous and non-cancerous cells. Targeted radionuclide therapy entails the use of molecular vectors to deliver radionuclides to tumours. Examples include radioimmunotherapy with antibody-based vectors,[68–71] radiolabelled nucleoside analogues that target DNA synthesis[72,73] and the use of mIBG (meta-iodobenzylguanidine) for the treatment of neuroendocrine tumours.[74–76]

Targeted therapy is fundamentally a systemic form of treatment. The main theoretical advantage is the ability to deliver an enhanced radiation dose to disease that is either too small to be localized by imaging modalities or too widespread to be treated by local means. For locally confined disease, targeted therapy should most appropriately be considered an adjunct to local forms of treatment such as surgery or external beam radiotherapy.

Interaction between targeting agents and their biological targets

SPECIFICITY

Enhanced radiation doses can be delivered to tumours even if they are too small to be detected by imaging modalities and thus not susceptible to local forms of therapy. This theoretical advantage of molecular targeting may be compromised by issues of cross-reactivity with other cell types, non-specific accumulation of radiolabelled molecules or their metabolites in excretory pathways, irradiation of normal tissues by activity in the systemic circulation and, in some cases, long-range photon irradiation of the whole body.

NON-UNIFORMITY

The uptake of targeting agents in tumours is characteristically heterogeneous, even in cases where the requisite molecular target[77] or biological differential[78] is expressed uniformly. A heterogeneous radionuclide distribution gives rise to a non-uniform dose distribution with the degree of correspondence depending on the range of emissions from the radionuclide.[79,80]

POTENCY

From a dosimetric perspective, the most important parameters of a radionuclide are its energy emission spectrum and half-life, $T_{1/2}$. If the number of radionuclide atoms per unit mass is N and the energy emitted per disintegration is E, then the absorbed dose rate is proportional to $N \times E/T_{1/2}$ for conditions of electronic equilibrium. The ratio $E/T_{1/2}$ is therefore a useful indicator of the intrinsic radiotherapeutic potency of the radionuclide. The actual potency of a radionuclide will also be influenced by the cellular conformation and radiobiological characteristics of the tumour target and the uniformity of the dose distribution.

RANGE

Radionuclides do not have to be internalized or in contact with every tumour cell in order to deliver effective treatment. Tumour cells in regions with restricted radionuclide uptake may be sterilized by 'cross-fire' radiation from activity in other parts of the tumour. The amount of cross-fire irradiation depends on the spatial configuration of tumour cells and the emission range of the radionuclide.[81,82] However, the finite emission range also means that radionuclides present in the blood pool can produce incidental irradiation of the entire body and particularly the bone marrow.

These four factors are interrelated and it is their interaction that determines the clinical utility of targeted radiotherapy in any particular instance.

Dose-rate effects

In targeted therapy, the absorbed dose rates experienced by both tumours and normal organs vary with time and are generally more complex than in other forms of radiation therapy. This is caused by biological processes of accumulation and clearance superimposed on a background of physical decay. In terms of the LQ model, several authors have provided RE formulae for targeted therapy-like dose-rate profiles.[56,57] For a simple monoexponentially decreasing dose rate that decays all the way to zero, the equation[54] for RE analogous to equation (6.4) is

$$\mathrm{RE} = 1 + \frac{r_0}{(\mu + k)\alpha/\beta} \qquad (6.14)$$

where r_0 is the initial dose rate, k is the effective decay rate, and μ is the monoexponential time constant for repair of radiation damage.

Values derived for the repair half-time for mammalian cells in culture and normal tissues in patients fall within a range of minutes to hours.[23,24] In contrast, most clinical applications of radionuclide therapy deliver radiation dose with an effective half-time of several days. In terms of equation (6.14) this means $\mu \gg k$. Comparing equation (6.14) with the corresponding equation (6.4) for the RE of fractionated external beam radiotherapy, one can see that r_0/μ plays an analogous role to that of the fraction size, d.

Tumour uptake of radiolabelled antibodies in solid disease is typically 0.01–0.02 per cent ID/g (injected doses/gram). For a typical administered activity of 3.7 GBq (100 mCi) of iodine-131, the corresponding initial absorbed dose rate would be 4–8 cGy/hour, assuming electronic equilibrium and ignoring photon irradiation. Therefore, for repair half-times of up to 2 hours ($\mu > 0.35\,h^{-1}$), the equivalent fraction sizes will generally be less than 0.2 Gy. This suggests that repair of radiation damage will be effectively complete for targeted therapy and that it is justifiable to use the approximation RE = 1 in most cases.

The intrinsic radiosensitivity of cells and their proliferation rate will be important determinants of response to the low dose rate irradiation produced by targeted radiotherapy.[83,84] Simplistically, radiosensitivity determines how the target cell survival depends on dose, while proliferation rate determines how it depends on treatment time. If cells are proliferating during treatment or are radio-resistant, then a higher proportion of the dose is 'wasted' because it is delivered at a dose rate that is too low to keep pace with the increasing cell number. This principle should be applicable to proliferating tumour cells and also proliferating normal cells such as those of the gastrointestinal epithelium or bone marrow. Radionuclides with short half-lives deliver their energy in a shorter time and may be the most appropriate choice if tumour localization is rapid. This may occur in therapy of highly accessible disease such as leukaemia or in multistep targeting.[85] In other cases, a short half-life may cause greater damage to bone marrow cells relative to tumour and act to reduce the therapeutic differential. The pharmacokinetic behaviour of the targeting agent is therefore an important determinant of the most suitable radionuclides for therapy.

Dosimetric factors

Modelling studies of targeted radiotherapy suggest that, for each potential therapeutic radionuclide, there will be a certain tumour size where the probability of cure is maximized.[86] This is a consequence of the size-dependent reduction in absorbed dose due to energy escape. In the case of the most widely used therapeutic radionuclide, ^{131}I, the maximum cure probability is predicted to occur at tumour diameters of several millimetres (Figure 6.9). This relationship between tumour size and the likelihood of cure differs significantly from that for external beam radiotherapy, where smaller tumours are generally less difficult to cure than larger ones. Optimal tumour sizes for higher energy beta-emitters are larger than for lower energy beta-emitters and range from centimetre dimensions for high-energy emitters such as ^{90}Y to sub-millimetre dimensions for low-energy emitters such as [199]Au.

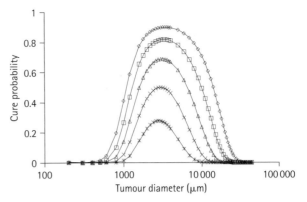

Figure 6.9 *Calculated relationship between tumour cure probability and tumour size for the radionuclide [131]I. Each curve corresponds to a different value of activity uptake in tumour. There is an apparent peak of tumour curability at around 3.4 mm diameter. (Modified from O'Donoghue et al.[86])*

These studies suggest that the anticipated size spectrum of disease is an important factor in the design of treatment strategies, especially with respect to the choice of therapeutic radionuclide. High-energy long-range emitters (such as ^{90}Y or [188]Re) will be poor choices for therapy of microscopic disease.

Another factor that has an impact on response to targeted radiotherapy is the characteristic non-uniformity of absorbed dose distributions in tumours. Modelling studies indicate that non-uniform absorbed dose distributions will produce inefficient tumour therapy.[87] They will 'under-dose' some elements of the tumour cell population and 'over-kill' others. Non-uniform dose distributions also become proportionately less effective as the mean dose increases, i.e. dose–response relationships have a concave-up shape. This means that simple 'dose escalation' may not lead to a significant increase in tumour response. To make matters worse, this effect is predicted to be most severe for radiosensitive tumours where targeted therapy would be anticipated to have the greatest likelihood of success. It is therefore important that therapeutic strategies be designed to reduce the adverse effects of dosimetric non-uniformity. Possible approaches include the use of 'cocktails' of radionuclides and targeting vectors,[86,88] combined modality therapy[89,90] and fractionation of targeted radiotherapy.[91,92,93]

KEY POINTS

- Ionizing radiation is a very biologically active form of energy and can cause cell death through mitotic or apoptotic pathways. The effectiveness per unit dose depends on the LET of the radiation.

The most important target molecule is DNA and the critical DNA lesions correspond to local multiply-damaged sites.

- Cell survival following irradiation can be assessed by clonogenic assays and expressed as survival curves. On a semi-logarithmic plot, cell survival curves have concave-downward curvature. The LQ fit is the most commonly used. The linear term (αD) is most important at low dose. The 'bendiness' of the survival curve can be described by the α/β ratio. Low values of α/β have more curvature.

- The '5 Rs' of radiobiology – radiosensitivity, repair, redistribution, repopulation and reoxygenation – govern the response of cell populations to ionizing radiation. In addition to these, normal tissue response is influenced by tissue organization, functional reserve and the kinetics of cellular renewal.

- The LQ model can be used to describe the radiation responses of normal tissues and tumours. Late effects in normal tissues have low α/β ratios and are highly dependent on fraction size but not irradiation time. Acute effects and tumour responses have high α/β ratios and are less dependent on fraction size but are dependent on time.

- The LQ model can generate iso-effect curves that are useful in analysing clinical data, designing altered fractionation schemes and correcting for scheduling problems that occur in treatment delivery.

- Items of concern for targeted radionuclide therapy include the specificity and uniformity of targeting and the range and therapeutic potency of the radionuclides. The selection of suitable treatment strategies requires knowledge of the pharmacokinetics of the targeting agent, the size spectrum of the disease target and the uniformity of targeting.

- Optimal therapeutic strategies for targeted radionuclide therapy may include the use of multiple molecular vectors and radionuclides, combined modality treatments and fractionation.

REFERENCES

1. Barendsen GW, Koot CJ, van Kersen GR et al. The effect of oxygen on impairment of the proliferative capacity of human cells in culture by ionizing radiations of different LET. Int J Radiat Biol 1966; 10: 317–27.

2. Munro TR. The relative radiosensitivity of the nucleus and cytoplasm of Chinese hamster fibroblasts. Radiat Res 1970; 42: 451–70.

3. Chan PC, Lisco E, Lisco H, Adelstein SJ. The radiotoxicity of iodine-125 in mammalian cells: II A comparative study on cell survival and cytogenetic responses to 125IUdR, 131IUdR and 3HTdR. Radiat Res 1976; 67: 332–43.

4. Kassis AI, Adelstein SJ, Haydock C et al. Lethality of Auger electrons from the decay of bromine-77 in the DNA of mammalian cells. Radiat Res 1982; 90: 362–73.

5. Bloomer WD, McLaughlin WH, Weichselbaum RR et al. The role of subcellular localization in assessing the cytotoxicity of iodine-125 labelled iododeoxyuridine, iodotamoxifen and iodoantipyrine. J Radioanal Chem 1981; 65: 209–21.

6. Narra VR, Howell RW, Harapanhalli RS et al. Radiotoxicity of some iodine-123, iodine-125 and iodine-131-labeled compounds in mouse testes: implications for radiopharmaceutical design. J Nucl Med 1992; 33: 2196–201.

7. Franken NAP, VanBree C, Kipp JBA, Barendsen GW. Modification of potentially lethal damage in irradiated Chinese hamster V79 cells after incorporation of halogenated pyrimidines. Int J Radiat Oncol Biol Phys 1997; 72: 101–9.

8. Marangoni E, Foray N, O'Driscoll M et al. Ku80 fragment with dominant negative activity imparts a radiosensitive phenotype to CHO-K1 cells. Nucleic Acids Res 2000; 28: 4778–82.

9. Foray N, Priestley A, Arlett CF, Malaise EP. Hypersensitivity of ataxia telangiectasia fibroblasts to ionizing radiation is associated with a repair deficiency of DNA double-strand breaks. Int J Radiat Biol 1997; 72: 271–83.

♦10. Pouget JP, Mather SJ. General aspects of the cellular response to low and high-LET radiation. Eur J Nucl Med 2001; 28: 541–61.

11. Lindahl T. Suppression of spontaneous mutagenesis in human cells by DNA base excision-repair. Mutat Res 2000; 462: 129–35.

12. Khanna KK, Jackson SP. DNA double-strand breaks: signaling, repair and the cancer connection. Nat Genet 2001; 27: 247–54.

13. Ward JF. The complexity of DNA-damage – relevance to biological consequences. Int J Radiat Biol 1994; 66: 427–32.

♦14. Kerr JFR, Winterford CM, Harmon BV. Apoptosis – its significance in cancer and cancer-therapy. Cancer 1994; 73: 2013–26.

15. Hengartner MO. The biochemistry of apoptosis. Nature 2000; 407: 770–6.

16. Kellerer AM, Rossi HM. A generalized formulation of dual radiation action. Radiat Res 1978; 75: 471–88.

17. Tobias CA. The repair misrepair model in radiobiology – comparison to other models. Radiat Res 1985; 104(2): S77–95.

18. Curtis SB. Lethal and potentially lethal lesions induced by radiation: a unified repair model. Radiat Res 1986; 106: 252–70.

19. Steel GG, McMillan TJ, Peacock JH. The 5Rs of radiobiology. Int J Radiat Biol 1989; 56: 1045–8.

♦20. Okunieff P, Morgan D, Niemerko A, Suit HD. Radiation dose-response of human tumors. Int J Radiat Oncol Biol Phys 1995; 32: 1227–37.

♦21. Deacon J, Peckham MJ, Steel GG. The radioresponsiveness of human-tumors and the initial slope of the cell-survival curve. *Radiother Oncol* 1984; **2**: 317–23.

♦22. Fertil B, Malaise EP. Intrinsic radiosensitivity of human cell lines is correlated with radioresponsiveness of human tumours: analysis of 101 published survival curves. *Int J Radiat Oncol Biol Phys* 1985; **11**: 1699–707.

23. Brenner DJ, Hall EJ. Conditions for the equivalence of continuous to pulsed low dose rate brachytherapy. *Int J Radiat Oncol Biol Phys* 1991; **20**: 181–90.

24. Bentzen SM, Saunders M, Dische S. Repair halftimes estimated from observations of treatment-related morbidity after CHART or conventional radiotherapy in head and neck cancer. *Radiother Oncol* 1999; **53**: 219–26.

25. Hall EJ. Radiation dose-rate: a factor of importance in radiobiology and radiotherapy. *Br J Radiol* 1972; **45**: 81–97.

26. Sinclair WK. Cyclic X-ray responses in mammalian cells *in vitro*. *Radiat Res* 1968; **33**: 620–43.

♦27. Steel GG. *The Growth Kinetics of Tumours*. Oxford: Oxford University Press, 1977.

28. Spratt JA, von Fournier D, Spratt JS, Weber EE. Decelerating growth and human breast cancer. *Cancer* 1993; **71**: 2013–19.

29. Withers HR, Taylor JM, Maciejewski B. The hazard of accelerated tumor clonogen repopulation during radiotherapy. *Acta Oncol* 1988; **27**: 131–46.

30. Trott KR. Cell repopulation and overall treatment time. *Int J Radiat Oncol Biol Phys* 1990; **19**: 1071–5.

31. Fowler JF. The phantom of tumor treatment – continually rapid proliferation unmasked. *Radiother Oncol* 1991; **22**: 156–8.

32. Taylor JMG, Withers HR, Mendenhall WM. Dose-time considerations of head and neck squamous cell carcinoma treated by irradiation. *Radiother Oncol* 1990; **17**: 95–102.

33. Bentzen SM, Johansen LV, Overgaard J, Thames HD. Clinical radiobiology of squamous cell carcinoma of the oropharynx. *Int J Radiat Oncol Biol Phys* 1991; **20**: 1197–206.

●34. Fowler JF, Harari PM. Confirmation of improved local-regional control with altered fractionation in head and neck cancer. *Int J Radiat Oncol Biol Phys* 2000; **48**: 3–6.

●35. Withers HR, Peters LJ. Transmutability of dose and time: commentary on the first report of RTOG 90003 (Fu KK *et al.*) *Int J Radiat Oncol Biol Phys* 2000; **48**: 1–2.

36. Denham JW, Kron T. Extinction of the weakest. *Int J Radiat Oncol Biol Phys* 2001; **51**: 807–19.

37. Thomlinson R, Gray LH. The histological structure of some human lung cancers and the possible implications for radiotherapy. *Br J Cancer* 1955; **9**: 539–49.

38. Hockel M, Knoop C, Schlenger K *et al.* Intratumoral pO2 predicts survival in advanced cancer of the uterine cervix. *Radiother Oncol* 1993; **26**: 45–50.

39. Nordsmark M, Bentzen SM, Overgaard J. Measurement of human tumour oxygenation status by a polarographic needle electrode. An analysis of inter- and intratumour heterogeneity. *Acta Oncol* 1994; **33**: 383–9.

40. Rasey JS, Koh WJ, Evans ML *et al.* Quantifying regional hypoxia in human tumors with positron emission tomography of [18F]fluoromisonidazole: a pretherapy study of 37 patients. *Int J Radiat Oncol Biol Phys* 1996; **36**: 417–28.

41. van Putten LM, Kallman RF. Oxygenation status of a transplantable tumour during fractionated radiation therapy. *J Natl Cancer Inst* 1968; **40**: 441–51.

42. Nordsmark M, Overgaard M, Overgaard J. Pretreatment oxygenation predicts radiation response in advanced squamous cell carcinoma of the head and neck. *Radiother Oncol* 1996; **41**: 31–9.

43. Brizel DM, Sibley GS, Prosnitz LR *et al.* Tumor hypoxia adversely affects the prognosis of carcinoma of the head and neck. *Int J Radiat Oncol Biol Phys* 1997; **38**: 285–9.

44. Brizel DM, Scully SP, Harrelson JM *et al.* Tumor oxygenation predicts for the likelihood of distant metastases in human soft tissue sarcoma. *Cancer Res* 1996; **56**: 941–3.

45. De Jaeger K, Kavanagh MC, Hill RP. Relationship of hypoxia to metastatic ability in rodent tumours. *Br J Cancer* 2001; **84**: 1280–5.

46. Rofstad EK, Rasmussen H, Galappathi K *et al.* Hypoxia promotes lymph node metastasis in human melanoma xenografts by up-regulating the urokinase-type plasminogen activator receptors. *Cancer Res* 2002; **62**: 1847–53.

47. Tubiana M, Dutreix J, Wambersie A. Introduction to radiobiology. London: Taylor & Francis, 1990.

♦ 48. Emami B, Lyman J, Brown A *et al.* Tolerance of normal tissues to therapeutic irradiation. *Int J Radiat Oncol Biol Phys* 1991; **21**: 109–22.

♦49. Michalowski A. Effects of radiation on normal tissues: hypothetical mechanisms and limitations of *in situ* assays of clonogenicity. *Radiat Environ Biophys* 1981; **19**: 157–72.

50. Wheldon TE, Michalowski AS. Alternative models for the proliferative structure of normal tissues and their response to irradiation. *Br J Cancer* 1986; **53** (Suppl. VII): 382–5.

51. Dörr W, Hendry JH. Consequential late effects in normal tissues. *Radiother Oncol* 2001; **61**: 223–31.

♦52. Barendsen GW. Dose fractionation, dose-rate and isoeffect relationships for normal tissue responses. *Int J Radiat Oncol Biol Phys* 1982; **8**: 1981–97.

53. Withers HR, Thames HD, Peters LJ. A new isoeffect curve for change in dose per fraction. *Radiother Oncol* 1983; **1**: 187–91.

♦54. Dale RG. The application of the linear-quadratic dose-effect equation to fractionated and protracted radiotherapy. *Br J Radiol* 1985; **58**: 515–28.

55. Dale RG. The application of the linear-quadratic model to fractionated radiotherapy when there is incomplete normal tissue recovery between fractions, and possible implications for treatments involving multiple fractions per day. *Br J Radiol* 1986; **59**: 919–27.

56. Millar WT. Application of the linear-quadratic model with incomplete repair to radionuclide directed therapy. *Br J Radiol* 1991; **64**: 242–51.

57. Howell RW, Goddu SM, Rao DV. Proliferation and the advantage of longer-lived radionuclides in radio-immunotherapy. *Med Phys* 1998; **25**: 37–42.

♦58. Thames HD, Hendry JH. *Fractionation in Radiotherapy*. London: Taylor & Francis, 1987.

♦59. Fowler JF. The linear-quadratic model and progress in fractionated radiotherapy. *Br J Radiol* 1989; **62**: 679–94.

60. Bentzen SM, Baumann M. The linear-quadratic model in clinical practice. In: Steel GG, ed. *Basic Clinical Radiobiology*, 3rd edn. London: Arnold, 2002.

●61. Dische S, Saunders M, Barrett A *et al.* A randomized multicentre trial of CHART versus conventional radiotherapy in head and neck cancer. *Radiother Oncol* 1997; **44**: 123–36.

●62. Saunders M, Dische S, Barrett A *et al.* Continuous hyperfractionated accelerated radiotherapy (CHART) versus conventional radiotherapy in non-small cell lung cancer: mature data from the randomized multicentre trial. *Radiother Oncol* 1999; **52**: 137–48.

63. Strandvist M. Studien über die kumulative Wirkung der Rontgenstrahlen bei Fraktionierung. *Acta Radiol* 1944; Suppl. 55.

64. Fowler JF, Stern BE. Dose-time relationships in radiotherapy and the validity of cell survival curve models. *Br J Radiol* 1963; **36**: 163–73.

65. Ellis F. Dose, time and fractionation: a clinical hypothesis. *Clin Radiol* 1969; **20**: 1–7.

◆66. Thames HD, Withers HR, Peters LJ, Fletcher GH. Changes in early and late radiation responses with altered dose fractionation: implications for dose survival relationships. *Int J Radiat Oncol Biol Phys* 1982; **8**: 219–26.

67. Hendry JH, Bentzen SM, Dale RG *et al.* A modelled comparison of the effects of using different ways to compensate for missed treatment days in radiotherapy. *Clin Oncol* 1996; **8**: 297–307.

●68. Press OW, Eary JF, Gooley T *et al.* A phase I/II trial of iodine-131-tositumomab (anti-CD20), etoposide, cyclophosphamide, and autologous stem cell transplantation for relapsed B-cell lymphomas. *Blood* 2000; **96**: 2934–42.

●69. Kaminski MS, Estes J, Zasadny KR *et al.* Radioimmunotherapy with iodine (131)I tositumomab for relapsed or refractory B-cell non-Hodgkin lymphoma: updated results and long-term follow-up of the University of Michigan experience. *Blood* 2000; **96**: 1259–66.

70. Kramer K, Cheung NK, Humm JL *et al.* Targeted radioimmunotherapy for leptomeningeal cancer using (131)I-3F8. *Med Pediatr Oncol* 2000; **35**: 716–18.

71. Divgi CR, Bander NH, Scott AM *et al.* Phase I/II radioimmunotherapy trial with iodine-131-labeled monoclonal antibody G250 in metastatic renal cell carcinoma. *Clin Cancer Res* 1998; **4**: 2729–39.

72. Kassis AI, Wen PY, Van den Abbeele AD *et al.* 5-[125I]iodo-2'-deoxyuridine in the radiotherapy of brain tumors in rats. *J Nucl Med* 1998; **39**: 1148–54.

73. Larsen RH, Vaidyanathan G, Zalutsky MR. Cytotoxicity of alpha-particle-emitting 5-[211At]astato-2'-deoxyuridine in human cancer cells. *Int J Radiat Biol* 1997; **72**: 79–90.

74. Lashford LS, Lewis IJ, Fielding SL *et al.* Phase I/II study of iodine 131 metaiodobenzylguanidine in chemoresistant neuroblastoma: a United Kingdom Children's Cancer Study Group investigation. *J Clin Oncol* 1992; **10**: 1889–96.

75. Hoefnagel CA. Nuclear medicine therapy of neuroblastoma. *Q J Nucl Med* 1999; **43**: 336–43.

76. Loh KC, Fitzgerald PA, Matthay KK *et al.* The treatment of malignant pheochromocytoma with iodine-131 metaiodobenzylguanidine (^{131}I-MIBG): a comprehensive review of 116 reported patients. *J Endocrinol Invest* 1997; **20**: 648–58.

77. Oosterwijk E, Bander NH, Divgi CR *et al.* Antibody localization in human renal cell carcinoma: A phase I study of monoclonal antibody G250. *J Clin Oncol* 1993; **11**: 738–50.

78. Moyes JS, Babich JW, Carter R *et al.* Quantitative study of radioiodinated metaiodobenzylguanidine uptake in children with neuroblastoma: correlation with tumor histopathology. *J Nucl Med* 1989; **30**: 474–80.

79. Yorke ED, Williams LE, Demidecki AJ *et al.* Multicellular dosimetry for beta-emitting radionuclides: Autoradiography, thermoluminescent dosimetry and three-dimensional dose calculations. *Med Phys* 1993; **20**: 543–50.

80. Humm JL, Macklis RM, Lu XQ *et al.* The spatial accuracy of cellular dose estimates obtained from 3D reconstructed serial tissue autoradiographs. *Phys Med Biol* 1995; **40**: 163–80.

◆81. Humm JL. Dosimetric aspects of radiolabelled antibodies for tumor therapy. *J Nucl Med* 1986; **27**: 1490–7.

82. Goddu SM, Rao DV, Howell RW. Multicellular dosimetry for micrometastases: dependence of self-dose versus cross-dose to cell nuclei on type and energy of radiation and subcellular distribution of radionuclides. *J Nucl Med* 1994; **35**: 521–30.

83. Fowler JF. Radiobiological aspects of low dose rates in radioimmunotherapy. *Int J Radiat Oncol Biol Phys* 1990; **18**: 1261–9.

84. O'Donoghue JA. The impact of tumor cell proliferation in radioimmunotherapy. *Cancer* 1994; **73**(Suppl): 974–80.

85. Paganelli G, Grana C, Chinol M *et al.* Antibody-guided three-step therapy for high grade glioma with yttrium-90 biotin. *Eur J Nucl Med* 1999; **26**: 348–57.

86. O'Donoghue JA, Bardiès M, Wheldon TE. Relationships between tumor size and curability for uniformly targeted therapy with β-emitting radionuclides. *J Nucl Med* 1995; **36**: 1902–9.

87. O'Donoghue JA. The implications of non-uniform tumor doses for radioimmunotherapy. *J Nucl Med* 1999; **40**: 1337–41.

88. Zweit J. Radionuclides and carrier molecules for therapy. *Phys Med Biol* 1996; **41**: 1905–14.

89. Buchegger F, Rojas A, Delaloye AB *et al.* Combined radioimmunotherapy and radiotherapy of human colon carcinoma grafted in nude mice. *Cancer Res* 1995; **55**: 83–9.

90. Vogel CA, Galmiche MC, Buchegger F. Radioimmunotherapy and fractionated radiotherapy of human colon cancer liver metastases in nude mice. *Cancer Res* 1997; **57**: 447–53.

91. Schlom J, Molinolo A, Simpson JF *et al.* Advantage of dose fractionation in monoclonal antibody-targeted radioimmunotherapy. *J Natl Cancer Inst* 1990; **82**: 763–71.

92. Buchsbaum D, Khazaeli MB, Liu T *et al.* Fractionated radioimmunotherapy of human colon carcinoma xenografts with ^{131}I-labeled monoclonal antibody CC49. *Cancer Res* 1995; **55**(Suppl): 5881–7s.

93. Goel A, Augustine S, Baranowska-Kortylewicz J *et al.* Single-dose versus fractionated radioimmunotherapy of human colon carcinoma xenografts using ^{131}I-labeled multivalent CC49 single-chain fvs. *Clin Cancer Res* 2001; **7**: 175–84.

7

Clinical applications of paediatric radiotherapy

JEAN-LOUIS HABRAND, B. ABDULKARIM & A. BERNARD

HISTORICAL BACKGROUND[1,2]

Radiation therapy was tested in cancer therapy soon after the discovery of X-rays by Wilhem Roentgen (1895/1896) and has been applied since the early 20th century. Nonetheless, for half a century, technological improvements have remained limited. Roentgentherapy was carried out using machines that produced photons of no more than 200–500 kV, with considerable cutaneous toxicity and limited penetration in biological tissues. These limitations favoured the extension of the use of radium 226, a natural radionuclide isolated by Pierre and Marie Curie, that could be readily implanted within the tumour. This allowed an improved sparing of surrounding tissues, when positioned according to strict rules of implantation. In parallel, observations that a relative sparing of normal tissues is induced by the fractionated administration of the dose were firmly documented in the 1930s and led to the 'dogmatic' delivery of the dose in four to five sessions per week.

The revolution in physics and technology which took place during the 1950s translated into considerable improvements in radiation-related tumour control and toxicity. This was mainly due to the introduction of megavoltage sources (cobalt 60, high-energy photons produced by electron accelerators), whose capabilities were further increased by the use of rotational 'isocentric' gantries. Maintenance of these sophisticated pieces of equipment along with the design and realization of increasingly complex personalized treatment planning gave rise to a completely new discipline – medical physics. One of its primary objectives was also to improve quality control and safety against radiation hazards. This explains the considerable interest in both the USA and Europe in artificial radionuclides (iridium 192, caesium 137, iodine 125), which overtook radium in the 1970s in their use in brachytherapy.

The emergence of radiobiology also dates back to the 1950s. This, the laboratory side of radiotherapy, helped to increase understanding of the basic mechanisms of action of ionizing radiation and also helped to formalize concepts applicable to clinical practice. Developments in medical physics and radiobiology also boosted the implementation of basic, and later clinical, research programmes dealing with 'exotic' particles (mainly protons and neutrons).[3–5]

Computer-based technology represents the most recent revolution. Introduced in the 1980s, it has had a profound impact on many aspects of radiotherapy, including three-dimensional modern imaging [computed tomography (CT) and magnetic resonance imaging (MRI)] used in treatment preparation,[6] fast and reliable dose calculations based on sophisticated algorithms, advances in linear accelerator equipment, and the development of new concepts in treatment planning (e.g. dose–volume correlations, biological modelling and intensity modulation).[7–10] Further rapid advances in these areas are expected.

BIOLOGICAL ASPECTS

Interaction of ionizing radiation with matter: from the atom to the tissue

PHYSICAL STAGE[1,11,12]

When photons such as X-rays or gamma rays strike biological material, they release mainly electrons and induce ionization. As they are not charged particles, their initial energy is progressively transferred in a random manner, which is responsible for the beam's attenuation along with energy absorption by the material. During collisions, photons are also deflected laterally. These processes explain depth–dose curve profiles that are measured experimentally, i.e. an initial build-up of the dose in relation to the path of secondary electrons, and then an exponentially decreasing dose and a lateral penumbra related to the scattering process.

The initial photon energy strictly conditions the beam's profile. Schematically, the higher this energy, the better the beam's penetration, the larger the build-up region (and so the lower the dose to the skin and subcutaneous tissues), and the lower the lateral penumbra (except at very high energies). For example, at 250 kV, a maximum dose (100 per cent) is deposited in the skin, 50 per cent is deposited at a depth of 7 cm, and the penumbra is of the order of 2 cm. At 4.5 MV, the depths for these doses are 1 and 13 cm, respectively, and the lateral penumbra is less than 1 cm.

Like photons, electrons can also be used therapeutically. As they are charged particles, they strongly interact with material all along their path and deposit a relatively uniform dose. In contrast to high-energy photons, their dose distribution profile exhibits a minimal initial build-up, quite a low penetration (no more than 5–6 cm at 20 MeV) and a large lateral penumbra (especially in depth).

The international unit of absorbed dose, the gray (Gy), is used as a measure of energy deposition in matter: 1 Gy corresponds to the absorption of 1 joule per kilogram (J/kg) of material. It is also defined as the amount of ionization produced by radiation in matter (1 Gy = 10^{17} ionizations/kg).

Heavier particles, such as neutrons, protons and stripped atomic nuclei, can also be used in more experimental radiotherapeutic programmes. Neutrons deposit a higher ionization energy along their path, and are considered high-LET (linear energy transfer) particles. They are of potential interest in radio-resistant tumours. Protons are low-LET particles, just as photons, but their dose-distribution, known as Bragg's curve, is radically different. This makes them of great interest in high-precision irradiation.[13] Theoretically, heavier ions combine both these biological and physical advantages. Depth–dose profiles for various types of ionizing radiation are shown in Figure 7.1.

MOLECULAR STAGE

Ionizing radiation generates peculiar ions called free radicals, which are characterized by the presence of single highly reactive electrons on their outer electronic layers. As soon as they are produced, free radicals profoundly affect the atomic environment, and therefore the molecular structures, of cellular components, especially DNA.

With photons, direct effects on DNA are less likely to occur than indirect ones, mediated by elements like oxygen (also found in water). The result is multiple single- and double-strand breaks (SSBs and DSBs, respectively). Enzymatic repair mechanisms are available, although they can be ineffective if they are overwhelmed by the intensity of damage, especially in DSBs. Generally they are considered to be more effective in normal cells than in tumour cells. They can also be defective if the patient has a disease such as xeroderma pigmentosum or ataxia telangiectasia, both of which affect sensitivity to radiation exposure. The time taken to achieve full recovery of

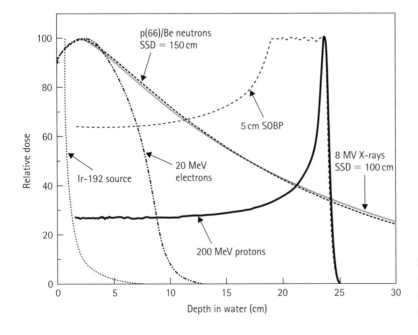

Figure 7.1 *Depth–dose characteristics for various types of ionizing radiation used in external beam radiotherapy. SSD, skin source distance; SOBP, spread out Bragg peak.*

reparable DNA damage (also called sublethal damage) is important in fractionated radiotherapy (see below).

CELLULAR STAGE, CELL SURVIVAL CURVES

At the dose level used commonly, most cell deaths are delayed until subsequent DNA replication (mitosis). Biological experiments have shown that mitotic blockade and cell death can even be delayed by several mitoses. This key concept explains the observation of slow tumour regression (by weeks or months) as well as late toxicity (up to decades). Recently, clinical observations have suggested that immediate cell death following very low doses of radiation could be mediated by apoptotic phenomena.[14]

Since the early 1960s, cellular sensitivity of mammalian cells to single doses of radiation has been extensively studied and fitted with mathematical models. The most documented of these, the linear quadratic formalism, describes the survival curves of mammalian cells as a function of dose:

$$S = \exp(-\alpha d + \beta d^2) \qquad (7.1)$$

where S is the proportion of cells surviving a dose d, and α and β are characteristic parameters of the survival curve. The α/β value is a reflection of the tissue radiosensitivity. The corresponding graphical representation (in semi-logarithmic coordinates) for late-responding normal tissues displays an initial 'shoulder' at low dose that corresponds to a relative inefficiency of radiation in this dose range (due to effective repair mechanisms; see below). This is followed by a straighter line at higher doses (Figure 7.2). In contrast, most acutely responding normal tissues as well as tumour tissues display straight curves throughout with a small or no initial shoulder.[15–17] This difference in the response to low doses of radiation for different cell lines has major implications in the design of multifractionated studies, dealing with reduced fraction doses.

TISSULAR STAGE

The classical 'law' by Bergogné and Tribondeau (1906) according to which tissue is more radiosensitive when it is made of undifferentiated and/or highly proliferative cells[18] has been revisited in the light of modern thinking on tissue organization. Numerous data have been accumulated indicating that both acute and late damage to normal tissues is caused by a combination of parenchymal, endothelial and stromal (also called 'supportive', e.g. glial cells in the brain) cell depletion following mitotic deaths.[19]

This could apply to tumour tissues as well. The parenchymal response, a depletion of parenchymal cells and, at a further stage, of clonogens, explains the acute toxicity (epidermitis, mucositis, pneumonitis). The non-parenchymal response can follow (but not necessarily) the parenchymal one and is responsible for late events such as submucosal or pulmonary fibrosis. There has been long-standing debate as to whether parenchymal and stromal cell depletion are the primary responses, with secondary vascular disturbances, or whether injuries to the microvasculature are primarily responsible for loss of oxygen and nutrient supply, and eventually for parenchymal cell depletion.

Factors that influence radiosensitivity

The biological response of tumours and normal tissues to ionizing radiation is governed by several factors.[1,20,21] Four 'classical' factors have been implicated: repair, repopulation, reoxygenation and reassortment. They are known as the 'four Rs of radiobiology'.

REOXYGENATION AND ANGIOGENESIS[22]

When partial oxygen pressure falls in tissues, a situation encountered in the depth of large tumours (and never physiologically in normal tissues), radiosensitivity falls as well (Figure 7.3). This 'oxygen effect' is due to the fact that radiation-induced free radicals are no longer 'fixed' by oxygen, an element that combines in highly toxic compounds such as hydrogen peroxide. This limitation of radiation efficacy on tumours is less pronounced with high-LET radiation that breaks DNA molecules directly. Unfortunately, clinical experience of high-LET particles or the use of oxidative drugs, or of the predictive value of hypoxia on tumour control, has remained very

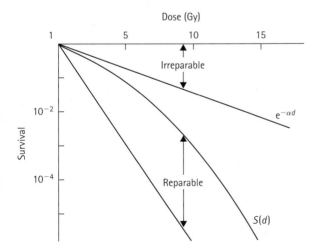

Figure 7.2 *Proportion of surviving cells following single doses of radiation. Middle curve: usual shape of curve in mammalian late-responding populations showing an initial 'shoulder' at low doses due to the effect of repair mechanisms. Curves on the left and right are hypothetical models without and with full repair of reparable damage. See text for details on S(d) and exp(−αd). (After Tubiana et al.[12])*

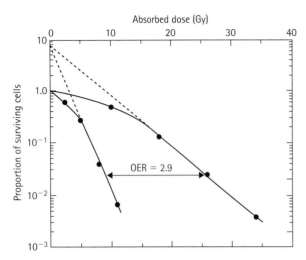

Figure 7.3 In vitro *survival curves in mouse mammary EMT6 cells under hypoxic (right curve) and aerobic (left curve) conditions. The photon dose needed to achieve a given surviving fraction is about three times greater under hypoxia. OER, oxygen enhancement ratio. (After Tubiana et al.[12])*

controversial.[23-25] New approaches are currently being investigated, such as the use of agents that act only at low oxygen pressure, that improve microvasculature or, conversely, that interfere with tumour angiogenesis.[26,27]

REPAIR

Effective physiological repair mechanisms can cope with DNA breakages by ionizing radiation (implicating enzymes such as DNA polymerase and DNA ligases). Nonetheless, some of them are irreparable or can only be poorly repaired, and this is called lethal damage (these breakages probably correspond to double-strand breaks that affect the same position in both DNA strands; they are much more difficult to repair as no complementary unaffected strand can be used as a model for repair). At low doses (i.e. ≤2 Gy), a substantial proportion of damage is still reparable and corresponds to single strand breaks. It is estimated that 6–8 hours [probably more as far as the central nervous system (CNS) is concerned] are necessary to achieve full recovery of this sublethal damage.[28] These considerations are important when multifractionated regimens are contemplated.

REPOPULATION

One possible means of improving the differential effect between tumour and normal tissues arises when cellular repopulation between two dose fractions is greater in the latter than in the former. For example, it has been shown that acutely responding normal tissues (i.e. skin and mucosae) are able to increase their cell turnover in order to limit acute toxicity. Unfortunately, some tumour types, such as Burkitt lymphoma, are known to have extremely fast repopulation, a situation better treated with accelerated regimens of dose delivery (see p. 137). Withers et al.[29] also showed in radiotherapy of head and neck carcinomas that an accelerated proliferation could be initiated at about the fourth week of treatment. These considerations explain the deleterious effect on local control of the 'split-course' technique, a regimen in which a gap is introduced into the course of treatment in order to alleviate acute toxicity and/or allow tumour (and therefore radiation field) shrinkage before boosting the residual disease.

REASSORTMENT

There is considerable variation in the cell killing achieved between various phases in the cell cycle. Most cells are more sensitive to radiation during the mitosis (M) and pre-mitotic (G2) phases than during the non-proliferative state (G0) or the synthesis phase (S). These differences can be explained by the amount of DNA present at the time of radiation (double in G2 and M), and also by differences in repair abilities (maximal in S phase).

Interactions between radiation and chemotherapy

Many drugs are radiosensitizing agents but to varying degrees.[30] The main mechanisms of interaction for common drugs are shown in Table 7.1. In practice, the effects can be minimized or enhanced by dose intensity of both agents, drug turnover, cell type, cell cycle duration and redistribution, and timing of the administration. For example, it has been shown that the presence of cisplatin adducts to DNA interferes seriously with subsequent radiation-induced repair mechanisms.

Dose and fractionation

The total dose required to achieve local control depends on the histological type of the tumour and its volume. Generally, the probability of local control as a function of dose exhibits a sigmoid-shaped curve, indicating that up to a certain threshold there is no clinically observable effect, which is followed by an abrupt increase in this probability with a small dose increment. A similar curve is reported for late toxicity.

As soon as the first clinical experiments in radiotherapy were conducted, it appeared that the administration of the dose in few sessions could improve the acute tolerance of normal tissues, especially the skin, and sometimes improve the effect on tumour tissues. This differential effect between normal and tumour tissues, as well as between normal tissues of different types, led to the standard fractionation of 10 Gy (1000 rad) per week, given in five daily sessions of 2 Gy. An acceptable alternative is four daily sessions of 2.5 Gy.

Table 7.1 *Possible mechanisms of interaction between drugs commonly used in adults and children and radiotherapy[30,63,64]*

Drugs	Interaction-type with radiotherapy
Actinomycin D	SD, PLD repair, ↑slope cell S curve
Adriamycin	PLD repair
Cis-platin	SD, PLD repair, oxygenation, ↑ slope oxic and hypoxic cell S curve
Methotrexate	Cell kinetics
Aracytine	SD, PLD repair, cell kinetics
5-Fluorouracil	Cell kinetics, ↑slope cell S curve
Vincristine	Cell kinetics
Nitrosourea (BCNU, CCNU)	SD repair, cell kinetics
CPT 11	PLD repair, oxygenation

↑, increase.

S, survival; SD, sublethal damage; PLD, potentially lethal damage.

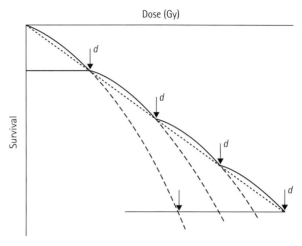

Figure 7.4 *Differential effect associated with fractionation. The fractionated dose (solid line on the right) provides a greater degree of protection than single doses (dashed lines on the left). d, dose per fraction. (After Tubiana et al.[12] and Peters et al.[66])*

In the 1940s, an attempt to rationalize the choice of a specific fractionation was conducted.[12] This corresponded to the need to alter the usual fractionation in unexpected situations (e.g. a gap in the treatment course due to an excessive toxicity, or breakdown of a machine), and also the need to compare different treatment modalities for similar tumour types in different institutions. The intensity of skin reactions and the regression of squamous cell carcinomas in the head and neck region were plotted independently as a function of total dose and number of sessions. This led to a highly convenient and popular set of curves, later formalized in the NSD (nominal standard dose) concept.[31]

Unfortunately, they were also perceived as universal models for the response of both normal and tumour tissues. The limitation of this approach became evident in the mid-1970s, when a late toxicity much more severe than that predicted by the models was recorded following slight increments of the dose per fraction. For example, it was reported by authors fractionating the usual dose rate of 10 Gy per week into three sessions of 3.3 Gy (330 rad) each, in order to alleviate patient overload in their department. Various types of late reaction were seen, including pericarditis after mantle irradiation, lung fibrosis in breast irradiation, and severe laryngeal oedema requiring tracheotomy in laryngeal cancers.[32] It also became evident that fractionation of the dose (i.e. the amount given per session) and protraction (i.e. the duration, in days, of the entire treatment course) should be considered as two separate entities.

Both biological and clinical data have shown that:

- *Fractionation of the dose* is associated with cell repair mechanisms following radiation, especially in sublethal damage, a process highly sensitive to the dose administered and inter-fraction interval (ideally ≥6–8 hours). As a consequence, fractionating the dose can preferentially protect late-responding tissues (heart, lung, kidney, retina) compared with acute-responding[33,34] or tumour tissues.

- *Protraction* is associated with cell repopulation velocity: the longer the treatment time, the better the protection of fast-growing cell populations. Increased protraction has been shown to improve acute tolerance of skin and mucosa, but unfortunately also to spare highly proliferating tumours with shorter doubling times.

Fractionation and protraction are also believed to favour oxygenation of hypoxic cells and cell-cycle redistribution.

Using the α/β formalism (see above), comparing one type of treatment delivering N fractions of d Gy each with a biologically isoeffective treatment of N' fractions of d' Gy each, one arrives at the following equation:

$$\frac{Nd}{N'd'} = \frac{(\alpha/\beta) + d'}{(\alpha/\beta) + d} \quad (7.2)$$

Practically speaking, the α/β value is estimated to be close to 2–3 in late-responding tissues, and 10 in acute-responding and tumour tissues. The differential effect induced by fractionation is most clearly evidenced on survival curves with marked initial curvature (i.e. low α/β ratio) (Figure 7.4).

There is some controversy concerning the repopulation pattern and velocity in both normal and tumour tissues. It is generally estimated that a 1-day gain (or loss) in treatment protraction is equivalent to a 0.3–0.5 Gy gain (loss) in total dose as far as tumours are concerned.

TECHNICAL ASPECTS

Radiation equipment

There are two techniques for delivering radiation therapy: external beam therapy and brachytherapy.

EXTERNAL BEAM RADIOTHERAPY

In external beam radiotherapy, the source of ionizing radiation is placed outside the patient and at a specific distance. Megavoltage equipment producing high-energy photons at several million electron-volts is preferred when tumours are located at depth. Compared with equipment of old (for roentgentherapy), which produced X-rays not exceeding 250–500 kV, current machines produce photons that range from around 1 MV (cobalt machines) up to 20–25 MV (linear accelerators). Electrons are also produced by linear accelerators. They deliver the dose superficially, which makes them appropriate for the irradiation of skin lesions or superficial lymphadenopathies. High-energy electrons that penetrate up to 6–7 cm may also be used in the management of spinal canal lesions, such as intramedullary gliomas or for spinal 'prophylaxis' in medulloblastomas.

Modern equipment also includes isocentric gantries, which can rotate around the patient quickly and accurately. They facilitate isocentric techniques, in which beams are directed from all angles to focus on the target located within the patient. A sophisticated couch (which can be isocentrically mounted) is also an integral part of the modern setup. Recent accelerators have online imaging capabilities (portal films), for immediate verification, and multileaf collimators (made of pairs of thin metallic leaves, electronically driven) that are progressively replacing conventional shielding blocks.

This enables delivery of coformal and intensity modulated radiation therapy, where the field can be adapted to tumour contour.

BRACHYTHERAPY

In brachytherapy, radioactive sources are placed near or implanted directly into the tumour. Sources can take the form of needles, wires or seeds. Iridium 192, caesium 137 and iodine 125 are the most common radionuclides employed. In the low-dose-rate approach (generally preferred in children), ~1 cGy is administered per minute, for a total of 2–6 days.[35] Although the total amount of radiation delivered to a tumour is similar to that in external beam radiotherapy, the dose administration is different since it is continuous. The biological advantages of continuous administration of a low dose of radiation include improved repair of sublethal injuries in normal tissues, efficacy in tumour hypoxic cells, and effectiveness in fast-growing tumours (due to shortening of treatment time, which avoids tumour clonogenic repopulation). Furthermore, brachytherapy offers the advantage of a high physical dose selectivity due to the rapid fall-off around the radioactive material. The disadvantages of the technique are the necessity of having to carry out one or two procedures in an operating room (usually under general anaesthetic in children), to implant and remove the material, and the need for hospitalization during irradiation with limited visitor contact (for safety reasons). Furthermore, only accessible sites can be treated in this way, more specifically anatomical cavities (mouth, oropharynx, vagina) and superficial soft part tumours. Large tumour sizes are also generally considered as contraindications. Brachytherapists involved in the management of paediatric tumours should have a high level of expertise and be able to cooperate effectively with paediatric surgeons, radiologists and paediatric oncologists.

Treatment simulation and planning[11]

To successfully treat a patient, the radiation oncologist must seek to maximize the dose delivered to the tumour and minimize that absorbed by normal tissues. As most tumours are deep-seated, and closely related to radiosensitive normal tissues, tailor-fit beam arrangements are necessary in most curative situations. The initial step includes a preparation called simulation. During this procedure, various immobilization devices are prepared, depending on the anatomical segment involved and the accuracy required.

Customized polystyrene moulds are easy to create and provide safe and comfortable positioning of large anatomical segments. For example, they allow fast and reproducible setup in radiotherapy of medulloblastoma which requires entire CNS coverage (Figure 7.5). Accuracy is of the order of a few millimetres if the patient is highly compliant. If not, additional accessories should be added, such as adhesive straps, plaster or foam moulages and thermoplastic sheets. Thermoplastic masks have gained wide acceptance in brain and head and neck conditions since they allow excellent control (even in non-compliant children) and are accurate to within a few millimetres; they are also relatively cheap (Figure 7.6). Stereotactic alignment generally requires the use of stereotactic frames inspired by neurosurgical appliances, since millimetric or submillimetric positioning is needed.[36] On the other hand, palliative treatment is commonly managed with simple devices such as rubber bands or sand or rice bags, especially in infants.

The second step in simulation is typically performed using a piece of radiological equipment called a simulator. The simulator is built up like a radiotherapy machine but can produce high-quality radiographs. During this procedure, many variables that are crucial for appropriate patient setup and treatment are recorded, including field size, angulation and positioning relative to anatomical

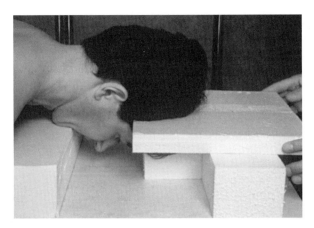

Figure 7.5 *Immobilization of a medulloblastoma patient using a polystyrene cast in preparation for radiotherapy.*

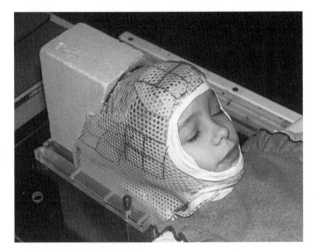

Figure 7.6 *Immobilization of a child with hemispheric glioma using a thermoplastic mask in preparation for radiotherapy.*

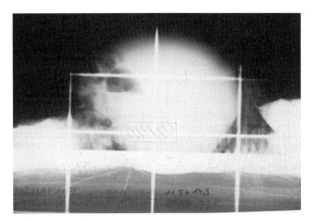

Figure 7.7 *Simulation film of a Pepper syndrome (4S neuroblastoma).*

realistic digitally reconstructed radiographs (similar to conventional radiographs) and 'beam's eye views' of the target along with surrounding anatomical structures. They also generate dose–volume histograms of the tumour and critical structures that help compare rival treatment plans and thus aid selection of the optimal one.

Treatment delivery

In the majority of children, radiation therapy can be administered without sedation. Treatment modalities should be clearly explained to children and their parents in appropriate language in order to receive optimal cooperation. It is wise to separate parents from their child as early as the simulation stage, something that becomes compulsory at the time of treatment. Portal films should be repeated as frequently as is necessary during treatment delivery, and at least once a week in the case of sophisticated planning. In children below 3 years of age, patient cooperation can be impossible to obtain. In these cases, conscious or deep sedation may be necessary.[37] General anaesthesia (using inhaled or intravenous medication) is usually reserved for children who are resistant to sedation or those requiring a high degree of immobilization, such as those with a retinoblastoma.

CLINICAL ASPECTS

Current place and mode of administration of radiotherapy in children

The mainstay of treatment (along with surgery) until the 1970s, radiation therapy is nowadays only part of an integrated management in which chemotherapy frequently plays the prominent role. Chemotherapy has proved particularly valuable in fast-growing processes that have a high propensity for early distant dissemination. Unlike radiotherapy, it is not known for interfering, in

landmarks (fiducial marks that help locate the beam's entry points are drawn on the skin or on the mask). The simulation films also allow drawing of customized blocks (generally made from lead-based alloys such as cerrobend) that shield normal tissues. Figure 7.7 shows the simulation film of opposed symmetrical lateral fields used in Pepper syndrome. The posterior limit of the beam is aligned with the anterior aspect of the spine, and a kidney block is added, in order to spare these structures.

A further important step is patient contour acquisition, a prerequisite for an accurate dose calculation, called dosimetry. Manual recording using simple paper transfer is still in use in urgent palliative situations. Otherwise, it is now routinely replaced by CT scan. High-definition CT scanning can provide the information necessary to perform three-dimensional treatment planning. The radiation oncologist, with the help of a biophysicist, can display organs and tumour contours on a workstation and design sophisticated beam arrangements (virtual simulation). Most recent software packages provide the long run, with normal tissue development (at least in terms of visible cosmetic sequelae). Chemotherapy has certainly been responsible for some of the major advances that have been recorded in the treatment of tumours during the past two decades (especially Burkitt lymphoma, osteosarcoma and nephroblastoma), with favourable long-term prognosis for about 70 per cent.

Nonetheless, radiotherapy still remains necessary in most therapeutic approaches for many reasons. Permanent local control of the primary is rarely maintained by chemotherapy alone (with or without surgical resection). This is the case for soft part sarcomas and advanced nephroblastomas, neuroblastomas and Ewing's sarcomas. Brain tumours, the most frequent solid neoplasms in childhood, have limited chemosensitivity, and radiotherapy remains the gold-standard treatment in most cases (with the notable exception of very young children). It is also noteworthy that radiotherapy has undergone considerable improvement, particularly during the past decade, which in most cases makes it acceptable to clinicians and parents in terms of long-term side-effects. These innovations include the possible dose and target volume adaptations to the response to an initial chemotherapy regimen (an approach largely investigated in Hodgkin's disease, 'low risk' medulloblastomas and resectable Ewing's sarcomas), and technical refinements such as conformal radiotherapy (especially in brain tumours),[38] brachytherapy (particularly in small-sized genitourinary neoplasms), hyperfractionation of the dose (e.g. in medulloblastomas and neuroblastomas) and heavy charged particles (mainly protons).[39] Table 7.2 shows the usual dose ranges for tumour control depending on tumour burden at the time of radiation (i.e. gross or microscopic invasion, such as is observed following effective chemotherapy or tumour resection). Table 7.3 gives the tolerance doses for late-responding normal tissues in children. Additional information is provided in the relevant chapters of this book.

Combined chemotherapy and radiotherapy

When chemotherapy and radiotherapy are combined, the therapeutic gain can result from a 'spatial' cooperation in which radiotherapy acts on the primary tumour and chemotherapy on distant metastases. There may also be an improved efficacy of the combination on the primary site, but this is generally achieved at the price of increased toxicity. As mentioned above, paediatric tumours represent a paradigm for such approaches.[40,41]

Historically speaking, the first clinical experiments were actually pioneered in this field in the early 1950s. Farber et al.[42] showed that a combination of actinomycin D injections and radiotherapy improved the outcome of nephroblastomas, and allowed a dose reduction of actinomycin D

Table 7.2 *Curative dose range (Gy, fractionated) of radiotherapy administered in common paediatric tumours*

Tumour type	Tumour burden	
	Microscopic invasion	Macroscopic invasion
Nephroblastoma	10–15	25–35
Acute lymphoblastic leukaemia	15–18	24–40
Seminoma	20–30	40–50
Neuroblastoma	20–25	35–40
Rhabdomyosarcoma	35–45	45–55
Benign glioma	45–50	50–55
Medulloblastoma	25–35	55–60
Ewing's sarcoma	40–45	55–60
Malignant glioma	50–55	55–60
Nasopharyngeal carcinoma	45–50	65–70

Table 7.3 *Tolerance doses of fractionated irradiation in children (from Bey,[65] and personal data)*

Tissue	Dose (Gy)	Type of lesion
Musculoskeletal system		
Growing cartilage	10	Hypoplasia
Vertebrae	10	Hypoplasia, asymmetrical growth
Soft tissues	20	Hypoplasia
Dental follicles	15–20	Hypoplasia
Endocrine glands		
Pituitary	20	Growth hormone failure
	40	Panhypopituitarism
Thyroid	25–30	Hypothyroidism
Gonads		
Ovaries	2–3	Infertility
	12	Primary amenorrhoea
Testicles	1–3	Infertility
	25	Leydig cell dysfunction
Whole brain	25	Intellectual impairments
Whole kidney	12	Renal failure
Whole lungs	15	Fibrosis

compared with the dosage of the drug administered alone. Later, the use of combined chemotherapy and radiotherapy largely contributed to the dramatic improvement in outcome for many tumour types (see above and chapters on specific tumours).

Unlike in their adult counterparts, in children the use of concomitant administration of both agents has remained limited, due to the concern of exacerbating the acute toxicity. Actinomycin D is still given along with radiation in nephroblastomas, anthracyclines in rhabdomyosarcomas, and cyclophosphamide in Ewing's sarcomas, but nowadays many protocols include the sequential administration of these agents, in which chemotherapy is followed by a 'tailor-fitted' local treatment. This approach does not avoid severe toxicity due to the interaction of both agents, as, for example, has occurred with the use of high-dose busulphan or cisplatinum followed by radiation.[43] Mathematical formalisms have been developed to evaluate the therapeutic gain of reducing local therapy according to the efficacy of systemic treatment. They have four scenarios, as highlighted by Fryer,[40] depending on whether chemotherapy is effective or ineffective:

- Effective chemotherapy plus conventional doses of radiation minimize the risk of local and distant recurrences, but at the price of severe sequelae in the young.
- Ineffective chemotherapy plus 'conventional' doses of radiation will probably lead to an excessive rate of early metastases.
- Effective chemotherapy and reduced doses of radiation can minimize the risk of local and distant failures at the price of a decreased toxicity, or lead to an excess of local failures.
- Ineffective chemotherapy combined with reduced doses of radiation will certainly lead to an increased risk of failure that can be purely local (at least initially).

In the last situation, the deleterious effect of chemotherapy on the outcome can sometimes be disregarded, and radiation alone erroneously incriminated. Some authors have also pointed out the risk of reducing radiation sensitivity by the prior administration of chemotherapeutic agents.[44]

Dose fractionation

The most commonly employed fractionations in children are somewhat below those employed in their adult counterparts: five sessions of 1.8 Gy/week are being recommended in many national/international studies. The dose per fraction can be lowered when large volumes of normal tissues are encompassed, in order to improve acute and, more markedly, late toxicity. It is also lowered in very young children, although the need to give treatment under general anaesthesia can require the adoption of some forms of hypofractionation (based on three to four weekly sessions only). Altered fractionation and/or protraction can be exploited to improve toxicity and/or efficacy.[45]

HYPERFRACTIONATION

Hyperfractionation (i.e. decreasing the dose per fraction) can be used to decrease late toxicity when the total dose is kept constant, or to increase the chances of local control when the total dose is increased in parallel (with supposedly equal toxicity). A typical example is represented by the American IRS IV study in rhabdomyosarcomas, in which a dose of 59.4 Gy was delivered in twice daily sessions of 1 Gy each. This was supposed to be equivalent to 45 Gy conventionally fractionated for late-responding tissues, and 55 Gy for tumour tissues.[46] Other studies dealing with pure hyperfractionation concerned the radiotherapeutic management of brainstem gliomas. Doses escalated up to 78 Gy were tested by the POG-CCSG group, in order to increase tumour-cell killing without excessive neurological toxicity.[47] Unfortunately, radiological and clinical symptoms of radionecrosis were observed above 75 Gy, without substantial improvement in tumour control. More encouraging are the preliminary experiments conducted in medulloblastomas.

ACCELERATED REGIMENS

These aim to shorten overall treatment duration and are generally indicated in fast-growing tumours. The safest way to deliver them is to administer two sessions of conventional doses of radiation (i.e. 2×2 Gy per day). Remarkable results were achieved in Burkitt's lymphoma before the advent of efficient polychemotherapy regimens.

ACCELERATED HYPERFRACTIONATED REGIMENS

These aim to shorten overall treatment time while maintaining the dose per fraction below the conventional level.[48] Such a regimen was tested in the MMT 89 SIOP study for paediatric soft tissue sarcomas, by delivering 45 Gy in twice daily fractions of 1.5 Gy each. Preliminary reports have failed to show any improvement in tumour control related to this acceleration.[49] Further evaluations should assess whether late tolerance has been influenced by the decreased fraction dose.

FACTORS THAT INFLUENCE LATE DAMAGE

Compared with chemotherapy, radiotherapy plays a major role in the genesis of late toxicity in children.[50] Cellular mechanisms of this toxicity include quiescent G1-phase cell injuries and vascular injuries. Many factors can influence late damage, and these are discussed below.

AGE AT THE TIME OF RADIATION

Highly proliferative tissues are more sensitive than others. In this respect, the younger the age, the higher the toxicity. In addition, some authors have suggested that rapid growth spurts are at higher risk. A typical example is the effect on skeletal development of radiation given during adolescence and pre-adolescence.[51]

TOTAL DOSE AND DOSE FRACTIONATION

Doses that are able to induce severe damage in childhood are far lower than those reported for adults. Animal models have shown that chondroblastic formation can be altered by doses as low as 10 Gy. Similarly, reduced dose per fraction seems to have a 'protective' effect on the growth of skeletal tissues, and possibly others.[28,52,53] Recent clinical studies on multiple fractions per day have been designed to confirm animal models. The low dose rate associated with brachytherapy seems to protect late-responding normal tissues as well.

VOLUME EFFECT

Most radiation oncologists have been intuitively aware since the early days of radiation therapy that damage to large amounts of irradiated normal tissue was less well tolerated by patients than damage to smaller amounts. However, it is only recently that tolerance of partial volumes has been studied extensively and on a scientific basis.[54] The analysis of clinical data available in the literature has shown that some organs (such as the liver and lungs) follow quite simple dose–volume correlations, while others (such as the spinal cord) are fairly 'insensitive' to a volume effect. Much effort is being expended today on modelling biological tolerance of individual organs using mathematical formalisms. In the near future, this might help to evaluate rival treatment plans produced by three-dimensional virtual simulations in terms of 'complication probability'. It should be noted, however, that none of the current models has been validated thus far by clinical studies in children.

TYPE OF RADIATION

Low-energy photons, such as those in the range 200–250 kV, are absorbed by bone to a greater degree than higher energy photons, and have a higher risk of sequelae.[55] High-LET particles, such as neutrons, which cause mainly 'lethal' (non-reparable) damage, are thought to be more active in radio-resistant malignancies,[56,57] but have a higher risk of late toxicity.[58] For this reason, neutrons have only very limited indications in children.

COMBINED TREATMENT MODALITIES

Concomitant chemoradiation combinations can substantially affect tolerance to one or both agents given alone. Evidence has been collected on both biological (see Table 7.1) and clinical grounds. For example, in acute lymphocytic leukaemia, the combination of 'prophylactic' intrathecal methotrexate and radiation to the brain has proven highly deleterious.[59] Under some circumstances, surgery performed prior to radiation can enhance radiation toxicity. This has been reported in liver injuries when partial hepatectomy was conducted a few weeks before radiation, and also in small-bowel injuries when one or multiple laparotomies were carried out months or years before radiation.[60]

CAN WE PREDICT THE INTENSITY OF SEQUELAE?

This is one of the most challenging issues of paediatric radiotherapy, because of the multiplicity of parameters involved: physiological, biological and technical. Valuable data in this area have been produced by the Philadelphia group, which has developed algorithms that aim to predict final height in children irradiated in the abdomen and the spine at various ages.[61]

OTHER FACTORS

Local inflammatory changes, which can be pre-existing or induced by radiation, have been incriminated in late damage. Radiation pneumonitis is a typical example since its intensity seems to be correlated with the endogenous production of interleukin-1 alpha and beta, tumour necrosis factor and transforming growth factor (TGF) beta levels. Better knowledge of individual cellular and molecular determinants (some of which are inherited) will certainly contribute to an improved understanding of the basic mechanisms of radiation toxicity and its management.[21,62]

KEY POINTS

- Nuclear DNA is the main target of radiation. Delayed mitotic death is the most common mode of action, although peculiar cell types can die earlier of apoptosis.
- Ionization of molecules leads to the production of free radicals. Radiolysis of intracellular water is one of the main phenomena.
- Mammalian cell survival curves generally display an initial 'shoulder' over the low-dose range. According to mathematical models, the shape of the survival curve can be represented by the α/β ratio.
- Low α/β values (≤ 3) have been recorded in cell populations responsible for late changes. High values (>5) have been reported in acute-responding tissues and in most tumours.
- The post-radiation effect on tissues (i.e. acute/late toxicity and tumour reduction) depends upon their growth velocity, and involves both parenchymal cell depletion and injury to the microvasculature (especially for late toxicity).
- Fractionation of the dose preferentially spares cell populations with efficient repair mechanisms; it

also allows repopulation and reoxygenation. Hyperfractionation of the dose offers promising avenues in terms of improved toxicity and tumour control.

- Improved physical dose distribution is one of the major advances of modern radiotherapy. It includes the use of high-energy X-ray beams, sophisticated equipment, advanced treatment-planning software, radionuclide implants and heavy charged particles.
- Some radiation types, such as neutrons, are more densely ionizing than photons along their track. These high-LET (linear energy transfer) particles can be three to 10 times more active on tumour as well as normal tissues.
- The presence of oxygen enhances the biological effect of radiation. When oxygen pressure within tissues falls, radiosensitivity falls as well (up to three times). Hypoxia is generally observed at depth in large tumours. Limitation of hypoxia and angiogenesis are being intensively investigated.
- Radiotherapy and chemotherapy are commonly administered in combination. In paediatric tumours they have brought about an impressive reduction of late toxicity when the dose intensity of each agent given together could be reduced.

REFERENCES

1. Nias AHW, ed. *An Introduction to Radiobiology*. Chichester: Wiley, 1998.
2. Mould RF. *A Century of X-rays and Radioactivity in Medicine*. Bristol: Institute of Physics, 1993.
3. Munzenrider JE, Liebsch NJ, Efird JT. Chordoma and chondrosarcoma of skull base: treatment with fractionated X-ray and proton radiotherapy. In: Johnson JT, Didolkar MS, eds. *Head and Neck Cancer*, vol III. Amsterdam: Elsevier, 1993; 649–54.
4. Noel G, Habrand JL, Helfre S *et al.* Proton beam therapy of central nervous system tumors in childhood: the preliminary Centre de Protontherapie d'Orsay experience. *Med Pediatr Oncol* 2003; **40**: 309–15.
5. Suit HD, Becht J, Leong J *et al.* Potential for improvement in radiation therapy. *Int J Radiat Oncol Biol Phys* 1988; **14**: 777–86.
6. Fraas BA, McShan DL, Diaz RF *et al.* Integration of magnetic resonance imaging into radiation therapy treatment planning: I. Technical considerations. *Int J Radiat Oncol Biol Phys* 1987; **13**: 1897–908.
7. Burman C, Kutcher GJ, Emami B, Goitein M. Fitting of normal tissue tolerance data to an analytical function. *Int J Radiat Oncol Biol Phys* 1991; **21**: 123–35.
8. Lyman JT, Wolbarst AB. Optimization of radiation therapy. III: a method of assessing complication probabilities from dose-volume histograms. *Int J Radiat Oncol Biol Phys* 1987; **13**: 103–9.
9. Verhey L. 3-D conformal therapy using beam intensity modulation. In: Meyer JL, Purdy JA, eds. *3-D Conformal Radiotherapy* (*Front Radiat Ther Oncol* **29**). Basel: Karger, 1996; 139–55.
10. Withers HR, Taylor JMG, Maciejewski B. Treatment volume and tissue tolerance. *Int J Radiat Oncol Biol Phys* 1988; **14**: 751–9.
11. Saw CB, ed. *Therapeutic Radiological Physics* (CD rom). Omaha, NE: CB Saw, Inc., 2002.
12. Tubiana M, Dutreix J, Wambersie A, eds. *Introduction to Radiobiology*. Taylor and Francis: London, 1990.
13. Miller DW. A review of proton beam radiation therapy. *Med Phys* 1995; **22**: 1943–54.
14. Fisher DE. Pathways of apoptosis and the modulation of cell death in cancer. *Hematol Oncol Clin North Am* 2001; **15**(5): 931–56.
15. Deacon CF, Wilson PA, Peckam MJ. The radiobiology of human neuroblastoma. *Radiother Oncol* 1985; **3**: 201–9.
16. Fertil B, Malaise EP. Intrinsic radiosensitivity of human cell lines is correlated with radioresponsiveness of human tumors: analysis of 101 published survival curves. *Int J Radiat Oncol Biol Phys* 1985; **11**: 1699–707.
17. Williams MV, Denekamp J, Fowler JF. A review of α/β ratios for experimental tumors: implications for clinical studies of altered fractionation. *Int J Radiat Oncol Biol Phys* 1985; **11**: 87–96.
18. Bergonié J, Tribondeau L. Actions des rayons x sur le testicule. *Archives d'Électricité Médicale* 1906; **14**: 779–91.
19. Schulte R. Early and late response to ion irradiation. In: Linz U, ed. *Ion Beams in Tumor Therapy*. London: Chapman and Hall, 1995; 53–62.
20. Rosen EM, Fan S, Goldbrerg ID, Rockwell S. Biological basis of radiation sensitivity. Part 1: factors governing radiation tolerance. *Oncology* 2000; **14**: 543–50.
21. Rosen EM, Fan S, Goldbrerg ID, Rockwell S. Biological basis of radiation sensitivity. Part 2: cellular and molecular determinants of radiosensitivity. *Oncology* 2000; **14**: 741–62.
22. Hockel M, Vaupel P. Tumor hypoxia: definitions and current clinical, biologic, and molecular aspects. *J Natl Cancer Inst* 2001; **93**: 266–76.
23. Girinski T, Pejovic MH, Haie C *et al.* Radical irradiation and misonidazole in the treatment of advanced cervical carcinoma: results of a phase II trial. *Int J Radiat Oncol Biol Phys* 1985; **11**: 1783–7.
24. Girinski T, Pejovic-Lenfant MH, Bourhis J *et al.* Prognostic value of hemoglobin concentrations and blood transfusions in advanced carcinoma of the cervix treated by radiation therapy: results of a retrospective study of 386 patients. *Int J Radiat Oncol Biol Phys* 1989; **16**: 37–42.
25. Overgaard J, Hansen HS, Overgaard M *et al.* A randomized double-blind phase III study of nimorazol as a hypoxic radiosensitizer of primary radiotherapy in supraglottic larynx and pharynx carcinoma. Results of the Danish Head And Neck Cancer Study (DAHANCA) Protocol 5-85. *Radiother Oncol* 1998; **46**: 135–46.
26. Del Rowe J, Scott C, Werner-Wasic M *et al.* Single-arm, open label phase II study of intravenously administered

tirapazamine and radiation therapy for glioblastoma multiforme. *J Clin Oncol* 2000; **18**: 1254–9.

27. Poon RTP, Fan ST, Wong J. Clinical implications of circulating angiogenic factors in cancer patients *J Clin Oncol* 2001; **19**: 1207–25.

28. Kian Ang K, Van der Kogel AJ, Van Dam J, Van Der Schueren E. The kinetics of repair of sublethal damage in the rat cervical spinal cord during fractionated irradiations. *Radiother Oncol* 1984; **1**: 247–53.

29. Withers HR, Taylor JMG, Maciejewski B. The hazards of accelerated tumor clonogenic repopulation during radiotherapy. *Acta Oncol* 1988; **27**: 131–46.

30. Fu KK. Interactions of chemotherapeutic agents and radiation. In: Meyer JL, Vaeth JM, eds. *Radiotherapy/Chemotherapy Interactions in Cancer Treatment* (*Front Radiat Ther Oncol* **26**) Karger: Basel, 1991; 162–71.

31. Orton CG, Ellis F. A simplification in the use of the NSD concept in practical radiotherapy. *Br J Radiol* 1973; **46**: 529–37.

32. Cosset JM, Henry-Amar M, Girinski T *et al.* Late toxicity of radiotherapy in Hodgkin's disease. The role of fraction size. *Acta Radiol* 1988; **27**: 123–30.

33. Eifel PJ. Decreased bone growth arrest in weanling rats with multiple fractions per day. *Int J Radiat Oncol Biol Phys* 1988; **15**: 141–5.

34. Hartsell WF, Hanson WR, Conterato DJ, Hendrickson FR. Hyperfractionation decreases the deleterious effects of conventional fractionation on vertebral growth in animals. *Cancer* 1989; **63**: 2452–5.

35. Gerbaulet A, Habrand JL. Brachytherapy in paediatric malignancies. In: Tobias JS, Thomas PRM, eds. *Current Radiation Oncology*, vol 3. London: Arnold, 1997; 299–311.

36. Meijer OW, Wolbers JG, Baayen JC, Slotman BJ. Fractionated stereotactic radiation therapy and single high-dose radiosurgery for acoustic neuroma: early results of a prospective clinical study. *Int J Radiat Oncol Biol Phys* 2000; **46**: 45–9.

37. Schulman SR. Anesthesia for external-beam radiotherapy. In: Halperin EC, Constine LS, Tarbell NJ, Kun LE, eds. *Pediatric Radiation Therapy*, 3rd edn. Philadelphia: Lippincott, 1999; 563–74.

38. Loeffler JS, Kooy HM, Tarbell NJ. The emergence of conformal radiotherapy: special implications for pediatric neuro-oncology. *Int J Radiat Oncol Biol Phys* 1999; **44**: 237–8.

39. Lin R, Hug EB, Schaefer RA *et al.* Conformal proton radiation therapy of the posterior fossa: a study comparing protons with three-dimensional planned photons in limiting dose to auditory structures. *Int J Radiat Oncol Biol Phys* 2000; **48**: 1219–26.

40. Fryer CJH. Pediatric oncology: the optimal model for evaluating radiation-chemotherapy interactions. In: Meyer JL, Vaeth JM, eds. *Radiotherapy/Chemotherapy Interactions in Cancer Treatment* (*Front Radiat Ther Oncol* **26**). Basel: Karger, 1991; 162–71.

41. Habrand JL, Oberlin O, Pein F *et al.* Chemoradiation in children with cancer. In: Mornex F, Mazeron JJ, Droz JP, Marty M, eds. *Concomitant Chemoradiation: Current Status and Future.* Amsterdam: Elsevier, 1999; 221–31.

42. Farber S, Pinkel D, Sears EM, Toch R. Advances in chemotherapy of cancer in man. *Adv Cancer Res* 1956; **4**: 1–71.

43. Vassal J, Hartman O, Habrand JL *et al.* Enhanced cutaneous radiation effects following high-dose busulfan therapy. *Cancer Chemother Pharmacol* 1989; **23**: 117–18.

44. Lehnert S, Green D, Batist G. Radiation response of drug-resistant variants of a human breast cancer cell line. *Radiat Res* 1989; **118**: 568–80.

45. Withers HR. Biologic basis for altered fractionation schemes. *Cancer* 1985; **55**: 2086–95.

46. Donaldson SS, Meza J, Breneman JC *et al.* Results from the IRS-IV randomized trial of hyperfractionated radiotherapy in children with rhabdomyosarcoma – a report from the IRSG. *Int J Radiat Oncol Biol Phys* 2001; **51**: 718–28.

47. Freeman CR, Kepner J, Kun LE *et al.* A detrimental effect of a combined chemotherapy-radiotherapy approach in children with diffuse intrinsic brain stem gliomas. *Int J Radiat Oncol Biol Phys* 2000; **47**: 561–4.

48. Saunders MI, Dische S, Rojas A. CHART (continuous, hyperfractionated, accelerated radiotherapy): a tale of two disciplines. *Br J Cancer* 1999; **80**: 110–15.

49. Habrand JL, Spooner D, Rey A *et al.* The role of radiation therapy (RT) in the management of localized soft tissue sarcomas (STS) in children. A report of the International Society of Pediatric Oncoogy (SIOP). *Int J Radiat Oncol Biol Phys* 1997; **39**(suppl, abstr 15): 142.

50. Donaldson S. Pediatric patients. Tolerance levels and effects of treatment. In: Meyer JL, Vaeth JM, ed. *Radiation Tolerance of Normal Tissues* (*Front Radiat Ther Oncol* **23**). Basel: Karger, 1989; **23**: 390–407.

51. Rubin P, Van Houtte P, Constine L. Radiation sensitivity and organ tolerance in pediatric oncology: a new hypothesis. *Front Radiother Oncol* 1982; **16**: 62–82.

52. Jordan SW, Anderson RE, Lane RG, Brayer JM. Fraction size and time dependance of X-ray induced late renal injury. *Int J Radiat Oncol Biol Phys* 1985; **11**: 1095–101.

53. Lauk S, Rüth S, Trott K-R. The effects of dose-fractionation on radiation-induced heart disease in rats. *Radiother Oncol* 1987; **8**: 363–7.

54. Emami B, Lyman J, Brown A *et al.* Tolerance of normal tissues to therapeutic irradiation. *Int J Radiat Oncol Biol Phys* 1991; **21**: 109–22.

55. Silber JH, Littman PS, Meadows AT. Stature loss following skeletal irradiation for childhod cancer. *J Clin Oncol* 1990; **8**: 304–12.

56. Laramore GE, Grifin TW. Fast neutron radiotherapy: where have we been and where are we going. The jury is still out. *Int J Radiat Oncol Biol Phys* 1995; **32**: 879–82.

57. Laramore GE, Griffith JT, Boesplflug M *et al.* Fast neuton radiotherapy for sarcomas of soft tissue, bone and cartilage. *Am J Clin Oncol* (*CCT*) 1989; **12**: 320–6.

58. Laramore GE, Martz KL, Nelson JS *et al.* Radiation Therapy Oncology Group (RTOG) survival data on anaplastic astrocytomas of the brain: does a more aggressive form of treatment adversely impact survival? *Int J Radiat Oncol Biol Phys* 1989; **17**: 1351–6.

59. Duffner PK. The long term effects of central nervous system therapy on children with brain tumors. In: Cohen ME, Duffner PK, eds. *Brain Tumors in Children* (*Neurol Clin* **9**). Philadelphia: WB Saunders, 1991; 479–95.

60. Gallez-Marchal D, Fayolle M, Henry-Amar M *et al.* Radiation injuries of the gastrointestinal tract in Hodgkin's disease: the

role of exploratory laparotomy and fractionation. *Radiother Oncol* 1985; **2**: 93–9.

61. Hogeboom EJ, Grosser SC, Guthrie KA *et al.* Stature loss following treatment for Wilms tumors. *Med Pediatr Oncol* 2001; **36**: 295–304.

62. Martin M, Lefaix J, Delanian S. TGF-beta and radiation fibrosis: a master switch and a specific therapeutic target. *Int J Radiat Oncol Biol Phys* 2000; **47**: 277–29.

63. Lamond JP, Wang M, Kinsella TJ, Bootman DA. Radiation lethality enhancement with 9-aminocamptothecine: topoisomerase I inhibitors. *Int J Radiat Oncol Biol Phys* 1996; **36**: 369–76.

64. Marchesini R, Colombo A, Caserini C *et al.* Interaction of ionizing radiation with topotecan in two human tumor cell lines. *Int J Cancer* 1996; **66**: 342–6.

65. Bey P. Particularités de la radiothérapie. In: Lemerle J, ed. *Cancers de l'Enfant (Encyclopédie des Cancers)*. Paris: Flammarion, 1989; 31–42.

66. Peters L, Brock WA, Travis EL. Radiation biology at clinically relevant fractions. In: De Vita VT, Hellman S, Rosenberg SA, eds. *Important Advances in Oncology*. Philadelphia: Lippincott, 1990; 65–83.

8

Cancer chemotherapy and mechanisms of resistance

ALAN V. BODDY

INTRODUCTION

Advances in the application of cancer chemotherapy to the treatment of childhood malignancies have been responsible for a dramatic improvement in cure rates over the last 20–30 years. Cure rates in some diseases, such as acute lymphoblastic leukaemia (ALL), have been particularly striking, whilst other tumours remain steadfastly resistant to treatment. Incremental gains in the tailoring of chemotherapy have been made by more refined classification of tumours, based on patient characteristics, tumour pathology or, increasingly, tumour genetics. Improvements have also been made in optimization of the timing, doses and scheduling of drugs so as to achieve the maximum anti-tumour effect.

In this chapter, the pharmacology of the major drugs used in paediatric oncology will be discussed, together with examples of how these agents are used to treat particular disease types. In this context, pharmacology encompasses the systemic pharmacology or pharmacokinetics (what the body does to the drug), cellular pharmacology (how the drug is modified by tumour and other cells) and pharmacodynamics (what the drug does to the body). Mechanisms of drug resistance will be described, as they relate to paediatric tumours, and methods to block or circumvent such resistance will also be covered.

GENERAL PRINCIPLES OF CANCER CHEMOTHERAPY

In order to exert an anti-tumour effect, chemotherapeutic agents must either block cell replication or induce cell death. As knowledge of the biochemical pathways that lead to cell death increases, it appears that many cytotoxic drugs with different immediate cellular targets ultimately kill cells by a common pathway of apoptosis.[1] The processes of cell division and apoptosis are intimately linked and thus cancer cells, and normal proliferating tissues, are most susceptible to the toxic effects of chemotherapeutic agents. Conversely, tumour cells which are characterized by disruption of cell-cycle control and may be deficient in apoptotic pathways may also be resistant to chemotherapy.[2]

A thorough description of the principles of cell-cycle control and apoptotic pathways[3] is beyond the scope of this chapter, but a basic knowledge of the major processes involved will aid in understanding the relationship between pharmacology and cellular effects.

The cell cycle can be divided into four phases (Figure 8.1), with an additional phase, G0, where cells are not dividing. After a round of cell division, cells enter a gap phase called G1. Cells must then initiate DNA synthesis in order to have sufficient material to replicate chromosomes (S-phase). Subsequently, cells enter a second gap

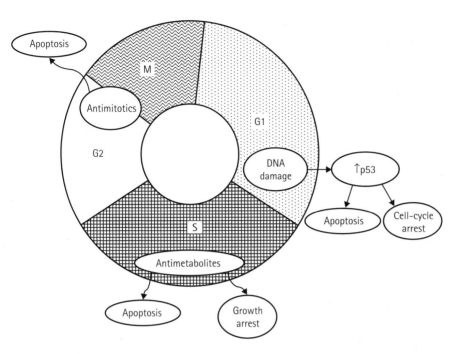

Figure 8.1 *The cell cycle and mechanisms of cell death and growth arrest.*

phase, G2. Mitosis (M-phase) follows G2 and results in cell division. Almost all current chemotherapeutic agents interfere with cell division indirectly, by damaging DNA, blocking DNA synthesis, interfering with DNA processing or disrupting mitosis. The pathway from these immediate drug–target interactions may be mediated by pro-apoptotic proteins such as p53,[4] or by inactivation of anti-apoptotic messengers such as Bcl-2[5] (Figure 8.1).

In many cases the precise mechanism leading from drug–target interaction to tumour cell death is not known. Further investigations of these mechanisms, even for drugs whose use has been established for decades, are continuing. Increased understanding of these processes should lead to more effective treatments and more selective drugs.

GENERAL PRINCIPLES OF PHARMACO-KINETICS AND PHARMACODYNAMICS

As there is such a close link between the anti-tumour and toxic effects of conventional chemotherapeutic agents, it is not surprising that the difference between an effective and a toxic dose is not large. Indeed, the ratio of these two doses, usually known as the therapeutic index, is often close to unity.

In the selection of drugs, schedules and doses, the primary concern is to obtain an anti-tumour effect with the minimum acceptable level of toxicity. The acceptable balance between the probability of anti-tumour effect and that of toxicity may be modulated by knowledge of the aggressiveness of the tumour, likely survival duration and other clinical factors. In order to determine such

probabilities, it is usually assumed that both anti-tumour effect and toxicity are related to the amount of drug in the tumour cell, and that plasma concentrations may reflect those attained at the target site of the drug.

The way in which the body acts to permit the entry of a drug, facilitate its distribution around the system and, ultimately, its removal, governs the pharmacokinetics of the drug. These processes may be related to the physiological characteristics of different organs, such as the gastrointestinal tract, liver and kidney, and to the perfusion of different tissues by the blood. The quantification of pharmacokinetics usually takes the form of measurements of drug concentrations in blood, and it is the interaction of the physiological processes that determines the amount of drug which may be measured in the blood, and the time-course. While such measurements may provide interesting scientific insight into the systemic pharmacology of a drug, it is the relationship between plasma concentrations and therapeutic outcome that is most relevant for the clinician. The term pharmacodynamics describes such relationships and may be applied to such downstream measurements of drug action as drug–target interactions, toxicity or time to relapse.

Drug absorption

Any drug that is administered by an extravascular route must overcome a number of physiological barriers before it can enter the systemic circulation. Thus, similar concerns apply to oral, subcutaneous and intramuscular routes of administration. The process of drug absorption is characterized by the rate at which drug appears in the blood following an extravascular dose, and the total proportion of that dose that enters the body. The latter is often referred to as the bioavailability of the drug or formulation.

Considering oral administration, there are several aspects of the oral formulation that govern the rate and extent of absorption.[6,7] Thus, small molecules, which are mostly un-ionized at the pH within the small intestine, are rapidly and completely absorbed. Conversely, larger molecules which contain charged ions may have very poor bioavailability as they cannot easily penetrate the lipid membranes lining the lumen of the small intestine. The formulation of orally administered drugs can also influence drug absorption, with the rate of dissolution controlling the concentration of drug in the intestine and thus the rate of absorption.

Drugs for which oral administration is common in chemotherapy include methotrexate, cyclophosphamide, temozolomide and 6-mercaptopurine. With the exception of etoposide, most natural product drugs are not administered orally. As substrates for p-glycoprotein, which is highly expressed in the luminal cells of the intestine, the absorption of these compounds is limited by their efflux.[6]

As well as the physical barriers to drug absorption, orally administered compounds must pass through the liver before entering the systemic circulation. Since the liver is the primary site for drug metabolism, the extent to which an oral dose is bioavailable may be limited by first-pass metabolism in the liver.[8]

Drug distribution

This is predominantly a passive process, governed by the perfusion of the different tissues within the body and by the relative degree of drug binding within the plasma and tissues. For some drugs, such as etoposide, binding to plasma protein limits elimination and toxic effects are more closely linked to unbound, rather than total, concentrations in plasma.[9] For drug delivery to tumours, further concerns may apply, as solid tumours have abnormal vasculature and may contain areas of poorly perfused tissue. Whether this poses a delivery problem for small, easily diffusible molecules has not been demonstrated, but for larger molecules, such as antibodies, there may be a limiting factor of drug distribution to the tumour.

Drug elimination

The main processes by which drugs are removed from the body are renal excretion, metabolism and biliary excretion. A brief description of these processes is given below.

RENAL EXCRETION

The removal of compounds in the urine is the aggregate of three processes. Glomerular filtration removes from the plasma small molecules (cut-off 60 000 Da) that are not bound to plasma protein. Carboplatin is mainly eliminated by this mechanism.[10] Renal secretion is an active process which can transfer both bound and unbound drugs from plasma and concentrate them in the urine. The renal elimination of etoposide and methotrexate is mediated to some extent by this mechanism.[11,12] Finally, tubular reabsorption is a passive process by which drugs move from a high concentration in the renal tubule, following reabsorption of water, to a relatively low concentration in the plasma. Reabsorption minimizes the renal excretion of small, un-ionized, lipophilic molecules, which are then eliminated by other mechanisms.

BILIARY EXCRETION

Drugs that are concentrated in the bile are those that have a high molecular weight ($>$500 Da) and/or are sufficiently hydrophilic that they are not reabsorbed following biliary secretion. Doxorubicin,[13] paclitaxel[14] and etoposide[15] are eliminated via biliary excretion. Although methotrexate is excreted in the bile, it is also subject to subsequent reabsorption, known as enterohepatic recycling.[16]

DRUG METABOLISM

For most drugs, chemical modification by metabolic enzymes is an effective means of elimination, as the metabolites are inactive and/or good substrates for renal or biliary excretion. For example, the reduced form of doxorubicin is more polar and has lower cytotoxic activity than the parent. For some compounds, e.g. cyclophosphamide, metabolism is required for activation, with reactive cytotoxic species generated by metabolism in the liver or in the tumour.[17]

Oxidative metabolism is perhaps the most common pathway of metabolism, often mediated by the cytochrome P450 family of microsomal enzymes.[18,19] The liver is the most common site of metabolism as it has the highest expression of drug-metabolizing enzymes. However, metabolism in other tissues, and in the tumour, may be pharmacologically significant for some drugs.

Pharmacokinetics and dosage regimen design

There are three pharmacokinetic parameters that are of interest for the design of dosage regimens, but these can only be used constructively with a knowledge of the pharmacodynamics of the agent.

CLEARANCE

The rate at which a drug is eliminated from the body is related to the plasma concentration by the parameter of clearance. For many drugs, overall plasma clearance is the sum of renal clearance and non-renal (often metabolism) clearance. The utility of clearance is that it describes the relationship between the dose administered and the area under the plasma concentration–time curve (AUC). The latter parameter is a measure of aggregate drug exposure and is often related to toxicity and, less closely, to anti-tumour effect. The best example of this pharmaco-dynamic relationship is with carboplatin. The clearance of carboplatin may be estimated from renal function and used to attain a target AUC which is known to be associated with an optimal probability of therapeutic effect, whilst minimizing toxicity.[20]

Clearance also links the rate of infusion to steady-state concentration during continuous intravenous administration. This is useful for drugs, such as etoposide, where an association between steady-state plasma concentration and toxicity, or efficacy, has been described.[21] When clearance is constant, the ratio of AUC values following an oral and an intravenous dose is the most common method of calculating bioavailability, as AUC reflects the total amount of drug entering the body.

VOLUME OF DISTRIBUTION

This parameter describes the relationship between the total amount of drug in the body and the concentration measured in plasma. As such, it reflects the degree of distribution of the drug outside the plasma. Although tissues may be grouped as being well perfused or poorly perfused and some drugs have volumes of distribution that map to physiological spaces, the value of volume of distribution is largely determined by drug binding in plasma and

tissues and often exceeds total body water. The clinical use of volume of distribution is in understanding the relationship between dose administered, which may be a loading dose in some instances, and the plasma concentration achieved.[22]

HALF-LIFE

As this term suggests, the half-life is the time taken for the plasma concentration to fall to half of its previous value. Under circumstances of linear elimination and pseudo-equilibrium of drug distribution, it also reflects the time for the amount of drug in the body to fall by half. As elimination is often a slower process than distribution, drug concentration–time curves may be characterized by more than one half-life, but it is the final or terminal phase of drug elimination that is of most interest. If drug action requires that a certain concentration be maintained in the plasma for the drug to be effective, the half-life determines how frequently a drug must be given. For drugs with a narrow therapeutic window between activity and toxicity, this may mean frequent or continuous administration if the half-life is short.

PHARMACODYNAMICS

The relationship between plasma concentrations of a drug and a clinical effect is described as the pharmacodynamics of the drug (Figure 8.2). For chemotherapeutic agents, this term is often applied to the relationship between plasma AUC and haematological toxicity.[23] Data in paediatric patients are relatively sparse,[24] perhaps because

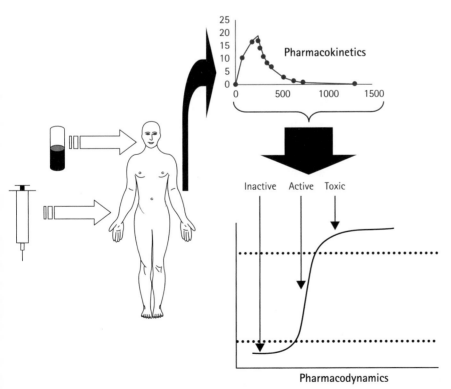

Figure 8.2 *Illustration of the relationship between drug administration, plasma drug concentration–time profiles (pharmacokinetics) and drug effects (pharmacodynamics).*

of the use of multi-agent regimens. Recently the term pharmacodynamics has been extended to include any measure of drug–target interaction.[25]

CANCER CHEMOTHERAPEUTIC AGENTS

The most useful method of classification of anti-tumour agents is by their mechanism of action, as shown in Table 8.1.

Antimetabolites

This class of drug blocks the synthesis of DNA by inhibiting enzymes that are crucial to the synthesis of purine or pyrimidine nucleotides. They may themselves act as false substrates for the enzymes, and some purine and pyrimidine analogues may be misincorporated into DNA. Since the primary mechanism is interference with DNA synthesis, antimetabolites act primarily on cells during the S-phase of the cell cycle. For this reason, antimetabolites exhibit the best example of schedule dependency in their actions. As most of the antimetabolites are close analogues of endogenous biochemical substrates, they are subject to extensive intracellular metabolism. Often such processing is required for activity.

METHOTREXATE

Methotrexate is the prototype for a number of folate analogues and can have activity against enzymes which require reduced folate as a cofactor. Thymidylate synthase (TS) is the rate-limiting enzyme in the synthesis of thymidylate (dTMP) from uracil precursors. In this reaction, methylene tetrahydrofolate acts as a methyl donor, resulting in the formation of dihydrofolate (Figure 8.3). In order to maintain a source of reduced folate cofactor, cells must reduce dihydrofolate back to tetrahydrofolate, a reaction mediated by dihydrofolate reductase (DHFR). This reaction is part of a larger folate cycle that includes the role of 10-formyl folates in purine synthesis (Figure 8.3).

The pharmacology of methotrexate is governed by its similarity to endogenous folates. As it is an ionized species at physiological pH, methotrexate is largely excreted unchanged in the urine, with a small amount of metabolism to 7-hydroxy-methotrexate.[26] In order to enter cells, ionized methotrexate requires a carrier-mediated process. This may be mediated by the reduced folate carrier, or folate receptor alpha. After gaining entry to the cell, methotrexate is subject to polyglutamation (Figure 8.4) with the higher-order polyglutamates having a greater affinity for DHFR. Polyglutamate derivatives also have a greater degree of intracellular retention, and so a longer duration of action, than the parent compound.[27]

In the treatment of ALL, methotrexate forms an important part of consolidation and maintenance

therapy. At conventional doses, the pharmacology of methotrexate is not so crucial. However, at the higher doses used in consolidation treatment, the probability of toxicity is such that pharmacological principles can be used to guide therapy.

Pharmacologically guided dosing of methotrexate has been used to optimize the treatment of ALL. In an initial study, patients treated with a continuous intravenous infusion were divided according to whether their steady-state plasma concentration fell above or below the median of 16 μM.[28] Those below the median were found to be at increased risk of relapse. The subsequent study showed that by titrating doses to achieve a plasma concentration of 12 μM, relapse rates could be improved in B-lineage leukaemia in comparison to a matched, but conventionally treated, control group.[29]

The principle of leucovorin (folinic acid) rescue is that host tissues that have accumulated and retain active polyglutamated methotrexate can salvage reduced folate from this exogenous source and so reverse the blockade of DNA synthesis before cell death occurs. This is particularly important following high-dose methotrexate, where the extent of formation of polyglutamates is reflected in the systemic pharmacology of the drug.[30] Thus, threshold plasma concentrations at 24 or 48 hours after a dose of methotrexate can trigger the administration of appropriate doses of leucovorin.

Methotrexate can be administered orally, with a high bioavailability, intravenously or intrathecally. Intravenous administration can be by bolus injection, resulting in triphasic elimination kinetics.

The toxicities of methotrexate include mucositis, haematological toxicity and hepatotoxicity. In order to avoid nephrotoxicity with high doses, hydration and alkalinization of the urine may be necessary.[31] In severe cases, and where plasma methotrexate concentrations show no sign of diminishing, administration of carboxypeptidase G_2 may be beneficial.[32] This enzyme severs the glutamate moiety from the methotrexate molecule (Figure 8.5), resulting in an ineffective and rapidly eliminated species.[33]

Resistance to methotrexate is related to its cellular pharmacology. Thus mutations in the reduced folate carrier, decreased folylpolyglutamate synthetase (FPGS) or increased gamma glutamyl hydrolase[34] have been associated with decreased sensitivity to methotrexate.[35] Elevated expression of TS and DHFR, together with decreased expression of FPGS underlie the difference between T- and B-cell lineages of ALL.[36]

Pyrimidine analogues

FLUOROPYRIMIDINES

As analogues of the pyrimidine bases of DNA, fluoropyrimidines may act by misincorporation into RNA or DNA, and may act as inhibitors of enzymes involved in DNA

Table 8.1 *Classification of the commonly used cytotoxic agents*

Class of agent	Drug name	Major clinical use	Common or dose–limiting toxicities	Rare toxicities
Antimetabolites				
Antifolate	Methotrexate	Leukaemia, lymphoma, CNS, osteosarcoma	BM, M, renal (HD)	Liver, lung, CNS
Pyrimidine analogue	5–Fluorouracil	Colorectal, liver	BM, M, diarrhoea	CNS, chest pain, conjunctivitis
	Cytarabine	Leukaemia, lymphoma, CNS	BM, M, N&V, diarrhoea	Liver, CNS, lung, conjunctivitis
Purine analogue	6–Mercaptopurine	Leukaemia, lymphoma,	BM	Liver
	6–Thioguanine	Leukaemia, lymphoma	BM	Liver
Alkylating agents				
Monofunctional	Temozolomide	CNS	BM, N&V	
	Nitrosoureas	CNS, lymphomas	BM (delayed), N&V	Lung, renal, C, sterility, liver
	DTIC (dacarbazine)	Sarcoma, Hodgkin's disease	N&V, BM, V	Flu-like syndrome, liver
	Procarbazine	Hodgkin's disease	N&V, BM, alcohol intolerance	N, hypersensitivity, C
Bifunctional	Thiotepa	CNS	BM, M	VOD, CNS
	Melphalan	Neuroblastoma, sarcomas, leukaemia, Hodgkin's disease	BM, A (HD), V	C, sterility
	Busulphan	Leukaemia, neuroblastoma	BM (cumulative), cutaneous	Lung, Addisonian–like state, sterility, liver
Bifunctional (oxazaphosphorine)	Cyclophosphamide	Leukaemia, lymphoma, neuroblastoma, rhabdomyosarcoma, Ewing's sarcoma, germ cell tumours	BM, N&V, A, haemorrhagic cystitis	SIADH, sterility, C, lung, heart (HD)
	Ifosfamide	Leukaemia, lymphoma, neuroblastoma, rhabdomyosarcoma, Ewing's sarcoma, germ cell tumours	BM, cystitis, A, N&V	CNS, kidney, SIADH, C, sterility
Platinum compounds	Cisplatin	Germ cell tumours, neuroblastoma, sarcomas, CNS, liver	N&V, diarrhoea, renal, N	BM (HD), hypersensitivity
	Carboplatin	Germ cell tumours, neuroblastoma, sarcomas, CNS, liver	BM, N&V (HD)	Renal (HD)

(continued)

Table 8.1 *Continued*

Class of agent	Drug name	Major clinical use	Common or dose-limiting toxicities	Rare toxicities
Tubulin-binding drugs	Vincristine	Leukaemia, lymphoma, Wilms' tumour, neuroblastoma, rhabdomyosarcoma	N, constipation, V, jaw pain	SIADH
	Vinblastine	Lymphoma	BM, V, jaw pain	N, M
	Vindesine	Sarcomas	BM, V	N
Topoisomerase II agents				
Epipodophyllotoxins	Etoposide	Leukaemia, lymphoma, neuroblastoma, germ cell tumours	BM, N&V (per os), A	N
	Teniposide	Leukaemia, lymphoma, neuroblastoma, germ cell tumours	BM, V, A	Lung
Anthracyclines	Doxorubicin	Leukaemia, lymphoma, neuroblastoma, rhabdomyosarcoma, Ewing's sarcoma, Wilms' tumour	BM, N&V, A, M, V	C, radiation recall
	Daunorubicin	Leukaemia	BM, N&V, A, M, V	C, radiation recall
	Epirubicin	Lymphoma, sarcoma	BM, A, V	C
	Amsacrine	Leukaemia	BM, V	C
Topoisomerase I agents	Topotecan	Investigational	BM, diarrhoea	N, N&V
	Irinotecan	Investigational	Diarrhoea, BM	A, N&V, M
Miscellaneous				
Antibiotic	Actinomycin D	Wilms' tumour, Ewing's sarcoma, rhabdomyosarcoma	BM, N&V, A, M, diarrhoea, V	Radiation recall, liver
	Bleomycin	Germ cell tumours, lymphoma	Fever chills, M, pigmentation	Lung, Raynaud's phenomenon, hypertension, hypersensitivity
Enzyme	L-Asparaginase	Leukaemia	Hypersensitivity, coagulopathy	Hypoalbuminaemia, hyperglycaemia, CNS, hyperamylasaemia, liver

A, alopecia; BM, bone marrow; C, cardiac; CNS, central nervous system; HD, high dose; M, mucositis; N&V, nausea and vomiting; N, neurotoxicity; SIADH, syndrome of inappropriate antidiuretic hormone; V, vesicant; VOD, veno-occlusive disease.

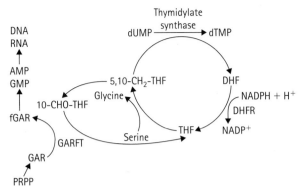

Figure 8.3 *Biochemistry of the folate cycle and thymidylate (dTMP) synthesis. AMP, adenosine monophosphate; DHFR, dihydrofolate reductase; dUMP, deoxyuridine monophosphate; fGAR, formyl glycinamide ribose; GAR, glycinamide ribose; GARFT, glycinamide ribosyl formyl transferase; GMP, guanosine monophosphate; PRPP, phosphoribosylpyrophosphate; THF, tetrahydrofolate.*

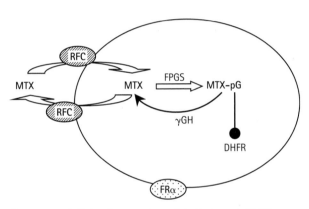

Figure 8.4 *Cellular pharmacology of methotrexate (MTX), including active uptake [by reduced folate carrier (RFC) and folate receptor α (FRα)], polyglutamation [by folylpolyglutamate synthetase (FPGS)] and hydrolysis [by γ-glutamyl hydrolase (γGH)]. Inhibition of dihydrofolate reductase (DHFR). MTX-pG, methotrexate polyglutamate.*

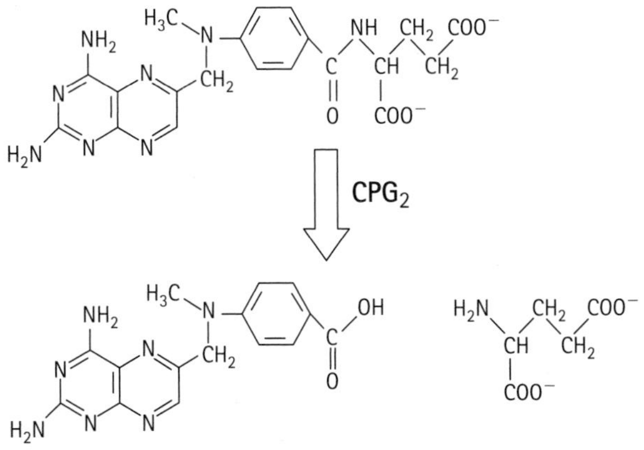

Figure 8.5 *Cleavage of methotrexate by carboxypeptidase G_2 (CPG$_2$).*

synthesis, such as thymidylate synthase. 5-Fluorouracil (5-FU) is the major drug in this class, and is used in the treatment of many solid tumours in adult patients, mainly breast, colorectal and head and neck. Recently gemcitabine has been developed as a treatment for pancreatic and lung cancers, but it also has activity in other solid tumours.[37]

The use of fluoropyrimidines in the treatment of paediatric malignancy is mainly confined to 5-FU treatment of nasopharyngeal carcinoma, with some use in the treatment of hepatoblastoma. These tumours may be analogous to adult malignancies where 5-FU is also active.

5-Fluorouracil requires metabolic activation to either ribose or deoxyribose nucleotides in order to exert its effects on DNA and RNA synthesis (Figure 8.6). 5-Fluorodeoxyuridine monophosphate (FdUMP) is also a potent inhibitor of TS, and this may be the primary mechanism of action of 5-FU.[38] In the presence of 5,10-methylene tetrahydrofolate, FdUMP forms a covalent ternary complex with TS. For this reason, 5-FU is combined with folinic acid (leucovorin) in the treatment of colorectal cancer.

The major route of elimination of 5-FU is metabolism by dihydropyrimidine dehydrogenase (DPD),[39] an enzyme which has a genetically determined deficiency in about 1 in 300 patients.[40] Inhibitors of DPD have been combined with 5-FU to optimize tumour delivery and permit oral administration.[41] Resistance to 5-FU has been associated with raised tumour DPD activity, but also with amplification of TS.[38]

CYTARABINE

Also known as cytidine arabinoside or ara-C, cytarabine is an analogue of the nucleoside cytosine and is activated by deoxycytidine kinase to the triphosphate form which is misincorporated into DNA, blocking transcription. The activating metabolic pathway must compete with the inactivating enzyme cytidine deaminase and the balance between these two enzymes in different tissues may influence the tumour selectivity of cytarabine. In leukaemic cell lines, formation of araCTP correlated well with sensitivity to cytarabine.[42]

After an intravenous dose of cytarabine, systemic concentrations fall rapidly due to deamination in the liver, with 70 per cent of the dose excreted in the urine as the inactive metabolite ara-U.[43] A prolonged infusion results in sustained concentrations of the active metabolite in tissues.[22] Doses vary according to clinical practice, from 100 mg/m² up to 3 g/m², usually administered 12-hourly for 5–7 days. In adult acute myeloid leukaemia patients, there was no correlation between clinical response and the systemic pharmacology of the parent drug,[44] and there is no correlation between araCTP concentrations in circulating leukaemic blasts and the plasma cytarabine concentrations.[45] Saturation of deoxycytidine kinase may

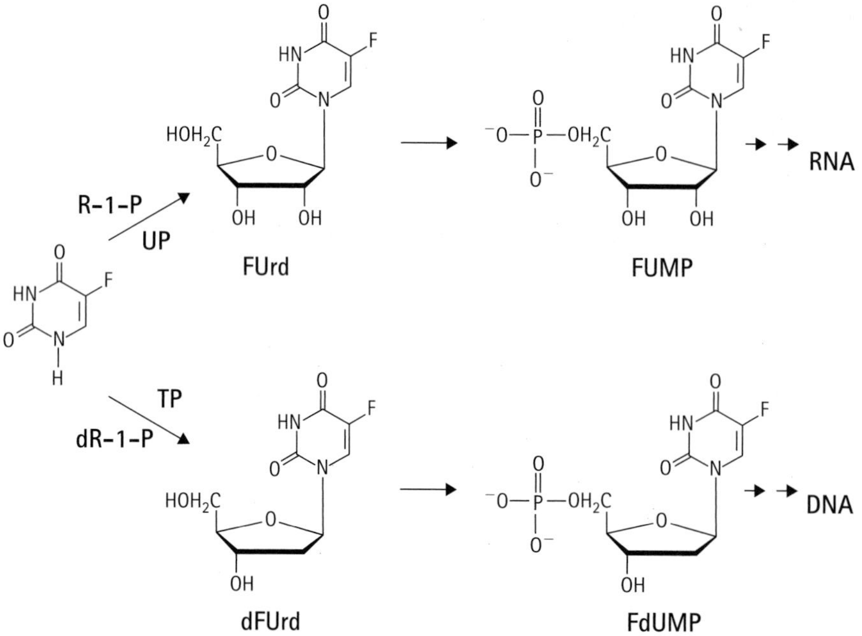

Figure 8.6 *Pathways of 5-fluorouracil anabolism to fluorouridine (FUrd), fluorouridine monophosphate (FUMP), using ribose-1-phosphate (R-1-P), resulting in RNA incorporation. The corresponding reaction involving deoxyribose-1-phosphate (dR-1-P)) leads to DNA analogues and the thymidylate synthase (TS) inhibitor fluorodeoxyuridine monophosphate (FdUMP). dFUrd, fluorodeoxyuridine; TP, thymidine phosphorylase; UP, uridine phosphorylase.*

occur at doses above 1 g/m^2, or if administration is by a shorter 1-hour infusion compared with a longer 4-hour infusion.[46] Higher doses may be associated with an increased risk of toxicity, as the deamination reaction is also saturated.[22] Resistance may be associated with low levels of deoxycytidine kinase. Methods for the detection of araCTP formation in clinical leukaemia samples have been described, but have not yet been applied to studies in paediatric patients.[47]

Purine analogues

6-MERCAPTOPURINE AND 6-THIOGUANINE

These purine analogues represent different precursors to a common pathway generating 6-thioguanine nucleotides (6-TGN) which are incorporated into DNA. They can also block *de novo* purine biosynthesis, presumably by competing for the relevant enzymes. 6-Mercaptopurine (6-MP) is the more commonly used compound, particularly in the treatment of ALL. The metabolism of 6-MP is mediated either by xanthine dehydrogenase[48] or, more importantly, by thiopurine methyltransferase (TPMT)[49] (Figure 8.7). The latter enzyme exhibits a genetic polymorphism,[50] such that individuals with a low activity of the enzyme benefit from dose adjustment to match the genotype.[51,52] Males tend to have higher activity of TPMT than females, perhaps contributing to poorer outcome in ALL.[49] 6-Thioguanine is also a substrate for TPMT.[53]

Either drug can be used in maintenance therapy of ALL. The bioavailability of both agents is high, but may be affected by food. Erythrocyte levels of TGNs correlate with

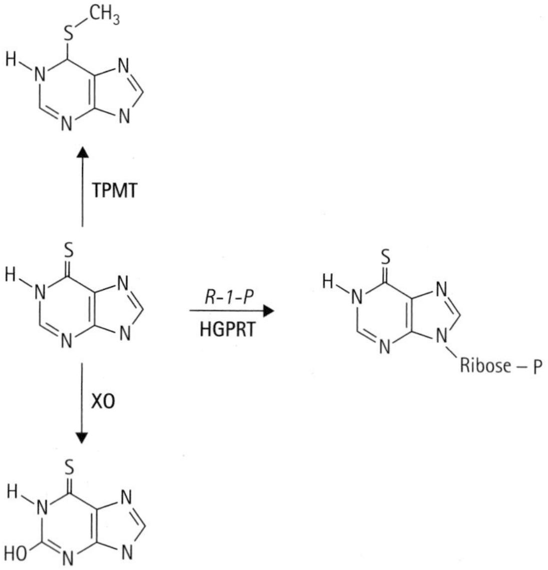

Figure 8.7 *Structure and metabolism of 6-mercaptopurine by xanthine oxidase (XO), thiopurine methyltransferase (TPMT) and hypoxanthine/guanine phosphoribosyltransferase (HGPRT). R-1-P, ribose-1-phosphate.*

clinical outcome, in terms of both toxicity and response to treatment.[52] Monitoring of 6-TGN in erythrocytes may aid compliance, as well as allowing dose adjustment.

Recently, evidence has emerged that methylation of 6-MP by TPMT may not simply inactivate the drug. This is based on observations that 6-MP is more cytotoxic to cells expressing TPMT than to matched cells lacking the enzyme.[53] Understanding of the influence of metabolism on the clinical response to 6-MP and 6-TG permits rational use of these important drugs, and it should be noted that maintaining an effective dose, whilst avoiding toxicity, is a critical determinant of response.[51]

Alkylating agents

Alkylating agents are drugs that react covalently with the nucleophilic purine bases of DNA to form alkylated adducts. For some agents, such as temozolomide, alkylation involves the simple transfer of an alkyl group to a base such as guanine. Other bifunctional agents can react at two positions, to give complex mixtures of cross-links between and within DNA strands.

Various mechanisms can recognize the formation of DNA adducts and trigger repair processes, which may result in resistance to alkylating agents, but can also act as a signal for the initiation of apoptosis.[2] Loss of function of the p53 tumour suppressor pathway is associated with resistance to many alkylating agents.[54] The alkylation of DNA has been linked to the mutagenic properties of these drugs, and may be associated with secondary malignancies.

MONOFUNCTIONAL ALKYLATING AGENTS

Temozolomide

This drug was introduced into clinical use relatively recently, and is used in the treatment of brain tumours and other solid tumours.[55] Temozolomide is an analogue of dacarbazine (DTIC), but does not require metabolic activation and reacts spontaneously at neutral pH to yield the alkylating species MTIC[56] and subsequently AIC (Figure 8.8). This methylating agent transfers a methyl group to the N^7 or O^6 of guanine, or the N^3 of adenine. These DNA lesions may be subject to repair by a number of mechanisms. Alkylation at the O^6 of guanine appears to be the primary cytotoxic lesion. Alkylated guanine is subject to inaccurate base-pairing during DNA replication, such that a mismatch of alkylated guanine with thymidine is obtained. Detection of such a lesion by mismatch repair (MMR) enzymes, which operate exclusively on the daughter strand, lead to a repeated mispairing with thymidine, thus forming a futile cycle of mismatch repair. It is the detection of this futile cycle that is thought to trigger apoptosis.[57] Cells with defective MMR enzyme pathways, which are commonly seen in tumours, are resistant to temozolomide.

An alternative pathway of repair of O^6 alkylation of guanine is by DNA alkyltransferase, which directly transfers the alkyl group to a cysteine residue on the enzyme itself, thus inactivating it.[58,59] Inhibitors of alkyltransferase, e.g. O^6-benzylguanine, have been developed to be combined with alkylating agents such as temozolomide and the nitrosoureas.[60] These combinations are still undergoing clinical evaluation, but their use is being

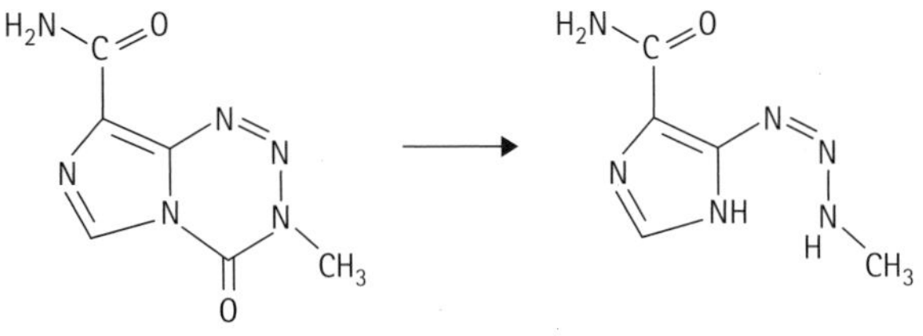

Figure 8.8 *Structure and anabolism of temozolomide.*

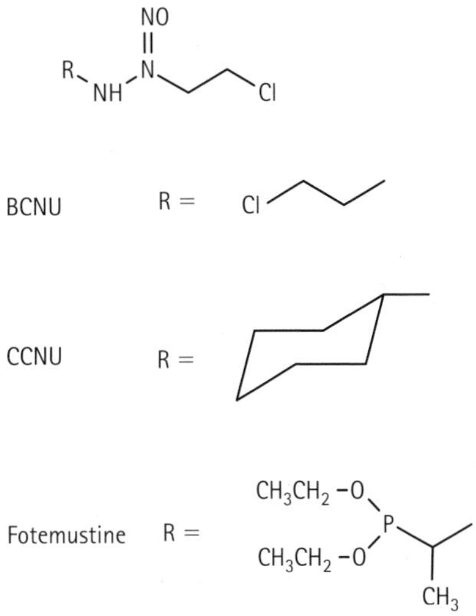

Figure 8.9 *Structure of nitrosoureas. BCNU, carmustine; CCNU, lomustine.*

targeted to tumours shown to express DNA alkyltransferase activity.[61,62]

Temozolomide has the clinical advantage that it is administered orally, at doses up to $200 \, \text{mg/m}^2$ per day over 5 days. Bioavailability is very high. As a drug that directly damages DNA, and a known mutagen,[63] the risk of secondary malignancies in long-term survivors should be evaluated. The major uses of temozolomide in adult malignancies are in brain tumours[64] and melanoma.[65] Response rates in paediatric patients with glioma have been modest.[66]

Nitrosoureas

This group of agents includes BCNU (carmustine), CCNU (lomustine) and fotemustine (Figure 8.9). These agents form carbamoyl adducts with proteins, but their primary mechanism of action is alkylation of DNA.[67,68] Although active in a number of tumour types, relatively little is known about the clinical pharmacology of the nitrosoureas due to their instability in aqueous media and their complex metabolism *in vivo*.[68] Alkylation is mediated by the formation of reactive carbonium ions, analogous to those formed by other chloroethyl-containing molecules. There is some indication that glutathione may play a role in tumour resistance to these drugs, although the clinical relevance of this is unknown.[69]

Absorption of BCNU is almost complete, with less than 1 per cent of a radiolabelled oral dose recovered in the faeces.[70] However, first-pass metabolism may limit the systemic availability of other nitrosoureas such as CCNU.[71] As small, lipid-soluble compounds, distribution of nitrosoureas is rapid and extensive. Volumes of distribution of 3–5 L/kg have been reported for BCNU,[72] while that of fotemustine is lower, at 31 L.[73] Nitrosoureas can penetrate the blood–brain barrier, with cerebrospinal fluid (CSF) concentrations around 30 per cent of those in plasma.[74]

Metabolism, either by dechlorination of fotemustine[75] or by hydroxylation of CCNU,[71] is mainly an inactivation mechanism, although relatively little is known about the primary route of elimination of these compounds.

Dacarbazine

Also known as DTIC, this compound is a forerunner to temozolomide. It requires hepatic oxidative metabolism to yield MTIC (Figure 8.8) and thus form an alkylating species.[76] Dacarbazine is given intravenously, and has some activity in central nervous system (CNS) tumours and melanoma.

Procarbazine

This is a non-classical, monofunctional alkylating agent that requires metabolic activation by aldehyde-oxidizing enzymes.[77]

BIFUNCTIONAL ALKYLATING AGENTS

Thiotepa

Thiotepa is a trisaziridino compound and thus potentially has three alkylating moieties (Figure 8.10). In practice, only two of these react, forming mono- or bifunctional DNA adducts. The oxidized metabolite, TEPA, retains some alkylating and cytotoxic activity.

Studies with thiotepa and TEPA in the presence or absence of a hepatic microsomal metabolizing system reveal that high concentrations of thiotepa are necessary to form DNA interstrand cross-links. In contrast, TEPA produces alkali labile DNA lesions, which are also seen when thiotepa is metabolized.[78] As for most alkylating agents, a role for glutathione (GSH) and glutathione-S-transferases (GSTs) in resistance to thiotepa has been suggested.[79] However, the clinical relevance of this remains unproven.

Thiotepa may be used as single doses, on cycles of 2–3 weeks. Recent studies have used higher doses with haema-

tological support,[80] and some protocols have advocated the use of continuous infusion.[81] Binding of thiotepa to plasma protein is not significant (10 per cent). After intravenous injection, thiotepa and TEPA can be found in the CSF at concentrations equivalent to those in plasma,[82] and the volume of distribution of thiotepa is close to total body water (0.7 ± 0.1 L/kg).[83]

Thiotepa is eliminated with a half-life of less than 2 hours after an intravenous dose. Elimination of TEPA is slower and concentrations of TEPA exceed those of the parent drug.[84] Excretion of parent drug in the urine is minimal (<6 per cent combined metabolites). The pharmacokinetics of thiotepa are dose-dependent, with less TEPA formed at higher doses of thiotepa (>55 mg/m^2).[85] Despite suggestions that TEPA is the active metabolite, haematological toxicity correlates most closely with AUC of thiotepa.[85]

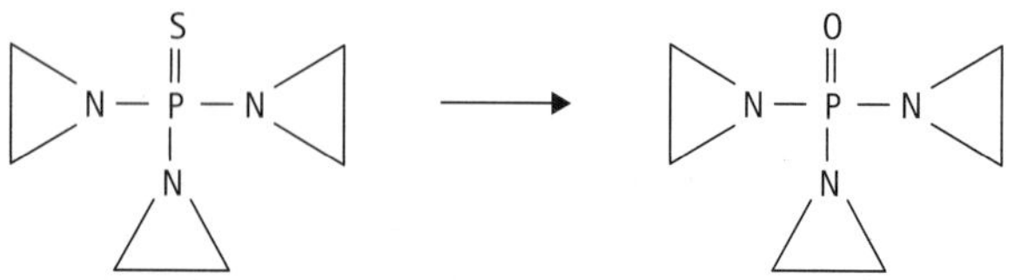

Melphalan

Melphalan is a nitrogen mustard attached to a phenylalanine moiety (Figure 8.11), which was synthesized in an attempt to exploit specific uptake of this amino acid by melanoma cells. Subsequently, melphalan has been shown to be active in a range of solid tumours and in multiple myeloma.

Melphalan forms mono- and bifunctional adducts with DNA. Like many alkylating agents, resistance to melphalan has been associated with glutathione and its associated transferase enzymes.[86] Clinical studies using buthionine sulphoximine, which depletes GSH, have been performed, but have failed to show any advantage over melphalan alone.[87]

Although both oral and intravenous preparations of melphalan may be used, the latter is more common. One of the major current uses is as myeloablative therapy prior to bone marrow transplant (BMT) or stem cell transplant. Doses of up to 220 mg/m^2 have been used, with the major non-haematological toxicity being mucositis.[88] Prolonged thrombocytopenia may also be a problem.

Oral dosing of melphalan results in a high degree of both inter- and intra-patient variability in plasma

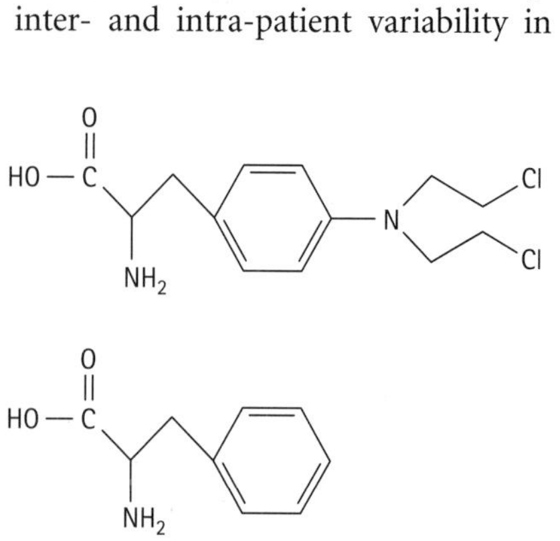

Figure 8.10 *Structure and metabolism of thiotepa.*

Figure 8.11 *Structure of melphalan, relative to that of phenylalanine.*

concentrations.[89] Appearance of drug in the plasma may be delayed for 1–4 hours,[90] with a half-life for absorption of 2–62 min.[91] Food also reduces the extent and rate of absorption, with bioavailability reduced from 85 to 58 per cent. Bioavailability may be as low as 28 per cent, or as high as 100 per cent,[91] as absorption may be dependent on active, energy-dependent processes. A volume of distribution of $20 \pm 4 \, L/m^2$ or $0.5 \pm 0.2 \, L/kg$ has been reported after intravenous administration.[92]

Melphalan is relatively stable, due to the aromatic ring that deactivates the mustard group. Most of the drug is eliminated via hydrolysis of the chloroethyl side-chains to mono- and dihydroxy- forms,[93] with relatively little elimination in urine.[94] Elimination of melphalan after oral administration correlates with renal function (glomerular filtration rate, GFR),[95] but this is not observed consistently.[96]

Plasma half-life after oral dosing is 0.9 ± 0.5 hours, but may range up to 552 min.[97] That after intravenous administration of low doses ($10–20 \, mg/m^2$) is 13–40 min or biphasic with half-lives of 8 ± 3 and 108 ± 21 min following higher doses.[93]

The elimination of melphalan is largely independent of renal and hepatic function. Dose reductions are often recommended in the renally impaired, based on an inverse correlation of AUC with GFR[98] and an increase in toxicity associated with renal insufficiency. However, studies of patients with creatinine clearance less than 40 mL/min show no difference in the pharmacokinetics of high-dose melphalan compared with patients with more normal renal function.[99] Pharmacokinetics of melphalan in children receiving 140 or $220 \, mg/m^2$ intravenously were comparable to those in adults.[99] Clearance ranges from 170 to 570 mL/min per m^2.

Busulphan

Busulphan (Figure 8.12) is a bifunctional alkylating agent forming both inter- and intra-strand cross-links in DNA. Mechanisms of resistance are similar to those cited for related alkylating agents. It is administered orally, either as intact or crushed tablets or as a suspension of the latter via a nasogastric tube. The dose is usually administered four times a day over four consecutive days.

The pharmacokinetics of busulphan are highly variable and depend on age, circadian variation[100] and disease type.[101] Dose adjustment based initially on body size (weight or surface area) and subsequently on plasma concentrations (trough plasma concentration or AUC) has been advocated.[102] Although the data suggesting a link between low plasma concentrations of busulphan and rejection of graft in BMT are relatively weak,[103] that between high concentrations and toxicity, particularly veno-occlusive disease (VOD), is very strong.[102] A threshold AUC for the occurrence of VOD has been identified at 1500 μM min, and dose adjustment to attain AUC values below this threshold is advocated.[102]

Reliable data on bioavailability are lacking. Estimates range from 20 to 120 per cent, and this variability probably underlies much of the reported variability in pharmacokinetics. Absorption is usually rapid, with maximum concentrations achieved in 30–120 min. Recent efforts towards formulating an intravenous preparation of busulphan will allow more precise dose individualization, as well as providing more reliable estimates of bioavailability.[104]

Busulphan enters the CNS easily, with CSF-to-plasma concentration ratios of 0.5–1.4.[105] Volume of distribution is estimated to be $27 \pm 11 \, L/m^2$ following oral administration in children.[105] The elimination of busulphan is rapid, with a half-life of less than 2 hours for children with inherited diseases, and 3 hours for children with leukaemia.[105] Pretreatment with anticonvulsants (phenytoin and phenobarbitone) may increase the rate of elimination of busulphan by about 20 per cent,[106] although this interaction is confounded by possible time-dependent pharmacokinetics. Similarly, concurrent treatment with cyclophosphamide may increase busulphan clearance.[103]

Busulphan clearance is faster in paediatric patients (200 mL/min per m^2) than in adults (95 mL/min per m^2),[107] and within the paediatric group it is fastest in patients below 5 years of age.[100] Also, volume of distribution in children is higher than that in adults.[108] Some, but not all, of the age dependence for elimination is removed by normalizing doses to surface area rather than weight and results in higher doses (mg/kg) in young children than in older patients.[104] This may be associated with a higher incidence of neurotoxicity.[109] Although liver involvement is a common feature of non-malignant syndromes treated with busulphan, there is no relation between the degree of pre-existing hepatic dysfunction and busulphan pharmacokinetics.

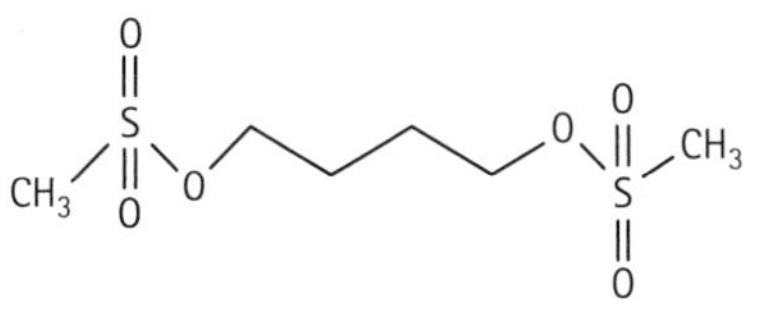

Chlorambucil

The attachment of an aromatic ring to a mustard group results in a more stable alkylating agent (Figure 8.13). Chlorambucil is an example of these aromatic mustards and is used primarily in the treatment of chronic lymphocytic leukaemia and lymphomas. Mutant p53[110] and multidrug resistance-associated protein[111] have also been proposed to play a role in resistance to chlorambucil, as has glutathione.[112]

Figure 8.12 *Structure of busulphan.*

The preferred route of administration for chlorambucil is oral, with rapid absorption resulting in a maximum plasma concentration after 15–30 min.[113] About 98 per cent of the drug in plasma is bound to protein[113] and only low concentrations are observed in the CSF.

Chlorambucil is metabolized to phenylacetic acid mustard. The metabolite has a longer half-life (approx. 150 min) and so has an AUC greater than or equal to that of the parent.[114] Phenylacetic acid has anti-tumour activity,[115] but may be more toxic to host tissues than is chlorambucil.[113] Like other mustards, chlorambucil may undergo oxidative N-dechloroethylation, which again may be linked to neurotoxicity.[116] Chlorambucil and its metabolite phenylacetic acid mustard are eliminated with half-lives of 1.0 and 1.9 hours, respectively.[114]

Cyclophosphamide and ifosfamide

The oxazaphosphorines, cyclophosphamide (CP) and ifosfamide (IFO), were among the first alkylating agents to be used therapeutically. Originally designed to exploit a postulated abundance of phosphoramidase enzymes in tumours compared with normal tissue, CP was thought to deliver nitrogen mustard selectively to malignant cells.[114] Although oxazaphosphorines do act as prodrugs,

the exact pharmacological route to DNA alkylation is more complex (Figure 8.14).

Both CP and IFO form bifunctional DNA adducts, through the action of their mustard metabolites (see below). Reaction occurs predominantly at the N^7 of guanine, via formation of a reactive aziridinium intermediate (Figures 8.14 and 8.15). The reaction of the second arm of the mustard leads to cross-links, with the differing configurations of the two mustards resulting in slightly different ranges of cross-linking. Subsequent processing or repair of these lesions is thought to result in cytotoxicity.

Because of the need for metabolic activation, and the potential for metabolic inactivation, oxazaphosphorines have a number of possible mechanisms for resistance.[17] While these have been described in pre-clinical models, relatively little evidence exists for their clinical relevance. As reactive alkylating species, oxazaphosphorines are able to form conjugates with other nucleophilic species such as glutathione.[117] The inactivation of oxazaphosphorine intermediates by aldehyde dehydrogenase (ALDH) enzymes may be a mechanism of clinical resistance.[118,119]

The clinical use of the oxazaphosphorines includes both haematological and non-haematological disease. Combination regimens including CP and IFO usually also comprise a topoisomerase II agent, vinca alkaloid or other drug. Cyclophosphamide is employed in high-dose regimens for two purposes: firstly, as a mobilizer of peripheral blood progenitor cells; and secondly, at higher doses, as a bone marrow ablative.[120]

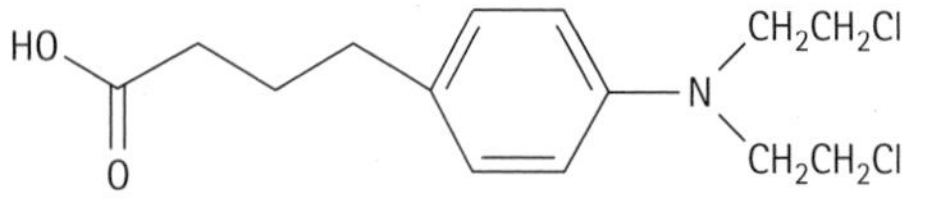

Figure 8.13 Structure of chlorambucil.

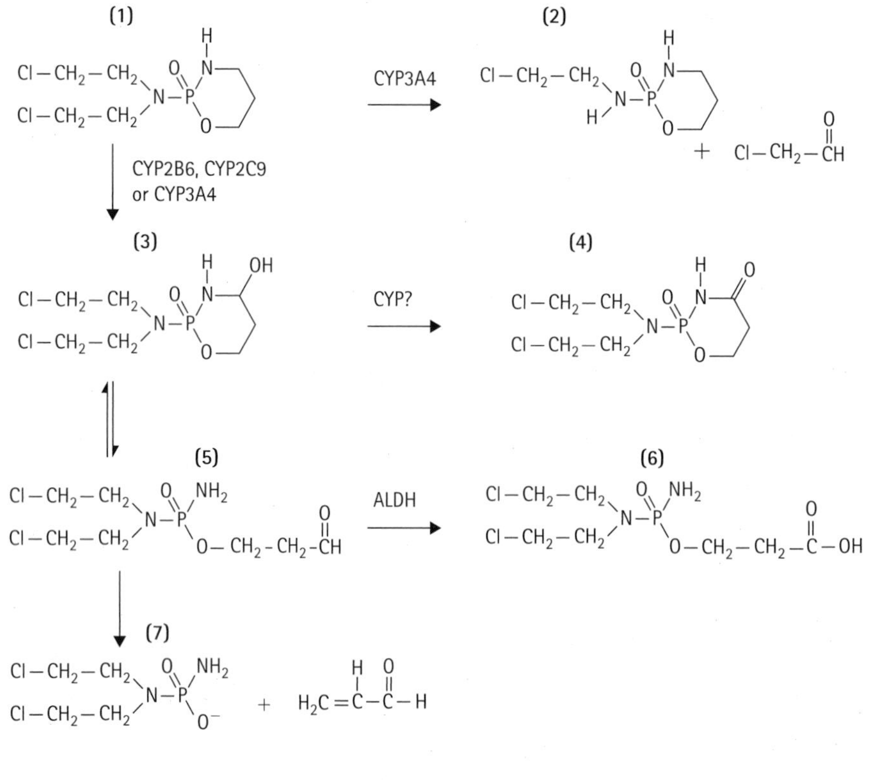

Figure 8.14 Metabolism of cyclophosphamide by cytochrome P450 (CYP) isoforms and aldehyde dehydrogenase (ALDH).

Ifosfamide, and CP at high doses, must be given with the uroprotective agent mesna. This prevents haemorrhagic cystitis, thought to be due to the toxic metabolites acrolein and chloroacetaldehyde. Mesna is usually given intravenously, but an oral formulation is also available.

When administered intravenously, CP and IFO have half-lives of 4–6 hours, with clearance values reported to be 5.4 L/hour for CP,[121] with a lower value for IFO of 2.5–4 L/hour.[122] Volume of distribution is hard to estimate due to the complex pharmacokinetics of these drugs, but is generally around 0.6 L/kg. The majority of elimination is by metabolism, with less than 20 per cent of a dose eliminated unchanged in the urine. There is no difference in pharmacokinetics between paediatric and adult patients.[123] While hepatic disease might be expected to reduce the activation of oxazaphosphorines, there are few clinical data available to confirm this.

Both CP and IFO are absorbed well following oral ingestion,[124,125] but bioavailability measures based on the parent drug may mask qualitative and quantitative effects, due to metabolism in the GI tract or first-pass metabolism. The pharmacology of IFO is different following oral administration with an unacceptably high incidence of encephalopathic episodes.[126]

The oxazaphosphorines distribute throughout the body, with a low degree of protein binding in the plasma.[121,122] Distribution of parent drug and metabolites has been determined in the CSF, with concentrations comparable to those seen in plasma.[127]

Oxazaphosphorines are prodrugs and require metabolic activation to form the DNA reactive mustard species PM (phosphoramide mustard) and IPM (isophosphoramide mustard).[17] As well as the activation pathway, CP and IFO may form inactive dechloroethylated, carboxy- and keto-metabolites (Figure 8.14). Dechloroethylation is much more significant for IFO, accounting for up to 50 per cent of a dose compared with less than 10 per cent for CP.[123] The formation of chloroacetaldehyde in this reaction and the different spectrum of toxicities observed with the two drugs suggest some causative role for chloroacetaldehyde in IFO nephro- or neurotoxicity.[128]

As oxazaphosphorines are dependent on metabolism for activity, drug interactions resulting in modification of metabolism are particularly important. Drugs which may inhibit activation of CP and IFO include antifungal agents (ketoconazole and fluconazole),[129] allopurinol and chlorpromazine.[130] Thiotepa may inhibit CP metabolism in high-dose chemotherapy.[131]

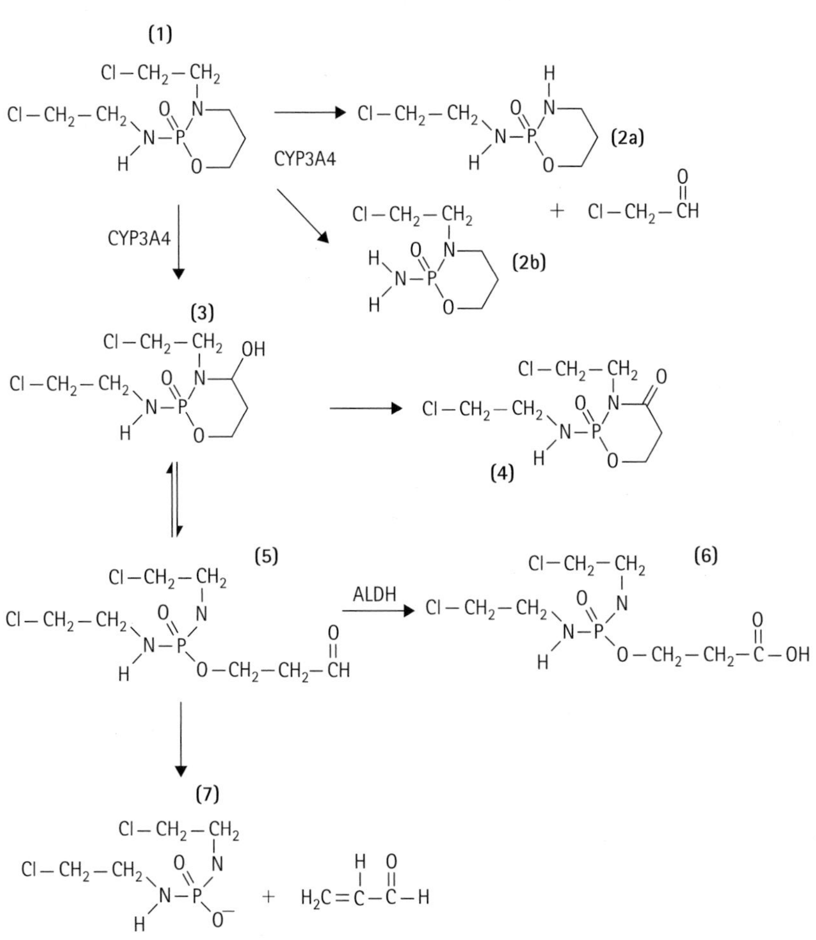

Figure 8.15 *Metabolism of ifosfamide by cytochrome P450 (CYP) isoforms and aldehyde dehydrogenase (ALDH).*

The most significant observation relating to the pharmacodynamics of oxazaphosphorines is that an inverse relationship exists between the AUC for parent CP and the likelihood of both response and cardiotoxicity.[132] Thus, less metabolism (presumably activating) is associated with a lower degree of pharmacologically active drug.

Platinum compounds

CISPLATIN AND CARBOPLATIN

These related agents both contain a tetravalent platinum atom, a reactive group that can be replaced by water in an aquation reaction, and two amino groups (Figure 8.16). The two labile chloride atoms of cisplatin are in the *cis*-configuration, and it should be noted that the *trans* isomer has no cytotoxic activity.[133] The positively charged aquated species formed by aquation reacts readily with nucleophiles such as DNA bases and proteins. As with bifunctional alkylating agents, the most cytotoxic lesions formed by the platinum compounds are intra- and interstrand cross-links within DNA.[134]

Carboplatin is similar to cisplatin, except that the dicarboxylate group is less readily displaced by aquation. This is reflected in a lower *in vitro* potency and in differences in the systemic and cellular pharmacology of the two agents.[135]

In paediatrics, platinum drugs are used in the treatment of neuroblastoma, Wilms' tumour, sarcomas and CNS tumours. Clinical regimens often include a combination with etoposide. The choice between cisplatin and carboplatin reflects the perceived differential activities of the two drugs and differences in toxicity.[136] The use of cisplatin may cause neurotoxicity, mainly deafness, and nephrotoxicity. Carboplatin administration is more commonly associated with haematological toxicity, although a syndrome of multiple organ failure has been described with very high doses or AUC values.[137]

Clinically, cisplatin is usually administered as a 24-hour infusion, although shorter durations, such as 4 or 6 hours, have been used. Despite the assumption that the higher peak plasma concentrations generated by shorter infusions might result in greater CNS penetration, clinical data indicate that the 24-hour schedule is more effective and that shorter infusions cause greater toxicity.[138] As cisplatin is usually measured as elemental platinum, it is important to distinguish between the pharmacokinetics of total platinum, much of which is bound to plasma proteins, and that of unbound platinum which largely reflects unchanged cisplatin.[139,140] The major route of elimination for cisplatin is by reaction with protein. Only 20–30 per cent of the dose (as platinum species) is excreted in the urine. The half-life of unchanged platinum following cisplatin administration is very short, while that of total platinum may be 10–20 hours.[141]

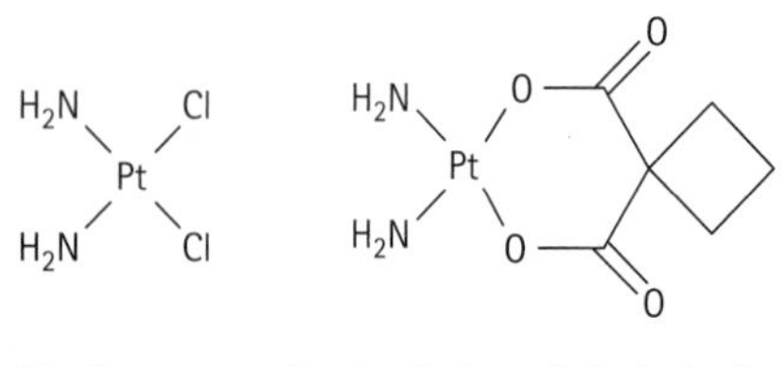

Carboplatin systemic pharmacology has been extensively studied. Since carboplatin is relatively stable in plasma, the major route of elimination is renal, with up to 80 per cent of a dose appearing in the urine within 24 hours.[142] The close relationship between carboplatin clearance from plasma and glomerular filtration rate has led to the concept of renal function-based dosing.[10,142] This approach uses a knowledge of the desired plasma exposure to the drug, or AUC, together with a well defined therapeutic window for AUC,[20] to administer doses aimed at producing a target AUC. A robust measure of renal function is required for this calculation. The clearance of EDTA has proved to be useful in dosing adult patients, and a similar calculation can be made for paediatric patients.[143] When high doses of carboplatin are employed (total AUC > 6 mg/mL min), the margin for error in the calculation of the appropriate dose is such that a therapeutic drug monitoring approach is justified. Limited sampling schemes have been proposed which allow rapid determination of AUC, and thus dose adjustments, to be made over several days of dosing.[144]

Resistance to platinum agents mirrors to some extent that associated with alkylating agents. There is some evidence of the involvement of glutathione-related pathways,[145,146] with a possible contribution from the multidrug resistance protein MRP,[147] which may act to export Pt-GSH conjugates from cells. At the level of DNA repair, nucleotide excision repair may mediate resistance to platinum agents,[148,149] and deficiency in MMR pathways may also result in insensitivity to this class of agents.[150,151] Inactivation or mutation in the p53 protein also results in resistance to platinum drugs.[152,153]

Tubulin binding drugs

VINCA ALKALOIDS

Originally isolated from the Madagascar periwinkle, vincristine (Figure 8.17) is included in combination therapies for a number of paediatric malignancies. Vinblastine is also used in the treatment of lymphomas. The vincas act by binding to α- and β-tubulin monomers, thus inhibiting their assembly to form the microtubular structures. The latter are necessary for mitosis and other functions related to cell structure.

Figure 8.16 *Structures of carboplatin and cisplatin. Pt, platinum.*

The dose-limiting toxicity of vincristine is neurotoxicity,[154] with well-documented fatal effects following inadvertent intrathecal administration. The major toxicity of vinblastine at clinically used doses is myelosuppression.

Both drugs are eliminated by metabolism, mediated by cytochrome P450 enzymes.[155] This may be accompanied by, or be followed by, glucuronidation. After intravenous administration, elimination is triphasic with an initial half-life of 5 min, an intermediate phase (half-life 2–3 hours) and an extended terminal elimination phase.[156] The latter is associated with extensive tissue binding. Most of the administered drug, including metabolites, is eliminated in the bile, and care must be taken when administering these drugs in the presence of obstructive jaundice or severe hepatic dysfunction.[157]

As with many agents derived from natural products, vinca alkaloids are subject to resistance associated with expression of p-glycoprotein or MRP.[158]

Although trials of taxanes, which promote assembly of tubulin monomers to form microtubules, continue in paediatric malignancies, activity has been disappointing.[159,160]

Topoisomerase II agents

ETOPOSIDE AND TENIPOSIDE

Podophyllotoxin, which is extracted from the mandrake plant, is a microtubular binding agent with cytotoxic properties. Etoposide and teniposide (Figure 8.18) are synthetic glycoside derivatives of podophyllotoxin, but these drugs act by binding to and stabilizing the complex formed between topoisomerase II enzymes and DNA.[161] Topoisomerase II facilitates the relaxation and unwinding of DNA by permitting the formation of a controlled break in double-stranded DNA, permitting another double strand to pass through the break. Normally, the topoisomerase-mediated double-strand break is resealed, but etoposide and other compounds (see below) act by stabilizing the topo II/DNA cleavable complex and prevent resealing of the double-strand break. The persistence of strand breaks can result in apoptosis and block DNA replication. Thus, cells are blocked in the S or early G2 phase of the cell cycle.

Etoposide is preferred over teniposide in most regimens. Combination therapy with a platinum compound

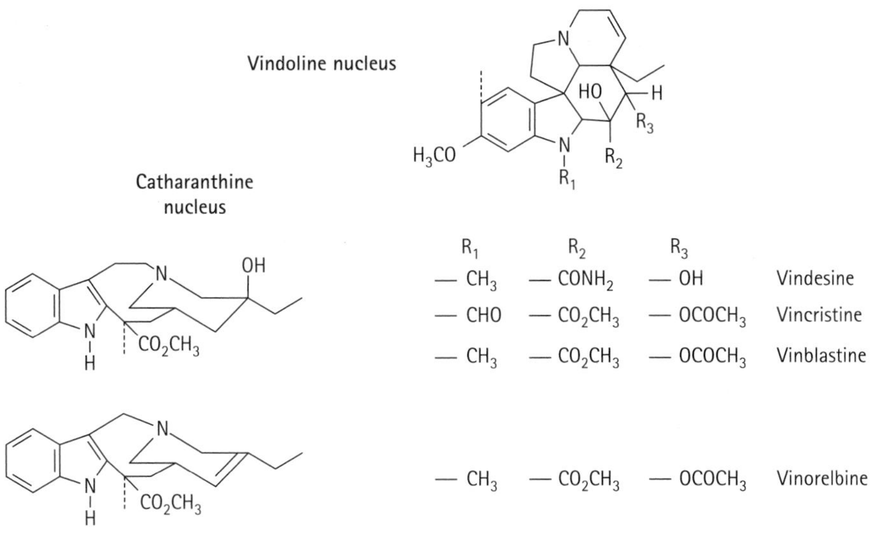

R$_1$	R$_2$	R$_3$	
— CH$_3$	— CONH$_2$	— OH	Vindesine
— CHO	— CO$_2$CH$_3$	— OCOCH$_3$	Vincristine
— CH$_3$	— CO$_2$CH$_3$	— OCOCH$_3$	Vinblastine
— CH$_3$	— CO$_2$CH$_3$	— OCOCH$_3$	Vinorelbine

Figure 8.17 *Structure of vincristine and analogues.*

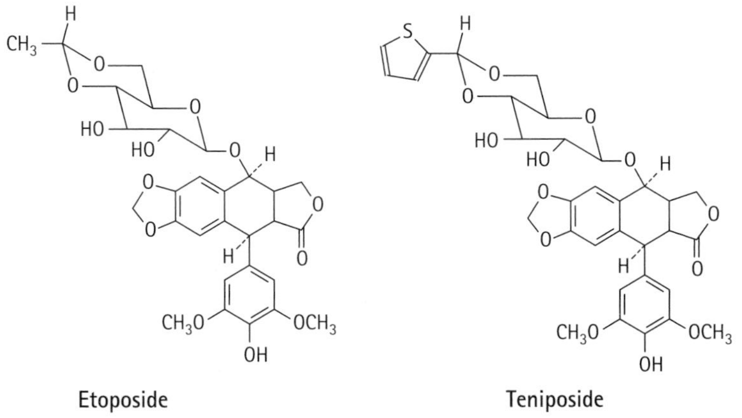

Etoposide

Teniposide

Figure 8.18 *Etoposide and teniposide.*

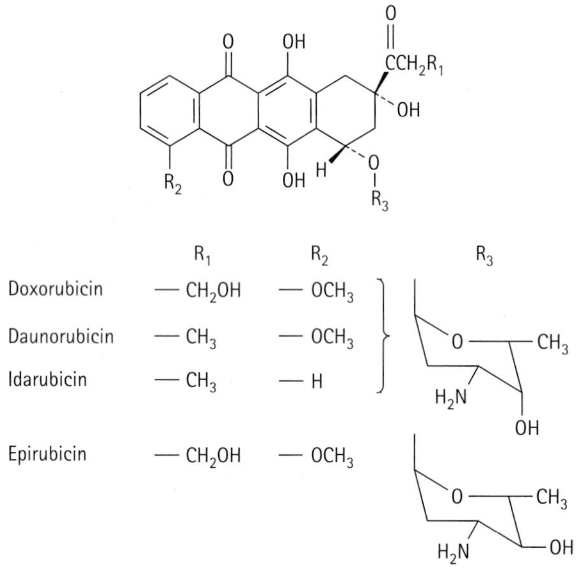

Figure 8.19 *Structures of anthracyclines.*

is common. Although the usual mode of administration is intravenous, etoposide may be administered orally.[162] However, the bioavailability of etoposide is low (less than 50 per cent) and variable both between individuals and between occasions in the same individual.[163] The intravenous formulation contains excipients which may be associated with hypersensitivity reactions. A prodrug form, etoposide phosphate, has been developed and releases etoposide rapidly and completely following intravenous administration.[164] The prodrug is much more water-soluble, permitting formulation in isotonic aqueous solutions.

Around 40 per cent of an intravenous dose is excreted unchanged in the urine and dose modification in patients with renal impairment has been advocated. The remainder of the drug is eliminated by metabolism, with only 10 per cent excreted in the bile.[161]

As with many natural products, etoposide and teniposide are substrates for p-glycoprotein-mediated multidrug resistance.[158] Clinical studies of etoposide combined with an inhibitor of p-glycoprotein, such as cyclosporin or PSC833, have shown a clear pharmacokinetic interaction, necessitating a marked reduction in the dose of etoposide administered.[165] However, the clinical benefit of such combinations is not yet proven. Resistance to etoposide has also been shown in cells with mutated or decreased topoisomerase II expression.[166]

ANTHRACYCLINES

Of the anthracyclines developed for clinical use (Figure 8.19), daunorubicin and doxorubicin are the two that are used most in paediatric malignancies. These compounds have been isolated from bacteria or are prepared semi-synthetically from such extracts and comprise a planar ring, combined with a sugar moiety. The intercalation of the planar ring into the major groove of the DNA helix may be stabilized by the binding of the amino sugar to the sugar-phosphate backbone of DNA. The affinity of anthracyclines for DNA may facilitate their primary cytotoxic mechanism, which may involve binding to the cleavable complex of topoisomerase II and DNA (as with etoposide),[167] or generation of reactive oxygen species (ROS). The latter mechanism involves reduction of the quinone to yield either a semiquinone or dihydroquinone by, respectively, one or two electron reductive enzymes.[168] The generation of ROS may underlie the cardiotoxicity of anthracyclines.[169]

Except for idarubicin, which has acceptable bioavailability, anthracyclines are administered intravenously. Care must be taken to avoid extravasation as these drugs are potent vesicants. The majority of an intravenous dose is eliminated by metabolism and biliary excretion.[170] The major alcohol metabolite is formed by carbonyl reductase enzymes, which reduce the ketone of the side-chain. Doxorubicinol is detectable in plasma at lower concentrations than the parent drug, but the concentrations of the corresponding metabolites for daunorubicin[171] and idarubicin[172] can exceed those of the parent. Idarubicinol retains significant cytotoxic activity, comparable to idarubicin.[173]

Mechanisms of resistance are similar to those for etoposide, with the addition of perturbations in the pathways resulting in ROS. Thus depletion of NADPH, a necessary cofactor for reductive enzymes, or chelation of iron, which promotes the formation of ROS, reduces the cytotoxicity of doxorubicin. Mutations in p53[174] and degree of expression of topoisomerase II isoforms[166] have also been associated with resistance to anthracyclines in tumour cell lines.

Although a number of schedules have been proposed for anthracycline administration, a short intravenous infusion is most common. After a rapid distribution phase, terminal half-lives of 20–30 hours have been reported.[170] Daunorubicin has a shorter half-life.[171] Recently, liposomal preparations of both daunorubicin[175] and doxorubicin[176] have been introduced. The clinical use of these agents suggests retention of anti-tumour activity with reduced toxicity.

AMSACRINE (mAMSA)

Amsacrine acts by binding to the cleavable complex formed between DNA and topoisomerase II. Cytotoxicity correlates closely with the formation of single and double-strand breaks in DNA.

Topoisomerase I agents

Relatively recently, agents based on the natural product camptothecin have been introduced into clinical use. While topotecan has been approved for the treatment of

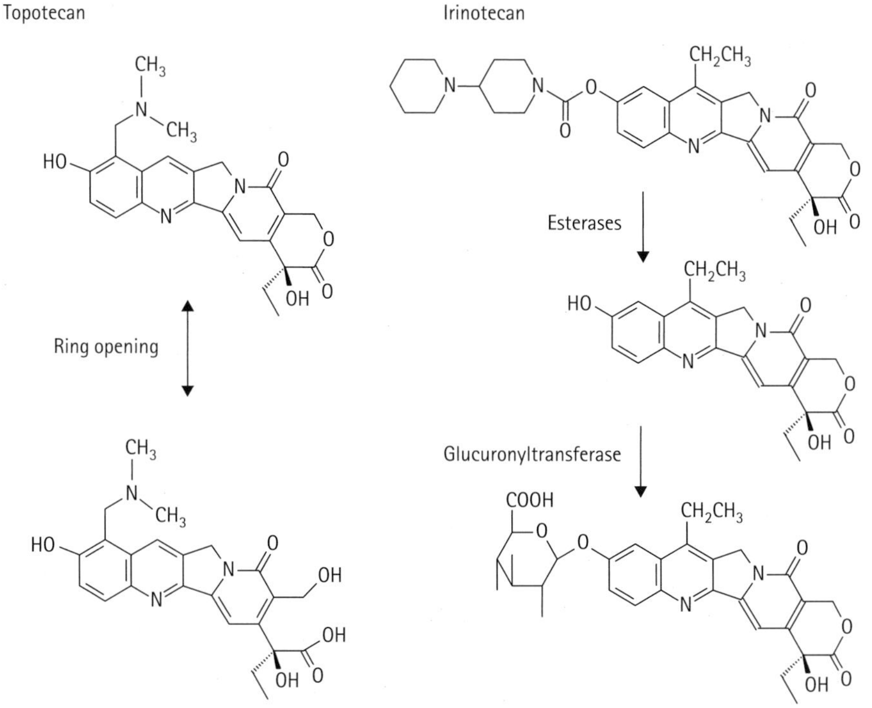

Topotecan

Irinotecan

Esterases

Ring opening

Glucuronyltransferase

Figure 8.20 *Structures and metabolism of topotecan, illustrating equilibrium between lactone and acid forms, and irinotecan, illustrating release of active SN38 from prodrug form and subsequent glucuronidation.*

some adult malignancies and is undergoing clinical studies in paediatrics,[177] irinotecan seems to possess a superior profile of activity and toxicity.[178]

The camptothecins act by binding to and stabilizing the cleavable complex formed between topoisomerase I and DNA.[179] Topoisomerase I acts in an analogous fashion to topoisomerase II, except that it binds to and causes a temporary break in single-stranded DNA, allowing the release of torsional strain within DNA. The 'untangling' of DNA in this manner is thought to be important for DNA repair and transcription.

All camptothecins exist in two forms when administered systemically, the intact lactone and a ring-opened carboxylic acid (Figure 8.20). The equilibrium between these two forms is pH-dependent and the lactone is thought to be the active form. Topotecan is usually administered by short intravenous infusion daily for 5 days. Oral dosing is possible as the bioavailability is around 40 per cent.[180] Irinotecan is a prodrug that rapidly releases the active moiety SN-38 by the action of plasma esterases.[181] Both repeated daily administration and single-dose, 3-weekly regimens have been used for irinotecan. Both drugs are metabolized to N-desmethyl metabolites, mediated by cytochrome P450 enzymes; the other main pathways of elimination are glucuronidation and renal excretion.[180] Camptothecins are active in neuroblastoma, brain tumours and Wilms' tumour. Diarrhoea and myelosuppression are the major dose-limiting side-effects of the camptothecins. The combination of topotecan with platinum drugs results in synergistic toxicity, although some activity of this combination has been noted.[182]

Resistance to camptothecins is associated with downregulation of expression or mutation in topoisomerase I.[183]

Miscellaneous agents

STEROIDS

The glucocorticoids dexamethasone and prednisolone are used in the treatment of leukaemias and lymphomas, as well as the treatment of nausea. The use of these two drugs varies between countries. In the UK, induction therapy for ALL uses 6.5 mg/m² per day dexamethasone, whereas the German BFM protocol uses 60 mg/m² per day prednisolone,[184] both given orally.

Glucocorticoids bind to the glucocorticoid receptor (GR) and cause apoptosis through inhibition of IL-2 production,[185] downregulation of c-myc[186] or repression of transcription factors such as AP1.[187] B-lineage malignancies are more sensitive,[188] possibly due to lower GR expression in T-lineage malignancies.[189]

When given at a dose of 0.3–2.5 mg/kg, the peak concentration of 0.01–2.4 μM occurs at around 2 hours, and the half-life is 2 hours.[190] Similarly, peak concentrations of 0.38–1.5 μM have been reported following doses of 13–17 mg/m², and the corresponding unbound concentrations of 0.28–0.55 μM are similar to those causing cytotoxicity *in vitro*.[191] An inverse correlation has been reported between clearance and age.[192] Concentrations of prednisolone in CSF are one-third the level of those in plasma.[193]

For dexamethasone, 0.1–0.3 mg/kg produced plasma concentrations of 0.13–0.67 μM. The half-life of dexamethasone is longer than that of prednisolone (2.4–9.5 hours), with a lower clearance and larger volume of distribution.[194]

Factors that influence the sensitivity of leukaemic cells to steroids include the expression of glucocorticoid receptors. *Ex vivo* studies using the MTT assay show correlation with clinical sensitivity[195] and indicate that resistance is associated with pro-B, T-cell and age less than 18 months or greater than 10 years.[196]

Toxicities associated with steroid treatment include avascular necrosis.[197]

ACTINOMYCIN D

This drug is a complex polypeptide with a central phenoxazone ring and is a product of a species of *Streptomyces*. It may act by intercalation, binding to DNA and so preventing DNA and RNA synthesis. By blocking DNA repair, actinomycin D is a potent radiosensitizer. Because of difficulties with the analysis of actinomycin D, only limited information is available on its systemic pharmacology.[198] Elimination appears to be rapid after intravenous administration. P-glycoprotein-mediated efflux is a major mechanism of resistance. VOD following actinomycin D administration has been reported, especially in Wilms' tumour patients.[199]

BLEOMYCIN

A complex antibiotic mixture derived from *Streptomyces* species, bleomycin consists primarily of the A2 polypeptide.[200] Bleomycin is often referred to as a radiomimetic, as it causes single- and double-strand breaks in DNA. Binding to DNA is mediated by a DNA-binding fragment with preferential affinity for A-T or G-C sequences. Iron, bound at a separate part of the polypeptide, is oxidized to yield ROS that can cause DNA strand breaks.

Following intravenous administration, elimination is biphasic with half-lives of 30 min and 3 hours. Elimination is primarily by renal excretion, and pulmonary toxicity may be enhanced in patients with renal dysfunction or in those who have had prior platinum treatment.

L–ASPARAGINASE

The rationale for the use of this drug was that malignant cells are unable to synthesize asparagine from aspartic acid as they lack L-asparagine synthetase, although this hypothesis is unproven. These cells are therefore dependent on extracellular sources of asparagine and so may be sensitive to depletion of this amino acid. L-asparaginase converts L-asparagine to aspartic acid and ammonia, depletes circulating L-asparagine from the body and so deprives the tumour cells of an essential nutrient. The main clinical use of L-asparaginase is in the induction of remission of leukaemia.[201]

There are three main forms of L-asparaginase available, which may not be used interchangeably, but may have useful complementary characteristics.[202] The *E. coli* form of L-asparaginase appears to be most active, but may also be associated with an increased risk of toxicity. Hypersensitivity reactions may occur and the presence of detectable antibodies to *E. coli* L-asparaginase may be associated with a failure of therapy.[203] Substitution of the *Erwinia*-derived enzyme may circumvent such an immune response and the pegylated form of the L-asparaginase may offer further advantages, such as an increase in half-life, more reliable depletion of L-asparagine and lower immunogenicity.[204]

Monitoring of L-asparaginase therapy may take the form of measurement of L-asparaginase activity in plasma or measurement of the depletion of L-asparagine. The latter is confounded by the relative lack of sensitivity of conventional assay methods and ignorance of the degree of depletion necessary for anti-tumour effect. Routine monitoring for the formation of antibodies to L-asparagine is also controversial, but detection of antibodies or hypersensitivity reactions may indicate the need for an alternative formulation or source of enzyme.

The half-life of L-asparaginase, which may be administered subcutaneously, intramuscularly or intravenously, is 12–24 hours, depending on the preparation used and the site of injection.[205] Intravenous administration is more reliable, but subcutaneous and intramuscular routes are often preferred.[206] Most regimens indicate administration every 2–3 days, although enzyme activity is often detectable for up to 3 weeks after large doses. A possible mechanism of resistance is increased expression of asparagine synthetase in tumour cells.[207]

APPLICATION OF PHARMACOLOGICAL PRINCIPLES IN PAEDIATRIC ONCOLOGY

Pharmacologically guided dosing

Due to the uncertain nature of the relationship between plasma concentrations and the clinical effects of most anti-tumour agents, there are few examples of the use of pharmacology to guide dosing in paediatrics. The situation in this patient group is particularly complicated, given that most regimens incorporate multiple agents. The primary examples of using a knowledge of pharmacology in order to optimize treatment are carboplatin and methotrexate, and in both cases this is particularly relevant when a high-dose regimen is used.

Carboplatin dosing according to renal function, with the aim of achieving a target AUC, is routine in the treatment of adult malignancies,[10] and is feasible for paediatrics.[143] The primary difficulty lies in obtaining a reliable estimate of GFR in young patients. In high-dose carbo-platin regimens, the dose is often split over 3 or 5 days, allowing an initial estimate of GFR to be used to calculate the dose for the first day, and carboplatin pharmacoki-netics to be used to adjust the dose on subsequent days.[144] Since there is a steepening of the relationship between toxicity and AUC at high doses, such adjustment can be crucial.

Dose adjustment of high-dose methotrexate in the treatment of paediatric B-cell ALL has also been demon-strated to be of benefit. Using a continuous infusion, with rapid monitoring and adjustment of the infusion rate, a target steady-state concentration can be maintained and provides an improvement in relapse-free survival.[29]

Although dose adjustment of etoposide has been applied in adults,[21] extension of this principle to pae-diatric patients is hampered by insufficient knowledge of the 'target' plasma concentration. Other drugs for which pharmacologically guided dosing has been pro-posed include melphalan, busulphan, L-asparagine and 6-mercaptopurine (as 6-TGN). In each case, the lack of a robust target end-point has deterred universal applica-tion of this approach, given the additional effort required to perform pharmacological studies.

High-dose chemotherapy

The rationale for the administration of high doses of chemotherapy is that drugs such as alkylating agents have steep dose–response curves in *in vitro* models. The toxici-ties associated with such high doses can be circumvented by the use of growth factors, a bone marrow transplant or stem cell support.

Of the component drugs used in paediatric high-dose regimens, the steepening of the toxicity curve with carboplatin has already been noted.[137] Similarly, thresh-olds for toxicity have been quoted for busulphan.[103] The addition of non-DNA-alkylating drugs, such as etoposide, has also been advocated, although the dose–response data for these agents are less consistent.

In terms of pharmacology, concerns regarding high-dose chemotherapy relate to saturation of drug-metabolizing enzymes or transport processes. This may result in disproportionately high plasma concentrations, if the enzymes are involved in drug elimination, or less than proportionate degrees of drug activation if metabo-lism is required for cytotoxic activity.

Combination chemotherapy

Treatment regimens for paediatric malignancies often contain a large number of component drugs. The selection of these components may be based on single agent activity or on theoretical considerations concerning mechanism of action and non-overlapping toxicities. In many cases, combinations have been arrived at based on empirical observations of activity and tolerability, with some evolu-tion over time of the doses, schedules and relative timing of administration of the component drugs. As our under-standing of the mechanism of action of different agents increases, the rationale underlying effective combinations becomes clear, e.g. the combination of a DNA-damaging agent such as cisplatin with a drug that interferes with DNA processing and repair, such as etoposide. New com-binations may also be indicated based on knowledge of established and novel mechanisms of cytotoxicity.

When drugs are administered simultaneously, inter-actions may occur at the level of the tumour, one drug blocking or augmenting the activity of another. Systemic drug interactions may also occur, often when drugs are either eliminated or activated by systemic metabolism. A number of drug interactions involving chemotherapeu-tic agents have been reported.[208] An apparently clinically relevant interaction between cisplatin and etoposide, where the former drug impeded the elimination of the latter, was suggested in a paediatric population.[209] A further study in adults did not replicate this finding, but did note a modest effect of platinum pretreatment on etoposide metabolism.[210]

A number of drugs have been shown to interact with the metabolism of cyclophosphamide, which is necessary for activation of this prodrug, but also contributes to its elimination. Fluconazole, given prophylactically against fungal infection, reduces the metabolism of cyclophos-phamide,[129] as do chlorpromazine and allopurinol.[130] Thiotepa, often combined with cyclophosphamide in high-dose regimens, also reduces cyclophosphamide metabo-lism.[131] Conversely, chronic treatment with steroids or anticonvulsants can increase the metabolism of both cyclophosphamide[130] and ifosfamide.[211] The impact of such interactions on the balance between activating and inactivating pathways of metabolism is unclear[212] and the clinical impact has not been fully elucidated.

Dose correction for body size

It seems intuitively obvious that the dose of a drug that is appropriate for an 18-year-old sarcoma patient will not be the same as that for a 6-month-old infant with neu-roblastoma. Yet the optimal method of adjusting doses to take account of age and body size is the subject of some debate.[213] Between the ages of 1 and 18 years, or for patients heavier than 10 kg, dose adjustment proportional to body surface area is almost universally applied, and appears to provide safe and effective chemotherapy regi-mens in many patients. In some cases, pharmacologically guided dosing or monitoring may be appropriate and there are almost certainly patients who are under- or over-treated by giving a constant dose per square metre.

However, it is those patients below 1 year or weighing less than 10 kg who have the biggest change in the relative dose of cytotoxic drug administered. Doses based on a per kilogram scale are commonly used in this population, often resulting in a substantial reduction in dose compared with the equivalent dose per square metre, as has been shown for etoposide.[214] Although both scales are open to criticism, it is this disjunction around 10 kg (or 12 kg in some protocols) that is most concerning. Also, infants who grow beyond 10 kg may be subject to sudden changes in the chemotherapy dose. A method for accurate calculation of body surface area based on weight has been advocated[215] to allow for uniformity of dosing in infants. This should be used only with the caveat that doses adjusted per square metre might be further reduced in infants, at the discretion of the paediatric oncologist.

CONCLUSION

There is an increasing appreciation of the role of pharmacology in drug selection, dosage regimen design and clinical management of paediatric malignancies. In the future, more target-based measures of tumour-specific pharmacology will become available, just as drugs more specific to paediatric tumours will be developed. Building on our current understanding of pharmacology should allow for the rational development of such novel agents.

KEY POINTS

- The difference between therapeutic and toxic doses is very small for most chemotherapeutic agents.
- Understanding of pharmacological principles can improve the clinical use of many agents, particularly with regard to the processes of:
  - absorption after oral dosing
  - drug distribution to tumour cells
  - drug metabolism
  - renal elimination of drug and metabolites.
- The following pharmacokinetic parameters are useful in designing drug dosage regimens:
  - clearance: directly related to the dose or rate of drug administration for a given target concentration of drug in the blood
  - half-life: determines the frequency of administration that is appropriate for a target profile of concentrations in the blood
  - volume of distribution: relates the dose to the observed concentration in blood or plasma.
- Although much can be determined with regard to the relationship between dose administered and concentrations of drug in blood or plasma (pharmacokinetics), the relationships between drug concentrations in body fluids and biochemical effects or clinical outcome (pharmacodynamics) are not well understood.
- The principles outlined above are used in paediatric oncology for a number of drugs in the following clinical settings:
  - pharmacologically guided dosing
  - high-dose chemotherapy
  - combination chemotherapy
  - dose correction for body size.
- Future developments in the pharmacology of drugs used in paediatric oncology are likely to include:
  - more direct measurements of drug–target interactions
  - pharmacogenetic investigations of drug-metabolizing enzymes and transport proteins
  - treatments tailored specifically to paediatric tumours.

REFERENCES

1. Konopleva M, Zhao SR, Xie Z et al. Apoptosis – molecules and mechanisms. In: Kaspers GJL, Pieters R, Veerman AJP, eds. Drug Resistance in Leukemia and Lymphoma III. The Netherlands: Kluwer/Plenum, 1999; 217–36.
♦ 2. Fisher DE. Apoptosis in cancer therapy: crossing the threshold. Cell 1994; 78: 539–42.
♦ 3. Grana X, Reddy EP. Cell cycle control in mammalian cells: role of cyclins, cyclin dependent kinases (CDKs), growth suppressor genes and cyclin-dependent kinase inhibitors (CDKIs). Oncogene 1995; 11: 211–19.
4. Ferreira CG, Tolis C, Giaccone G. p53 and chemosensitivity. Ann Oncol 1999; 10: 1011–21.
5. Ruvolo PP, Deng X, May WS. Phosphorylation of Bcl2 and regulation of apoptosis. Leukemia 2001; 15: 515–22.
6. Bardelmeijer HA, van Tellingen O, Schellens JHM, Beijnen JH. The oral route for the administration of cytotoxic drugs: strategies to increase the efficiency and consistency of drug delivery. Invest New Drugs 2000; 18: 231–41.
7. Singh BN. Effects of food on clinical pharmacokinetics. Clin Pharmacokinet 1999; 37: 213–55.
8. Sparreboom A, vanAsperen J, Mayer U et al. Limited oral bioavailability and active epithelial excretion of paclitaxel (Taxol) caused by P-glycoprotein in the intestine. Proc Natl Acad Sci USA 1997; 94: 2031–5.
9. Stewart CF, Arbuck SG, Fleming RA, Evans WE. Relation of systemic exposure to unbound etoposide and hematologic toxicity. Clin Pharmacol Ther 1991; 50: 385–93.
●10. Calvert AH, Newell DR, Gumbrell LA et al. Carboplatin dosage: prospective evaluation of a simple formula based on renal function. J Clin Oncol 1989; 7: 1748–56.

11. Liegler DG, Henderson ES, Hahn MA, Oliverio VT. The effect of organic acids on renal clearance of methotrexate in man. *Clin Pharmacol Ther* 1969; **10**: 849–57.

12. Pflüger K-H, Hahn M, Holz J-B *et al*. Pharmacokinetics of etoposide: correlation of pharmacokinetic parameters with clinical conditions. *Cancer Chemother Pharmacol* 1993; **31**: 350–6.

13. Camaggi CM, Comparsi R, Strocchi E *et al*. Epirubicin and doxorubicin comparative metabolism and pharmacokinetics – a crossover study. *Cancer Chemother Pharmacol* 1988; **21**: 221–8.

14. Ellis AG, Webster LK. Inhibition of paclitaxel elimination in the isolated perfused rat liver by Cremophor EL. *Cancer Chemother Pharmacol* 1999; **43**: 13–18.

15. Creaven PJ. The clinical pharmacology of VM26 and VP16–213. *Cancer Chemother Pharmacol* 1982; **7**: 133–40.

16. Hendel J, Brodthagen H. Entero-hepatic cycling of methotrexate estimated by use of the D-isomer as a reference marker. *Eur J Clin Pharmacol* 1984; **26**: 103–7.

♦17. Sladek N. Metabolism of oxazaphosphorines. *Pharmacol Ther* 1988; **37**: 301–55.

♦18. Nebert DW. Suggestions for the nomenclature of human alleles: relevance to ecogenetics, pharmacogenetics and molecular epidemiology. *Pharmacogenetics* 2000; **10**: 279–90.

19. Ingelman-Sundberg M, Oscarson M, Daly AK *et al*. Human cytochrome P-450 (CYP) genes: A web page for the nomenclature of alleles. *Cancer Epidemiol Biomarker Prev* 2001; **10**: 1307–8.

●20. Jodrell DI, Egorin MJ, Canetta RM *et al*. Relationships between carboplatin exposure and tumor response and toxicity in patients with ovarian cancer. *J Clin Oncol* 1992; **10**: 520–8.

●21. Joel SP, Ellis P, O'Byrne K *et al*. Therapeutic monitoring of continuous infusion etoposide in small-cell lung cancer. *J Clin Oncol* 1996; **14**: 1903–12.

22. Avramis VI, Weingberg KI, Sato JK *et al*. Pharmacology studies of 1-beta-D-arabinofuranosylcytosine in pediatric patients with leukemia and lymphoma after a biochemically optimal regimen of loading bolus plus continuous infusion of the drug. *Cancer Res* 1989; **49**: 241–7.

23. Karlsson MO, Molnar V, Bergh J *et al*. A general model for time-dissociated pharmacokinetic-pharmacodynamic relationships exemplified by paclitaxel myelosuppression. *Clin Pharmacol Ther* 1998; **63**: 11–25.

24. Newell DR, Pearson ADJ, Balmanno K *et al*. Carboplatin pharmacokinetics in children: the development of a pediatric dosing formula. *J Clin Oncol* 1993; **11**: 2314–23.

25. Dowlati A, Haaga J, Remick SC *et al*. Sequential tumor biopsies in early phase clinical trials of anticancer agents for pharmacodynamic evaluation. *Clin Cancer Res* 2001; **7**: 2971–6.

26. Jacobs SA, Stoller RG, Chabner BA, Johns DG. 7-hydroxymethotrexate as a urinary metabolite in human subjects and rhesus monkeys receiving high dose methotrexate. *J Clin Invest* 1976; **57**: 534–8.

27. Jolivet J, Cowan KH, Curt GA *et al*. The pharmacology and clinical use of methotrexate. *N Engl J Med* 1983; **309**: 1094–104.

28. Evans W, Crom W, Abromowitch M *et al*. Clinical pharmacodynamics of high-dose methotrexate in acute lymphocytic leukemia. Identification of a relation between concentration and effect. *N Engl J Med* 1986; **314**: 471–7.

●29. Evans WE, Relling MV, Rodman JH *et al*. Conventional compared with individualised chemotherapy for childhood acute lymphoblastic leukemia. *N Engl J Med* 1998; **338**: 499–505.

30. Wolfrom C, Hepp R, Hartmann R *et al*. Pharmacokinetic study of methotrexate, folinic acid and their serum metabolites in children treated with high-dose methotrexate and leucovorin rescue. *Eur J Clin Pharmacol* 1990; **39**: 377–83.

31. Relling MV, Fairclough D, Ayers D *et al*. Patient characteristics associated with high-risk methotrexate concentrations and toxicity. *J Clin Oncol* 1994; **12**: 1667–72.

32. Mohty M, Peyriere H, Guinet C *et al*. Carboxypeptidase G2 rescue in delayed methotrexate elimination in renal failure. *Leuk Lymphoma* 2000; **37**: 441–3.

33. Widemann BC, Sung E, Anderson L *et al*. Pharmacokinetics and metabolism of the methotrexate metabolite 2,4-diamino-N-10-methylpteroic acid. *J Pharmacol Exp Ther* 2000; **294**: 894–901.

34. Panetta JC, Wall A, Pui CH *et al*. Methotrexate intracellular disposition in acute lymphoblastic leukemia: A mathematical model of gamma-glutamyl hydrolase activity. *Clin Cancer Res* 2002; **8**: 2423–9.

35. van der Laan F, Jansen G, Kathmann I *et al*. Mechanisms of acquired resistance to methotrexate in a human squamous carcinoma cell line of the head and neck, exposed to different treatment schedules. *Eur J Cancer* 1991; **27**: 1274–8.

36. Rots MG, Willey JC, Jansen G *et al*. mRNA expression levels of methotrexate resistance-related proteins in childhood leukemia as determined by a standardized competitive template-based RT-PCR method. *Leukemia* 2000; **14**: 2166–75.

♦37. Noble S, Goa KL. Gemcitabine – a review of its pharmacology and clinical potential in non-small cell lung cancer and pancreatic cancer. *Drugs* 1997; **54**: 447–72.

♦38. Pinedo HM, Peters GJ. Fluorouracil: biochemistry and pharmacology. *J Clin Oncol* 1988; **6**: 1653–64.

39. Fleming RA, Milano G, Thyss A *et al*. Correlation between dihydropyrimidine dehydrogenase-activity in peripheral mononuclear-cells and systemic clearance of fluorouracil in cancer-patients. *Cancer Res* 1992; **52**: 2899–902.

40. Diasio RB, Harris BE, Song R. Diurnal-variation of human dihydropyrimidine dehydrogenase (dpd) activity – potential effect on plasma 5-fluorouracil (fu) levels and resultant toxicity in patients treated with protracted infusions of fu. *Clin Pharmacol Ther* 1989; **45**: 135.

41. Baccanari D, Davis S, Knick V, Spector T. 5-ethynyluracil (776c85) – a potent modulator of the pharmacokinetics and antitumor efficacy of 5-fluorouracil. *Proc Natl Acad Sci USA* 1993; **90**: 11064–8.

42. Kohl U, Schwabe D, Montag E *et al*. Formation of cytosine arabinoside-5'-triphosphate in different cultured lymphoblastic leukaemic cells with reference to their drug sensitivity. *Eur J Cancer* 1995; **31a**: 209–14.

43. Ho DHW, Frei E. Clinical pharmacology of 1-B-D-arabinofuranosyl cytosine. *Clin Pharmacol Ther* 1971; **12**: 944–54.

44. Harris AL, Potter C, Bunch C *et al*. Pharmacokinetics of cytosine arabinoside in patients with acute myeloid leukaemia. *Br J Clin Pharmacol* 1979; **8**: 219–27.

45. Avramis VI, Biener R, Krailo M et al. Biochemical pharmacology of high dose 1-b-D-arabinofuranosylcytosine in childhood acute leukaemia. Cancer Res 1987; 47: 6786–92.

46. Plunkett W, Liliemark JO, Adams TM, Nowak B, Estey E, Kantarjan H et al. Saturation of 1-β-D-arabinofuranosylcytosine 5′-triphosphate accumulation in leukaemia cells during high-dose 1-β-D-arabino-furanosylcytosine therapy. Cancer Res 1987; 47: 3005–11.

47. Yamauchi T, Ueda T, Nakamura T. A new and sensitive method for determination of intracellular 1-β-D-arabinofuranosylcytosine 5′-triphosphate content in human materials in vivo. Cancer Res 1996; 56: 1800–4.

48. Rowland K, Lennard L, Lilleyman JS. In vitro metabolism of 6-mercaptopurine by human liver cytosol. Xenobiotica 1999; 29: 615–28.

♦49. Lennard L. The clinical pharmacology of 6-mercaptopurine. Eur J Clin Pharmacol 1992; 43: 329–39.

♦50. Krynetski EY, Evans WE. Genetic polymorphism of thiopurine S-methyltransferase: Molecular mechanisms and clinical importance. Pharmacology 2000; 61: 136–46.

51. Lennard L. Clinical implications of thiopurine methyltransferase – optimization of drug dosage and potential drug interactions. Ther Drug Monit 1998; 20: 527–31.

52. Relling MV, Hancock ML, Boyett JM et al. Prognostic importance of 6-mercaptopurine dose intensity in acute lymphoblastic leukemia. Blood 1999; 93: 2817–23.

53. Dervieux T, Blanco JG, Krynetski EY et al. Differing contribution of thiopurine methyltransferase to mercaptopurine versus thioguanine effects in human leukemic cells. Cancer Res 2001; 61: 5810–16.

54. O'Connor PM, Jackman J, Bae I et al. Characterization of the p53 tumor suppressor pathway in cell lines of the National Cancer Institute anticancer drug screen and correlations with the growth-inhibitory potency of 123 anticancer agents. Cancer Res 1997; 57: 4285–300.

♦55. Stupp R, Gander M, Leyvraz S, Newlands ES. Current and future developments in the use of temozolomide for the treatment of brain tumours. Lancet Oncol 2001; 2: 552–60.

56. Newlands ES, Stevens MFG, Wedge SR et al. Temozolomide: a review of its discovery, chemical properties and clinical trials. Cancer Treat Rev 1997; 23: 35–61.

57. Liu LL, Markowitz S, Gerson SL. Mismatch repair mutations override alkyltransferase in conferring resistance to temozolomide but not to 1,3-bis(2-chloroethyl)nitrosourea. Cancer Res 1996; 56: 5375–9.

58. Bobola MS, Tseng SH, Blank A et al. Role of O-6-methylguanine-DNA methyltransferase in resistance of human brain-tumor cell-lines to the clinically relevant methylating agents temozolomide and streptozotocin. Clin Cancer Res 1996; 2: 735–41.

59. Middlemas DS, Stewart CF, Kirstein MN et al. Biochemical correlates of temozolomide sensitivity in pediatric solid tumor xenograft models. Clin Cancer Res 2000; 6: 998–1007.

♦60. Pegg AE. Repair of O-6-alkylguanine by alkyltransferases. Mutat Res 2000; 462: 83–100.

61. Kokkinakis DM, Bocangel DB, Schold SC et al. Thresholds of O-6-alkylguanine-DNA alkyltransferase which confer significant resistance of human glial tumor xenografts to treatment with 1,3-bis(2-chloroethyl)-1-nitrosourea or temozolomide. Clin Cancer Res 2001; 7: 421–8.

62. Esteller M, Garcia-Foncillas J, Andion E et al. Inactivation of the DNA-repair gene MGMT and the clinical response of gliomas to alkylating agents. N Engl J Med 2000; 343: 1350–4.

63. Cai YN, Wu MH, Xu-Welliver M et al. Effect of O-6-benzylguanine on alkylating agent-induced toxicity and mutagenicity in Chinese hamster ovary cells expressing wild-type and mutant O-6-alkylguanine-DNA alkyltransferases. Cancer Res 2000; 60: 5464–9.

64. Friedman HS, Kerby T, Calvert H. Temozolomide and treatment of malignant glioma. Clin Cancer Res 2000; 6: 2585–97.

65. Middleton MR, Grob JJ, Aaronson N et al. Randomized phase III study of temozolomide versus dacarbazine in the treatment of patients with advanced metastatic malignant melanoma. J Clin Oncol 2000; 18: 158–66.

66. Nicholson HS, Krailo M, Ames MM et al. Phase I study of temozolomide in children and adolescents with recurrent solid tumors: a report from the children's cancer group. J Clin Oncol 1998; 16: 3037–43.

67. Reed DJ. 2-chloroethylnitrosoureas. In: Powis G, Prough RA, eds. Metabolism and Actions of Anti-cancer Drugs. London: Taylor and Francis; 1987.

♦68. Lemoine A, Lucas C, Ings RMJ. Metabolism of chloroethylnitrosoureas. Xenobiotica 1991; 21: 775–91.

69. Smith MT, Evans CG, Doane-Setzer P et al. Denitrosation of 1,3-bis(2-chloroethyl)-1-nitrosourea by class mu glutathione transferases. Cancer Res 1989; 49: 2621–5.

70. DeVita VT, Denham C, Davidson JD, Oliverio VT. The physiological disposition of the carcinostatic 1,3 bis(2-chloroethyl)-1-nitrosourea(BCNU) in man and animals. Clin Pharmacol Ther 1967; 8: 566–77.

71. Lee FYF, Workman P, Roberts JJ, Bleehen NM. Clinical pharmacokinetics of oral CCNU (lomustine). Cancer Chemother Pharmacol 1985; 14: 125–31.

72. Levin VA, Hoffman W, Weinkam RJ. Pharmacokinetics of BCNU in man: preliminary study of 20 patients. Cancer Treat Rep 1978; 62: 1305–12.

73. Tranchand B, Lucas C, Biron P et al. Phase I pharmaco-kinetics study of high-dose fotemustine and its metabolite 2-chloroethanol in patients with high-grade gliomas. Cancer Chemother Pharmacol 1993; 32: 46–52.

74. Sponzo RW, DeVita VT, Oliverio VT. Physiologic disposition of 1-(2-chloroethyl)-3-cyclohexyl-1-nitrosourea (CCNU) and 1-(2-chloroethyl(-3-(4-methyl cyclohexyl)-1-nitrosourea)) (MeCCNU) in man. Cancer 1973; 31: 1154–9.

75. Ings RMJ, Gray AJ, Taylor AR et al. Disposition, pharmacokinetics and metabolism of ^{14}C-fotemustine in cancer patients. Eur J Cancer 1990; 26: 838–42.

76. Tsang LLH, Quarterman CP, Gescher A, Slack JA. Comparison of the cytotoxicity in vitro of temozolomide and dacarbazine, prodrugs of 3-methyl-(triazen-1yl)imidazole-4-carboxamide. Cancer Chemother Pharmacol 1991; 27: 342–6.

77. Tweedie DJ, Fernandez D, Spearman ME et al. Metabolism of azoxy derivatives of procarbazine by aldehyde dehydrogenase and xanthine oxidase. Drug Metab Dispos 1991; 19: 793–803.

78. Cohen NA, Egorin MJ, Snyder SW et al. Interaction of N, N′, N′-triethylenethiophosphoramide and N, N′, N′-triethylenephosphoramide with cellular DNA. Cancer Res 1991; 51: 4360–6.

79. Dirven HAAM, Dictus ELJT, Broeders NLHL *et al.* The role of human glutathione S-transferase isoenzymes in the formation of glutathione conjugates of the alkylating cytostatic drug thiotepa. *Cancer Res* 1995; **55**: 1701–6.

80. Hara J, Osugi Y, Ohta H *et al.* Double-conditioning regimens consisting of thiotepa, melphalan and busulfan with stem cell rescue for the treatment of pediatric solid tumors. *Bone Marrow Transplant* 1998; **22**: 7–12.

81. Henner WD, Shea TC, Furlong EA *et al.* Pharmacokinetics of continuous-infusion high-dose thiotepa. *Cancer Treat Rep* 1987; **71**: 1043–7.

82. Heideman RL, Cole DE, Balis F *et al.* Phase I and pharmacokinetic evaluation of thiotepa in the cerebrospinal fluid and plasma of pediatric patients: evidence for dose-dependent plasma clearance of thiotepa. *Cancer Res* 1989; **49**: 736–41.

83. Cohen BE, Egorin MJ, Kohlhepp EA *et al.* Human plasma pharmacokinetics and urinary excretion of thiotepa and its metabolites. *Cancer Treat Rep* 1986; **70**: 859–64.

84. Hagen B, Neverdal G, Walstad RA, Nilsen OG. Long-term pharmacokinetics of thio-TEPA, TEPA and total alkylating activity following i. v. bolus administration of thio-TEPA in ovarian cancer patients. *Cancer Chemother Pharmacol* 1990; **25**: 257–62.

85. O'Dwyer PJ, LaCreta F, Engstrom PF *et al.* Phase I/Pharmacokinetic re-evaluation of ThioTEPA. *Cancer Res* 1991; **51**: 3171–6.

86. Alaoui-Jamali MA, Panasci L, Centurioni GM *et al.* Nitrogen mustard-DNA interaction in melphalan-resistant mammary carcinoma cells with elevated intracellular glutathione and glutathione-S-transferase activity. *Cancer Chemother Pharmacol* 1992; **30**: 341–7.

87. O'Dwyer PJ, Hamilton TC, Lacreta FP *et al.* Phase-I trial of buthionine sulfoximine in combination with melphalan in patients with cancer. *J Clin Oncol* 1996; **14**: 249–56.

88. Moreau P, Kergueris M-F, Milpied N *et al.* A pilot study of 220 mg/m^2 melphalan followed by autologous stem cell transplantation in patients with advanced haematological malignancies: pharmacokinetics and toxicity. *Br J Haematol* 1996; **95**: 527–30.

89. Choi KE, Ratain MJ, Williams SF *et al.* Plasma pharmacokinetics of high dose oral melphalan in patients treated with trialkylator chemotherapy and autologous bone marrow reinfusion. *Cancer Res* 1989; **49**: 1318–21.

90. Taha IA-K, Ahmad RA, Rogers DW *et al.* Pharmacokinetics of melphalan in children following high-dose intravenous injection. *Cancer Chemother Pharmacol* 1983; **10**: 212–16.

91. Bosanquet AG, Gilby ED. Pharmacokinetics of oral and intravenous melphalan during routine treatment of multiple myeloma. *Eur J Cancer Clin Oncol* 1982; **18**: 355–62.

92. Zucchetti M, D'Incalci M, Willems Y *et al.* Lack of effect of cisplatin on i.v. L-PAM plasma pharmacokinetics in ovarian cancer patients. *Cancer Chemother Pharmacol* 1988; **22**: 87–9.

93. Alberts DS, Chang SY, Chen H-SG *et al.* Kinetics of intravenous melphalan. *Clin Pharmacol Ther* 1979; **26**: 73–80.

94. Reece PA, Hill HS, Green RM *et al.* Renal clearance and protein binding of melphalan in patients with cancer. *Cancer Chemother Pharmacol* 1988; **22**: 348–52.

95. Adair C, Bridges J, Desai Z. Renal function in the elimination of oral melphalan in patients with multiple myeloma. *Cancer Chemother Pharmacol* 1986; **17**: 185–8.

96. Kergueris M, Milpied N, Moreau P *et al.* Pharmacokinetics of high-dose melphalan in adults: influence of renal function. *Anticancer Res* 1994; **14**: 2379–82.

97. Alberts DS, Chang SY, Chen H-SG *et al.* Oral melphalan kinetics. *Clin Pharmacol Ther* 1979; **26**: 737–45.

98. Osterborg A, Ehrsson H, Eksborg S *et al.* Pharmacokinetics of oral melphalan in relation to renal function in multiple myeloma patients. *Eur J Cancer Clin Oncol* 1989; **25**: 899–903.

99. Tricot G, Alberts DS, Johnson C *et al.* Safety of autotransplants with high-dose melphalan in renal failure. A pharmacokinetic and toxicity study. *Clin Cancer Res* 1996; **2**: 947–52.

100. Hassan M, Oberg G, Bekassy AN *et al.* Pharmacokinetics of high dose busulphan in relation to age and chronopharmacology. *Cancer Chemother Pharmacol* 1991; **28**: 130–4.

101. Vassal G, Fischer A, Challine D *et al.* Busulfan disposition below the age of three: Alteration in children with lysosomal storage disease. *Blood* 1993; **82**: 1030–4.

102. Grochow LB. Busulphan disposition: the role of therapeutic drug monitoring in bone marrow transplantation induction regimens. *Semin Oncol* 1993; **20**(Suppl 4): 18–25.

● 103. Slattery JT, Sanders JE, Buckner CD *et al.* Graft rejection and toxicity following bone marrow transplantation in relation to busulfan pharmacokinetics. *Bone Marrow Transplant* 1995; **16**: 31–42.

104. Shaw P, Scharping C, Brian R, Earl J. Busulfan pharmacokinetics using a single daily high-dose regimen in children with acute leukemia. *Blood* 1994; **84**: 2357–62.

105. Vassal G, Gouyette A, Hartmann O *et al.* Pharmacokinetics of high-dose busulfan in children. *Cancer Chemother Pharmacol* 1989; **24**: 386–90.

106. Hassan M, Oberg G, Bjorkholm M *et al.* Influence of prophylactic anticonvulsant therapy on high-dose busulphan kinetics. *Cancer Chemother Pharmacol* 1993; **33**: 181–6.

107. Pawlowska AB, Blazar BR, Angelucci E *et al.* Relationship of plasma pharmacokinetics of high-dose oral busulfan to the outcome of allogeneic bone marrow transplantation in children with thalassemia. *Bone Marrow Transplant* 1997; **20**: 915–20.

108. Grochow LB, Krivit W, Whitley CB, Blazar B. Busulfan disposition in children. *Blood* 1990; **75**: 1723–7.

♦ 109. Vassal G, Deroussent A, Hartmann O *et al.* Dose-dependent neurotoxicity of high-dose busulfan in children: a clinical and pharmacological study. *Cancer Res* 1990; **50**: 6203–7.

110. Morabito F, Filangeri M, Callea I *et al.* Bcl-2 protein expression and p53 gene mutation in chronic lymphocytic leukemia: correlation with in vitro sensitivity to chlorambucil and purine analogs. *Haematologica* 1997; **82**: 16–20.

111. Barnouin K, Leier I, Jedlitschky G *et al.* Multidrug resistance protein-mediated transport of chlorambucil and melphalan conjugated to glutathione. *Br J Cancer* 1998; **77**: 201–9.

112. Yang WZ, Begleiter A, Johnston JB *et al.* Role of glutathione and glutathione-S-transferase in chlorambucil resistance. *Mol Pharmacol* 1992; **41**: 625–30.

113. Newell DR, Calvert AH, Harrap KR, McElwain TJ. Studies on the pharmacokinetics of chlorambucil and prednimustine in man. *Br J Clin Pharmacol* 1983; **15**: 253–8.

114. Hartvig P, Simonsson B, Oberg G *et al*. Inter- and intraindividual differences in oral chlorambucil pharmacokinetics. *Eur J Clin Pharmacol* 1988; **35**: 551–4.

115. Godeneche D, Madelmont JC, Moreau MF *et al*. Comparative physico-chemical properties, biological effects, and disposition in mice of four nitrogen mustards. *Cancer Chemother Pharmacol* 1980; **5**: 1–9.

116. Lee FYF, Coe P, Workman P. Pharmacokinetic basis for the comparative antitumour activity and toxicity of chlorambucil, phyenylacetic acid mustard and β,β-difluorochlorambucil (CB7103) in mice. *Cancer Chemother Pharmacol* 1986; **17**: 21–9.

117. Dirven HAAM, van Ommen B, van Bladeren PJ. Involvement of human glutathione-S-transferase isoenzymes in the conjugation of cyclophosphamide metabolites with glutathione. *Cancer Res* 1994; **54**: 6215–20.

118. Dockham PA, Lee M-O, Sladek NE. Identification of human liver aldehyde dehydrogenases that catalyze the oxidation of aldophosphamide and retinaldehyde. *Biochem Pharmacol* 1992; **43**: 2453–69.

119. Sreerama L, Sladek NE. Identification of the class-3 aldehyde dehydrogenases present in human MCF-7/0 breast adenocarcinoma cells and normal human breast tissue. *Biochem Pharmacol* 1994; **48**: 617–20.

120. Savarese DMF, Hsieh C, Stewart MF. Clinical impact of chemotherapy dose escalation in patients with hematologic malignancies and solid tumors. *J Clin Oncol* 1997; **15**: 2981–95.

121. Moore MJ. Clinical pharmacokinetics of cyclophosphamide. *Clin Pharmacokinet* 1991; **20**: 194–208.

♦122. Kaijser GP, Beijnen JH, Bult A, Underberg WJM. Ifosfamide metabolism and pharmacokinetics (review). *Anticancer Res* 1994; **14**: 517–32.

♦123. Boddy AV, Yule SM. Metabolism and pharmacokinetics of oxazaphosphorines. *Clin Pharmacokinet* 2000; **38**: 291–304.

♦124. Lind MJ, McGown AT, Hadfield JA *et al*. The effect of ifosfamide and its metabolites on intracellular glutathione levels in vitro and in vivo. *Biochem Pharmacol* 1989; **38**: 1835–40.

125. Struck RF, Alberts DS, Horne K *et al*. Plasma pharmacokinetics of cyclophosphamide and its cytotoxic metabolites after intravenous versus oral administration in a randomized, crossover trial. *Cancer Res* 1987; **47**: 2723–6.

126. Cerny T, Küpfer A. The enigma of ifosfamide encephalopathy. *Ann Oncol* 1992; **3**: 679–81.

127. Yule SM, Price L, Pearson ADJ, Boddy AV. Cyclophosphamide and ifosfamide metabolites in the cerebrospinal fluid of children. *Clin Cancer Res* 1997; **3**: 1985–92.

128. Goren MP, Wright RK, Pratt CB, Pell FE. Dechloroethylation of ifosfamide and neurotoxicity. *Lancet* 1986; **ii**: 1219–20.

129. Yule SM, Walker D, Pearson ADJ. Potential inhibition of alkylating agent metabolism by fluconazole. *Eur J Clin Microbiol Infect Dis* 1994; **13**: 1086–7.

130. Yule SM, Boddy AV, Cole M *et al*. Cyclophosphamide metabolism in children. *Cancer Res* 1995; **55**: 803–9.

131. Rae JM, Desta Z, Soukhova NV, Flockhart DA. Thiotepa is a specific inhibitor of cytochrome P4502B6: implications for cyclophosphamide metabolism. *Drug Metab Dispos* 2002; **30**: 525–30

132. Ayash LJ, Wright JE, Tretyakov O *et al*. Cyclophosphamide pharmacokinetics: Correlation with cardiac toxicity and tumor response. *J Clin Oncol* 1992; **10**: 995–1000.

●133. Connors TA, Cleare MJ, Harrap KR. Structure activity relationships of the antitumor platinum coordination complexes. *Cancer Treat Rep* 1979; **63**: 1499–502.

134. Drobnik J. Antitumor activity of platinum complexes. *Cancer Chemother Pharmacol* 1983; **10**: 145–9.

135. Go RS, Adjei AA. Review of the comparative pharmacology and clinical activity of cisplatin and carboplatin. *J Clin Oncol* 1999; **17**: 409–22.

♦136. Doz F, Pinkerton R. What is the place of carboplatin in paediatric oncology? *Eur J Cancer* 1994; **30A**: 194–201.

137. Grigg A, Szer J, Skov K, Barnett M. Multi-organ dysfunction associated with high-dose carboplatin therapy prior to autologous transplantation. *Bone Marrow Transplant* 1996; **17**: 67–74.

138. Reece PA, Staffod I, Abbott RL *et al*. Two- versus 24-hour infusion of cisplatin: pharmacokinetic considerations. *J Clin Oncol* 1989; **7**: 270–5.

139. Reece PA, Stafford I, Davy M *et al*. Influence of infusion time on unchanged cisplatin disposition in patients with ovarian cancer. *Cancer Chemother Pharmacol* 1989; **24**: 256–60.

140. Peng B, English MW, Boddy AV *et al*. Cisplatin pharmacokinetics in children with cancer. *Eur J Cancer* 1997; **33**: 1823–8.

141. Dominici C, Petrucci F, Caroli S *et al*. A pharmacokinetic study of high-dose continous infusion cisplatin in children with solid tumors. *J Clin Oncol* 1989; **7**: 100–7.

142. Egorin M, Van Echo D, Olman E *et al*. Prospective validation of a pharmacokinetically based dosing scheme for the cis-diamminedichloroplatinum(II) analogue diamminecyclobutanedicarboxylatoplatinum. *Cancer Res* 1985; **45**: 6502–6.

143. Thomas HD, Boddy AV, English MW *et al*. Prospective validation of renal function-based carboplatin dosing in children with cancer: a United Kingdom Children's Cancer Study Group trial. *J Clin Oncol* 2000; **18**: 3614–21.

●144. Veal GJ, Foot A, McDowell H *et al*. Optimization of high dose carboplatin treatment in children with stage IV soft tissue sarcoma (SIP/UKCCSG MMT98 study) by real-time pharmacokinetic monitoring. (Abs 1364) San Francisco, CA: American Association for Cancer Research, 2002; 275.

145. Kartalou M, Essigmann JM. Mechanisms of resistance to cisplatin. *Mutat Res* 2001; **478**: 23–43.

146. Zhang K, Chew M, Yang EB *et al*. Modulation of cisplatin cytotoxicity and cisplatin-induced DNA cross-links in HepG2 cells by regulation of glutathione-related mechanisms. *Mol Pharmacol* 2001; **59**: 837–43.

147. Hinoshita E, Uchiumi T, Taguchi K *et al*. Increased expression of an ATP-binding cassette superfamily transporter, multidrug resistance protein 2, in human colorectal carcinomas. *Clin Cancer Res* 2000; **6**: 2401–7.

148. Ferry KV, Hamilton TC, Johnson SW. Increased nucleotide excision repair in cisplatin-resistant ovarian cancer cells – role of ERCC1-XPF. *Biochem Pharmacol* 2000; **60**: 1305–13.

149. Stoehlmacher J, Ghaderi V, Iqbal S *et al*. A polymorphism of the XRCC1 gene predicts for response to platinum based

treatment in advanced colorectal cancer. *Anticancer Res* 2001; **21**: 3075–9.

150. Plumb JA, Strathdee G, Sludden J *et al.* Reversal of drug resistance in human tumor xenografts by 2′-deoxy-5-azacytidine-induced demethylation of the hMLH1 gene promoter. *Cancer Res* 2000; **60**: 6039–44.

151. Pepponi R, Graziani G, Falcinelli S *et al.* hMSH3 overexpression and cellular response to cytotoxic anticancer agents. *Carcinogenesis* 2001; **22**: 1131–7.

152. Shiga H, Heath EI, Rasmussen AA *et al.* Prognostic value of p53, glutathione S-transferase pi, and thymidylate synthase for neoadjuvant cisplatin-based chemotherapy in head and neck cancer. *Clin Cancer Res* 1999; **5**: 4097–104.

153. Lin XJ, Ramamurthi K, Mishima M *et al.* P53 modulates the effect of loss of DNA mismatch repair on the sensitivity of human colon cancer cells to the cytotoxic and mutagenic effects of cisplatin. *Cancer Res* 2001; **61**: 1508–16.

154. Desai ZR, van den Berg HW, Bridges JM, Shanks RG. Can severe vincristine neurotoxicity be prevented? *Cancer Chemother Pharmacol* 1982; **8**: 211–14.

155. Zhou X-J, Zhou-Pan X-R, Gauthier T *et al.* Human liver microsomal cytochrome P450 3A isozymes mediated vindesine biotransformation. *Biochem Pharmacol* 1993; **45**: 853–61.

156. de Graaf SSN, Bloemhof H, Vendrig DEMM, Uges DRA. Vincristine disposition in children with acute lymphoblastic leukemia. *Med Pediatr Oncol* 1995; **24**: 235–40.

157. van Tellingen O, Sips JHM, Beijnen JH *et al.* Pharmacology, bio-analysis, and pharmacokinetics of the vinca alkaloids and semi-synthetic derivatives. *Anticancer Res* 1992; **12**: 1699–716.

158. Bradshaw DM, Arceci RJ. Clinical relevance of transmembrane drug efflux as a mechanism of multidrug resistance. *J Clin Oncol* 1998; **16**: 3674–90.

♦159. Hurwitz CA, Strauss LC, Kepner J *et al.* Paclitaxel for the treatment of progressive or recurrent childhood brain tumors: a pediatric oncology phase II study. *J Pediatr Hematol Oncol* 2001; **23**: 277–81.

160. Doz F, Gentet JC, Pein F *et al.* Phase I trial and pharmacological study of a 3-hour paclitaxel infusion in children with refractory solid tumours: a SFOP study. *Br J Cancer* 2001; **84**: 604–10.

161. Clark P, Slevin M. The clinical pharmacology of etoposide and teniposide. *Clin Pharmacokinet* 1987; **12**: 223–52.

♦162. Davidson A, Gowing R, Lowis S *et al.* Phase II study of 21 day schedule oral etoposide in children. *Eur J Cancer* 1997; **33**: 1816–22.

163. Harvey VJ, Slevin ML, Joel SP *et al.* Variable bioavailability following repeated oral doses of etoposide. *Eur J Cancer Clin Oncol* 1985; **21**: 1315–19.

164. Millward MJ, Newell DR, Mummaneni V *et al.* Phase I and pharmacokinetic study of a water-soluble etoposide prodrug, etoposide phosphate (BMY-40481). *Eur J Cancer* 1995; **31A**: 2409–11.

165. Bisogno G, Cowie F, Boddy A *et al.* High-dose cyclosporin with etoposide – toxicity and pharmacokinetic interaction in children with solid tumours. *Br J Cancer* 1998; **77**: 2304–9.

166. Brown GA, McPhaerson JP, Gu L *et al.* Relationship of DNA topoisomerase IIa and b expression to cytotoxicity of antineoplastic agents in human acute lymphoblastic leukemia cell lines. *Cancer Res* 1995; **55**: 78–82.

167. Drlica K, Franco RJ. Inhibitors of DNA topoisomerases. *Biochemistry* 1988; **27**: 2253–8.

♦168. Peters JH, Gordon GR, Kashiwase D *et al.* Redox activities of antitumor anthracyclines determined by microsomal oxygen consumption and assays for superoxide anion and hydroxyl radical generation. *Biochem Pharmacol* 1986; **35**: 1309–23.

169. Lipshultz SE, Colan SD, Gelber RD *et al.* Late cardiac effects of doxorubicin therapy for acute lymphoblastic leukemia in childhood. *N Engl J Med* 1991; **324**: 808–15.

170. Mross K, Maessen P, Vandervijgh W *et al.* Pharmacokinetics and metabolism of epidoxorubicin and doxorubicin in humans. *J Clin Oncol* 1988; **6**: 517–26.

171. Kokenberg E, Sonneveld P, Sizoo W *et al.* Cellular pharmacokinetics of daunorubicin: relationships with the response to treatment in patients with acute myeloid leukemia. *J Clin Oncol* 1988; **6**: 802–12.

172. Cammaggi CM, Carisi P, Strocchi E, Pannuti F. High-performance liquid chromatographic analysis of idarubicin and fluorescent metabolites in biological fluids. *Cancer Chemother Pharmacol* 1992; **30**: 303–6.

173. Tidefelt U, Prenkert M, Paul C. Comparison of idarubicin and daunorubicin and their main metabolites regarding intracellular uptake and effect on sensitive and multidrug-resistant HL60 cells. *Cancer Chemother Pharmacol* 1996; **38**: 476–80.

174. Aas T, Borresen A-L, Geisler S *et al.* Specific p53 mutations are associated with de novo resistance to doxorubicin in breast cancer patients. *Nat Med* 1996; **2**: 811–14.

●175. Bellott R, Auvrignon A, Leblanc T *et al.* Pharmacokinetics of liposomal daunorubicin [DaunoXome] during a phase I-II study in children with relapsed acute lymphoblastic leukaemia. *Cancer Chemother Pharmacol* 2001; **47**: 15–21.

176. Marina NM, Cochrane D, Harney E *et al.* Dose escalation and pharmacokinetics of pegylated liposomal doxorubicin (Doxil) in children with solid tumors: a pediatric oncology group study. *Clin Cancer Res* 2002; **8**: 413–18.

177. Pratt CB, Stewart C, Santana VM *et al.* Phase I study of topotecan for pediatric patients with solid tumours. *J Clin Oncol* 1994; **12**: 539–43.

178. Blaney S, Berg SL, Pratt C *et al.* A Phase I study of irinotecan in pediatric patients: A Pediatric Oncology Group study. *Clin Cancer Res* 2001; **7**: 32–7.

179. Costin D, Potmesil M. Preclinical and clinical development of camptothecins. *Adv Pharmacol* 1994; **29B**: 51–72.

♦180. Herben VMM, ten Bokkel Huinink WW, Beijnen JH. Clinical pharmacokinetics of topotecan. *Clin Pharmacokinet* 1996; **31**: 85–102.

♦181. Rivory LP, Chatelut E, Canal P *et al.* Kinetics of the in vivo interconversion of the carboxylate and lactone forms of irinotecan (CPT-11) and of its metabolite SN-38 in patients. *Cancer Res* 1994; **54**: 6330–3.

182. Athale UH, Stewart C, Kuttesch JF *et al.* Phase I study of topotecan and carboplatin in pediatric solid tumors. *J Clin Oncol* 2002; **20**: 88–95.

183. Slichenmyer WJ, Rowinsky EK, Donehower RC, Kaufmann SH. The current status of camptothecin analogues as antitumor agents. *J Natl Cancer Inst* 1993; **85**: 271–91.

184. Reiter A, Schrappe M, Ludwig W-D et al. Chemotherapy in 998 unselected childhood acute lymphoblastic leukaemia patients. Results and conclusions of the multi-centre trial ALL-BFM 86. Blood 1994; 84: 3122–33.

185. Arya SK, Wong-Staal F, Gallo RC. Dexamethasone-mediated inhibition of human T-cell growth factor and gamma-interferon messenger RNA. J Immunol 1984; 133: 273–6.

186. Thulasi R, Harbour DV, Thompson EB. Suppression of c-myc is a critical step in glucocorticoid-induced human leukemic cell lysis. J Biol Chem 1993; 268: 18 306–12.

187. Jonat C, Rahmsdorf HJ, Park K-K et al. Antitumor promotion and anti-inflammation: down-modulation of AP-1(Fos/Jun) activity by glucocorticoid hormone. Cell 1990; 62: 1189–204.

188. Ito C, Evans WE, McNinch L et al. Comparative cytotoxicity of dexamethasone and prednisolone in childhood acute lymphoblastic leukemia. J Clin Oncol 1996; 14: 2370–6.

189. Quddus FF, Levenathal BG, Boyett JM et al. Glucocorticoid receptors in immunological subtypes of childhood acute lymphocytic leukemia cells: a pediatric oncology group study. Cancer Res 1985; 45: 6482–6.

190. Green OC, Winter JJ, Kawahara FS et al. Plasma levels, half-life values and correlation with physiologic assays for growth and immunity. J Pediatr 1978; 93: 299–303.

191. Choonara I, Wheeldon J, Rayner P et al. Pharmacokinetics of prednisolone in children with acute lymphoblastic leukemia. Cancer Chemother Pharmacol 1989; 23: 392–4.

192. Hill MR, Szefler SJ, Ball BD et al. Monitoring glucocorticoid therapy: a pharmacokinetic approach. Clin Pharmacol Ther 1990; 48: 390–8.

193. Bannwarth B, Schaeverbeke T, Pehourcq F et al. Prednisolone concentrations in cerebrospinal fluid after oral prednisone. Preliminary data. Rev Rhumat 1997; 64: 301–4.

194. Richter O, Ern B, Reinhardt D, Becker B. Pharmacokinetics of dexamethasone in children. Pediatr Pharmacol 1983; 3: 329–37.

195. Kaspers GJ, Pieters R, Van Zantwijk ER et al. Prednisolone resistance in childhood acute lymphoblastic leukemia: in vitro-in vivo correlations and cross-resistance to other drugs. Blood 1998; 92: 259–66.

196. Pieters R, den Boer ML, Durian M et al. Relation between age, immunophenotype and in vitro drug resistance in 396 children with acute lymphoblastic leukemia – implications for treatment of infants. Leukemia 1998; 12: 1344–8.

197. Gaynon PS, Lustig RH. The use of glucocorticoids in acute lymphoblastic-leukemia of childhood – molecular, cellular, and clinical considerations. J Pediatr Hematol Oncol 1995; 17: 1–12.

198. Brothman AR, Davis TP, Duffy JJ, Lindell TJ. Development of an antibody to actinomycin D and its application for the detection of serum levels by radioimmunoassay. Cancer Res 1982; 42: 1184–7.

199. D'Antiga L, Baker A, Pritchard J et al. Veno-occlusive disease with multi-organ involvement following actinomycin-D. Eur J Cancer 2001; 37: 1141–8.

200. Dorr RT, Meyers R, Snead K, Liddil JD. Analytical and biological inequivalence of two commercial formulations of the antitumor agent bleomycin. Cancer Chemother Pharmacol 1998; 42: 149–54.

201. Oettgen HF, Old LJ, Boyese EA et al. Inhibition of leukemias in man by L-asparaginase. Cancer Res 1967; 27: 2619–31.

202. Asselin BL. The three asparaginases – comparative pharmacology and optimal use in childhood leukemia. In: Kaspers GJL, Pieters R, Veerman AJP, eds. Drug Resistance in Leukemia and Lymphoma III. The Netherlands: Kluwer/Plenum, 1999; 621–9.

203. Muller HJ, Beier R, Loning L et al. Pharmacokinetics of native Escherichia coli asparaginase (Asparaginase medac) and hypersensitivity reactions in ALL-BFM 95 reinduction treatment. Br J Haematol 2001; 114: 794–9.

204. Kurre HA, Ettinger AG, Veenstra DL et al. A pharmaco-economic analysis of pegaspargase versus native Escherichia coli L-asparaginase for the treatment of children with standard-risk, acute lymphoblastic leukemia: The Children's Cancer Group Study (CCG-1962). J Pediatr Hematol Oncol 2002; 24: 175–81.

205. Albertsen BK, Schroder H, Ingerslev J et al. Comparison of intramuscular therapy with Erwinia asparaginase and asparaginase Medac: pharmacokinetics, pharmacodynamics, formation of antibodies and influence on the coagulation system. Br J Haematol 2001; 115: 983–90.

206. Albertsen BK, Jakobsen P, Schroder H et al. Pharmacokinetics of Erwinia asparaginase after intravenous and intramuscular administration. Cancer Chemother Pharmacol 2001; 48: 77–82.

207. Dubbers A, Wurthwein G, Muller HJ et al. Asparagine synthetase activity in paediatric acute leukaemias: AML-M5 subtype shows lowest activity. Br J Haematol 2000; 109: 427–9.

208. Loadman P, Bibby M. Pharmacokinetic drug interactions with anticancer drugs. Clin Pharmacokinet 1994; 26: 486–500.

♦209. Relling M, McLeod H, Bowman L, Santana V. Etoposide pharmacokinetics and pharmacodynamics after acute and chronic exposure to cisplatin. Clin Pharmacol Ther 1994; 56: 503–11.

210. Thomas HD, Porter DJ, Bartelink I et al. Randomized cross-over clinical trial to study potential pharmacokinetic interactions between cisplatin or carboplatin and etoposide. Br J Clin Pharmacol 2002; 53: 83–91.

211. Boddy AV, Yule SM, Wyllie R et al. Pharmacokinetics and metabolism in children of ifosfamide administered as a continuous infusion. Cancer Res 1993; 53: 3758–64.

212. Rodman J, Murry D, Madden T, Santana V. Altered etoposide pharmacokinetics and time to engraftment in pediatric patients undergoing autologous bone marrow transplantation. J Clin Oncol 1994; 12: 2390–7.

213. Gurney H. Dose calculation of anticancer drugs: a review of the current practice and introduction of an alternative. J Clin Oncol 1996; 14: 2590–611.

♦214. Boos J, Krumplemann S, Schulze-Westhoff P et al. Steady-state levels and bone marrow toxicity of etoposide in children and infants: does etoposide require age-dependent dose calculation? J Clin Oncol 1995; 13: 2954–60.

●215. Sharkey I, Boddy AV, Wallace H et al. Body surface area estimation in children using weight alone: application in paediatric oncology. Br J Cancer 2001; 85: 23–8.

9

Serum markers in tumour diagnosis and treatment

STEWART J. KELLIE

INTRODUCTION

The range and clinical applications of biological tumour-associated compounds found in the serum or urine of children with cancer have been refined and expanded during the past three decades. Tumour markers comprise molecules secreted into the circulation by tumour tissue, or represent host tissue-derived metabolic or immunological products in response to neoplasia. This heterogeneous group of biological compounds consists of oncofetal proteins (alpha-fetoprotein, carcinoembryonic antigen), enzymes (neuron-specific enolase, alkaline phosphatase), hormones (human chorionic gonadotrophin, catecholamines and their metabolites), carbohydrate antigens (CA125, CA19.9) and others, including neopterin and related compounds, neurotensin and transcobalamin I.

Biological tumour markers have clinical utility in the differential diagnosis of paediatric tumours, in detecting residual disease following apparent complete resection, thereby confirming clinical staging, and as a means of evaluating response to therapy following surgery, chemotherapy or irradiation. Additionally, the detection of an elevated biological marker may indicate tumour recurrence before this is detected clinically or investigationally. However, tumour markers that are absolutely specific for a particular type of cancer, organ or tissue of origin, or markers which may identify tumour-bearing individuals do not exist. For this reason, the clinical applications of serum markers have been restricted largely to monitoring response to therapy or detecting recurrence. The specificity and sensitivity of commonly used tumour markers in general use in children are suboptimal; the observation of 'false-positive' results in a number of non-malignant conditions and the variable rate of 'false-negative' results in children with cancer underline the importance of carefully evaluating marker results. The clinical applications of tumour markers in screening for cancer in adult or paediatric populations are controversial. Recently, the usefulness of screening whole populations of well infants for occult neuroblastoma using urinary catecholamine metabolites has generated a spirited debate on the economic, social and medical implications of mass screenings.

This chapter reviews the range and clinical utility of biological tumour markers found in serum and urine, the role of physiological hormones and 'so-called' prognostic factors in paediatric tumour diagnosis and monitoring. The current status and opposing scientific viewpoints surrounding the controversial issue of screening infant populations for the presence of occult neuroblastoma are presented.

ALPHA-FETOPROTEIN (AFP)

Historical background

Hirszfeld and Halber[1] first suggested the existence of an immunological relationship between embryonic antigens and cancer tissue in 1932. AFP is the most thoroughly characterized oncodevelopmental antigen and serves as an important model of carcinofetal alteration in humans.

Alpha-fetoprotien was first described during the investigation of serum proteins in the human fetus by Bergstrand and Czar.[2] Abelev et al.'s[3] description in 1963 of an oncofetal antigen arising in an experimental liver tumour which was immunologically identical to a normal fetal protein represented the introduction of a potential 'cancer marker' into modern medicine and refocused attention on the broad issue of carcinofetal reversion in malignancy. However, the biological reasons for observed changes in the structure, or concentration, of carcinofetal or oncodevelopmental gene products remain poorly understood, although gene activation, gene depression and other regulatory abnormalities of protein synthesis have all been suggested. Tatarinov[4] reported high serum AFP concentrations in a patient with hepatocellular carcinoma. Human AFP was subsequently purified and characterized,[5,6] and immunochemical studies by Ruoslahti and Seppälä have shown that serum AFP isolated from human fetuses and from patients with liver tumours is immunologically identical.[7] Since these early studies, the relationship between AFP production in humans and various physiological states and pathological alterations has been well documented.

Method of AFP measurement have undergone considerable refinement since Abelev et al.[3] first used the double diffusion method in 1963. The evolution of increasingly sensitive assays of serum AFP has paralleled this marker's expanding clinical role during the past three decades. Counter electrophoresis with a sensitivity of 0.25–0.5 μg/mL was described in 1971, followed by a latex agglutination inhibition technique with a sensitivity of 250 ng/mL in 1974, and immunoautoradiography with a sensitivity of 50 ng/mL in 1971. Radioimmunoelectrophoresis (1976), enzyme-linked immunosorbent assay (ELISA) (1976) and radioimmunoassay (1971) have improved the sensitivity of AFP detection to 20, 3 and 0.5 ng/mL respectively.[7] These developments have been reflected in improved methods of measurement of other tumour markers.

Physiology

Physiological synthesis of AFP occurs in all three fetal tissues. Synthesis occurs in the human fetal yolk sac, hepatocytes and gastrointestinal mucosa during the early first trimester, but AFP synthesis takes place predominantly in the hepatocytes after the eighth week.[7,8] AFP reaches a peak serum concentration of 3.0×10^6 ng/mL by the 15th week of gestation and declines thereafter, in part due to the rapid increase in fetal size. The AFP level ranges from 2.0×10^4 to 5.0×10^4 ng/mL at birth, falling

to normal adult levels (<20 ng/mL) by approximately 8 months of age.[9,10]

The rapid physiological fall in serum AFP concentration during the first 8 months of postnatal life is a potential source of false-positive error in interpretation in well infants in whom physiological elevations of AFP up to 200 times the normal adult range may be observed. The clinician's dilemma is heightened by the high age-specific incidence of hepatoblastoma, testicular or sacrococcygeal teratomas observed during the first year of life. Fortunately, these neoplasms are most commonly associated with massive elevations of serum markers, which facilitate differentiation of these tumours from physiological elevations. Wu et al.[11] monitored serum AFP levels in 32 normal babies consecutively from 2–3 days to 4 months after birth, and also measured serum AFP concentrations in 116 random specimens from infants with normal liver enzymes to establish age-related normal ranges. This study demonstrated that the half-life of AFP was approximately 5.5 days between birth and 2 weeks of age, 11 days between 2 weeks and 2 months of age, and 33 days between 2 and 4 months of age. Although the rate of decline was similar among patients of a similar age (Figure 9.1), individual levels were highly variable and found to be independent of gestational age, weight or type of milk feed (Table 9.1). The results indicate that AFP reaches adult levels after 8 months of age. The change in the rate of AFP degradation during the first month of life implies that a considerable amount of AFP synthesis exists after birth. These results, which extend and confirm work by Masseyeff et al.,[12] are important in

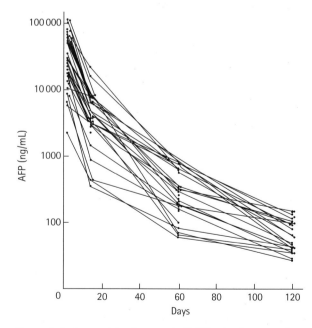

Figure 9.1 *Serum alpha-fetoprotein (AFP) levels of 32 normal babies measured consecutively at 2 or 3 days, 2 weeks, and 2 and 4 months after birth. (Reproduced with permission from Wu et al.[11])*

interpreting moderate elevations of serum AFP during the first year of life.

The biological half-life of AFP has been estimated to range from 3.5 to 7 days by serial measurements in children following complete resection of AFP-producing tumours.[13,14] Figure 9.2 represents the expected rate of fall of serum AFP based on a half-life of 7 days, plotted on a logarithmic scale. Irrespective of the pretreatment concentration, the expected rate of fall following successful tumour treatment should be parallel to the line, and deviation away from the expected rate of fall should be regarded as evidence of persisting or recurrent AFP-secreting tumour.

AFP is neither specific for cancer of a particular site or histology, nor restricted to tumour-bearing individuals. Non-neoplastic conditions during infancy or later in life may result in elevated AFP concentrations. Elevated levels have been observed during the first 6 months of life in children with neonatal hepatitis, hepatic injury from biliary atresia or congestive hepatomegaly.[15] Significant elevations of AFP beyond 6 months of age have been seen in children with viral hepatitis,[16] ataxia-telangiectasia[17] and congenital tyrosinosis.[18] AFP values in children with benign hepatic disorders tend to be higher than those found in adults with similar pathology.[19,20] AFP is not an acute-phase reactant, and, as expected, elevated values following hepatic trauma or toxic injury have not been observed.[21]

BETA–HUMAN CHORIONIC GONADOTROPHIC HORMONE

Human chorionic gonadotrophin (hCG) is a glycoprotein hormone that comprises two dissimilar subunits, designated α and β. The α subunit of hCG shares structural homology with the α subunit of anterior pituitary hormones, including luteinizing hormone, follicle-stimulating hormone and thyroid-stimulating hormone. However, the recognition of antigenically distinct carboxyl terminals on the β chains of these hormones has enabled the development of a specific radioimmunoassay for the determination of the β subunit of hCG without interference from other hormones or the α subunit.[22] The sensitivity of the widely available radioimmunoassay is approximately to 0.5–1 ng/mL. The normal serum half-life of β-hCG is approximately 24 hours,[23,24] indicating that blood levels should rapidly return to normal after complete resection of an hCG-producing tumour (Figure 9.3).

Table 9.1 *Average normal serum alpha-fetoprotein (AFP) of infants at various ages (Reproduced with permission from Wu et al.[11])*

Age	No.	Mean ± SD (ng/mL)
Premature	11	134 734 ± 41 444
Newborn	55	48 406 ± 34 718
Newborn to 2 weeks	16	33 113 ± 32 503
2 weeks to 1 month	43	9452 ± 12 610
1 month	12	2654 ± 3080
2 months	40	323 ± 278
3 months	5	88 ± 87
4 months	31	74 ± 56
5 months	6	46.5 ± 19
6 months	9	12.5 ± 9.8
7 months	5	9.7 ± 7.1
8 months	3	8.5 ± 5.5

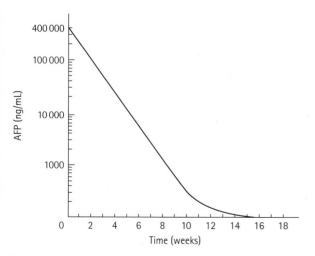

Figure 9.2 *Serum alpha-fetoprotein (AFP) levels following complete resection of an AFP-secreting tumour. The line depicts the expected rate of fall based on a half-life of 7 days. (Reproduced with permission from Wu et al.[11])*

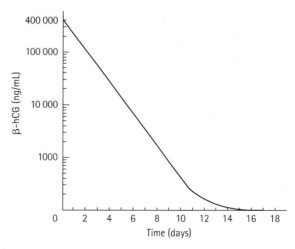

Figure 9.3 *Serum beta-human chorionic gonadotrophin (β-hCG) levels following complete resection of a β-hCG-secreting tumour. The line depicts the expected rate of fall based on a half-life of 24 hours.*

CLINICAL APPLICATIONS OF AFP AND β-hCG

The totipotential and pluripotential capabilities of germ cell tumours are phenotypically expressed by their diverse clinical, pathological and prognostic features. Pathologically, this group of tumours comprises germinomas, embryonal carcinomas, endodermal sinus tumours (yolk sac), choriocarcinomas, teratomas, polyembryomas and gonadoblastomas. Most of the current classifications of germ cell tumours arising in both gonadal and extragonadal sites are essentially modifications of Teilum's concepts.[25] The schema illustrated in Figure 9.4 restricts the term 'embryonal carcinoma' to tumours composed of undifferentiated, totipotential embryonal cells, with the potential to differentiate into extra-embryonal neoplasms (endodermal sinus tumours and choriocarcinomas) and tumour derived from all three germ layers (teratomas). Two-thirds of germ cell tumours in children are located in extragonadal sites; the majority of these are in the sacrococcygeal region in infants, the anterior mediastinum, and midline sites within the central nervous system (CNS), particularly the hypothalamic and pineal regions.

Germinomas

Germinoma is a general term used to designate a malignant germ cell tumour arising from the gonads or in an extragonadal site. Seminomas and dysgerminomas refer to germinomas arising in the testis and ovary, respectively, and are terms that have been replaced by the more generic term, germinoma. These tumours comprise approximately 15 per cent of all paediatric germ cell tumours, and 11 per cent of all ovarian tumours in children.[26] Germinomas in children are most commonly found in the ovary in girls or the pineal region in adolescent boys. Pure germinomas of the testis or anterior mediastinum are uncommon during the first two decades of life. Both immunohistochemical analysis of tumour tissue for AFP and serum AFP levels are negative in pure germinomas. Although β-hCG positivity has been noted, and elevated cerebrospinal fluid (CSF) levels of hCG have been demonstrated, findings that probably relate to the presence of multinucleated syncytiotrophoblasts in patients with mixed germ cell tumours rather than representing β-hCG secretion by 'pure germinoma'. Admixtures of other germ cell tumour types within germinomas are a more common observation than pure germinomas, underlining the importance of detailed histological examination of tumour material, and caution in interpreting raised biomarkers in patients with supposedly pure germinomas. Markers for AFP and β-hCG should be negative if there are no other malignant germ cell elements.

Embryonal carcinomas

The clinical and histological relationships between embryonal carcinomas and endodermal sinus tumours (yolk sac carcinomas) are close but poorly defined. Embryonal carcinoma is a highly malignant neoplasm comprising germ cells which may be regarded as the stem cells of teratomas, endodermal sinus tumours and choriocarcinomas. Pure embryonal carcinoma is an uncommon finding in infants and children. This histological pattern is most frequently observed in association with other germ cell tumour elements, including teratoma and endodermal sinus tumour. Endodermal carcinoma is found most frequently in the testes of young adults and commonly demonstrates positive immunostaining for AFP,[27] and raised serum AFP levels have been documented in up to 70 per cent of these patients.[28] Raised serum and CSF β-hCG levels and immunopositivity for β-hCG have been demonstrated in patients with embryonal carcinoma.[29] However, it is possible that this represents an analogous situation to patients with so-called pure germinomas with raised hCG. It is probable that patients with embryonal carcinoma and

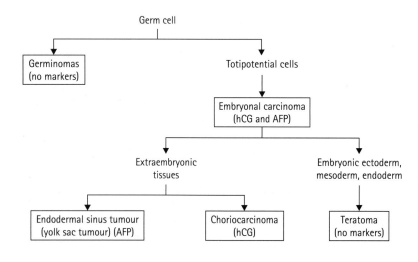

Figure 9.4 *Classification scheme of germ cell tumours, based on Teilum's[25] classification. AFP, alpha-fetoprotein; hCG, human chorionic gonadotrophin.*

immunopositivity for hCG or raised serum levels have tumours containing areas of syncytiotrophoblastic differentiation within embryonal carcinoma.

Endodermal sinus tumours (yolk sac tumours)

Endodermal sinus tumours occur almost exclusively in children, and represent the most common malignant germ cell tumour in this age group. The ovary, testis and sacrococcygeal region are the commonest sites of involvement, with less common primary sites being the anterior mediastinum, the pineal region of the CNS, vagina, vulva and liver in paediatric patients.[29–31] AFP synthesis in children with endodermal sinus tumours is analogous to the physiological AFP synthesis by the fetal yolk sac originally described by Gitlin and Boseman.[13] Endodermal sinus tumours represent the commonest testicular tumours in boys aged less than 3 years. Serum AFP is elevated in approximately 75 per cent of patients with endodermal sinus tumours. The serum levels of β-hCG are normal in patients with pure endodermal sinus tumours but may be elevated in patients with mixed germ cell tumours.

Choriocarcinomas

These tumours are uncommon, highly malignant germ cell tumours characterized by syncytiotrophoblastic differentiation, the presence of multinucleated giant cells and immunopositivity for β-hCG. Choriocarcinomas occur in both gestational and non-gestational forms, and the possibility of pregnancy mimicking an abdominal tumour in an adolescent female with a raised serum β-hCG must be considered before investigations with potentially hazardous ionizing radiation are pursued. Most choriocarcinomas in the paediatric age range are non-gestational and arise in the gonads, mediastinum, retroperitoneum or brain. Almost all extragonadal choriocarcinomas occur in males. Rarely, choriocarcinoma may present in infancy with evidence of disseminated tumour, features of gonadotrophic stimulation and raised β-hCG as a complication of maternal-placental choriocarcinoma.[32] Patients with choriocarcinoma show strong tumour immunopositivity for β-hCG. Virtually all patients will show elevated levels of β-hCG, but not of AFP.[28]

Germ cells arising within the CNS

Approximately 6 per cent of germ cell tumours are found within the CNS and comprise 1–2 per cent of all intracranial malignancies. The majority are located in midline sites with a preponderance in the pineal region. Tumours in this location often present with signs and symptoms of raised intracranial pressure, isosexual precocious puberty and Parinaud's syndrome (paralysis of upward gaze, absent or diminished pupillary reaction to light but not accommodation, and retraction nystagmus). These tumours may encompass a wide histological spectrum, making biopsy desirable. However, the risk of open or stereotactic biopsy in patients with highly vascular, deeply located midline tumours may be unacceptable. In this situation, the assay of AFP and β-hCG in serum and CSF may identify the presence of immature germ cell elements. Although raised CSF biomarkers lack diagnostic specificity in the absence of tissue diagnosis, they provide the opportunity to monitor tumour response to irradiation or chemotherapy.[33,34]

Marker level monitoring

The detection and quantitation of AFP and β-hCG in tumour tissue and the serum of patients with gonadal and extragonadal germ cell tumours are important for diagnosis and to monitor the response to therapy. Raised levels of AFP and/or β-hCG indicate the presence of endodermal sinus tumour elements or trophoblastic elements. Because of their relatively brief half-lives, the measurement of pre- and post-surgery levels have been useful in minimizing clinical staging errors. Although the majority of children with germ cell tumours have elevations of either AFP or β-hCG, there is a group in whom these markers are negative at the time of initial diagnosis and remain so throughout follow-up. A large group of patients with initially positive markers demonstrate falling serum levels of AFP and β-hCG in response to therapy. These biomarkers serve a particularly useful purpose in monitoring response to therapy and in the early detection of recurrent disease, often weeks or months before recurrence is apparent using modern diagnostic imaging techniques. The role of serum biomarkers in determining the duration of chemotherapy for children with germ cell tumours has not been resolved. Some groups, reporting excellent long-term outcome in patients with advanced germ cell tumours, continue treatment with cisplatin based chemotherapy combinations for only 2 to 3 courses after complete remission, defined clinically, radiologically and with serum markers.[35] This approach, relying heavily on normalization of markers, contrasts with the traditional model of determining duration of therapy in advance, based on histology and stage without reference to individual patient characteristics. Tumour recurrence unassociated with raised biomarkers in patients with raised serum AFP or β-hCG estimations at diagnosis have been documented in children.[35]

Hepatic malignancies

Primary malignant liver tumours in children comprise up to 3 per cent of paediatric malignancies.[36] Over 90 per cent of malignant liver tumours in children are hepatoblastomas or hepatocellular carcinomas.[37] Diagnostic elevations of serum AFP or β-hCG are not seen in children with other types of primary malignant liver tumours, including rhabdomyosarcoma, fibrosarcoma, angiosarcoma or secondary involvement by metastatic tumour or haemopoietic malignancy. Less than one-half of all liver tumours in children are benign;[38] of these, mesenchymal hamartomas and vascular tumours, particularly haemangiomas and haemangioendotheliomas, are observed most frequently.

HEPATOBLASTOMA

Hepatoblastomas are malignant tumours arising from the hepatic blastema and may contain both epithelial and/or mesenchymal elements. Ninety per cent are diagnosed within the first 3 years of life at a median age of 1 year. The AFP level is raised, often to massive levels, in 90–95 per cent of patients with hepatoblastoma and provides a reliable marker of complete resection when the fall in the serum AFP concentration is compared with the normal fall-off (Figure 9.2).[37] Approximately 3 per cent of patients with hepatoblastoma secrete β-hCG[39–41] and may develop isosexual precocious puberty as a result of gonadotrophic stimulation. These patients may demonstrate recurrence of their clinical endocrine abnormalities, in addition to raised tumour markers, at the time of recurrence.

HEPATOCELLULAR CARCINOMA

The annual incidence of hepatocellular carcinoma in children is less than the incidence of hepatoblastoma. Histopathologically, hepatocellular carcinoma resembles its counterpart in adults. Hepatocellular carcinoma shows two age peaks during childhood and adolescence; the first before the age of 4 years and the second between the ages of 12 and 15 years.[42] This tumour is associated with cirrhosis significantly less frequently than in adults, but retains its strong aetiological association with hepatitis B infection.[43,44] Serum AFP is elevated in up to 50 per cent of children with hepatocellular carcinoma, and provides a valuable marker for monitoring the response to surgery or chemotherapy. Unfortunately, AFP is of limited value in patients with the fibrolamellar variant of hepatocellular carcinoma because levels of this biomarker are not usually informative.[45,46] The level of unsaturated vitamin B_{12} binding protein, (transcobalamin I) is elevated in most children with the fibrolamellar variant, and may be a useful marker of disease progression.[47]

Other neoplasms with informative AFP or β-hCG levels

The value of AFP estimations in children with hepatic malignancies or germ cell tumours is well established.

One of the major advantages of AFP is its high level of specificity (i.e. its low false-positive rate). Elevated levels of AFP have been reported infrequently in association with malignant tumours of the gastrointestinal tract, most commonly in adult patients with tumours of the pancreas, biliary tract or stomach, and less frequently in patients with colorectal carcinoma, but not in association with oesophageal or small-bowel carcinomas.[48] These gastrointestinal neoplasms are seen commonly in the elderly, but rarely in adolescents. Mild elevations of AFP outside the normal range may be observed in some patients with non-malignant conditions, including a variety of hepatobiliary disorders (Box 9.1). Elevated β-hCG levels have been reported in neoplasms involving the gastrointestinal tract (stomach, liver, pancreas), lung, breast and ovary and rarely in lymphoproliferative disorders.[49–52] These tumours are rare in adolescents and are usually associated with serum concentrations of less than 10 ng/mL. Rarely, mild elevations of β-hCG may be seen in patients with non-malignant disorders (Box 9.1). In contrast to North America, where paediatric oncologists care for patients aged up to 18–21 years, European and Australian oncologists rarely see newly diagnosed patients aged over 15 years and are even less likely to come across these typically 'adult' neoplasms.

Box 9.1 *Raised alpha-fetoprotein (AFP) and beta-human chorionic gonadotrophin (β-hCG) in non-malignant conditions (Adapted from Schneider et al.[15])*

Raised AFP in non-malignant conditions

Hepatic pathology
- Extrahepatic biliary atresia
- Neonatal hepatitis
- Viral hepatitis, acute or chronic
- Liver cirrhosis
- Liver abscess

Hereditary disorders
- Hereditary AFP persistence
- Ataxia telangiectasia
- Hereditary tyrosinaemia, type 1

Other
- Systemic lupus erythematosus
- Hirschsprung's disease
- Pregnancy
- Infancy

Raised β-hCG in benign disorders
- Very uncommon
- Chronic renal insufficiency
- Systemic lupus erythematosus

CATECHOLAMINE METABOLITES IN NEURAL CREST TUMOURS

Normal catecholamine metabolism

Adrenaline, noradrenaline and dopamine, the principal catecholamines found in the body, are synthesized by a sequence of hydroxylation and decarboxylation steps from the amino acids phenylalanine and tyrosine. Tyrosine is converted to dopa and then to dopamine following transportation into the neuronal cytoplasm. Dopamine enters the granulated vesicles and is converted to noradrenaline by dopamine β-hydroxylase. Synthesis is regulated by feedback inhibition of tyrosine hydroxylase by noradrenaline and dopamine, so that synthesis of dopa is coupled to catecholamine release. Noradrenaline is subsequently N-methylated by the phenylethanolamine N-methyltransferase to adrenaline. Both adrenaline and noradrenaline are metabolized by O-methylation to biologically inactive products with the enzyme catechol-O-methyltransferase (COMT) and by oxidative deamination with monoamine oxidase (MAO). The metanephrines and 3-methyoxy-4-hydroxymandelic acid (MHMA) are the major metabolic end-products of noradrenaline and adrenaline metabolism. Homovanillic acid (HVA) is the major end-product of dopamine metabolism (Figure 9.5).

Untimed versus 24-hour urine collections

Twenty-four-hour urine collections have the advantage of taking into account diurnal variation in the rate of metabolite excretion and do not rely on a normal serum creatinine for interpretation. However, one of the issues not often discussed in the debate concerning the accuracy of a 24-hour urine collection versus an untimed collection is the assumption that the former is complete. The difficulty in obtaining a reliable 24-hour collection, particularly in young children, is well known, leading to delays and inaccuracies. Untimed collections are rapid, easy to collect, and provide a result that makes a correction for the rate of urine production, but not for diurnal variation of catecholamine metabolite or creatinine secretion.[53] Although the adequacy of this approach has been questioned recently,[54] results obtained by Gitlow *et al.* in 1970[55] have been confirmed by others.[56,57] Analysis of the reliability of untimed urine specimens in the diagnosis of neural crest tumours has produced results that are as good as, or better than, previously published data. This demonstrates the practical value of using catecholamine metabolite determinations expressed as 'creatinine equivalents' on untimed urine specimens in the diagnosis of these tumours.[56,57] Physiological factors, medication and dietary factors may influence the measurement of catecholamine metabolite excretion regardless of collection technique.

Factors affecting urinary catecholamine metabolite excretion

PHYSIOLOGICAL FACTORS

The 24-hour urinary excretion of catecholamines and their metabolites increases with age up to about 16 years, when the adult range is obtained. The ratio of urinary MHMA and HVA excretion, expressed as micrograms per milligram of creatinine, decreases steadily with age from infancy through to early adulthood. Increased physiological levels of adrenaline and noradrenaline secretion have been noted in ambulant subjects compared with hospitalized, recumbent patients. Moreover, increased noradrenaline secretion has been noted in response to raised autonomic sympathetic nervous activity related to physical stress, pain or cold, whereas mental stress may lead to increased secretion of adrenaline. Overall, the influence of physiological factors on the urinary excretion of

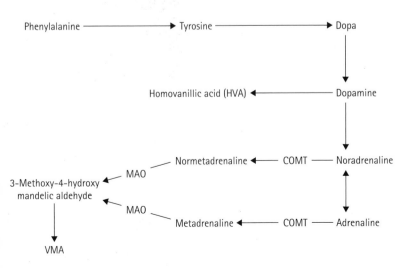

Figure 9.5 *Biosynthesis and catabolism of circulating of catecholamines. COMT, catechol-O-methyltransferase; MAO, monoamine oxidase; VMA, vanillylmandelic acid.*

catecholamines appears to be insignificant and does not appear to result in false-positive elevations of catecholamine metabolite excretion in patients with suspected neural crest tumours.

PATHOPHYSIOLOGICAL FACTORS

Essential hypertension has been associated with a slight to moderate elevation of noradrenaline secretion related to increased sympathetic tone. Patients with poorly controlled diabetes mellitus may excrete increased amounts of catecholamines, probably related to severe ketoacidosis and hypoglycaemia. Occasionally, traumatic injury may result in pathophysiological secretion of catecholamines. Patient medications may increase or decrease catecholamine metabolite excretion. A number of antihypertensive drugs that affect catecholamine binding and release may produce a decrease in catecholamine secretion. Antihypertensive treatment with guanethidine, debrisoquin and the rauwolfia alkaloids may artificially diminish catecholamine metabolite excretion, whereas increased excretion may occur during treatment with catecholamine-containing drugs or sympathomimetics. Drugs in the former category include theophylline, L-dopa, chlorpromazine, prochlorperazine and caffeine. Treatment with sympathomimetics, including dextroamphetamine, ephedrine and methylphenidate, may elevate catecholamine excretion. A number of these agents are used commonly in children with asthma, severe vomiting or behaviour disorders, and represent a potential source of false-positive error, depending on the analytical method used for assaying metabolite excretion.

DIETARY FACTORS

The relevance of dietary restriction whilst assessing urinary biogenic amine excretion has been the source of controversy. Dietary restrictions were once widely recommended and are still used by some centres today when a 24-hour urine collection for diagnostic purposes is in progress, because of concerns relating to possible false-positive results due to the concentration of catecholamines in certain foods. Classically, children with neural crest tumours completing a 24-hour urine collection have avoided a variety of foods for 2 days before and on the day of collection. The degree of dietary restriction varies greatly between centres. Common items of restricted foods include avocados, bananas, plums, pineapples, walnuts, chocolate, vanilla-flavoured foods, vitamins and coffee. Feldman et al.[58] investigated the dopamine, adrenaline, noradrenaline and serotonin content in 30 varieties of fruits and vegetables using a radioenzymatic assay technique. High concentrations of dopamine were identified in red and yellow bananas. Seven healthy volunteers consumed 1.6 kg of banana pulp

in addition to their conventional diet; a mean increase in HVA excretion of 46 ± 9.8 per cent over baseline values was observed; however, actual HVA excretion beyond the normal range was observed in only one of the seven volunteers. The impact of banana consumption on MHMA excretion was not determined due to the low adrenaline and noradrenaline concentrations in banana pulp. The absence of significant increases in MHMA or HVA excretion, which may result in a false-positive test result among children and young adults eating normal diets, has been confirmed by others.[59–61] More recently, dietary interference in the determination of biogenic amines has been virtually eliminated by the development of specific and sensitive high-performance liquid chromatographic (HPLC) methods.[62]

Clinical applications

NEUROBLASTOMA

Neuroblastoma is the commonest extracranial solid tumour in children and is derived from sympathetic neural crest tissue. Neuroblastoma is one of the 'small blue round' cell tumours of childhood and demonstrates a spectrum of maturation ranging from differentiated ganglioneuromas to highly undifferentiated neuroblastomas. The cells comprising neuroblastoma lack the ability to store quantities of dopamine for further metabolism to noradrenaline. As a consequence, the major urinary metabolites are dopamine and its metabolite HVA, although some MHMA is produced. A review of urinary excretion of these analytes using HPLC in 35 children with advanced neuroblastoma confirmed HVA to be the diagnostic analyte of choice. In this study HVA was elevated in 34 patients, with dopamine and MHMA elevations in 29 patients.[63] The usefulness of urinary dopamine and/or HVA compared with MHMA in the diagnosis of neuroblastoma has been documented by others.[64–67] Urinary MHMA, HVA, dopamine and 3-methoxy-4-hydroxy-phenylglycol (MHPG) are usually elevated beyond the normal range in almost 100 per cent of patients with neuroblastoma.[55] HPLC measurement of HVA, the primary metabolite of dopamine, has shown this to be the most useful analyte for the detection of small primary tumours (Evans stages I and II), in addition to being the most consistently elevated analyte in children with disseminated abdominal tumours.[63]

LaBrosse et al.[68] have examined the interrelationships between the excretion of catecholamine metabolites, age at diagnosis, stage of disease, site of primary tumour and prognosis. They found elevated levels of MHMA excretion in 71 per cent of patients and HVA excretion in 75 per cent. Additionally they observed significantly higher levels of MHMA excretion in patients with stages IV and IV-S compared with patients with stages I, II, or III disease.

They found no significant relationship between MHMA or HVA excretion and the primary site of the tumour, but noted that the MHMA/HVA ratio was significantly related to survival in stage IV patients, although no correlation between levels of MHMA or HVA excretion and prognosis was observed. Both LaBrosse et al.[68] and Laug et al.[69] have demonstrated a statistically significant relationship between a high MHMA/HVA ratio and a more favourable prognosis. However, this ratio does not reliably predict outcome in children with other stages of neuroblastoma.

False-positive elevations of catecholamine metabolite excretion, suggesting the presence of a neural crest tumour in a patient without additional evidence of malignancy, are rare. Gitlow et al.[70] noted elevated HVA excretion, but diminished or normal excretion of other catecholamine metabolites in children with familial dysautonomia. Rosano[63] reported elevated urinary catecholamine metabolites in two children with Duchenne-type muscular dystrophy without evidence of neural crest tumour. The elevated levels (expressed as milligrams per gram of creatinine) in these patients may reflect the effect of muscular dystrophy on muscle mass and creatinine excretion. The high level of specificity (i.e. the low false-positive rate) of urinary catecholamine excretion for patients with neural crest tumours has reinforced the value of these assays for both diagnosis and follow-up. Refined assay techniques and broadening clinical applications, including mass screening of infants, ensure these markers will remain clinically useful, as well as a potential source of controversy in the years to come.

The potential diagnostic roles of plasma catecholamines or their metabolites have received relatively little attention. Schuman et al.[71] described the use of venous catecholamine sampling via selective vena caval catheterization in an infant with an occult ganglioneuroma secreting vasoactive intestinal peptide and catecholamines, resulting in intractable diarrhoea. Elevated levels of plasma noradrenaline, adrenaline and dopamine localized the otherwise unidentifiable tumour, permitting curative surgery. More recently, assays of plasma catecholamines in children with neuroblastoma have been reported.[72] Boomsma et al.[72] investigated the relationships of noradrenaline, adrenaline, dopa, dopamine, and aromatic L-amino acid decarboxylase (ALAAD) to disease activity. The wide variation of plasma levels of noradrenaline, adrenaline and dopamine reported underscore the inconsistent relationship between these markers and disease activity. However, plasma dopa and ALAAD activity were clearly elevated in 10 out of 10 patients with active untreated neuroblastoma. ALAAD, and to a lesser extent dopa levels fell with successful treatment and increased with relapse. The future role of these plasma markers in monitoring disease activity remains to be determined.

PHAEOCHROMOCYTOMA

Phaeochromocytoma is a rare tumour in children, and fewer than 10 per cent of cases are malignant. The majority are associated with paroxysmal headache, sweating, palpitations and arterial hypertension. The metabolites of choice for the diagnosis of phaeochromocytoma are noradrenaline and adrenaline.[63,73] MHMA alone should not be relied upon for diagnosis or monitoring, as this metabolite is normal in approximately 10 per cent of patients.[73] HPLC and mass spectroscopy, combined with gas chromatography, are both highly sensitive and specific methods, although the latter is compromised by the high cost of instrumentation and the need for specialized support. Fluorescence techniques are subject to interference (and false-positive results) from a variety of drugs and B group vitamins. Urinary dopamine and HVA are usually normal in patients with these tumours.

CARCINOID TUMOUR

Carcinoid tumours arise from enterochromaffin cells, which are thought to migrate from the neural crest to their final location in diverse organs. These tumours may be benign or malignant, with the benign varieties most commonly found in the appendix. Extra-appendiceal carcinoids are rare in children.[74] Carcinoid tumours and their metastases produce excessive amounts of 5-hydroxytryptamine (serotonin), histamine and other vasoactive peptides, resulting in the 'carcinoid syndrome', characterized by tachycardia, hyperperistalsis, frequent watery stools, patchy cyanosis or vasodilatation of the skin, asthma and valvular heart disease. Urinary excretion of a serotonin metabolite, 5-hydroxyindolacetic acid (5-HIAA), is elevated. At present there is a general consensus that the measurement of 5-HIAA in a 24-hour urine sample is the most appropriate initial test.[75] Although urinary serotonin excretion is not elevated in all carcinoid tumours, both this and urinary 5-HIAA may have a role in monitoring disease progress in some patients. The relative importance of various diagnostic markers for carcinoid tumours has been examined in some detail elsewhere.[76]

OTHER TUMOUR MARKERS

A large group of interesting tumour-derived molecules produced by cancer cells and tumour-associated metabolic or immunological products from normal tissues have been described. These products include oncofetal antigens, such as carcinoembryonic antigen (CEA), carbohydrate antigens (CA125, CA19.9 and CA15.3), host response markers such as soluble interleukin-2, neopterin and related compounds, transcobalamin I, neurotensin and elements detected by proton nuclear magnetic resonance spectroscopy. In comparison to the tumour markers discussed earlier in this chapter, the remainder are of limited clinical application in paediatric oncology at the present time, although their roles are being examined in specialized centres.

Neuron–specific enolase

The enolases are a group of glycolytic enzymes which exist as dimers composed of three immunologically distinct subunits designated alpha, beta and gamma. The most acidic isoenzyme is composed of two gamma subunits, and is termed neuron-specific enolase (NSE). NSE is distributed widely throughout the body in both neuronal and neuroendocrine cells, and has also been identified in non-neuronal tissue. NSE has been demonstrated, using immunostaining techniques, in all types of neurons, as well as pinealocytes, pituitary glandular peptide-secreting cells, thyroid parafollicular cells, adrenal medullary chromaffin cells, neuroendocrine cells found in lung and in other tissues which derive from the embryological neural crest. The diversity of mature tissues expressing NSE has proven to be the major factor limiting its use in diagnosing malignancies arising from specific tissues.

The major clinical application of serum NSE concentrations in paediatric oncology has been this marker's relationship with stage and treatment outcome in children with neuroblastoma.[76,77] Zeltzer et al.[77] demonstrated a significant relationship between disease stage and NSE levels in 61 children with neuroblastoma. The median serum NSE values in patients with stages I, II, III, IV and

IV-S disease were 13, 23, 40, 214 and 40 ng/mL, respectively. Although NSE is widely described as being a 'tumour marker', its greatest utility appears to be as a prognostic factor in patients with a confirmed diagnosis of neuroblastoma. Zeltzer et al.'s study confirmed that infants with stage IV-S disease have significantly lower NSE levels than patients with stage IV disease, despite their extensive tumour burden. Zeltzer et al. reported a significantly inferior outcome for patients with pre-treatment NSE levels >100 ng/mL (2-year disease-free survival of 10 per cent) compared with those with values <100 ng/mL (2-year disease-free survival of 79 per cent).

Elevated NSE levels have recently been documented in a variety of paediatric tumours.[77,78] Cooper et al.[78] demonstrated elevated NSE levels at the time of diagnosis in a variety of neoplasms including neuroblastoma, especially advanced disease, and less frequently in children with Wilms' tumour, acute leukaemia, non-Hodgkin's lymphoma, Ewing's sarcoma and soft tissue sarcomas (Table 9.2). Zeltzer et al.[77] demonstrated significant NSE elevations in patients with leukaemia, hepatoblastoma and primitive neuroectodermal tumour (PNET). NSE has also been suggested as a marker for immature ovarian teratoma and dysgerminoma;[79] four of eight patients with ovarian teratoma had values between 10 and 50 ng/mL, whereas four of six patients with dysgerminoma had NSE values >50 ng/mL. Raised serum NSE in patients with immature teratoma may reflect enzyme synthesized and released by neural components contained in these tumours. However, dysgerminomas are not generally considered to be of neural origin and the

Table 9.2 *Neuron-specific enolase (NSE) levels at diagnosis in children with cancer (Reproduced with permission from Cooper et al.[78])*

Tumour	Number	Serum NSE (ng/mL)			
		<25	25–50	51–100	100
Controls[a]					
a	27	27			
b	11	11			
Neuroblastoma					
Stages I and II	9	6	1	1	1
Stages III and IV	63	9	7	16	31
Stage IVs	3	2	1		
Ganglioneuroma	4	4			
Retinoblastoma	4	4			
Wilms' tumour					
Stages I and II	15	13	2		
Stages II and IV	14	5	3	4	2
Lymphoma	15	9	5	1	
Acute lymphoblastic leukaemia	23	20	2	–	1
Acute myeloblastic leukaemia	2	1	1		
Ewing's sarcoma	11	10	1		
Soft tissue sarcoma	23	19	3	1	

[a] Controls: a, Hospital for Sick Children, London; b, Service d'Hematologie Pediatrique, Cliniques Universitaires St Luc Brussels.

marked elevation of NSE is these patients is surprising. The value of serial NSE estimations in the subsequent management of these patients is not known.[79] The presence of raised NSE in children with neuroblastoma and Wilms' tumour and the recent demonstration of raised serum NSE in adults with renal cell carcinoma confirm this marker's lack of specificity in differentiating between these tumours.[80]

Raised serum levels in a variety of tumours have been reflected by immunohistochemical studies which have demonstrated NSE in neuroblastomas, ganglioneuroblastomas, neurogangliomas, phaeochromocytomas, retinoblastomas and CNS tumours, including medulloblastomas, PNETs, paragangliomas, olfactory neuroblastomas, capillary haemangioblastomas, Merkel cell tumours and medullary thyroid carcinomas.[81–83]

The clinical relevance of increased NSE concentration in CSF has been studied recently. Jacobi and Reiber[84] detected NSE levels >20 ng/mL in the CSF of 33 out of 172 patients with a variety of neurological disorders, including CNS tumours, cerebral infarctions, cerebral ischaemia, CNS inflammatory diseases and epilepsy. They confirmed that raised levels of NSE in CSF were not specific for a particular type of neurological disorder. Although the CSF NSE estimation may help identify patients with pathological organic CNS pathology, it lacks diagnostic usefulness.[84]

Carcinoembryonic antigen

Carcinoembryonic antigen is a glycoprotein moiety first described in fetal intestine, liver and pancreas during the first 6 months of gestation. CEA is elevated in approximately 70 per cent of adult patients with adenocarcinoma of the colon. CEA concentration is more likely to be of assistance in determining tumour bulk at diagnosis and adequacy of initial therapy, particularly if surgical resection is thought to be complete, and in monitoring response to subsequent therapy. The introduction of sensitive radioimmunoassays has shown that serum CEA may be elevated in diverse malignant and benign conditions. Elevated serum CEA levels have been described in children with colon cancer[85,86] and less frequently in children with Wilms' tumour, histiocytic lymphoma, hepatoblastoma, hepatocellular carcinoma, stage IV neuroblastoma with hepatic involvement, germ cell tumour, pulmonary blastoma and retinoblastoma.[87–91] Howell et al.[92] demonstrated tissue CEA immunoreactivity in 68 per cent of patients with ameloblastoma; however, serum CEA levels were not reported. Although rare in paediatric neoplasms, CEA immunoreactivity may have potential value in diagnosis and follow-up. CEA has also been reported to be elevated in a variety of non-neoplastic conditions, including hepatic cirrhosis, hepatitis,

inflammatory bowel disease and bronchitis.[88,90] This lack of specificity severely limits the utility of this marker in the diagnosis of paediatric malignancy and in differentiating malignant from non-malignant conditions.

Soluble interleukin-2

The interleukin-2 (IL-2) receptor is expressed on the cytoplasmic membrane of T lymphocytes, on some B cells, and on monocytes following their activation. The same receptor has also been found on cell membranes in several lymphoproliferative disorders, including T-cell leukaemia, non-Hodgkin's lymphoma, hairy cell leukaemia, B-cell chronic lymphocytic leukaemia and Hodgkin's disease. Increased serum IL-2 receptor levels have been described in adults with various leukaemias, non-Hodgkin's lymphoma and Hodgkin's disease. Pui et al.[93] and Wagner et al.[94] have correlated raised serum IL-2 receptor levels with advanced diseased, increased tumour burden and an unfavourable prognosis in patients with non-Hodgkin's lymphoma. These findings have more recently been extended to children with non-T, non-B acute lymphoblastic leukaemia,[95] where higher interleukin-2 levels were also associated with a poorer prognosis.[95] More recently, Pui et al.[96] have demonstrated that higher levels of IL-2 receptor in children with Hodgkin's disease are associated with advanced disease and, more importantly, were found to be an independent predictor of treatment outcome after adjustment for other co-variables (Figure 9.6). Raised levels of serum IL-2 have also been found in patients with immunological disorders, such as the acquired immunodeficiency syndrome and infectious mononucleosis.[97] At the present time, the application of this marker in detecting residual tumour or for monitoring the course of malignant disease has not been studied prospectively.

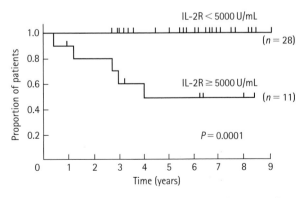

Figure 9.6 *Comparison of time-to-failure durations according to serum interleukin-2 receptor (IL-2R) levels for patients with stage III or IV Hodgkin's disease. Significantly worse treatment results were evident for patients with higher levels (≥5000 U/mL). (Reproduced with permission from Pui et al.[96])*

Transcobalamin I and neurotensin

The fibrolamellar variant of hepatocellular carcinoma is seen more commonly in older adolescents and young adults than in younger children. In contrast to patients with classical hepatocellular carcinoma, the serum AFP is usually normal in patients with the fibrolamellar variant;[48,49] however, the serum concentration of total, unsaturated transcobalamin-binding capacity is often raised in such patients, and has been shown to rise in response to recurrent disease prior to clinical or radiological evidence of recurrence.[49,50] Transcobalamin I alone appears to be a more sensitive and specific tumour marker than the total unsaturated vitamin B_{12} binding capacity. Carmel and Eisenberg,[98] in a retrospective survey of 139 patients, found that half of the patients with cancer had some abnormality of serum vitamin B_{12} or its binding proteins, although the highest levels were most commonly observed in patients with primary or secondary liver involvement. These investigations are of limited value in diagnosis because of low selectivity and specificity. Elevated concentrations of neurotensin, a polypeptide hormone found in the gastrointestinal tract and CNS, have been found in four out of four patients with the fibrolamellar variant, but in only one of 16 patients with classic hepatocellular carcinoma.[99] Neurotensin may have a role as a tumour marker at diagnosis or recurrence in patients with AFP-negative fibrolamellar hepatocellular carcinoma.

Nuclear magnetic resonance (NMR) spectroscopy

Controversy surrounds the value of water-suppressed proton NMR spectroscopy for cancer detection.[100–102] Differences in the T1 and T2 values of the composite proton NMR signal between malignant and non-malignant tissues have prompted investigation into the application of this modality as a means of identifying patients with cancer using a sensitive and specific blood test. Fossel et al.[100] analysed plasma from 337 people using water-suppressed proton NMR spectroscopy. Patients with malignant tumours were distinguished from normal controls reliably ($P < 0.0001$). Patients with benign tumours had statistically significant wider line widths compared with those with malignant tumours ($P < 0.0001$). Although the preliminary results demonstrated the potential value of this approach, other factors, including fasting, alcohol consumption, lactic acidosis and diabetic ketoacidosis, may interfere with lipoprotein peaks, possibly invalidating the results. Wilding et al.[102] investigated proton NMR spectra in healthy patients, patients with overt malignancy and those with hypertriglyceridaemia. Contrary to the findings of Fossel et al., Wilding et al. were unable to distinguish normal individuals from those with malignant tumours. The future of

NMR spectral information as a general marker for cancer remains to be determined by specialized groups of investigators. Further work involving larger groups of patients with malignancies and non-malignant disorders, using NMR spectral information obtained from body fluids including urine, CSF and amniotic fluid, is necessary to determine whether this modern technology can provide specific and sensitive identification of tumour-bearing individuals in the future.

Neopterin and related compounds

Of the pterins, neopterin, first described in 1979 by Watcher et al.,[103] has been shown to be the most consistently raised in several malignancies, including the lymphoproliferative disorders. Neopterin is a metabolite derived from human macrophages following induction by gamma interferon and is produced in increased amounts by activated and rapidly proliferating cells. It appears to be a sensitive and specific activation marker of T-cell/ macrophage interplay and can be detected in measurable quantities in plasma and urine. Abate et al.[104] demonstrated raised urinary neopterin excretion above the upper limit of normal in 85 per cent of a series of adult patients with non-Hodgkin's lymphoma and found a relationship between the level of neopterin excretion with disease stage and the presence of constitutional symptoms. Regardless of stage, patients with lower neopterin excretion fared better than those with higher levels of excretion. Neopterin appeared to have prognostic significance, particularly in patients with limited disease. Raised neopterin levels in patients appeared to be a consequence of activation of the host immune system rather than a product of malignant cells. Unfortunately, raised levels have also been demonstrated in patients with viral infections and other malignant tumours, thereby diminishing its role as a specific tumour marker. Neopterin has not demonstrated clinical utility in patients with colorectal carcinoma.

Carbohydrate antigens (CA125, CA19.9, CA15.3)

CA125 is a glycoprotein associated with non-mucinous ovarian cancer. Elevated levels have also been found in adult patients with carcinoma of the endometrium and fallopian tube and breast cancer. Elevated levels have been found during the first trimester of pregnancy, possibly reflecting CA125-associated glycoprotein production by the fetus, and also in patients with endometriosis, hepatitis and pelvic inflammatory disease, and in menstruating females.[105,106] Although the majority of ovarian tumours in children and adolescents are germ cell tumours, approximately one-third of malignant ovarian tumours occurring after the age of 15 years are of epithelial origin. Elevated

CA125 is found in over 80 per cent of patients with mucinous or non-mucinous ovarian carcinomas, and it is likely that this serum tumour marker will retain utility in diagnosis, assessing response to treatment and as a marker for early pre-clinical recurrence in a restricted number of adolescent patients.

CA19.9 is a carbohydrate cell surface antigen, found in the sera of patients with colorectal, gastric or pancreatic cancer.[107] Unfortunately, elevated concentrations of this carbohydrate antigen have been found in a variety of non-malignant conditions, including inflammatory bowel disease, biliary disease, pancreatitis and hepatitis.[108] CA15.3 and CA50 are carbohydrate antigens found predominantly in adults with breast and other carcinomas. They appear to be of little relevance to paediatric oncologists at present and are hampered, like the other carbohydrate antigens, by low specificity and sensitivity.

PROGNOSTIC FACTORS

Prognostic factors are indices derived from clinical and laboratory data that provide a prospective measure of the success of treatment. Traditionally, stage, site and extent of disease have provided the basis for prognostic classification. More recently, the value of tumour histology, immunological techniques, and cytogenetic and molecular analysis have been studied. The importance of individual prognostic factors may change with therapeutic refinement, with some previously important risk factors losing their predictive value and new prognostic factors appearing. Circulating serum markers, including lactate dehydrogenase (LDH), alkaline phosphatase (ALP) and ferritin, lack both sensitivity and specificity for the presence of cancer in children, but retain clinical utility both as prognostic factors and as markers of tumour activity.

Lactate dehydrogenase, an enzyme that favours the reduction of pyruvate to lactate, is widely distributed throughout body tissue. Elevated serum levels have been reported in children with solid tumours including germ cell tumours, Ewing's sarcoma, neuroblastoma, non-Hodgkin's lymphoma and osteosarcoma.[109–112] Although LDH lacks tumour specificity, it has recently been found to be useful for following disease activity in patients with neuroblastoma, Ewing's sarcoma and osteosarcoma.[109–111]

Serum ALP is a biological marker derived from the cell membrane of osteoblasts, and its value in diagnosis and monitoring response to therapy in adolescents with osteosarcoma remains unclear because of a lack of specificity. Elevated serum concentrations have been described in patients with liver disease, healing fractures in association with normal growth and may be elevated in patients receiving long-term parenteral nutrition therapy. Serum ALP levels may be elevated during treatment with antifungal agents, chlorothiazide, diazepam, gentamicin, phenytoin, phenobarbital, propranolol, sulphamethoxazole and aspirin. The prognostic significance of serum ALP levels was investigated in 116 children and adolescents with osteosarcoma treated at St Jude Children's Research Hospital. Although a white blood cell count $>8 \times 10^9$ L and LDH >300 U/L at diagnosis were correlated with shortened disease-free survival, no prognostic significance was attached to pre-therapy ALP levels.[113]

Ferritin is an iron storage protein present in most eukaryotic cells. Ferritin concentrations are particularly high in the liver, spleen and bone marrow. Raised serum ferritin levels may occur in association with a diversity of benign and malignant conditions, including acute-phase reactions to tissue injury, necrosis, inflammation or infection, liver disease, megaloblastic anaemia, haemolytic anaemia, sideroblastic anaemia, thalassaemia and iron overload (haemochromatosis, haemosiderosis). Raised levels have also been observed in children with Hodgkin's disease, hepatocellular carcinoma, neuroblastoma and germ cell tumours. Hann et al.[114] investigated serum ferritin levels in 58 children with neuroblastoma and demonstrated that increased levels correlated with active disease, confirming these findings in a longitudinal study. The ferritin levels were noted to return to normal in patients achieving remission. Their study suggested that increased serum ferritin in patients with neuroblastoma was tumour-derived and estimations of this marker could potentially provide a measure of disease activity. Almost 100 per cent of children with hepatocellular carcinoma have elevated serum ferritin levels: the importance of this observation is nullified by the fact that more than three-quarters of patients with uncomplicated cirrhosis also have elevated levels. Although the serum ferritin level is of limited value diagnostically, it appears to fall with tumour response and rise with tumour recurrence or progression.

HORMONAL TUMOUR MARKERS

The endocrine manifestations of cancer in children and adolescents may result from the production of excessive amounts of hormone from a benign or malignant tumour arising in a gland normally associated with physiological synthesis. Ectopic hormone production may occur in tumours arising in endocrine glands which normally produce other hormones, or from hormones synthesized and secreted by tumours unrelated to endocrine tissue (Table 9.3). Biologically active hormones are found in age-related levels in the serum of normal persons. However, elevated levels provide a valuable biological marker in patients with functioning endocrine tumours due to the relative specificity for the organ of origin. Serial estimations offer a means of monitoring response to therapy and of detecting pre-clinical recurrence. Endocrine tumours in childhood are rare, comprising approximately 5 per cent of neoplasms in this age group. The majority are non-functioning. The presence of elevated hormone levels and the degree of elevation have generally been unhelpful in differentiating benign adenomas from their malignant counterparts.

SCREENING FOR NEUROBLASTOMA IN INFANCY

Screening for disease offers the opportunity for early recognition, intervention and initiation of treatment in patients with pre-clinical disease. Successful screening programmes for phenylketonuria, galactosaemia and neonatal hypothyroidism have encouraged paediatricians to critically examine a wide variety of childhood diseases for their suitability for early detection through screening programmes. In order to develop an effective screening programme, a number of principles and recommendations require consideration:

- The human and economic cost of the condition being investigated should be sufficiently serious to warrant justification of screening on a cost/benefit basis.

Table 9.3 *Hormones as tumour markers in paediatric oncology*

Hormone tumour marker	Syndrome	Tumour type	Ectopic production
Cortisol, aldosterone, androgen, oestrogen	Cushing's, Crohn's Virilization Feminization	Adrenal hyperplasia Adrenal adenoma Adrenal carcinoma	Adrenal rests (liver, testis, ovary)
Androgen	Isosexual precocity (male) Virilism (female)	Leydig cell tumour (testis) Sertoli–Leydig cell tumour (ovary)	
Oestrogen	Isosexual precocity (female) Feminization (male)	Granulosa cell tumour (ovary) Sertoli cell tumour (testis)	
Adrenaline, dopamine, noradrenaline	Hypertension	Adrenal hyperplasia Adrenal adenoma Adrenal carcinoma	
Erythropoietin	Erythrocytosis	Wilms' tumour Renal carcinoma Adrenal carcinoma	Cerebral haemangioblastomatosis Hepatoma Phaeochromocytoma
Renin	Hypertension	Wilms' tumour	
Thyrocalcitonin	Parathyroid hyperplasia Diarrhoea MEN IIa, IIb	Medullary (C-cell) thyroid carcinoma	Carcinoid
T3/T4	Hyperthyroidism	Thyroid adenoma Thyroid carcinoma	Thyrotropin (pituitary)
PTH	MEN I, IIa	Parathyroid hyperplasia Parathyroid adenoma Parathyroid carcinoma	Hepatoma Renal carcinoma
Prolactin, ACTH, growth hormone, LH, FSH, TSH	Galactorrhoea Cushing's syndrome Gigantism Precocious puberty Hyperthyroidism	Hormone-secreting adenomas	Neuroblastoma Phaeochromocytoma Hepatoblastoma Choriocarcinoma
Insulin	Hypoglycaemia	Insulinoma	Carcinoid
Gastrin	Zollinger–Ellinson syndrome	Gastrinoma	
Glucagon	Hyperglycaemia	Glucagonoma	Carcinoid
VIP	Watery diarrhoea $\downarrow K^+$	VIPoma	
Somatostatin	Hyperglycaemia	Somatostatinoma	

ACTH, adrenocorticotrophic hormone; FSH, follicle-stimulating hormone; LH, luteinizing hormone; MEN, multiple endocrine neoplasia; PTH, parathyroid hormone; T3, tri-iodothyronine; T4, thyroxine; TSH, thyroid-stimulating hormone; VIP, vasoactive intestinal polypeptide.

- Diagnostic screening tests should be sufficiently sensitive (i.e. have a low false-negative rate) in identifying affected individuals, and also have high specificity (i.e. a low false-positive rate) whereby non-affected individuals are not identified as having pre-clinical disease.
- Pre-clinical detection should be expected to be associated with improved outcome. This principle is well illustrated by newborn screening for metabolic disorders which, left untreated, may be associated with disastrous neurodevelopmental consequences.
- Effective treatment for the condition being screened for should be readily available.
- The condition should be relatively prevalent in the selected population, as an inverse relationship exists between the prevalence of the condition and the cost of case finding.
- Sufficient facilities should be available for the diagnosis, counselling and treatment of patients identified by the screening programme.

Historical background – the Japanese experience

With the exception of screening for neuroblastoma, introduced by Japanese workers in 1973, the principal applications for tumour markers in paediatric oncology have been to assist in differential diagnosis, predict outcome or monitor therapy. Controversy regarding screening infants for neuroblastoma has increased recently with the initiation of selective screening of infants for neuroblastoma in Europe, North America and Australia by a number of paediatric oncology groups. Interest in this approach has been stimulated by the results of the Japanese neuroblastoma mass screening programme.

In 1973, Sawada et al.[115] first developed a 'mass' screening system involving 6- to 7-month-old infants in Kyoto City, Japan. Assaying only vanillylmandelic acid (VMA) using a spot test method, a comparison was drawn between patients with neuroblastoma diagnosed before screening became available with those detected after. Their results indicated a striking increase in the proportion of infants aged less than 12 months with neuroblastoma (12/22 patients, 54.6 per cent) and a decrease in the proportion aged over 2 years at diagnosis (7/22 patients, 31.8 per cent) during the 8 years after initiation of mass screening in 1973 compared with the 12 years before 1973. These changes were reflected in improved survival after screening; before mass screening only 17.1 per cent (6/35) survived, whereas 72.7 per cent (16/22) of those diagnosed after 1973 were alive at the time of reporting in 1983. The authors claimed the improved prognosis was dependent on early diagnosis.

Nishi et al.[116] evaluated the impact of screening 6-month-old infants from Sapporo City, Hokkaido, for neuroblastoma using HPLC determinations of MHMA and HVA in filter paper urine. Improvement in three parameters after the initiation of mass screening were noted:

- age at diagnosis
- clinical stage
- survival.

A significant increase in the proportion of cases diagnosed before 12 months of age was reported – 14.3 per cent (5/35) before screening compared with 66.7 per cent (12/18) after initiation of screening. In addition, they observed a significant increase in the number of patients with stages I, II and IV-S disease after 1981. Their findings are reflected in a statistically significant improvement in survival comparing patients diagnosed before screening became available with those diagnosed more recently. Parallel analysis of age, clinical stage at diagnosis and survival rate in the remainder of the Hokkaido Prefecture, where neuroblastoma screening had not been available, showed no change in these parameters compared with the period before 1981. The programme in Hokkaido was expanded in October 1987 to include the entire island. Naito et al.,[117] reporting on the expanded experience in Hokkaido, noted that the proportion of patients with neuroblastoma aged less than 12 months had increased from 17 to 66 per cent, and the proportion of stage I and stage II patients had increased from 9 to 26 per cent and from 9 to 32 per cent, respectively. These findings were reflected by an improvement in the 5-year survival rate from 23 to 66.7 per cent.

Current controversies

Advocates in Europe, North America and Australia for the development and implementation of mass screening programmes of infants for neuroblastoma point to the Japanese data to justify international expansion of the screening programme. Proponents of mass screening emphasize the statistically significant survival advantage enjoyed by infants aged less than 12 months compared with older children, and also to the increasing proportion of infants with limited stage disease, who have a more favourable prognosis compared with older children with disseminated disease at diagnosis. Do infants with 'good prognosis', lower-stage disease evolve into 'poor prognosis', symptomatic children with disseminated neuroblastoma? Clearly, if such a hypothesis could be proven, the benefits of early detection and treatment would justify mass screening of infants for neuroblastoma, and could be expected to be associated with a reduction in later mortality from this disease. Neuroblastoma is neither clinically nor biologically a homogeneous disorder, and evidence suggesting that infants detected by mass screening programmes may not necessarily be those who present at a later time with poor prognosis disease has promoted vigorous debate concerning the presuppositions and methods of screening programmes.

Hayashi et al.[118] recently studied solid tumour cytogenetics in 15 infants with neuroblastoma initially identified by urinary MHMA mass screening. Interestingly, near triploidy or hyperdiploidy was found in each infant, a prognostic feature that Look et al.[119] had previously demonstrated to be strongly predictive for a favourable outcome. Hayashi et al.'s results differed from the cytogenetic patterns commonly observed in neuroblastomas in children aged over 1 year. In this latter age group, diploidy or near diploidy, homogeneously staining regions, double minutes and translocations of chromosome 1 were most commonly found. These cytogenetic features identify a subgroup of patients with a poor prognosis. One can speculate, therefore, that the cytogenetic abnormalities identified in infants diagnosed by mass screening further define a subgroup of patients who already have a favourable prognosis. Both Hayashi et al.[118] and Nishi et al.[116] have reported improved prognosis in children with neuroblastoma detected as a result of pre-clinical screening. Further population-based investigation will be required to determine whether screening is detecting good-prognosis patients whose tumours may spontaneously regress. It may be that the tumour cell molecular biology, and patterns of metastasis and drug resistance are fundamentally different in these patients compared with children aged over 1 year at diagnosis. To date, there is no evidence supporting the hypothesis that infants with good-prognosis disease develop poor-prognosis disease with the passage of time if they remain undetected during their first year of life. A preliminary report from the Quebec neuroblastoma screening project has examined the impact of screening infants for pre-clinical neuroblastoma on this tumour's population-based mortality.[120] A high rate of compliance during the first months (92 per cent) and provision for a 5-year study may permit answers to these important questions. Unfortunately, data from Japan thus far have focused on survival of the screened population, and population-based studies will be necessary to determine whether the increased number of infants detected by screening during the first year of life will be offset by a corresponding reduction in the prevalence of poor-prognosis neuroblastomas amongst children aged over 2 years, and whether such a difference will be associated with a 'down-staging' of the tumour.

The impact of spontaneous remission of neuroblastoma during the first year of life has been explored by Carlsen.[121] This study, undertaken with the dual aims of determining the frequency of spontaneous regression of neuroblastoma and also the impact this has on the assessment of the benefits of screening, indicated that spontaneous regression occurred in less than 2 per cent of cases. However, Carlsen's epidemiological findings of increased incidence and survival rates in association with an unchanged mortality raised the possibility that the inclusion of 'borderline' lesions among the pool of 'real' neuroblastomas has occurred during recent decades in Denmark, possibly as a result of tumours diagnosed incidentally by abdominal palpation or routine chest radiograph.

Selection of metabolites and methods of analysis have been developed and refined since Sawada et al.[115] first assayed MHMA using a qualitative spot test for screening in 1973. Sequential studies have determined the relative importance of MHMA or HVA, or both, or the MHMA/HVA ratio as the optimal metabolite, or combination, for evaluation. Overall, HVA is regarded as a better tumour marker than MHMA for the presence of neuroblastoma. Pritchard et al.[122] have demonstrated that approximately one-third of patients with low-stage disease have no evidence of raised urinary excretion of either MHMA or HVA. Interestingly, these researchers suggested that MHMA may be the preferred urinary marker for neuroblastoma in infancy. This observation has recently been supported by Tuchman et al.[120] Refinements in assay techniques have reduced the rate of false-positive detection of neuroblastoma from 3.8 per cent of infants after initial evaluation using the MHMA spot test, to 0.016 per cent using a quantitative HPLC assay for MHMA and HVA.[123,124] More recently, the development of HPLC, thin layer chromatography, gas chromatography/mass spectrometry and enzyme-linked immunoassay has improved both the sensitivity and specificity of screening tests. The selection of screening method depends on the regional availability of the method in question as much as on the philosophy regarding the cost/effectiveness ratio. The Quebec neuroblastoma study, for example, uses a two-step approach employing initial qualitative screening with thin layer chromatography followed by gas chromatography/mass spectrometry in selected cases.[120]

A neuroblastoma screening programme hinges on the acceptance of screening by the infants' parents. Compliance rates ranging from 50–75 to 92 per cent for population-based infant screening programmes have been reported. Information and education regarding the objectives of neuroblastoma screening are best introduced during the antenatal period and reinforced shortly after delivery to maximize the overall level of compliance. Although compliance is likely to be higher in studies where urine is collected prior to initial discharge from hospital, later testing may be more appropriate if the hypothesis that screening at 6 months of age is likely to detect infants at risk of poor-prognosis disease is correct.

Whether or not the fundamental goals of screening infants at birth, 6 months or even later will result in the pre-clinical detection of poor-prognosis neuroblastoma remains to be determined. Expanding clinical interest in neuroblastoma screening in Europe, North America and Australia, coupled with the continued refinement of neuroblastoma screening in Japan, will provide a novel insight into the overall significance of screening for malignancy in a paediatric population. In the meantime, controversy will continue, until current projects yield mature data and important epidemiological, clinical and biological questions can be answered in a scientifically and statistically valid way.

Recently published results from the USA and Germany have indicated that the pendulum may be swinging away from conclusions supporting the value of screening for neuroblastoma at age 3 weeks, 6 months or 12 months of age.[125,126] These studies emphasize that screening programmes overdiagnose neuroblastoma, but that the overdiagnosis rate represents children who had neuroblastoma but who would not benefit from earlier detection or treatment.

KEY POINTS

- CSF normal ranges of β-hCG and AFP require better characterization, especially in the neonatal age range. These data will become increasingly important in the diagnosis and monitoring of patients with intracranial germ cell tumours.
- Can abnormal serum and/or CSF AFP and/or β-hCG substitute for tissue diagnosis in patients with unequivocal radiological evidence of suspected intracranial germ cell tumours? The diagnostic value of s-kit, the soluble form of the proto-oncogene c-*kit* in the CSF and serum of patients with intracranial germinomas without elevations of AFP or β-hCG is currently under investigation.
- Clinical studies correlating the rate of fall of tumour markers with survival are indicated. Prospective collection of serial tumour marker data in response to treatment is to be incorporated into current international CNS germ cell studies.
- Is there a role for neuroblastoma screening in healthy infants: USA versus European perspective? The balance in this debate appears to have swung away from widespread support for community screening of all infants in the absence of evidence of a significant change in mortality and because of evidence that many of the tumours detected in screening programmes demonstrate biological markers more commonly associated with an excellent prognosis.
- Can the sensitivity and specificity of tumour markers be improved by using molecular and immunological methods on fresh or fixed tissue rather than less precise serum markers?
- A new era of biological and molecular prognostic factors has arrived and the methods commonly used during the past 20–30 years are likely to be overtaken, although availability and cost will become a health care issue.

REFERENCES

1. Hirszfeld L, Halber W. Untersuchungen über Verwandtschaftsreaktionen Zwischen Embryonal – und Krebsgewebe. I Mitteilung. Rattenembryonen und Menschentumoren. *Z Immunitätsforsch* 1932; **75**: 193–208.
2. Bergstrand CG, Czar B. Demonstration of a new protein fraction in serum from the human fetus. *Scand J Clin Lab Invest* 1956; **8**: 174.
3. Abelev GI, Perova SD, Khramkova NI *et al.* Production of embryonal alpha-globulin by the transplantable mouse hepatomas. *Transplantation* 1963; **1**: 174–80.
4. Tatarinov YS. Detection of embryospecific alpha-globulin in the blood sera of patients with primary liver tumours. *Vop Med Khim* 1964; **10**: 90–1.
5. Nishi S. Isolation and characterization of a human fetal α-globulin from the sera of fetuses and a hepatoma patient. *Cancer Res* 1970; **30**: 2507–13.
6. Alpert E, Drysdale JW, Isselbacher KJ *et al.* Isolation, characterization and demonstration of microheterogeneity. *J Biol Chem* 1972; **247**: 3792–8.
7. Ruoslahti E, Seppälä M. α-Fetoprotein in cancer and fetal development. *Adv Cancer Res* 1979; **29**: 275–346.
♦8. Gitlin D, Perricelli A, Gitlin GM. Synthesis of α-fetoprotein by liver, yolk sac and gastrointestinal tract of the human conceptus. *Cancer Res* 1972; **32**: 979–82.
9. Brock DJ, Scrimgeour JB, Nelson MM. Amniotic fluid alpha fetoprotein measurements in the early diagnosis of central nervous system disorders. *Clin Genet* 1975; **7**: 163–9.
10. Gitlin D. Normal biology of α fetoprotein. *Ann NY Acad Sci* 1975; **259**: 7–16.
●11. Wu JT, Book L, Sudar K. Serum alpha fetoprotein (AFP) levels in normal infants. *Pediatr Res* 1981; **15**: 50–2.
12. Masseyeff R, Gilli J, Krebs B *et al.* Evolution of α-fetoprotein serum levels throughout life in humans and rats, and during pregnancy in the rat. *Ann NY Acad Sci* 1975; **259**: 17.
13. Gitlin D, Boseman M. Serum AFP, albumin and G-globulin in the human conceptus. *J Clin Invest* 1966; **45**: 1826–38.
14. Walhof CM, Van Sonderen L, Voûte PA, Delemarre JFM. Half-life of alpha-fetoprotein in patients with a teratoma, endodermal sinus tumor or hepatoblastoma. *Pediatr Hematol Oncol* 1988; **5**: 217–27.

◆15. Schneider DT, Calaminus G, Gobel U. Diagnostic value of alpha₁-fetoprotein and beta-human chorionic gonadotrophin in infancy and childhood. *Pediatr Hematol Oncol* 2001; **18**: 11–26.

16. Masopust J, Radl J, Houstek J. Occurrence of alpha-1-fetoprotein in some infants suffering from hepatopathy. *Protides Biol Fluids* 1970; **18**: 239–42.

17. Waldmann TA, McIntire KR. Serum AFP levels in patients with ataxia telangiectasia. *Lancet* 1972; **2**: 1112–15.

18. Belanger C, Belanger M, Larochelle J. Existence of d'alpha-foetoprotein circulate chez 8 patients sonffrant de tyrosinemia hereditare. *Tame* 1972; **101**: 877–8.

19. Bloomer JR, Waldmann TA, McIntire KR, Klatskin G. α-Fetoprotein in nonneoplastic hepatic disorders. *J Am Med Assoc* 1975; **233**: 38–41.

20. Kew MC, Purves LR, Bersohn I. Serum alpha-fetoprotein levels in acute viral hepatitis. *Gut* 1973; **14**: 939–42.

21. Alpert E, Starzl TE, Schur PH, Isselbacher J. Serum AFP in hepatoma patients after liver transplantation. *Gastroenterology* 1971; **61**: 144–8.

●22. Rosen SW, Weintraub DB, Vaitukaitis JL *et al.* Placental proteins and their subunits as tumor markers. *Ann Intern Med* 1975; **82**: 71–83.

23. Vaitukaitis JL, Braunstein GD, Ross GT. A radioimmunassay which specifically measures human chorionic gonadotrophin in the presence of human luteinizing hormone. *Am J Obstet Gynecol* 1972; **113**: 751–8.

24. Zarate A, MacGregor C. Beta subunit hCG and the control of trophoblastic disease. *Semin Oncol* 1982; **9**: 187–90.

25. Teilum G. Classification of endodermal sinus tumour (mesoblastoma vitellinum) and so-called 'embryonal carcinoma' of the ovary. *Acta Pathol Microbiol Scand* 1965; **64**: 407–29.

◆26. Dehner LP. Gonadal and extragonadal germ cell neoplasia of childhood. *Hum Pathol* 1983; **14**: 493–511.

27. Sharry A, Janzer RC, Von Hochstelter AR *et al.* Primary intracranial germ-cell tumours – a clinicopathologic study of 14 cases. *J Neurosurg* 1985; **62**: 826.

28. Javadpour N. The role of biologic tumor markers in testicular cancer. *Cancer* 1980; **45**: 1755–61.

29. Packer RJ, Sutton LN, Rorke LB *et al.* Intracranial embryonal cell carcinoma. *Cancer* 1984; **54**: 520–4.

30. Huntington RW, Bullock WK. Yolk sac tumors of extragonadal origin. *Cancer* 1970; **25**: 1368–76.

◆31. Green DM. The diagnosis and treatment of yolk sac tumors in infants and children. *Cancer Treat Rev* 1983; **10**: 265–88.

32. Uctzelsen CL, Bruninga G. Infantile choriocarcinoma. A characteristic syndrome. *J Pediatr* 1968; **73**: 374–8.

33. Edwards MSB, Davis RL, Laurent JP. Tumor markers and cytologic features of cerebrospinal fluid. *Cancer* 1985; **56**(Suppl): 1773–7.

34. Allen JC, Nisselbaum J, Epstein F *et al.* Alpha-fetoprotein and human chorionic gonadotrophin determination in cerebrospinal fluid. An aid to the diagnosis and management of intracranial germ-cell tumors. *J Neurosurg* 1979; **51**: 368–74.

35. Pinkerton CR, Pritchard J, Spitz L. High complete response rate in children with advanced germ cell tumours using cisplatin–containing combination chemotherapy. *J Clin Oncol* 1986; **4**: 194–9.

36. Alagille D, Odievre M. Liver and biliary tract disease in children. New York: John Wiley, 1979; 311.

37. Weinberg AG, Feinegold MJ. Primary hepatic tumors in childhood. *Hum Pathol* 1983; **14**: 512–37.

38. Mahour GH, Wogu GV, Siegal SE, Isaacs H. Improved survival in infants and children with primary malignant liver tumors. *Am J Surg* 1983; **146**: 236–40.

39. McArthur JW, Toll GD, Russfeld AB *et al.* Sexual precocity attributable to ectopic gonadotropin secretion by hepatoblastoma. *Am J Med* 1973; **54**: 390–403.

40. Murthy ASK, Vawter GF, Lee ABH *et al.* Hormonal bioassay of gonadotropin producing hepatoblastoma. *Arch Pathol Lab Med* 1980; **104**: 513–17.

41. Nakagawara A, Ikeda K, Tsuneyoshi M *et al.* Hepatoblastoma producing both alpha-fetoprotein and human chorionic gonadotropin. *Cancer* 1985; **56**: 1636–42.

42. Exelby PR, Filler RM, Grosfeld JL. Liver tumors in children with particular reference to hepatoblastoma and hepatocellular carcinoma. American Academy of Pediatrics Surgical Section Survey 1974. *J Pediatr Surg* 1974; **10**: 329–37.

43. Lack EE, Neave C, Vawter GF. Hepatocellular carcinoma. Review of 32 cases of childhood and adolescence. *Cancer* 1983; **52**: 1510–15.

44. Ohaki Y, Misugi K, Sasaki Y, Tsunoda A. Hepatitis B surface antigen positive hepatocellular carcinoma in children. Report of a case and review of the literature. *Cancer* 1983; **51**: 822–8.

45. Maltz C, Lightdale CJ, Winawer SJ. Hepatocellular carcinoma. New directions in etiology. *Am J Gastroenterol* 1980; **74**: 361–5.

46. Paradinas FJ, Melia WM, Wilkinson ML *et al.* High serum vitamin B12 binding capacity as a marker of the fibrolamellar variant of hepatocellular carcinoma. *Br Med J* 1982; **285**: 840–2.

●47. Wheeler K, Pritchard J, Luck W, Rossiter M. Transcobalamin I as a 'marker' for fibrolamellar hepatoma. *Med Pediatr Oncol* 1986; **14**: 227–9.

48. McIntire KR, Waldmann TA, Moertel CG, Go VLW. Serum α-fetoprotein in patients with neoplasms of the gastrointestinal tract. *Cancer Res* 1975; **35**: 991–6.

49. Vaitukaitis JL, Ross GT, Braunstein GD, Rayford PL. Gonadotropins and their subunits: basic and clinical studies. *Recent Prog Horm Res* 1976; **32**: 289–331.

50. Kahn CR, Rosen SW, Weintraub BD *et al.* Ectopic production of chorionic gonadotropin and its subunits by islet cell tumors. *N Engl J Med* 1977; **297**: 565–9.

51. Gailani S, Chu TM, Nussbaum A *et al.* Human chorionic gonadotrophins (hCG) in non-trophoblastic neoplasms. *Cancer* 1976; **38**: 1684–6.

52. Tormey DC, Waalkes TP, Snyder JJ, Simon RM. Biological markers in breast carcinoma II. Clinical correlations with human chorionic gonadotrophin. *Cancer* 1977; **39**: 2391–6.

53. Mautalen CA. Circadian rhythm of urinary total and free hydroxyproline excretion and its relation to creatinine excretion. *J Lab Clin Med* 1970; **75**: 8–11.

54. Soldin SJ, Hill JG. Liquid chromatographic analysis for urinary 4-hydroxy-3-methoxymandelic acid and 4-hydroxy-3-methoxyphenylacetic acid, and its use in the investigation of neural crest tumours. *Clin Chem* 1981; **27**: 503–4.

55. Gitlow SE, Bertani LM, Rausen A *et al.* Diagnosis of neuroblastoma by qualitative and quantitative determination

of catecholamine metabolites in urine. *Cancer* 1970; **25**: 1377–83.

56. Tuchman M, Morris CL, Ramnaraine ML *et al.* Value of random urinary homovanillic acid and vanillylmandelic acid levels in the diagnosis and management of patients with neuroblastoma. Comparison with 24-hour urine collections. *Pediatrics* 1985; **75**: 324–8.

57. Kellie SJ, Clague AE, McGeary HM, Smith PJ. The value of catecholamine metabolite determination on untimed urine collections in the diagnosis of neural crest tumours in children. *Aust Paediatr J* 1986; **22**: 313–15.

58. Feldman JM, Lee EM, Castleberry CA. Catecholamine and serotonin content of foods: effect on urinary excretion of homovanillic acid and 5-hydroxyindoleacetic acid. *J Am Diet Assoc* 1987; **87**: 1031–3.

59. Muscettola G, Wehr T, Goodwin FK. Effect of diet on urinary MHPG excretion in depressed patients and normal control subjects. *Am J Psychiatry* 1997; **134**: 914–16.

60. Rayfield EJ, Cain JP, Casey MP *et al.* Influence of diet on urinary VMA excretion. *J Am Med Assoc* 1972; **221**: 704–5.

61. Weetman RM, Rider PS, Oei TO *et al.* Effect of diet on urinary excretion of VMA, HVA, metanephrine, and total free catecholamine in normal preschool children. *J Pediatr* 1976; **88**: 46–50.

62. Potezny N, Rosenblatt AL. The effects of various dietary constituents on the urinary excretion of biogenic amines and their metabolites. In: Sampson DC, ed. *The Clinical Biochemist.* AACB Monograph. Dee Why, Australia: AACB Publications, 1986; 52–3.

63. Rosano TG. Liquid-chromatographic evaluation of age-related changes in the urinary excretion of free catecholamines in pediatric patients. *Clin Chem* 1984; **30**: 301–3.

64. Earl J. Measurement of the acidic metabolites of biogenic amines. In: Sampson DC, ed. *The Clinical Biochemist.* Monograph. Dee Why, Australia: AACB Publications, 1986; 57–62.

65. Brewster MA, Berry DH, Moriarty M. Urinary 3-methoxy-4-hydroxyphenylacetic (homovanillic) and 3-methoxy-4-hydroxymandelic (vanillylmandelic) acids: gas-liquid chromatographic methods and experience with 13 cases of neuroblastoma. *Clin Chem* 1977; **23**: 2247–9.

66. Kaser H. Catecholamine-producing neural tumors other than pheochromocytoma. *Pharmacol Rev* 1965; **18**: 659–64.

67. Hinterberger H, Bartholomew RJ. Catecholamines and their acidic metabolites in urine and in tumour tissue in neuroblastoma, ganglioneuroma and phaechromocytoma. *Clin Chim Acta* 1969; **23**: 169–75.

68. LaBrosse EH, Com-Nougué C, Zucker J-M *et al.* Urinary excretion of 3-methoxy-4-hydroxymandelic acid and 3-methoxy-4-hydroxyphenylacetic acid by 288 patients with neuroblastoma and neural crest tumors. *Cancer Res* 1980; **40**: 1995–2001.

69. Laug WE, Siegel SE, Shaw KNF *et al.* Initial urinary catecholamine metabolite concentrations and prognosis in neuroblastoma. *Pediatrics* 1978; **62**: 77–83.

70. Gitlow SE, Bertain LM, Wilk E *et al.* Excretion of catecholamine metabolites by children with familial dysautonomia. *Pediatrics* 1970; **46**: 513–22.

71. Schuman AJ, Alario AJ, Pitel PA. Occult gangioneuroma with diarrhea: localization by venous catecholamines. *Med Pediatr Oncol* 1984; **12**: 93–6.

72. Boomsma F, Ausema L, Hakvoort-Cammel FGA *et al.* Combined measurements of plasma aromatic L-amino acid decarboxylase and DOPA as tumour markers in diagnosis and follow-up of neuroblastoma. *Eur J Cancer Clin Oncol* 1989; **25**: 1045–52.

73. Stenstrom G, Sjogren B, Waldenstrom J. Excretion of adrenalin, noradrenaline, vanilmandelic acid and metanephrins in 64 patients with phaeochromaytoma. *Acta Med Scand* 1983; **214**: 145–52.

74. Anderson A, Bergdahl L. Carcinoid tumors of the appendix in children: a report of 25 cases. *Acta Chir Scand* 1977; **143**: 173–5.

75. Sampson D. Biochemical methods for diagnosis of carcinoid tumour: what should we really be measuring? *Clin Biochem Rev* 1987; **8**: 87–94.

76. Odelstad L, Pahlman S, Lackgren G *et al.* Neurone-specific enolase: a marker for differential diagnosis of neuroblastoma and Wilms' tumour. *J Pediatr Surg* 1982; **17**: 381–5.

●77. Zeltzer PM, Marangos PJ, Evans AE, Schneider SL. Serum neuron-specific enolase in children with neuroblastoma. Relationship to stage and disease course. *Cancer* 1986; **57**: 1230–4.

●78. Cooper EH, Pritchard J, Bailey CC, Ninane J. Serum neuron-specific enolase in children's cancer. *Br J Cancer* 1987; **56**: 65–7.

79. Kawata M, Sekiya S, Hatakeyama R, Takamizawa H. Neuron-specific enolase as a serum marker for immature teratoma and dysgerminoma. *Gynecol Oncol* 1989; **32**: 191–7.

80. Takashi M, Haimoto H, Tanaka J *et al.* Evaluation of gamma-enolase as a tumor marker for renal cell carcinoma. *J Urol* 1989; **141**: 830–4.

81. Touitou Y, Heshmati HM. Neurone-specific enolase in medullary thyroid carcinoma. *Clin Chem* 1988; **34**: 2375–6.

82. Feldenzer JA, McKeever PE. Selective localization of gamma-enolase in stromal cells of cerebellar hemangioblastomas. *Acta Neuropathol (Berl)* 1987; **72**: 281–5.

83. Burger PC, Grahmann FC, Bliestle A, Kleihues P. Differentiation in the medulloblastoma. A histological and immunohistochemical study. *Acta Neuropathol (Berl)* 1987; **73**: 115–23.

84. Jacobi C, Reiber H. Clinical relevance of increased neuron-specific enolase concentration in cerebrospinal fluid. *Clin Chim Acta* 1988; **177**: 49–54.

♦85. Rao BN, Pratt CB, Fleming ID *et al.* Colon carcinoma in children and adolescents: a review of thirty cases. *Cancer* 1985; **55**: 1322–6.

86. Pratt CB, Rivera G, Shanks E *et al.* Colorectal carcinoma in adolescents – implications regarding etiology. *Cancer* 1977; **40**(Suppl): 2464–72.

87. Felberg NT, Michelson JB, Shields JA. CEA family syndrome. Abnormal carcinoembryonic antigen (CEA) levels in asymptomatic retinoblastoma family members. *Cancer* 1976; **37**: 1397–402.

88. Mann JR, Lakin GE, Leonard JC *et al.* Clinical applications of serum carcinoembryonic antigen and alpha-fetoprotein levels in children with solid tumours. *Arch Dis Child* 1978; **53**: 366–74.

89. Maeda M, Tozuka S, Kanayama M, Uchida T. Hepatocellular carcinoma producing carcinoembryonic antigen. *Dig Dis Sci* 1988; **33**: 1629–31.

90. Sculier JP, Body JJ, Jacobowitz D, Fruhling J. Value of CEA determination in biological fluids and tissues. *Eur J Cancer Clin Oncol* 1987; **23**: 1091–3.

91. Melia WM, Johnson PJ, Carter S *et al*. Plasma carcinoembryonic antigen in the diagnosis and management of patients with hepatocellular carcinoma. *Cancer* 1981; **48**: 1004–8.

92. Howell RE, Handlers JP, Aberle AM *et al*. CEA immunoreactivity in odontogenic tumors and keratocysts. *Oral Surg Oral Med Oral Pathol* 1988; **66**: 576–80.

93. Pui C-H, Ip SH, Kung P *et al*. High serum interleukin-2 receptor levels are related to advanced disease and a poor outcome in childhood non-Hodgkin's lymphoma. *Blood* 1987; **70**: 624–8.

94. Wagner DK, Kiwanuka J, Edwards BK *et al*. Soluble interleukin-2 receptor levels in patients with undifferentiated and lymphoblastic lymphomas: correlation with survival. *J Clin Oncol* 1987; **5**: 1262–74.

♦95. Pui C-H, Ip SH, Iflah S, *et al*. Serum interleukin-2 receptor levels in childhood acute lymphoblastic leukemia. *Blood* 1988; **71**: 1135–7.

♦96. Pui C-H, Ip SH, Thompson E *et al*. High serum interleukin-2 receptor levels correlate with a poor prognosis in children with Hodgkin's disease. *Leukemia* 1989; **3**: 481–4.

97. Kloster BE, John PA, Miller LE *et al*. Soluble interleukin-2 receptors are elevated in patients with AIDS or at risk of developing AIDS. *Clin Immunol Immunopathol* 1987; **45**: 440–6.

98. Carmel R, Eisenberg L. Serum vitamin B_{12} and transcobalamin abnormalities in patients with cancer. *Cancer* 1977; **40**: 1348–53.

99. Collier NA, Weinbren K, Broom SG *et al*. Neurotensin secretion by fibrolamellar carcinoma of the liver. *Lancet* 1984; **1**: 538–40.

100. Fossel ET, Carr JM, McDonagh J. Detection of malignant tumours. Water-suppressed proton nuclear magnetic resonance spectroscopy of plasma. *N Engl J Med* 1986; **315**: 1369–76.

101. Berger S, Pflüger K-H, Etzel WA, Fischer J. Detection of tumours with nuclear magnetic resonance spectroscopy of plasma. *Eur J Cancer Clin Oncol* 1989; **25**: 535–43.

102. Wilding P, Senior MB, Innbushi T, Ludwick ML. Assessment of proton nuclear magnetic resonance spectroscopy for detection of malignancy. *Clin Chem* 1988; **34**: 505–11.

103. Watcher H, Hausen A, Grassmayr K. Erhote Ausscheidung von Neopterin im Harn von Patienten mit Malignen Tumoren und mit Viruserkrankungen. *Hoppe Seylers Z Physiol Chem* 1979; **360**: 1957–60.

104. Abate G, Comella P, Marfella A *et al*. Prognostic relevance of urinary neopterin in non-Hodgkin's lymphomas. *Cancer* 1989; **63**: 484–9.

●105. Ruibal A, Encabo G, Martinez-Miralles E *et al*. CA-125 serum levels in non-malignant pathologies. *Bull Cancer* (*Paris*) 1984; **71**: 145–8.

106. Pittaway DE, Foyez JA. Serum CA-125 antigen levels increase during menses. *Am J Obstet Gynecol* 1987; **156**: 75.

●107. Herlyn M, Sears HF, Steplewski Z *et al*. Monoclonal antibody detection of a circulating tumor associated antigen. I.

Presence of antigen in sera of patients with colorectal, gastric and pancreatic carcinoma. *J Clin Immunol* 1982; **2**: 135–41.

108. Touitou Y, Bogdan A. Tumor markers in non-malignant diseases. *Eur J Cancer Clin Oncol* 1988; **24**: 1083–91.

109. Bacci G, Avella M, McDonald D *et al*. Serum lactate dehydrogenase (LDH) as a tumor marker in Ewing's sarcoma. *Tumori* 1988; **74**: 649–55.

110. Quin JJ, Altman AJ, Frantz CN. Serum lactic dehydrogenase: an indicator of tumor activity in neuroblastoma. *J Pediatr* 1980; **97**: 88–91.

111. Link MP, Shuster JJ, Goorin AM *et al*. Adjuvant chemotherapy in the treatment of osteosarcoma: Results of the Multi-Institutional Osteosarcoma Study. In: Ryan JR, Baker LH, eds. *Recent Concepts in Sarcoma Treatment*. Proceedings of the International Symposium on Sarcomas. Dordrecht: Kluwer Academic, 1988.

112. Von Eyben FE, Blaabjerg O, Petersen PH *et al*. Serum lactate dehydrogenase isoenzyme 1 as a marker of testicular germ cell tumor. *J Urol* 1988; **140**: 986–90.

113. Liddell RHA, Meyer WH, Dodge RK *et al*. Prognostic indicators for patients with osteosarcoma (OS) treated with adjuvant chemotherapy. *Proc Am Assoc Clin Res* 1988; **29**: 226.

114. Hann H-WL, Levy HM, Evans AE. Serum ferritin as a guide to therapy in neuroblastoma. *Cancer Res* 1980; **40**: 1411–13.

115. Sawada T, Kidowaki T, Sakamoto I *et al*. Neuroblastoma. Mass screening for early detection and its prognosis. *Cancer* 1984; **53**: 2731–5.

116. Nishi M, Miyake H, Takeda T *et al*. Effects of the mass screening of neuroblastoma in Sapporo City. *Cancer* 1987; **60**: 433–6.

117. Naito H, Sasaki M, Yamashiro K *et al*. Improvement in prognosis of neuroblastoma through mass population screening. *J Pediatr Surg* 1990; **25**: 245–8.

118. Hayashi Y, Inaba T, Hanada R, Yamamoto K. Chromosome findings and prognosis in 15 patients with neuroblastoma found by VMA mass screening. *J Pediatr* 1988; **112**: 567–71.

●119. Look AT, Hayes A, Nitschke R *et al*. Cellular DNA content as a predictor of response to chemotherapy in infants with unresectable neuroblastoma. *N Engl J Med* 1984; **311**: 231–5.

120. Tuchman M, Lemieux B, Avray-Blias C *et al*. Screening for neuroblastoma at 3 weeks of age: methods and preliminary results from the Quebec Neuroblastoma Screening Project. *Pediatrics* 1990; **86**: 765–73.

121. Carlsen NLT. How frequent is spontaneous remission of neuroblastomas? Implications for screening. *Br J Cancer* 1990; **61**: 441–6.

122. Pritchard J, Barnes J, Germond S *et al*. Stage and urinary catecholamine metabolite excretion in neuroblastoma. *Lancet* 1989; **2**: 514–15.

123. Sawada T, Nakata T, Takasugi N *et al*. Mass screening for neuroblastoma in infants in Japan. *Lancet* 1984; **2**: 271–3.

124. Matsumoto M, Anazawa A, Zuzuki K *et al*. Urine mass screening for neuroblastoma by high performance liquid chromatography (HPLC). *Pediatr Res* 1985; **19**: 625.

●125. Schilling FH, Spix C, Berthold F *et al*. Neuroblastoma screening at one year of age. *N Engl J Med* 2002; **346**: 1047–53.

●126. Woods WG, Gao R-N, Shuster JJ *et al*. Screening of infants due to neuroblastoma. *N Engl J Med* 2002; **346**: 1041–6.

10

Design and role of clinical trials

RICHARD SPOSTO

INTRODUCTION

A clinical trial is 'any form of planned experiment which involves patients and is designed to elucidate the most appropriate treatment of future patients with a given medical condition'.[1] This concise definition encompasses several types of clinical trial, each differing in their objectives, complexity, target population, duration and number of patients, but all of which are necessary to advance the understanding of the prognosis and treatment of paediatric cancer. Clinical trials are usually classified as phase I, phase II or phase III. In their simplest form, phase I trials are preliminary studies of new single agents or combination treatments to establish a maximum tolerated dose (MTD); phase II trials look for preliminary evidence of efficacy of the drug or combination at the MTD using short-term or surrogate efficacy end-points; and phase III trials provide evidence of (lack of) efficacy compared with a control or standard treatment based on long-term efficacy end-points. Very often, there are advantages to combining the objectives and features of more than one of these traditional types into a single trial, so that a trial cannot be so simply classified. However, it is useful to discuss clinical trials within this traditional framework.

The important issues in the design and analysis of clinical trials in adult and paediatric cancer are similar, and have been discussed extensively in the statistical and medical literature.[2–24] There are additional challenges in the design of clinical trials in childhood paediatric cancer. Many paediatric cancers are rare, so that adequately sized studies are not possible in a single institution, but rather must be conducted through large cooperative groups, such as the United Kingdom Children's Cancer Study Group (UKCCSG), the French Society of Pediatric Oncology (SFOP) and the Children's Oncology Group (COG) in the United States. Cancers such as medulloblastoma/ primitive neuroectodermal tumour (PNET) and neuroblastoma occur primarily in children, so that information about treatment efficacy is not available from studies already conducted in adults with similar tumours. In many childhood cancers, cures (i.e. eradication of the malignancy) are achieved in a majority of patients, but at the cost of often significant long-term morbidity.[25] As treatment efficacy improves, the objectives of clinical trials gradually shift towards reducing the morbidity of treatment while maintaining treatment efficacy.

This chapter describes the role and design of clinical trials in oncology, with an emphasis on their application to research in paediatric cancer. No attempt will be made to present a comprehensive discussion of all aspects of the design and analysis of clinical trials in paediatric oncology, but the major issues and methods in the design of clinical trials will be highlighted, and references provided to two excellent books[1,26] and numerous articles that will assist the interested reader in further examination of the subtler issues.

PHASE I TRIALS

A phase I clinical trial establishes the MTD of treatment, and the frequency and types of toxicity, using a minimum number of patients. Phase I trials precede phase II efficacy trials of treatment, which usually will use the highest dose that can be administered safely, namely the MTD.[27]

Successive cohorts of patients are enrolled in a phase I trial and treated with increasing doses of the treatment until unacceptable rates of toxicity are observed. 'Dose' can literally refer to the dose of a single therapeutic agent, but it can also refer to any successive change in dose, schedule, infusion rate, etc. of a drug, treatment modality or combination that can increase efficacy but can also increase toxicity. A dose escalation study design with well understood statistical properties ensures that a minimum number of patients are treated at inappropriately low dose levels or at unacceptably high dose levels.

In many cases, the MTD has already been determined in adults before a phase I study is performed in children, so that problems associated with under-dosing patients enrolled early in the trial are less of a concern.[27] When the MTD has not been determined in adults, accelerated escalation designs can be used to minimize the number of patients treated at presumably sub-therapeutic doses, without compromising the precision of MTD estimates or placing more patients at risk for excess toxicity.[17]

The number of patients used in phase I trials is small by design, so that the estimate of the MTD is imprecise.[28] Investigation of the toxicity of treatment at the MTD will continue in the subsequent phase II trial.

Eligible patient population

The study population for a phase I trial should include only patients who have adequate physiological status, so that the toxicities that are observed can be attributed to the treatment rather than to a patient's poor condition.[27] Since the primary goal of phase I trials is to determine a safe dose rather than to establish efficacy, it is not necessary to restrict the trial to patients with a specific histological diagnosis or tumour location, unless the toxicity of the treatment is likely to be affected by these considerations. Because phase I trials are sometimes performed without prior human data on toxicity or efficacy, they are restricted to patients for whom all known available treatments have been attempted and failed, or to newly diagnosed patients whose prognosis is known to be extremely grave because no known effective treatment exists (e.g. intrinsic brainstem glioma).

Definitions of dose–limiting toxicity and MTD

Dose-limiting toxicities (DLTs) are toxicities whose occurrence in a large fraction of patients is unacceptable. DLT should be defined explicitly and precisely as part of the study design. For example, with myelosuppressive therapy, expected haematological toxicities would typically not be considered DLTs unless they resulted in unacceptable risk

of death or unacceptable delays in therapy administration. Serious non-haematological toxicities would be included. The following definition of DLT may be applicable to many situations: 'Dose limiting toxicity (DLT) is defined as the occurrence of any of the following:

- toxic death, which is death attributable to treatment
- any grade 4 non-haematological toxicity
- any grade 3 non-haematological toxicity that does not resolve within 7 days after appropriate intervention (grade 3 nausea and vomiting is not included in this definition)
- failure to recover to absolute neutrophil count $>500/\mu L$ and platelets $>25\,000/\mu L$ within 7 days of the last dose of therapy in any cycle.'

Often, the listed toxicities are qualified with the requirement that they are possibly, probably or definitely attributable to the treatment.

There is some confusion and inconsistency in the literature and textbooks about the definition of MTD (see, for example, Smith et al.[27] and Arbuck[29]). The MTD is an unobservable population quantity that represents the dose above which the DLT rate will exceed the tolerable rate in a hypothetical, very large group of patients like those in the trial. For example, we may define the MTD as the dose at which 20 per cent of patients would experience a DLT. The study design and data collected in a phase I trial provide an estimate of the MTD. Because of statistical variation, it is possible, and in fact likely, that the estimate of the MTD will differ from the true population value of the MTD.

Standard three-patient cohort design

In the most common type of phase I study, cohorts of three to six patients are treated at each dose in a predetermined sequence of escalating doses.[30] Up to six patients are treated at each dose level, but three at a time, starting with the lowest dose level. If none of the first three patients at a dose level experiences a DLT, the next three patients are treated at the next higher dose level. If exactly one of the three experiences a DLT, the next three patients are treated with the same dose. If no further DLTs are observed, three patients are treated at the next higher dose level. However, if two or more patients experience DLTs at a dose level, the dose is reduced (if possible) and three more patients are treated (to a maximum of six). The estimated MTD is the highest dose level at which six patients are treated and no more than one patient experiences a DLT.

The estimated MTD from the standard design is *not* likely to be a dose at which DLTs occur rarely. On average, this design picks MTDs that have DLT rates of 15–20 per cent. This is illustrated in Figure 10.1, which is based on a simulation of 1000 identical phase I trials using

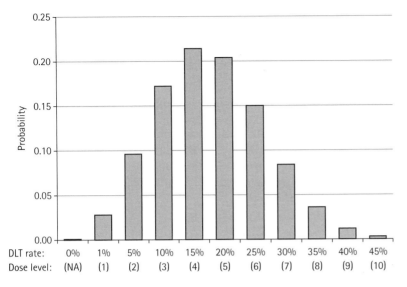

Figure 10.1 *Probability of selection of different dose levels as the maximum tolerated dose. DLT, dose-limiting toxicity; NA, not applicable.*

the standard design. The figure shows dose levels used in the trials (starting dose 1), the true DLT rates at each dose level in the target population of patients (abscissa), and the probability that different dose levels are selected as the MTD (ordinate).

Note that the modal estimate of MTD is dose level 4, which has a population DLT rate of 15 per cent. The average DLT rate of the selected MTD in these 1000 trials is 18 ± 9 per cent (mean ± SD), with DLT rates of ≥25 per cent occurring with a combined probability of 0.29, and those with rates of ≥35 per cent occurring with a probability of 0.051. Hence, if 20 per cent is the acceptable rate for the DLT, then this rule will significantly under-dose (≤10 per cent DLT rate) with a probability of 0.30, and significantly overdose (DLT rate ≥30 per cent) with a probability of 0.14. On the other hand, if 10 per cent were the highest acceptable DLT rate, then this rule would significantly overdose (≥20 per cent) with a probability of 0.49.

Other phase I designs

The above example illustrates a deficiency in the standard phase I design. Although this design is ubiquitous, simple and intuitive, its statistical rationale is weak.[16,31] One cannot target a different DLT rate even when this is desired because of the type and severity of toxicity likely to be encountered. The design also ignores the information about the MTD that is available from patients treated around the selected dose.[10] The design can also result in the treatment of many patients at therapeutically sub-optimal doses when low starting doses are required. This creates an ethical concern, since many patients go into these trials with at least some expectation of deriving therapeutic benefit from the treatment.[16] In recent years, phase I trial designs have been proposed to address many of these perceived deficiencies, including multi-stage designs[16,17,30] and continual reassessment methods (CRMs).[7,32,33] A very good comparison of the properties

of a number of proposed designs is provided by Ahn.[19] Designs where the starting dose and escalation scheme are guided by pharmacokinetic parameters have been used,[31,34–36] which is important when one considers inter-patient variability in drug metabolism and distribution, especially in the context of variable doses of steroid or other supportive care agents.

Study coordination and patient safety monitoring

The staged designs used in phase I trials ensure that no patient is treated at the next higher dose before the current dose has been reasonably demonstrated to be safe. For example, if a DLT can occur during a 3-week course of treatment or during the 2-week rest before the start of the next course, then no more than the three patients needed to fill the current cohort should be enrolled until each patient in this cohort has either been observed for the entire 5-week period or experienced a DLT. After each cohort is completed, a deliberate effort should be made to collect all relevant toxicity data, to review these data within a small committee of coordinating investigators, and decide which patients satisfy the definition of DLT. Procedures should be in place in the study coordinating office to suspend the study when all patients needed for a cohort have been enrolled, and to reopen the study only after the review committee has authorized it.

PHASE II TRIALS

Phase II trials are used to obtain preliminary evidence of treatment efficacy. Most phase II studies use a multi-stage design. An initial small cohort of patients is enrolled and treated. Enrolment of additional cohorts depends on whether sufficient numbers of tumour responses are observed in the first cohort. In this way, large numbers of patients are not exposed to obviously ineffective treatments. Designs that utilize this philosophy are described by Chang et al.[2] and Simon.[37]

Eligible patient population

Patients enrolled in phase II studies are similar to those in phase I studies, but with some exceptions. First, phase II studies target (histologically, biologically) similar tumours to establish treatment efficacy within each type. Second, when response is an end-point, patients must have (radiographically) measurable disease that can be assessed periodically to measure response to treatment.

Definition of response

The primary end-point for most phase II trials is tumour response. In the past, response has typically been defined in terms of the reduction in maximum cross-sectional area by computed tomography (CT) or magnetic resonance imaging (MRI). In the last few years, the RECIST (Response Evaluation Criteria in Solid Tumors) criteria have been proposed to simplify and standardize assessment of response. RECIST uses maximum tumour diameter, which is easier to obtain, is more reproducible and results in similar conclusions about treatment efficacy compared with cross-sectional area or tumour volume.[38–41]

In RECIST criteria, individual tumour lesions are either measurable (in at least one dimension) or nonmeasurable [e.g. positive cerebrospinal fluid (CSF) cytology, malignant pleural effusion, elevated human chorionic gonadotrophin (hCG), or other lesions that cannot be quantified but which can be described as 'positive' or 'negative']. Some or all of the measurable lesions are called 'target' lesions. The sum of the largest diameter (SLD) of the target lesions is calculated and used as the reference (baseline) measurement. All other lesions are non-target lesions and are not measured, although their presence or absence is noted. After one or more courses of treatment, the response in target lesions is defined as follows:

- complete response (CR) – complete disappearance of tumour
- partial response (PR) – 30 per cent reduction in the SLD compared with the baseline measurements
- progressive disease (PD) – 20 per cent increase in SLD compared with its smallest value during treatment, or appearance of new lesions
- stable disease (SD) – all other situations.

Non-target lesions are classified as follows:

- CR – complete disappearance

- incomplete response/SD – less than complete disappearance, no new lesions
- PD – appearance of new lesions.

The overall response to treatment is a synthesis of response in target lesions, response in non-target lesions, and the appearance of new lesions. For example, CR in both target and non-target lesions without any new lesions would be considered an overall CR, whereas CR in target lesions but incomplete response/SD in non-target lesions without new lesions would be considered overall PR. Complete details of the RECIST criteria can be found in Therasse et al.[38]

Standard two-stage design

The most common phase II study design is the two-stage design. An initial small number of patients are enrolled and treated, response is measured, and then a second cohort is enrolled provided that there is sufficient evidence that the treatment is effective in the first cohort. In order to design the study, a low response rate (p_0), which is not of interest, and a higher response rate (p_1), which is of interest, are selected. Both CR and PR are included as responses. One then devises criteria for rejecting or accepting a treatment, based on statistical principles, that have only a small chance of accepting a treatment that has poor efficacy (i.e. its response rate p is less than p_0) but a good chance of accepting a treatment with good efficacy (i.e. its response rate p is at least p_1). This is usually expressed in terms of a statistical hypothesis test:[42]

$$H_0: p \leqslant p_0 \text{ vs. } H_A: p > p_0$$

with appropriate values for the α error (type I error, false-positive) rate and β error (type II error, false-negative) rate corresponding to p_0 and p_1, respectively. Typically, $\alpha = 0.05$ and $\beta = 0.80$. However, it is hard to appreciate the properties of the design in these terms. It is best instead to consider the entire operating characteristic (i.e. power curve) of the design.

Figure 10.2 shows the operating characteristic for three different two-stage designs as described by Simon.[37] The designs were derived using the computer program OPT.[26] In this hypothetical study, a treatment that produces responses in fewer than 20 per cent of patients is considered ineffective. Therefore, all three designs have $\alpha \leqslant 0.05$ when $p_0 = 0.20$, meaning that an ineffective treatment will rarely be accepted mistakenly. Designs 1 and 2 were set so that $\beta \leqslant 0.20$ when $p_1 = 0.35$, so treatments that produce response with probability 0.35 or more will be rejected with probability $\leqslant 0.20$ (i.e. they will be accepted with probability >0.80). Both designs will accept nearly 100 per cent of treatments that have a response rate of 0.45 or more. Both will also only identify 50 per cent of treatments that have a response rate of 0.30, even though

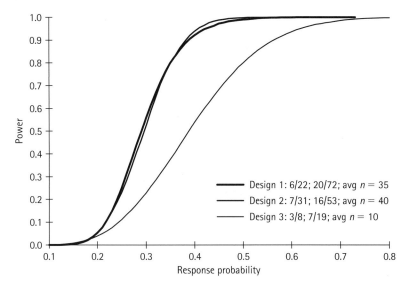

Figure 10.2 *Operating characteristics for two-stage phase II designs.*

Legend in figure:
— Design 1: 6/22; 20/72; avg $n = 35$
— Design 2: 7/31; 16/53; avg $n = 40$
— Design 3: 3/8; 7/19; avg $n = 10$

these may be of clinical interest. The designs differ in the average number of patients that will be treated.

Design 1 minimizes the average number of patients treated with poor treatments. Twenty-two patients are treated at first, then 50 more patients if at least six of these 22 respond. At least 20/72 responses are required to call the treatment effective. Design 2 minimizes the maximum number of patients treated. It requires at least 7/31 responses in the first stage, and 16/53 responses ultimately. Design 3 uses $\beta = 0.20$ when $p_1 = 0.50$. It requires many fewer patients, but as a result is less likely to accept a treatment with even a large response rate. Whereas designs 1 and 2 will identify a treatment with a 0.35 response rate 80 per cent of the time, design 3 will identify such a treatment only 40 per cent of the time.

Other phase II designs

The study design described above is appropriate when the treatment is cytotoxic, since the expected treatment effect is that the tumour shrinks. When the treatment is cytostatic (e.g. anti-angiogenesis agents, differentiation agents), neither the RECIST criteria nor this common design is appropriate.[43,44] Phase II trials of cytostatic treatments use longer-term end-points, such as time to tumour progression, and will resemble single arm screening trials that compare, for example, 1-year progression-free survival percentage to an historical or hypothetical baseline.[43,44]

In paediatric cancer, where the number of patients that are available is limited, it is important to utilize patients efficiently in phase II trials.[11] Randomized phase II trials can be used to conduct concurrent phase II evaluations of several therapies, and can also be used to screen treatment when there are more treatments to study than there are patients to evaluate them with traditional designs.[45–47] Hybrid phase I/II studies,[48] possibly with intra-patient dose escalation[49] to enhance dose intensity, and designs

which simultaneously evaluate both toxicity and efficacy end-points[3,50] are also possible.

PHASE III TRIALS

Phase III, or confirmatory, trials enrol large numbers of patients, assign them randomly to two or more treatments, and then follow them for outcome. Randomized trials minimize or eliminate bias that occurs with non-randomized, historically controlled trials or reports of case series. All patients are treated and followed in contemporary time, so that changes in patient selection criteria or referral patterns, improvements in imaging or supportive care measures, and any other factors that can affect the composition of the study cohort or the evaluation of outcome are represented equally in all treatment groups. Random allocation avoids inadvertent preferential selection of patients with better or worse prognosis for a particular treatment.

There is a continuing debate about the necessity of randomized trials to demonstrate the efficacy of new treatments.[18,51,52] Non-randomized, historically controlled trials are sometimes attractive in paediatric cancer research because these diseases are rare, and 'traditionally' sized (by adult cancer standards) phase III randomized trials could take an extraordinarily long time to complete, even in a cooperative group setting. Ironically, it is the fact that paediatric cancers are rare that can make historical controls unattractive – sufficiently large historical cohorts accumulated over many years will probably not be comparable to similarly sized cohorts treated prospectively over a similar number of years. Well designed, randomized clinical trials provide the most convincing evidence of which of several alternative treatments is best. Nevertheless, when outcome with the best available treatment is predictably grave, such as for paediatric brainstem tumours,[53] a randomized trial will be less ethically justifiable or practically feasible, since randomization to a known ineffective treatment is unattractive to patients and physicians.[54]

Eligible patient population

The patients included in a phase III trial should be those for whom the scientific question is relevant, and for whom the therapies being studied are appropriate and safe. In other ways, the patient cohort should mimic clinical practice by enrolling any patient for whom the treatments in the study would be appropriate.[55] One should never exclude patients from analysis based on events (e.g. deviations from protocol therapy, toxicity) that occur after the patient has been enrolled and the treatment has started. It is best to assume that events that occur after the start of treatment are possibly related to the treatment. To do otherwise distorts the patient population and reduces the generalizability of the study, since patients are excluded based on information that will not be available to a physician who is deciding which treatment course to take for a new patient. For example, patients who are found not to be able to tolerate an assigned treatment, and who must therefore receive a significantly modified treatment or alternative treatment, must be included because they inform about the practical efficacy of the treatment in the general population. The outcome in only those patients who can complete the therapy is irrelevant to a physician who must decide whether to use the treatment.

End-points for phase III trials

Phase III trials in paediatric cancer are almost always designed to decide which treatment can most effectively eradicate cancer. In contrast to phase I and phase II studies, where the primary end-points – toxicity and tumour response – are observed quickly, phase III trials use end-points that measure treatment effectiveness in the long term. Two common end-points for phase III trials are:

- event-free survival (EFS) – the time from start of treatment to (radiographically or pathologically) confirmed disease progression or recurrence, death from any cause, or occurrence of a second malignant neoplasm (SMN), whichever comes first
- survival (S) – the time from the start of treatment to death from any cause.

The definition of EFS includes all possible events that can be considered treatment failures, whether they are related directly to disease recurrence or indirectly to the side effects of the treatment. Non-cancer-related events are included because to exclude these would lead to biased comparisons. If one compares a 'mild' treatment that cures 50 per cent of patients with an aggressive one that results in toxic death in 16 per cent of patients but cures 60 per cent of those patients who survive the treatment, the second treatment would look superior if the toxic deaths were not counted, but would be nearly identical in terms of EFS, and would be inferior overall when one also considers the toxicity of the treatment.

Other end-points can also be used. For example, it would be important to distinguish recurrences in sites of original disease from recurrences outside of original sites, if, for example, the study involved a reduction in the dose of radiation to involved fields in the treatment of Hodgkin's disease. Specific end-points like this should be analysed as components of more general, primary end-points, such as EFS, which reflect overall treatment success.[56]

Randomization and stratification

In a randomized study, one of several treatments is assigned to patients without influence from the patient, the treating physician or the study investigators. A randomized trial cannot be ethically proposed to a patient who prefers a treatment that is available outside of the study. Nor should a physician participate who cannot recommend any of the study treatments with clinical equipoise or substantial uncertainty as to which, if any, of the treatments is better.[57–60]

The simplest way to assign treatment in a randomized trial is simple random allocation. For a two-treatment randomized trial, this is equivalent to flipping a coin and assigning 'heads' to one treatment and 'tails' to another. In practice, the coin would be replaced with a computer that generates pseudo-random numbers. Randomization between one of three treatments is achieved by generating a random number between, say, 1 and 999 inclusive and assigning treatment 1 if the number is 1–333, treatment 2 if it is 334–666, and treatment 3 otherwise. However, in most randomized trials, blocked randomization or stratified/blocked randomization is used. These methods allocate treatments so that similar numbers of patients are allocated to each treatment, and important patient characteristics are approximately balanced in all treatment groups. These schemes can simplify data presentation and increase statistical precision.[13,26]

There are several rules that should be followed in randomization. First, randomization only occurs for patients who can appropriately be treated with any of the possible treatments. Patients who cannot receive one or more of the treatments should be screened out before randomization. Second, treatment assignments are final and irrevocable. For example, if a patient is randomized in the wrong stratum (say, in the age <10 stratum as opposed to the age ≥11 stratum), there is no option to re-randomize the patient within the 'correct' stratum. (Besides, correcting the stratum is not necessary, since occasional stratum mistakes are inconsequential to the analysis.) Allowing re-randomization opens the process to manipulation that can introduce bias. Third, randomization should be performed by a central coordinating office that will screen out ineligible patients and assure unbiased treatment assignment. The archaic practices of distributing envelopes to individual centres, or allowing centres to perform their own randomizations, can be manipulated and therefore are unacceptable. Fourth, randomization should occur as closely as possible to the time when the experimental treatments differ. For treatments that differ early, the randomization can occur at the time of study entry. For treatments that differ later on (e.g. a randomization to receive radiation therapy or not after 6 months of chemotherapy for Hodgkin's disease), the randomization should also occur late in treatment. A separate screening for eligibility for randomization should be undertaken[61] (for instance, in the Hodgkin's disease example, patients with active residual disease after chemotherapy should all receive radiation therapy, and hence would not be eligible for the randomization).

Methods for survival analysis

The most commonly used statistical methods for phase III oncology clinical trials are the product limit (PL, Kaplan–Meier) estimate, the log-rank (LR) test, and Cox regression analysis. The PL estimate is used to compute the percentage of patients who survive, or survive event-free (e.g. 5-year S, or 3-year EFS, etc.). The LR test and Cox analysis are used to compare S and EFS between treatment and/or prognostic groups.[14,62] These methods are used because they correctly account for patient censoring. A patient is called 'censored' when the primary end-point has not been observed for that patient at the most recent follow-up – the patient was alive and the disease had not recurred or progressed. Censoring is common in phase III trials in paediatric oncology because many patients do not experience a treatment failure during the trial period, either because they have been cured or because they have not yet been followed long enough. Common statistical methods, such as t-tests or simple linear regression,[42] do not take censoring into account and will be misleading if used.

The LR test and Cox regression analysis are based on the simple assumption that a treatment that produces a higher S or EFS percentage in the long term will also do so at all earlier times, so that if treatment A has a higher 10-year EFS than treatment B, it will also have higher 1-, 2- and 5-year EFS. Another way to think of this is in terms of the failure rate per unit time – if treatment B results in X times more failures per month than treatment A 1 year after the start of treatment, this will also be true 2, 5 and 10 years after the start of treatment. This test is most sensitive to these so-called 'proportional hazards' (PH) differences. There may not always be compelling biological reasons to believe the PH assumption absolutely, and there are examples where it does not

hold.[63,64] However, it is usually true to the extent that use of the LR test and Cox analysis is appropriate. The term used to describe PH differences is the 'relative failure rate' (RFR). RFR is unity when two treatments are equally effective. RFR is 0.5 when one treatment results in half the failure rate of another treatment.

How big should a phase III trial be?

In statistical hypothesis testing, one asks whether the data provide evidence that a parameter (in this case RFR) is different from a hypothesized value. Typically, the null (H_0) hypothesis is the state of nature that is not of interest, and the alternative hypothesis (H_A) is of interest. For the LR test, the null and alternative hypotheses are:

$$H_0:\text{RFR} = 1 \quad \text{vs.} \quad H_A:\text{RFR} \neq 1.$$

To set up the test, a critical value is chosen, which is the LR chi-squared value above which one concludes that the treatments are different. The critical value is chosen so that the α error rate under H_0 has the desired, small value. The number of patients in the study is set so that the β error rate is sufficiently low for the smallest treatment difference of practical clinical interest. Usually, $\alpha = 0.05$ and $\beta = 0.20$. $1 - \beta$ is called the 'power' of the test.

A unique feature of the LR test is that the real determinant of the power of the test is the average number of events observed during the trial, and not the number of patients enrolled. A trial with 43 patients in each of two treatments, one with long-term EFS of 0.25 and the other with long-term EFS of 0.50, will have about the same power for RFR = 2 as a study with 185 patients per treatment with EFS rates of 0.81 and 0.90, respectively. Even though RFR = 0.5 in both cases, in absolute terms the first study detects a 0.25 difference in long-term EFS (0.50 vs. 0.25), while the second detects a 0.09 difference (0.90 vs. 0.81). (An algebraic consequence of the proportional-hazards assumption is that $\text{EFS}_B = \text{EFS}_A^{\text{RFR}}$, where EFS_B and EFS_A are the event-free survival percentages for treatments B and A, respectively, and RFR is the relative failure rate in group B compared with group A.) As a rule of thumb, for a two-sided LR test with $\alpha = 0.05$, one has to observe 70 failures during the trial to detect RFR = 0.5 with a power of 0.80, 100 events to detect RFR = 0.56, 200 events to detect RFR = 0.67, and 350 events to detect RFR = 0.75. A method for computing sample size in paediatric cancer trials, where a fraction of patients will be cured, is described by Sposto and Sather.[65]

A dilemma that sometimes occurs in rare paediatric cancers is that, even with large, multi-institutional collaborations, it may be impossible to design a trial that can be accomplished in a reasonable time (e.g. <10 years) that has a sufficient number of patients to detect the smallest difference of clinical interest with traditionally small α and β errors. The only available options in these cases seem to be:

- to conduct a large and long randomized study, the results from which may be irrelevant when the study is complete
- to perform a small randomized trial that is well controlled but has higher error rates
- to perform a single-treatment, historically controlled study that is precise but may be biased
- to conclude that the study question can never be answered adequately.

While there is no uniformly best choice, the use of small, randomized trials is a preferable strategy in situations where a good historical control series is not available.[23]

Intent-to-treat analysis

There is an accepted convention of 'intent-to-treat' analysis in randomized trials. Sometimes a patient will agree to be randomized, but after randomization will switch or be switched to another of the available treatments on the study, or the patient or physician may opt for an entirely different treatment, either because of preference or because the treatment cannot be tolerated. The 'intent-to-treat' principle says that patients who deviate or switch from the assigned treatment should be neither excluded nor censored from the analysis. They should be included in the primary analysis according to the randomly assigned treatment. This principle may seem counterintuitive, but unpredictable bias will be introduced if it is not followed. Decisions to change treatment are often influenced by factors that also influence prognosis, and excluding or censoring these patients can cause incomparability of the randomized groups.[66] A randomized trial is really a comparison of similar groups of patients treated with different initial intents but who may unavoidably deviate from the intended treatment. It is not a comparison of artificially constructed, 'pure' groups of patients who receive only the treatment exactly as described, since such groups of patients do not exist in practice.

Interim safety monitoring and criteria for early stopping

Phase III trial designs include scheduled, interim analyses to discover early, compelling evidence that one treatment is superior or inferior to the others. These interim analyses may be performed semi-annually, annually or at one or two key times during the study. Interim analyses are used to avoid the unacceptable situation where an extremely large benefit for one treatment is found that would have been obvious early in the trial if one had looked. Statistical methods have been developed to

conduct interim analyses in a way that preserves the statistical properties of the study design.[67,68]

Reduction in treatment (equivalence) trials

As treatments for paediatric cancer improve, or as homogeneous subsets of patients with better long-term prognosis are identified, the objectives of randomized trials shift from improving EFS to decreasing morbidity with minimal decrease in efficacy. These so-called 'reduction-in-therapy' or 'equivalence' trials will include primary end-points that reflect both efficacy (e.g. EFS) and morbidity (e.g. quality of life, cognitive function). These studies will be designed to protect against clear reductions in efficacy while simultaneously detecting important improvements in long-term morbidity.[24,69–71]

SOME GENERAL ISSUES IN CLINICAL TRIALS

The study protocol document

All clinical trials should be described in a protocol document. The protocol describes the objectives of the research, the rationale and background for performing the research, the details of treatment and patient management, guidelines for surgery, radiology, radiation therapy, chemotherapy, pathology and any other medical disciplines in the study. It should also describe which patients are eligible for the study, the study design, including the number of patients required, the duration of the study, the primary and secondary end-points, planned statistical analyses, interim safety monitoring rules, the data that are to be collected, and enrolment and randomization procedures. This is by no means a comprehensive list. The protocol document should contain any information that is required by physicians involved in treating or managing patients in the study, or staff involved in coordinating or administering the study, or reviewers charged with scientific, methodological, patient safety or ethical review of the study. An excellent discussion of the required contents of protocol documents can be found in Piantadosi.[26]

Data acquisition, quality assurance and security

The data needed to analyse and administer a clinical trial should be identified before the study begins. These will include data to establish eligibility, other pre-treatment data that will be used in analysis, and follow-up data that include toxicity, details of treatment administration, tumour response, disease recurrence, and follow-up and life status. The level of detail necessary in each of these categories of data depends on whether the focus of the study is toxicity (phase I), short-term efficacy (phase II) or long-term efficacy (phase III). The data collection should be parsimonious. The goal is to include only those data necessary to answer the research questions and coordinate the study. The goal is not to computerize the medical record.

One should maintain a regular schedule for reviewing and updating the trial data. For single-institution studies, a weekly or monthly review of patient charts should be conducted, and the new data entered in the database. For larger, multi-institutional studies, paper forms or, preferably, computer- or web-based data entry should be used. Computer-generated data reports should be produced at frequent intervals to identify missing or contradictory data or delinquent follow-up. It is important to keep data accurate and up to date, because an important part of the trial coordination is the protection of patient safety through periodic monitoring and analysis. Monitoring will be ineffective if the data are not current and accurate.

Data should be routinely and securely backed up. Large institutions usually have centrally administered computer networks with a sophisticated back-up system for data kept on the network. They also have firewalls to protect the network from external snooping, vandalism or computer viruses. In this kind of environment, data should be stored on the network volumes rather than on individual computer workstations to take advantage of these sophisticated protections. If a centrally administered computer environment is not available, then procedures for routine back-up, anti-virus protection and security will have to be provided on the computer or computers where the data are stored.

Guidelines for reporting the results of clinical trials

Careful, thorough, and concise reporting of the results of clinical trials is important in getting the result of the trials accepted, and in allowing others to compare the results of the trial to other research and to their own experience. Recently, detailed guidelines for the reporting of randomized clinical trials have been described (the CONSORT statement[72,73]). In addition, an excellent, detailed discussion of reporting of all types of clinical trials is given by Piantadosi.[26]

ETHICAL ISSUES IN THE CONDUCT OF CLINICAL TRIALS

The important difference between clinical trials and other types of experimental science is the involvement of humans, and the resulting requisite care on the part of the investigators to ensure that patients are fully informed of their participation in an experiment and that there are risks as well as possible benefits that derive from such participation.

Declaration of Helsinki

Virtually all countries that perform clinical trials adhere to the Declaration of Helsinki, the international agreement that outlines ethical principles in the conduct of medical research.[59,74] This agreement reaffirms the duty of physicians to safeguard the welfare of patients, to participate only in research that is scientifically sound, that is sufficiently important that benefits to society can outweigh risks to subjects, that is conducted with the full knowledge and voluntary participation of the subjects, and that is independently reviewed for adherence to accepted ethical and safety conventions. The most recent version of the declaration includes revisions designed to address the issue of randomized trials conducted in developing nations, and adds a statement that the results of the medical research must have a reasonable likelihood of benefiting the population in which the research was conducted.[74]

Institutional review board or research ethics committee

Study protocols should be reviewed by special ethical review committees that are independent of the investigators or sponsors of the research. The composition of these committees will differ depending on the laws and regulations of the country where the research is performed. The charge of this committee is to ensure that the research adheres to accepted ethical and patient safety practices. Most major institutions participating in clinical research have a standing research ethics committee that reviews all research conducted at the institutions, whether the institution has originated the research or is simply participating in it.

Informed consent

All patients should be aware that they will be participating in scientific research, that there may be risks as well as benefits to participating in this research, and that they can decline to participate in the research or withdraw from participation in the research at any time without compromising the care that they will receive. These rights should be explained to patients and their parents in person, by either the treating physician or another member of the medical team who is familiar with the research. In addition, the parents and patients should be provided with an 'informed consent' document that describes in detail, but in understandable language, the risks and benefits of participating in the research, and their rights and expectations as patients. An informed consent document should be signed by the patient or patient's guardian prior to enrolment in the study and prior to the start of any part of the treatment that can be considered experimental.[75]

Patient confidentiality

Patient confidentiality must be maintained as (or more) stringently for the data collected in clinical trials as would be the case for patients' medical records. Since clinical trial data will be reviewed and analysed by non-medical personnel (e.g. statisticians, study coordinators) who are not primarily responsible for the patient's care, the research charts should be available only to those persons who need to see them. In addition, the computerized research data should be stored without patients' names, and instead be identified with unique patient identification numbers. There will be a need to link these at times to patients' names, but the correspondence between identifiers and patients' names should be kept in a separate, secure computer file with restricted access.

Data and safety monitoring board

In randomized, phase III clinical trials, it is an accepted practice that a data and safety monitoring board (DSMB) or data monitoring committee (DMC) be constituted.[76–78] The rationale for these committees is that investigators who are directly involved in the trial are probably not in the best position impartially to evaluate the accumulating evidence as to whether or not treatments differ, and to weigh this information against the risks and benefits to future patients of continuing the trial. The membership of the DSMB should include at least several physicians who are expert in research into the treatment of paediatric cancer as well as a non-affiliated biostatistician, and may also include an expert on ethics and a lay patient advocate. The DSMB will usually meet 6-monthly or annually, depending on the study and the details of the interim statistical monitoring. Members will be provided with a detailed report of treatment toxicities and other side-effects, deaths and treatment failures that have occurred, as well as a formal interim statistical analysis of the results to date. These will be provided in a report produced by the study biostatistician, which will also include a discussion by the study's physician coordinator of problems with occurrence and management of toxicities. In most instances, the physician coordinator will be blinded to any of the interim statistical analysis. It should be said that there is not uniform agreement on the need for an independent monitoring committee.[79]

MULTIDISCIPLINARY COLLABORATION IN THE DESIGN OF CLINICAL TRIALS

As this chapter has highlighted, there are many important aspects of clinical trials that can affect the ability of the trial to answer the scientific question being posed. It is important, therefore, that the design of clinical trials be developed amid close collaboration between representatives of all medical and non-medical disciplines (e.g. surgery, pathology, radiology, biostatistics, pharmacy, nursing) that will be instrumental to the conduct of the trial, the care of patients enrolled in the trial, and the analysis and publication of results. Multidisciplinary collaboration ensures that:

- studies address well defined hypotheses and objectives
- end-points for achieving these objectives are clearly defined
- data necessary to evaluate the objectives are collected
- patients are treated and managed according to the treatment as described in the protocol
- study design is efficient
- statistical analyses provide a clear answer
- statistically valid patient safety monitoring rules are in place.

KEY POINTS

- Clinical trials in paediatric cancer share many features of trials in adults, but also are unique in several respects.
- The size, design and key end-points of a clinical trial depend on whether the primary objective is toxicity and feasibility, short-term tumour response, or long-term disease control and cure.
- The design of clinical trials in paediatric cancer should arise amid close collaboration between all of the medical and non-medical disciplines that will be instrumental in the conduct of the study, the care of patients, and the analysis and reporting of the study results.
- All clinical trials, regardless of their objectives, require scrupulous attention to protection of patient rights and to monitoring of patient safety.

REFERENCES

1. Pocock SJ. *Clinical Trials: A Practical Approach.* New York: John Wiley, 1983.

2. Chang MN, Therneau TM, Wieand HS, Cha SS. Designs for group sequential phase II clinical trials. *Biometrics* 1987; **43**: 865–74.

3. Conaway MR, Petroni GR. Bivariate sequential designs for phase II trials. *Biometrics* 1995; **51**(2): 656–64.

4. Jennison C, Turnbull BW. Sequential equivalence testing and repeated confidence-intervals, with applications to normal and binary responses. *Biometrics* 1993; **49**(1): 31–43.

5. Lin DY, Shen L, Ying Z, Breslow NE. Group sequential designs for monitoring survival probabilities. *Biometrics* 1996; **52**: 1033–41.

6. Liu PY, Dhlberg S, Crowley J. Selection designs for pilot studies based on survival. *Biometrics* 1993; **49**: 391–8.

7. O'Quigley J, Pepe M, Fisher L. Continual reassessment method: a practical design for phase 1 clinical trials in cancer. *Biometrics* 1990; **46**(1): 33–48.

8. Pocock SJ. Interim analyses for randomized clinical trials: the group sequential approach. *Biometrics* 1982; **38**(1): 153–62.

9. Slud EV. Analysis of factorial survival experiments. *Biometrics* 1994; **50**: 25–38.

10. Storer BE. Design and analysis of phase I clinical trials. *Biometrics* 1989; **45**(3): 925–37.

11. Whitehead J. Designing Phase II Studies in the context of a programme of clinical research. *Biometrics* 1985; **41**(2): 373–83.

12. Kramar A, Potvin D, Hill C. Multistage designs for phase II clinical trials: statistical issues in cancer research. *Br J Cancer* 1996; **74**(8): 1317–20.

13. Peto R, Pike MC, Armitage P *et al.* Design and analysis of randomized clinical trials requiring prolonged observation of each patient. I. Introduction and design. *Br J Cancer* 1976; **34**(6): 585–612.

14. Peto R, Pike MC, Armitage P *et al.* Design and analysis of randomized clinical trials requiring prolonged observation of each patient. II. Analysis and examples. *Br J Cancer* 1977; **35**(1): 1–39.

15. Piantadosi S, Fisher JD, Grossman S. Practical implementation of a modified continual reassessment method for dose-finding trials. *Cancer Chemother Pharmacol* 1998; **41**(6): 429–36.

16. Ratain MJ, Mick R, Schilsky RL, Siegler M. Statistical and ethical issues in the design and conduct of phase I and II clinical trials of new anticancer agents [see comments]. *J Natl Cancer Inst* 1993; **85**(20): 1637–43.

17. Simon R, Freidlin B, Rubinstein L *et al.* Accelerated titration designs for phase I clinical trials in oncology. *J Natl Cancer Inst* 1997; **89**(15): 1138–47.

18. Concato J, Shah N, Horwitz RI. Randomized, controlled trials, observational studies, and the hierarchy of research designs [see comments]. *N Engl J Med* 2000; **342**(25): 1887–92.

19. Ahn C. An evaluation of phase I cancer clinical trial designs. *Stat Med* 1998; **17**(14): 1537–49.

20. Brittain E, Wittes J. Factorial designs in clinical trials: the effects of non-compliance and subadditivity. *Stat Med* 1989; **8**: 161–71.

21. Piantadosi S, Liu G. Improved designs for dose escalation studies using pharmacokinetic measurements. *Stat Med* 1996; **15**(15): 1605–18.

22. Simes RJ. Application of statistical decision theory to treatment choices: implications for the design and analysis of clinical trials. *Stat Med* 1986; **5**: 411–50.

23. Sposto R, Stram DO. A strategic view of randomized trial design in low-incidence cancer. *Stat Med* 1999; **18**(10): 1183–97.

24. Whitehead J. Sequential designs for equivalence studies. *Stat Med* 1996; **15**: 2703–15.

25. Meadows AT. Curing cancer in children: minimizing price, maximizing value. *J Clin Oncol* 1995; **13**: 1837–9.

26. Piantadosi S. *Clinical Trials: A Methodologic Perspective.* New York: John Wiley; 1997.

27. Smith M, Bernstein M, Bleyer WA *et al.* Conduct of phase I trials in children with cancer. *J Clin Oncol* 1998; **16**(3): 966–78.

28. Christian MC, Korn EL. The limited precision of phase I trials [editorial; comment]. *J Natl Cancer Inst* 1994; **86**(22): 1662–3.

29. Arbuck SG. Workshop on phase I study design. Ninth NCI/EORTC New Drug Development Symposium, Amsterdam, March 12, 1996. *Ann Oncol* 1996; **7**(6): 567–73.

30. Korn EL, Midthune D, Chen TT *et al.* A comparison of two phase I trial designs. *Stat Med* 1994; **13**: 1799–806.

31. Mick R, Ratain MJ. Model-guided determination of maximum tolerated dose in Phase I clinical trials: evidence for increased precision. *J Natl Cancer Inst* 1993; **85**(3): 217–23.

32. Miller S. An extension of the continual reassessment methods using a preliminary up-and-down design in a dose finding study in cancer patients, in order to investigate a greater range of doses. *Stat Med* 1995; **14**(9–10): 911–22 (discussion, p. 923).

33. Rinaldi DA, Burris HA, Dorr FA *et al.* Initial phase I evaluation of the novel thymidylate synthase inhibitor, LY231514, using the modified continual reassessment method for dose escalation. *J Clin Oncol* 1995; **13**(11): 2842–50.

34. Gianni L, Vigano L, Surbone A *et al.* Pharmacology and clinical toxicity of 4′-iodo-4′-deoxydoxorubicin: an example of successful application of pharmacokinetics to dose escalation in phase I trials. *J Natl Cancer Inst* 1990; **82**(6): 469–77.

35. Collins JM, Grieshaber CK, Chabner BA. Pharmacologically guided phase I clinical trials based upon preclinical drug development. *J Natl Cancer Inst* 1990; **82**(16): 1321–6.

36. Berlin J, Stewart JA, Storer B *et al.* Phase I clinical and pharmacokinetic trial of penclomedine using a novel, two-stage trial design for patients with advanced malignancy. *J Clin Oncol* 1998; **16**(3): 1142–9.

37. Simon R. Optimal two-stage designs for phase II clinical trials. *Control Clin Trials* 1989; **10**(1): 1–10.

38. Therasse P, Arbuck SG, Eisenhauer EA *et al.* New guidelines to evaluate the response to treatment in solid tumors. European Organization for Research and Treatment of Cancer, National Cancer Institute of the United States, National Cancer Institute of Canada [see comments]. *J Natl Cancer Inst* 2000; **92**(3): 205–16.

39. James K, Eisenhauer E, Christian M *et al.* Measuring response in solid tumors: unidimensional versus bidimensional measurement [see comments]. *J Natl Cancer Inst* 1999; **91**(6): 523–8.

40. Hilsenbeck SG, Von Hoff DD. Measure once or twice – does it really matter? [editorial; comment] [see comments]. *J Natl Cancer Inst* 1999; **91**(6): 494–5.

41. Gehan EA, Tefft MC. Will there be resistance to the RECIST (Response Evaluation Criteria in Solid Tumors)? [editorial; comment]. *J Natl Cancer Inst* 2000; **92**(3): 179–81.

42. Dixon WJ, Massey FJ. *Introduction to Statistical Analysis,* 3rd edn. New York: McGraw-Hill, 1969.

43. Mick R, Crowley JJ, Carroll RJ. Phase II clinical trial design for noncytotoxic anticancer agents for which time to disease progression is the primary endpoint. *Control Clin Trials* 2000; **21**(4): 343–59.

44. Korn EL, Arbuck SG, Pluda JM *et al.* Clinical trial designs for cytostatic agents: are new approaches needed? *J Clin Oncol* 2001; **19**(1): 265–72.

45. Simon R, Wittes RE, Ellenberg SS. Randomized phase II clinical trials. *Cancer Treat Rep* 1985; **69**(12): 1375–81.

46. Strauss N, Simon R. Investigating a sequence of randomized phase II trials to discover promising treatments. *Stat Med* 1995; **14**: 1479–89.

47. Thall PF, Estey EH. A Bayesian strategy for screening cancer treatments prior to phase II clinical evaluation. *Stat Med* 1993; **12**(13): 1197–211.

48. Thall PF, Russell KE. A strategy for dose-finding and safety monitoring based on efficacy and adverse outcomes in phase I/II clinical trials. *Biometrics* 1998; **54**(1): 251–64.

49. Blaney SM, Needle MN, Gillespie A *et al.* Phase II trial of topotecan administered as 72-hour continuous infusion in children with refractory solid tumors: a collaborative Pediatric Branch, National Cancer Institute, and Children's Cancer Group Study. *Clin Cancer Res* 1998; **4**(2): 357–60.

50. Conaway MR, Petroni GR. Designs for phase II trials allowing for a trade-off between response and toxicity. *Biometrics* 1996; **52**(4): 1375–86.

51. Pocock SJ, Elbourne DR. Randomized trials or observational tribulations? [editorial; comment]. *N Engl J Med* 2000; **342**(25): 1907–9.

52. Benson K, Hartz AJ. A comparison of observational studies and randomized, controlled trials [see comments]. *N Engl J Med* 2000; **342**(25): 1878–86.

53. Mandell LR, Kadota R, Freeman C *et al.* There is no role for hyperfractionated radiotherapy in the management of children with newly diagnosed diffuse intrinsic brainstem tumors: results of a Pediatric Oncology Group phase III trial comparing conventional vs. hyperfractionated radiotherapy. *Int J Radiat Oncol Biol Phys* 1999; **43**(5): 959–64.

54. Emanuel EJ, Patterson WB. Ethics of randomized clinical trials [see comments]. *J Clin Oncol* 1998; **16**(1): 365–6 (discussion, pp. 366–71).

55. George SL. Reducing patient eligibility criteria in cancer clinical trials. *J Clin Oncol* 1996; **14**(4): 1364–70.

56. Prentice RL, Kalbfleisch JD, Peterson AV Jr *et al.* The analysis of failure times in the presence of competing risks. *Biometrics* 1978; **34**(4): 541–54.

57. Sackett DL. Uncertainty about clinical equipoise. There is another exchange on equipoise and uncertainty. *Br Med J* 2001; **322**(7289): 795–6.

58. Lilford RJ. Uncertainty about clinical equipoise. Clinical equipoise and the uncertainty principles both require further scrutiny. *Br Med J* 2001; **322**(7289): 795.

59. Lilford RJ, Djulbegovic B. Declaration of Helsinki should be strengthened. Equipoise is essential principle of human experimentation. *Br Med J* 2001; **322**(7281): 299–300.

60. Weijer C, Shapiro SH, Cranley Glass K. For and against: clinical equipoise and not the uncertainty principle is the moral underpinning of the randomised controlled trial. *Br Med J* 2000; **321**(7263): 756–8.

61. Durrleman S, Simon R. When to randomize? *J Clin Oncol* 1991; **9**(1): 116–22.

62. Kalbfleisch J, Prentice R. *The statistical analysis of failure time data.* New York: John Wiley; 1980.

63. Matthay KK, Villablanca JG, Seeger RC *et al.* Improved outcome for high risk neuroblastoma with high dose therapy and purged autologous bone marrow transplantation and with subsequent 13-cis-retinoic acid. *N Engl J Med* 1999; **341**(16): 1165–73.

64. Nesbit ME, Buckley JD, Feig SA *et al.* Chemotherapy for induction of remission of childhood acute myeloid leukemia followed by marrow transplantation or multiagent chemotherapy: A report from the Children's Cancer Group. *J Clin Oncol* 1994; **12**: 127–35.

65. Sposto R, Sather HN. Determining the duration of comparative clinical trials while allowing for cure. *J Chronic Dis* 1985; **38**(8): 683–90.

66. Lee YJ, Ellenberg JH, Hirtz DG, Nelson KB. Analysis of clinical trials by treatment actually received: is it really an option? *Stat Med* 1991; **10**(10): 1595–605.

67. Lan KK, Rosenberger WF, Lachin JM. Use of spending functions for occasional or continuous monitoring of data in clinical trials. *Stat Med* 1993; **12**(23): 2219–31.

68. Betensky RA. Conditional power calculations for early acceptance of H0 embedded in sequential tests. *Stat Med* 1997; **16**: 465–77.

69. Durrleman S, Simon R. Planning and monitoring of equivalence studies. *Biometrics* 1990; **46**: 329–36.

70. Fleming TR. Design and interpretation of equivalence trials. *Am Heart J* 2000; **139**(4): S171–6.

71. Com-Nougue C, Rodary C, Patte C. How to establish equivalence when data are censored: a randomized trial of treatments for B nonHodgkin's lymphoma. *Stat Med* 1993; **12**: 1353–64.

72. Altman DG, Begg C, Cho M *et al.* Better reporting of randomised controlled trials: the CONSORT statement [editorial] [see comments]. Improving the quality of reporting of randomized controlled trials. The CONSORT statement [see comments]. *Br Med J* 1996; **313**(7057): 570–1.

73. Begg C, Cho M, Eastwood S *et al.* Improving the quality of reporting of randomized controlled trials. The CONSORT statement [see comments]. *J Am Med Assoc* 1996; **276**(8): 637–9.

74. Reynolds T. Declaration of Helsinki revised. *J Natl Cancer Inst* 2000; **92**(22): 1801–3.

75. Grossman SA, Piantadosi S, Covahey C. Are informed consent forms that describe clinical oncology research protocols readable by most patients and their families? *J Clin Oncol* 1994; **12**(10): 2211–15.

76. Wittes J. Behind closed doors: the data monitoring board in randomized clinical trials. *Stat Med* 1993; **12**(5–6): 419–24.

77. Whitehead J. On being the statistician on a data and safety monitoring board. *Stat Med* 1999; **18**(24): 3425–34.

78. DeMets DL, Pocock SJ, Julian DG. The agonising negative trend in monitoring of clinical trials. *Lancet* 1999; **354**(9194): 1983–8.

79. Harrington D, Crowley J, George SL *et al.* The case against independent monitoring committees. *Stat Med* 1994; **13**(13–14): 1411–14.

PART 2

Diagnosis and management of individual cancers

11

Acute myeloid leukaemia

MARRY VAN DEN HEUVEL-EIBRINK

INTRODUCTION

Acute myeloid leukaemia (AML) is a clonal disease that is characterized by a maturation arrest during the differentiation of the haemopoietic cells to normal mature myeloid blood cells.[1–3] AML includes a heterogeneous group of disorders of which the diversity is characterized by differences in morphological, immunophenotypic and genotypic features. In childhood, AML is a rare disease, with an incidence of 1–3 per 100 000 persons each year. In most countries, it accounts for 15–20 per cent of childhood leukaemias, although there are exceptions, such as Japan and some parts of Africa, where AML seems to be more common than acute lymphoblastic leukaemia (ALL) during childhood.[4,5]

At present, the cause of AML is not known. In adults, some environmental factors have consistently been linked to the origin of the disease, i.e. exposure to radiation, alkylating agents, chronic benzene exposure and cigarette smoking, and also exposure to radioactive irradiation as illustrated by long-term survival studies of those exposed to the atomic bomb.[6–16] Leukaemia is the result of a multi-step malignant transformation of a haematological clone in the bone marrow, and several hits, which in children may even start *in utero*, are necessary to develop AML.[17–23] Over the past decades, treatment results have improved markedly. Several groups have reported a 80–90 per cent complete remission (CR) rate after intensive induction chemotherapy, resulting in 50–60 per cent disease-free survival (Table 11.1).[24–34] This chapter outlines

Table 11.1 *Outcome in recent paediatric acute myeloid leukaemia studies*

Reference	Study	Accrual period	Patients (*n*)	Age (years)	CR rate (%)	pEFS (5 year)	pDFS* (5 year)	pOS (5 year)
Amadori et al.[30]	AIOEP-LAME87	1987–90	161	<14	79	25	31	42
Lie et al.[24,54]	NOPHO93	1993–2000	219	<18	91	49 (7 year)	54 (7 year)	64 (7 year)
Chang et al.[29,35]	POG 8821	1988–93	560	<21	85	32 (4 year)	NS	NS
Webb et al.[33]	MRC10/12	1988–2000	698	<15	92	52	58	61
Woods et al.[27,57]	CCG 2891	1989–93	887	<21	74	27–42 (3 year)	37–55	42–52 (3 year) from CR
Creutzig et al.[53,65]	BFM93	1993–98	471	<17	82	51	62	60
Perel et al.[184]	LAME89/91	1988–96	268	<20	90	48 (6 year)	53	60 (6 year)
Krance et al.[189]	St. Judes AML-91	1991–96	73	<21	78	40	NS	NS
Behar et al.[25]	EORTC	1988–91	108	<18	77	41 (3 year)	52 (3 year)	56 (3 year)

*From CR rate.

CR, complete remission; DFS, disease-free survival; EFS, event-free survival; NS, not specified; OS, overall survival.

the diagnostic issues, prognostic factors and current treatment modalities for children with AML.

DIAGNOSTIC ISSUES

The clinical presentation of AML is determined by leukaemic infiltration of the bone marrow, which causes a reduction in the number and impairment of the function of the blood cells from the three haemopoietic cell lines. The presenting symptoms may be non-specific and usually include anaemia, fever, infections and haemorrhagic diathesis. Extramedullary leukaemic infiltration is reported in 4–10 per cent in the central nervous system (CNS).[24,28,30,33,35,36] Also, infiltration of the liver, spleen and lymph nodes is reported in a variable number of patients. Infiltration of the skin is mainly found in infants and/or patients with monocytic subtypes of AML.

The morphological classification used until recently is the French-American-British (FAB) classification described by Bennet et al.[37] It distinguishes FAB types M0–7 by morphological and histochemical characteristics. For initial cytochemical staining of peripheral blood and bone marrow slides, myeloperoxidase (MPO) and Sudan black B (SBB) are valuable, which stain negative in ALL and positive in M1–4 and some M5 cases. Non-specific esterase differentiates between M4 and M5 cases, as it stains monoblasts selectively (see also Chapter 4). The immunophenotype represents the stage at which the maturation arrest has occurred during haemopoietic development. The panmyeloid markers CD13 and CD33 are expressed in more than 90 per cent of paediatric AML patients. AML M7 (megakaryoblastic leukaemia) often shows CD41 and CD42 expression, whereas M4/5 express CD14, CD15 and CD11b. In patients with AML M2 with t(8;21), CD34 and CD19 expression is often found.[38,39]

The karyotype, which reveals the numerical and/or structural abnormalities of the chromosomes in the leukaemic blast cells, reflects the clonal character of the disease.[40]

A close correlation between morphological, immunophenotypic and genotypic characterizations of AML has been described in recent decades (see also Chapter 4). Recently, a new classification of myeloid haematological malignancies based on morphological, immunophenotypic and cytogenetic features has been proposed by the World Health Organization (WHO).[41–43] Paediatric approaches to this classification were reported recently to distinguish AML from the other myeloproliferative diseases in paediatric patients (Box 11.1).[44,45] Currently, the main difference between adult and childhood classification is that patients with refractory cytopenia with excess of blasts (RAEBt) are considered to have myelodysplastic syndrome (MDS) in most paediatric protocols if the blast percentage remains

---

Box 11.1 *Classification of acute myeloid leukaemia (AML)/myelodysplastic syndrome (MDS) in children according to the WHO classification and its paediatric approach*[41,44]

Acute myeloid leukaemia

AML with recurrent genetic abnormalities
- AML with t(8;21)(q22;q22), (AML1/ETO)*)
- AML with inv(16)(p13q22) or t(16;16)(p13;q22) (CBFβ/MYH11)*)
- AML with (15;17)(q22;q12), (PML/RARα) and variants (acute promyelocytic leukaemia or promyelocytic leukaemia*) (APL or PML)
- AML met 11q23 (MLL) abnormalities (*regardless of blast percentage)

AML not otherwise categorized (blast percentage >30%)
- AML minimally differentiated
- AML without maturation
- AML with maturation
- Acute myelomonocytic leukaemia
- Acute monocytic leukaemia
- Acute erythroid leukaemia
- Acute megakaryoblastic leukaemia (in non-Down's syndrome)
- Myeloid/granulocytic sarcoma (chloroma)

Myelodysplastic/myeloproliferative diseases

Myelodysplastic/myeloproliferative disease
- Juvenile myelomonocytic leukaemia (JMML)
- Chronic myelomonocytic leukaemia (CMML) (secondary only)
- BCR-ABL-negative chronic myeloid leukaemia (Ph⁻CML)

Down's syndrome (DS) disease
- Transient abnormal myelopoiesis (TAM)
- Myeloid leukaemia in DS

Myelodysplastic syndrome (MDS)
- Refractory cytopenia (RC) (PB $\leqslant$ 2% and BM $\leqslant$ 5% blasts)
- Refractory anaemia with excess of blasts (RAEB) (PB, 2–19%; or BM, 5–19% blasts)
- RAEB in transformation (RAEBt) (PB or BM, 20–29% blasts)

BM, bone marrow; PB, peripheral blood.

---

between 20 and 30 per cent after repeated bone marrow investigations, whereas adults will be treated with AML therapy if the blast percentage exceeds 20 per cent. Apart from percentages of blasts, karyotype is important for stratification of patients. For example, in *de novo* AML patients with inv(16)/t(16;16), t(8;21) and t(15;17), it is recommended to follow AML treatment regimens, regardless of blast percentage. As the prognosis is excellent with chemotherapy only, these patients should not be considered for MDS treatment, i.e. bone marrow transplantation (BMT). On the other hand, monosomy 7 patients are more likely to have dysplastic features with a poor prognosis and should be considered MDS-related AML, and therefore BMT should consequently always be an up-front consideration.

IMPORTANT CLINICAL FACTORS

Acute myeloid leukaemia is a heterogeneous disease. A variety of parameters have been examined which discriminate clinical and biological subgroups.[27,28,35,36,46–48]

Age

Ten to 15 per cent of children with AML present in infancy.[28,33] Younger children are more likely to have FAB type M7, whereas older children are more likely to have FAB types M0 and M3.[33] The prognostic value of age in childhood AML has been investigated by several study groups.[28,33,35,49–52] Until recently, younger age reflected a dismal prognosis.[35,49,53] More recently, some reports have shown that infants have a 60–70 per cent long-term event-free survival (EFS) and may reflect an even better prognostic subgroup of patients than older children.[28,33,35,48,49,51,52,54–58] Subgroup analysis in this young age group identified FAB M4/M5 and t(9;11) translocation as favourable prognostic factors, whereas CNS involvement, male gender, FAB M7 and high white blood cell count (WBC) were associated with adverse outcome.[49] Others have shown that prognostic factors in subgroups of infant AML patients disappear by intensifying induction treatment.[49,51] The contribution of high-dose Ara-C (HDAC) and anthracyclines in the currently used intensive chemotherapy induction schedules is likely to be responsible for the relatively higher cure rate in infants. Also, regimens with etoposide are highly effective, especially in monoblastic leukaemia, which is frequently seen in infant AML.[59] Recent studies have shown the feasibility of stem cell transplantation in infant AML patients.[52,60,61] However, at present, the additional role of allogeneic stem cell transplantation is still unclear in infants with AML who receive intensive chemotherapy, as randomized studies are not available.

In general, as age increases, prognosis worsens, especially over the age of 10 years.[28,33,36] It is not known what mechanism is responsible for this. In the past, it has been suggested that poor compliance in adolescents and teenagers may be an important factor in chemotherapy failure.[36,62] However, since in AML most chemotherapy is administered intravenously, this does not seem to play a major role. It is more likely that with increased age, the biology of the leukaemia develops into a more aggressive type, which is partly reflected by the differences in incidence of certain FAB subtypes, cytogenetic abnormalities and presence of extramedullary disease in the different age groups.[49] In teenagers, prognostic analyses of subgroups have been performed, showing that a leucocyte count $<50 \times 10^9$/L and t(9;11) conferred a favourable prognostic group.[49] Although a higher cure rate is achieved overall with currently available high-dose chemotherapy, in several studies on paediatric AML, patients over the age of 10 years still represented a poor prognostic subgroup for survival.[28,33,36] Some studies have reported a poor outcome for boys as compared with girls, although in most recent reports this difference has vanished, especially in multivariate analyses.[24,49,63]

Extramedullary disease

Extramedullary leukaemic infiltration may affect spleen, liver, skin, gingiva, lymph nodes and the CNS. CNS infiltration is reported in 4–10 per cent of children with de novo AML.[28,30,33,35,36,48,64] CNS-positive patients at diagnosis do not represent a poor prognostic group.[35,36] Currently, therapy protocols usually include cranial irradiation in case of CNS disease at diagnosis, above the age of 2–3 years. However, children with de novo AML without CNS infiltration who are treated with intensive chemotherapy, including intrathecal chemotherapy, have a very low CNS relapse rate, indicating that these treatment regimens without CNS irradiation are sufficient to prevent CNS relapse.[33] Randomized studies to show the benefit of CNS irradiation are not yet available. One randomized study by Creutzig et al.[65] suggested that CNS irradiation was of benefit during maintenance. However, these patients were randomized between intravenous etoposide and CNS irradiation, and the numbers of patients were too small to give a conclusive answer.

Hepatosplenomegaly is reported in 5–15 per cent of patients with AML and is a reflection of the leukaemic tumour burden. Hurwitz et al.[36] reported that splenomegaly was an important prognostic factor for EFS in a multivariate analysis, whereas hepatomegaly was not. Another study in 560 paediatric AML patients showed that non-CNS extramedullary disease was correlated with a lower EFS.[35] Skin and gingiva infiltration in young children is mainly found in monocytic leukaemia. No data are available on the prognostic value of isolated skin infiltration in paediatric AML. Chloromas, myeloid sarcomas and granulocytic sarcomas are extramedullary accumulations of AML blasts most often localized in lymph nodes, skin and soft tissue, but also in the brain, gastrointestinal tract (GI) tract and reproductive system.[66–68] Chloromas are associated with the FAB M2 and the genotype t(8;21) and usually have a high CD56 expression.[69–72] Supported by results of cell line studies, the current hypothesis is that the cell adhesion molecules CD56/NCAM may be involved in the homing and invasion of these leukaemic cells into certain tissues in the body.[36,72,73] Chloromas are very often the presenting symptom of the disease. They can occur without any bone marrow involvement and should be regarded as full-blown AML and thus treated with systemic chemotherapy even in the case of a localized skin lesion, because of the high probability of local, and more importantly systematic, relapse in cases of inadequate therapy.[74]

White blood cell count

In a large cohort of paediatric AML patients, a WBC higher than 10×10^9/L was found to be an independent unfavourable prognostic factor ($P < 0.002$).[36] These results were confirmed by other studies where WBC thresholds were set at 50 or 100×10^9/L.[28,33,35,36,48,49,65] The prognostic significance varies among the different FAB subtypes, which reflects the heterogeneity of the disease and underscores the need for multivariate analyses. For instance, patients with AML M3 usually present with a low WBC, but have a higher risk of early death caused by diffuse intravascular coagulation (DIC), whereas children with AML M7 are at higher risk for treatment failure, even without an initial increased WBC.[28,33,35,36,48]

Treatment response

One of the most important clinical prognostic factors is the response to induction chemotherapy. Berlin–Frankfurt–Münster (BFM) studies, for instance, have shown that CR rate and disease-free survival (DFS) were significantly better for children with a substantial blast reduction on day 15 (<15 per cent blasts) compared with those with >15 per cent blasts.[75] In the NOPHO-AML 93 study the response to the first cycle of chemotherapy was the most powerful prognostic factor for CR and survival.[24] This early response to one or two cycles of chemotherapy reflects the *in vivo* sensitivity of the leukaemic blasts to chemotherapy. In contrast to childhood ALL studies, *in vitro* drug sensitivity studies have not shown a correlation with clinical response and outcome in paediatric AML.[76,77] Thirty to 40 per cent of children with AML will eventually relapse. The prognosis of patients who relapse within 18 months after primary diagnosis is less favourable than that of patients with a longer duration of first CR.[78–82]

BIOLOGICAL FACTORS

Morphology

Morphology and karyotype are closely correlated in certain subgroups of AML (see Chapter 4). Patients with FAB type M4Eo most often present with inv(16), FAB M2 with t(8;21), and acute promyelocytic leukaemia (APL) patients (FAB M3) with t(15;17). These subgroups represent AML patients with a very favourable prognosis. FAB types M5 and M7 are more often seen in younger children, whereas the incidence of M0, M1 and M2 increases with rising age.[33] One study showed an unfavourable outcome in FAB M5 patients.[35] Patients with M1/M2 FAB types with Auer rods have been reported to have a better CR rate,[36,48] although a better EFS was not always reached.[36] In most studies, FAB M7 in non-Down's patients is predictive for a poor outcome.[35,48] Recent studies show that using the current intensive chemotherapy regimens based on cytogenetic stratification, the independent prognostic significance of FAB types vanishes.[27,28,33]

In contrast, morphological features, such as the occurrence of dysplasia, have been reported to be of prognostic importance.[46] This myelodysplastic syndrome-related AML (MDR-AML) presentation is rarely seen in children, and, if so, it is most often associated with monosomy 7. In these patients, stem cell transplantation should be considered, especially if the dysplastic features remain after CR has been reached.

Immunophenotype

Several reports suggested a relationship between certain antigens [CD11b, CD13, CD14, CD34, CD56 and TdT (terminal deoxynucleotidyl transferase)] and poor prognosis in AML patients.[83–92] In contrast to children, in adults most studies confirm the correlation of the expression of the immature phenotypes, such as CD34-positive AML with poor prognosis, whereas the expression of panmyeloid markers was associated with a better outcome. However, subsequent studies have produced conflicting results.[47,49,84–89,91,93]

Cytogenetics and gene aberrations

CONSTITUTIONAL GENETIC DISORDERS

Hereditary diseases such as Fanconi's anaemia, Down's syndrome (DS) and Bloom's syndrome are associated with an increased risk of development of AML.[94–96] Infrequently, families with an unexplained high risk of AML have been described.[97] Trisomy 21 is the most frequently occurring constitutional disorder associated with paediatric AML and has a 20-fold higher risk of leukaemia compared with other children. In Scandinavia, 13 per cent of all AML cases were patients with DS,[28] whereas an incidence of 104/1114 (9 per cent) was reported in the Children's Cancer Group (CCG),[27] and 35/688 (5 per cent) in the Medical Research Council (MRC) trials.[33] The peak incidence of AML in DS is under the age of 4 years.[98,99] Because the disease is very often preceded by a MDS-like phase, it may be difficult to classify the AML according to the FAB criteria. Therefore this disease is a separate category in the new paediatric approach of the WHO classification (Box 11.1).[44] Most cases reveal the megakaryoblastic subtype and the maturation arrest most often affects a common progenitor for platelets and erythroid cells, but all morphological subtypes have been described.[100–102] This morphological heterogeneity can be shown by clone-specific markers that are present in both lineages in interphase cytogenetic analysis.[103] M7 in DS is different from M7 in non-DS patients, mainly infants, of whom the latter frequently reveal t(1;22).

It appears that the development of AML M7 is associated with a critical period of prenatal or perinatal haemopoiesis in children with DS. This interpretation is supported by the occurrence of transient myeloproliferative disorders (TMDs) in neonates with DS and the observation that most AML cases in DS children occur in the first years of life.[104,105] Recently, acquired activating mutations in exon 2 of *GATA1*, an X-linked gene encoding a transcription factor that promotes megakaryocytic differentiation, were found in DS patients with TMD and AML, establishing the genetic basis of unique prenatal collaboration between genes on chromosome 21 and a mutated gene on chromosome X.[22] Although in most DS patients with TMD a spontaneous regression occurs within 2–3 months, 20–30 per cent will develop AML in early childhood. DS children with AML M7 have a high cure rate with chemotherapy only.[99,103] This is the result of a better response to chemotherapy and especially an increased intracellular turnover from Ara-C to Ara-CTP in DS.[106] This clinical drug sensitivity is in concordance with relatively high *in vitro* sensitivity of the DS AML blasts for Ara-C and anthracyclines.[77,107] Bone marrow transplantation is therefore not recommended in DS patients in first CR. Caution is needed in the treatment of DS patients, as the increased sensitivity to Ara-C is also followed by more toxicity.[108] The current BFM childhood AML protocol therefore even recommends adjustment of dosages for DS patients with the intention to decrease toxicity while retaining good prognosis.

ACQUIRED SOMATIC GENETIC ABERRATIONS

Recently, Gilliland *et al.*[132] proposed that two classes of mutations are both necessary to develop AML, a suggestion which links to the general 'two-hit hypothesis' in leukaemia.[20,109–111] Class I mutations confer a proliferative signal [e.g. a RTK (receptor tyrosine kinase) or RAS mutation], which leads to a survival advantage of the leukaemic cells. Class II aberrations include, for instance, core binding factor (CBF) fusion genes, such as in leukaemias with t(15;17)-, t(8;21)- and inv(16)/t(16;16)-induced impairment of haemopoietic differentiation. This two-hit hypothesis, which leads to the maturation arrest and proliferation advantage, is supported by the FLT3 Asp835 and c-KIT Asp816 activating loop mutations, which have been reported in CBF AML.[111–114]

Clonal chromosomal abnormalities and associated class II genetic aberrations

Numerical and structural abnormalities are found in 70–80 per cent of children with AML (Figure 11.1).[47,115,116] Patients with t(15;17), t(8;21) and inv(16)/t(16;16) comprise a group with relatively favourable prognosis, characterized by low rates of clinical drug resistance and superior overall survival (OS) (61–69 per cent) associated with a lower relapse rate (RR).[47,115–119] In the most recent

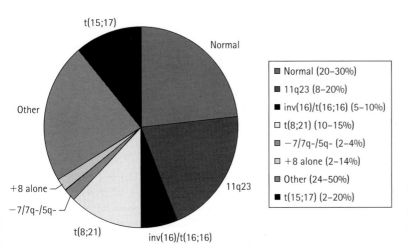

Legend:
- Normal (20–30%)
- 11q23 (8–20%)
- inv(16)/t(16;16) (5–10%)
- t(8;21) (10–15%)
- −7/7q-/5q- (2–4%)
- +8 alone (2–14%)
- Other (24–50%)
- t(15;17) (2–20%)

Figure 11.1 *Cytogenetic abnormalities in paediatric acute myeloid leukaemia (AML). (Data are from Raimondi et al.,[47] Grimwade et al.,[115] Jahns-Streubel et al.[116])*

Table 11.2 *Most common structural cytogenetic abnormalities and fusion genes in acute myeloid leukaemia*

Structural cytogenetic abnormality	Breakpoint	Fusion transcript
t(8;21)	q22;q22	AML1-ETO
t(15;17)	q22;q12	PML-RARα
inv(16)	p13;q22	CBFβ-MYH11
t(16;16)	p13;q22	CBFβ-MYH11
t(9;11)	p22;q23	MLL-AF9
t(6;9)	p23;q34	DEK-CAN

UK-MRC AML12 study, a 3-year EFS of 80 per cent from CR was reached in these three subgroups of patients without stem cell transplantation.[34] In these patients, additional cytogenetic aberrations have not been found to have a large impact on prognosis.[115]

The incidence of APL characterized by t(15;17) varies from 2 to 20 per cent in children.[30,47,115] The highest incidence is found in Mediterranean countries. APL, or AML M3, has unique molecular and clinical characteristics. The t(15;17) carries the fusion protein PML-RARα which causes an arrest of myeloid differentiation at the promyeloid stage followed by abnormal proliferation of promyelocytes (Table 11.2).[120] Treatment with all-*trans*-retinoic acid (ATRA), which induces differentiation, is currently added to standard chemotherapy. The outcome of APL, even if not treated with ATRA, was found to be better than in patients with normal cytogenetics.[47,115] In contrast, in the past, CR rates in t(15;17) patients usually did not differ from patients with normal cytogenetics, reflecting the clinical problems at diagnosis, especially the propensity of haemorrhagic diathesis.

The t(8;21)(q22;q22) has been reported in 10–15 per cent of paediatric AML cases, making it the most frequent cytogenetic abnormality.[30,47,115] The reciprocal translocation involving the *ETO* gene on chromosome 8 and the *AML-1* gene on chromosome 21 results in a fusion gene whose product behaves as an aberrant transcription factor. AML M2 with t(8;21) is usually associated with Auer rods, bone marrow eosinophilia and sex chromosome loss (-Y in males and -X in females). The CR rate in these patients is very high with intensive chemotherapy regimens (95–98 per cent), with a 4-year OS of more than 60 per cent.[24,34,35] This outcome may be treatment protocol-related as other authors have reported a poor outcome for t(8;21) AML in the past.[121,122]

Inversion 16(p13;q22)(inv(16)), or t(16;16) (p13;q22) associated with FAB type M4Eo is found in 5–10 per cent of paediatric AML patients.[47,115] The inversion involves the fusion of the *CBF-β* gene, a transcription factor and the myosin heavy-chain (*MYH11*) gene. AMLM4Eo, is associated with a high WBC at diagnosis, accounting for more disease-related morbidity and mortality in the past. However, with current supportive care regimens, patients with inv(16)/t(16;16) have proved to have an excellent outcome.[47,115]

Unquestionably, paediatric AML patients with inv(16)/t(16;16), t(8;21) and t(15;17) represent a favourable subgroup of patients. Recently, the UK-MRC10 trial showed a 10-year survival rate of 76 per cent from CR in this good risk group.[34] Currently, in most paediatric trials, BMT is no longer recommended in first CR for patients with inv(16)/t(16;16), t(8;21) and t(15;17). Preliminary data, such as a 3-year EFS of 80 per cent from CR in the most recent UK-MRC12 study, show that without stem cell transplantation, but with intensive chemotherapy, this stratification is feasible and effective in paediatric AML.[123]

In 8–20 per cent of children with AML, 11q23 abnormalities are found.[47,58,115] Most frequently, they involve t(9;11)(p22;q23) and t(11;19)(q23;p13.1), and less frequently t(10;11)(p11;q23) and t(6;11)(q25;q23). A poorer outcome in patients with t(10;11)(p11;q23) compared with patients with t(9;11)(p22;q23) was reported in the MRC10 trial; however, the subgroups of paediatric patients are very small.[34] Raimondi *et al.*[47] reported poor outcome in patients with any 11q23 abnormality, with an overall 4-year survival of 24 per cent. Studies in infant AML showed that 11q23 abnormalities with *MLL* rearrangements were correlated with M4 and M5 FAB subtypes and hyperleucocytosis, and did not show a correlation with treatment response or outcome.[49,51,124–126] It is very likely that subgroups of patients with 11q23 abnormalities represent favourable prognostic subgroups, such as, for instance, patients with t(9;11).[124,127,128] One study reported t(9;11) to be an independent favourable prognostic factor in children less than 24 months of age.[49] Also, in teenagers, a leucocyte count $<50 \times 10^9$/L and t(9;11) were associated with favourable outcome.[49,124] The uniqueness of this translocation coding for the *MLL-AF9* fusion gene transcript is underscored by recently reported *in vitro* studies, which showed that in contrast to other *MLL*-positive AML patients, t(9;11) patients are far more sensitive to cytarabine, etoposide, anthracyclines and 2-cdA.[76] Currently, t(9;11) cases are stratified into a favourable risk group, e.g. by the NOPHO and the St Jude group.

Abnormalities of chromosomes 5 and 7 are very rare in children (<3 per cent of all cases).[30,47,115] In adults, the presence of complex cytogenetic changes, -5/(5q-), and monosomy 7 predicts poorer outcome with a CR rate of 60–75 per cent, an OS of 13–29 per cent, and a RR of 70–100 per cent.[115] Patients with 7q- did not reveal a different outcome to standard risk patients.[115,129] However, because of low numbers of paediatric patients with monosomy 7 and 7q-, it is difficult to evaluate the outcome of this cytogenetic subgroup separately. In some studies, abnormalities of chromosome 7 have been established as adverse prognostic factors in childhood AML, but monosomy 7 is not yet generally used for stratification of therapy.[27,47,57,117–119,123,130] Collaboration between the international study groups will be necessary to evaluate the prognostic significance of monosomy 7 and 7q- in childhood AML. To date, there is no explanation for the extremely poor outcome in adult AML patients with monosomy 7. Monosomy 7 patients are more likely to have secondary leukaemias and MDR-AML, which form a group of biologically more resistant leukaemias. It has been hypothesized that expression of the classical multidrug resistance gene (MDR-1 gene) on chromosome 7q21 is involved in the poor prognosis of these patients. However, no evidence of selection of a specific MDR-1-related allelic variant in monosomy 7 could be identified.[131] In vitro these cases are less sensitive to Ara-C.[76]

Two studies report clonal complex cytogenetic abnormalities, defined by the presence of a clone with at least five unrelated cytogenetic abnormalities as an adverse prognostic factor.[47,115]

The most common numerical abnormality in paediatric AML is trisomy 8, with an incidence of 8–10 per cent of all cases.[30,47,115] However, the effect on outcome is difficult to assess, as most cases show hyperdiploidy, which is associated with several known recurrent chromosomal abnormalities.[30,47,115]

Class I genetic aberrations

These aberrations involve mutations and epigenetic changes in genes that are involved in the biological behaviour of the leukaemic cells. Some of these class 1 aberrations are frequently found in patients with CBF AML, supporting Gilliland's pathogenetic model hypothesis.[20,109–111]

The fms-like tyrosine kinase 3 (FLT3) is a RTK expressed on haemopoietic progenitor cells and is involved in the proliferation and differentiation of haemopoietic stem cells. The receptor has an extracellular domain and a cytoplasmic domain that carries a tyrosine kinase motif.[132] Internal tandem duplications of FLT3 (FLT3/ITD), first described by Nakao et al.,[133] lead to ligand-independent FLT3 dimerization and consecutive activation through autophosphorylation.[132] This results in a proliferation and survival advantage of the leukaemic cell. FLT3/ITDs are found in 20–30 per cent of adult AML patients.[113,134–139] These FLT3/ITDs are found in only 10–15 per cent of paediatric patients with AML.[139–144] They are associated with high WBC at diagnosis, have a higher incidence in M1/M2 cases, and are associated with induction failure and a poor outcome.[145] The incidence is higher in patients with normal cytogenetics[139–144] and, interestingly, a very low incidence is found in paediatric AML patients with 11q23 abnormalities and DS. FLT3/ITDs are found in

8 per cent of patients with a MLL translocation, but in 30 per cent with intragenic MLL abnormalities in adult AML.[146] Also, recently a strong correlation was found between FLT3/ITDs and partial tandem duplication of the MLL gene.[147] In adults, not only ITDs but also point mutations D835 and D516 have shown a prognostic significance.[148] In 6 per cent of the adult t(8;21) cases, FLT3 mutations were found.[114] So far, no information is available on these point mutations in childhood AML. As AML patients with FLT3/ITDs and mutations represent poor risk groups, especially within the standard and intermediate risk groups according to standard cytogenetics, this may very well be an important diagnostic tool for risk group stratification in children with AML in the future. Moreover, targeted therapy like FLT3 targeted tyrosine kinase inhibitors may be of clinical benefit for this selected group of patients.[149–151]

In adult AML patients with t(8;21), c-KIT exon 8 mutations are reported in only 2 per cent of cases, and Asp 816 mutations in 8 per cent. Recently, in patients with inv(16) c-KIT, exon 8 mutations were found in more than 20 per cent, whereas Asp 816 mutations were found in only 8 per cent.[112,114,152] FLT3 and c-KIT mutations were mutually exclusively expressed in these CBF AML patients, i.e. 40 per cent of the AML patients possessed either a c-KIT or a FLT3 mutation.[114] Recently, a subgroup analysis revealed that adult AML patients with inv(16) with c-KIT exon 8 mutations are at higher risk of relapse.[114] This suggests that molecular characterization of these CBF AMLs may allow the identification of a subset of AML patients with a more aggressive disease.

Another example of a gene that has proved to be an important biological determinant of outcome in adult AML is EVI1 expression. EVI1, a zinc-finger transcription factor, is one of the genes involved in 3q21 and 3q26 defects.[153–155] The most commonly reported abnormality, inv(3)(q21q26), is associated with overexpression of EVI1, and is postulated to deregulate haemopoiesis. EVI1 is also expressed in patients lacking 3q abnormalities.[156] A high expression of EVI1 predicts poor survival in adult AML.[157,158]

Furthermore, bi-allelic mutations in the CCAAT/enhancer binding protein α (CEBPα gene) were recently described as prognostic markers in adult AML.[159] CEBPα is an essential transcription factor for granulocytic differentiation, and low CEBPα levels were found to be associated with poor outcome. Another potentially interesting gene, identified by viral insertion mutagenesis, is the peripheral cannabinoid receptor Cb2, a novel oncoprotein which induces a reversible block in neutrophilic differentiation.[160–163] The role of these and many more recently identified genetic aberrations, some of which have already been shown to be of prognostic importance in adult AML, needs to be established in future prospective studies in paediatric AML.

Drug resistance proteins

The prognostic value of expression of drug resistance genes, e.g. in *de novo* AML, has been studied mostly in adult AML.[90,92,164–175] Expression of the *MDR-1* gene on chromosome 7, encoding p-glycoprotein, a drug efflux pump, has been identified as an independent unfavourable prognostic factor for response and survival in large cohorts of adult AML patients. The prognostic value of the other drug resistance proteins, such as the multi-drug resistance-related protein (MRP-1), lung resistance-related protein (LRP) and breast cancer resistance protein (BCRP), is more debatable. In children, the role of drug resistance proteins has been studied less extensively, but so far there is no evidence of prognostic value of these proteins in paediatric AML.[176–178] A single arm study in relapsed/refractory AML in which *MDR-1* reversing agents were used showed equal CR rates in *MDR-1*-positive and -negative patients.[179] A prognostic role has been suggested for MRP3, but this needs to be confirmed by other groups.[178]

Minimal residual disease

As CR rates are very high using current treatment strategies in paediatric AML, reducing relapse risk is an important challenge for future therapy protocols. One method of identifying patients with a higher risk of future relapse is the assessment of minimal residual disease (MRD). Recently, sensitive immunological and molecular genetic methods have been developed to detect MRD. One study in 252 children treated according to CCG-2941 and CCG-2961 showed that MRD detected by immunophenotypic multidimensional flow cytometry at the end of consolidation predicted for the occurrence of relapse.[180] Others showed that four different risk groups could be identified by MRD detection after induction in patients who were morphologically in CR.[178] In addition to immunophenotyping, promising targets for detection of MRD in AML patients are *WT1* and *FLT3*.[181,182]

In the future, MRD detection may be used for treatment stratification in post-remission therapy. Moreover, MRD detection pre- and post-transplant may become important prognosticators for the outcome of individual cases after BMT.[183] However, the clinical significance of the MRD-positive clone at certain time points during therapy with respect to outcome requires further evaluation and may very well be dependent on treatment protocol. Also, the clinical relevance of methodological problems such as immunophenotypic shifts, using leukaemia-associated phenotypes, and stability of the *FLT3* mutations needs to be established before MRD can be used for stratification of treatment in paediatric AML.

Prognostic factors

From the above, it can be concluded that WBC, early response to chemotherapy, structural cytogenetic abnormalities such as t(8;21), t(15;17) and inv(16)/t(16;16), complex karyotype and numerical abnormalities such as monosomy 7 are important prognostic factors in paediatric AML, and therefore are used for stratification of therapy. In the near future, it is very likely that identification of class I genetic aberrations will enable identification of subgroups of patients within the CBF AML cases who may benefit from more targeted therapy.

TREATMENT

In recent decades, treatment of childhood AML has improved considerably, with a CR rate of 75–92 per cent and an overall survival of 50–60 per cent (Table 11.1). The (estimated) EFS rates at 5 years have been reported to be 48–67 per cent in recent paediatric AML studies.[27,28,31–35,51,65,184] In addition to the use of effective combinations of intensive chemotherapeutic agents, CNS prophylaxis and identification of risk groups, improved supportive care regimens and BMT conditions have contributed to a better outcome for paediatric AML patients (Figure 11.2).

Induction chemotherapy

Treatment of AML focuses on eradication of the malignant clone followed by recovery of normal haemopoiesis. Induction treatment in AML is intensive and will always be followed by bone marrow aplasia. The aim is to achieve complete remission (CR) as soon as possible. The definition of CR is still based on morphological criteria and is defined as less than 5 per cent of leukaemic blasts in the bone marrow at a time point when bone marrow cellularity is restored after induction chemotherapy. According to National Cancer Institute criteria, bone marrow cellularity of >20 per cent and a circulating neutrophil count of $1500/mm^3$ are required to confirm CR.[185] To reach CR, intensive chemotherapy is necessary, of which anthracyclines and cytosine-arabinoside (Ara-C) have proved to be the most powerful drugs in AML so far. Classically, this has been done by combining 7 days of Ara-C with a 3-day anthracycline schedule, the so-called 7 + 3 regimen. In patients with APL, the differentiating agent ATRA is added to conventional chemotherapy to induce cell differentiation and maturation.[120,186]

The most recently performed trials, by several groups (UK-MRC, POG, BFM), differed from their previous treatment protocols by a more intensified induction therapy (Figure 11.2). UK-MRC found that the DAT regimen [daunomycin (DNR), Ara-C and 6-TG] with 3 days of DNR + 10 days of 6-TG, as compared with 1 day of DNR and 5 days of 6-TG, resulted in a higher CR rate (66 vs. 61 per cent) and a shorter time to reach CR (34 vs. 46 days). The most recent MRC (10 + 12) trials show a CR rate of 80–90 per cent after two courses of ADE (high-dose Ara-C, daunomycin and etoposide).[34] In study POG 8498, high-dose Ara-C (HDAC) in the second induction course did not result in a higher CR rate than the standard DAT regimen (85 per cent in both groups); however, the HDAC patients showed an improved EFS (34 vs. 29 per cent) and DFS (42 vs. 34 per cent) as compared with the standard induction treatment group. The same was found in the BFM group. After intensification of induction treatment in treatment protocols 83 and 88, a CR rate was reached that was comparable with the BFM 78 protocol (75–80 per cent), but an increase in EFS from 38 per cent in BFM 78 to 47 per cent in BFM 83 was found.[48] The NOPHO AML studies 88 and 93 showed CR rates of 87 and 91 per cent, respectively, after two induction cycles. In the NOPHO-AML93 trial, the Ara-C dose was increased from 800 mg/m^2 to 12.5 g/m^2 in patients in which the blast percentage was not below 5 per cent at day 16 of induction.[24] In the US-Children's Cancer Group (CCG), timing intensification rather than therapy intensification was pursued. In protocol CCG-2891, therapy consisted of dexamethasone, cytarabine, 6-thioguanine, etoposide and rubidomycine and the patients were randomized between giving the second cycle after haemopoietic recovery or after 6 days of rest. Although no differences were seen in CR rate, the 8-year EFS rate for the intensive timing group was 42 per cent, whereas that for the other group was 27 per cent.[57]

In general, current induction treatment schedules consist of one or two short courses of intensive chemotherapy. Combined with either etoposide or 6-thioguanine, anthracyclines and Ara-C are the important agents of the induction regimen. The question as to which anthracycline will provide the best efficacy still remains unanswered. To date, idarubicin and mitoxantrone have not proven to be superior to daunorubicin.[31,65,187] Recently, cladribine was introduced into the treatment regimen of newly diagnosed patients, and may, in combination with other drugs, become an important agent in achieving complete remission in paediatric AML.[188–190]

Post-induction therapy

In this phase, the aim is to consolidate the CR state (consolidation phase) and to prevent the recurrence of AML. Further intensive treatment is needed to eradicate MRD. Consolidation of the chemotherapy consists of repeated administration of drugs already administered during the induction phase. Intensification of therapy is mainly performed by adding other chemotherapeutic agents to prevent therapy failure due to clinical drug resistance. The ultimate intensification consists of myeloablative therapy with stem cell transplantation.

No general conclusion as to how many cycles of chemotherapy should be administered to provide an adequate consolidation and intensification can be drawn. Intensive chemotherapy schedules, even of a short duration, seem to be of greater value than a less intensive regimen over a longer maintenance period. This was shown in a randomized study, CCG-213, in which the more intensive regimen had a 5-year survival rate of 68 per cent, while the less intensive arm had a 44 per cent survival from the end of consolidation.[191] In BFM AML 93, a randomization between two and three cycles of HAM (high-dose Ara-C and mitoxantrone) showed no difference in survival. Also, preliminary results of the recent MRC-AML12 trial, a randomization between two and three intensive post-induction chemotherapy cycles, showed no advantage of either regimen.[34] In the NOPHO studies 88 and 93, extremely high dosages of Ara-C were applied, up to 50 g/m^2, administered in four blocks. The studies in which HDAC was administered revealed a lower relapse rate compared with schedules without HDAC.[28,31,192,193] Again, as for induction chemotherapy, the intensity of schedules of chemotherapy seems to be of more value than the length of the period over which the therapy is given. The therapeutic efficacy of maintenance therapy in paediatric AML has not been proven until now.[191,194] Currently, APL is the only AML subgroup in which treatment is successfully amended according to the presence of the molecular reminiscence of the fusion protein, as this persistence predicts a high relapse rate.[195–199] In children, collaborative studies will be necessary to prove the efficacy of maintenance treatment based on molecular residual disease.[120]

CNS prophylaxis and therapy

By 1978 it had become clear that CNS prophylaxis is necessary in paediatric AML, as the number of CNS relapses decreases impressively with adequate CNS prophylaxis. However, the relative contribution of intrathecal therapy, intravenous HDAC and cranial irradiation is not clear. Only one study (BFM 87) has randomized patients to receive cranial irradiation versus intravenous etoposide.[200] Interestingly, patients who did not receive cranial irradiation were more likely to relapse, not only in the CNS but also in the bone marrow. However, as the randomization stopped early, full conclusions could not be drawn from this study. Most current intensive chemotherapy protocols contain intrathecal chemotherapy without CNS irradiation, providing an adequate CNS prophylaxis

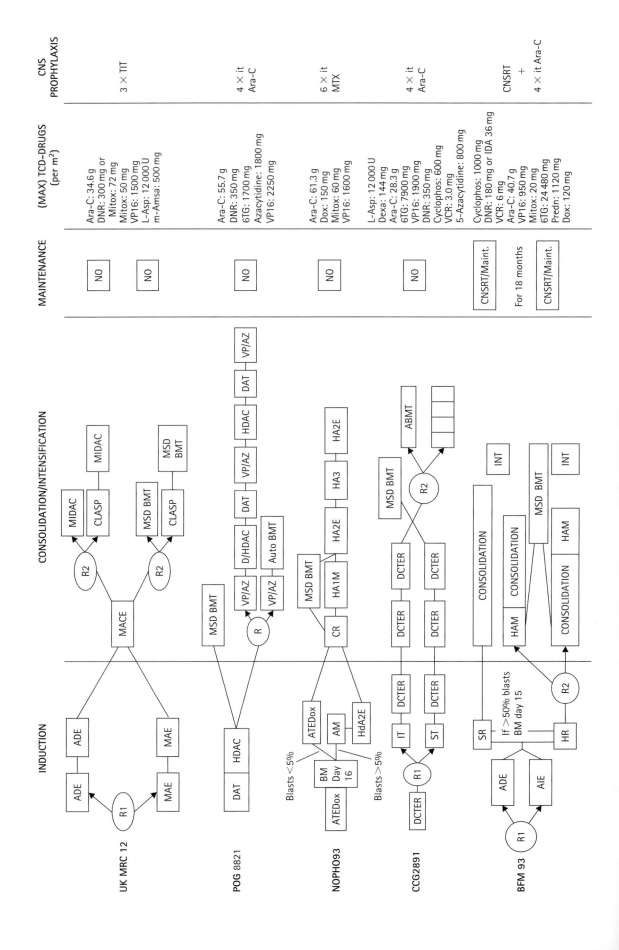

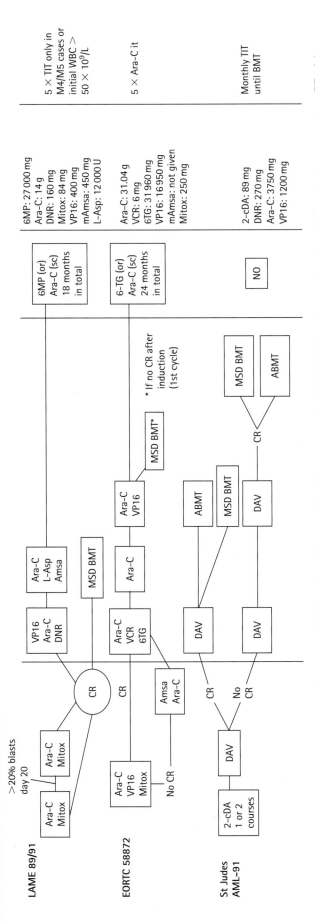

Figure 11.2 *Recent paediatric acute myeloid leukaemia (AML) studies with reasonable follow-up time (Table 11.1). TCD, total cumulative doses; CNS, central nervous system; TIT, triple intrathecal chemotherapy, i.e. prednisolone, MTX and Ara-C; Ara-C, cytosine arabinoside; MTX, methotrexate; it, intrathecal; IT, intensive timing; ST, standard timing; CNSRT, cranial irradiation; DNR, daunorubicin; VP16, etoposide; L-asp, L-asparaginase; m-Amsa, amsacrine; 6TG, 6-thioguanine; Dox, doxorubicin; Mitox, mitoxantrone; Dexa, dexamethasone; Cyclophos, cyclophosphamide; Predn, prednisolone; VCR, vincristine; 6MP, 6-mercaptopurine; 2-cDA, 2-chlorodeoxycytidine; HDAC, high-dose Ara-C; MSD, matched sibling donor; ABMT, autologous BMT; CR, complete remission; R, randomization; R1, R2, first and second consecutive randomizations; SR, standard risk; HR, high risk; ADE, Ara-C + DNR + VP16; MAE, Ara-C + Mitox + VP16; MACE, Ara-C + m-Amsa + VP16; MIDAC, Mitox + HDAC; CLASP, HDAC + L-Asp; VP/A2, etoposide + azacytidine; DAT, DNR + Ara-C + 6TG; ATEDox, Ara-C + 6TG + VP16 + Dox; AM, Ara-C + Mitox; HA2E, HDAC + VP16; HA1M, HDAC + Mitox; HA3, HDAC; DCTER, Dexa + Ara-C + 6TG + VP16 + DNR; HAM, AIE, Ara-C + VP16 + idarubicin; DAV, DNR + Ara-C + VP16. (For references, see Table 11.1.)*

with outcome comparable to the BFM 87 studies (Figure 11.2). This indicates that intrathecal therapy in combination with HDAC provides an adequate CNS prophylaxis. Most CNS-positive patients >2 years of age have been treated with CNS irradiation in the past in most treatment schedules, apart from patients for whom early BMT was considered.[33,184] In one protocol, radiotherapy was avoided and replaced by extra intrathecal injections.[30] Most studies do not report how CNS-positive patients have been treated and it is likely that 'doctor's choice' plays an important role in these patients. As patients younger than 2 years of age are mainly treated with extra intrathecal injections, and are doing reasonably well, it would be reasonable to reconsider the role of additional intrathecal therapy in CNS-positive patients with avoidance of radiotherapy.

Stem cell transplantation

Myeloablative therapy and/or total body irradiation with subsequent stem cell transplantation has proven to be of value in the total eradication of the leukaemic clone in AML patients. In cases of allogeneic BMT (allo-BMT), in addition to restoration of normal haemopoiesis, the 'graft-versus-leukaemia' (GvL) effect is an important element of the treatment. This phenomenon was first described in 1956 by Barnes and Loutit,[201] and was confirmed after the excess of relapses after full T-cell depletions of the donor grafts in the 1970s and 1980s.[202] Currently, this principle is further adapted by donor lymphocyte infusions (DLIs), which are used to re-induce remission in patients who relapse after allo-BMT.[203,204]

ALLOGENEIC BMT

In the past, multiple studies have shown the efficacy of allogeneic stem cell transplantation from an HLA-identical sibling donor for children with *de novo* AML in first remission. POG 8821 conducted a randomized trial in which patients with an HLA-identical sibling were transplanted while patients without such a donor received autologous BMT (ABMT) or chemotherapy. This so-called biological randomization showed that patients treated with allogeneic BMT had a 3-year EFS of 52 per cent, whereas patients treated with chemotherapy or ABMT had an EFS of 37 per cent.[29] A similar result was reported by the CCG2891 study in which, respectively, 60 and 48–53 per cent survival rates were found in patients treated with allo-BMT and ABMT/chemotherapy. The EORTC trial 18A showed a long-term DFS of 46 per cent from the time of CR for allo-BMT patients, as compared with 33 per cent for non-transplanted patients.[27,80] Recently, preliminary results of the UK-MRC10 and 12, in which biological randomization was performed between allo-BMT in *de novo* paediatric AML patients with an HLA-identical sibling versus intensive chemotherapy for patients without a sibling donor, showed no difference in survival, even if only two (instead of three) intensification blocks were administered.[34,123] There was a lower risk of relapse after allo-BMT, but this was offset by the somewhat increased risk of regimen-related mortality.[31] Current protocols, such as the UK MRC-AML15 and the NOPHO 2003 trials, therefore do not include allo-BMT for the so-called good risk patients, i.e. Down's syndrome, t(8;21), t(15;17), t(9;11) and inv(16)/t(16;16), nor for the standard risk group of paediatric AML patients without cytogenetic abnormalities, even if a HLA-identical sibling is available.

MATCHED UNRELATED DONOR BMT

Stem cell transplantation with a matched unrelated donor (MUD) or a (mis)matched family donor (MFD) used to carry a higher risk of graft-versus-host disease (GvHD) and subsequent treatment-related morbidity and mortality. This is illustrated by the Seattle update on 161 patients (adults and children), which reported a 30 per cent leukaemia-free survival rate for patients transplanted with a MUD donor in first CR.[205] The Italian Bone Marrow Transplant Group reported a 31 per cent DFS in AML patients, but a 44 per cent transplant-related mortality rate with a MUD transplantation. The University of Minnesota reported 23 per cent of acute GvHD and 50 per cent incidence of chronic GvHD in children with AML after MUD transplantation in CR1.[206] Interestingly, a comparison between autologous BMT and MUD-BMT in paediatric AML patients showed that the patients with an autologous transplant had a superior outcome, reflecting the toxicity of the MUD regimens in the past. Currently, MUD-BMT is considered as effective as, and not necessarily more toxic than, a HLA-identical family donor transplantation and therefore feasible for a small group of *de novo* AML patients who are thought to benefit from allogeneic BMT. This is mainly due to the improvement of graft preparations, which reduces GvHD while conserving GvL, together with improved supportive care facilities. Moreover, the current development of pre-emptive testing and treatment of post-BMT Epstein–Barr virus lymphoproliferative disease by pre-emptive B-cell depletion using anti-CD20 has contributed to the improvement of MUD transplant results.[207] Furthermore, preliminary data on new developments in transplant regimens, such as ideal mismatch transplantations based on mHag-A2 class I HLA typing, using killing inhibitory receptor (KIR) mismatch or 'smart mismatch transplantation', which provides the GvL effect but reduces the GvHD, show promising results, especially in AML, and may improve outcome in children in AML particularly after MUD transplantation in the future.[208]

ABMT

Autologous bone marrow transplant (ABMT) is less toxic than allo-BMT, but it is also less effective, most probably because of the lack of GvL effect and the risk of re-infusion of minimal residual clonogenic disease. It has been suggested that novel purging regimens may lower the risk of MRD in the graft.[209,210] However, the benefit of ABMT over conventional intensive chemotherapy has not been proven overall, as reported by US-CCG2891, the POG8821, UK-MRC10 and the AIOEP/LAM87 paediatric AML groups.[27,29–31,57,211,212]

In conclusion, the results overall show that the indication for allo-BMT in a paediatric patient with AML in first CR has become debatable and in most cases can be replaced by the use of high-dose intensive chemotherapy. Only subgroups with a poor response to induction chemotherapy, and patients with MDS-related AML and/or MDS-related clonal abnormalities like monosomy 7/7q- and complex karyotype are currently considered for allo-BMT in first CR. If allo-BMT is indicated, transplantation with a HLA-identical sibling remains the treatment of first choice, but with current transplant regimens and supportive care, allo- and MUD- regimens might be considered for this selected small group of AML patients in which BMT is considered to be of advantage over chemotherapy only.

Supportive care regimens

More intensive chemotherapy regimens have resulted in improved survival, but the counterpart of intensifying treatment is increased toxicity. Clearly, a balance must be found between therapeutic efficacy and regimen-related morbidity and mortality.

TUMOUR LYSIS SYNDROME AND HYPERLEUCOCYTOSIS

Tumour lysis syndrome prevention is an important part of the induction supportive care regimen, especially in the rare cases of paediatric AML (mainly AML M4 and M5) that present with high WBC at diagnosis. The problems of high potassium levels, hyperphosphataemia and hypocalcaemia are often accompanied by haemorrhage and leucostasis. The large size of the monocytic cells and their adhesive properties lead to plugging of small blood vessels in lungs and brain, potentially causing acute respiratory distress syndrome, bleeding, convulsions and encephalopathy, which can lead to life-threatening conditions and results in a relatively high treatment-related mortality in paediatric AML as compared with ALL. Reduction of the high WBC by effective antileukaemic treatment, together with regimens that reduce the risk of urate nephropathy, such as allopurinol and rasburicase, and adequate fluid intake, will in most patients be effective to overcome these temporary problems, and only incidentally is leukapheresis and/or haemodialysis required.

HAEMORRHAGE

Bleeding problems are due to low numbers of platelets, and in occasional cases to diffuse intravascular clotting disorders, such as occur in some cases of M3, M4 and M5 AML. During induction therapy it is recommend to keep the platelet count above $15–20 \times 10^9/L$ to avoid intracranial and GI bleeding, especially in cases of fever. Also, in APL patients it is recommended to start ATRA as soon as possible as this has proved to reduce the haemorrhage risk significantly.[186,213]

INFECTION

In AML, risk of infection is increased because the disease itself impairs the normal granulopoiesis and lymphopoiesis, and therefore humoral and cellular immunity is compromised. Central venous lines, which are necessary for the administration of chemotherapy, form a predilection site for infection. Moreover, natural barriers such as GI and oral mucosal layers are injured after HDAC and anthracyclines. AML treatment should include broad-spectrum antibiotics in case of neutropenic fever, covering Gram-positive and Gram-negative sepsis, while anaerobic infectious agents should also be covered in case of serious bowel and mucosal problems. There is an elevated risk of streptococcal infections, especially after HDAC, for which prophylactic use of penicillin is recommended.

Fungal origin of infections should always be considered in AML, especially in the case of pulmonary and cerebral infections. The antigen test galactomannan (GM) has recently been introduced as a marker for invasive *Aspergillus* infections. This antigen can be detected in serum and bronchoalveolar lavage fluid,[214] and may be important especially for the follow-up of patients during antifungal treatment.[214,215] Where there is a suspicion of a pulmonary fungal infection in a child with AML on high-resolution computed tomography scan, it is recommended that a bronchoalveolar lavage be performed, and in the case of a solid mass a biopsy should be performed.[216] *Aspergillus fumiginatus* and *Candida albicans* are the most frequently found fungal infections in children with AML. In the last decade, promising new agents, such as liposomal amphotericin, broad-spectrum azoles and echocandinens, have become available which have shown good efficacy and lower toxicity.[217] Also, as neutropenia is one of the most important risk factors for mortality in invasive fungal infections, granulocyte colony-stimulating factor (G-CSF) should be considered in order to mobilize granulocytes, to shorten the neutropenic period. Unfortunately, there are no randomized

Table 11.3 *Reports on response in paediatric acute myeloid leukaemia patients at first relapse*

References	Patients (*n*)	Age (years)	CR (%)	Therapy (after CR)	OS (%) (2 years)	DFS (%)
Vignetti et al.[218]	50	9–54	68	18CT/16BMT	30	25
Steuber et al.[219]	126	0–18	33	29CT/27BMT	NS	NS
Stahnke et al.[78]	102	1–19	51	12CT/50BMT	26	40
Webb et al.[82]	88	0–15	69	17CT/44BMT	23	53

DFS, disease-free survival; NS, not specified; OS, overall survival.

trials available that prove the efficacy of G-CSF in AML patients with invasive fungal infections. In the past, the concern has been that this may mobilize leukaemic cells as well, but so far there is no evidence that the use of G-CSF causes a higher risk of relapse. In case of hypogammaglobulinaemia, intravenous gammaglobulin infusions might be useful during infectious periods in aplasia. In addition to fungal and bacterial infections, life-threatening infections due to viruses, *Mycoplasma pneumoniae* and *Pneumocystis carinii* (PCP) should be feared. Adenovirus, respiratory syncytial virus and influenza infections in AML patients all lead to life-threatening pulmonary infections.

To prevent bacterial, fungal and PCP infections, adequate prophylaxis is recommended until the patient is well beyond the last neutropenic period after discontinuation of therapy. Furthermore, it is recommended that paediatric AML patients be treated by experienced medical and nursing staff in paediatric oncology centres with advanced and intensive care facilities.

NUTRITION

The treatment of AML is very intensive and mucosal problems of the GI tract and mouth are frequently observed. Even when these problems do not occur, patients with AML are at risk of anorexia at an early stage. The great majority of patients require nasogastric tube or parenteral feeding after intensive chemotherapy courses.

RELAPSED AML

A relapse rate of 30–50 per cent is still the main cause of treatment failure in children with AML. Over 90 per cent of relapses occur in the bone marrow, whereas CNS relapse is very uncommon. The survival of relapsed patients is determined by the time of relapse. In cases of early relapse, within 1–1.5 years after diagnosis, the CR rate is 50 per cent and the OS is 0–10 per cent. If relapse occurs after 1.5 years, the CR rate is 80–90 per cent and the OS is up to 30–50 per cent.[78–82] Successful reinduction of a relapsed AML is possible in a substantial

proportion of patients with combinations of chemotherapy (Table 11.3). Most protocols so far have used combinations of anthracyclines with cytarabine, asparaginase and etoposide. Fludarabine and 2-chloro-deoxyadenosine combined with HDAC with or without anthracyclines and/or G-CSF have also been used, with a relatively good second CR rate.[78,82,191,218–228]

To date, multicentre randomized trials investigating the advantages of the chosen drug combinations have been scarce. After reaching second CR, stem cell transplantation is the treatment of choice to eradicate the leukaemic clone completely.[53,81,82] No studies are available which compare ABMT with allogeneic BMT in second CR in children. Second relapse remains the major cause of treatment failure in relapsed AML patients, but the risk of relapse has been shown to be lower in children after BMT in comparison with chemotherapy alone, and the survival rate in transplanted children is higher.[53,81,82] In addition to the development of new targeted drugs, in the future, relapsed AML patients may benefit from developments of immunosuppressive regimens, immunomodulatory regimens such as interleukin-2 and greater experience with donor lymphocyte infusions in transplant settings.[229–232]

LATE EFFECTS OF TREATMENT OF PAEDIATRIC AML

As more and more children with AML are cured, the issue of late sequelae will become more important. But since it is only during recent decades that long-term survivors have been registered, it is still difficult to assess the very long-term sequelae in people who suffered from AML in childhood.

Endocrine disorders

The effect of AML treatment on height is mainly determined by whether the patient received radiation of the cerebrum or total body irradiation. Both have been documented to cause growth hormone (partial or complete) deficiency and impaired growth in long-term survivors. The younger the patient at the time of treatment, the more obvious these problems are, particularly if the patient was below the age of 1 year.[233–237] Impairment of gonadal function is also a concern, especially in transplanted patients who received CNS and total body irradiation.[233]

Cardiotoxicity

As anthracyclines play a key role in the better survival rates nowadays, the occurrence of heart failure in later life is one of the main concerns for patients with AML. Five to 10 per cent of long-term survivors have clinical or sub-clinical cardiotoxicity, measured by decreasing left ventricular shortening fractions, especially if in the past the total cumulative dose exceeded 300 mg/m^2.[233,235,236] It has to be considered that drugs like cyclophosphamide and amsacrine might potentiate the risk of later cardiomyopathy.

Second malignancies

Since the survival rate in paediatric AML has increased dramatically over recent decades, the number of reports on second malignancies after AML therapy is increasing. Special caution is warranted in patients after radiation therapy, and especially after BMT, where radiotherapy is combined with immunosuppressive agents. Of the chemotherapeutic agents, topoisomerase-II inhibitors are the most important drugs that induce leukaemias, mostly AML with *MLL* rearrangements.[238,239] Haematological malignancies have been reported to have a relatively short latency, within less than 10 years after completion of AML therapy.[233,235,240] Second solid malignant tumours have been reported mainly in very long survivors after more than 10 years. Also benign solid tumours, such as uterine fibroids, fibroadenomas of the breast, angiomas and osteochondromas, have been reported after treatment for AML in childhood.[233,240]

Hepatitis B (HBV) and C (HVC)

Patients treated before 1990 are potentially at higher risk for the development of transfusion-related virus infection. In a recent study involving 77 survivors at St Judes, 74 were transfused with a median of 24 (2–10) times.[233] Among the 44 survivors tested for HBV, two were seropositive (5 per cent). In addition, 15 out of 53 patients tested for HVC (28 per cent) were seropositive. The two patients with HBV were co-infected with HVC. Of the 15 HVC-positive patients, 10 became chronic carriers.

Neurocognitive function

As in other paediatric oncological diagnoses, late effects on psychological and cognitive function are mainly determined by past irradiation of the CNS. Recently, a study involving 77 long-term survivors of AML showed that 66 of the patients did not have any academic problems in school. The other patients needed extra educational classes, but showed surprisingly minor problems. CNS irradiated patients had more problems than non-irradiated patients.[233]

DEVELOPMENT OF MOLECULAR TARGETED THERAPY

Identification of better prognostic subgroups, based on biological characteristics, may lead to more specific therapy by developing new drugs focused on biological targets. Moreover, early and late toxicity prevention should be part of the up-front treatment considerations. Current developments in gene expression microarray analyses, retroviral insertion mutagenesis and other biological studies have identified novel genes which are important in leukaemogenesis, and may be important for risk stratification in childhood AML in the future. These studies are improving the understanding of the biological heterogeneity of AML and will lead to a more optimal risk-adapted treatment strategy for children with AML.

Receptor tyrosine kinase inhibitors

The high frequency and poor outcome of AML cases with *FLT3* mutations make *FLT3* a highly interesting target for therapy. *In vitro*, several drugs are active against *FLT3*, such as herbimycin A, AG1296, CT 53518, CEP-701 and PKC 412. Herbimycin A was shown to inhibit tyrosine phosphorylation of the mutant but not the wild-type (wt) *FLT3* and prevented leukaemic progression in mice transplanted with mutant *FLT3*-transformed 32D cells.[241] AG1296 shows inhibitory activity of wt-*FLT3* and also other kinases such as platelet-derived growth factor (PDGF) and c-KIT. The autophosphorylation of *FLT3*/ITD was inhibited by AG1296 and AG1295 in primary AML cells.[242,243] For AG1296 and CT53518, it was shown that the phosphorylation of downstream targets of *FLT3* were also inhibited.[242,243] CT53518 appeared to be an effective drug both *in vitro* and in a mouse model.[244] CEP-701 overcomes the differentiation block[245] in primary AML cells and appeared to be a very potent cytotoxic drug against autophosphorylated wt-*FLT3* and constitutively activated mutant *FLT3 in vitro*.[243] In a murine model of *FLT3*/ITD leukaemia, inhibition of *FLT3* phosphorylation by CEP-701 was shown, as well as prolonged survival.[243] Different compounds from Sugen have shown activity against *FLT3* and related RTKs such as VEGFR2, PDGFR and KIT both *in vitro* and *in vivo*.[246] Finally, PKC412 has shown significant activity against *FLT3* that is activated by mutation or overexpression of the wild-type receptor in AML.[247] For both diseases, the activity of the drug was shown in mouse models, and target-validating experiments were performed which showed that *FLT3* was the target of the drug.

Phase I/II clinical studies of several *FLT3* inhibitors are underway.[248] The first published trial with SU5416 showed biological but only modest clinical activity in AML patients, and toxicities that were mainly attributable to drug formulation.[249] In the near future, we will get answers to the question of whether *FLT3* inhibition is indeed more than just a promising target for AML therapy, and if so, future studies should make clear how to combine *FLT3* inhibitors with other drugs for AML. Another tyrosine kinase inhibitor is imatinib, developed as a specific BCR-ABL TK inhibitor for chronic myelogenous leukaemia (CML).[250] Imatinib is toxic for AML cells by interfering with the activity of c-KIT. Ongoing trials will assess the efficacy of imatinib in AML.

Farnesyltransferase inhibitors

Farnesyltransferase inhibitors (FTIs) are small-molecule inhibitors that selectively inhibit farnesylation of a number of intracellular substrate proteins such as Ras, mitogen-activated protein kinase (MAPK) and phosphatidyl inositol-3 kinase (PI3K)/AKT.[251] Recently, it has been reported that these biological targets are expressed in childhood AML following activating mutations.[252] Compounds such as R115777 are currently being evaluated in phase I/II studies in AML patients.[253]

Angiogenesis inhibitors

Vascular endothelial growth factor (VEGF) is elevated in 66 per cent of AML patients.[254,255] Angiogenesis inhibitors have a broad spectrum of anti-tumour activity and lack of documented resistance, are relatively non-toxic, and are potentially synergistic with other anti-tumour therapies. Phase I/II studies are being performed with VEGF inhibitors such as thalidomide and SU5416 in leukaemia.[256] Until now, the clinical value of these agents has not been assessed for paediatric AML.

Histone deacetylation and demethylating agents

Recently, the concepts of histone acetylation and DNA methylation have become familiar[257] as epigenetic phenomena in AML. Histone acetylation modulates higher-order chromatin structure through the acetylation of lysine tails.[258] Deacetylating agents, such as trichostatin A, butyrates and depsipeptide, are available, which can overcome transcriptional repression in leukaemic cells.[256] DNA methylation is related to histone acetylation. DNA methylation of the CPG islands of the promoter regions recruits the histone deacetylase to block gene expression during transcription. This is mediated by binding of the protein MeCP2.[259,260] Preclinical data from Cameron *et al*.[261] have shown that DNA demethylation using decitabine plus the deacetylating agent trichostatin A synergized in re-expressing genes that were silenced in cancer. Phase I/II trials for this combination of drugs in clinical settings are now being performed at doses that presumably result in the maximum hypomethylation of inappropriately methylated genes.[256,262,263]

Differentiating agents

The most prominent example of differentiation therapy is the use of ATRA for the treatment of APL. Other agents with similar differentiation-inducing effect are currently under investigation, such as arsenic trioxide (ATO) and the high-dose demethylating agent 5′-azacitidine.[264,265]

Apoptosis inducers

Protein kinase C (PKC) inhibitors such as bryostatin and UCN-01 have been shown to influence phosphorylation of the anti-apoptotic gene *BCL*-2 and subsequently promote apoptosis.[266] Preclinical trials have shown that these drugs can restore Ara-C-induced apoptosis in resistant cells.[266] In leukaemia and myelodysplastic syndromes, ongoing phase I trials are studying the combination of bryostatin with cytarabine, fludarabine and 2-chlorodeoxyadenosine, and a phase II study is looking at its combination with ATRA.[266] Another approach to overcoming leukaemic cell resistance to chemotherapy is downregulation of *BCL*-2 activity by antisense oligonucleotides. Preclinical and pilot studies using this approach in AML patients have shown promising results.[267,268] Another way to induce chemotherapy-induced apoptosis is to activate signal transduction function by inhibition of STAT3 (a signal transducer and activator of transcription), which is activated in approximately 50 per cent of adult AML patients. Arsenic trioxide has been proven to inhibit STAT3 *in vitro* and is currently used in phase I clinical trials.[269]

Immunotherapy

Immunotherapy for AML consists of several toxin-conjugated antibodies and tumour vaccines. The best developed drug for clinical use is the calicheamicin-conjugated anti-CD33 monoclonal antibody CMA 676.[270–273] CD33 is expressed on the vast majority of AML blasts and is therefore an attractive target for antibody-mediated therapy.[274,275] CMA 676 or gemtuzumab ozogamicin (Mylotarg) is a monoclonal antibody directed against CD33 conjugated with a cytotoxic antibiotic, calicheamicin.[276] *In vitro* and *in vivo* studies in adult AML patients have made it clear that, after binding of Mylotarg to CD33, the drug is rapidly internalized and hydrolysed in the cytoplasm. Calicheamicin then enters the nucleus and binds to DNA, leading to double-stranded DNA breaks and finally cell death.[276–278] A phase I study by Sievers *et al.*[270] showed that $9\,mg/m^2$ of Mylotarg was the saturating dose but the MTD was not reached. This led to several phase II trials with a schedule of Mylotarg as a 2-hour infusion at this dose at 2-week intervals for two doses in patients with relapsed AML.[279] About 30 per cent of patients achieved CR and a relatively favourable toxicity profile for the drug was found. Despite relatively high levels of myelosuppression and grade III/IV hyperbilirubinaemia and elevated transaminases in about one-fifth of the patients, the incidences of mucositis and infections were low (4 and 28 per cent, respectively). The drug was administered on an outpatient basis in about 40 per cent of patients. The only major concern is the fact that Mylotarg induces severe liver toxicity in some cases, especially in veno-occlusive disease (VOD).[280–283] In a comparison between relapsed AML patients treated with Mylotarg and a historical control group treated with conventional chemotherapy, the survival of both groups appeared to be similar, while there were fewer hospitalization days in the Mylotarg-treated group.[284] In elderly patients with relapsed AML, the CR rate was 13 per cent and CR with incomplete platelet recovery was 15 per cent, resulting in an overall remission rate of 28 per cent.[285] Mylotarg was approved by the FDA for use in elderly CD33-positive AML patients.[286] Recently published and ongoing studies involving younger and elderly patients with AML focus on the combination of Mylotarg with standard AML chemotherapy such as fludarabine, cytarabine and cyclosporin, idarubicin and cytarabine, and topotecan and cytarabine.[287–289] Clinical trials using Mylotarg in combination with conventional chemotherapy in paediatric AML patients have begun and the initial results are promising.[270,272,290]

Some studies have suggested that leukaemic cells *in vitro* can be cultured with cytokines to induce at least partial differentiation into dendritic cells. Since dendritic cells are the most efficient antigen-presenting cells, it is likely that induction of differentiation *in vivo* would make these cells highly immunogenic and that this might be the basis for effective tumour vaccines in the future.[291] Preclinical studies showed that interleukin (IL)-2 had a significant anti-tumour effect. Clinical studies post-BMT showed a significant immunomodulatory effect, but without any effect on outcome.[292] Also, IL-2 has been used in maintenance therapy to eradicate MRD by immunomodulation.[293] The first studies evaluating IL-2 with respect to outcome are awaited.[294]

KEY POINTS

- Three to four courses of very intensive chemotherapy without BMT form the treatment of choice for the majority of paediatric AML patients. Therapy should be stratified according to cytogenetic risk groups and response to induction chemotherapy. In the future, class I gene aberrations may be of value to improve stratification based on biological characteristics of the AML patients.
- Using current intensive chemotherapy, there is no benefit of maintenance therapy in childhood AML.
- With CR rates for AML already high, reducing relapse rates as a way to improve survival should gain special interest.
- Detection of MRD may be of help in identifying AML subgroups that need alternative treatment strategies.
- CNS involvement at diagnosis has, in the past, generally been treated with CNS irradiation in most treatment schedules for patients over 2 years of age. It would be reasonable to reconsider the role of extra intrathecal therapy with avoidance of radiotherapy, as is currently recommended in some studies in ALL.
- The role of allo-BMT in regimens using intensive chemotherapy has become questionable, and there is no role for ABMT in paediatric AML. Only patients with a poor response to induction chemotherapy, using high-dose induction regimens, and those with MDR-AML and/or unfavourable cytogenetics, such as complex karyotypes or monosomy 7/7q-, may benefit from additional allo-BMT. If BMT is indicated, MUD transplantation should equally be considered in cases where there is no available matched sibling donor.
- Targeting new identified genes and proteins that have proved to be of prognostic significance for subgroups of AML should be the focus of future research. Development of new treatment protocols should focus on risk-adapted therapy, based on these molecular targets.
- In order to reduce toxicity, a special focus should be the risk of cardiotoxicity, and already in some

protocols the total cumulative anthracycline dosages have been decreased, especially during consolidation therapy. In addition to efficacy and toxicity studies on liposomal anthracyclines, cardioprotectants such as cardioxane and ICRF 187 are under investigation. Both agents might decrease the risk of heart failure while maintaining efficacy.

- Patients with Down's syndrome should be considered for reduction of therapy, as results of treatment are excellent with chemotherapy alone and the risk of toxicity and especially infections is considerable.

REFERENCES

1. Griffin JD, Lowenberg B. Clonogenic cells in acute myeloblastic leukemia. *Blood* 1986; **68**: 1185–95.
2. Fialkow PJ, Singer JW, Adamson JW *et al.* Acute nonlymphocytic leukemia: heterogeneity of stem cell origin. *Blood* 1981; **57**: 1068–73.
3. Fialkow PJ, Singer JW, Raskind WH *et al.* Clonal development, stem-cell differentiation, and clinical remissions in acute nonlymphocytic leukemia. *N Engl J Med* 1987; **317**: 468–73.
4. Linet M. The leukemias:epidemiological aspects. In: Likenfield AM, ed. *Monographs in Epidemiology and Biostatistics.* Oxford: Oxford University Press, 1985; 1–295.
5. Linet MS, Devesa SS. Descriptive epidemiology of the leukemias. In: Henderson ES, Lister TA, eds. *Leukemia*, 5th edn. Philadelphia: WB Saunders, 1990; 207–24.
6. Darby SC, Nakashima E, Kato H. A parallel analysis of cancer mortality among atomic bomb survivors and patients with ankylosing spondylitis given X-ray therapy. *J Natl Cancer Inst* 1985; **75**: 1–21.
7. Hempelmann LH, Hall WJ, Phillips M *et al.* Neoplasms in persons treated with X-rays in infancy: fourth survey in 20 years. *J Natl Cancer Inst* 1975; **55**: 519–30.
8. Curtis RE, Boice JD Jr, Stovall M *et al.* Risk of leukemia after chemotherapy and radiation treatment for breast cancer. *N Engl J Med* 1992; **326**: 1745–51.
9. Brown LM, Blair A, Gibson R *et al.* Pesticide exposures and other agricultural risk factors for leukemia among men in Iowa and Minnesota. *Cancer Res* 1990; **50**: 6585–91.
10. Rodella S, Ciccone G, Rege-Cambrin G, Vineis P. Cytogenetics and occupational exposures in acute nonlymphocytic leukemia and myelodysplastic syndrome. Working Group on the Epidemiology of Hematolymphopoietic Malignancies in Italy. *Scand J Work Environ Health* 1993; **19**: 369–74.
11. Ciccone G, Mirabelli D, Levis A *et al.* Myeloid leukemias and myelodysplastic syndromes: chemical exposure, histologic subtype and cytogenetics in a case-control study. *Cancer Genet Cytogenet* 1993; **68**: 135–9.
12. Sandoval C, Pui CH, Bowman LC *et al.* Secondary acute myeloid leukemia in children previously treated with alkylating agents, intercalating topoisomerase II inhibitors, and irradiation. *J Clin Oncol* 1993; **11**: 1039–45.
13. Garfinkel L, Boffetta P. Association between smoking and leukemia in two American Cancer Society prospective studies. *Cancer* 1990; **65**: 2356–60.
14. Severson RK, Davis S, Heuser L *et al.* Cigarette smoking and acute nonlymphocytic leukemia. *Am J Epidemiol* 1990; **132**: 418–22.
15. Brill AB, Tomonoga M, Heyssel RM. Leukemia in man following exposure to Hiroshima and Nagasaki and comprison to other human experience. *Ann Intern Med* 1962; **56**: 590–609.
16. Inskip PD, Kleinerman RA, Stovall M *et al.* Leukemia, lymphoma, and multiple myeloma after pelvic radiotherapy for benign disease. *Radiat Res* 1993; **135**: 108–24.
17. Hunger SP, Cleary ML. What significance should we attribute to the detection of MLL fusion transcripts? *Blood* 1998; **92**: 709–11.
18. Greaves MF. Aetiology of acute leukaemia. *Lancet* 1997; **349**: 344–9.
19. Gale KB, Ford AM, Repp R *et al.* Backtracking leukemia to birth: identification of clonotypic gene fusion sequences in neonatal blood spots. *Proc Natl Acad Sci USA* 1997; **94**: 13950–4.
20. Greaves MF. Speculations on the cause of childhood acute lymphoblastic leukemia. *Leukemia* 1988; **2**: 120–5.
21. Mundschau G, Gurbuxani S, Gamis AS *et al.* Mutagenesis of GATA1 is an initiating event in Down syndrome leukemogenesis. *Blood* 2003; **101**: 4298–300.
22. Rainis L, Bercovich D, Strehl S *et al.* Mutations in exon 2 of GATA1 are early events in megakaryocytic malignancies associated with trisomy 21. *Blood* 2003; **102**: 981–6.
23. Hitzler JK, Cheung J, Li Y *et al.* GATA1 mutations in transient leukemia and acute megakaryoblastic leukemia of Down syndrome. *Blood* 2003; **101**: 4301–4.
24. Lie SO, Abrahamsson J, Clausen N *et al.* Treatment stratification based on initial in vivo response in acute myeloid leukaemia in children without Down's syndrome: results of NOPHO-AML trials. *Br J Haematol* 2003; **122**: 217–25.
25. Behar C, Suciu S, Benoit Y *et al.* Mitoxantrone-containing regimen for treatment of childhood acute leukemia (AML) and analysis of prognostic factors: results of the EORTC Children Leukemia Cooperative Study 58872. *Med Pediatr Oncol* 1996; **26**: 173–9.
26. Hann IM, Stevens RF, Goldstone AH *et al.* Randomized comparison of DAT versus ADE as induction chemotherapy in children and younger adults with acute myeloid leukemia. Results of the Medical Research Council's 10th AML trial (MRC AML10). Adult and Childhood Leukaemia Working Parties of the Medical Research Council. *Blood* 1997; **89**: 2311–18.
27. Woods WG, Neudorf S, Gold S *et al.* A comparison of allogeneic bone marrow transplantation, autologous bone marrow transplantation, and aggressive chemotherapy in children with acute myeloid leukemia in remission: a report from the Children's cancer group. *Blood* 2001; **97**: 56–62.
28. Lie SO, Jonmundsson G, Mellander L *et al.* A population-based study of 272 children with acute myeloid leukaemia treated on two consecutive protocols with different intensity: best outcome in girls, infants, and children with Down's syndrome. Nordic Society of Paediatric Haematology and Oncology (NOPHO). *Br J Haematol* 1996; **94**: 82–8.

29. Ravindranath Y, Yeager AM, Chang MN et al. Autologous bone marrow transplantation versus intensive consolidation chemotherapy for acute myeloid leukemia in childhood. Pediatric Oncology Group. N Engl J Med 1996; **334**: 1428–34.

30. Amadori S, Testi AM, Arico M et al. Prospective comparative study of bone marrow transplantation and postremission chemotherapy for childhood acute myelogenous leukemia. The Associazione Italiana Ematologia ed Oncologia Pediatrica Cooperative Group. J Clin Oncol 1993; **11**: 1046–54.

31. Stevens RF, Hann IM, Wheatley K, Gray RG. Marked improvements in outcome with chemotherapy alone in paediatric acute myeloid leukaemia: results of the United Kingdom Medical Research Council's 10th AML trial. MRC Childhood Leukaemia Working Party. Br J Haematol 1998; **101**: 130–40.

32. Creutzig U, Ritter J, Zimmermann M et al. Idarubicin improves blast cell clearance during induction therapy in children with AML: results of study AML-BFM 93. AML-BFM Study Group. Leukemia 2001; **15**: 348–54.

33. Webb DK, Harrison G, Stevens RF et al. Relationships between age at diagnosis, clinical features, and outcome of therapy in children treated in the Medical Research Council AML 10 and 12 trials for acute myeloid leukemia. Blood 2001; **98**: 1714–20.

34. Gibson B, Webb D, de Graaf S, Wheatley K. Improved outcome in MRC 12 pediatrics: Has the limit of conventional chemotherapy been reached? Blood 2002; **100**: 37a, 124a.

35. Chang M, Raimondi SC, Ravindranath Y et al. Prognostic factors in children and adolescents with acute myeloid leukemia (excluding children with Down syndrome and acute promyelocytic leukemia): univariate and recursive partitioning analysis of patients treated on Pediatric Oncology Group (POG) Study 8821. Leukemia 2000; **14**: 1201–7.

36. Hurwitz CA, Schell MJ, Pui CH et al. Adverse prognostic features in 251 children treated for acute myeloid leukemia. Med Pediatr Oncol 1993; **21**: 1–7.

37. Bennett JM, Catovsky D, Daniel MT et al. Criteria for the diagnosis of acute leukemia of megakaryocyte lineage (M7). A report of the French-American-British Cooperative Group. Ann Intern Med 1985; **103**: 460–2.

38. Kita K, Nakase K, Miwa H et al. Phenotypical characteristics of acute myelocytic leukemia associated with the t(8;21)(q22;q22) chromosomal abnormality: frequent expression of immature B-cell antigen CD19 together with stem cell antigen CD34. Blood 1992; **80**: 470–7.

39. Smith FO, Lampkin BC, Versteeg C et al. Expression of lymphoid-associated cell surface antigens by childhood acute myeloid leukemia cells lacks prognostic significance. Blood 1992; **79**: 2415–22.

40. Mittelman F, ed. An International System for Human Cytogenetic Nomenclature (ISCN). Basel: Karger, 1995.

41. Vardiman JW, Harris NL, Brunning RD. The World Health Organization (WHO) classification of the myeloid neoplasms. Blood 2002; **100**: 2292–302.

42. Jaffe ES HN, Stein H, Vardiman JW, eds. World Health Organization Classification of Tumours: Pathology and Genetics of Tumours of Haematopoietic and Lymphoid Tumours. Lyon: IARC, 2001.

43. Harris NL, Jaffe ES, Diebold J et al. The World Health Organization classification of neoplastic diseases of the hematopoietic and lymphoid tissues. Report of the Clinical Advisory Committee meeting, Airlie House, Virginia, November, 1997. Ann Oncol 1999; **10**: 1419–32.

44. Hasle H, Niemeyer CM, Chessells JM et al. A pediatric approach to the WHO classification of myelodysplastic and myeloproliferative diseases. Leukemia 2003; **17**: 277–82.

45. Mandel K, Dror Y, Poon A, Freedman MH. A practical, comprehensive classification for pediatric myelodysplastic syndromes: the CCC system. J Pediatr Hematol Oncol 2002; **24**: 596–605.

46. Buchner T, Heinecke A. The role of prognostic factors in acute myeloid leukemia. Leukemia 1996; **10**(Suppl 1): S28–9.

47. Raimondi SC, Chang MN, Ravindranath Y et al. Chromosomal abnormalities in 478 children with acute myeloid leukemia: clinical characteristics and treatment outcome in a cooperative pediatric oncology group study-POG 8821. Blood 1999; **94**: 3707–16.

48. Creutzig U, Zimmermann M, Ritter J et al. Definition of a standard-risk group in children with AML. Br J Haematol 1999; **104**: 630–9.

49. Pui CH, Raimondi SC, Srivastava DK et al. Prognostic factors in infants with acute myeloid leukemia. Leukemia 2000; **14**: 684–7.

50. Chessells JM, Harrison CJ, Kempski H et al. Clinical features, cytogenetics and outcome in acute lymphoblastic and myeloid leukaemia of infancy: report from the MRC Childhood Leukaemia working party. Leukemia 2002; **16**: 776–84.

51. Kawasaki H, Isoyama K, Eguchi M et al. Superior outcome of infant acute myeloid leukemia with intensive chemotherapy: results of the Japan Infant Leukemia Study Group. Blood 2001; **98**: 3589–94.

52. Marco F, Bureo E, Ortega JJ et al. High survival rate in infant acute leukemia treated with early high-dose chemotherapy and stem-cell support. Groupo Español de Trasplante de Medula Osea en Ninos. J Clin Oncol 2000; **18**: 3256–61.

53. Creutzig U, Ritter J, Zimmermann M et al. Improved treatment results in high-risk pediatric acute myeloid leukemia patients after intensification with high-dose cytarabine and mitoxantrone: results of Study Acute Myeloid Leukemia – Berlin-Frankfurt-Münster 93. J Clin Oncol 2001; **19**: 2705–13.

54. Lie SO, Jonmundsson GK, Mellander L et al. Chemotherapy of acute myelocytic leukemia in children. Ann NY Acad Sci 1997; **824**: 84–90.

55. Ravindranath Y, Steuber CP, Krischer J et al. High-dose cytarabine for intensification of early therapy of childhood acute myeloid leukemia: a Pediatric Oncology Group study. J Clin Oncol 1991; **9**: 572–80.

56. Satake N, Maseki N, Nishiyama M et al. Chromosome abnormalities and MLL rearrangements in acute myeloid leukemia of infants. Leukemia 1999; **13**: 1013–17.

57. Woods WG, Kobrinsky N, Buckley JD et al. Timed-sequential induction therapy improves postremission outcome in acute myeloid leukemia: a report from the Children's Cancer Group. Blood 1996; **87**: 4979–89.

58. Hilden JM, Smith FO, Frestedt JL et al. MLL gene rearrangement, cytogenetic 11q23 abnormalities, and expression of the NG2 molecule in infant acute myeloid leukemia. Blood 1997; **89**: 3801–5.

59. Cassileth PA, Harrington DP, Appelbaum FR et al. Chemotherapy compared with autologous or allogeneic bone

marrow transplantation in the management of acute myeloid leukemia in first remission. *N Engl J Med* 1998; **339**: 1649–56.

60. Bostrom B. Relapse after bone marrow transplantation for acute leukaemia. *Lancet* 1985; **2**: 44.

61. Woolfrey AE, Gooley TA, Sievers EL *et al.* Bone marrow transplantation for children less than 2 years of age with acute myelogenous leukemia or myelodysplastic syndrome. *Blood* 1998; **92**: 3546–56.

62. Smith SD, Rosen D, Trueworthy RC, Lowman JT. A reliable method for evaluating drug compliance in children with cancer. *Cancer* 1979; **43**: 169–73.

63. Pui CH, Ribeiro RC, Campana D *et al.* Prognostic factors in the acute lymphoid and myeloid leukemias of infants. *Leukemia* 1996; **10**: 952–6.

64. Bisschop MM, Revesz T, Bierings M *et al.* Extramedullary infiltrates at diagnosis have no prognostic significance in children with acute myeloid leukaemia. *Leukemia* 2001; **15**: 46–9.

65. Creutzig U, Berthold F, Boos J *et al.* [Improved treatment results in children with AML: Results of study AML- BFM 93]. *Klin Padiatr* 2001; **213**: 175–85.

66. Neiman RS, Barcos M, Berard C *et al.* Granulocytic sarcoma: a clinicopathologic study of 61 biopsied cases. *Cancer* 1981; **48**: 1426–37.

67. Eshghabadi M, Shojania AM, Carr I. Isolated granulocytic sarcoma: report of a case and review of the literature. *J Clin Oncol* 1986; **4**: 912–17.

68. Meis JM, Butler JJ, Osborne BM, Manning JT. Granulocytic sarcoma in nonleukemic patients. *Cancer* 1986; **58**: 2697–709.

69. Tallman MS, Hakimian D, Shaw JM *et al.* Granulocytic sarcoma is associated with the 8;21 translocation in acute myeloid leukemia. *J Clin Oncol* 1993; **11**: 690–7.

70. Hagihara M, Kobayashi H, Miyachi H, Ogawa T. Clinical heterogeneity in acute myelogenous leukemia with the 8;21 translocation. *Keio J Med* 1991; **40**: 90–3.

71. Swirsky DM, Li YS, Matthews JG *et al.* 8;21 translocation in acute granulocytic leukaemia: cytological, cytochemical and clinical features. *Br J Haematol* 1984; **56**: 199–213.

72. Krishnan K, Ross CW, Adams PT *et al.* Neural cell-adhesion molecule (CD 56)-positive, t(8;21) acute myeloid leukemia (AML, M-2) and granulocytic sarcoma. *Ann Hematol* 1994; **69**: 321–3.

73. Byrd JC, Weiss RB. Recurrent granulocytic sarcoma. An unusual variation of acute myelogenous leukemia associated with 8;21 chromosomal translocation and blast expression of the neural cell adhesion molecule. *Cancer* 1994; **73**: 2107–12.

74. Pui MH, Fletcher BD, Langston JW. Granulocytic sarcoma in childhood leukemia: imaging features. *Radiology* 1994; **190**: 698–702.

75. Creutzig U, Ritter J, Schellong G. Identification of two risk groups in childhood acute myelogenous leukemia after therapy intensification in study AML-BFM-83 as compared with study AML-BFM-78. AML-BFM Study Group. *Blood* 1990; **75**: 1932–40.

76. Zwaan CM, Kaspers GJ, Pieters R *et al.* Cellular drug resistance in childhood acute myeloid leukemia is related to chromosomal abnormalities. *Blood* 2002; **100**: 3352–60.

77. Zwaan CM, Kaspers GJ, Pieters R *et al.* Different drug sensitivity profiles of acute myeloid and lymphoblastic leukemia and normal peripheral blood mononuclear cells in children with and without Down syndrome. *Blood* 2002; **99**: 245–51.

78. Stahnke K, Boos J, Bender-Gotze C *et al.* Duration of first remission predicts remission rates and long-term survival in children with relapsed acute myelogenous leukemia. *Leukemia* 1998; **12**: 1534–8.

79. Thalhammer F, Geissler K, Jager U *et al.* Duration of second complete remission in patients with acute myeloid leukemia treated with chemotherapy: a retrospective single-center study. *Ann Hematol* 1996; **72**: 216–22.

80. Keating MJ, Smith TL, Kantarjian H *et al.* Cytogenetic pattern in acute myelogenous leukemia: a major reproducible determinant of outcome. *Leukemia* 1988; **2**: 403–12.

81. Webb DK. Management of relapsed acute myeloid leukaemia [see comments]. *Br J Haematol* 1999; **106**: 851–9.

82. Webb DK, Wheatley K, Harrison G *et al.* Outcome for children with relapsed acute myeloid leukaemia following initial therapy in the Medical Research Council (MRC) AML 10 trial. MRC Childhood Leukaemia Working Party. *Leukemia* 1999; **13**: 25–31.

83. Rowe JM, Liesveld JL. Treatment and prognostic factors in acute myeloid leukaemia. *Bailliere's Clin Haematol* 1996; **9**: 87–105.

84. Creutzig U, Harbott J, Sperling C *et al.* Clinical significance of surface antigen expression in children with acute myeloid leukemia: results of study AML-BFM-87. *Blood* 1995; **86**: 3097–108.

85. Venditti A, Del Poeta G, Buccisano F *et al.* Prognostic relevance of the expression of Tdt and CD7 in 335 cases of acute myeloid leukemia. *Leukemia* 1998; **12**: 1056–63.

86. Kita K, Miwa H, Nakase K *et al.* Clinical importance of CD7 expression in acute myelocytic leukemia. The Japan Cooperative Group of Leukemia/Lymphoma. *Blood* 1993; **81**: 2399–405.

87. Bradstock K, Matthews J, Benson E *et al.* Prognostic value of immunophenotyping in acute myeloid leukemia. Australian Leukaemia Study Group. *Blood* 1994; **84**: 1220–5.

88. De Nully Brown P, Jurlander J, Pedersen-Bjergaard J *et al.* The prognostic significance of chromosomal analysis and immunophenotyping in 117 patients with de novo acute myeloid leukemia. *Leuk Res* 1997; **21**: 985–95.

89. Campos L, Guyotat D, Archimbaud E *et al.* Surface marker expression in adult acute myeloid leukaemia: correlations with initial characteristics, morphology and response to therapy. *Br J Haematol* 1989; **72**: 161–6.

90. Del Poeta G, Stasi R, Venditti A *et al.* Prognostic value of cell marker analysis in de novo acute myeloid leukemia. *Leukemia* 1994; **8**: 388–94.

91. Solary E, Casasnovas RO, Campos L *et al.* Surface markers in adult acute myeloblastic leukemia: correlation of CD19+, CD34+ and CD14+/DR–phenotypes with shorter survival. Groupe d'Etude Immunologique des Leucemies (GEIL). *Leukemia* 1992; **6**: 393–9.

92. Van den Heuvel-Eibrink MM, van der Holt B, te Boekhorst PA *et al.* MDR 1 expression is an independent prognostic factor for response and survival in de novo acute myeloid leukaemia. *Br J Haematol* 1997; **99**: 76–83.

93. Legrand O, Perrot JY, Baudard M *et al.* The immunophenotype of 177 adults with acute myeloid leukemia: proposal of a prognostic score. *Blood* 2000; **96**: 870–7.

94. Sandler DP. Epidemiology of acute myelogenous leukemia. *Semin Oncol* 1987; **14**: 359–64.

95. Neglia JP, Robison LL. Epidemiology of the childhood acute leukemias. *Pediatr Clin North Am* 1988; **35**: 675–92.

96. Hardnen DG. Inherited factors in leukemia and lymphoma. *Leukemia Res* 1985; **9**: 705–8.

97. Snyder AL, Henderson ES, Li FP *et al*. Possible inherited leukaemogenic factors in familial acute myelogenous leukaemia. *Lancet* 1970; **1**: 586–9.

98. Robison LL, Nesbit ME Jr, Sather HN *et al*. Down syndrome and acute leukemia in children: a 10-year retrospective survey from Childrens Cancer Study Group. *J Pediatr* 1984; **105**: 235–42.

99. Ravindranath Y, Abella E, Krischer JP *et al*. Acute myeloid leukemia (AML) in Down's syndrome is highly responsive to chemotherapy: experience on Pediatric Oncology Group AML Study 8498. *Blood* 1992; **80**: 2210–14.

100. Richards M, Welch J, Watmore A *et al*. Trisomy 21 associated transient neonatal myeloproliferation in the absence of Down's syndrome. *Arch Dis Child Fetal Neonatal Ed* 1998; **79**: F215–17.

101. Litz CE, Davies S, Brunning RD *et al*. Acute leukemia and the transient myeloproliferative disorder associated with Down syndrome: morphologic, immunophenotypic and cytogenetic manifestations. *Leukemia* 1995; **9**: 1432–9.

102. Lange BJ, Kobrinsky N, Barnard DR *et al*. Distinctive demography, biology, and outcome of acute myeloid leukemia and myelodysplastic syndrome in children with Down syndrome: Children's Cancer Group Studies 2861 and 2891. *Blood* 1998; **91**: 608–15.

103. Zipursky A, Thorner P, De Harven E *et al*. Myelodysplasia and acute megakaryoblastic leukemia in Down's syndrome. *Leuk Res* 1994; **18**: 163–71.

104. Homans AC, Verissimo AM, Vlacha V. Transient abnormal myelopoiesis of infancy associated with trisomy 21. *Am J Pediatr Hematol Oncol* 1993; **15**: 392–9.

105. Yumura-Yagi K, Hara J, Tawa A, Kawa-Ha K. Phenotypic characteristics of acute megakaryocytic leukemia and transient abnormal myelopoiesis. *Leuk Lymphoma* 1994; **13**: 393–400.

106. Taub JW, Huang X, Matherly LH *et al*. Expression of chromosome 21-localized genes in acute myeloid leukemia: differences between Down syndrome and non-Down syndrome blast cells and relationship to in vitro sensitivity to cytosine arabinoside and daunorubicin. *Blood* 1999; **94**: 1393–400.

107. Taub JW, Stout ML, Buck SA *et al*. Myeloblasts from Down syndrome children with acute myeloid leukemia have increased in vitro sensitivity to cytosine arabinoside and daunorubicin. *Leukemia* 1997; **11**: 1594–5.

108. Creutzig U, Ritter J, Vormoor J *et al*. [Transient myeloproliferation and acute myeloid leukemia in infants with Down's syndrome]. *Klin Padiatr* 1990; **202**: 253–7.

109. Gilliland DG. Hematologic malignancies. *Curr Opin Hematol* 2001; **8**: 189–91.

110. Deguchi K, Gilliland DG. Cooperativity between mutations in tyrosine kinases and in hematopoietic transcription factors in AML. *Leukemia* 2002; **16**: 740–4.

111. Gupta R, Knight CL, Bain BJ. Receptor tyrosine kinase mutations in myeloid neoplasms. *Br J Haematol* 2002; **117**: 489–508.

112. Beghini A, Peterlongo P, Ripamonti CB *et al*. C-kit mutations in core binding factor leukemias. *Blood* 2000; **95**: 726–7.

113. Kottaridis PD, Gale RE, Frew ME *et al*. The presence of a FLT3 internal tandem duplication in patients with acute myeloid leukemia (AML) adds important prognostic information to cytogenetic risk group and response to the first cycle of chemotherapy: analysis of 854 patients from the United Kingdom Medical Research Council AML 10 and 12 trials. *Blood* 2001; **98**: 1752–9.

114. Care RS, Valk PJ, Goodeve AC *et al*. Incidence and prognosis of c-KIT and FLT3 mutations in core binding factor (CBF) acute myeloid leukaemias. *Br J Haematol* 2003; **121**: 775–7.

115. Grimwade D, Walker H, Oliver F *et al*. The importance of diagnostic cytogenetics on outcome in AML: analysis of 1,612 patients entered into the MRC AML 10 trial. The Medical Research Council Adult and Children's Leukaemia Working Parties. *Blood* 1998; **92**: 2322–33.

116. Jahns-Streubel G, Braess J, Schoch C *et al*. Cytogenetic subgroups in acute myeloid leukemia differ in proliferative activity and response to GM-CSF. *Leukemia* 2001; **15**(3): 377–84.

117. Kalwinsky DK, Raimondi SC, Schell MJ *et al*. Prognostic importance of cytogenetic subgroups in de novo pediatric acute nonlymphocytic leukemia. *J Clin Oncol* 1990; **8**: 75–83.

118. Martinez-Climent JA, Lane NJ, Rubin CM *et al*. Clinical and prognostic significance of chromosomal abnormalities in childhood acute myeloid leukemia de novo. *Leukemia* 1995; **9**: 95–101.

119. Leverger G, Bernheim A, Daniel MT *et al*. Cytogenetic study of 130 childhood acute nonlymphocytic leukemias. *Med Pediatr Oncol* 1988; **16**: 227–32.

120. Gregory J, Feusner J. Acute promyelocytic leukaemia in children. *Best Pract Res Clin Haematol* 2003; **16**: 483–94.

121. Martinez A, San Miguel JF, Valverde B *et al*. Functional expression of MDR-1 in acute myeloid leukemia: correlation with the clinical-biological, immunophenotypical, and prognostic disease characteristics. *Ann Hematol* 1997; **75**: 81–6.

122. Leblanc T, Auvrignon A, Michel G *et al*. Prognosis of cytogenetics in 250 children with acute myeloid leukemia treated in the LAME 89/91 protocol. *Blood* 1996; **88**: 634a.

123. Gibson BE, Webb D, Wheatley K. Does transplant in first CR have a role in pediatric AML? A review of the MRC10 & 12 trials. *Blood* 2000; **96**: 522a.

124. Rubnitz JE, Raimondi SC, Tong X *et al*. Favorable impact of the t(9;11) in childhood acute myeloid leukemia. *J Clin Oncol* 2002; **20**: 2302–9.

125. Sorensen PH, Chen CS, Smith FO *et al*. Molecular rearrangements of the MLL gene are present in most cases of infant acute myeloid leukemia and are strongly correlated with monocytic or myelomonocytic phenotypes. *J Clin Invest* 1994; **93**: 429–37.

126. Cimino G, Rapanotti MC, Elia L *et al*. ALL-1 gene rearrangements in acute myeloid leukemia: association with M4-M5 French-American-British classification subtypes and young age. *Cancer Res* 1995; **55**: 1625–8.

127. Rubnitz JE, Behm FG, Downing JR. 11q23 rearrangements in acute leukemia. *Leukemia* 1996; **10**: 74–82.

128. Rubnitz JE, Behm FG, Pui CH *et al.* Genetic studies of childhood acute lymphoblastic leukemia with emphasis on p16, MLL, and ETV6 gene abnormalities: results of St. Jude Total Therapy Study XII. *Leukemia* 1997; **11**: 1201–6.

129. Swansbury J. Cytogenetic studies in hematologic malignancies: an overview. *Methods Mol Biol* 2003; **220**: 9–22.

130. Hasle H, Arico M, Basso G *et al.* Myelodysplastic syndrome, juvenile myelomonocytic leukemia, and acute myeloid leukemia associated with complete or partial monosomy 7. European Working Group on MDS in Childhood (EWOG-MDS). *Leukemia* 1999; **13**: 376–85.

131. van den Heuvel-Eibrink MM, Wiemer EA, de Boevere MJ *et al.* MDR1 expression in poor-risk acute myeloid leukemia with partial or complete monosomy 7. *Leukemia* 2001; **15**: 398–405.

132. Gilliland DG, Griffin JD. The roles of FLT3 in hematopoiesis and leukemia. *Blood* 2002; **100**: 1532–42.

133. Nakao M, Yokota S, Iwai T *et al.* Internal tandem duplication of the flt3 gene found in acute myeloid leukemia. *Leukemia* 1996; **10**: 1911–18.

134. Stirewalt DL, Kopecky KJ, Meshinchi S *et al.* FLT3, RAS, and TP53 mutations in elderly patients with acute myeloid leukemia. *Blood* 2001; **97**: 3589–95.

135. Kelly LM, Liu Q, Kutok JL *et al.* FLT3 internal tandem duplication mutations associated with human acute myeloid leukemias induce myeloproliferative disease in a murine bone marrow transplant model. *Blood* 2002; **99**: 310–18.

136. Kiyoi H, Naoe T, Nakano Y *et al.* Prognostic implication of FLT3 and N-RAS gene mutations in acute myeloid leukemia. *Blood* 1999; **93**: 3074–80.

137. Schnittger S, Schoch C, Dugas M *et al.* Analysis of FLT3 length mutations in 1003 patients with acute myeloid leukemia: correlation to cytogenetics, FAB subtype, and prognosis in the AMLCG study and usefulness as a marker for the detection of minimal residual disease. *Blood* 2002; **100**: 59–66.

138. Rombouts WJ, Blokland I, Lowenberg B, Ploemacher RE. Biological characteristics and prognosis of adult acute myeloid leukemia with internal tandem duplications in the Flt3 gene. *Leukemia* 2000; **14**: 675–83.

139. Meshinchi S, Woods WG, Stirewalt DL *et al.* Prevalence and prognostic significance of Flt3 internal tandem duplication in pediatric acute myeloid leukemia. *Blood* 2001; **97**: 89–94.

140. Kondo M, Horibe K, Takahashi Y *et al.* Prognostic value of internal tandem duplication of the FLT3 gene in childhood acute myelogenous leukemia. *Med Pediatr Oncol* 1999; **33**: 525–9.

141. Xu F, Taki T, Yang HW *et al.* Tandem duplication of the FLT3 gene is found in acute lymphoblastic leukaemia as well as acute myeloid leukaemia but not in myelodysplastic syndrome or juvenile chronic myelogenous leukaemia in children. *Br J Haematol* 1999; **105**: 155–62.

142. Iwai T, Yokota S, Nakao M *et al.* Internal tandem duplication of the FLT3 gene and clinical evaluation in childhood acute myeloid leukemia. The Children's Cancer and Leukemia Study Group, Japan. *Leukemia* 1999; **13**: 38–43.

143. Liang P, Pardee AB. Differential display of eukaryotic messenger RNA by means of the polymerase chain reaction [see comments]. *Science* 1992; **257**: 967–71.

144. Whitman SP, Archer KJ, Feng L *et al.* Absence of the wild-type allele predicts poor prognosis in adult de novo acute myeloid leukemia with normal cytogenetics and the internal tandem duplication of FLT3: a cancer and leukemia group B study. *Cancer Res* 2001; **61**: 7233–9.

145. Thiede C, Steudel C, Mohr B *et al.* Analysis of FLT3-activating mutations in 979 patients with acute myelogenous leukemia: association with FAB subtypes and identification of subgroups with poor prognosis. *Blood* 2002; **99**: 4326–35.

146. Libura M, Asnafi V, Tu A *et al.* FLT3 and MLL intragenic abnormalities in AML reflect a common category of genotoxic stress. *Blood* 2003; **102**: 2198–204.

147. Steudel C, Wermke M, Schaich M *et al.* Comparative analysis of MLL partial tandem duplication and FLT3 internal tandem duplication mutations in 956 adult patients with acute myeloid leukemia. *Genes Chromosomes Cancer* 2003; **37**: 237–51.

148. Yamamoto Y, Kiyoi H, Nakano Y *et al.* Activating mutation of D835 within the activation loop of FLT3 in human hematologic malignancies. *Blood* 2001; **97**: 2434–9.

149. Armstrong SA, Kung AL, Mabon ME *et al.* Inhibition of FLT3 in MLL. Validation of a therapeutic target identified by gene expression based classification. *Cancer Cell* 2003; **3**: 173–83.

150. Levis M, Allebach J, Tse KF *et al.* A FLT3-targeted tyrosine kinase inhibitor is cytotoxic to leukemia cells in vitro and in vivo. *Blood* 2002; **99**: 3885–91.

151. Kelly LM, Yu JC, Boulton CL *et al.* CT53518, a novel selective FLT3 antagonist for the treatment of acute myelogenous leukemia (AML). *Cancer Cell* 2002; **1**: 421–32.

152. Gari M, Goodeve A, Wilson G *et al.* c-kit proto-oncogene exon 8 in-frame deletion plus insertion mutations in acute myeloid leukaemia. *Br J Haematol* 1999; **105**: 894–900.

153. Khanna-Gupta A, Lopingco MC, Savinelli T *et al.* Retroviral insertional activation of the EVI1 oncogene does not prevent G-CSF-induced maturation of the murine pluripotent myeloid cell line 32Dcl3. *Oncogene* 1996; **12**: 563–9.

154. Lopingco MC, Perkins AS. Molecular analysis of Evi1, a zinc finger oncogene involved in myeloid leukemia. *Curr Top Microbiol Immunol* 1996; **211**: 211–22.

155. Zent C, Kim N, Hiebert S *et al.* Rearrangement of the AML1/CBFA2 gene in myeloid leukemia with the 3;21 translocation: expression of co-existing multiple chimeric genes with similar functions as transcriptional repressors, but with opposite tumorigenic properties. *Curr Top Microbiol Immunol* 1996; **211**: 243–52.

156. Russell M, List A, Greenberg P *et al.* Expression of EVI1 in myelodysplastic syndromes and other hematologic malignancies without 3q26 translocations. *Blood* 1994; **84**: 1243–8.

157. Barjesteh van Waalwijk van Doorn-Khosrovani S, Erpelinck C, van Putten WL *et al.* High EVI1 expression predicts poor survival in acute myeloid leukemia: a study of 319 de novo AML patients. *Blood* 2003; **101**: 837–45.

158. Valk PJ, Vankan Y, Joosten M *et al.* Retroviral insertions in Evi12, a novel common virus integration site upstream of Tra1/Grp94, frequently coincide with insertions in the gene

encoding the peripheral cannabinoid receptor Cnr2. *J Virol* 1999; **73**: 3595–602.

159. Van Waalwijk Van Doorn-Khosrovani SB, Erpelinck C, Meijer J *et al.* Biallelic mutations in the CEBPA gene and low CEBPA expression levels as prognostic markers in intermediate-risk AML. *Hematol J* 2003; **4**: 31–40.

160. Joosten M, Valk PJ, Vankan Y *et al.* Phenotyping of Evi1, Evi11/Cb2, and Evi12 transformed leukemias isolated from a novel panel of cas-Br-M murine leukemia virus-infected mice. *Virology* 2000; **268**: 308–18.

161. Joosten M, Valk PJ, Jorda MA *et al.* Leukemic predisposition of pSca-1/Cb2 transgenic mice. *Exp Hematol* 2002; **30**: 142–9.

162. Jorda MA, Lowenberg B, Delwel R. The peripheral cannabinoid receptor Cb2, a novel oncoprotein, induces a reversible block in neutrophilic differentiation. *Blood* 2003; **101**: 1336–43.

163. Valk PJ, Delwel R. The peripheral cannabinoid receptor, Cb2, in retrovirally-induced leukemic transformation and normal hematopoiesis. *Leuk Lymphoma* 1998; **32**: 29–43.

164. Campos L, Guyotat D, Archimbaud E *et al.* Clinical significance of multidrug resistance P-glycoprotein expression on acute nonlymphoblastic leukemia cells at diagnosis. *Blood* 1992; **79**: 473–6.

165. Del Poeta G, Stasi R, Aronica G *et al.* Clinical relevance of P-glycoprotein expression in de novo acute myeloid leukemia. *Blood* 1996; **87**: 1997–2004.

166. Hunault M, Zhou D, Delmer A *et al.* Multidrug resistance gene expression in acute myeloid leukemia: major prognostic significance for in vivo drug resistance to induction treatment. *Ann Hematol* 1997; **74**: 65–71.

167. Del Poeta G, Venditti A, Stasi R *et al.* P-glycoprotein and terminal transferase expression identify prognostic subsets within cytogenetic risk classes in acute myeloid leukemia. *Leuk Res* 1999; **23**: 451–65.

168. Willman CL. The prognostic significance of the expression and function of multidrug resistance transporter proteins in acute myeloid leukemia: studies of the Southwest Oncology Group Leukemia Research Program. *Semin Hematol* 1997; **34**: 25–33.

169. Leith CP, Kopecky KJ, Godwin J *et al.* Acute myeloid leukemia in the elderly: assessment of multidrug resistance (MDR1) and cytogenetics distinguishes biologic subgroups with remarkably distinct responses to standard chemotherapy. A Southwest Oncology Group study. *Blood* 1997; **89**: 3323–9.

170. Legrand O, Simonin G, Perrot JY *et al.* Pgp and MRP activities using calcein-AM are prognostic factors in adult acute myeloid leukemia patients. *Blood* 1998; **91**: 4480–8.

171. Legrand O, Zittoun R, Marie JP. Role of MRP1 in multidrug resistance in acute myeloid leukemia. *Leukemia* 1999; **13**: 578–84.

172. Legrand O, Simonin G, Zittoun R, Marie JP. Lung resistance protein (LRP) gene expression in adult acute myeloid leukemia: a critical evaluation by three techniques. *Leukemia* 1998; **12**: 1367–74.

173. Ross DD, Karp JE, Chen TT, Doyle LA. Expression of breast cancer resistance protein in blast cells from patients with acute leukemia. *Blood* 2000; **96**: 365–8.

174. Ross DD. Novel mechanisms of drug resistance in leukemia. *Leukemia* 2000; **14**: 467–73.

175. Van den Heuvel-Eibrink MM, Wiemer EA, Prins A *et al.* Increased expression of the breast cancer resistance protein (BCRP) in relapsed or refractory acute myeloid leukemia (AML). *Leukemia* 2002; **16**: 833–9.

176. Sievers EL, Smith FO, Woods WG *et al.* Cell surface expression of the multidrug resistance P-glycoprotein (P-170) as detected by monoclonal antibody MRK-16 in pediatric acute myeloid leukemia fails to define a poor prognostic group: a report from the Children's Cancer Group. *Leukemia* 1995; **9**: 2042–8.

177. Van den Heuvel-Eibrink MM, Sonneveld P, Pieters R. The prognostic significance of membrane transport-associated multidrug resistance (MDR) proteins in leukemia. *Int J Clin Pharmacol Ther* 2000; **38**: 94–110.

178. Steinbach D, Furchtbar S, Sell W *et al.* Contrary to adult patients, expression of the multidrug resistance gene (MDR1) fails to define a poor prognostic group in childhood AML. *Leukemia* 2003; **17**: 470–1.

179. Dahl GV, Lacayo NJ, Brophy N *et al.* Mitoxantrone, etoposide, and cyclosporine therapy in pediatric patients with recurrent or refractory acute myeloid leukemia. *J Clin Oncol* 2000; **18**: 1867–75.

180. Sievers EL, Lange BJ, Alonzo TA *et al.* Immunophenotypic evidence of leukemia after induction therapy predicts relapse: results from a prospective Children's Cancer Group study of 252 patients with acute myeloid leukemia. *Blood* 2003; **101**: 3398–406.

181. Kottaridis PD, Gale RE, Langabeer SE *et al.* Studies of FLT3 mutations in paired presentation and relapse samples from patients with acute myeloid leukemia: implications for the role of FLT3 mutations in leukemogenesis, minimal residual disease detection, and possible therapy with FLT3 inhibitors. *Blood* 2002; **100**(7): 2393–8.

182. Trka J, Kalinova M, Hrusak O *et al.* Real-time quantitative PCR detection of WT1 gene expression in children with AML: prognostic significance, correlation with disease status and residual disease detection by flow cytometry. *Leukemia* 2002; **16**(7): 1381–9.

183. Bader P, Hancock J, Kreyenberg H *et al.* Minimal residual disease (MRD) status prior to allogeneic stem cell transplantation is a powerful predictor for post-transplant outcome in children with ALL. *Leukemia* 2002; **16**: 1668–72.

184. Perel Y, Auvrignon A, Leblanc T *et al.* Impact of addition of maintenance therapy to intensive induction and consolidation chemotherapy for childhood acute myeloblastic leukemia: results of a prospective randomized trial, LAME 89/91. Leucamie Aique Myeloide Enfant. *J Clin Oncol* 2002; **20**: 2774–82.

185. Cheson BD, Horning SJ, Coiffier B *et al.* Report of an international workshop to standardize response criteria for non-Hodgkin's lymphomas. NCI Sponsored International Working Group. *J Clin Oncol* 1999; **17**: 1244.

186. Warrell RP Jr, de The H, Wang ZY, Degos L. Acute promyelocytic leukemia [see comments]. *N Engl J Med* 1993; **329**: 177–89.

187. Berman E, Heller G, Santorsa J *et al.* Results of a randomized trial comparing idarubicin and cytosine arabinoside with daunorubicin and cytosine arabinoside in adult patients with newly diagnosed acute myelogenous leukemia. *Blood* 1991; **77**: 1666–74.

188. Santana VM, Hurwitz CA, Blakley RL et al. Complete hematologic remissions induced by 2-chlorodeoxyadenosine in children with newly diagnosed acute myeloid leukemia. Blood 1994; **84**: 1237–42.

189. Krance RA, Hurwitz CA, Head DR et al. Experience with 2-chlorodeoxyadenosine in previously untreated children with newly diagnosed acute myeloid leukemia and myelodysplastic diseases. J Clin Oncol 2001; **19**: 2804–11.

190. Kearns CM, Blakley RL, Santana VM, Crom WR. Pharmacokinetics of cladribine (2-chlorodeoxyadenosine) in children with acute leukemia. Cancer Res 1994; **54**: 1235–9.

191. Wells RJ, Woods WG, Buckley JD et al. Treatment of newly diagnosed children and adolescents with acute myeloid leukemia: a Children's Cancer Group study. J Clin Oncol 1994; **12**: 2367–77.

192. Bloomfield CD, Lawrence D, Byrd JC et al. Frequency of prolonged remission duration after high-dose cytarabine intensification in acute myeloid leukemia varies by cytogenetic subtype. Cancer Res 1998; **58**: 4173–9.

193. Cassileth PA, Lynch E, Hines JD et al. Varying intensity of postremission therapy in acute myeloid leukemia. Blood 1992; **79**: 1924–30.

194. Ritter J, Vormoor J, Creutzig U, Schellong G. Prognostic significance of Auer rods in childhood acute myelogenous leukemia: results of the studies AML-BFM-78 and -83. Med Pediatr Oncol 1989; **17**: 202–9.

195. Lo-Coco F, Breccia M, Diverio D. The importance of molecular monitoring in acute promyelocytic leukaemia. Best Pract Res Clin Haematol 2003; **16**: 503–20.

196. Diverio D, Pandolfi PP, Biondi A et al. Absence of reverse transcription-polymerase chain reaction detectable residual disease in patients with acute promyelocytic leukemia in long-term remission. Blood 1993; **82**: 3556–9.

197. Lemons RS, Keller S, Gietzen D et al. Acute promyelocytic leukemia. J Pediatr Hematol Oncol 1995; **17**: 198–210.

198. Lemons DS, Lackman J, Jones ME, Winske D. Noise-induced instability in self-consistent Monte Carlo calculations. Phys Rev E: Stat Phys Plasmas Fluids Related Interdisc Topics 1995; **52**: 6855–61.

199. Bucy RP, Karr L, Huang GQ et al. Single cell analysis of cytokine gene coexpression during CD4+ T-cell phenotype development. Proc Natl Acad Sci USA 1995; **92**: 7565–9.

200. Creutzig U, Ritter J, Zimmermann M, Schellong G. Does cranial irradiation reduce the risk for bone marrow relapse in acute myelogenous leukemia? Unexpected results of the Childhood Acute Myelogenous Leukemia Study BFM-87. J Clin Oncol 1993; **11**: 279–86.

201. Barnes DWH, Loutit JF. Treatment of murine leukemia with X-rays and homologous bone marrow. Br Med J 1956; **ii**: 626–7.

202. Apperley JF, Rassool F, Parreira A et al. Philadelphia-positive metaphases in the marrow after bone marrow transplantation for chronic granulocytic leukemia. Am J Hematol 1986; **22**: 199–204.

203. Kolb HJ, Schattenberg A, Goldman JM et al. Graft-versus-leukemia effect of donor lymphocyte transfusions in marrow grafted patients. European Group for Blood and Marrow Transplantation Working Party Chronic Leukemia. Blood 1995; **86**: 2041–50.

204. Kolb HJ, Mittermuller J, Clemm C et al. Donor leukocyte transfusions for treatment of recurrent chronic myelogenous leukemia in marrow transplant patients. Blood 1990; **76**: 2462–5.

205. Sierra J, Storer B, Hansen JA et al. Transplantation of marrow cells from unrelated donors for treatment of high-risk acute leukemia: the effect of leukemic burden, donor HLA- matching, and marrow cell dose. Blood 1997; **89**: 4226–35.

206. Davies SM, Wagner JE, Shu XO et al. Unrelated donor bone marrow transplantation for children with acute leukemia. J Clin Oncol 1997; **15**: 557–65.

207. van Esser JW, Niesters HG, van der Holt B et al. Prevention of Epstein–Barr virus-lymphoproliferative disease by molecular monitoring and preemptive rituximab in high-risk patients after allogeneic stem cell transplantation. Blood 2002; **99**: 4364–9.

208. Goulmy E. Human minor histocompatibility antigens: new concepts for marrow transplantation and adoptive immunotherapy. Immunol Rev 1997; **157**: 125–40.

209. Ball ED, Wilson J, Phelps V, Neudorf S. Autologous bone marrow transplantation for acute myeloid leukemia in remission or first relapse using monoclonal antibody-purged marrow: results of phase II studies with long-term follow-up. Bone Marrow Transplant 2000; **25**: 823–9.

210. Smith BD, Jones RJ, Lee SM et al. Autologous bone marrow transplantation with 4-hydroperoxycyclophosphamide purging for acute myeloid leukaemia beyond first remission: a 10-year experience. Br J Haematol 2002; **117**: 907–13.

211. Hahlen K, Weening RS, Postma A et al. Results of DCLSG protocol ANLL94, BFM oriented intensive chemotherapy, followed by allogeneic or autologous bone marrow transplantation. Med Pediatr Oncol 2000; **35**: 251:121a.

212. Ortega JJ, Olive T. Haematopoietic progenitor cell transplant in acute leukaemias in children: indications, results and controversies. Bone Marrow Transplant 1998; **21**(Suppl 2): S11–16.

213. Biondi A, Rovelli A, Cantu-Rajnoldi A et al. Acute promyelocytic leukemia in children: experience of the Italian Pediatric Hematology and Oncology Group (AIEOP). Leukemia 1994; **8**: S66–70.

214. Salonen J, Lehtonen OP, Terasjarvi MR, Nikoskelainen J. Aspergillus antigen in serum, urine and bronchoalveolar lavage specimens of neutropenic patients in relation to clinical outcome. Scand J Infect Dis 2000; **32**: 485–90.

215. Maertens J, Vrebos M, Boogaerts M. Assessing risk factors for systemic fungal infections. Eur J Cancer Care (Engl) 2001; **10**: 56–62.

216. Ruhnke M, Bohme A, Buchheidt D et al. Diagnosis of invasive fungal infections in hematology and oncology. Guidelines of the Infectious Diseases Working Party (AGIHO) of the German Society of Hematology and Oncology (DGHO). Ann Hematol 2003; **82**(Suppl. 2): S141–8.

217. Bohme A, Ruhnke M, Buchheidt D et al. Treatment of fungal infections in hematology and oncology. Guidelines of the Infectious Diseases Working Party (AGIHO) of the German Society of Hematology and Oncology (DGHO). Ann Hematol 2003; **82**(Suppl. 2): S133–40.

218. Vignetti M, Orsini E, Petti MC et al. Probability of long-term disease-free survival for acute myeloid leukemia patients

after first relapse: A single-centre experience. *Ann Oncol* 1996; **7**: 933–8.

219. Steuber CP, Krischer J, Holbrook T *et al.* Therapy of refractory or recurrent childhood acute myeloid leukemia using amsacrine and etoposide with or without azacitidine: a Pediatric Oncology Group randomized phase II study. *J Clin Oncol* 1996; **14**(5): 1521–5.

220. Estey EH. Use of colony-stimulating factors in the treatment of acute myeloid leukemia. *Blood* 1994; **83**: 2015–19.

221. Kornblau SM, Estey E, Madden T *et al.* Phase I study of mitoxantrone plus etoposide with multidrug blockade by SDZ PSC-833 in relapsed or refractory acute myelogenous leukemia. *J Clin Oncol* 1997; **15**: 1796–802.

222. Fleischhack G, Hasan C, Graf N *et al.* IDA-FLAG (idarubicin, fludarabine, cytarabine, G-CSF), an effective remission-induction therapy for poor-prognosis AML of childhood prior to allogeneic or autologous bone marrow transplantation: experiences of a phase II trial. *Br J Haematol* 1998; **102**: 647–55.

223. Archimbaud E, Thomas X, Leblond V *et al.* Timed sequential chemotherapy for previously treated patients with acute myeloid leukemia: long-term follow-up of the etoposide, mitoxantrone, and cytarabine-86 trial. *J Clin Oncol* 1995; **13**: 11–18.

224. Capizzi RL, Poole M, Cooper MR *et al.* Treatment of poor risk acute leukemia with sequential high-dose ARA-C and asparaginase. *Blood* 1984; **63**: 694–700.

225. Kern W, Schoch C, Haferlach T *et al.* Multivariate analysis of prognostic factors in patients with refractory and relapsed acute myeloid leukemia undergoing sequential high-dose cytosine arabinoside and mitoxantrone (S-HAM) salvage therapy: relevance of cytogenetic abnormalities. *Leukemia* 2000; **14**: 226–31.

226. Whitlock JA, Wells RJ, Hord JD *et al.* High-dose cytosine arabinoside and etoposide: an effective regimen without anthracyclines for refractory childhood acute non-lymphocytic leukemia. *Leukemia* 1997; **11**: 185–9.

227. Santana VM, Mirro J Jr, Kearns C *et al.* 2-Chlorodeoxyadenosine produces a high rate of complete hematologic remission in relapsed acute myeloid leukemia. *J Clin Oncol* 1992; **10**: 364–70.

228. Vahdat L, Wong ET, Wile MJ *et al.* Therapeutic and neurotoxic effects of 2-chlorodeoxyadenosine in adults with acute myeloid leukemia. *Blood* 1994; **84**: 3429–34.

229. Meloni G, Vignetti M, Andrizzi C *et al.* Interleukin-2 for the treatment of advanced acute myelogenous leukemia patients with limited disease: updated experience with 20 cases. *Leuk Lymphoma* 1996; **21**: 429–35.

230. Higano CS, Brixey M, Bryant EM *et al.* Durable complete remission of acute nonlymphocytic leukemia associated with discontinuation of immunosuppression following relapse after allogeneic bone marrow transplantation. A case report of a probable graft-versus-leukemia effect. *Transplantation* 1990; **50**: 175–7.

231. Falkenburg JH, Smit WM, Willemze R. Cytotoxic T-lymphocyte (CTL) responses against acute or chronic myeloid leukemia. *Immunol Rev* 1997; **157**: 223–30.

232. Collins RH Jr, Shpilberg O, Drobyski WR *et al.* Donor leukocyte infusions in 140 patients with relapsed malignancy after

allogeneic bone marrow transplantation. *J Clin Oncol* 1997; **15**: 433–44.

233. Leung W, Hudson MM, Strickland DK *et al.* Late effects of treatment in survivors of childhood acute myeloid leukemia. *J Clin Oncol* 2000; **18**: 3273–9.

234. Leung W, Hudson M, Zhu Y *et al.* Late effects in survivors of infant leukemia. *Leukemia* 2000; **14**: 1185–90.

235. Leahey AM, Teunissen H, Friedman DL *et al.* Late effects of chemotherapy compared to bone marrow transplantation in the treatment of pediatric acute myeloid leukemia and myelodysplasia. *Med Pediatr Oncol* 1999; **32**: 163–9.

236. Michel G, Socie G, Gebhard F *et al.* Late effects of allogeneic bone marrow transplantation for children with acute myeloblastic leukemia in first complete remission: the impact of conditioning regimen without total-body irradiation – a report from the Societe Francaise de Greffe de Moelle. *J Clin Oncol* 1997; **15**: 2238–46.

237. Sanders JE, Pritchard S, Mahoney P *et al.* Growth and development following marrow transplantation for leukemia. *Blood* 1986; **68**: 1129–35.

238. Pui CH, Ribeiro RC, Hancock ML *et al.* Acute myeloid leukemia in children treated with epipodophyllotoxins for acute lymphoblastic leukemia. *N Engl J Med* 1991; **325**: 1682–7.

239. Pui CH. Epipodophyllotoxin-related acute myeloid leukaemia. *Lancet* 1991; **338**: 1468.

240. Socie G, Curtis RE, Deeg HJ *et al.* New malignant diseases after allogeneic marrow transplantation for childhood acute leukemia. *J Clin Oncol* 2000; **18**: 348–57.

241. Naoe T, Kiyoe H, Yamamoto Y *et al.* FLT3 tyrosine kinase as a target molecule for selective antileukemia therapy. *Cancer Chemother Pharmacol* 2001; **48**(Suppl 1): S27–30.

242. Tse KF, Allebach J, Levis M *et al.* Inhibition of the transforming activity of FLT3 internal tandem duplication mutants from AML patients by a tyrosine kinase inhibitor. *Leukemia* 2002; **16**: 2027–36.

243. Levis M, Allebach J, Tse KF *et al.* A FLT3-targeted tyrosine kinase inhibitor is cytotoxic to leukemia cells in vitro and in vivo. *Blood* 2002; **99**: 3885–91.

244. Kelly LM, Liu Q, Kutok JL *et al.* FLT3 internal tandem duplication mutations associated with human acute myeloid leukemias induce myeloproliferative disease in a murine bone marrow transplant model. *Blood* 2002; **99**: 310–18.

245. Zheng R, Friedman AD, Small D. Targeted inhibition of FLT3 overcomes the block to myeloid differentiation in 32Dcl3 cells caused by expression of FLT3/ITD mutations. *Blood* 2002; **100**: 4154–61.

246. Yee KW, O'Farrell AM, Smolich BD *et al.* SU5416 and SU5614 inhibit kinase activity of wild-type and mutant FLT3 receptor tyrosine kinase. *Blood* 2002; **100**: 2941–9.

247. Weisberg E, Boulton C, Kelly LM *et al.* Inhibition of mutant FLT3 receptors in leukemia cells by the small molecule tyrosine kinase inhibitor PKC412. *Cancer Cell* 2002; **1**: 433–43.

248. Sawyers CL. Finding the next Gleevec: FLT3 targeted kinase inhibitor therapy for acute myeloid leukemia. *Cancer Cell* 2002; **1**: 413–15.

249. Giles FJ, Stopeck AT, Silverman LR *et al.* SU5416, a small molecule tyrosine kinase receptor inhibitor, has biologic

activity in patients with refractory acute myeloid leukemia or myelodysplastic syndromes. *Blood* 2003; **102**: 795–801.

250. Heinrich MC, Griffith DJ, Druker BJ *et al.* Inhibition of c-kit receptor tyrosine kinase activity by STI 571, a selective tyrosine kinase inhibitor. *Blood* 2000; **96**: 925–32.

251. Cortes J, Albitar M, Thomas D *et al.* Efficacy of the farnesyl transferase inhibitor R115777 in chronic myeloid leukemia and other hematologic malignancies. *Blood* 2003; **101**(5): 1692–7.

252. Meshinchi S, Stirewalt DL, Alonzo TA *et al.* Activating mutations of RTK/ras signal transduction pathway in pediatric acute myeloid leukemia. *Blood* 2003; **102**(4): 1474–9.

253. Lancet JE, Karp JE. Farnesyltransferase inhibitors in hematologic malignancies: new horizons in therapy. *Blood* 2003; **102**(12): 3880–9.

254. Fiedler W, Graeven U, Ergun S *et al.* Vascular endothelial growth factor, a possible paracrine growth factor in human acute myeloid leukemia. *Blood* 1997; **89**: 1870–5.

255. Folkman J. Tumor angiogenesis: therapeutic implications. *N Engl J Med* 1971; **285**: 1182–6.

256. Zwiebel JA. New agents for acute myelogenous leukemia. *Leukemia* 2000; **14**: 488–90.

257. Lin RJ, Nagy L, Inoue S *et al.* Role of the histone deacetylase complex in acute promyelocytic leukaemia. *Nature* 1998; **391**: 811–14.

258. Collins SJ. Acute promyelocytic leukemia: relieving repression induces remission. *Blood* 1998; **91**: 2631–3.

259. Nan X, Ng HH, Johnson CA *et al.* Transcriptional repression by the methyl-CpG-binding protein MeCP2 involves a histone deacetylase complex. *Nature* 1998; **393**: 386–9.

260. Jones PL, Veenstra GJ, Wade PA *et al.* Methylated DNA and MeCP2 recruit histone deacetylase to repress transcription. *Nat Genet* 1998; **19**: 187–91.

261. Cameron EE, Bachman KE, Myohanen S *et al.* Synergy of demethylation and histone deacetylase inhibition in the re-expression of genes silenced in cancer. *Nat Genet* 1999; **21**: 103–7.

262. Singal R, Ginder GD. DNA methylation. *Blood* 1999; **93**: 4059–70.

263. Estey EH. How I treat older patients with AML. *Blood* 2000; **96**: 1670–3.

264. Niu C, Yan H, Yu T *et al.* Studies on treatment of acute promyelocytic leukemia with arsenic trioxide: remission induction, follow-up, and molecular monitoring in 11 newly diagnosed and 47 relapsed acute promyelocytic leukemia patients. *Blood* 1999; **94**: 3315–24.

265. Issa JP, Baylin SB, Herman JG. DNA methylation changes in hematologic malignancies: biologic and clinical implications. *Leukemia* 1997; **11**(Suppl 1): S7–11.

266. Wang S, Vrana JA, Bartimole TM *et al.* Agents that down-regulate or inhibit protein kinase C circumvent resistance to 1-beta-D-arabinofuranosylcytosine-induced apoptosis in human leukemia cells that overexpress Bcl-2. *Mol Pharmacol* 1997; **52**: 1000–9.

267. Cheson BD, Zwiebel JA, Dancey J, Murgo A. Novel therapeutic agents for the treatment of myelodysplastic syndromes. *Semin Oncol* 2000; **27**: 560–77.

268. Pepper C, Hooper K, Thomas A *et al.* Bcl-2 antisense oligonucleotides enhance the cytotoxicity of chlorambucil in B-cell chronic lymphocytic leukaemia cells. *Leuk Lymphoma* 2001; **42**: 491–8.

269. Benekli M, Xia Z, Donohue KA *et al.* Constitutive activity of signal transducer and activator of transcription 3 protein in acute myeloid leukemia blasts is associated with short disease-free survival. *Blood* 2002; **99**: 252–7.

270. Sievers EL, Appelbaum FR, Spielberger RT *et al.* Selective ablation of acute myeloid leukemia using antibody-targeted chemotherapy: a phase I study of an anti-CD33 calicheamicin immunoconjugate. *Blood* 1999; **93**: 3678–84.

271. Appelbaum FR. Antibody-targeted therapy for myeloid leukemia. *Semin Hematol* 1999; **36**: 2–8.

272. Sievers EL. Targeted therapy of acute myeloid leukemia with monoclonal antibodies and immunoconjugates. *Cancer Chemother Pharmacol* 2000; **46**: S18–22.

273. Sievers EL. Clinical studies of new 'biologic' approaches to therapy of acute myeloid leukemia with monoclonal antibodies and immunoconjugates. *Curr Opin Oncol* 2000; **12**: 30–5.

274. Larson RA. Current use and future development of gemtuzumab ozogamicin. *Semin Hematol* 2001; **38**: 24–31.

275. Giles FJ. Gemtuzumab ozogamicin: promise and challenge in patients with acute myeloid leukemia. *Expert Rev Anticancer Ther* 2002; **2**: 630–40.

276. Hinman LM, Hamann PR, Wallace R *et al.* Preparation and characterization of monoclonal antibody conjugates of the calicheamicins: a novel and potent family of antitumor antibiotics. *Cancer Res* 1993; **53**: 3336–42.

277. van Der Velden VH, te Marvelde JG, Hoogeveen PG *et al.* Targeting of the CD33-calicheamicin immunoconjugate Mylotarg (CMA-676) in acute myeloid leukemia: in vivo and in vitro saturation and internalization by leukemic and normal myeloid cells. *Blood* 2001; **97**: 3197–204.

278. Voutsadakis IA. Gemtuzumab ozogamicin (CMA-676, Mylotarg) for the treatment of CD33+ acute myeloid leukemia. *Anticancer Drugs* 2002; **13**: 685–92.

279. Sievers EL, Linenberger M. Mylotarg: antibody-targeted chemotherapy comes of age. *Curr Opin Oncol* 2001; **13**: 522–7.

280. Leopold LH, Berger MS, Feingold J. Acute and long-term toxicities associated with gemtuzumab ozogamicin (mylotarg) therapy of acute myeloid leukemia. *Clin Lymphoma* 2002; **2**(suppl. 1): S29–34.

281. Cohen AD, Luger SM, Sickles C *et al.* Gemtuzumab ozogamicin (Mylotarg) monotherapy for relapsed AML after hematopoietic stem cell transplant: efficacy and incidence of hepatic veno-occlusive disease. *Bone Marrow Transplant* 2002; **30**: 23–8.

282. Rajvanshi P, Shulman HM, Sievers EL, McDonald GB. Hepatic sinusoidal obstruction after gemtuzumab ozogamicin (Mylotarg) therapy. *Blood* 2002; **99**: 2310–14.

283. Stadtmauer EA. Gemtuzumab ozogamicin in the treatment of acute myeloid leukemia. *Curr Oncol Rep* 2002; **4**(5): 375–80.

284. Lang K, Menzin J, Earle CC, Mallick R. Outcomes in patients treated with gemtuzumab ozogamicin for relapsed acute myelogenous leukemia. *Am J Health Syst Pharm* 2002; **59**(10): 941–8.

285. Larson RA, Boogaerts M, Estey E *et al.* Antibody-targeted chemotherapy of older patients with acute myeloid leukemia

in first relapse using Mylotarg (gemtuzumab ozogamicin). *Leukemia* 2002; **16**(9): 1627–36.

286. Berger MS, Leopold LH, Dowell JA *et al*. Licensure of gemtuzumab ozogamicin for the treatment of selected patients 60 years of age or older with acute myeloid leukemia in first relapse. *Invest New Drugs* 2002; **20**(4): 395–406.

287. Tsimberidou A, Estey E, Cortes J *et al*. Gemtuzumab, fludarabine, cytarabine, and cyclosporine in patients with newly diagnosed acute myelogenous leukemia or high-risk myelodysplastic syndromes. *Cancer* 2003 **97**(6): 1481–7.

288. Alvarado Y, Tsimberidou A, Kantarjian H *et al*. Pilot study of Mylotarg, idarubicin and cytarabine combination regimen in patients with primary resistant or relapsed acute myeloid leukemia. *Cancer Chemother Pharmacol* 2003; **51**(1): 87–90.

289. Cortes J, Tsimberidou AM, Alvarez R *et al*. Mylotarg combined with topotecan and cytarabine in patients with refractory acute myelogenous leukemia. *Cancer Chemother Pharmacol* 2002; **50**(6): 497–500.

290. Zwaan Ch M, Reinhardt D, Jurgens H *et al*. Gemtuzumab ozogamicin in pediatric CD33-positive acute lymphoblastic leukemia: first clinical experiences and relation with cellular sensitivity to single agent calicheamicin. *Leukemia* 2003; **17**: 468–70.

291. Cignetti A, Bryant E, Allione B *et al*. CD34(+) acute myeloid and lymphoid leukemic blasts can be induced to differentiate into dendritic cells. *Blood* 1999; **94**: 2048–55.

292. Guillaume T, Rubinstein DB, Symann M. Immune reconstitution and immunotherapy after autologous hematopoietic stem cell transplantation. *Blood* 1998; **92**: 1471–90.

293. Wiernik PH, Dutcher JP, Todd M *et al*. Polyethylene glycolated interleukin-2 as maintenance therapy for acute myelogenous leukemia in second remission. *Am J Hematol* 1994; **47**: 41–4.

294. Sievers EL, Lange BJ, Sondel PM *et al*. Children's cancer group trials of interleukin-2 therapy to prevent relapse of acute myelogenous leukemia. *Cancer J Sci Am* 2000; **6**(Suppl 1): S39–44.

12

Acute lymphoblastic leukaemia

MARTIN SCHRAPPE & ROB PIETERS

INTRODUCTION

Acute lymphoblastic leukaemia (ALL) is the most prevalent malignancy in children and adolescents. It accounts for approximately 25 per cent of all cancers in this age group and for almost 75 per cent of childhood leukaemias.[1,2] Treatment of childhood ALL is a true success story of modern clinical oncology, with an overall cure rate of 65 per cent to almost 80 per cent by application of intensive multiagent chemotherapeutic regimens.[1–17] However, only a few study groups worldwide present data on unselected patient populations, thus limiting outcome comparisons of different treatment protocols. Most published reports address specific patient subsets only. In the most recently completed therapy study within the Berlin–Frankfurt–Münster (BFM) study group, ALL-BFM 90, the overall probability of event-free survival (EFS) at 6 years for all 2178 patients ($\leqslant$18 years) was 78 per cent (standard error, 1 per cent).[15] In the recent British UKALL-X study,[5] a 5-year disease-free survival (DFS) of 62 per cent was achieved in 1612 patients (0–14 years). Patients randomized to receive two intensification treatments fared best in that trial, with a 5-year DFS of 71 per cent. Investigators from the Dana-Farber Cancer Institute (DFCI) reported excellent treatment results in two subsequent trials that included patients of the same age range as in the ALL-BFM 90 trial: their EFS was 72 per cent in trial 81-01, and 78 per cent for 220 patients in trial 85-01.[11,14] The last two treatment programmes of the St Jude Children's Research Hospital resulted in a 4-year probability of EFS of 73 per cent ($n = 358$; 0–18 years) in study XI, and in a 5-year EFS of 67 per cent ($n = 188$) in study XII.[7,12] In the latter trial, patients with

B-lineage ALL who received pharmacologically adapted doses of methotrexate, cytarabine and VP-16 (etoposide) achieved a 5-year EFS of 76 per cent, as compared with 66 per cent for patients with standard medication.

Important principles of diagnostic work-up and treatment of childhood ALL are presented with a summary of the important steps that have led to these concepts. Apologies are made to those whose research may have been omitted. Also, this chapter excludes mature B-cell ALL or French-American-British (FAB) classification L3, as it is now successfully treated by a non-Hodgkin's lymphoma (NHL) therapy-based approach.[18–20]

The aetiology of childhood ALL is not yet fully understood. Genetic predisposition is likely, due to the increased incidence among subjects with constitutional karyotypic aberrations (e.g. in patients with trisomy 21), genetic instability or genetic disease. Epidemiological data suggest that there might be some impact of environmental factors (radiation, nutrition, living conditions, electromagnetic fields).[21] It was also suggested that infections in early childhood might play a role.[22] This could be one of the factors that are responsible for the non-concordant onset of an otherwise molecularly concordant ALL as demonstrated for a pair of identical twins with *TEL/AML1*-positive ALL.[23] In 1997, a very interesting publication[24] directly demonstrated for the first time that ALL with the *MLL-AF4* fusion gene is initiated *in utero*, as neonatal blood spots on Guthrie cards already contained leukaemia-specific sequences even though the disease was not diagnosed before 5–24 months later. Very recently, it was demonstrated that typical leukaemia fusion genes can be found in 1 out of every 1000–10 000 nucleated cells in cord blood of healthy newborns at a 100-fold higher frequency than what would be expected from the incidence of acute leukaemia. This indicates that additional postnatal events or cofactors are necessary to produce the final leukaemic transformation.[25]

DIAGNOSTIC ISSUES

The clinical presentation of a child with ALL largely depends on the extent of the leukaemic infiltration of the bone marrow and extramedullary sites. Typical clinical signs are fever, pallor, fatigue, bruises, enlargement of liver, spleen and lymph nodes, and pain (e.g. bone pain). In most patients, blood cell counts show anaemia, thrombocytopenia and granulocytopenia with or without concomitant leucocytosis. Even leucopenia can be present. On average, the initial white blood cell (WBC) count is approximately $10\,000/\mu L$. In all cases, the diagnosis of ALL has to be confirmed by bone marrow aspiration, and in some cases by Jamshidi needle biopsy. Additional diagnostics include lumbar puncture, chest X-ray and ultrasound examination to exclude extramedullary involvement. Computed tomography (CT) or MRI scan of the brain may be done if there are neurological symptoms such as cranial nerve palsy and testis biopsy with non-symmetrical testis enlargement.

Morphology

The diagnosis of ALL is established when at least 25 per cent lymphoblasts are present in the bone marrow (BM), or when leukaemic blasts are present in the peripheral blood (PB) or the cerebrospinal fluid (CSF). BM and blood smears, as well as CSF cytospin preparations, are usually stained using a modified Wright staining technique and evaluated according to FAB criteria.[26] Cytochemistry reactions, in particular, are useful in separating ALL from acute myeloid leukaemia (AML) (alpha naphthyl butyrate positive in monoblasts, and myeloperoxidase positive in myeloblasts and monoblasts) or to separate different subtypes of ALL (acid phosphatase positive in T-ALL, rarely in B-precursor). Certainly, cytomorphology plays a smaller role today than it did previously, but it is still necessary for the diagnosis of leukaemia, especially in diagnostically difficult cases with atypical clinical presentations. Therefore, it is helpful to realize the more frequent associations of morphological presentation (subtype by FAB classification) and immunophenotype and genotype (Table 12.1).

Central nervous system disease

Central nervous system involvement stage 3 (CNS3) is diagnosed if more than 5 cells/μL are counted in a non-blood-contaminated CSF sample and if lymphoblasts are identified unequivocally, or if intracerebral infiltrates are detected on cranial CT.[27] CNS2 refers to an intermediate state in which fewer than 5 cells/μL CSF are detected, but blasts are unequivocally identified. CNS1 describes negativity for CNS disease (<5 cells/μL CSF, no blasts). CSF samples should be carefully analysed after cytospin preparation, a method through which cellular components within the CSF are concentrated by centrifugation. The definition of CNS involvement is difficult if the lumbar puncture was traumatic (TLP+). The ratio of blasts to erythrocytes in CSF as compared with the ratio in the blood can be used for differentiation. In most clinical trials, only CNS3 is defined as CNS involvement with therapeutic consequences, although this has been a subject of debate.[28,29]

Immunophenotype

Immunophenotyping procedures have been extensively described elsewhere.[30–32] Briefly, surface antigens are considered positive if 20 per cent or more of the leukaemic cells express the antigen with more than 98 per cent fluorescence intensity, as compared with negative control cells. Positivity for terminal deoxynucleotide

Table 12.1 *Association of acute lymphoblastic leukaemia (ALL) immunophenotypes with FAB subtypes and some of the most frequently detected leukaemia genes derived from chromosomal translocations*

	FAB subtype	L1 or L2	L3
Precursor B-cell			
Pro-B	CD19+, CD10−	*MLL-AF4, MLL-ENL*	
Common	CD19+, CD10+	*TEL/AML1, BCR/ABL*	
Pre-B	CD19+, cy μ+	*E2A/PBX1*	
(Mature) B-cell			*MYC*
B	CD19+, sur μ+		
T-cell	CD19−, cyCD3+, CD7+	*HOX11, TCRα/β/δ*	

cy, cytoplasmatic; sur, surface; μ+, immunoglobulin detected.

transferase (TdT) and cytoplasmic (cy) antigens is defined as more than 10 per cent of the cells exhibiting nuclear (TdT) or intracytoplasmatic (cyIgM, cyCD3) fluorescence. In the early 1990s, two-colour flow cytometric analysis with appropriate monoclonal antibodies directly conjugated to fluorescein isothiocyanate or phycoerythrin was introduced. In many trials, immunophenotypic subgroups are defined according to the European Group for the Immunological Characterization of Leukaemias (EGIL), as follows: [30]

- pro-B ALL: TdT+, CD19+, CD10−, cyIgM−, surface immunoglobulin (sIg)−
- common (c) ALL: TdT+, CD19+, CD10+, cyIgM−, sIg−
- pre-B ALL: TdT+, CD19+, CD10+/−, cyIgM+, sIg−
- T-ALL: TdT+, cyCD3+, CD7+.

Coexpression of myeloid antigen(s) is defined as simultaneous expression of one or more of the myeloid lineage-associated molecules tested (CD13, CD33 and CD65s) on at least 20 per cent of the lymphoblasts.

DNA index

Cellular DNA content is determined by flow cytometry.[33,34] The DNA index of leukaemic blasts is defined as the ratio of DNA content in leukaemic G0/G1 cells to that of normal diploid lymphocytes. In this assay, a widely accepted cut-off point at 1.16, which correlates with more than 50 chromosomes per cell, is used to distinguish prognostic categories.

Cytogenetic and molecular genetic analysis

Most leukaemias are characterized by structural genetic abnormalities, usually translocations and/or deletions. A large variety of abnormalities have been described.[35,36] During the 1990s, the role of the genes affected by the chromosomal translocations was analysed; the most important translocations are shown in Table 12.1. Molecular genetics also allowed the screening for the BCR/ABL, different MLL, and TEL/AML1 fusion products by reverse transcription-polymerase chain reaction (RT-PCR) or fluorescence in situ hybridization (FISH) in most of the large study groups on childhood ALL.[3,37–41] Thus, today, a combined approach using cytogenetic and molecular genetic techniques is often employed at initial diagnosis. These techniques, as well as flow cytometry, are also used to monitor disease burden during therapy by detecting, for example, leukaemia clone-specific characteristics such as immunoglobulin or T-cell receptor gene rearrangements.[42]

RISK ASSESSMENT BY IDENTIFICATION OF PROGNOSTIC FACTORS

One of the most difficult challenges in treatment of childhood ALL is the adjustment of therapy according to the risk of treatment failure (standard/low, intermediate or high). The identification of prognostic factors has become an essential element in the design, conduct and analysis of clinical trials in childhood leukaemia over the last two decades, but also in the clinical management of childhood ALL. These factors mostly include clinical and biological characteristics that are assessable at diagnosis.[1–3] In addition, several study groups evaluated early response to treatment as a prognostic factor for treatment allocation. There has been some variation with regard to timing and type of response evaluation.[9,15,43–51] The significance of prognostic factors can certainly not be generalized for a uniform risk classification system for all study groups, since virtually all of these factors are associated with the type and intensity of treatment administered. Furthermore, additional differences between study groups (e.g. eligibility criteria and ethnic or racial composition of study populations) have to be taken into account when the relevance of specific prognostic factors is discussed.

In an initiative to develop a uniform approach to risk classification in childhood ALL, the National Cancer Institute (NCI) sponsored a concerted publication of major US study groups that described the so-called NCI criteria. In this 1996 publication, the major risk groups in B-precursor (B-pc) ALL (standard and high), excluding infants, were defined by age at diagnosis and initial leucocyte count (WBC) based on criteria developed during an international workshop in Rome in 1985. Standard-risk ALL was defined by the presence of less than 50 000 leucocytes/μL and age at diagnosis of 1–9 years. High-risk ALL was defined as ≥50 000 WBC, or age ≥10 years.[52,53] The definition did not include infant ALL and T-cell ALL. This easily applicable method of risk group classification also allows the outcome of different treatment protocols for these subgroups to be compared, as described below. The disadvantage of this classification is the disregard of early response as the leading prognostic factor, but this can be explained by the lack of systematic assessment of early response in some of the US studies.

Intensive research on the clinical, biological, immunological and genetic aspects of ALL has identified numerous features with prognostic potential, several of which have been extensively evaluated in large patient populations, although not uniformly in all subgroups. These prognostic factors include characteristics such as gender, race, CNS status at diagnosis and particular immunological or genetic features (e.g. structural and numerical chromosomal aberrations) of the leukaemic clone.[1–3] Table 12.2 shows a minimum list of prognostic variables

Table 12.2 *Prognostic factors recommended to be assessed in patients with childhood acute lymphoblastic leukaemia (ALL)*

	Favourable	Unfavourable	References[e]
Age at diagnosis (years)	≥1 and <10 years	<1 or ≥10 years	Group A
Sex	Female	Male	Group B
WBC[a] count at diagnosis (×10⁹/L)	<50	≥50	Group C
Immunophenotype	Common ALL	Pro-B-ALL, T-ALL	Group D
CNS disease[b]	No (CNS 1)	Yes (CNS 3)	Group E
Genetic features[c]	DNA index[d] > 1.16, TEL/AML1 positivity, hyperploidy	DNA index ≤ 1.0, hypoploidy, t(9;22) or BCR/ABL positivity, t(4;11) or MLL/AF4 positivity	Group F
Early response to treatment (peripheral blood)	<1 × 10⁹/L blood blasts after 7 days' induction with daily prednisone and a single intrathecal dose of methotrexate on treatment day 1	≥1 × 10⁹/L blood blasts after 7 days' induction with daily prednisone and a single intrathecal dose of methotrexate on treatment day 1	Group G
Early response to treatment (bone marrow)	<5% leukaemic blasts in the bone marrow (M1) on days 7 and 15 of induction treatment	>25% leukaemic blasts in the bone marrow (M3) on day 7 and/or day 15 of induction treatment or 5–25% leukaemic blasts in the bone marrow (M2 or M3) on day 15 of induction treatment	Group H
Remission status after induction therapy	Remission bone marrow (M1) (BFM treatment day 33)	No response to treatment exemplified through ≥5% blasts in the bone marrow (M2 or M3) after induction therapy	Group I

[a] White blood cell count.
[b] For patients with CNS 2 status, see the section on 'Consolidation/extramedullary therapy'.
[c] Assessed by flow cytometry, cytogenetic techniques or molecular genetic techniques.
[d] Defined as the ratio of DNA content in leukaemic G0/G1 cells to that of normal diploid lymphocytes.
[e] Reference groups: A[6,15,52,53]; B[15,16,183]; C[6,15,52,53]; D[15,184–186]; E[187]; F[15,74,75,188–195]; G[9,15,43,44]; H[45–47]; I[15,51].

that, today, are recommended to be assessed in childhood ALL. Since treatment strategies differ among study groups, it is difficult to make uniformly applicable statements about these factors. Therefore, the majority of study groups now assess the most promising of these features in prospective trials in order to demonstrate their prognostic strength in the corresponding patient populations. Inevitably, this is dependent on the availability of funding, appropriate technology and expertise. This approach allows valid comparisons of different treatments for specific patient subgroups defined by the features in question, and, therefore, may help to identify treatment components that are beneficial for certain subgroups. The success of these cooperative ventures strongly depends on the quality of communication among the large study groups and the ability to arrive at a consensus. In this way it should be possible to generate the tools needed to develop a more uniform approach for risk assessment in childhood ALL.

Biological subclasses and risk assessment

Based upon the biological factors age, immunophenotype and genetic abnormalities, biological subclasses of ALL can be discriminated with clinical and prognostic consequences (Table 12.2). It is essential to realize that these so-called biological entities are not really homogeneous entities, and within one subclass the response to therapy, and therefore also the outcome, may largely differ (Table 12.3). Also, the prognostic relevance of biological subclasses depends on the treatment given. Finally, because many factors are interrelated, only proper multivariate analyses elucidate which factors have independent relevance in which protocol.

AGE

Infants have the worst outcome, which is associated with the high incidence of the unfavourable pro-B ALL phenotype with MLL gene rearrangements in about 80 per cent of all cases. This type of ALL usually presents with a very high tumour load.[54–60] In experimental systems, infant ALL cells show autonomous cell growth *in vitro* and cell proliferation when inoculated in mice,[61] and are more resistant *in vitro* to steroids and L-asparaginase, compared with other ALL cells.[62] Infant ALL shows a poor response to prednisone *in vivo* three times more often than other types of ALL.[63] An increased *in vitro* sensitivity to ara-C is striking.[62] Older children with ALL also

Table 12.3 *Event-free survival (EFS) according to prednisone good response and prednisone poor response in specific patient subsets (data from recent ALL-BFM trials)*

	Prednisone good response		Prednisone poor response		
	n	% EFS ± SE	*n*	% EFS ± SE[a]	Reference
NCI risk group[a]					
Standard	1324	87 ± 1	48	45 ± 7	Schrappe *et al.*[15]
High	564	73 ± 2	143	31 ± 4	
Immunophenotype					
Pro-B ALL	80	68 ± 6	19	0	Schrappe *et al.*[15]
Common ALL	1274	84 ± 1	67	46 ± 6	
Pre-B ALL	338	79 ± 2	13	31 ± 13	
T-ALL	180	78 ± 3	101	32 ± 5	
Genetic aberrations					
t(9;22) or *BCR/ABL*-positive	37	55 ± 8	20	10 ± 7	Schrappe *et al.*[80]
Infants					
All infants	78	53 ± 6	27	15 ± 7	Dördelmann *et al.*[63]
Infants with 11q23 rearrangement	17	41 ± 12	11	9 ± 9	
Infants t(4;11) or *MLL/AF4*-positive	9	33 ± 16	7	0 ± 0	

ALL, acute lymphoblastic leukaemia; *n*, no. of patients; NCI, National Cancer Institute; SE, standard error.
[a] For explanation of NCI risk groups, see section on 'Risk assessment by identification of prognostic factors'.

have a relatively poor outcome. This is especially true for children over 10 years of age, but above this age, the outcome decreases with increasing age. This is associated with the age-dependent incidence of favourable (*TEL/AML1*, hyperdiploidy) and unfavourable (*BCR/ABL*, T-ALL, pro-B ALL) characteristics.[3] Cells from children >10 years are more drug-resistant than cells from younger children.[62] Adult ALL has the poorest outcome and is characterized by an even higher resistance to (in particular) steroids.[64,65] Furthermore, the tolerance to side-effects of drugs increases with age. Examples are the age-dependent incidences of allergic reactions to L-asparaginase and avascular necrosis of bone due to steroids.[66]

IMMUNOPHENOTYPE

Mature B-ALL has a poor outcome when treated with regular ALL protocols. However, treatment by B-NHL schedules has been very successful.[18,20] Pro-B ALL and T-ALL are characterized by a relatively poor prognosis compared with common/pre-B ALL, even though this, again, is strictly treatment-dependent.[9,16,67] For pro-B ALL this might be related to the association with *MLL* gene rearrangements.[60,68] T-ALL is characterized by specific genetic abnormalities and usually presents clinically with a mediastinal mass and a relatively high WBC compared with common/pre-B ALL.[69,70] T-ALL cells accumulate fewer methotrexate polyglutamates and less araCTP (cytarabinetriphosphate) *in vitro* and *in vivo* and are less sensitive to a large variety of drugs compared with common/pre-B ALL.[62,71,72] Both pro-B and T-ALL show a relatively high percentage of patients with a poor response

to prednisone *in vivo* (Table 12.3).[9] In many protocols, T-ALL and pro-B ALL are treated as high-risk ALL. Common/pre-B ALL is the most favourable type of ALL in which prognostically good genetic features can be found.

GENETIC ABNORMALITIES

Hyperdiploidy (DNA index >1.16 or number of chromosomes >50) is associated with a good outcome (Table 12.2).[33,34,72] In particular, extra copies of chromosomes 4, 10, 17 and 21 have been found to be associated with this favourable outcome.[73,74] Hyperdiploid ALL cells show an increased tendency to apoptosis, an increased capacity to form methotrexate polyglutamates and a relatively high sensitivity to antimetabolites and L-asparaginase.[75] *TEL/AML1* fusion is also detected in about 25 per cent of common/pre-B ALL but is usually not associated with hyperdiploidy and therefore depicts another group of common/pre-B ALL with a favourable outcome.[76,77] This relatively good outcome depends on the treatment given and is suggested to be associated with a high sensitivity to L-asparaginase.[78,79] Three features related to a poor outcome are hypodiploidy, 11q23 abnormalities and the presence of the Philadelphia chromosome, t(9;22). Hypodiploidy is very rare, and particular characteristics are hard to describe. Prognosis in patients with 11q23 abnormalities depends strongly on age at diagnosis, as shown in a large meta-analysis.[68] In infants with ALL, reactivity of leukaemic cells with the antibody 7.1 can specifically identify patients with 11q23/MLL rearrangements.[59] The translocation t(9;22) leading to the *BCR/ABL* fusion is seen in fewer than 5 per cent of cases of common/pre-B ALL. Children with a *BCR/ABL*-positive

ALL more often show a poor response to prednisone (Table 12.3)[80] and have high levels of minimum residual disease (MRD) after induction therapy. They are usually treated according to high-risk therapy and may benefit from bone marrow transplantation (BMT) (see below).[81] The incidence of *BCR/ABL* positivity rises with age while, in contrast, the *TEL/AML1* fusion gene is not seen in those over 10 years of age.[3]

Of interest are recently developed gene expression profiling studies. It appears that, as expected, specific biological subclasses such as *MLL* gene rearrangement, *TEL/AML1* and *BCR/ABL* have specific gene expression profiles.[82] Also, the first study looking at the prognostic value of this gene profile revealed a very high power to discriminate between patients who will, and those who will not, relapse.[83] Because this can be studied at initial diagnosis, making it possible to change treatment early if required, the gene profile seems a very promising tool for risk assessment in the future but its value has to be confirmed.

The value of early response to treatment for risk assessment

Several study groups have evaluated a variety of early response estimates as prognostic factors for treatment allocation in childhood ALL.[43–50]

The BFM study group started as early as 1983 to assess the value of the 'prednisone response'[43] (see Box 12.1 for a definition of this and other measures of early response to treatment) and has used this for patient stratification since 1986.[9,84] Within the BFM studies, including 3735 childhood ALL patients from 1983 to 1995, the *in vivo* response to prednisone has consistently been one of the strongest prognostic factors for the prediction of treatment outcome.[84] The prognostic significance of inadequate reduction of leukaemic blasts in peripheral blood by multiagent remission induction was confirmed retrospectively in the St Jude Total Therapy Study XI.[49] Children's Cancer Group (CCG) investigators have also utilized early response (as measured in the BM on days 7 and 14 of induction) to identify patients at higher risk of failure.[47] In UKALL-X, after stratification for age, gender and WBC, the most significant prognostic factor was also early response, as measured in the BM on day 14.[5] The specificity of response evaluation might vary with the composition of the induction regimen and the time of response evaluation.[47,48,85]

The morphological evaluation of peripheral blood smears in a central setting yields highly reproducible results, while BM morphology is far more susceptible to bias introduced through, for example, technical variability related to the marrow aspiration procedure (see Box 12.1). Nevertheless, there are also limitations with regard to the

Box 12.1 *Analysis of early response to treatment in childhood ALL*

Prednisone response (BFM study group)
In current BFM trials for ALL, therapy for all patients starts with a 7-day monotherapy with prednisone and one intrathecal dose of methotrexate on day 1. The first day of treatment is the day of the first administration of prednisone. The dosage of prednisone is increased steadily to 60 mg/m² daily according to leukaemic cell mass, and renal and metabolic parameters in order to circumvent complications of acute cell lysis. The number of leukaemic blasts in the blood on day 8 is calculated from the absolute leucocyte count and the percentage of blasts in peripheral blood smears as determined by central review in the study centre. The presence of $\geq 1000/\mu L$ blasts in the blood on day 8 is defined as a 'prednisone poor response'; a count of leukaemic cells in blood of $< 1000/\mu L$ is required for the diagnosis of a 'prednisone good response'.

Bone marrow day 7 and day 14 (as evaluated, for example, by the Children's Cancer Group)
On treatment days 7 and 14 of remission induction therapy, bone marrow aspirates are obtained from the patient. The early response to therapy in the bone marrow is rated M1, M2 or M3. M1 represents a bone marrow aspirate displaying less than 5 per cent residual leukaemic blasts and signs of recovering haemopoiesis. M2 refers to a bone marrow aspirate with the presence of leukaemic blasts in the range of 5–25 per cent, while an M3 rating describes all bone marrow aspirates where the percentage of leukaemic blasts exceeds 25 per cent. Extremely hypocellular marrow aspirates are generally regarded as less than 5 per cent residual blasts (M1). At both time points, an M1 rating confers a good prognosis, while M2 and M3 ratings are associated with a poorer prognosis. The group of patients with M2 or M3 marrow on day 7 can be further separated into patients with an intermediate or poor prognosis by using the day 14 marrow score. Those with an M2 or M3 marrow on day 14 comprise the subset of patients with a poor prognosis.

prednisone response. One such limitation addresses the patient population with an initial leukaemic blast count of less than 1000/μL (~15 per cent of the patient population). Even though these patients arguably cannot be evaluated accurately for the kinetics of their leukaemic cell reduction, their assignment to the group of prednisone good-responders (defined by blast counts <1000/μL on treatment day 8) does not result in a difference in treatment results when compared with 'true' prednisone good-responders.[86] In contrast, patients with very high initial blast counts and impressive leukaemic cell mass reduction under prednisone (to blast counts $\geq 1000/\mu L$ on treatment day 8) may be subject to overtreatment. Figure 12.1(a) shows the most recent results with the prednisone response as a clinical tool for risk assessment and therapy stratification in patients with B-precursor ALL from trial ALL-BFM 90.[15] While the 1694 prednisone good-responders had a 6-year EFS rate of 81 per cent, the 99 prednisone poor-responders during the same time period only reached an EFS of 33 per cent. For comparative purposes, Figure 12.1(b) shows the subset of patients from the same patient population that had

data on morphological bone marrow evaluation on treatment day 15 available at the reference laboratory. In addition to the above-mentioned advantages of the prednisone response compared with bone marrow analysis for the evaluation of early response to treatment, it is apparent that prednisone response is, at the least, not a worse predictor of treatment outcome in ALL-BFM studies than is BM evaluation at day 15. The BM response of day 15 can also provide some extra information on top of the risk groups which are based on WBC, age and prednisone response. For example, patients with a poor response to prednisone and M3 BM at day 15 have a particularly poor prognosis.

Predictive value of biological risk factors as compared with response parameters

With regard to the prognostic relevance of markers used for risk assessment in childhood ALL, Figures 12.2(a) and (b) show data from the ALL-BFM study group on a variety of variables separated by good or poor prognostic impact on treatment outcome. In a hypothetical scenario of a patient population experiencing 20 per cent therapy failure rate, for example, a prognostic marker would ideally be applicable to all patients, but would identify

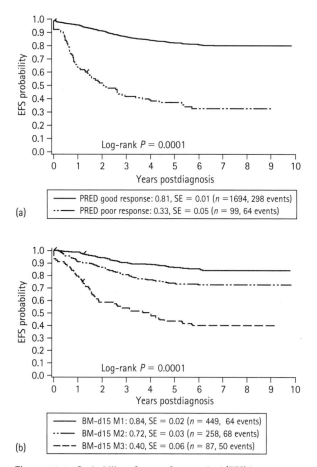

(a)

(b)

Figure 12.1 *Probability of event-free survival (EFS) in B-precursor cell acute lymphoblastic leukaemia (ALL), according to response to treatment. (a) Response to a 7-day prednisone pre-phase (and one intrathecal methotrexate on day 1) as defined by < 1000 leukaemic blasts (PRED good response) or > 1000 blasts on day 8 of treatment (PRED poor response). (b) Response to 14 days of BFM induction (including prednisone pre-phase) as defined by bone marrow analysis on day 15 (BM-d15, centralized): M1, < 5% blasts; M2, 5–25% blasts; and M3, ≥25% blasts. SE, standard error; n, number of cases.*

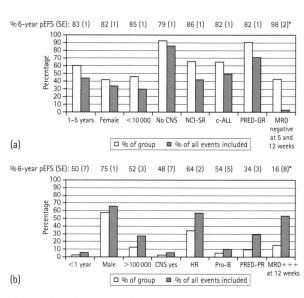

(a)

(b)

Figure 12.2 *The prognostic relevance of important presenting features and response in childhood acute lymphoblastic leukaemia (ALL). (a) Best risk category: except for the early negativity of minimal residual disease (MRD) the specific prognostic relevance of these variables is low. (b) Worst risk category: the highest proportion of recurrences is found among patients with a prednisone poor response (PRED-PR) and high MRD positivity (MRD+ + +) at 12 weeks. c-ALL, common ALL; NCI-SR, standard risk by National Cancer Institute criteria; pEFS, probability of event-free survival; HR, high risk by NCI criteria; PRED-GR, prednisone good response; *RFS, relapse-free survival.*

only those patients who will fail conventional treatment (or those who can expect cure). Thus, a marker for relapse should test positive in 20 per cent of the population. Although such markers with 100 per cent sensitivity and specificity do not exist in real life, Figure 12.2 exemplifies that in ALL-BFM patients, the prednisone poor response identifies 10 per cent of the patient population, which accounts for almost 30 per cent of all events. This excellent model of sensitivity and specificity is exceeded only by a molecular method of monitoring response to treatment, namely, by the detection of MRD with a leukaemic clone-specific immunoglobulin or T-cell receptor rearrangement.[42,87–94] Genetic markers such as chromosomal translocations are not displayed in Figure 12.2, as the majority of patients do not have informative genetics with known prognostic significance. The prognostic specificity of translocations t(9;22) and t(4;11) is certainly high, but it is limited to a very small proportion of the patients. The majority of relapses occur in patients with normal cytogenetics or undetectable genetic lesions. Table 12.3 indicates that the predictive prognostic value of most given biological factors depends on unknown additional features controlling the responsiveness of the disease. Even within genetically or immunophenotypically defined subgroups, differences in treatment responsiveness (based on prednisone response) can be found. To understand this heterogeneity, a thorough analysis of host factors is required.

A large number of relapses still appear to be unpredictable with currently available clinical, genetic and immunological markers. For this patient subset, the careful monitoring of microscopically, immunologically or molecular genetically detectable *in vivo* treatment responses might provide the means to target more intensive therapy to the patient at true risk of relapse.[46,63,80,90]

Evaluation of treatment response by measurement of MRD

Conventional methods of risk classification in childhood ALL are not sufficient to identify the patient at true risk of relapse. Even though the inadequate early response to prednisone is highly predictive of treatment failure, the majority of recurrences are still observed in the large group of patients with an adequate early response to treatment.[9,15] Therefore, based on the first results with regard to early response to treatment generated by the ALL-BFM study group and the findings from molecular detection of minimal residual leukaemic disease, a prospective MRD study was initiated by the International BFM study group in 1991.[90] In that study, patients from Austria, Germany, Italy and the Netherlands were enrolled. Treatment was based on the strategy of the ALL-BFM 90 and the very similar AIEOP-91 protocol.[6,15]

It appeared that the individual response to treatment, as measured by MRD analysis by PCR-based detection of leukaemic clone-specific immunoglobulin and/or T-cell receptor gene rearrangements, was by far the strongest predictor of outcome. For the first time, it was possible to identify patients with basically no risk of relapse, and to define patients who had a more than 80 per cent probability of relapse while on current treatment protocols. The new and unique result was that this high-risk group comprised two-thirds of all relapses if the prednisone response was also utilized. Furthermore, the group of patients with almost no risk of relapse was as large as about 40 per cent of all patients. The remaining intermediate-risk patients were defined by measurable but decreasing levels of MRD, and were found to have a prognosis of approximately 75 per cent relapse-free survival. Similar results on the value of MRD in childhood ALL could also be demonstrated by others.[92,93] Flow-cytometric analysis of MRD by detection of specific antigen patterns of the leukaemic clone yields sensitive and reliable results comparable to PCR-based approaches.[89,93–95]

The first important aim for clinical research utilizing MRD information will be to confirm the prognostic value of MRD in large prospective therapy studies. Such studies should clarify whether different tools to analyse MRD will complement each other. They also should set standards with regard to clinical, methodological, logistical and financial issues. The results will improve our understanding of the importance of disease kinetics in childhood ALL and might lead to new molecular definitions for remission and relapse.[96] Variability in the kinetics of the treatment response is probably dependent not only on the leukaemic subtype but also on the number and dosage of drugs being used, indicating the impact of the treatment protocol.[97,98] More importantly, MRD analysis at pre-defined time points with standardized methods may be used for stratification. A large international study group formed by the Italian AIEOP and the German-Austrian-Swiss ALL-BFM Study Group has decided to largely replace conventional risk variables with the use of response evaluation (on the basis of prednisone response and/or PCR-based MRD detection at two informative time points) for selecting postconsolidation treatment intensity. The trial will not only allow controlled treatment reduction in MRD low-risk patients but will also apply treatment intensifications to MRD intermediate- and high-risk patients. Only if treatment results after such MRD-based reassignment of patients demonstrate that less intensive therapy is uniformly efficacious in low-risk patients, and more intensive or alternative therapy can reduce the number of recurrences in patients identified by MRD as being more resistant, will there be justification to introduce this technique as an essential management tool. There may be a desire among clinicians to use this sensitive test more frequently throughout therapy, in particular if relapse is suspected. This might produce a large number of treatment deviations, and the more heterogeneous these deviations are, the more difficult it will be to derive prognostic information from future trials.

TREATMENT

Overall cure rates of 65 per cent to almost 80 per cent can be achieved in childhood ALL by application of intensive multiagent chemotherapeutic regimens.[1–17,84] It is very difficult to compare the outcome of different protocols because of differences in patient selection and risk group classification.[99] By using the NCI risk criteria mentioned above, in 2002 many study groups presented the treatment results of the protocols being used in the late 1980s and early 1990s in a uniform way. These results are summarized in Table 12.4. As an example, Figure 12.3 displays updated results of four trials of the ALL-BFM study group performed from 1981 to 1995. With the exception of trial ALL-BFM 83, a steady improvement in prognosis was achieved.[15,84]

Table 12.4 *Five-year event-free survival in recent major childhood acute lymphoblastic leukaemia (ALL) treatment protocols*[99]

Group	Study protocol	n	All patients (%)	B-lineage (%)	T-lineage (%)
DFCI	91–01	377	83	84	79
BFM	90	2178	78	80	61
NOPHO	92–98	1143	78	79	61
POG	86–96	NI	NI	71	51
COALL	92	538	77	78	71
St Jude	13A	165	77	80	61
CCG	89–95	5121	75	75	73
DCLSG	ALL8	467	73	73	71
EORTC	58881	2065	71	72	64
AIEOP	91	1194	71	75	40
DCLSG	ALL7	174	68	71	58
UKALL	XI	2090	63	65	51
Tokyo	92–13	347	63	63	59

NI, not indicated.
Study groups: AIEOP, Associazione Italiana Ematologia Oncologia Pediatrica; BFM, Berlin–Frankfurt–Münster; CCG, Children's Cancer Group; COALL, Co-operative Study Group for Childhood Acute Lymphoblastic Leukemia; DCLSG, Dutch Childhood Leukemia Study Group; DFCI, Dana-Farber Cancer Institute; EORTC, European Organisation for Research and Treatment of Cancer; NOPHO, Nordic Society of Paediatric Haematology and Oncology; POG, Pediatric Oncology Group; St Jude, St Jude Children's Research Hospital; UKALL, Medical Research Council Acute Lymphoblastic Leukaemia Trial; Tokyo, Tokyo Children's Cancer Study Group.

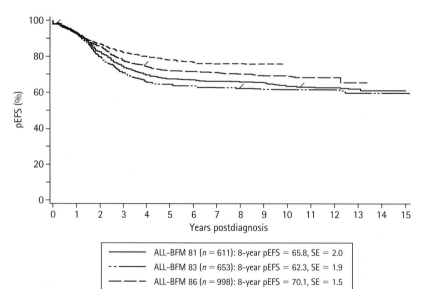

Figure 12.3 *Event-free survival (EFS) in four consecutive trials of the ALL-BFM study group. n, number of cases; pEFS, probability of event-free survival; SE, standard error.*

Modern regimens consist of at least four elements, including:

- an induction phase aiming at an initial remission induction within approximately 4–6 weeks through the use of multiple cancer chemotherapeutic drugs
- a consolidation segment to eradicate residual leukaemic blasts in patients who are in remission by morphological criteria
- extracompartment therapy such as CNS directed therapy
- a maintenance period to further stabilize remission by suppressing re-emergence of a drug-resistant clone through continuing reduction of residual leukaemic cells.

In the second half of the 1970s, the ALL-BFM study group introduced an additional treatment element, a so-called reinduction or delayed reintensification phase.[16,100] For certain patient populations, cranial radiotherapy may be needed as an additional treatment component in order to specifically target leukaemic cells in the CNS. For clinical practice, but also for evaluation of study results, the definitions of complete remission (CR) and relapse are important:[9,15,27] CR is defined as the absence of leukaemic blasts in blood and CSF, fewer than 5 per cent lymphoblasts in marrow aspiration smears, and no evidence of localized disease. Relapse is defined as recurrence of lymphoblasts or localized leukaemic infiltrates at any site. There is some debate as to whether definition of remission or relapse can be based purely on molecular evidence of disease. If prospective studies have unequivocally demonstrated the prognostic significance of such findings, it would be logical to adapt the definitions accordingly.

Risk–adapted therapy

The intensive multimodal treatment regimens used in ALL are usually tailored according to a patient's individual risk profile, as described in the risk assessment section of this chapter. Each therapy administered to an ALL patient is potentially life-threatening where serious complications are encountered. The risk assessment procedures applied by the different study groups mainly translate into the definition of two or three risk groups (standard/low, intermediate, high).[1–3,6,9–15] As an example of a risk-adapted modern clinical protocol, Figure 12.4 shows an outline of the treatment strategy applied in the ALL-BFM 95 study (1995–2000), in which patients were assigned to standard-risk (SR), medium-risk (MR) and high-risk (HR) subgroups. The main criteria for stratification were the early response to treatment (prednisone response), initial WBC count and age at diagnosis. Additional criteria included the presence of T-cell

immunophenotype, a BCR/ABL rearrangement or t(9;22) translocation, and a MLL/AF4 rearrangement or t(4;11) translocation (Box 12.2). As can be seen in Figure 12.4, all patients who did not qualify for the HR therapy received induction protocol I (with a reduced anthracycline dose in SR patients, protocol I′), consolidation/extracompartment protocol M, reinduction (delayed intensification) protocol II and maintenance therapy. HR patients were treated with a shorter induction, and continued on a more intensive rotational consolidation schedule consisting of three different 6-day-long pulses of intensive chemotherapy (HR-1′, 2′, 3′), which were repeated twice and followed by reinduction (delayed intensification) protocol II. Maintenance therapy was initiated 2 weeks after the end of reinduction (protocol II). Drugs in maintenance therapy were orally administered: daily 6-mercaptopurine and methotrexate once per week. Total therapy duration was 24 months for all patients, except for boys in the SR subgroup, who received 36 months of maintenance therapy.

Remission induction

Contemporary treatment approaches for childhood ALL aim at an initial remission induction within approximately 4–6 weeks through the use of multiple cancer chemotherapeutic drugs.[1–17] In most of the study groups, this is generally achieved through the systemic application of three drugs (glucocorticoid, vincristine, L-asparaginase), to which an anthracycline may be added as a fourth. Applying such a treatment strategy, more than 95 per cent of the childhood ALL patients usually achieve remission (in study ALL-BFM 90, 98.3 per cent CR rate); the remaining patients will either have died of treatment- or disease-related complications or display non-responsive disease.[9,15,17,51] The latter group includes patients who will achieve only delayed remission or show resistant disease. Because of the poor prognosis of this minor non-responsive patient population, alternative therapeutic approaches should be considered early during the disease process.

Within the ALL-BFM strategy, remission induction is initiated with a 7-day monotherapy with orally administered prednisone (and one intrathecal dose of methotrexate on day 1), which is complemented by intravenous application of three additional drugs (vincristine, daunorubicin, L-asparaginase) starting on treatment day 8. The prolonged initiation of induction therapy through the 7-day prednisone pre-phase is particularly useful for avoiding complications related to extensive tumour cell lysis. In the BFM group, this first phase of induction treatment is subsequently followed by an early intensification phase, including intravenous cyclophosphamide and cytarabine, intrathecal methotrexate and

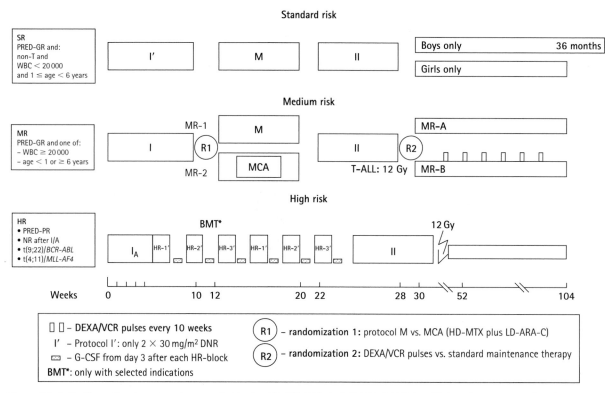

Figure 12.4 *Outline of treatment strategy applied in the ALL–BFM 95 study (1995–2000), in which patients were assigned to standard-risk (SR), medium-risk (MR) and high-risk (HR) subgroups. BMT, bone marrow transplantation; DEXA, dexamethasone; DNR, daunorubicin; G-CSF, granulocyte colony-stimulating factor; HD-MTX, high-dose methotrexate; I/A, protocol I, phase A; LD-ARA-C, low-dose cytarabine; NR, no response ; PRED-GR, prednisone good response; PRED-PR, prednisone poor response; VCR, vincristine; WBC, white blood cell count.*

Box 12.2 *Stratification criteria in trial ALL-BFM 95 by risk group: standard, medium and high*

- *Standard risk (SR)* – prednisone good response, and initial WBC <20 × 10⁹/L, and age at diagnosis >1 to <6 years, no HR cytogenetics, and no T-ALL (all criteria to be fulfilled)
- *Medium risk (MR)* – prednisone good response, no HR cytogenetics, and one of the following: initial WBC >20 × 10⁹/L, or age at diagnosis <1 or >6 years
- *High risk (HR)* – prednisone poor response, prednisone good response but ≥5 per cent marrow blasts on treatment day 33 (M2 or M3 marrow), t(9;22)- or *BCR/ABL* positivity, t(4;11)- or *MLL/AF4* positivity

oral 6-mercaptopurine. The outlined strategy of prolonged induction/early intensification proved to be successful in several BFM trials, as well as trials performed by other study groups.[4,6,9,15–17,84,100–102]

Glucocorticoids and drug combinations during induction treatment

In contrast to adult ALL, where a four-drug remission induction therapy including an anthracycline seems almost mandatory, the necessity of such a four-drug induction regimen in specific subgroups of paediatric ALL is subject to debate. It is unclear if addition of an anthracycline to a three-drug induction regimen is of benefit to certain low- or intermediate-risk groups. In a study of the CCG for intermediate-risk patients, it appeared that patients ≥10 years of age fared best if they received the full four-drug BFM induction/consolidation and reintensification (and cranial radiotherapy), whereas children <10 years old fared equally well if induction contained only prednisone, vincristine and asparaginase.[101] The dose intensity of the induction phase can also have a major impact on the overall results, as was demonstrated by the result of the ALL-BFM 83 study, which was significantly inferior to ALL-BFM 86 and 90.[9,15,43] In ALL-BFM 83, the induction phase was 14 days longer than in ALL-BFM 90, with the same cumulative dose of the four drugs used (prednisone, vincristine, daunorubicin, L-asparaginase). In some regimens, the first 4 weeks of treatment are based on only two or three drugs. In the Dutch Study VI for non-high-risk patients, treatment is initiated with vincristine and dexamethasone only before L-asparaginase is added.[102] In the COALL regimen, the first 4 weeks of treatment also omit L-asparaginase. Preliminary data from that group indicate that the number of drugs, as much as the time used for induction therapy, has an impact on the response (as detected by analysis of MRD) but not necessarily on the final outcome.[103] Addition of high-dose methotrexate early in a three-drug induction regimen, as shown in a limited number of patients by the DFCI consortium, can improve disease control but also strongly enhances toxicity.[104]

The choice of the corticosteroid for optimal induction therapy is still being debated.[105] Dexamethasone appears to have a stronger antileukaemic effect, which can be demonstrated *in vitro*.[106] However, both *in vivo* and *in vitro* resistance of ALL cells to prednisolone is also associated with increased resistance to dexamethasone.[50] One study in the Netherlands (Dutch Study VI) for non-high-risk patients demonstrated the feasibility of 4 weeks of dexamethasone (at $6 \, mg/m^2$ per day) when combined only with vincristine, whereas a pilot study performed by the DFCI group indicated severe complications, including toxic deaths, when dexamethasone was combined with doxorubicin, vincristine and L-asparaginase.[102,107] Later data from the DFCI group suggested that the dose of corticosteroid had an impact on final outcome.[108] Currently, several study groups are evaluating the role of the glucocorticoids in induction therapy in randomized trials. CCG investigators recently reported that in standard-risk ALL, dexamethasone, when given in induction therapy at $6 \, mg/m^2$ per day, can provide a better EFS than prednisone at $40 \, mg/m^2$ per day.[109]

Consolidation/extramedullary therapy

Eradication of residual leukaemic blasts in patients who are in remission by morphological criteria is the primary aim of consolidation treatment. This treatment is necessary, as patients successfully induced into remission but not given additional treatment usually relapse within months.[1] Today, most study groups use 6-mercaptopurine and methotrexate to maintain remission. A few groups use continuous infusion cycles of high-dose methotrexate (combined with leucovorin rescue). The contribution of high-dose methotrexate in consolidation/extramedullary therapy is probably largely due to its CNS effect, as cytotoxic methotrexate levels are also achieved in the CSF during high-dose methotrexate application.[110,111] Another systemically administered drug that is discussed in the context of CNS disease prevention is dexamethasone,

which has been shown to be superior to prednisolone.[102,112] The importance of this finding is currently being evaluated by several study groups. For further extramedullary disease prevention, repeated intrathecal injections of methotrexate throughout the treatment period and cranial radiotherapy in defined subsets of patients are used.[6,8,9,15,113] Instead of the sole application of intrathecal methotrexate, some study groups add additional drugs to this treatment (a glucocorticoid, either hydrocortisone or prednisolone, and cytarabine, mostly restricted to high-risk patients).[15,114] It remains unclear whether triple-drug intrathecal injections are of any benefit to any patient subset.

In the BFM trial ALL-BFM 81,[115] low- and intermediate-risk patients were randomized to compare the efficiency of 18-Gy cranial radiotherapy with intermediate-dose methotrexate ($0.5 \, g/m^2$) given as four 24-hour infusions, together with intrathecal methotrexate every 2 weeks during consolidation. The higher incidence of relapses found in those patients who did not receive cranial radiotherapy was due to the higher number of relapses with CNS involvement. Only 'standard risk' ALL patients with a low initial cell mass were protected from CNS-related relapses with intermediate-dose methotrexate without cranial radiotherapy (1.6 per cent isolated and 3.2 per cent combined CNS relapses).[116–118] Nevertheless, the rate of relapse after long-term observation of low-risk patients from trial ALL-BFM 81 demonstrated an advantage for the irradiated subset of patients (12.9 per cent relapses overall as compared with 22.2 per cent in the non-irradiated group).[84]

In the subsequent trial, ALL-BFM 83, the strong impact of intensive reintensification on the rate of systemic and extramedullary relapses was found in a randomized study on low-risk patients.[84,116] All patients received intermediate-dose methotrexate during consolidation, but low-risk patients were then randomized to receive or not receive postconsolidation reinduction therapy in an attempt to decrease the toxicity of treatment in the group of patients with the lowest risk of relapse. Patients of both treatment arms were not irradiated under the protection of intermediate-dose methotrexate. The number of isolated CNS relapses was low in both groups, but the rate of combined CNS and bone marrow relapses, and especially of isolated systemic relapses, was significantly higher in patients who had not been exposed to reinduction therapy. When the results were compared with the corresponding subset of patients from ALL-BFM 81, the rate of combined CNS/bone marrow relapses was also three times higher in patients not receiving reinduction therapy. This provided evidence that reinduction therapy is important not only for systemic, but also for extramedullary, disease control.[84,111]

The first reduction of cranial radiotherapy from 18 to 12 Gy in patients other than those with low-risk ALL was performed on a randomized basis in trial ALL-BFM 83.[43,84,111] Intermediate-risk patients were treated with either 12 or 18 Gy cranial radiotherapy, with patients receiving intermediate-dose methotrexate during consolidation and a total of eight intrathecal methotrexate injections throughout treatment. With regard to CNS relapse rates, the two cranial radiotherapy regimens were equally effective. The comparison of these intermediate-risk patients with the corresponding subset of patients from ALL-BFM 81 who had received systemic methotrexate but not presymptomatic radiotherapy confirmed the large difference in the number of CNS-related relapses found in the randomized comparison in the earlier trials, indicating that intermediate-dose methotrexate without cranial radiotherapy does not provide adequate CNS protection.[84,111,117] In the subsequent ALL-BFM 86 and ALL-BFM 90 trials,[9,15] additional reduction of cranial radiotherapy was performed under the protection of intensified intrathecal methotrexate therapy as well as systemic application of high-dose methotrexate ($5 \, g/m^2 \times 4$ in consolidation). In ALL-BFM 86, high-risk patients were treated with 18 instead of 24 Gy. In ALL-BFM 90, cranial radiotherapy was only 12 Gy for intermediate- and high-risk patients. The results of these two trials showed that identical subsets of intermediate-risk patients defined by prednisone good response and B-precursor ALL had CNS-related relapse frequencies below 3 per cent. In the ALL-BFM 90 trial, even in cases of B-precursor ALL with an increased initial cell mass but adequate early response to prednisone, no increase in CNS-related relapses could be demonstrated after the dose of cranial radiotherapy had been decreased from 18 to 12 Gy.[15] Also, in T-cell ALL patients in both the ALL-BFM 86 and 90 trials, the relapse incidence could be reduced, especially among prednisone good responders, by the introduction of high-dose methotrexate in consolidation therapy.[9,15] A dose of 12 Gy of cranial radiotherapy for T-cell ALL patients with a prednisone good response provided effective control at both systemic and CNS sites.[15]

In ALL-BFM 86,[9] only the small group of high-risk patients, mainly due to an inadequate corticosteroid response (10 per cent of the total study population), had an increased incidence (11.6 per cent) of relapses with CNS involvement. The overall outcome, as well as the cumulative incidence of CNS relapses (CI CNS), was not significantly improved in patients with a prednisone poor response in ALL-BFM 86 compared with those in ALL-BFM 83.[84] The introduction of a modified approach to the high-risk group in ALL-BFM 90, utilizing a postinduction series of intensified consolidation elements (containing high-dose methotrexate, high-dose cytarabine and nine doses of intrathecal triple therapy), decreased the number of relapses with CNS involvement to 5 per cent, even though the dose of cranial radiotherapy had been decreased to 12 Gy in patients without CNS involvement. On the other hand, this approach was not successful in reducing the rather high rate of systemic relapses: the 8-year EFS for patients with a prednisone poor response was 31.8 per cent.[15,84]

With regard to the influence of methotrexate dose during consolidation/extramedullary therapy on the incidence of testicular relapse in boys with ALL, 1144 boys with newly diagnosed ALL, enrolled in the ALL-BFM 81, 83 or 86 trials, were retrospectively evaluated for the influence of methotrexate on the testicular relapse-free interval.[119] The cumulative incidence of isolated testicular relapses was significantly higher in the group receiving cranial radiotherapy (without intravenous methotrexate) than in the groups receiving intermediate-dose methotrexate ($0.5 \, g/m^2$ per 24 hours $\times$ 4) and high-dose methotrexate ($5 \, g/m^2$ per 24 hours $\times$ 4) (6.7 vs. 2.5 and 2.3 per cent, respectively). High-dose methotrexate did not lower the rate of isolated testicular relapse any further.

A study on the long-term outcome of 596 children and adolescents with ALL (CALGB 7611 study) who were randomized between 1976 and 1979 to receive intermediate-dose methotrexate plus intrathecal methotrexate or cranial radiation plus intrathecal methotrexate showed that radiotherapy offered better CNS protection but intermediate methotrexate offered better haematological and better testicular protection.[120] A study of the Paediatric Oncology Group on T-cell ALL suggested that intravenous methotrexate in combination with triple intrathecal therapy and rotational chemotherapy can be as effective as a combination of chemotherapy with cranial radiotherapy but will result in a higher incidence of CNS recurrences.[121]

Indications for preventive cranial radiotherapy

The majority of CNS relapses of ALL are observed within 24 months of the initiation of treatment, indicating the importance of effective and early CNS prevention. Since cranial radiotherapy does cause acute and late side-effects and may cause secondary malignant glioma, it was hoped that this treatment could be eliminated from ALL therapy, at least for low- and intermediate-risk patients. This possibility was tested by randomized evaluation of patients in the ALL-BFM 81 trial, but failed, as described above.[84,115,116] Adjustments of CNS-directed chemotherapy in several consecutive clinical trials performed thereafter have led to a successful strategy in which preventive radiotherapy is restricted to a well-defined patient group with an increased risk of CNS or systemic recurrence. This well-defined patient subset in the BFM study group is represented by all patients aged 1 year or over with T-cell ALL (intermediate- and high-risk), and all high-risk ALL cases (see Box 12.2 for stratification criteria in

ALL-BFM 95). With regard to intermediate-risk T-ALL, an intergroup analysis performed by the Italian ALL study group AEIOP and the BFM study group revealed the importance of cranial radiotherapy in cases of prednisone good-responding T-cell ALL for the prevention of CNS as well as systemic relapses.[122] The main difference between these regimens was the lack of cranial radiotherapy in the Italian study, which was replaced by nine doses of intrathecal methotrexate/cytarabine/prednisolone (intrathecal triple therapy) during maintenance. T-cell ALL patients treated in AIEOP 91 had two times more systemic and five times more CNS relapses than patients treated in BFM 90. Another study for intermediate-risk patients of the CCG demonstrated that extended intrathecal methotrexate therapy is as effective as cranial radiotherapy if systemic therapy comprises a more intensive regimen with delayed intensification.[113] This study group also demonstrated that, in high-risk patients, no significant difference in outcome can be found between cranial radiotherapy and intrathecal methotrexate for CNS prevention. The latter treatment provided less effective CNS control but better protection from marrow relapse.[123] This study underscores the fact that the contribution of cranial irradiation to prevention of relapse depends on the underlying systemic chemotherapy. A Dutch study using the BFM regimen from trial ALL-BFM 86 was successful in preventing CNS recurrence without the use of cranial radiotherapy.[9,17]

The comparative long-term toxicity of cranial radiotherapy versus CNS-directed chemotherapy with respect to the development of neuropsychological functioning, hormonal disturbances and secondary malignancies remains to be determined. Cranial irradiation, in particular, is associated with the development of secondary brain tumours.[124–127] The results of randomized comparisons between patients treated with chemoprophylaxis based on systemic high-dose methotrexate and intrathecal methotrexate (or intrathecal triple therapy) and those treated with radiotherapy (especially the lower dose of 12 Gy), or combinations of both, should settle the issue of which regimen has less long-term toxicity.[128,129]

Reinduction

Reinduction or delayed intensification of childhood ALL treatment was introduced by the BFM group in ALL-BFM 76.[100] In the second half of the 1970s, this new therapeutic approach was limited to high-risk patients who were characterized by large leukaemic cell mass (mainly based on an initial WBC count of $>25 \times 10^9$/L). The timing of reinduction was either directly after induction or at 5 months after diagnosis. From these studies it was learned that patients receiving this type of treatment (protocol II) fared significantly better with regard to

outcome than did patients from ALL-BFM 70, in particular if reinduction was delayed: the 10-year EFS rate for these patients was 70 per cent (delayed) compared with 60 per cent (given shortly after induction) and 38 ± 4 per cent in ALL-BFM 70 (no reinduction). Therefore, overall outcome was significantly better in BFM 76/79 than in the first BFM study: the 10-year EFS was 67 per cent compared with 54 per cent in BFM 70.[116] Figure 12.4 illustrates how reinduction treatment (protocol II) is incorporated into a modern clinical treatment protocol, the treatment strategy of the ALL-BFM 95 trial, in which reinduction or delayed intensification treatment is given 2–3 weeks after completion of consolidation/extracompartment therapy protocol M/MCA. Similar to induction protocol I, two treatment phases (induction and intensification) can be distinguished in protocol II: phase 1 includes systemic applications of dexamethasone ($10 \, \text{mg/m}^2$ per day $\times$ 21), vincristine, L-asparaginase and doxorubicin. Phase 2 of reinduction comprises cyclophosphamide, 6-thioguanine and cytarabine.

The first randomized clinical trials that proved the value of reinduction for the successful therapy of non-high-risk childhood ALL were conducted in parallel by the BFM group and the CCG in the first half of the 1980s.[43,100,101,116] In the ALL-BFM 83 study, patients in the low-standard-risk group (low leukaemic cell mass and absence of mediastinal mass or CNS disease) were randomized to receive or not receive reintensification with so-called protocol III after interim maintenance with intermediate-dose methotrexate. Protocol III is similar to protocol II but comprises only two doses of vincristine and doxorubicin each (instead of four), only 2 weeks of dexamethasone, and no cyclophosphamide. Patients did not receive cranial radiotherapy. Patients treated on protocol III showed a significantly better EFS, mainly due to the lower incidence of systemic recurrences: the 8-year EFS was 81.8 per cent, compared with 58.3 per cent for protocol II. In addition, patients receiving reintensification had a cumulative incidence of CNS recurrences of 3.8 per cent, compared with 12.3 per cent in patients treated without reinduction.[84]

In ALL-BFM 86, a very similar observation was made in a non-randomized comparison between standard-risk patients (defined by a low tumour load and a prednisone good response) who were treated in the first part of trial ALL-BFM 86 without reinduction and patients treated with the so-called reinduction protocol II after amendment of the protocol.[9,84] Despite the use of high-dose methotrexate during consolidation in that study, reinduction with protocol II had a major impact on the number of relapses.[18] This was also found in the Dutch trial 'Study 7'.[17] The difference in relapse incidence between these patient groups was due to systemic relapses, and not to the number of CNS relapses. Interestingly, a recent randomized study by the CCG, applying an augmented BFM protocol in high-risk patients with a slow initial response, showed that intensified consolidation and further reinduction or double-delayed reintensification can further improve outcome for this patient subset, even though the effect appeared to be limited to patients less than 10 years of age.[130] Unfortunately, this approach was associated with a high incidence of avascular bone necrosis. The Italian AIEOP study group successfully utilized two reintensifications with protocol II in the high-risk group, which resulted in an improved EFS of 56.5 per cent.[131]

Maintenance therapy

Maintenance treatment aims at a further stabilization of remission by suppressing the re-emergence of a drug-resistant clone through consistently reducing the pool of residual leukaemic cells. The current standard of maintenance therapy consists of treatment with daily oral mercaptopurine and weekly oral methotrexate for a total duration of 2–3 years (sometimes 3 years only for boys). Dose adjustments of 6-mercaptopurine and methotrexate are usually made according to WBC count. On some protocols, additional pulsed applications of vincristine and a glucocorticoid, and eventually intrathecal therapy are administered.[132] It is important to note that reduction of maintenance below 2 years has been associated with an increased frequency of leukaemic relapses.[116,133,134]

An overview of all randomized trials that began before 1987 and studied the effects on long-term outcome of the duration and intensity of maintenance chemotherapy was published by the Childhood ALL Collaborative Group in 1996.[133] Data were studied from 3900 children to compare longer (in particular 3 years) and shorter (in particular 2 years) maintenance durations; from 3700 children to analyse the contribution of intensive reinduction chemotherapy during maintenance; and from 1300 children to study the role of pulses of vincristine and prednisone during maintenance. Increased death rates in remission were due to longer maintenance (2.7 vs. 1.2 per cent), VCR/prednisone pulses (4.0 vs. 3.2 per cent) and intensive reinduction (4.8 vs. 3.3 per cent). These increases in death rates were, however, counterbalanced by lower relapse rates. The total number of leukaemic events was significantly reduced by longer maintenance (23.3 vs. 27.6 per cent), vincristine/prednisone pulses (31.2 vs. 40.4 per cent) and intensive reinduction (27.8 vs. 35.8 per cent). Because many of the patients who relapsed could be treated successfully afterwards, the overall survival of children with ALL improved significantly only for intensive reinduction (18.5 vs. 22.3 per cent). Based upon these results, it was concluded that intensive reinduction chemotherapy led

to a 4 per cent increase in long-term survival. For each individual treatment schedule, it is, of course, important to realize that potential improvements of outcome by introducing certain therapy elements or longer duration of maintenance therapy depend on the therapy that is given before maintenance therapy starts, and on the subgroup of patients studied. It is not clear whether extended maintenance of up to 2.5 or 3 years for boys, as used by, for example, CCG and BFM study groups, offers any beneficial effect in the context of current treatment strategies. Other issues that have to be resolved in the future include differences in requirements for maintenance therapy in specific childhood ALL patient subsets (e.g. those defined immunophenotypically or genetically).

Haemopoietic stem cell transplantation

Allogeneic bone marrow transplantation from a matched related donor has been shown to improve the survival of children with ALL in second remission.[135,136] The main reasons for this improvement are most probably further intensification of treatment and the graft-versus-leukaemia (GvL) effect. However, with decreasing transplant-related mortalities through progress in the understanding and management of graft-versus-host disease and the GvL effect, as well as increasing numbers of registered donors, allogeneic bone marrow or peripheral stem cell transplantations are more and more becoming a therapeutic option for specific high-risk patient subsets with ALL in first remission. Because the number of well designed randomized clinical trials on the value of bone marrow or peripheral stem cell transplantation in patients with ALL in first remission is small, it will be a major task of current and future trials to identify clearly those patient subsets that truly benefit from these therapeutic approaches compared with innovative high-dose chemotherapy regimens.[137–144]

Indications for BMT in first complete remission

All study groups reserve BMT for defined high-risk groups that differ slightly between protocols. For example, current BFM guidelines restrict matched related or unrelated donor bone marrow or peripheral stem cell transplantation in first complete remission to specific subsets of high-risk patients. These guidelines include patients not in remission at the end of induction treatment (M2 or M3 marrow at treatment day 33), patients with the non-random chromosomal translocations t(9;22) or t(4;11) (or positivity for the respective fusion RNAs: *BCR/ABL* and *MLL/AF4*), as well as prednisone poor responders with a T-cell or pro-B-cell immunophenotype. Recent collaborative analyses of the data of ALL study groups suggest that BCR/ABL-positive ALL, but not MLL gene-rearranged ALL, did benefit from allogeneic BMT.[68,81] However, considering the risk of transplant-related mortality as well as late treatment-related morbidity, it will be important in the future to develop strategies for the identification of 'highest-risk' patients within the high-risk subset of children with ALL. One potential approach is shown in Table 12.3, which presents the EFS of patients with high-risk features, such as age less than 1 year or the t(9;22) separated by initial response to treatment.[63,80] A combined approach of initial patient or genetic characteristics with early response to treatment can distinguish patients with a very high risk of relapse. Analysis of MRD has further improved the development of eligibility criteria for transplantation. In the current AIEOP-BFM study, a high level of MRD after 12 weeks of treatment is used for the indication of a matched family or matched unrelated donor stem cell transplantation.

Toxicity and supportive care

Quality of treatment will increasingly be the focus of attention and will be tested for its impact on the quality of life, as defined by short- and long-term toxicity. This issue has become more important as the best major study groups have reached comparable rates of long-term EFS. Supportive care, mainly through prevention of infectious complications such as cotrimoxazol for Pneumocystis carinii pneumonia prophylaxis, antimycotic treatment of mucous membranes and prophylaxis for varicella zoster virus infection, as well as aggressive treatment of potential bacterial and/or fungal infections, has contributed in part to the above-described increases in EFS. An adequate supply of blood components and maintenance of nutritional status are essential in the management of children with ALL, as is appropriate psychosocial support for the patient and the family.

Early mortality in ALL-BFM trials 83 to 90 ranged from 0.3 to 1.7 per cent of patients, with the main cause of treatment-related fatalities being infections during neutropenia, occasionally combined with organ dysfunction.[15] With regard to post-remission toxicity, fatality rates of 1.3 and 1.6 per cent were noted in trials ALL-BFM 86 and 90, respectively.[15,51] These fatalities were mainly due to infectious complications, but also involved bleeding and organ failure. The described mortality observed in BFM trials is comparable to mortalities observed in trials by other study groups.[5–8,14,17,84,101]

With overall improvements in survival, the long-term adverse effects of treatment have become apparent as well. These include secondary neoplasms such as acute myeloid leukaemia (e.g. associated with etoposide treatment) and radiotherapy-associated brain tumours, cardiac late effects (anthracycline therapy-associated cardiomyopathy), avascular necrosis of bone, and neuropsychological (e.g. methotrexate therapy-associated) and endocrinological deficits.[66,128,129,145–150]

The rate of secondary leukaemias varies between different study protocols, from 0.3 per cent in ALL-BFM 90[15] to 6 per cent in US studies.[146,151,152] Epipodophyllotoxins are thought to be responsible, to a large extent, for these secondary malignancies. Secondary brain tumours are due to CNS radiation as mentioned above, although the use of thiopurines in combination with an increased susceptibility of the host might also play a role.[126] This observation might, however, be dependent on the combination and timing of chemotherapy and radiotherapy.[153] Cardiac late effects depend on the dose of anthracyclines administered. Continuous infusions of anthracyclines are not protective for cardiomyopathy.[154–157] Avascular necrosis of bone is associated mainly with the use of steroids and is seen especially in older children (>10 years in particular) and adults with ALL.[66,148,149,158] In most but not all studies, neurocognitive functioning is impaired by cranial radiotherapy at a dose of 18 Gy or higher.[159–163] Dexamethasone might have long-term neurocognitive side-effects.[164]

PERSPECTIVE: HOST AND TUMOUR GENETIC VARIABILITY

If one applies the epidemiological triangle explaining the interrelationships among host, disease and environment in childhood ALL,[165] it becomes clear that host factors potentially contribute in large part to the variability in treatment outcome observed in uniformly treated specific disease entities (Table 12.3). The heterogeneity of response observed in childhood Ph+ ALL can serve as an example.[80] It is possible, however, that unknown tumour genetic variation is also contributing to this heterogeneity. Until recently, host factors in the relationship with childhood ALL were mostly represented by patient characteristics such as race or gender. However, with technological advances over the past two decades, research into the identification and contribution of potential genetic and biochemical host factors has markedly increased. In particular, tremendous efforts within the Human Genome Project have already resulted in a large pool of genetic information that is continuously growing and will help to untangle the impact of a patient's genetic background on treatment effect and toxicity. In this context, the fields of pharmacogenetics and immunogenetics are of particular current interest to researchers working in the field of ALL.

Pharmacogenetics refers to research in which associations between genetic differences and variability in drug response are studied in defined populations.[166,167] The ultimate goal of pharmacogenetic studies is to develop genetic profiles for patients to optimize drug dosing, resulting in a maximum treatment effect with minimum toxicity. With regard to immunogenetics, the genetic characterization of molecular complexes such as the major histocompatibility complex (MHC), cytokines and cellular receptors has produced a large amount of information on the role of host immunogenetic variability in disease processes.[166,167] The latter studies will be of particular importance for profiling susceptibility towards treatment-related infectious complications and for problems associated with, for example, BMT procedures. A major tool for the development of such genetic profiles is the single nucleotide polymorphism (SNP, pronounced 'snip').[166,167] SNPs describe positions within the genome where two alternative bases are observed in a population at a frequency of more than 1 per cent. SNPs are observed in every 500–1000 base pairs. This frequency in the entire human genome, approximately 3 billion base pairs, translates into an expected number of three to six million SNPs. It is assumed that SNPs may be responsible for as much as 90 per cent of the genetic diversity in mankind and, therefore, are suggested to play an important role in the observed phenotypic variations among individuals.

Numerous candidate genes may be of importance in childhood ALL.[167] With regard to treatment, most of the research on genetic variability in patient populations conducted to date has focused on drug-metabolizing enzymes. The most extensively studied of these enzymes is thiopurine methyltransferase (TPMT) which catalyses the S-methylation of thiopurines (e.g. 6-mercaptopurine, 6-thioguanine).[168] The TPMT locus is subject to genetic polymorphism, with heterozygous individuals (about 10 per cent of the Caucasian population) having intermediate TPMT activity, and homozygous individuals (about only 0.33 per cent of Caucasians) having low TPMT activity.[169,170] The TPMT genotype shows excellent concordance with TPMT phenotype[169] and is associated with toxicity and outcome in childhood ALL.[126,168,171–175] A recent study at St Jude Children's Research Hospital found that patients with lower TPMT activity fared significantly better than those with higher TPMT activity.[126] However, as maintenance therapy with antimetabolites is an essential element of all treatment regimens for childhood ALL, and there is no uniform approach with regard to dose, dose-adjustment procedures and scheduling of drugs during this treatment period, it will be important to confirm the St Jude findings in further prospective trials and to develop strategies for implementing them in future therapeutic strategies.[153]

Within the BFM study group, we have conducted preliminary research on the genetic variability of glutathione S-transferase (GST) genes and their potential impact on the clinical course of childhood ALL. GSTs are a family of cytosolic enzymes involved in the detoxification of various exogenous as well as endogenous reactive species.[176] In two case–control studies with BFM patients, we found protective effects of specific GST genotypes on the risk of relapse in childhood ALL.[177,178] The most pronounced effect was observed for the GSTT1 null genotype. These findings were not confirmed in the only other study addressing the association of GST genotypes and outcome in childhood ALL, from researchers at St Jude Children's Research Hospital.[179] These divergent results imply that host genetic variability may have different impacts depending on treatment characteristics.

An important focus for future studies will be the contribution of individual genotypic profiles to leukaemia outcome, taking into account cytogenetic and/or molecular genetic as well as immunophenotypic features of patient populations. Certain host cell genotypes may be associated with leukaemogenesis in specific cytogenetically and/or molecular genetically defined leukaemia subsets.[165,180] Hence, when genotypic profiles are related to leukaemia outcome, it will be important to consider information associated with the aetiology of the disease. Also, specific subtypes of leukaemia so far characterized by classic cytogenetic and molecular genetic techniques, such as those with BCR/ABL, MLL gene rearrangement, hyperdiploidy and different T-ALL subtypes, appear to have specific profiles on gene expression profiling studies.[82,83,181,182] These gene expression profiles may lead to key genes involved in leukaemogenesis but also to new targets for therapy.[82] Also, differences in gene profiles between drug-responsive and drug-resistant cases may found to be important for clinical practice. In addition, the first study showed that the gene profile had a very strong prognostic value, comparable to measuring MRD, but this finding has to be confirmed.[83] Finally, when proteomic studies begin to develop with the same speed as genomic studies have in the last decade, this field may also lead to important developments for childhood ALL.

KEY POINTS

- Diagnostics in childhood ALL must determine the clinical dissemination of the disease (CNS involvement?) and must include immunophenotyping and molecular genetics, in order to provide therapy adapted to the risk of relapse.
- Results of molecular genetics at diagnosis are prerequisites for monitoring disease, either by RT-PCR of fusion genes (e.g. BCR/ABL) or by

quantitative PCR of rearranged leukaemia-specific T-cell receptor and immunglobulin genes.

- Careful monitoring of *in vivo* response to treatment can provide fairly specific prognostic information. Detection of MRD is a highly sensitive technology which allows prospective evaluation of treatment response in the submicroscopic range.
- The prognostic impact of MRD at some point in therapy depends on the composition of each treatment protocol and should be prospectively determined.
- Multiagent chemotherapy, including repetitive intrathecal methotrexate, can provide continuous first remission (CR1) in 75 per cent of patients. Contemporary treatment protocols provide the same level of cure for precursor-B-cell and T-cell ALL. Subgroups can be defined in which 5-year EFS is approaching 90 per cent.
- Only a minority of patients require cranial radiotherapy: according to most studies, this comprises patients with CNS involvement, inadequate treatment response, and those with T-cell ALL (and high WBC).
- A small subgroup of patients with ALL in CR1 are eligible for allogeneic haemopoietic stem cell transplantation. Briefly, these are patients with poor response to therapy and those with high-risk cytogenetics (e.g. *BCR/ABL*).
- Inadequate treatment response is the combined consequence of drug resistance of the leukaemic cell and of host mechanisms such as altered drug metabolism.

REFERENCES

1. Margolin J, Poplack D. Acute lymphoblastic leukaemia. In: Pizzo P, Poplack D, eds. *Principles and Practice of Pediatric Oncology*, 3rd edn. Philadelphia: Lippincott-Raven, 1997; 409–62.
2. Ritter J, Schrappe M. Clinical features and therapy of lymphoblastic leukaemia. In: Lilleyman JS, Hann IM, Blanchette VS, eds. *Paediatric Hematology*, 2nd edn. London: Churchill Livingstone, 1999; 537–63.
♦3. Pui CH, Evans WE. Acute lymphoblastic leukaemia. *N Engl J Med* 1998; **339**(9): 605–15.
4. Riehm H, Gadner H, Henze G et al. The Berlin childhood acute lymphoblastic leukemia therapy study, 1970–1976. *Am J Pediatr Hematol Oncol* 1980; **2**: 299–306.
5. Chessells JM, Bailey C, Richards SM. Intensification of treatment and survival in all children with lymphoblastic leukaemia: results of UK Medical Research Council trial UKALL X. *Lancet* 1995; **345**: 143–8.
6. Conter V, Arico M, Valsecchi MG et al. Intensive BFM chemotherapy for childhood ALL: interim analysis of the AIEOP-ALL 91 study. Associazione Italiana Ematologia Oncologia Pediatrica. *Haematologica* 1998; **83**(9): 791–9.
7. Evans WE, Relling MV, Rodman JH et al. Conventional compared with individualized chemotherapy for childhood acute lymphoblastic leukemia. *N Engl J Med* 1998; **338**: 499–505.
8. Gustafsson G, Kreuger A, Clausen N et al. Intensified treatment of acute childhood lymphoblastic leukaemia has improved prognosis, especially in non-high-risk patients: the Nordic experience of 2648 patients diagnosed between 1981 and 1996. Nordic Society of Paediatric Haematology and Oncology (NOPHO). *Acta Paediatr* 1998; **87**(11): 1151–61.
9. Reiter A, Schrappe M, Ludwig W-D et al. Chemotherapy in 998 unselected childhood acute lymphoblastic leukemia patients. Results and conclusions of the multicenter trial ALL-BFM 86. *Blood* 1994; **84**: 3122–33.
10. Gaynon PS, Steinherz PG, Bleyer WA et al. Improved therapy for children with acute lymphoblastic leukemia and unfavorable presenting features: a follow-up report of the Children's Cancer Group Study CCG-106. *J Clin Oncol* 1993; **11**: 2234–42.
11. Niemeyer CM, Reiter A, Riehm H et al. Comparative results of two intensive treatment programs for childhood acute lymphoblastic leukemia: the Berlin-Frankfurt-Munster and Dana-Farber Cancer Institute protocols. *Ann Oncol* 1991; **2**: 745–9.
12. Rivera GK, Raimondi SC, Hancock ML et al. Improved outcome in childhood acute lymphoblastic leukaemia with reinforced early treatment and rotational combination chemotherapy. *Lancet* 1991; **337**: 61–6.
13. Sackmann-Muriel F, Felice MS, Zubizarreta PA et al. Treatment results in childhood acute lymphoblastic leukemia with a modified ALL-BFM'90 protocol: lack of improvement in high-risk group. *Leuk Res* 1999; **23**: 331–40.
14. Schorin MA, Blattner S, Gelber RD et al. Treatment of childhood acute lymphoblastic leukemia: Results of Dana-Farber Cancer Institute/Children's Hospital Acute Lymphoblastic Leukemia Consortium Protocol 85-01. *J Clin Oncol* 1994; **12**: 740–7.
15. Schrappe M, Reiter A, Ludwig W-D et al. Improved outcome in childhood ALL despite reduced use of anthracyclines and of cranial radiotherapy: Results of trial ALL-BFM 90. *Blood* 2000; **95**(11): 3310–22.
16. Henze G, Langermann HJ, Kaufmann U et al. Thymic involvement and initial white blood count in childhood acute lymphoblastic leukemia. *Am J Pediatr Hematol Oncol* 1981; **3**(4): 369–76.
17. Kamps WA, Bökkerink JPM, Hählen K et al. Intensive treatment of children with acute lymphoblastic leukemia according to ALL-BFM 86 without cranial radiotherapy: Results of DCLSG protocol ALL-7 (1988–1991). *Blood* 1999; **94**(4): 1226–36.
18. Reiter A, Schrappe M, Ludwig WD et al. Favorable outcome of B-cell acute lymphoblastic leukemia in childhood: a report of three consecutive studies of the BFM group. *Blood* 1992; **80**: 2471–8.
19. Reiter A, Schrappe M, Tiemann M et al. Improved treatment results in childhood B-cell neoplasms with tailored intensification of therapy: a report of the Berlin-Frankfurt-Munster Group Trial NHL-BFM 90. *Blood* 1999; **94**(10): 3294–306.

20. Patte C, Philip T, Rodary C et al. High survival rate in advanced-stage B-cell lymphomas and leukemias without CNS involvement with a short intensive polychemotherapy: results from the French pediatric oncology society of a randomized trial of 216 children. J Clin Oncol 1991; 9: 123–32.
21. Skinner J, Mee TJ, Blackwell RP et al. Exposure to power frequency electric fields and the risk of childhood cancer in the UK. Br J Cancer 2002; 87: 1257–66.
22. Greaves MF. Aetiology of acute leukaemia. Lancet 1997; 349: 344–9.
23. Ford AM, Bennett CA, Price CM et al. Fetal origins of the TEL-AML1 fusion gene in identical twins with leukemia. Proc Natl Acad Sci USA 1998; 95(8): 4584–8.
24. Gale KB, Ford AM, Repp R et al. Backtracking leukemia to birth: identification of clonotypic gene fusion sequences in neonatal blood spots. Proc Natl Acad Sci USA 1997; 94(25): 13950–4.
25. Mori H, Colman SM, Xiao Z et al. Chromosome translocations and covert leukemic clones are generated during normal fetal development. Proc Natl Acad Sci USA 2002; 99(12): 8242–47.
26. Bennett JM, Catovski D, Daniel MT et al. Proposals for the classification of the acute leukaemias. French-American-British (FAB) cooperative group. Br J Haematol 1976; 33: 451–8.
27. van der Does van den Berg A, Bartram CR, Basso G et al. Minimal requirements for the diagnosis, classification, and evaluation of the treatment of childhood acute lymphoblastic leukemia (ALL) in the 'BFM Family' Cooperative Group. Med Pediatr Oncol 1992; 20: 497–505.
28. Pui CH. Toward optimal central nervous system-directed treatment in childhood acute lymphoblastic leukemia. J Clin Oncol 2003; 21: 179–81.
29. Burger B, Zimmermann M, Mann G et al. Diagnostic cerebrospinal fluid (CSF) examination in children with acute lymphoblastic leukemia (ALL): significance of low leukocyte counts with blasts or traumatic lumbar puncture. J Clin Oncol 2003; 21: 184–8.
30. Ludwig WD, Rieder H, Bartram CR et al. Immunophenotypic and genotypic features, clinical characteristics, and treatment outcome of adult pro-B acute lymphoblastic leukemia: results of the German multicenter trials GMALL 03/87 and 04/89. Blood 1998; 92(6): 1898–909.
31. Weir EG, Borowitz MJ. Flow cytometry in the diagnosis of acute leukemia. Semin Hematol 2001; 38: 124–38.
32. Bene MC, Castoldi G, Knapp W et al. Proposals for the immunological classification of acute leukaemias. European group for the immunological characterisation of leukaemias (EGIL). Leukemia 1995; 9: 1783–6.
33. Look AT, Roberson PK, Williams DL et al. Prognostic importance of blast cell DNA content in childhood acute lymphoblastic leukemia. Blood 1985; 65: 1079–86.
34. Hiddemann W, Wörmann B, Ritter J et al. Frequency and clinical significance of DNA aneuploidy in acute leukemia. Ann NY Acad Sci 1986; 468: 227–40.
35. Harbott J, Ritterbach J, Ludwig W-D et al. Clinical significance of cytogenetic studies in childhood acute lymphoblastic leukemia: experience of the BFM trials. Recent Results Cancer Res 1993; 131: 123–32.
♦36. Pui C-H, Crist WM, Look AT. Biology and clinical significance of cytogenetic abnormalities in childhood acute lymphoblastic leukemia. Blood 1990; 76: 1449–63.
♦37. Rubnitz JE, Crist WM. Molecular genetics of childhood cancer: implications for pathogenesis, diagnosis, and treatment. Pediatrics 1997; 100: 101–8.
38. Schlieben S, Borkhardt A, Reinisch I et al. Incidence and clinical outcome of children with BCR/ABL-positive acute lymphoblastic leukemia (ALL). A prospective RT-PCR study based on 673 patients enrolled in the German pediatric multicenter therapy trials ALL-BFM 90 and CoALL-05-92. Leukemia 1996; 10: 957–63.
39. van der Burg M, Beverloo HB, Langerak AW et al. Rapid and sensitive detection of all types of MLL gene translocations with a single FISH probe set. Leukemia 1999; 13: 2107–13.
♦40. Avet-Loiseau H. FISH analysis at diagnosis in acute lymphoblastic leukemia. Leuk Lymphoma 1999; 33: 441–9.
♦41. Harrison CJ. The genetics of childhood acute lymphoblastic leukaemia. Baillieres Best Pract Res Clin Haematol 2000; 13: 427–39.
42. Foroni L, Harrison CJ, Hoffbrand AV, Potter MN. Investigation of minimal residual disease in childhood and adult acute lymphoblastic leukaemia by molecular analysis. Br J Haematol 1999; 105: 7–24.
43. Riehm H, Reiter A, Schrappe M et al. Die Corticosteroid-abhängige Dezimierung der Leukämiezellzahl im Blut als Prognosefaktor bei der akuten lymphoblastischen Leukämie im Kindesalter (Therapiestudie ALL-BFM 83) [The in vivo response on corticosteroid therapy as an additional prognostic factor in childhood acute lymphoblastic leukemia (therapy study ALL-BFM 83)]. Klin Pädiatr 1987; 199: 151–60.
44. Arico M, Basso G, Mandelli F et al. Good steroid response in vivo predicts a favorable outcome in children with T-cell acute lymphoblastic leukemia. Cancer 1995; 75: 1684–93.
45. Gaynon PS, Desai AA, Bostrom BC et al. Early response to therapy and outcome in childhood acute lymphoblastic leukemia: a review. Cancer 1997; 80: 1717–26.
46. Gaynon PS, Bleyer WA, Steinherz PG et al. Day 7 marrow response and outcome for children with acute lymphoblastic leukemia and unfavorable presenting features. Med Pediatr Oncol 1990; 18: 273–9.
47. Steinherz PG, Gaynon PS, Breneman JC et al. Cytoreduction and prognosis in acute lymphoblastic leukemia – the importance of early marrow response: report from the Children's Cancer Group. J Clin Oncol 1996; 14(2): 389–98.
48. Schrappe M, Reiter A, Riehm H. Cytoreduction and prognosis in childhood acute lymphoblastic leukemia. J Clin Oncol 1996; 14(8): 2403–5.
49. Gajjar A, Ribeiro R, Hancock ML et al. Persistence of circulating blasts after 1 week of multiagent chemotherapy confers a poor prognosis in childhood acute lymphoblastic leukemia. Blood 1995; 86(4): 1292–5.
50. Kaspers GJ, Pieters R, Van Zantwijk CH et al. Prednisolone resistance in childhood acute lymphoblastic leukemia: Vitro-vivo correlations and cross-resistance to other drugs. Blood 1998; 92(1): 259–66.
51. Janka-Schaub GE, Stührk H, Kortüm B et al. Bone marrow blast count at day 28 as the single most important

prognostic factor in childhood acute lymphoblastic leukemia. *Haematol Blood Transfus* 1992; **34**: 233–7.

52. Smith M, Arthur D, Camitta B *et al.* Uniform approach to risk classification and treatment assignment for children with acute lymphoblastic leukemia. *J Clin Oncol* 1996; **14**: 18–24.

53. Mastrangelo R, Poplack DG, Bleyer WA *et al.* Report and recommendations of the Rome Workshop Concerning Poor-Prognosis Acute Lymphoblastic Leukemia in Children: biologic bases for staging, stratification, and treatment. *Med Pediatr Oncol* 1986; **14**: 191–4.

54. Reaman GH, Steinherz PG, Gaynon PS *et al.* Improved survival of infants less than 1 year of age with acute lymphoblastic leukemia treated with intensive multiagent chemotherapy. *Cancer Treat Rep* 1987; **71**: 1033–8.

55. Ludwig W, Bartram CR, Harbott J *et al.* Phenotypic and genotypic heterogeneity in infant acute leukemia. *Leukemia* 1989; **3**: 431–9.

56. Pui C-H, Frankel LS, Carroll AJ *et al.* Clinical characteristics and treatment outcome of childhood acute lymphoblastic leukemia with the t(4;11)(q21;23): a collaborative study of 40 cases. *Blood* 1991; **77**: 440–7.

57. Pui CH, Kane JR, Crist WM. Biology and treatment of infant leukemias. *Leukemia* 1995; **9**: 762–9.

58. Reaman GH, Sposto R, Sensel MG *et al.* Treatment outcome and prognostic factors for infants with acute lymphoblastic leukemia treated on two consecutive trials of the Children's Cancer Group. *J Clin Oncol* 1999; **17**(2): 445–55.

59. Silverman LB, McLean TW, Gelber RD *et al.* Intensified therapy for infants with acute lymphoblastic leukemia: results from the Dana-Farber Cancer Institute Consortium. *Cancer* 1997; **80**: 2285–95.

60. Borkhardt A, Wuchter C, Viehmann S *et al.* Infant acute lymphoblastic leukemia – combined cytogenetic, immunophenotypical and molecular analysis of 77 cases. *Leukemia* 2002; **16**: 1685–90.

♦61. Biondi A, Cimino G, Pieters R, Pui CH. Biological and therapeutic aspects of infant leukemia. *Blood* 2000; **96**(1): 24–33.

62. Pieters R, den Boer ML, Durian M *et al.* Relation between age, immunophenotype and in vitro drug resistance in 395 children with acute lymphoblastic leukemia – implications for treatment of infants. *Leukemia* 1998; **12**(9): 1344–8.

63. Dördelmann M, Reiter A, Borkhardt A *et al.* Prednisone response is the strongest predictor of treatment outcome in infant acute lymphoblastic leukemia. *Blood* 1999; **94**(4): 1209–17.

64. Styczynski J, Pieters R, Huismans DR *et al.* In vitro drug resistance profiles of adult versus childhood acute lymphoblastic leukaemia. *Br J Haematol* 2000; **110**: 813–18.

65. Maung ZT, Reid MM, Matheson E *et al.* Corticosteroid resistance is increased in lymphoblasts from adults compared with children: preliminary results of in vitro drug sensitivity study in adults with acute lymphoblastic leukaemia. *Br J Haematol* 1995; **91**: 93–100.

66. Mattano LA, Sather HN, Trigg ME, Nachman JB. Osteonecrosis as a complication of treating acute lymphoblastic leukemia in children: a report from the Children's Cancer Group. *J Clin Oncol* 2000; **18**(18): 3262–72.

67. Pullen J, Shuster JJ, Link M *et al.* Significance of commonly used prognostic factors differs for children with T cell acute lymphocytic leukemia (ALL), as compared to those with B-precursor ALL. A Pediatric Oncology Group (POG) study. *Leukemia* 1999; **13**(11): 1696–707.

68. Pui CH, Gaynon PS, Boyett JM *et al.* Outcome of treatment in childhood acute lymphoblastic leukaemia with rearrangements of the 11q23 chromosomal region. *Lancet* 2002; **359**(9321): 1909–15.

69. Heerema NA, Sather HN, Sensel MG *et al.* Frequency and clinical significance of cytogenetic abnormalities in pediatric T-lineage acute lymphoblastic leukemia: a report from the Children's Cancer Group. *J Clin Oncol* 1998; **16**(4): 1270–8.

70. Steinherz PG, Gaynon PS, Breneman JC *et al.* Treatment of patients with acute lymphoblastic leukemia with bulky extramedullary disease and T-cell phenotype or other poor prognostic features: randomized controlled trial from the Children's Cancer Group. *Cancer* 1998; **82**(3): 600–12.

71. Evans WE, Pui CH, Relling MV. Defining the optimal dosage of methotrexate for childhood acute lymphoblastic leukemia. New insights from the lab and clinic. *Adv Exp Med Biol* 1999; **457**(23): 537–41.

72. Whitehead VM, Vuchich MJ, Cooley L *et al.* Translocations involving chromosome 12p11-13, methotrexate metabolism, and outcome in childhood B-progenitor cell acute lymphoblastic leukemia: a Pediatric Oncology Group study. *Clin Cancer Res* 1998; **4**: 183–8.

73. Heerema NA, Sather HN, Sensel MG *et al.* Prognostic impact of trisomies of chromosomes 10, 17, and 5 among children with acute lymphoblastic leukemia and high hyperdiploidy (>50 chromosomes). *J Clin Oncol* 2000; **18**(9): 1876–87.

74. Harris MB, Shuster JJ, Carroll A *et al.* Trisomy of leukemic cell chromosomes 4 and 10 identifies children with B-progenitor cell acute lymphoblastic leukemia with a very low risk of treatment failure: a pediatric oncology group study. *Blood* 1992; **79**: 3316–24.

75. Kaspers GJ, Smets LA, Pieters R *et al.* Favorable prognosis of hyperdiploid common acute lymphoblastic leukemia may be explained by sensitivity to antimetabolites and other drugs: results of an in vitro study. *Blood* 1995; **85**(3): 751–6.

76. Romana SP, Poirel H, Leconiat M *et al.* High frequency of t(12;21) in childhood B-lineage acute lymphoblastic leukemia. *Blood* 1995; **86**(11): 4263–9.

77. Borkhardt A, Cazzaniga G, Viehmann S *et al.* Incidence and clinical relevance of TEL/AML1 fusion genes in children with acute lymphoblastic leukemia enrolled in the German and Italian multicenter therapy trials. *Blood* 1997; **90**(2): 571–7.

78. Kaspers GJ, Veerman AJ, Pieters R *et al.* In vitro cellular drug resistance and prognosis in newly diagnosed childhood acute lymphoblastic leukemia. *Blood* 1997; **90**: 2723–9.

79. Ramakers-van Woerden NL, Pieters R, Loonen AH *et al.* TEL/AML1 gene fusion is related to in vitro drug sensitivity for L- asparaginase in childhood acute lymphoblastic leukemia. *Blood* 2000; **96**: 1094–9.

80. Schrappe M, Arico M, Harbott J *et al.* Ph+ childhood acute lymphoblastic leukemia: good initial steroid response allows early prediction of a favorable treatment outcome. *Blood* 1998; **92**(8): 2730–41.

81. Arico M, Valsecchi MG, Camitta B *et al.* Outcome of treatment in children with Philadelphia chromosome-positive acute lymphoblastic leukemia. *N Engl J Med* 2000; **342**(14): 998–1006.

82. Armstrong SA, Staunton JE, Silverman LB *et al.* MLL translocations specify a distinct gene expression profile that distinguishes a unique leukemia. *Nat Genet* 2002; **30**: 41–7.

83. Yeoh EJ, Ross ME, Shurtleff SA *et al.* Classification, subtype discovery, and prediction of outcome in pediatric acute lymphoblastic leukemia by gene expression profiling. *Cancer Cell* 2002; **1**: 133–43.

84. Schrappe M, Reiter A, Zimmermann M *et al.* Long-term results of four consecutive trials in childhood ALL performed by the ALL-BFM study group from 1981 to 1995. *Leukemia* 2000; **14**(12): 2205–22.

85. Thyss A, Suciu S, Bertrand Y *et al.* Systemic effect of intra-thecal methotrexate during the initial phase of treatment of childhood acute lymphoblastic leukemia. The European Organization for Research and Treatment of Cancer Children's Leukemia Cooperative Group. *J Clin Oncol* 1997; **15**: 1824–30.

86. Lauten M, Stanulla M, Zimmermann M *et al.* Clinical outcome of patients with childhood acute lymphoblastic leukaemia and an initial leukaemic blood blast count of less than 1000 per microliter. *Klin Padiatr* 2001; **213**: 169–74.

87. Hansen-Hagge TE, Yokota S, Bartram CR. Detection of minimal residual disease in acute lymphoblastic leukemia by in vitro amplification of rearranged T-cell receptor d chain sequences. *Blood* 1989; **74**(5): 1762–7.

88. Yokota S, Hansen-Hagge TE, Ludwig W-D *et al.* Use of polymerase chain reactions to monitor minimal residual disease in acute lymphoblastic leukemia patients. *Blood* 1991; **77**: 331–9.

89. Campana D, Coustan-Smith E, Janossy G. The immunologic detection of residual disease in acute leukemia. *Blood* 1990; **76**: 163–71.

90. van Dongen JJM, Seriu T, Panzer-Grumayer ER *et al.* Prognostic value of minimal residual disease in childhood acute lymphoblastic leukemia: a prospective study of the International BFM Study Group. *Lancet* 1998; **352**: 1731–8.

91. Panzer-Grumayer ER, Schneider M, Panzer S *et al.* Rapid molecular response during early induction chemotherapy predicts a good outcome in childhood acute lymphoblastic leukemia. *Blood* 2000; **95**(3): 790–4.

92. Cave H, van der Werff ten Bosch J, Suciu S *et al.* Clinical significance of minimal residual disease in childhood acute lymphoblastic leukemia. European Organization for Research and Treatment of Cancer–Childhood Leukemia Cooperative Group [see comments]. *N Engl J Med* 1998; **339**(9): 591–8.

93. Coustan-Smith E, Behm FG, Sanchez J *et al.* Immunological detection of minimal residual disease in children with acute lymphoblastic leukaemia. *Lancet* 1998; **351**: 550–4.

94. Neale GA, Coustan-Smith E, Pan Q *et al.* Tandem application of flow cytometry and polymerase chain reaction for comprehensive detection of minimal residual disease in childhood acute lymphoblastic leukemia. *Leukemia* 1999; **13**(8): 1221–6.

95. Dworzak MN, Froschl G, Printz D *et al.* Prognostic significance and modalities of flow cytometric minimal residual disease detection in childhood acute lymphoblastic leukemia. *Blood* 2002; **99**(6): 1952–8.

96. Pui CH, Campana D. New definition of remission in childhood acute lymphoblastic leukemia. *Leukemia* 2000; **14**(5): 783–5.

97. Willemse MJ, Seriu T, Hettinger K *et al.* Detection of minimal residual disease identifies differences in treatment response between T-ALL and precursor B-ALL. *Blood* 2002; **99**(12): 4386–93.

98. zur Stadt U, Harms DO, Schluter S *et al.* MRD at the end of induction therapy in childhood acute lymphoblastic leukemia: outcome prediction strongly depends on the therapeutic regimen. *Leukemia* 2001; **15**(2): 283–5.

99. Schrappe M, Camitta B, Pui CH *et al.* Long-term results of large prospective trials in childhood acute lymphoblastic leukemia. *Leukemia* 2000; **14**(12): 2193–4.

100. Riehm H, Gadner H, Henze G *et al.* Acute lymphoblastic leukemia: treatment results in three BFM Studies (1970–1981). In: Murphy SB, Gilbert JR, eds. *Leukemia Research: Advances in Cell Biology and Treatment.* Amsterdam: Elsevier Science Publishing, 1983; 251–63.

101. Tubergen DG, Gilchrist GS, O'Brien RT *et al.* Improved outcome with delayed intensification for children with acute lymphoblastic leukemia and intermediate presenting features: a Children's Cancer Group phase III trial. *J Clin Oncol* 1993; **11**: 527–37.

102. Veerman AJ, Hahlen K, Kamps WA *et al.* High cure rate with a moderately intensive treatment regimen in non-high-risk childhood acute lymphoblastic leukemia. Results of protocol ALL VI from the Dutch Childhood Leukemia Study Group. *J Clin Oncol* 1996; **14**(3): 911–18.

103. zur Stadt U, Harms DO, Schluter S *et al.* [Minimal residual disease analysis in acute lymphoblastic leukemia of childhood within the framework of COALL Study: results of an induction therapy without asparaginase]. *Klin Padiatr* 2000; **212**(4): 169–73.

104. Niemeyer CM, Gelber RD, Tarbell NJ *et al.* Low-dose versus high-dose methotrexate during remission induction in childhood acute lymphoblastic leukemia (Protocol 81-01 update). *Blood* 1991; **78**: 2514–19.

105. Gaynon PS, Lustig RH. The use of glucocorticoids in acute lymphoblastic leukemia of childhood. Molecular, cellular, and clinical considerations [Review]. *J Ped Hemat Oncol* 1995; **17**(1): 1–12.

106. Kaspers GJ, Veerman AJ, Popp-Snijders C *et al.* Comparison of the antileukemic activity in vitro of dexamethasone and prednisolone in childhood acute lymphoblastic leukemia. *Med Pediatr Oncol* 1996; **27**(2): 114–21.

107. Hurwitz CA, Silverman LB, Schorin MA *et al.* Substituting dexamethasone for prednisone complicates remission induction in children with acute lymphoblastic leukemia. *Cancer* 2000; **88**(8): 1964–9.

108. Schwartz CL, Thompson EB, Gelber RD *et al.* Improved response with higher corticosteroid dose in children with acute lymphoblastic leukemia. *J Clin Oncol* 2001; **19**: 1040–6.

109. Bostrom BC, Sensel MR, Sather HN *et al.* Dexamethasone versus prednisone and daily oral versus weekly intravenous mercaptopurine for patients with standard-risk acute lymphoblastic leukemia: a report from the Children's Cancer Group. *Blood* 2003; **101**: 3809–17.

110. Milano G, Thyss A, Debeauvais FS *et al.* CSF drug levels for children with acute lymphoblastic leukemia treated by $5\,g/m^2$ methotrexate. *Eur J Cancer* 1990; **26**(4): 492–5.

111. Schrappe M, Reiter A, Riehm H. Prophylaxis and treatment of meningeosis in childhood acute lymphoblastic leukemia. *J Neurooncol* 1998; **38**: 159–65.

112. Jones B, Freeman AI, Shuster JJ et al. Lower incidence of meningeal leukemia when prednisone is replaced by dexamethasone in the treatment of acute lymphocytic leukemia. *Med Pediatr Oncol* 1991; **19**(4): 269–75.

113. Tubergen DG, Gilchrist GS, O'Brien RT et al. Prevention of CNS disease in intermediate-risk acute lymphoblastic leukemia: comparison of cranial radiation and intrathecal methotrexate and the importance of systemic therapy: a Children's Cancer Group report. *J Clin Oncol* 1993; **11**: 520–6.

114. Pullen J, Boyett J, Shuster J et al. Extended triple intrathecal chemotherapy trial for prevention of CNS relapse in good-risk and poor-risk patients with B-progenitor acute lymphoblastic leukemia: a Pediatric Oncology Group study. *J Clin Oncol* 1993; **11**: 839–49.

115. Schrappe M, Beck J, Brandeis WE et al. Die Behandlung der akuten lymphoblastischen Leukämie im Kindes- und Jugendalter: Ergebnisse der multizentrischen Therapiestudie ALL-BFM 81. *Klin Pädiatr* 1987; **199**: 133–50.

116. Riehm H, Gadner H, Henze G et al. Results and significance of six randomized trials in four consecutive ALL-BFM trials. *Haematol Blood Transfus* 1990; **33**: 439–50.

117. Buhrer C, Henze G, Hofmann J et al. Central nervous system relapse prevention in 1165 standard-risk children with acute lymphoblastic leukemia in five BFM trials. *Hamatol Bluttransfus* 1990; **33**: 500–3.

118. Schrappe M, Reiter A, Henze G et al. Prevention of CNS recurrence in childhood ALL: Results with reduced radiotherapy combined with CNS-directed chemotherapy in four consecutive ALL-BFM trials. *Klin Pädiatr* 1998; **210**: 192–9.

119. Doerdelmann M, Reiter A, Zimmermann M et al. Intermediate dose methotrexate is as effective as high dose methotrexate in preventing isolated testicular relapse in childhood ALL. *J Pediatr Hematol Oncol* 1998; **20**(5): 444–50.

120. Freeman AI, Boyett JM, Glicksman AS et al. Intermediate-dose methotrexate versus cranial irradiation in childhood acute lymphoblastic leukemia: a ten-year follow-up. *Med Pediatr Oncol* 1997; **28**(2): 98–107.

121. Laver JH, Barredo JC, Amylon M et al. Effects of cranial radiation in children with high risk T cell acute lymphoblastic leukemia: a Pediatric Oncology Group report. *Leukemia* 2000; **14**(3): 369–73.

122. Conter V, Schrappe M, Arico M et al. Role of cranial radiotherapy for childhood T-cell acute lymphoblastic leukemia with high WBC count and good response to prednisone. *J Clin Oncol* 1997; **15**(8): 2786–91.

123. Nachman J, Sather HN, Cherlow JM et al. Response of children with high-risk acute lymphoblastic leukaemia treated with and without cranial irradiation: a report from the Children's Cancer Group. *J Clin Oncol* 1998; **16**(3): 920–30.

124. Langer T, Martus P, Ottensmeier H et al. CNS late-effects after ALL therapy in childhood. Part III: neuropsychological performance in long-term survivors of childhood ALL: impairments of concentration, attention, and memory. *Med Pediatr Oncol* 2002; **38**: 320–8.

125. Löning L, Kaatsch P, Riehm H, Schrappe M. Secondary neoplasms subsequent to acute lymphoblastic leukemia in childhood – experience of the BFM study group. *Blood* 1998; **92**(Suppl.1): 679a.

126. Relling MV, Rubnitz JE, Rivera GK et al. High incidence of secondary brain tumours after radiotherapy and antimetabolites. *Lancet* 1999; **354**(9172): 34–9.

127. Walter AW, Hancock ML, Pui CH et al. Secondary brain tumors in children treated for acute lymphoblastic leukemia at St Jude Children's Research Hospital. *J Clin Oncol* 1998; **16**(12): 3761–7.

128. Ochs J, Mulhern R, Fairclough D et al. Comparison of neuropsychologic functioning and clinical indicators of neurotoxicity in long-term survivors of childhood leukemia given cranial radiation or parenteral methotrexate: a prospective study. *J Clin Oncol* 1991; **9**: 145–51.

129. Butler RW, Hill JM, Steinherz PG et al. Neuropsychological effects of cranial irradiation, intrathecal methotrexate, and systemic methotrexate in childhood cancer. *J Clin Oncol* 1994; **12**: 2621–9.

130. Nachman JB, Sather HN, Sensel MG et al. Augmented post-induction therapy for children with high-risk acute lymphoblastic leukemia and a slow response to initial therapy. *N Engl J Med* 1998; **338**(23): 1663–71.

131. Arico M, Valsecchi MG, Conter V et al. Improved outcome in high-risk childhood acute lymphoblastic leukemia defined by prednisone-poor response treated with double Berlin-Frankfurt-Munster protocol II. *Blood* 2002; **100**(2): 420–6.

132. Chessels JM. Maintenance treatment and care in lymphoblastic leukaemia. *Arch Dis Child* 1995; **73**: 368–78.

133. Group CAC. Duration and intensity of maintenance chemotherapy in acute lymphoblastic leukaemia: overview of 42 trials involving 12 000 randomised children. Childhood ALL Collaborative Group. *Lancet* 1996; **347**: 1783–8.

134. Toyoda Y, Manabe A, Tsuchida M et al. Six months of maintenance chemotherapy after intensified treatment for acute lymphoblastic leukemia of childhood. *J Clin Oncol* 2000; **18**(7): 1508–16.

135. Chao N, Forman SJ. Allogeneic bone marrow transplantation for acute lymphoblastic leukemia. In: Forman SJ, Blume KG, Thomas ED, eds. *Bone Marrow Transplantation*. Cambridge, MA: Blackwell Scientific Publications, 1994; 618–28.

136. Barrett AJ, Horowitz MM, Pollock BH et al. Bone marrow transplants from HLA-identical siblings as compared with chemotherapy for children with acute lymphoblastic leukemia in a second remission. *N Engl J Med* 1994; **331**: 1253–8.

137. Chessells JM, Bailey C, Wheeler K, Richards SM. Bone marrow transplantation for high-risk childhood lymphoblastic leukaemia in first remission: experience in MRC UKALL X. *Lancet* 1992; **340**: 565–8.

138. Locatelli F, Zecca M, Rondelli R et al. Graft versus host disease prophylaxis with low-dose cyclosporine-A reduces the risk of relapse in children with acute leukemia given HLA-identical sibling bone marrow transplantation: results of a randomized trial. *Blood* 2000; **95**(5): 1572–9.

139. Woolfrey AE, Anasetti C, Storer B et al. Factors associated with outcome after unrelated marrow transplantation for treatment of acute lymphoblastic leukemia in children. *Blood* 2002; **99**(6): 2002–8.

140. Moussalem M, Esperou Bourdeau H, Devergie A et al. Allogeneic bone marrow transplantation for childhood acute lymphoblastic leukemia in second remission: factors predictive of survival, relapse and graft-versus-host disease. Bone Marrow Transplant 1995; 15: 943–7.

141. Oakhill A, Pamphilon DH, Potter MN et al. Unrelated donor bone marrow transplantation for children with relapsed acute lymphoblastic leukaemia in second complete remission. Br J Haematol 1996; 94: 574–8.

142. Passweg JR, Tiberghien P, Cahn JY et al. Graft-versus-leukemia effects in T lineage and B lineage acute lymphoblastic leukemia. Bone Marrow Transplant 1998; 21: 153–8.

143. Saarinen UM, Mellander L, Nysom K et al. Allogeneic bone marrow transplantation in first remission for children with very high-risk acute lymphoblastic leukemia: a retrospective case-control study in the Nordic countries. Nordic Society for Pediatric Hematology and Oncology (NOPHO). Bone Marrow Transplant 1996; 17: 357–63.

144. Uderzo C, Valsecchi MG, Bacigalupo A et al. Treatment of childhood acute lymphoblastic leukemia in second remission with allogeneic bone marrow transplantation and chemotherapy: ten-year experience of the Italian Bone Marrow Transplantation Group and the Italian Pediatric Hematology Oncology Association. J Clin Oncol 1995; 13(2): 352–8.

145. Neglia JP, Meadows AT, Robison LL et al. Second neoplasms after acute lymphoblastic leukemia in childhood. N Engl J Med 1991; 325: 1330–6.

146. Winick NJ, McKenna RW, Shuster JJ et al. Secondary acute myeloid leukemia in children with acute lymphoblastic leukemia treated with etoposide. J Clin Oncol 1993; 11: 209–17.

147. Lipshultz SE, Lipsitz SR, Mone SM et al. Female sex and drug dose as risk factors for late cardiotoxic effects of doxorubicin therapy for childhood cancer. N Engl J Med 1995; 332(26): 1738–43.

148. Pieters R, van Brenk AI, Veerman AJ et al. Bone marrow magnetic resonance studies in childhood leukemia. Evaluation of osteonecrosis. Cancer 1987; 60(12): 2994–3000.

149. Ribeiro RC, Fletcher BD, Kennedy W et al. Magnetic resonance imaging detection of avascular necrosis of the bone in children receiving intensive prednisone therapy for acute lymphoblastic leukemia or non-Hodgkin lymphoma. Leukemia 2001; 15: 891–7.

150. Löning L, Zimmermann M, Reiter A et al. Secondary neoplasms subsequent to Berlin-Frankfurt-Münster therapy of childhood acute lymphoblastic leukemia: significantly lower risk without cranial radiotherapy. Blood 2000; 95(9): 2770–5.

151. Pui CH, Behm FG, Raimondi SC et al. Secondary acute myeloid leukemia in children treated for acute lymphoid leukemia. N Engl J Med 1989; 321: 136–42.

152. Pui C-H, Ribeiro R, Hancock ML et al. Acute myeloid leukemia in children treated with epipodophyllotoxins for acute lymphoblastic leukemia. N Engl J Med 1991; 325: 1682–7.

153. Stanulla M, Loning L, Welte K, Schrappe M. Secondary brain tumours in children with ALL. Lancet 1999; 354: 1126–7.

154. Lipshultz SE, Giantris AL, Lipsitz SR et al. Doxorubicin administration by continuous infusion is not cardioprotective: the Dana-Farber 91–01 Acute Lymphoblastic Leukemia protocol. J Clin Oncol 2002; 20: 1677–82.

155. Rammeloo LA, Postma A, Sobotka-Plojhar MA et al. Low-dose daunorubicin in induction treatment of childhood acute lymphoblastic leukemia: no long-term cardiac damage in a randomized study of the Dutch Childhood Leukemia Study Group. Med Pediatr Oncol 2000; 35: 13–19.

156. Nysom K, Holm K, Lipsitz SR et al. Relationship between cumulative anthracycline dose and late cardiotoxicity in childhood acute lymphoblastic leukemia. J Clin Oncol 1998; 16: 545–50.

157. Sorensen K, Levitt G, Bull C et al. Anthracycline dose in childhood acute lymphoblastic leukemia: issues of early survival versus late cardiotoxicity. J Clin Oncol 1997; 15(1): 61–8.

158. Chan-Lam D, Prentice AG, Copplestone JA et al. Avascular necrosis of bone following intensified steroid therapy for acute lymphoblastic leukaemia and high-grade malignant lymphoma. Br J Haematol 1994; 86(1): 227–30.

159. Precourt S, Robaey P, Lamothe I et al. Verbal cognitive functioning and learning in girls treated for acute lymphoblastic leukemia by chemotherapy with or without cranial irradiation. Dev Neuropsychol 2002; 21(2): 173–95.

160. Hill JM, Kornblith AB, Jones D et al. A comparative study of the long term psychosocial functioning of childhood acute lymphoblastic leukemia survivors treated by intrathecal methotrexate with or without cranial radiation. Cancer 1998; 82: 208–18.

161. Hertzberg H, Huk WJ, Ueberall MA et al. CNS late effects after ALL therapy in childhood. Part I: Neuroradiological findings in long-term survivors of childhood ALL – an evaluation of the interferences between morphology and neuropsychological performance. Med Pediatr Oncol 1997; 28: 387–400.

162. MacLean WEJ, Noll RB, Stehbens JA et al. Neuropsychological effects of cranial irradiation in young children with acute lymphoblastic leukemia 9 months after diagnosis. The Children's Cancer Group. Arch Neurol 1995; 52: 156–60.

163. Jankovic M, Brouwers P, Valsecchi MG et al. Association of 1800 cGy cranial irradiation with intellectual function in children with acute lymphoblastic leukaemia. ISPACC. International Study Group on Psychosocial Aspects of Childhood Cancer. Lancet 1994; 344: 224–7.

164. Waber DP, Carpentieri SC, Klar N et al. Cognitive sequelae in children treated for acute lymphoblastic leukemia with dexamethasone or prednisone. J Pediatr Hematol Oncol 2000; 22(3): 206–13.

165. Shpilberg O, Dorman JS, Shahar A, Kuller LH. Molecular epidemiology of hematological neoplasms – present status and future directions. Leuk Res 1997; 21: 265–84.

♦166. Roses AD. Pharmacogenetics and the practice of medicine. Nature 2000; 405: 857–65.

♦167. Evans WE, Relling MV. Pharmacogenomics: translating functional genomics into rational therapeutics. Science 1999; 286(5439): 487–91.

168. McLeod HL, Krynetski EY, Relling MV, Evans WE. Genetic polymorphism of thiopurine methyltransferase and its clinical relevance for childhood acute lymphoblastic leukemia. Leukemia 2000; 14(4): 567–72.

169. Yates CR, Krynetski EY, Loennechen T et al. Molecular diagnosis of thiopurine S-methyltransferase deficiency: genetic basis for azathioprine and mercaptopurine intolerance [see comments]. Ann Intern Med 1997; **126**: 608–14.

170. Otterness D, Szumlanski C, Lennard L et al. Human thiopurine methyltransferase pharmacogenetics: gene sequence polymorphisms. Clin Pharmacol Ther 1997; **62**: 60–73.

171. Lennard L, Lilleyman JS, Van Loon J, Weinshilboum RM. Genetic variation in response to 6-mercaptopurine for childhood acute lymphoblastic leukaemia. Lancet 1990; **336**: 225–9.

172. Relling MV, Hancock ML, Rivera GK et al. Mercaptopurine therapy intolerance and heterozygosity at the thiopurine S-methyltransferase gene locus [see comments]. J Natl Cancer Inst 1999; **91**(23): 2001–8.

173. Bo J, Schroder H, Kristinsson J et al. Possible carcinogenic effect of 6-mercaptopurine on bone marrow stem cells: relation to thiopurine metabolism. Cancer 1999; **86**: 1080–6.

174. Relling MV, Hancock ML, Boyett JM et al. Prognostic importance of 6-mercaptopurine dose intensity in acute lymphoblastic leukemia. Blood 1999; **93**(9): 2817–23.

175. McLeod HL, Coulthard S, Thomas AE et al. Analysis of thiopurine methyltransferase variant alleles in childhood acute lymphoblastic leukaemia. Br J Haematol 1999; **105**: 696–700.

176. Ketterer B. Protective role of glutathione and glutathione transferases in mutagenesis and carcinogenesis. Mutat Res 1988; **202**: 343–61.

177. Stanulla M, Schrappe M, Brechlin AM et al. Polymorphisms within glutathione S-transferase genes (GSTM1, GSTT1, GSTP1) and risk of relapse in childhood B-cell precursor acute lymphoblastic leukemia: a case-control study. Blood 2000; **95**(4): 1222–8.

178. Anderer G, Schrappe M, Mueller-Brechlin A et al. Polymorphisms within glutathione S-transferase genes and initial response to glucocorticoids in childhood acute lymphoblastic leukaemia. Pharmacogenetics 2000; **10**: 715–26.

179. Chen CL, Liu Q, Pui CH et al. Higher frequency of glutathione S-transferase deletions in black children with acute lymphoblastic leukemia. Blood 1997; **89**(5): 1701–7.

180. Krajinovic M, Labuda D, Richer C et al. Susceptibility to childhood acute lymphoblastic leukemia: influence of CYP1A1, CYP2D6, GSTM1, and GSTT1 genetic polymorphisms. Blood 1999; **93**: 1496–501.

181. Golub TR, Slonim DK, Tamayo P et al. Molecular classification of cancer: class discovery and class prediction by gene expression monitoring. Science 1999; **286**: 531–7.

182. Ferrando AA, Neuberg DS, Staunton J et al. Gene expression signatures define novel oncogenic pathways in T cell acute lymphoblastic leukemia. Cancer Cell 2002; **1**: 75–87.

183. Pui CH, Boyett JM, Relling MV et al. Sex differences in prognosis for children with acute lymphoblastic leukemia. J Clin Oncol 1999; **17**: 818–24.

184. Uckun FM, Sensel MG, Sun L et al. Biology and treatment of childhood T-lineage acute lymphoblastic leukemia. Blood 1998; **91**(3): 735–46.

185. Pui CH, Rivera GK, Hancock ML et al. Clinical significance of CD10 expression in childhood acute lymphoblastic leukemia. Leukemia 1993; **7**: 35–40.

186. Ludwig W-D, Harbott J, Bartram CR et al. Incidence and prognostic significance of immunophenotypic subgroups in childhood acute lymphoblastic leukemia: Experience of the BFM study 86. Recent Results Cancer Res 1993; **131**: 269–82.

187. Pinkel D, Woo S. Prevention and treatment of meningeal leukemia in children. Blood 1994; **84**: 355–66.

188. Trueworthy R, Shuster J, Look T et al. Ploidy of lymphoblasts is the strongest predictor of treatment outcome in B-progenitor cell acute lymphoblastic leukemia of childhood: a Pediatric Oncology Group study. J Clin Oncol 1992; **10**: 606–13.

189. Heerema NA, Nachman JB, Sather HN et al. Hypodiploidy with less than 45 chromosomes confers adverse risk in childhood acute lymphoblastic leukemia: a report from the children's cancer group. Blood 1999; **94**(12): 4036–45.

190. Pui CH, Williams DL, Raimondi SC et al. Hypodiploidy is associated with a poor prognosis in childhood acute lymphoblastic leukemia. Blood 1987; **70**: 247–53.

191. Trka J, Zuna J, Hrusak O et al. Impact of TEL/AML1-positive patients on age distribution of childhood acute lymphoblastic leukemia in Czech Republic. Leukemia 1998; **12**: 996–1007.

192. Loh ML, Silverman LB, Young ML et al. Incidence of TEL/AML1 fusion in children with relapsed acute lymphoblastic leukemia. Blood 1998; **92**(12): 4792–7.

193. Fletcher JA, Lynch EA, Kimball VM et al. Translocation (9;22) is associated with extremely poor prognosis in intensively treated children with acute lymphoblastic leukemia. Blood 1991; **77**(3): 435–9.

194. Behm FG, Raimondi SC, Frestedt JL et al. Rearrangement of the MLL gene confers a poor prognosis in childhood acute lymphoblastic leukemia, regardless of presenting age. Blood 1996; **87**(7): 2870–7.

195. Rubnitz JE, Link MP, Shuster JJ et al. Frequency and prognostic significance of HRX rearrangements in infant acute lymphoblastic leukemia: a Pediatric Oncology Group study. Blood 1994; **84**: 570–3.

13

Non-Hodgkin's lymphoma

CATHERINE PATTE

INTRODUCTION

Lymphomas are malignant proliferations of lymphoid cells at various stages of differentiation and activation. They occur at all ages, but some categories occur more frequently in certain age groups. In children, only a few subtypes of non-Hodgkin's lymphoma (NHL) are seen, predominantly lymphoblastic and Burkitt lymphoma. Clinical presentation is predominantly characterized by the presence of extranodal disease with very rapid growth and dissemination that is not contiguous, and in particular involves the bone marrow and central nervous system (CNS).

Recent biological studies have contributed greatly to a better classification of NHL. The prognosis for a child with widespread disease has also changed in the last 20 years as a result of better understanding of the pathological process and better use of intensive chemotherapeutic regimens.[1,2]

EPIDEMIOLOGY

Non-Hodgkin's lymphoma has a peak incidence between 7 and 10 years of age, and is uncommon before 2 years of age. A male predominance is evident, with a male:female ratio of between 2.5:1 and 3:1. An annual incidence of approximately seven cases per million children makes it the third most common childhood malignancy.

A few familial cases have been described. Certain individuals with an increased risk of developing NHL have also been identified. These include heritable conditions associated with immunodeficiency, such as ataxia telangiectasia, Wiskott–Aldrich syndrome and conditions where immunodeficiency has been acquired, such as post-organ transplantation or acquired immuno-deficiency syndrome (AIDS). Purtilo et al.[3] also described an X-linked syndrome characterized by a particular sensitivity to Epstein–Barr virus (EBV) and the occurrence of malignant lymphomas, especially of the Burkitt type, and fatal infectious mononucleosis. Specific geographical areas are also recognized for particular types of lymphoma, e.g. 'endemic' (African) Burkitt lymphoma.

The aetiology has been particularly linked with EBV, after it was noted that EBV particles were present in the nucleus of malignant cells in endemic Burkitt lymphoma. Human T-cell leukaemia/lymphoma virus (HTLV-1) is also thought to play a role in the genesis of adult T-cell malignancy in Japan. Although these viruses are known to have transforming and immortalizing properties on B and T cells *in vitro*, and are inferred as having a role in the oncogenic process, other events are also needed to establish a malignant state. Furthermore, primary evidence of viral participation in oncogenesis is rare, EBV being found in only 20 per cent of cases of non-endemic Burkitt lymphoma, and to date no viral particles have been found in childhood T-cell lymphoma.

BIOLOGY

Histology

The classification of NHL has changed many times over the years and became clearer with the understanding of the differentiation pathways of the normal lymphocytes and with the explosion of new diagnostic tools (immunophenotyping, cytogenetics, molecular biology and now gene sequencing). In many cases, these new tools 'confirmed' subtypes already recognized by pathologists, but they gave important information about the pathogenesis of lymphomas. For example, the clinical and histopathological particularities of the anaplastic large-cell lymphoma were recognized around 1975 but it was named 'malignant histiocytosis'. Later on, immunophenotypic characteristics [CD30+ (Ki1+), EMA+, T or 'null lineage'], cytogenetics [t(2;5)] and molecular biology (*NPM/ALK* fusion gene leading to a fusion protein) allowed the entity to be named more appropriately (anaplastic large-cell lymphoma) and to produce antibodies for the recognition of the fusion protein on paraffin sections (ALK antibody).

Similarly, Burkitt lymphoma was recognized early in the 1960s and its specific translocation described in the 1970s. But in one classification its name changed to 'small non-cleaved cell', and in another it was classified among the 'immature' 'lymphoblastic' lymphomas. Now it is clear that it is a 'mature' (peripheral) B-cell lymphoma originating from the germinal centre.

In the majority of cases, only four categories of lymphoma occur in children: Burkitt, lymphoblastic, large B-cell and anaplastic large-cell. Table 13.1 gives their characteristics. The indicated frequency is an average (that of western Europe) which depends on geography (Burkitt represents the majority of lymphomas in equatorial Africa and is less frequent in northern Europe and Japan) and age (frequency of large-cell lymphomas increases among adolescents).

DNA microarray technology allows the study of the expression of many genes at once. As for each new technique, we have to learn and determine its implication for diagnosis and prognosis and its further utility in clinical practice.

Cytogenetics and molecular biology

Cytogenetic and molecular biological studies have contributed to our knowledge of the fundamental processes in NHL, but have not yet contributed to therapy. In Burkitt lymphoma, tumour cells are characterized by a translocation involving the long arm of chromosome 8, region q23-q24, and the majority of cases exhibit a

Table 13.1 *Different types of lymphomas encountered in children and their biological features*

	Burkitt (50%)	Precursor T/B-lymphoblastic (30%)		Large B-cell (10%)	Anaplastic large-cell (10%)
Corresponding stage of development	Germinal centre	Immature		Germinal centre	Mature T-cell
Histology					
Cell size	Medium	Medium		Large	Voluminous
Cytoplasm	Narrow, basophilic, with vacuoles	Narrow, pale			Abundant and clear, erythrophagocytosis
Nucleus	Round	Convoluted +/−		Cleaved +/− vesicular	Irregular, clear
Nucleoli	Several nucleoli	Poorly discernible nucleoli		Distinct, often adherent to nucleus membrane	Voluminous
Chromatin	Coarse and irregular	Finely stippled			
FAB equivalent	L3	L1, L2			
Immunophenotyping	CD20+	TdT+		CD20+	CD30+
	CD79a+	B lineage	T lineage	CD79a+	EMA+
	S Ig+	CD19+	CD7+	S If +/−	ALK+
	Ki 67+, >95%	CD 79a+	CD2+	bcl 6 +/−	(T or 'null' markers)
		S Ig−	CD3c+	Ki 67, 60–90%	
		cμ −/+			
Cytogenetics	t(8;14)(q24;q32) or variant t(2;8) (p11;q24) t(8;22) (q24;q11)	No specific abnormalities		Occasional t(8;14) (q24;q32) der (3)(q27) (bcl 6)	t(2;5) (p23;q35) or variant
Result	Transcriptional deregulation of c-MYC			Transcriptional deregulation of bcl 6	NPM/ALK fusion protein ALK is a tyrosine kinase receptor ALK located on 2p23

translocation of t(8;14)(q24;q32). Variant translocations include t(2;8)(p12;q24) and t(8;22)(q24;q11). In the translocation t(8;14), the oncogene c-*myc* moves from its normal position on chromosome 8 and is rearranged with the gene for heavy-chain immunoglobulin. In the variant translocations, c-*myc* remains on chromosome 8, but the kappa and lambda immunoglobulin light-chain genes translocate from their normal positions on chromosomes 2 and 22, respectively, to a region distal to the c-*myc* oncogene. Transcriptional deregulation of the c-*myc* gene results, and this leads to elevated expression, something that is thought to play a crucial role in the genesis and/or maintenance of this malignancy.[4]

In T-cell tumours, chromosomal abnormalities are more heterogeneous. They can involve chromosome 14, at the locus of the gene for the alpha-chain of the T-cell receptor, or chromosome 7, at the locus of the gene for the beta chain of the T-cell receptor.

CLINICAL FEATURES

Abdomen

The abdomen is the most common primary site (30–45 per cent). Intussusception leading to the discovery of a small excisable abdominal tumour is a rare presentation; the more common clinical picture is that of a large and rapidly growing abdominal mass often associated with ascites. Ultrasound scanning objectively assesses the intraperitoneal mass and defines precisely any intra-abdominal spread. Laparotomy should be avoided, except in the event of an abdominal emergency, and the diagnosis should be made by cytological examination of ascites or percutaneous needle biopsy of the tumour. Surface markers invariably show B-cell phenotype, and histology shows Burkitt lymphoma in the majority of cases, others being large B-cell lymphoma.

Mediastinum

Mediastinal tumours (25–35 per cent) are, typically, T-cell lymphoblastic lymphomas, but in rare cases they can be large B-cell or Burkitt lymphomas. Mediastinal compression and/or cervical or axillary lymphadenopathy clarify the diagnosis. Chest X-ray shows a localized thymic mass often associated with pleural or pericardial effusions (Figures 13.1a and b). Patients are at particular risk of developing respiratory distress, worsened or provoked by general anaesthesia. Diagnosis should therefore be made using cytological examination of effusions or bone marrow smears. If a tumour biopsy is needed, then this should be done by percutaneous needle biopsy or mediastinoscopy.

Other sites

The third most common site is that of the head and neck, including Waldeyer's ring and the facial bones (10–20 per cent), followed by the superficial lymph nodes (5–10 per cent) (Figure 13.1c). The remaining 5–10 per cent includes tumours that arise from less common sites such as bone, skin, thyroid, orbit, eyelid, kidney and epidural space. Diagnosis is confirmed by tissue biopsy with immunophenotyping since no particular type of lymphoma is associated with these sites. Bone lymphoma can be localized, but it can also be generalized and is often associated with hypercalcaemia. Kidney lymphoma can be confused with nephroblastoma, but suspicion should be aroused where the tumour is bilateral, the infiltration multinodular or diffuse, or when renal failure is present. Subcutaneous lymphoma particularly occurs in young children aged under 2 years, and is of precursor B-cell phenotype.

Clinical particularities of anaplastic large-cell lymphomas

This disease has some characteristic clinical features, as follows:

- usually node involvement, which is often painful
- frequent skin involvement: inflammatory symptoms of the involved nodes, distant macular lesions, or generalized skin changes resembling ichthyosis
- frequency of systemic symptoms with widely fluctuating fever
- 'wax and wane' evolution in a few cases with previous episode(s) of spontaneous regression.

INITIAL WORK-UP AND STAGING

Once the diagnosis of NHL has been made, a speedy assessment of diagnosis, staging and general evaluation must be done in order that appropriate treatment can be commenced as soon as possible.

Diagnosis

A diagnosis can be obtained utilizing biopsy material including tumour-touch preparations, cytological examination of effusion fluids and bone marrow smears. Surgical procedures can be avoided in diffuse disease. Also recommended are immunological studies (preferentially obtained on suspended cells from fresh tumours or on frozen sections, but immunohistochemistry on paraffin sections is of value) and cytogenetic studies.

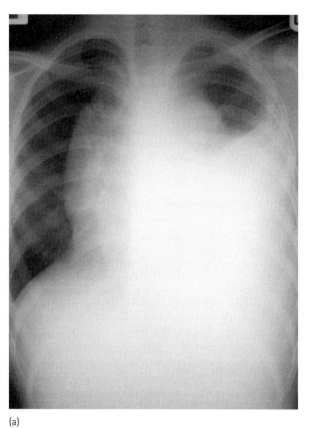

(a)

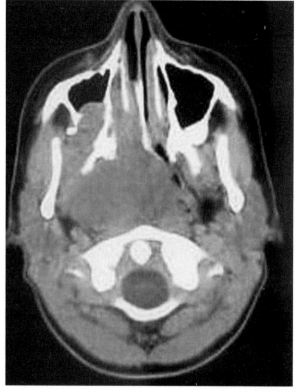

(c)

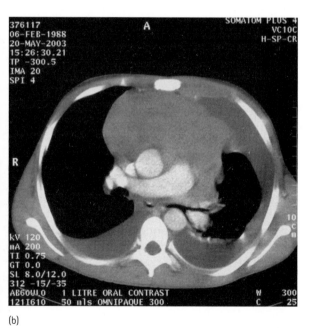

(b)

Figure 13.1 *(a) Chest X-ray in a child with precursor T-lymphoblastic lymphoma of mediastinum; (b) computed tomography (CT) scan in child with precursor T-lymphoblastic lymphoma of mediastinum; (c) CT scan in a child with peripheral B-cell lymphoma of nasopharynx.*

Staging

Due to the predominance of extranodal primaries and the unpredictable pattern of spread, the Ann Arbor classification is not adapted to childhood NHL. Several classifications have been proposed, but the system most commonly used is that of Murphy[5] (see Box 13.1).

Certain problems still remain with these systems: the size and number of tumours and the fact that the histopathological and immunohistological characteristics are not taken into account. Within the same stage, there may be a different prognosis depending on the localization or previous excision; in stage I, orbital or Waldeyer's ring tumours appear to have a worse prognosis than excised

Box 13.1 *St Jude's staging for childhood non-Hodgkin's lymphoma*

Stage I

A single tumour (extranodal) or single anatomical area (nodal) with the exclusion of the mediastinum or abdomen

Stage II

A single tumour (extranodal) with regional node involvement

Two or more nodal areas on the same side of the diaphragm

Two single (extranodal) tumours with or without regional node involvement on the same side of the diaphragm

A primary gastrointestinal tract tumour, usually in the ileocaecal area, with or without involvement of associated mesenteric nodes only, grossly completely resected

Stage III

Two single tumours (extranodal) on opposite sides of the diaphragm

Two or more nodal areas above and below the diaphragm

All the primary intrathoracic tumours (mediastinal, pleural, thymic)

All extensive primary intra-abdominal disease, unresectable

All paraspinal or epidural tumours, regardless of other tumour site(s)

Stage IV

Any of the above with initial CNS and/or bone marrow involvement

Box 13.2 *Initial work-up*

Mandatory

Physical examination
Chest and nasopharyngeal X-rays
Abdominal ultrasound
Bilateral bone marrow aspirations
CSF examination
Complete blood count
LDH, serum electrolytes, BUN, creatinine, uric acid levels

Optional, depending on clinical circumstances

Bone scan and skeletal survey
Local CT scan (head and neck tumours)
Magnetic resonance imaging (CNS disease)
Abdominal CT scan (stage I or abdominal stage II)
Thoracic CT scan
Bone marrow biopsy in large-cell NHL

BUN, blood urea nitrogen; LDH, lactate dehydrogenase.

General evaluation

Patients often have other problems, such as malnutrition, infection, post-surgical complications and respiratory and metabolic abnormalities; these may be life-threatening or compromise the onset of therapy. Hypercalcaemia, which is not always related to bone marrow involvement, requires treatment as a separate entity.

The tumour lysis syndrome may be present prior to treatment or may develop during treatment. Preventive measures must therefore always be instituted, i.e. hyperhydration and uricolytic drug. Classically allopurinol has been used in most countries, except in France and Italy, where urate oxidase (Uricozyme®) was available. Urate-oxidase transforms uric acid into allantoin, which is highly soluble in urine. It has been shown that urate oxidase is more efficient at promptly reducing serum uric acid level, to prevent uric acid nephropathy and to preserve renal function, allowing a better excretion of the other cell metabolites, such as potassium and phosphorus.[6] A recombinant urate oxidase is now available.[1,7,8] This has eliminated the need for alkalinization, but hydration and strict monitoring of patients during the lysis phase remain essential.

Potential factors causing renal failure must also be defined (uric acid nephropathy, tumour infiltration or urinary obstruction), in order that prompt and appropriate treatment can be started; this may include dialysis or transcutaneous pyelostomy. In order to minimize these complications, both the French and German protocols commence with low-dose therapy that produces a tumour regression. This is then followed a week later by a more intensive regimen.

local nodal disease. In stage II, abdominal tumours have a better prognosis than a large nasopharyngeal tumour invading the base of the skull.

The traditional boundary between leukaemia and lymphoma has been arbitrarily defined by more or less than 25 per cent blast cells in the bone marrow, but this does not correspond to either clinical or biological differences.

CNS involvement is defined on the basis of unequivocal malignant cells in a cytocentrifuged specimen of spinal fluid and/or the presence of obvious neurological deficits, such as cranial nerve palsies.

Staging procedures are outlined in Box 13.2. Abdominal ultrasound is adequate for abdominal disease; computed tomographic (CT) scanning is not necessary in the primary investigation of abdominal and mediastinal disease.

TREATMENT

Until the 1970s, childhood NHL had a poor prognosis, with only a few localized tumours being cured by surgery and radiotherapy. The majority of children died within weeks of diagnosis of local progression or, if local control was achieved, from marrow or CNS disease. Considerable therapeutic improvements have been achieved in the past 20 years as a result of better use of chemotherapy in prospective multicentre studies.

Surgery

Indications for elective surgery are very few. A small localized tumour may be completely excised. In the case of abdominal tumours, diagnosis will often be the fortuitous result of surgery for intestinal intussusception or 'acute appendicitis' that unexpectedly reveals lymphoma. Primary surgical excision or debulking of abdominal, head and neck, and mediastinal tumours should not be attempted. Extensive surgery is uselessly mutilating and is often followed by tumour regrowth. Moreover, it delays and may complicate chemotherapy.

Rarely, abdominal surgery is needed during treatment for complications such as intestinal perforation. If this occurs during a neutropenic period, mortality is high. At the time of remission evaluation, a residual mass may be removed or widely biopsied for careful pathological excision before determining whether a complete or partial remission has been obtained.

Radiotherapy

Radiotherapy can be highly efficacious in lymphoma, but it is a local therapy and NHL should always be regarded as a potentially generalized disease. It provides no advantage over chemotherapy alone and adds both immediate and long-term toxicity to the treatment. Consequently, indications for radiotherapy are now rare. It may be warranted in emergency situations, such as spinal cord compression, although chemotherapy is often as effective. Mediastinal localized residual tumours may benefit from radiotherapy.

Chemotherapy

Chemotherapy is the treatment of choice in childhood NHL, even in the presence of apparently localized disease. The conclusions from protocols carried out in the 1970s were as follows:

- Although complete remission was obtained in 85–95 per cent of all patients and survival rates were improved, results were disappointing in advanced stages, survival being 30–50 per cent.

- Despite CNS treatment with intrathecal therapy, often accompanied by cranial radiotherapy, CNS relapses were frequent (10–20 per cent).
- Treatment results were different for peripheral B-cell and peripheral T-cell lymphomas. B-cell lymphomas benefit from intensive short pulse chemotherapy such as COMP[9] or COPAD,[10] whereas T-cell and precursor B disease benefit from a 'leukaemic' regimen that is continuous and prolonged, such as in LSA2L28,[11] or the BFM protocols.[12]
- Relapses show differing patterns, occurring in the first year in Burkitt lymphoma and generally within the first 2 years, but up to 5 years, in precursor T disease.
- Phase II studies have shown the efficacy of high-dose methotrexate, both on systemic disease and CNS disease.[13]
- After relapses, some patients could be salvaged by high-dose chemotherapy with bone marrow transplantation.[14]

Localized NHLs are much less common than non-localized lymphomas and require less intensive treatment. CNS prophylaxis can be avoided in B-cell stage I and abdominal stage II.[15] Until recently, in the USA, localized NHLs have been treated with the same protocol, whatever the histology.[16,17] These studies and one in the UK have decreased the intensity and the duration of treatment but kept event-free survival (EFS) >85 per cent. Radiotherapy appeared not to be beneficial. However, the Pediatric Oncology Group (POG) had worse EFS in precursor B and T diseases, even if relapsed patients could be salvaged by second-line leukaemia-like treatment (EFS = 61 per cent).[17] These findings support the SFOP (Société Française D'Oncologie Pédiatrique) and BFM (Berlin–Frankfurt–Münster) approaches, where treatment is adapted to histology and immunophenotype, as in the advanced stages.

There is a similar controversy in large-cell lymphomas. Should they all be treated the same way as in the USA,[1,18,19] or should they have different treatment depending on histology and phenotype (large B-cell vs. anaplastic CD30+) as in Europe? Results of the last POG study showed that in large B-cell lymphoma there was benefit from the addition of HD MTX/Ara-C (high-dose methotrexate/cytosine arabinoside) to the APO regimen [Adriamycin (doxorubicin) prednisone, Oncovin], whereas this was not the case in anaplastic large-cell lymphoma. These data are in favour of treating these two subtypes of lymphoma differently.[20]

Peripheral B-cell lymphomas

Most studies concern Burkitt lymphoma, but in some recent European studies, large B-cell lymphomas were included (the latter represent 10–15 per cent of the cases).[21,22] Fractionated cyclophosphamide (CPM), intermediate-dose (ID) or high-dose (HD) MTX and Ara-C are the most important drugs in Burkitt NHL. Vincristine (VCR), adriamycin (ADR), etoposide (VP-16), ifosfamide (IFO) and prednisone are also effective. Drugs are administered in various combinations, but usually as short pulsed courses.

Since 1981, the largest studies have taken place in Europe, in both France (LMB protocols) and Germany (BFM protocols), and as a result of these well organized multicentre studies, there has been considerable improvement in outcome.

LMB PROTOCOLS

The general scheme of the LMB protocols is a cytoreductive phase (COP course) with low doses of VCR, CPM, and prednisone the week before the intensive induction based on HD MTX and fractionated CPM (two courses of COPAD M), followed by a consolidation phase based on Ara-C in continuous infusion. CNS directed therapy is given using HD MTX and intrathecal (IT) MTX. The SFOP conducted several consecutive multicentre studies in France, Belgium and the Netherlands (LMB81, 84, 86, 89).[21,23,24] In the course of the first three studies, which took into consideration advanced stage Burkitt disease, EFS was increased up to 75–90 per cent for NHL CNS− patients, whereas duration of treatment was progressively reduced from 12 to 4 months, and toxicity, especially toxic death rate, was decreased parallel to the investigators' experience. CNS directed therapy by HD MTX (3 g/m^2 in a 4-hour infusion) and IT MTX was efficient (CNS relapse rate < 2 per cent in patients). It appeared that partial remission (with documented viable cells in the residual mass) at the end of induction could be cured by treatment intensification with autologous bone marrow transplantation and that the absence of tumour reduction after the COP was indicative of a poor prognosis (EFS = 22 per cent). For patients with initial CNS involvement whose EFS was only 19 per cent in the LMB81 protocol, the pilot LMB86 study based on a higher dose of MTX (8 g/m^2 in 4 h), triple IT and a consolidation with continuous infusion and HD Ara-C and VP-16 (CYVE courses)[25] succeeded in improving EFS to 75 per cent.

In the LMB89 study (1989–96), all B-cell disease (Burkitt and large B-cell, NHL and ALL), whatever the stage, was included. Patients were stratified in three therapeutic groups:

- group A (resected stage I and abdominal stage II) received two courses of COPAD (VCR, CPM, ADR and prednisone)
- group B (patients not eligible for groups A or C) received a 3.5-month treatment identical to the short arm of the LMB84 protocol

- group C (patients with CNS involvement and ALL with >70 per cent of blasts in bone marrow) received a more intensive treatment similar to that of the LMB86 protocol.

Treatment was further intensified for patients who did not respond to COP in group B and any patient with residual viable cells after the consolidation phase. A total of 561 patients were enrolled. Five-year survival was 92 per cent and EFS was 91 per cent. EFS was 98 per cent for stage I + II, 91 per cent for stage III and 87 per cent for stage IV and B-ALL. The outcome was similar for Burkitt and large B-cell disease (EFS rates of 92 and 89 per cent, respectively). In group B, multivariate analysis of prognostic factors showed that a lactate dehydrogenase (LDH) level greater than twofold the normal value (89.5 per cent for LDH > N × 2 vs. 95 per cent for LDH ≤ N × 2), no response after COP (EFS = 72 per cent) and age ≥ 15 years were associated with a lower EFS. CNS involvement was the only prognostic factor in group C (79 per cent for CNS+ vs. 90 per cent for CNS−).[21]

The next study, the FAB LMB96 (May 1996–June 2001), was a randomized international trial with the participation of the SFOP, the UKCCSG (United Kingdom Children's Cancer Study Group) from Great Britain and the CCG (Children's Cancer Group) from the USA. It was an attempt to reduce treatment further, especially cyclophosphamide dosage, to avoid sterility in boys,[26] to reduce its duration, and to suppress cranial irradiation in patients with initial CNS involvement.

BFM PROTOCOLS

In the course of the four consecutive BFM studies (81, 83, 86, 90),[22,27,28] treatment intensity was progressively increased, treatment duration reduced and CNS irradiation withdrawn. In the BFM 90 study (1990–1995), treatment was stratified into three risk groups (a little different from those of the French study). It consists of two, four or six 5-day courses including dexamethasone, MTX 5 g/m^2 (or 0.5 g/m^2 in the lowest risk group) in a 24-hour infusion and intrathecal injections in each course, and alternating IFO, cytarabine and etoposide with cyclophosphamide and doxorubicin. The 6-year EFS was 89 per cent for the 413 patients, and 97, 98, 88, 73 and 74 per cent for stages I, II, III, IV and ALL, respectively.[22]

The most remarkable data are the increase of EFS from 50 to 80 per cent for patients with stage IV and L3-ALL (study 86) and those with abdominal stage III and LDH > 500 (study 90) when MTX was increased from 0.5 to 5 g/m^2. In the following BFM 95 study, the duration of the MTX infusion was randomized (24 h vs. 4 h).

UKCCSG PROTOCOLS

After 1990, the LMB scheme was used. In the 9002 study (treatment similar to group B of LMB89), EFS of the 112 patients (90 stage III and 42 stage IV CNS− up to 70 per cent blasts in bone marrow) was 83 per cent.[29] In the 9003 protocol (similar to the group C of LMB89), 63 patients with stage IV CNS+ and B-ALL were enrolled, 33 of whom had CNS disease. EFS was 69 per cent.[30] Contrary to the LMB89, LDH level was not found to be prognostic (but it was not known in 30 per cent of the patients), and neither was CNS disease. In the 9003 series, a higher rate of early metabolic complications and toxic deaths, probably due to the absence of availability of urate-oxidase, might explain the poorer results compared with LMB89 group C.

POG PROTOCOLS

The third largest series of Burkitt lymphomas is that of the Pediatric Oncology Group in the USA. EFS rates obtained in the 86 series with the total-therapy-B (Ara-C in a 48-hour infusion in stage III and replaced by HD Ara-C in stage IV and B-ALL) were: 79 per cent in 57 stage III; 79 per cent in 40 stage IV; 65 per cent in 51 L3-ALL patients; and 52 per cent in 24 CNS+ patients.[31,32] In study 9317 for advanced stages, there were two randomizations on the total-therapy-B backbone: (i) administration of Ara-C in either a 48-hour infusion or four high-dose boluses; (ii) the addition of one course of IFO/VP16 (CNS+ patients were not randomized and received the course). Although it was concluded that EFS of CNS+ patients was increased (79 per cent, $n = 48$ patients),[33] the analysis of the second randomization showed that IFO/VP-16 did not improve EFS (83 per cent for 141 CNS− patients receiving IFO/VP-16 vs. 79 per cent for 136 not receiving IFO/VP-16).[34]

OTHER PROTOCOLS

Other studies have reported interesting results, especially the NCI series, in which adults and children with Burkitt and large B-cell lymphoma have the same outcome;[35] but they have involved a smaller number of patients who generally came from single institutions.

In countries that have limited resources but where Burkitt lymphoma is common, therapeutic improvements have also been achieved thanks to the adaptation of therapy to the local environment and to better management of the initial, especially metabolic, problems.

Precursor T and B lymphoblastic lymphomas

Patients with these lymphomas have to be treated with a protocol similar or identical to those used in high-risk forms of ALL. Most are T-lineage, but a few are B-lineage.[36] Although their biology is not similar, they are generally treated by the same protocols.

THE LSA2L2 PROTOCOL AND DERIVED PROTOCOLS

In 1979, the LSA2L2 protocol was published.[11] It consisted of a 2- or 3-year 10-drug intensive regimen administering drugs 5 days a week during consolidation and every 2 weeks during maintenance to 39 patients. With CNS directed therapy based on IT MTX, isolated CNS relapse rate was 8–15 per cent. As shown by the CCSG randomized trial, it appeared to be most effective in mediastinal or lymphoblastic lymphoma.[9]

Some tried to improve CNS control by the addition of cranial irradiation or HD MTX. At the Institut Gustave Roussy in France, the original protocol was modified by the addition of 10 HD MTX ($3\,g/m^2$ in a 3-hour infusion). The EFS was 79 per cent for 33 stage III patients and 72 per cent for 43 stage IV patients (24 of whom had more than 25 per cent bone marrow involvement). Only one isolated CNS relapse occurred among the 69 patients without CNS involvement.[37]

However, this protocol appears to be inferior to the BFM regimen, which is now the reference protocol.

BFM AND DERIVED PROTOCOLS

Since 1976, lymphomas, other than peripheral B-cell lymphomas, have been treated using the same protocol as that for ALL. The induction (protocol I: prednisone, VCR, daunorubicin, L-asparaginase followed by CPM, Ara-C, 6-MP [6-mercaptopurine] and associated with IT MTX) and the reinduction (protocol II: same drugs, but lower total doses and with dexamethasone replacing prednisone) underwent very few modifications during studies 76, 81, 83, 86 and 90.[28,38] These phases are followed by a maintenance with daily 6-MP and weekly MTX. Four courses of ID MTX ($0.5\,g/m^2$) were introduced in study 83, and replaced by HD MTX ($5\,g/m^2$ in a 24-hour infusion) in study 86. In parallel, cranial irradiation was reduced from 18 to 12 Gy. Since 1976, the results have been similar: EFS was 78 per cent for 42 stage III and IV patients treated in study 76, and 79 per cent for 71 patients treated in study 86. However, in study 90, which enrolled 101 patients, EFS improved to 90 per cent without a significant change in the chemotherapy regimen.[28,38] This might be due to the long experience of the investigators with the protocol. In the now closed BFM 95 study, cranial irradiation is deleted in CNS− patients.

Several European groups and centres that have adopted the BFM protocol, or a slightly modified protocol, for treatment of leukaemia now use the same protocol to treat precursor lymphoblastic lymphoma.[39]

OTHER PROTOCOLS

Dahl et al.[40] published a series of 22 patients with stage III and IV lymphoblastic lymphomas, using a protocol based on early and intermittent reinductions with VM-26 (teniposide), Ara-C in addition to VCR, prednisone, asparaginase, triple IT and maintenance with 6-MP and MTX. The EFS was 73 per cent with a regimen containing no CPM and no anthracyclines, but these results have never been confirmed on a larger series of patients.[40]

In the UK, lymphoblastic T-NHLs have been treated with a continuous intensive leukaemia-like regimen. In study 8503, the EFS of 95 patients with stage III and IV T-cell lymphoblastic lymphoma was 65 per cent.[41] In the following study, HD MTX + IT MTX was introduced with omission of cranial irradiation.

In the POG studies, all T-cell malignancies, lymphoma and leukaemia, were treated according to the same protocol. In the 8704 (T3) protocol, after achieving complete remission, patients were randomized to receive HD intensive asparaginase consolidation (25 000 IU/m^2) given weekly for 20 weeks. Outcome was improved in the more intensive treatment (EFS of NHL: 78 vs. 64 per cent), demonstrating the effectiveness of asparaginase.[42] The following POG study 9404 randomized the addition of four doses of HD MTX (5 g/m^2) to a multi-agent chemotherapy backbone modified from the DFCI (Dana–Farber Leukemia consortium). In the interim analysis, 3-year EFS was 86 per cent in the more intensive treatment, clearly demonstrating the effectiveness of HD MTX in lymphoblastic lymphoma, by reducing the occurrence of initial failure and CNS relapse.[43]

Anaplastic large-cell lymphomas

This disease is rare, so the largest series include only about 10 patients per year, which causes obvious difficulties. In the USA, these lymphomas have been included in the same protocol as other large-cell lymphomas. In Europe, they are considered as a specific entity and generally treated by 'B-cell-like' rather than 'T-cell-like' protocols. Overall survival rate was at 70–80 per cent.[44–49] EFS is often lower, indicating that relapses can be salvaged, particularly if the first treatment was not very intensive. In relapse, weekly vinblastine has been shown to be effective.[50] The analysis of the pooled data of the German, French and UK series showed that the BFM regimen was at least as efficient as the others with a lower dose of drugs, especially CPM and ADR. It also revealed the following prognostic factors: mediastinal, visceral (lung, liver, spleen) and skin involvement.[51] This analysis is the basis of the ongoing international European study ALCL 99, which asks two questions using the BFM protocol: (i) the best modality of administration of HD MTX (1 g/m^2 in a 24-hour infusion with IT MTX vs. 3 g/m^2 in a 3-hour infusion without IT); (ii) the role of vinblastine as maintenance therapy in higher-risk patients.

Indications for high-dose chemotherapy and haemopoietic stem cell transplantation

The need for HD chemotherapy with haemopoietic stem cell transplantation has greatly diminished in parallel with the improvement in survival using intensive conventional regimens, and indications are restricted to initial poor responders and relapses which respond to a second-line treatment.[52,53] However, relapses that have occurred under the present protocols are more 'resistant' than those used previously, and to find an effective second-line chemotherapy has become a challenge.[54]

CURRENT CONTROVERSIES

THE ROLE OF SURGERY AND RADIOTHERAPY

With the exception of the rare localized primary tumour that is amenable to complete resection, surgery has no real role beyond biopsy for a histological diagnosis. There is no place for debulking surgery in extensive thoracic or abdominal disease. In the case of abdominal B-cell disease where there is a residual mass post-chemotherapy, a second-look laparotomy may be necessary: if there is residual disease at this time, the patient may still be cured by intensification of treatment.

Radiotherapy may have a role in lymphoblastic and large-cell lymphoma (there is no evidence of efficacy in Burkitt's lymphoma). The only indication for radiotherapy is refractory localized disease, or as consolidation of second remission following local recurrence. For these subtypes, cranial irradiation is still generally used when there is initial lymphoma of the CNS, but not as part of routine early CNS-directed therapy. Testis and bone irradiation are still used where these are initial sites of disease, although this is probably unnecessary in most cases.[55]

WHAT IS THE PLACE OF A PET SCAN IN DISEASE EVALUATION?

Experience with PET (positron emission tomography) scans in childhood NHL is very limited, but it is hoped that this investigation will help to predict active tumour in a residual mass.[36,49] Further evaluation is required.

CAN G-CSF DECREASE NEUTROPENIA AND THE RELATED COMPLICATIONS?

As most of the chemotherapy regimens used to treat childhood NHL are intensive and followed by pancytopenia, especially neutropenia, great hope was placed in G-CSF (granulocyte colony-stimulating factor) to decrease the frequency of neutropenia and the related complications. But the two randomized studies – one in

T-lymphoblastic lymphoma,[56] the other in SFOP protocols following COPADM courses[57] – did not show any clinical advantage of the use of G-CSF.

CAN CNS THERAPY BE IMPROVED?

Central nervous system therapy has been improved by the use of HD MTX, which has advantageously replaced cranial irradiation whose neurological and endocrinological damage is well known. Questions remain about the optimal dosage of HD MTX, infusion duration, number of courses and route of folinic rescue, and the usefulness or otherwise of combined IT injections.

CNS involvement in B-cell NHL, usually regarded as a bad prognostic indicator, is nowadays curable with intensive conventional chemotherapy: HD MTX and HD Ara-C are the drugs of choice along with triple IT injections. The BFM studies indicate (and we await the results of the FAB LMB96 study) that CNS irradiation can be avoided. However, patients with CNS disease still have the worst results, and in the LMB89 study it is the only bad prognostic factor in group C.[21] Is it correlated with more advanced disease, as suggested by two studies,[58,59] or is it a bad prognostic factor *per se*? How to intensify treatment in the group of patients who have the highest rate of toxic death remains uncertain.

ARE THERE PROGNOSTIC FACTORS WITHIN MURPHY STAGE III AND IV PATIENTS TO INDICATE THOSE WHO REQUIRE MORE/LESS TREATMENT?

Since relatively high survival rates have now been reached, the question posed is how to decrease treatment intensity without jeopardizing these. To do so, it is necessary to find new prognostic factors, which is proving more and more difficult, as they change depending on the therapeutic regimens employed.

In lymphoblastic lymphoma, no one to date has succeeded in finding prognostic factors. Response to corticosteroids, which is such a powerful factor in T-ALL, could not be demonstrated in NHL. This might be due in part to the difficulty in response assessment equivalent and a simple blast count in blood.

In peripheral B-cell disease, the absence of tumour regression 1 week after COP, which was a factor for bad prognosis in the LMB84 study, was taken into account in order to intensify earlier chemotherapy in the subsequent studies. Outcome was improved from 22 to 70 per cent in the LMB89 study, but it remains among the bad prognostic factors.[21]

Is age a prognostic factor? Age >15 years was found to be prognostic for EFS in the LMB89 study, but not for survival, and the number of patients was small.[21] Age was not prognostic in two small series of patients with B-cell NHL.[35,60] Very few data are available on patients between

15 and 20 years old, because many are treated on different protocols in adult departments, and often are not registered in studies. An effort should be made to clarify this question.

With new technologies, such as DNA microarray, there is some hope of identifying biological features that would emerge as prognostically independent factors. However, it should be noted that all therapeutic improvement has been obtained independently of understanding the biology of lymphoma.

Controversies regarding localized tumours persist. Treating these lymphomas with the same protocol whatever their histology and phenotype does not seem appropriate in the view of European investigators, nor is the equal treatment of stages I and II whatever the localization, tumour size and extent of previous excision. On the other hand, treatment intensity could be further decreased for some patients. This is being done for B-cell resected stage I and abdominal stage II, which were treated in the French LMB89 study by only two courses of COPAD,[21] and for resected tumours by two courses of chemotherapy in BFM90.[22] However, when treatment is thought not to have immediate life-threatening consequences or major long-term sequelae, the rationale behind a further decrease in therapy is debatable.

Within the advanced stages, it is necessary to find prognostic subgroups to try and decrease therapy for the better prognostic types, noting that prognostic factors identified in one study might not be relevant in another. Bone marrow involvement was not a prognostic factor in the LMB studies, unlike most other studies. An attempt to reduce treatment has been made in the FAB LMB96 study. Results are not yet known, but the study had to be stopped in group C because the third interim analysis showed an inferior EFS in the reduced arm.

One of the aims of decreasing treatment is to decrease long-term sequelae such as infertility, especially in boys. Cyclophosphamide given above a cumulative dose of $9 \, g/m^2$ produces male sterility,[26] so reaching this dosage should be avoided, at least for patients who have no bad prognostic factors. In fact, it would be preferable not to exceed $5 \, g/m^2$ because there are individual susceptibilities, and factors such as age at treatment or modality of drug administration remain undetermined.

HOW SHOULD POST-TRANSPLANT B-CELL NHL BE MANAGED?

With the increasing use of organ transplantation, there is an awareness of both polyclonal and monoclonal B-cell lymphomas developing in patients profoundly immunosuppressed by drugs. Such patients, usually recipients of cardiac or renal transplants, will develop 'high-grade' tumours that are histologically indistinguishable from true malignant disease. In some patients there may be a clear viral pathogen, such as EBV, in which case a poly-clonal tumour may be demonstrable.

The outcome of these tumours is generally good, and with reduction or cessation of cyclosporin they often resolve spontaneously. However, in a number of patients, the disease will be more aggressive and may require therapy. Therapy by monoclonal antibodies such as anti-CD20 may be effective in B-cell lymphoproliferative disease.[61,62]

IS THERE A ROLE FOR TUMOUR-SPECIFIC TARGETED THERAPY IN B-CELL NHL?

Monoclonal antibody targeted therapy for B-cell lymphoma in adults has produced encouraging results. The anti-CD20 antibody, rituximab, has been studied in large cohorts of patients. Its efficacy has been proved in follicular lymphoma, and in large B-cell lymphoma in elderly patients in association with chemotherapy.[63–65] It is now being studied in large B-cell lymphoma in younger adults. Except in post-transplant lymphoproliferative disease, it has not yet been evaluated in paediatric practice. The therapy seems to have only minor side-effects but is very expensive. Taking into account the high survival rate now obtained, its place in the treatment of Burkitt lymphoma in children will be difficult to assess. However, it is necessary to evaluate such a specific therapy, and to date no phase II studies have been performed.

KEY POINTS

- NHL in children is a fast-growing tumour which disseminates widely, especially in bone marrow and in the CNS.
- Appropriate management of tumour lysis syndrome is essential. Urate-oxidase is more effective than allopurinol.
- Treatment differs according to the histological subtype (Burkitt, large B-cell, T-lymphoblastic, anaplasic large-cell).
- Burkitt and large B-cell NHL are treated with intensive, pulsed chemotherapy, the major drugs being cyclophosphamide, HD MTX and Ara-C. Vincristine, doxorubicin and VP16 are also used. The cure rate is 80–90 per cent.
- T-lymphoblastic NHL is treated with intensive semi-continuous and prolonged chemotherapy. The cure rate is 75–90 per cent.
- In Burkitt and T-lymphoblastic NHL, CNS directed therapy is essential and based on intrathecal injections, HD MTX ± Ara-C. Cranial irradiation is not necessary.

- Optimal treatment for anaplasic large-cell lymphoma is still debated. The cure rate is 70–80 per cent.
- The place of rituximab (anti-CD20) is not yet determined.
- The value of the PET scan in residual mass has to be studied.

REFERENCES

♦1. Patte C. Non-Hodgkin's lymphoma. *Eur J Cancer* 1998; **34**: 359–62.

♦2. Sandlund JT, Downing JR, Crist WM. Non-Hodgkin's lymphoma in childhood. *N Engl J Med* 1996; **334**: 1238–48.

3. Purtilo DT, Szymanski I, Bhawan J *et al.* Epstein–Barr virus infections in the X-linked recessive lymphoproliferative syndrome. *Lancet* 1978; **15**: 798–801.

♦4. Hecht JL, Aster JC. Molecular biology of Burkitt's lymphoma. *J Clin Oncol* 2000; **18**: 3707–21.

5. Murphy SB. Classification, staging and end results of treatment of childhood non-Hodgkin's lymphomas: dissimilarities from lymphomas in adults. *Semin Oncol* 1980; **7**: 332–9.

6. Patte C, Sakiroglu C, Ansoborlo S *et al.* Urate-oxidase in the prevention and treatment of metabolic complications in patients with b-cell lymphoma and leukemia, treated in the Société Française D'Oncologie Pédiatrique LMB89 Protocol. *Ann Oncol* 2002; **13**: 789–95.

7. Pui CH, Mahmoud HH, Wiley JM *et al.* Recombinant urate oxidase for the prophylaxis or treatment of hyperuricemia in patients with leukemia or lymphoma. *J Clin Oncol* 2001; **19**: 697–704.

8. Goldman SC, Holcenberg JS, Finklestein JZ *et al.* A randomized comparison between rasburicase and allopurinol in children with lymphoma or leukemia at high risk for tumor lysis. *Blood* 2001; **97**: 2998–3003.

9. Anderson JR, Wilson JF, Jenkin DT *et al.* Childhood non-Hodgkin's lymphoma: the results of a randomized therapeutic trial comparing a 4-drug regimen (COMP) with a 10-drug regimen (LSA2-L2). *N Engl J Med* 1983; **308**: 559–65.

10. Patte C, Rodary C, Sarrazin D *et al.* [Results of treatment of 178 pediatric non-Hodgkin's malignant lymphomas between 1973 and 1978]. *Arch Fr Pediatr* 1981; **38**: 321–7.

11. Wollner N, Exelby PR, Lieberman PH. Non-Hodgkin's lymphoma in children: a progress report on the original patients treated with the LSA2-L2 protocol. *Cancer* 1979; **44**: 1990–9.

12. Muller-Weihrich S, Henze G, Jobke A *et al.* [BFM Study 1975/81 for treatment of non-Hodgkin lymphoma of high malignancy in children and adolescents]. *Klin Padiatr* 1982; **194**: 219–25.

13. Patte C, Bernard A, Hartmann O *et al.* High-dose methotrexate and continuous infusion ara-c in children's non-Hodgkin's lymphoma: phase ii studies and their use in further protocols. *Pediatr Hematol Oncol* 1986; **3**: 11–18.

14. Hartmann O, Pein F, Beaujean F et al. High-dose polychemotherapy with autologous bone marrow transplantation in children with relapsed lymphomas. J Clin Oncol 1984; **2**: 979–85.

15. Murphy SB, Hustu HO, Rivera G, Berard CW. End results of treating children with localized non-Hodgkin's lymphomas with a combined modality approach of lessened intensity. J Clin Oncol 1983; **1**: 326–30.

16. Meadows AT, Sposto R, Jenkin RD et al. Similar efficacy of 6 and 18 months of therapy with four drugs (COMP) for localized non-Hodgkin's lymphoma of children: a report from the Children's Cancer Study Group. J Clin Oncol 1989; **7**: 92–9.

17. Link MP, Shuster JJ, Donaldson SS et al. Treatment of children and young adults with early-stage non-Hodgkin's lymphoma [see comments]. N Engl J Med 1997; **337**: 1259–66.

18. Laver JH, Mahmoud H, Pick TE et al. Results of a randomized phase III trial in children and adolescents with advanced stage diffuse large cell non-Hodgkin's lymphoma: a Pediatric Oncology Group Study. Leuk Lymphoma 2001; **42**: 399–405.

19. Sposto R, Meadows AT, Chilcote RR et al. Comparison of long-term outcome of children and adolescents with disseminated non-lymphoblastic non-Hodgkin lymphoma treated with COMP or daunomycin-COMP: a report from the Children's Cancer Group. Med Pediatr Oncol 2001; **37**: 432–41.

20. Laver JH, Weinstein HJ, Hutchison RE et al. Lineage specific differences in outcome for advanced stage diffuse large cell lymphoma in children and adolescents: results of a randomized phase III Pediatric Oncology Group Trial. (Abstract ASH no. 1455.) Blood 2001; **98**: 11.

●21. Patte C, Auperin A, Michon J et al. The Société Française D'Oncologie Pédiatrique LMB89 protocol: highly effective multiagent chemotherapy tailored to the tumor burden and initial response in 561 unselected children with B-cell lymphomas and L3 leukemia. Blood 2001; **97**: 3370–9.

●22. Reiter A, Schrappe M, Tiemann M et al. Improved treatment results in childhood B-cell neoplasms with tailored intensification of therapy: a report of the Berlin-Frankfurt-Munster Group Trial NHL-BFM 90. Blood 1999; **94**: 3294–306.

23. Patte C, Philip T, Rodary C et al. Improved survival rate in children with stage III and IV B cell non-Hodgkin's lymphoma and leukemia using multi-agent chemotherapy: results of a study of 114 children from the French Pediatric Oncology Society. J Clin Oncol 1986; **4**: 1219–26.

●24. Patte C, Philip T, Rodary C et al. High survival rate in advanced-stage B-cell lymphomas and leukemias without CNS involvement with a short intensive polychemotherapy: results from the French Pediatric Oncology Society of a randomized trial of 216 children. J Clin Oncol 1991; **9**: 123–32.

25. Gentet JC, Patte C, Quintana E et al. Phase II study of cytarabine and etoposide in children with refractory or relapsed non-Hodgkin's lymphoma: a Study of the French Society of Pediatric Oncology. J Clin Oncol 1990; **8**: 661–5.

26. Aubier F, Patte C, Oberlin O et al. Influence on male fertility of chemotherapy treatment for non-Hodgkin's lymphoma (abstract). Med Pediatr Oncol 1997; **29**: 425.

27. Muller-Weihrich S, Beck J, Henze G et al. [BFM Study 1981/83 of the treatment of highly malignant non-Hodgkin's lymphoma in children: results of therapy stratified according to histologic immunological type and clinical stage]. Klin Padiatr 1984; **196**: 135–42.

28. Reiter A, Schrappe M, Parwaresch R et al. Non-Hodgkin's lymphomas of childhood and adolescence: results of a treatment stratified for biologic subtypes and stage – a report of the Berlin-Frankfurt-Munster Group. J Clin Oncol 1995; **13**: 359–72.

29. Atra A, Imeson JD, Hobson R et al. Improved outcome in children with advanced stage B-cell non-Hodgkin's lymphoma (B-NHL): results of the United Kingdom Children Cancer Study Group (UKCCSG) 9002 Protocol. Br J Cancer 2000; **82**: 1396–402.

30. Atra A, Gerrard M, Hobson R et al. Improved cure rate in children with B-cell acute lymphoblastic leukaemia (B-ALL) and stage IV B-cell non-Hodgkin's lymphoma (B-NHL) – results of the UKCCSG 9003 protocol. Br J Cancer 1998; **77**: 2281–5.

31. Brecher ML, Schwenn MR, Coppes MJ et al. Fractionated cylophosphamide and back to back high dose methotrexate and cytosine arabinoside improves outcome in patients with stage III high grade small non-cleaved cell lymphomas (SNCCL): a randomized trial of the Pediatric Oncology Group. Med Pediatr Oncol 1997; **29**: 526–33.

32. Bowman WP, Shuster JJ, Cook B et al. Improved survival for children with B-cell acute lymphoblastic leukemia and stage IV small noncleaved-cell lymphoma: a Pediatric Oncology Group Study. J Clin Oncol 1996; **14**: 1252–61.

33. Schwenn MR, Mahmoud H, Bowman PW et al. Successful treatment of small noncleaved cell lymphoma and B cell ALL with CNS involvement: a Pediatric Oncology Group (POG) study. (Proceedings of the 36th ASCO meeting, abstract no 2282.) J Clin Oncol 2000; **19**: 580a.

34. Schwenn MR, Mahmoud H, Bowman PW et al. The addition of VP-ifosfamide did not improve EFS for CNS negative patients with advanced-stage small noncleaved lymphoma or B-cell ALL: a POG study. (Proceedings of the 37th ASCO meeting, abstract no. 1465.) J Clin Oncol 2001; **21**:367a.

35. Magrath I, Adde M, Shad A et al. Adults and children with small non-cleaved-cell lymphoma have a similar excellent outcome when treated with the same chemotherapy regimen. J Clin Oncol 1996; **14**: 925–34.

36. Neth O, Seidemann K, Jansen P et al. Precursor B-cell lymphoblastic lymphoma in childhood and adolescence: clinical features, treatment, and results in trials NHL-BFM 86 and 90. Med Pediatr Oncol 2000; **35**: 20–7.

37. Patte C, Kalifa C, Flamant F et al. Results of the LMT81 protocol, a modified LSA2L2 protocol with high dose methotrexate, on 84 children with non-B-cell (lymphoblastic) lymphoma. Med Pediatr Oncol 1992; **20**: 105–13.

●38. Reiter A, Schrappe M, Ludwig WD et al. Intensive ALL-type therapy without local radiotherapy provides a 90% event-free survival for children with T-cell lymphoblastic lymphoma: a BFM Group Report. Blood 2000; **95**: 416–21.

39. Uyttebroeck A, Suciu S, Bertrand Y et al. Treatment of childhood T-cell lymphoblastic lymphoma according to the strategy for acute lymphoblastic leukemia: long term results

of the EORTC 58881 trial. (Abstract ASH no. 3350.) *Blood* 2001; **98**: 11.

40. Dahl GV, Rivera G, Pui CH *et al*. A novel treatment of childhood lymphoblastic non-Hodgkin's lymphoma: early and intermittent use of teniposide plus cytarabine. *Blood* 1985; **66**: 1110–14.

41. Eden OB, Hann I, Imeson J *et al*. Treatment of advanced stage T cell lymphoblastic lymphoma: results of the United Kingdom Children's Cancer Study Group (UKCCSG) Protocol 8503. *Br J Haematol* 1992; **82**: 310–16.

●42. Amylon MD, Shuster J, Pullen J *et al*. Intensive high-dose asparaginase consolidation improves survival for pediatric patients with T cell acute lymphoblastic leukemia and advanced stage lymphoblastic lymphoma: a Pediatric Oncology Group Study. *Leukemia* 1999; **13**: 335–42.

43. Asselin B, Shuster J, Amylon MD *et al*. Improved EFS with HD MTX in T-cell lymphoblastic leukemia and advanced lymphoblastic lymphoma: a POG study. (Proceedings of the 37th ASCO meeting.) *J Clin Oncol* 2001; **20**: 367a.

44. Brugieres L, Caillaud JM, Patte C *et al*. Malignant histiocytosis: therapeutic results in 27 children treated with a single polychemotherapy regimen. *Med Pediatr Oncol* 1989; **17**: 193–6.

45. Brugieres L, Deley MC, Pacquement H *et al*. CD30(+) anaplastic large-cell lymphoma in children: analysis of 82 patients enrolled in two consecutive studies of the French Society of Pediatric Oncology. *Blood* 1998; **92**: 3591–8.

46. Reiter A, Schrappe M, Tiemann M *et al*. Successful treatment strategy for Ki-1 anaplastic large-cell lymphoma of childhood: a prospective analysis of 62 patients enrolled in three consecutive Berlin-Frankfurt-Munster group studies. *J Clin Oncol* 1994; **12**: 899–908.

47. Seidemann K, Tiemann M, Schrappe M *et al*. Short-pulse B-non-Hodgkin lymphoma-type chemotherapy is efficacious treatment for pediatric anaplastic large cell lymphoma: a report of the Berlin-Frankfurt-Munster Group Trial NHL-BFM 90. *Blood* 2001; **97**: 3699–706.

48. Sandlund JT, Pui CH, Santana VM *et al*. Clinical features and treatment outcome for children with CD30+ large-cell non-Hodgkin's lymphoma. *J Clin Oncol* 1994; **12**: 895–8.

49. Spaepen K, Stroobants S, Dupont P *et al*. Prognostic value of positron emission tomography (PET) with fluorine-18 fluorodeoxyglucose ([18F]FDG) after first-line chemotherapy in non-Hodgkin's lymphoma: is [18F]FDG-PET a valid alternative to conventional diagnostic methods? *J Clin Oncol* 2001; **19**: 414–19.

50. Brugieres L, Quartier P, Le Deley MC *et al*. Relapses of childhood anaplastic large-cell lymphoma: treatment results in a series of 41 children – a report from the French Society of Pediatric Oncology. *Ann Oncol* 2000; **11**: 53–8.

51. Le Deley MC, Reiter A, Williams D *et al*. Prognostic factors in childhood anaplastic large cell lymphoma: results of the European Intergroup study. *Ann Oncol* 1999; **10**(Suppl. 3): 6.

52. Philip T, Hartmann O, Pinkerton R *et al*. Curability of relapsed childhood B-cell non-Hodgkin's lymphoma after intensive first line therapy: a report from the Société Française D'Oncologie Pédiatrique. *Blood* 1993; **81**: 2003–6.

53. Ladenstein R, Pearce R, Hartmann O *et al*. High-dose chemotherapy with autologous bone marrow rescue in children with poor-risk Burkitt's lymphoma: a report from the European Lymphoma Bone Marrow Transplantation Registry. *Blood* 1997; **90**: 2921–30.

54. Atra A, Gerrard M, Hobson R *et al*. Outcome of relapsed or refractory childhood B-cell acute lymphoblastic leukaemia and B-cell non-Hodgkin's lymphoma treated with the UKCCSG 9003/9002 protocols. *Br J Haematol* 2001; **112**: 965–8.

55. Dalle JH, Mechinaud F, Michon J *et al*. Testicular disease in childhood B-cell non-Hodgkin's lymphoma: the French Society of Pediatric Oncology Experience. *J Clin Oncol* 2001; **19**: 2397–403.

56. Laver J, Amylon M, Desai S *et al*. Randomized trial of R-MetHu granulocyte colony-stimulating factor in an intensive treatment for T-cell leukemia and advanced-stage lymphoblastic lymphoma of childhood: a Pediatric Oncology Group Pilot Study. *J Clin Oncol* 1998; **16**: 522–6.

57. Patte C, Laplanche A, Bertozzi AI *et al*. Granulocyte colony-stimulating factor in induction treatment of children with non-Hodgkin's lymphoma: a randomized study of the French Society of Pediatric Oncology. *J Clin Oncol* 2002; **20**: 441–8.

58. Gururangan S, Sposto R, Cairo MS *et al*. Outcome of CNS disease at diagnosis in disseminated small noncleaved-cell lymphoma and B-cell leukemia: a Children's Cancer Group Study. *J Clin Oncol* 2000; **18**: 2017–25.

59. Haddy TB, Adde MA, Magrath IT. CNS involvement in small noncleaved-cell lymphoma: is CNS disease per se a poor prognostic sign? *J Clin Oncol* 1991; **9**: 1973–82.

60. Todeschini G, Tecchio C, Degani D *et al*. Eighty-one percent event-free survival in advanced Burkitt's lymphoma/leukemia: no differences in outcome between pediatric and adult patients treated with the same intensive pediatric protocol. *Ann Oncol* 1997; **8**(Suppl 1): 77–81.

61. Faye A, Quartier P, Reguerre Y *et al*. Chimaeric anti-CD20 monoclonal antibody (rituximab) in post-transplant b-lymphoproliferative disorder following stem cell transplantation in children. *Br J Haematol* 2001; **115**: 112–18.

62. Serinet MO, Jacquemin E, Habes D *et al*. anti-CD20 monoclonal antibody (rituximab) treatment for Epstein–Barr virus-associated, B-cell lymphoproliferative disease in pediatric liver transplant recipients. *J Pediatr Gastroenterol Nutr* 2002; **34**: 389–93.

63. McLaughlin P, Grillo-Lopez AJ, Link BK *et al*. Rituximab chimeric anti-CD20 monoclonal antibody therapy for relapsed indolent lymphoma: half of patients respond to a four dose treatment program. *J Clin Oncol* 1998; **16**: 2825–33.

64. Czuczman MS, Grillo-Lopez AJ, White CA *et al*. Treatment of patients with low-grade B-cell lymphoma with the combination of chimeric anti-CD20 monoclonal antibody and CHOP chemotherapy. *J Clin Oncol* 1999; **17**(1): 268–76.

65. Coiffier B, Lepage E, Brière J *et al*. CHOP chemotherapy + rituximab compared to CHOP alone in elderly patients with diffuse large B-cell lymphoma. *N Engl J Med* 2002; **346**: 235–42.

14

Hodgkin's disease

HEATHER P. McDOWELL, BOO MESSAHEL & ODILE OBERLIN

AETIOLOGY AND EPIDEMIOLOGY

The true nature of Hodgkin's disease may still be obscure, but the concept of Hodgkin's disease as a neoplasm of the lymphatic system has prevailed, based on the presence of a putative malignant cell population. The mononucleated Hodgkin's cells (and their polynucleated derivatives, the Reed–Sternberg cells) are consistently found in Hodgkin's disease and, despite their relative paucity, are now considered to be the neoplastic component of this condition.

The possible progenitor for these cells remains unclear, although the majority of opinion supports the view that Hodgkin's and Reed–Sternberg cells are lymphocytic in origin and may be derived from an immature stage of differentiation of B or T cells.[1]

The cause(s) of Hodgkin's disease remain(s) unknown. Reports of case clustering among relatives of patients or student groups suggest an environmental or infectious aetiology.[2] The finding that children in low socioeconomic groups with large sibship, as well as young adults with a high socioeconomic standard and small family, have a high risk for Hodgkin's disease resembles remarkably the epidemiology of poliovirus infection, and supports the hypothesis of the pathogenetic role of an infectious agent.[3]

Several findings argue for the role of an Epstein–Barr virus (EBV) infection. In advanced socioeconomic countries, Hodgkin's disease is more prevalent in patients with a preceding history of infectious mononucleosis,[4] and elevated antibody titres against various antigens of EBV are found in the serum of these patients.[5] There is now evidence that Reed–Sternberg cells harbour the EBV genome in many cases.[6–8] Two large studies comparing the rates of EBV positivity in Hodgkin's tumour cells with histological subtypes and epidemiological data found EBV positivity more commonly linked to the mixed cellularity subtype.

In 277 patients from 10 countries, developing countries were found to have a higher proportion of EBV-positive cases (100 per cent in Kenya, 50 per cent in the UK), with both relative prevalence and EBV strain type reflecting each of the respective general populations.[9] In the second study of 1500 patients (including 224 children), age, sex, ethnicity, histological subtype and regional economic status were all independent significant factors for EBV-positive cases. Children under 14 years of age, lower economic development and Asian origin were significant predictors of EBV positivity.[10]

The present hypothesis for pathogenesis of Hodgkin's disease is a chronic antigen stimulation, and EBV seems to be involved in that process in a significant number of cases. The gene rearrangement occurring secondarily to chronic stimulation may result in the expression or amplification of normal genes controlling the production of cytokines, which are responsible for the presence of nonmalignant cells around Hodgkin's and Reed–Sternberg cells.

Although Hodgkin's disease is less common than non-Hodgkin's lymphoma (NHL) among patients with congenital or acquired immunodeficiencies, the incidence appears to be increasing. Four cases of Hodgkin's disease in patients with ataxia telangiectasia have been registered on the SIOP Hodgkin's study. Wiskott–Aldrich syndrome and Bloom's syndrome have also been reported.[11] There is some evidence that Hodgkin's disease occurring in

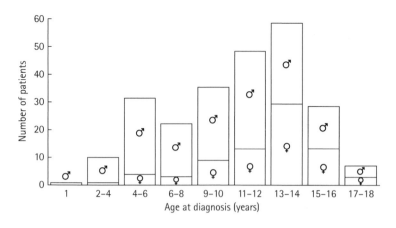

Figure 14.1 *Age and sex distribution of 220 children with Hodgkin's disease included in the first French cooperative study (personal communication).*

Table 14.1 *Sex ratio, stages, mediastinal involvement and histology by age group in HD*

	Total	≤7 years	8–11 years	≥12 years
Number	238	49	76	114
Sex ratio (male:female)	2.2	9	3	1.2
Stages I and II	74%	80%	78%	71%
Mediastinal involvement	54%	37%	43%	68%
Histology				
Nodular sclerosis	37%	15%	30%	50%
Mixed cellularity	40%	60%	41%	32%

association with immunodeficiency is more often of mixed cellularity than nodular sclerosing subtype, reinforcing the theory of EBV-driven malignancy.[12] No clear relation exists between Hodgkin's disease and the particular distribution of HLA histocompatibility antigens HLA A1, B5 and B15.[13] There are some data that suggest an increased risk of developing the disease in parents and siblings of the same family, which could indicate either environmental or genetic influence.[14] A population-based cancer study of twins in the UK showed a significant risk of Hodgkin's disease among persons with a same-sex twin, especially among males.[15] A similar study in America showed increased concordance rates among monozygotic twins, with a standardized incidence ratio of about 100.[16]

Over the last two decades, a rise in the incidence of Hodgkin's disease has been recorded. An increase from 3.6 to 4.5 per million has been reported in the UK registry, and an increase from 5.7 to 6.0 per million in the USA.[17] The age-specific incidence curve is bimodal, with one peak in young adults aged 15–30 years, and the second at age 45–55 years. Paediatric cases represent the beginning of the first peak and explain the increased incidence with advancing age through childhood. The disease is uncommon before 5 years and very rare under 2 years of age (Figure 14.1).

There is wide international variation in the incidence of Hodgkin's disease. In undeveloped countries, Hodgkin's disease occurs more frequently among children younger than 10 years. In Asia, North Africa and South America the incidence exceeds 7 per million, with 70 per cent of childhood cases occurring below the age of 10 years.[18] This gives further support to the theory that an infective agent has an aetiological role in this disease.

With progressing age, the male:female incidence ratio changes, being 10:1 under 7 years of age, with the male preponderance falling to as low as 1.1 after the age of 12 (Table 14.1).

PATHOLOGY

A correct diagnosis is only possible with adequate tissue samples from an open surgical nodal biopsy. Needle biopsies and frozen section material are not suitable for the examination of lymph node architecture and the stromal cellular elements.

Central to the diagnosis of Hodgkin's disease is the identification of the characteristic Reed–Sternberg cell: large multinucleated giant cells with inclusion-like nucleoli surrounded by a clear halo. Variants of the Reed–Sternberg cell may exist, such as the mononuclear Hodgkin's cell or a lacunar Reed–Sternberg cell, the latter being characteristic of nodular sclerosing Hodgkin's disease. The presence of these cells alone, although necessary for diagnosis, is not sufficient for a histological diagnosis of Hodgkin's disease since cells of similar appearance may also be found in reactive processes, infectious mononucleosis, phenytoin-induced 'pseudolymphoma', graft-versus-host reactions and even NHL.

Table 14.2 *Distribution of various histological subtypes in children with Hodgkin's disease[a]*

Series	No. of patients	Lymphocytic predominance (%)	Nodular sclerosis (%)	Mixed cellularity (%)	Lymphocyte depletion (%)	Unclassified (%)
Stanford	55	9	62	20	2	7
Australia	53	11	68	17	4	–
Memphis	88	12.5	33	34	20.5	–
Turkey	40	7.5	17.5	67.5	7.5	–
France	238	13	37	40	0.5	9.5
UK	331	21	47	22	<1	8

[a]Data from Shankar et al.,[20] Ekert et al.,[43] Oberlin et al.,[95] Donaldson and Link,[89] Smith and Rivera,[118] and Cavdar et al.[119]

The lymph node architecture is usually disrupted by the accumulation of reactive cells: lymphocytes of various sizes, histiocytes, eosinophils, plasma cells and fibroblasts. Collagen bands and diffuse fibrosis are the two different types of connective tissue proliferation. The relative proportions of Reed–Sternberg cells, lymphocytes and both sclerosis and fibrosis are taken into account when using the Rye histopathological classification.[19]

The frequency of the different histological subtypes varies according to different paediatric series. These discrepancies may be due in part to the lack of comparability with respect to age and sex distribution, but may also be due to disagreement about histopathological interpretation among the various pathologists concerned (Table 14.2).

Certain patterns of disease are consistent with their histological subtype. The lymphocytic type is often associated with localized cervical or inguinal disease, while nodular sclerosis commonly presents with mediastinal involvement in the adolescent age group. Mixed cellularity and the rare cases of lymphocyte depletion may be associated with a more diffuse disease occurring above and below the diaphragm.

The introduction of an effective multimodal therapy in the treatment of Hodgkin's disease has erased the previous prognostic difference between the two more frequent types: nodular sclerosis and mixed cellularity. A study reported by Shankar et al.[20] on 331 patients failed to show a difference in outcome dependent on histological subtype. There was a high relapse rate in stage I mixed cellularity subtype, reflecting a more aggressive biological behaviour. However, in 2000, Landman-Parker et al.[21] reported on the French study MDH90, and stated that significant predictors of event-free survival (EFS) were haemoglobin <10.5 g/dL, 'B' biological class and nodular sclerosis histology. Clinical and pathological experience over the past two decades also suggests that the two original subtypes of lymphocyte (nodular and diffuse) predominant forms proposed by Lukes and Butler[22] should be distinguished, as the nodular form presents at a single nodal site, and even without therapy progresses extremely slowly over a period of many years. A proportion of these patients may later develop either another type of Hodgkin's disease or large-cell NHL, even if untreated.[23]

Box 14.1 *Constitutional symptoms in the Ann Arbor classification*

- Presence of unexplained fever
- Night sweats
- Unexplained loss of 10 per cent or more of body weight in the 6 months before admission

No constitutional symptoms = A; one or more of these = B

Cytogenetic studies are difficult to perform and interpret owing to the scarcity of the Hodgkin's/Reed–Sternberg cells and the low number of mitoses. Forty cases were well documented by Thangavelu and LeBeau.[24] No constant change of karyotype has been identified, such as the translocation 8/14 in Burkitt lymphoma, although some aberrations appeared to occur non-randomly in a number of chromosomes, including 1, 2, 7, 11, 14, 15 and 21. Two of these chromosomes (7 and 11) have also been observed to be abnormal in secondary leukaemias, and the question arises as to whether a genetically determined chromosome instability is inherent in patients with Hodgkin's disease.[25]

CLINICAL PRESENTATION AND STAGING MODALITIES

Painless cervical lymphadenopathy is the most frequent presenting symptom (in 80 per cent of children), often with a pain-free and fluctuating course, which causes a delay in diagnosis. About 60 per cent have concomitant, mostly asymptomatic, involvement of the mediastinum; disease limited to the mediastinum, however, is very rare (1 per cent), as confirmed in our French series.

An evaluation of constitutional symptoms, such as those described in Box 14.1, should be made. The presence of one of these symptoms is of prognostic significance and confers a disease classification 'B' in the staging procedure. B symptoms were noted in 32 per cent of the children registered in the French study. Their frequency increases with advanced stages of the disease (5 per cent in stage I, 28 per cent in stage II, 64 per cent in stage III and 81 per cent in stage IV). In terms of diagnosis, isolated splenomegaly, hepatomegaly and symptoms relating to lung or pleural involvement often pose the most difficult challenges in diagnosis.

Clinical staging procedures

On the basis of past experience, the goal of a detailed staging procedure at diagnosis is to tailor treatment to the extent of the disease.

INITIAL PHYSICAL EXAMINATION

This should include careful evaluation of all peripheral nodal areas. Doubtful nodes should be explored by cytology or even biopsy if disease in that site leads to a change of stage and/or therapy. Evaluation of the liver and spleen can be difficult as they are often normally palpable in young children. However, abnormal clinical findings are, for the most part, in concordance with those ascertained using imaging techniques.

THORACIC IMAGING

Mediastinal involvement is present in around 60 per cent of cases, but this incidence varies with age, from 40 per cent before 8 years to 70 per cent after 12 years (Table 14.1). Posteroanterior and lateral chest X-rays evaluate mediastinal involvement, but computed tomography (CT) scanning has replaced conventional tomography and is now essential for recognizing lymphatic spread to the diaphragmatic region, and extralymphatic extension to the pericardium, pleura or pulmonary parenchyma. To evaluate the response to therapy, serial CTs are also used; the impact of this procedure has still to be evaluated. Both CT and magnetic resonance imaging (MRI) can now detect previously unevaluated mediastinal disease and may result in some patients receiving mediastinal irradiation when, in the past, none was given. Any benefit from this is questionable. In the post-therapy setting MRI provides better morphological details than CT, but is not significantly different in identifying disease sites.[26]

Gallium scanning (Ga-67) has been readopted as an imaging tool to delineate mediastinal involvement.[27] However, when comparing CT with Ga-67 for initial staging, Devizzi et al.[28] showed Ga-67 to have less sensitivity than CT or MRI (90 vs. 96 and 100 per cent, respectively).

More recently, fluorine-18 fluorodeoxyglucose positron emission tomography (FDG-PET) has been evaluated for initial staging and post-therapy.[29–31] At diagnosis,

Kostakoglu et al.[32] showed FDG-PET to have a significantly higher sensitivity to detect disease than Ga-67 scintigraphy (100 vs. 71.5 per cent for site, and 100 vs. 80.3 per cent for patient sensitivity). In the post-therapy setting, where there is possible residual disease, Naumann et al.[33] showed, in a study of 58 patients, an increased likelihood of relapse if FDG-PET was positive ($P = 0.004$). FDG-PET appears to be highly sensitive in detecting residual disease indicative of future relapse, but as yet it has not been evaluated in the paediatric population.

Both clinical and radiological examinations are required to exclude nasopharyngeal and oropharyngeal disease. Any suspicious areas should be biopsied to confirm the diagnosis, especially as disease involving Waldeyer's ring is exceptionally uncommon (only one case out of 220 children in a French series).

ABDOMINAL INVESTIGATION

The most effective way of imaging abdominal lymph nodes in children remains controversial. Correlation between the results of lymphography and those of histological examination in children is excellent, with a 95 per cent accuracy rate,[34] and this has been the reference method of imaging the retroperitoneal lymph nodes. In comparison with CT scanning, it can evaluate better both the size and abnormal architecture of pelvic and para-aortic lymph nodes. However, general anaesthesia is necessary for the procedure in very young children, and patients with massive mediastinal and pulmonary involvement should be excluded on account of a high-risk morbidity.

Abdominopelvic CT scans in children are an easier and less invasive procedure than lymphography, and appear to be complementary to the latter since they can visualize the enlarged nodes of the coeliac axis, porta hepatis, splenic pedicle and mesenteric nodes. MRI imaging can give a more accurate morphological definition of lymph nodes than CT and is replacing it in some centres.

Ultrasound imaging is also non-invasive, relatively simple to carry out, and inexpensive. Visualization of the same nodal areas as seen on CT scans can be carried out, but in addition a high degree of accuracy in the determination of splenic size and intrahepatic masses can be obtained. It remains a useful tool in the follow-up of patients, provided a baseline investigation is done at diagnosis.

In the hands of an expert with modern equipment, abdominopelvic CT scanning and ultrasound imaging are both now considered to be reliable and allow lymphography to be avoided in most cases. The increased use of combined modality therapy allows the clinician to rely on imaging by CT scan or ultrasound to detect the areas involved that will need irradiation after chemotherapy.

Surgical staging procedures

Should surgery play a role in staging at all? Advocates for surgery argue that accurate anatomical verification of disease extent is obtainable by surgery but is unavailable from the investigations described above. This can alter the clinical stage of approximately one-third of the patients with localized disease IA–IIA with the finding of occult subdiaphragmatic involvement.[35,36] Historically, surgery was essential in order to calculate radiation fields when radiotherapy was the only mode of therapy, and in itself this improved the relapse-free survival rate of children.[36]

Laparotomy is, however, a major surgical procedure, requiring the assessment of all the lymph node regions of the abdomen. It is painful, costly and delays the beginning of the treatment. Moreover, surgical procedures are not without risk to the patient. Although perioperative mortality or severe morbidity, in experienced hands, is minimal, there is the late postoperative complication of intestinal obstruction: a 1–10 per cent incidence as reviewed by Jenkin and Berry.[37]

Serious regard should also be given to the risk of overwhelming post-splenectomy sepsis. A review of the data from four large series of patients splenectomized for Hodgkin's disease and lymphoma reveals an incidence rate of serious bacterial infection ranging from 1 to 10 per cent, with a mortality of 0–5 per cent.[38–41] In the Stanford experience, the rate of bacterial infection was related to the intensity of treatment, and significantly increased when chemotherapy was given compared with radiotherapy alone.[41] Acquisition of antibody response following pneumococcal vaccination is variable, particularly in view of the haste often needed to make a diagnosis and commence treatment.[42] Consequently, lifelong antibiotic prophylaxis against *Streptococcus pneumoniae* has been recommended for these patients. The exact role of vaccination against *Haemophilus influenzae* remains unclear; efficacious prophylaxis already exists in the form of rifampicin given after close contact.

The decision about the use of laparotomy relates directly to the treatment options. When treatment with radiation alone is to be considered, laparotomy may be indicated, but this option applies to a very limited group of children. On the other hand, if chemotherapy alone is used, an accurate evaluation of subdiaphragmatic disease may not be essential. Laparotomy has been avoided in an Australian study and by the UK group.[43,44] Many investigators now recommend combined-modality treatment. In such programmes, comparison of the two staging strategies (clinical only or clinical plus surgical) before similar treatment (four to six cycles of multiagent chemotherapy plus involved field radiotherapy) does not show any superiority of surgical staging.[45]

The use of laparotomy was abandoned in France in 1975. Although there is a risk of failing to detect subdiaphragmatic disease, the incidence of abdominal relapses in patients clinically staged IA–IIA and treated by chemotherapy before involved field radiation therapy is very low: 4.4 per cent in an adult series,[35] 0 per cent in children treated with the MOPP regimen before involved field radiotherapy,[46] and 2 per cent in a recent French cooperative study.[47] Chemotherapy has thus cured radiologically undetectable disease in the majority of this group of patients.

The Italian national group observed similarly good results in clinically staged patients.[48] Three consecutive German paediatric studies have, in a step by step fashion, reduced the indications of laparotomy and splenectomy. In the last study, indications were restricted to patients with abnormal abdominal imaging or enlargement of pulmonary hilar nodes.[49]

At Stanford, the previously routinely performed pathological staging during earlier paediatric studies is now omitted for stage IA patients with high cervical nodes of lymphocytic-predominant histology and patients with positive lymphography or with isolated mediastinal involvement or stage IV disease.[50] In the UK, irradiation alone is used for clinically staged high cervical stage IA patients. Virtually all those with undetected disease are cured with subsequent chemotherapy (UKCCSG, unpublished data).

The necessity to perform oophoropexy in girls before pelvic irradiation does not warrant systematic laparotomy, and radiotherapy is not always necessary since iliac node involvement is rare (<10 per cent of cases). If required, oophoropexy can be performed prior to radiation therapy.

SEARCH FOR EXTRANODAL INVOLVEMENT

In children, the differential diagnosis of multiple pulmonary parenchymal nodular lesions is seldom difficult, although infection and Hodgkin's disease may coexist. Most commonly, lung involvement is associated with mediastinal and hilar lymphadenopathies and a nodular sclerosing pathology.

In the presence of hepatomegaly, where distinct intrahepatic nodules are present, needle biopsy can be undertaken using radiographic guidance. However, unless atypical, these lesions can be clinically considered as lymphoma. In the case of diffuse hepatic enlargement, in accordance with the SIOP Study Group, a 'mini-laparotomy' is adequate in order to inspect the organ, define the most likely regions involved, and take an adequate biopsy. Possible microscopic involvement of the liver can remain undetected in clinically staged patients who have an apparently normal hepatic size. However, the fact that relapse in the liver after combined treatment is now very rare demonstrates the efficacy of chemotherapy in sterilizing occult involvement.

Box 14.2 *Recommendations for diagnostic work-up of children with Hodgkin's disease*

Mandatory procedures
- Surgical biopsy reviewed by experienced pathologist
- History with special attention to fever, sweating and weight loss
- Physical examination with cytology or biopsy of doubtful nodes
- Complete blood count and erythrocyte sedimentation rate
- Chest X-ray (posteroanterior and lateral views)
- Lymphogram or CT scan in the younger child

Procedures required under certain conditions
- Chest CT scan if mediastinal, hilar or pulmonary involvement is present or suspected
- Abdominal ultrasound or CT scan if lymphogram is equivocal or if the child has hepatomegaly or splenomegaly or systemic symptoms with normal lymphogram
- Postnasal space X-ray if cervical nodes are involved
- Bone marrow biopsy if systemic symptoms are associated with stage II–IV
- Liver biopsy if hepatomegaly is homogeneous
- Radioisotopic bone scan if stage IV
- Pleural cytology if there is a pleural effusion

Promising research procedures
- Positron emission tomography
- Mediastinal magnetic resonance imaging
- Interleukin-2 receptor and CD8 serum levels

Box 14.3 *Ann Arbor staging classification*

Stage I
Involvement of a single lymph node region (I) or a single extralymphatic organ or site (IE)

Stage II
Involvement of two or more lymph node regions on the same side of the diaphragm (II) or solitary involvement of an extralymphatic organ or site and one or more lymph node regions on the same side of the diaphragm (IIE)

Stage III
Involvement of lymph node regions on both sides of the diaphragm (III) which may be accompanied by localized involvement of extralymphatic organ or site (IIIE) or by involvement of the spleen (IIIS), or both (IIISE)

Stage IV
Diffuse or disseminated involvement of one or more extralymphatic organs or tissues with or without associated lymph node enlargement

Box 14.2 summarizes the procedures for diagnostic work-up of children with Hodgkin's disease. On completion of these diagnostic investigations, the stage of the disease can be assigned, as shown in Box 14.3, according to the 'Ann Arbor Classification'.[52]

The modality of staging used influences the stage distribution of patients, and this is shown in Table 14.3. If staging is only clinical, the incidence of localized stages (I and II) reaches 70 per cent. When investigations include laparotomy, half the children are in stages I and II, and one-third are in stage III. This distribution should be taken into account when comparing the intensity of treatment in children treated by a protocol stratified according to stage.

LABORATORY STUDIES

Laboratory studies must include a complete blood count and measurement of the ESR. Neutrophilia is frequently found and eosinophilia occurs in 15 per cent of patients. Lymphopenia is a sign of advanced disease. An elevated ESR is closely related to stage and the presence of systemic symptoms; its prognostic importance was recognized early and highlighted in multivariate analysis.[53] However, the introduction of chemotherapy to many paediatric protocols and adaptation of treatment to stage and systemic symptoms have eliminated its prognostic impact.

Bone marrow involvement is infrequent in children: 3 per cent in the French study. These patients were found to differ significantly from those without marrow involvement with regard to B symptoms, clinical stage, haemoglobin level and erythrocyte sedimentation rate (ESR). Bone marrow biopsies should therefore always be performed in the presence of advanced disease, systemic symptoms, abnormal blood count or local bone involvement. They are not usually needed in stage I and II disease. In the rare cases of bone involvement at diagnosis, lesions are usually located in the spine and the pelvis. Marrow involvement may be the single site of extranodal involvement and MRI seems to be a valuable non-invasive procedure to evaluate this.[51] In the event of relapse, initial bone marrow involvement may be an indication for high-dose chemotherapy with bone marrow rescue. Involvement of other extranodal sites (e.g. kidney, skin and central nervous system) is seldom present at diagnosis.

Table 14.3 *Stage distribution according to the staging modality[a]*

Series	Staging	n	I (%)	II (%)	I + II (%)	III (%)	IV (%)
Stanford	Pathological	55	15	35	50	40	11
Memorial Hospital	Pathological	110	29	33	62	32	12
German group	Pathological	170	24	29	53	39	8
	Selective laparotomy	207	24	36	60	31	9
Australia	Clinical	53	32	40	72	19	9
France	Clinical	238	32	42	74	17	9
UK	Clinical	331	30	38	68	24	8

[a]Data are from Shankar *et al.*,[20] Ekert *et al.*,[43] Brämswig *et al.*,[49] Donaldson and Link,[89] Oberlin *et al.*[95] and Tan *et al.*[120]

Elevated serum copper levels have been described as a non-specific biochemical indicator in adults, predominantly useful as a predictive indicator of relapse.[54]

Recent studies have shown that increased serum levels of interleukin-2 (IL-2) receptors and of CD8 antigen (a surface membrane component of suppressor/cytotoxic T cells) correlate with a poor prognosis. They are higher in patients with advanced disease and with B symptoms retain significance in multivariate analysis.[55] Poor outcome has also been linked to elevated IL-10 levels, a cytokine thought to be involved in the pathogenesis of Hodgkin's disease.[56]

TREATMENT METHODS

There is universal agreement that cure for this disease should be achieved with the minimum amount of therapy. Progress in this respect is due to a review of past clinical experience. Appropriate treatment depends on both the extent of the disease and the age of the patient since, despite the similarity of the disease between adults and children, it is now obvious that the sequelae of therapy, and especially those of radiotherapy, are of paramount importance in children. The therapeutic regimens that will enable this goal to be attained remain the subject of debate.

Radiotherapy

Kaplan[57] was the first to point out that a radiation dose ranging from 40 to 44 Gy was the optimal tumoricidal dose to cure Hodgkin's lymphoma. He also described the definition of the fields to treat multiple lymph node chains in continuity, thus avoiding junctions within the field and the risk of overlapping in that plane. The 'mantle field' includes all the main lymph node chains above the diaphragm: the two cervical and supraclavicular areas, the two axillary areas and the mediastinum with lung hilus. The 'inverted Y field' encompasses all the major abdominal lymph node chains: para-aortic, iliac and inguinal lymph

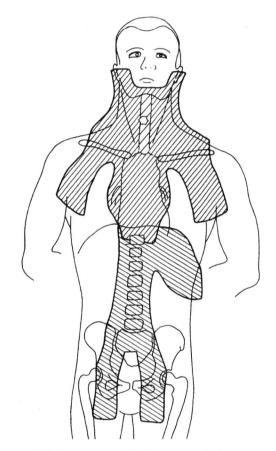

Figure 14.2 *Total nodal irradiation – mantle field and inverted Y.*

nodes, with spleen extension often being added. These two fields require a single junction and represent the so-called TNI (total nodal irradiation) method (Figure 14.2).

Extended field radiotherapy covers the treatment of apparently uninvolved lymphatic regions and the extent of the field varies greatly from study to study and from stage to stage. For a cervical stage II, for example, it may encompass the ipsilateral axillary areas, a complete mantle, or even a complete mantle and a lumbosplenic field (Figure 14.3).

'Involved fields' should be employed only for treatment limited to the involved lymph node chain. However, the definition of 'involved' field varies from one group of workers to another: for example, some groups do not consider that the axillary area constitutes an anatomical continuity to be irradiated if only cervical nodes are involved (Figures 14.4a and 14.5a); this is at variance with the definition of the Rye Symposium, which concluded that if cervical, infraclavicular or axillary nodes are involved, all three regions should be treated (Figures 14.4b and 14.5b). We consider that bilateral radiation of the neck in unilateral disease is only indicated to avoid later cosmetic problems of asymmetry. In the French study, the limited fields employed also varied in single node disease (Figure 14.6).

The late effects of high-dose radiotherapy are now well recognized as a result of the increasing number of cured patients and the longer follow-up times. These effects correlate closely to the dose, the fields irradiated and the age at the time of treatment, being more detrimental when delivered to younger patients. Radiation induces soft tissue and skeletal growth impairment that may result in abnormally short sitting and standing heights.[58] A mantle field results in a thin chin and neck, a narrow chest with short clavicles and high spinal kyphosis (Figure 14.7). These so-called cosmetic deficits severely impair the quality of life of these children when they become young adults.

The frequency of radiation-induced thyroid dysfunction is around 30 per cent.[59] Hypothyroidism is the most common disturbance with a relative risk of 17.1 ($P < 0.0001$) compared with siblings. Hyperthyroidism occurs in 5 per cent, which is eightfold greater than in the normal population ($P < 0.0001$), and thyroid cancer is 18 times what is expected at 20 years from diagnosis. Both dose of radiotherapy and gender influence this – higher doses and female gender carry a higher risk.

Controversies still exist concerning the role of lymphography in the incidence of hypothyroidism. Some studies have demonstrated that pre-irradiation lymphography significantly increased the incidence of hypothyroidism,[60] contrasting with the series from Green et al.[61] showing a protective effect for lymphography. This investigation is now rarely carried out.

The treatment of thyroid dysfunction is also the subject of some debate. Low levels of thyroxine obviously

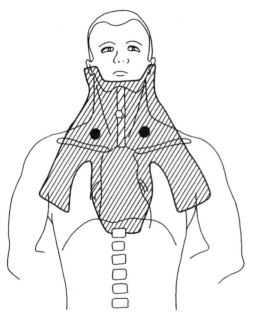

Figure 14.3 *An example of an extended field for cervical stage II.*

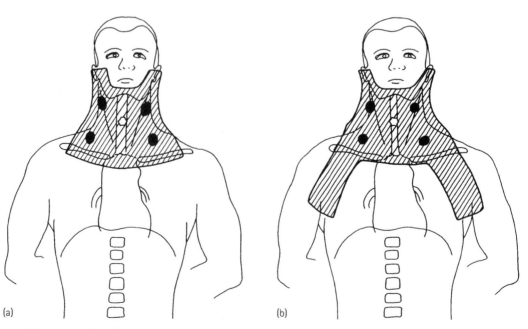

(a)

(b)

Figure 14.4 *(a) Limited involved field for cervical stage II. (b) Limited field according to the Rye symposium for the same stage.*

require thyroid replacement therapy. Animal studies show that there is a predisposition to thyroid adenoma or carcinoma through chronic stimulation of the thyroid by high levels of thyroid-stimulating hormone (TSH), and this is an argument to treat even those patients with compensated hypothyroidism. However, the incidence of thyroid carcinoma after irradiation for Hodgkin's disease is very low: four cases among 979 children with 2–29 years'

follow-up.[62] The long latency of these tumours makes difficult any prospective randomized study to answer this question fully in children.

High-dose radiation may induce late pleural or pericardial effusion (Figure 14.8). In long-term survivors, we have observed constrictive pericarditis occurring more than 10 years after the treatment. An increased incidence of coronary artery disease has also been shown in data

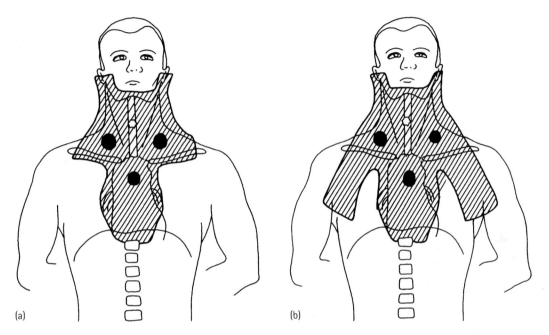

(a)   (b)

Figure 14.5 *(a) Limited involved field with mediastinal involvement. (b) Limited involved field with mediastinal involvement as defined by the Rye symposium.*

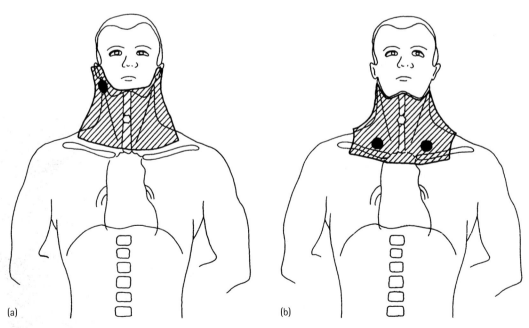

(a)   (b)

Figure 14.6 *(a) Limited field, excluding the clavicles, for a single upper cervical node. (b) Limited field, excluding the mandible, for a lower single supraclavicular node.*

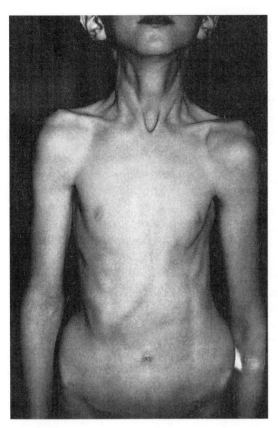

Figure 14.7 *Thoracic and abdominal musculoskeletal abnormalities in a boy who received 40 Gy in a mantle and lumbosplenic field at the age of 4 years.*

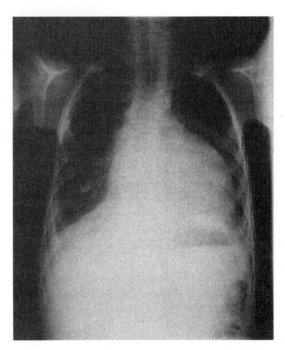

Figure 14.8 *Pericarditis that occurred 11 years after a 40 Gy mantle field received at the age of 15 years.*

Table 14.4 *MOPP, ABVD, OPPA and ChlVPP chemotherapy regimens*

Regimen	Dose (mg/m²)	Administration	
		Route	Timing
MOPP			
Mechlorethamine	6	i.v.	Days 1 and 8
Vincristine	1.5	i.v.	Days 1 and 8
Procarbazine	100	p.o.	Days 1–14
Prednisone	40	p.o.	Days 1–14
ABVD			
Adriamycin	25	i.v.	Days 1 and 15
Bleomycin	10	i.v.	Days 1 and 15
Vinblastine	6	i.v.	Days 1 and 15
DTIC	375	i.v.	Days 1 and 15
OPPA			
Vincristine	1.5	i.v	Days 1, 8 and 15
Prednisolone	60	p.o.	Days 1–15
Procarbazine	100	p.o.	Days 1–15
Doxorubicin	40	i.v.	Days 1–15
ChlVPP			
Chlorambucil	6	p.o.	Days 1–14
Vinblastine	6	i.v	Days 1 and 8
Procarbazine	100	p.o.	Days 1–14
Prednisolone	40	p.o.	Days 1–14

i.v., intravenous; p.o., per os.

from the Institut Gustave-Roussy.[63] In the same study, late functional pulmonary involvement was related to the total dose of radiation and a fraction size greater than 200 rads (2 Gy). Green *et al.*[64] also found a high incidence of asymptomatic pericardial thickening on echocardiogram in long-term survivors after childhood Hodgkin's disease. The clinical significance of these findings remains to be assessed with longer follow-up.

The risk of chronic radiation enteritis with subacute obstruction and malabsorption is increased by staging laparotomy and extensive intra-operative investigation. Soft-tissue fibrosis may also induce limb lymphoedema or retroperitoneal fibrosis with ureteric obstruction. As a final point, oophoropexy should be performed in all girls receiving pelvic irradiation in order to protect ovarian function. A lateral transposition technique reduces the scattered dose received by the ovaries.

Chemotherapy

The MOPP regimen was first described in 1967 by Carbone[65] and consists of a combination of drugs (mechlorethamine, vincristine, procarbazine and prednisone) (Table 14.4). It achieved dramatic results in advanced disease that was not previously curable.[66] Several modifications were made to the MOPP programme, vinblastine being substituted for vincristine nd/or cyclophosphamide, or chlorambucil being substituted for mechlorethamine.[67,68] None of these combinations has proved to be significantly better than the MOPP regimen. A new four-drug combination (ABVD) was developed in 1974 with totally different components from those in MOPP: adriamycin, bleomycin, vinblastine and DTIC (Table 14.4). The efficacy of ABVD has been tested in randomized studies versus MOPP and the usefulness of alternating non-cross-resistant regimens has been validated. Adult studies have shown that a hybrid regimen (MOPP/ABVD) is more effective than a single regimen (MOPP).[69–71] In addition to improved efficacy, a 10-year follow-up has reported a low incidence of late effects.[72]

The late effects of chemotherapy are increasingly well defined as the number of long-term survivors grows. Gonadal injury is of particular importance. All boys develop normal puberty after MOPP, even if they are azoospermic. Recent data regarding male fertility after chemotherapy did not confirm that prepubertal testes are less sensitive to alkylating agents than adult testes. As in adults, six cycles of MOPP will result in azoospermia; however, azoospermia was also observed in two boys who received two and three cycles of MOPP. The toxic doses of procarbazine and mechlorethamine still require assessment.[73] In the same study, elevated follicle-stimulating hormone (FSH) correlated well with azoospermia. German paediatric data show a relationship between FSH level and the dose of procarbazine.[49] The significance of these findings still has to be assessed with longer follow-up since we, for example, have seen patients with normal FSH despite azoospermia. A reduced long-term toxicity has been reported by Schellong et al.,[74] where etoposide was substituted for procarbazine in the combination vincristine, etoposide, prednisolone and doxorubicin (OPPA) (Table 14.4), used in the German study DAL-HD-90. There was no difference in overall survival (OS). In contrast, the Milan studies showed a preservation of fertility in most of the men who received ABVD chemotherapy as adults.[69]

MOPP chemotherapy may also induce ovarian damage, but young age at the time of treatment is associated with less gonadal damage even if the incidence of premature ovarian ageing is not well known.[75] The use of gonadotrophin-releasing hormone (GnRH) analogues for functional protection of the ovary and preservation of fertility during polychemotherapy in adolescents has recently been reported but needs further investigation.[76]

Pulmonary function tests have been sequentially evaluated in patients treated as adults with high-dose mantle irradiation and six cycles of either ABVD or MOPP. The mean vital capacity at the end of treatment was statistically lower in the ABVD group with incomplete recovery at 2 years.[77] The paediatric experience of three cycles of ABVD alternating with three of MOPP in conjunction with low-dose radiation shows that, with a 27.5-month mean

follow-up, out of 20 patients, 40 per cent had abnormal lung volumetric measures. Out of 11 patients, six had a low value of carbon monoxide diffusion capacity (DL_{CO}), while two out of 14 asymptomatic patients were considered to have an abnormal cardiac nuclear gated angiogram.[50] Villani et al.[78] have shown that, after four cycles of ABVD and a median dose of 36 Gy mediastinal radiotherapy, there is a significant reduction in forced expiratory volume in 1 second (FEV_1), vital capacity and DL_{CO}, indicating a restrictive pattern of lung defect. These worrying results need longer follow-up.

Data concerning the late effects of treatment are now accumulating.[79–82] Hudson et al.[83] documented the increased risk of death following treatment for Hodgkin's disease. In the largest cohort to date of 5925 patients treated for Hodgkin's disease in childhood and adolescence, 157 second solid tumours (SSTs) and 26 acute leukaemias were documented.[84] The risk of developing a SST remained significantly higher among the 20-year survivors (cumulative risk, 6.5 per cent) and persisted for 25 years (cumulative risk, 11.7 per cent). Temporal trends for cancers of the thyroid, female breast, bone/connective tissue, stomach and oesophagus were all consistent with past radiotherapy exposure. There was a greater than 50-fold increased risk of thyroid and respiratory tract malignancies if treatment was prior to 10 years of age. Although this study reports on treatment modalities employed many years ago, it underscores the importance of long term follow-up and the challenges of reducing treatment. The risk of developing leukaemia is associated with the dose of alkylating agents received.[85] The outcome with ABVD in children remains to be reported, but in adults the risk of leukaemia seems to be very small or absent.[86] The German-Austrian Group have substituted mechlorethamine in the MOPP regimen with doxorubicin in OPPA since 1978 for stage IA/IB and IIA patients.[87] Advanced-stage disease cases also received OPPA, but, in addition, varying numbers of courses of cyclophosphamide, vincristine methotrexate and prednisolone (COMP). The estimated cumulative risk for leukaemia was 1.1 per cent at 15 years, which is less than has been reported with MOPP.

Experiences in reducing therapy

The potential sequelae and mechanisms discussed above have been taken into account in designing paediatric protocols since the late 1970s. Since both radiotherapy and chemotherapy are characterized by their well known efficacy and late effects, the problem is to retain the former while avoiding the latter. In discussing the strategies for decreasing treatment, experience differs from one team or group to another; this is summarized in Table 14.5.

CLINICAL STAGING

As has been stated, we now assume laparotomy and splenectomy to be unnecessary procedures, taking into consideration cost and the efficacy of chemotherapy to treat occult infradiaphragmatic disease.

THE REDUCTION OF RADIATION FIELDS

The introduction of effective primary chemotherapy has allowed limitation of the volume of irradiation. In the Intergroup Study of Hodgkin's disease in children with pathological stage I or II, a randomized three-arm study

Table 14.5 *Experiences in reducing therapy*

Institution	No. of patients	Dates	Staging	Therapy OS (%)	Results FFS	(%)
Series with high-dose involved field radiotherapy + chemotherapy						
Intergroup Hodgkin's disease study	279	1975–81	PS I–II	IF RT		41
				EF RT	93	67
				IF RT + 6 MOPP		95
France Villejuif	60	1975–80	CS I–IV	6 MOPP + IF RT	93	86
Series with low-dose radiotherapy + MOPP or procarbazine-containing chemotherapy						
Stanford	55	1970–83	PS I–II	6 MOPP + modif IF	100	96
			PS III–IV	+ EF	78	84
Toronto	57	1973–79	CS I–III	6 MOPP + EF RT	92	88
			CS IV	6 MOPP + EF RT	85	65
France SFOP	67	1982–88	CSIA–IIA	2 MOPP + 2 ABVD + 20 Gy IF	92	88
	71		CS IB–IIB–III	3 MOPP + 3 ABVD + 20 Gy IF	95	86
	21		CS IV	3 MOPP + 3 ABVD + 20 Gy IF	73	62
Italy	87	1983–87	CS IIA (M/T > 0.33)	3 MOPP + 3 ABVD + 20/25 Gy EF		81
			CS III	3 MOPP + 3 ABVD + 20/25 Gy EF		
			CS IIIB–IV	5 MOPP + 5 ABVD + 20/25 Gy EF		
Germany HD82	207	1982–84	Selective splenectomy		95	
			CS I–IIA	2 OPPA + 35 Gy IF		98
			CS IIB–III	2 OPPA + 2 COPP + 30 Gy IF		94
			CS III–IV	2 OPPA + 4 COPP + 20 Gy IF		86
Germany DAL- HD90	578	1990-1995	CS I–IIA	2 OPPA + 25 Gy IF	91	95
			CS IIA–IIIA	2 OPPA + 2 COPP + 25 Gy		96
			CS IIB–IV	2 OPPA + 4 COPP + 20 Gy		89
Philadelphia	29	1991–1994	CS I–IIA	4 COPP/ABV + 20–24 Gy	93	82
			CS IIB–III	6 COPP/ABV + 20–24 Gy		
			CS IV	8 COPP/ABV		
Series with radiotherapy + chemotherapy without alkylating agents						
France SFOP	66	1982–88	CS IA–IIA	4 ABVD + 20 Gy IF	100	91
Italy	83	1983–89	CS IA–IIA (M/T < 0.33)	3 ABVD + 20/25 Gy IF	97	95
Milan	39	1979–85	CS IA–IIA	3 ABVD + 30/35 Gy EF		97
			CS IB–IIB–III	6 ABVD + 30/35 Gy EF		
Germany HD85	98	1985–86	Selective laparotomy		93	
			CS I–IIA2	OPA + 35 Gy IF		85
			CS IIB–IIIA	2 OPA + 2 COMP + 30 Gy IF		55
			CS IIIB–IV	2 OPA + 4 COMP + 25 Gy IF		49
French HDH90	202	1990–96	CS IA–IIB	4 VBVP + 20 Gy IF		91
Series with chemotherapy alone						
Holland	21	1975–84	CS I–III (<4 cm)	6–12 MOPP	100	90
UKCCSG	282	1982–84	CS I–IV	6–8 ChlVPP (+RT large med.)	91	73
Australia	53	1978	CS I–IV	4–12 ChlVPP or MOPP	94	92
Holland	21	1988–93	CS I–IV	3 MOPP + 3 ABVD		90

ABVD, adriamycin + bleomycin + vinblastine + DTIC; ChlVPP, chlorambucil + vinblastine + procarbazine + prednisone; COMP, cyclophosphamide + Oncovin + methotrexate + prednisone; COPP, cyclophosphamide + Oncovin + procarbazine + prednisone; CS, clinically staged; EF, extended field; FFS, failure-free survival; for IB–IIB–III, total lymphoid RT; IF, involved field; M/T, mediastinum/thoracic ratio; modif IF, for IA–IIA: IF 'according to Rye symposium'; MOPP, mechlorethamine + Oncovin + procarbazine + prednisone; OPA, Oncovin + prednisone + adriamycin; OPPA, Oncovin + procarbazine + prednisone + adriamycin; PS, pathologically staged; RT, radiotherapy; OS, overall survival.
Data are from Landman-Parker et al.,[21] Ekert et al.,[43] Radford et al.,[67] Vecchi et al.,[71] Schellong et al.,[74,93] Gehan et al.,[88] Oberlin et al.,[46,95] Donaldson and Link,[89] Jenkin et al.,[90] Hamilton et al.,[91] Fossati-Bellani et al.,[96] Behrendt et al.,[98] van den Berg et al.[99]

compared involved-field radiotherapy, extended-field radiotherapy and involved-field radiotherapy followed by six courses of MOPP.[88] There was no significant difference in survival; however, the disease-free survival (DFS) in the MOPP arm was excellent (93 per cent) at 5 years, contrasting with 67 per cent for the first arm and 41 per cent for extended-field radiation therapy. In the first paediatric study by the Institut Gustave-Roussy, 60 children were treated by involved-field radiation after three or six courses of MOPP. In the group of 60 patients, the 5-year survival was 93 per cent, and the DFS was 86 per cent with only two relapses outside the irradiated area.[46]

THE REDUCTION OF RADIATION DOSES

This was first proposed by both the Stanford group and the Toronto team. In Stanford, after systematic splenectomy, 54 children were given six courses of MOPP; radiation doses were then decided according to the age [ranging from 1500 to 2500 rads (15 to 25 Gy)] and the response to treatment, with boosts often being added. Radiation ports were determined by the pathological staging: involved-field irradiation was given in stages IA–IIA; fields were more extended for patients with extranodal extension; and total nodal irradiation was given to children with B symptoms or stage III disease.[89] In the

Canadian series reported by Jenkin *et al.*,[90] radiation was given in extended fields with six courses of MOPP. Both these series had the same good results as those using high-dose radiotherapy.

Other national studies in Italy and France, on larger groups of patients, have confirmed the efficacy of low-dose radiation.[91] In these studies, radiation doses were tailored according to the response to primary chemotherapy. A dose of 20 Gy was given if complete remission was achieved or if the mass reduction was estimated to be at least 70 per cent of the initial mass. As is now clear, residual mass does not always indicate active disease. In the French study, radiation volume was limited to the areas strictly involved in stages IA–IIA–III and IV, but also encompassed a lumbosplenic field in stages IB–IIB (Table 14.5). With a median follow-up ranging from 1 to 7.5 years (median 4 years) the updated results show that at 5 years, OS is 92 per cent, and DFS is 86.5 per cent (Figure 14.9). According to the stage, the DFS is 90 per cent for stages IA–IIA, 86 per cent for stages IB–IIB–III, and 62 per cent for stage IV (Figure 14.10). A subsequent larger European cooperative study carried out by the International Society of Paediatric Oncology (SIOP) has confirmed these results, limiting the radiation dose to 20 Gy for good responders.[92]

In the Italian protocol, involved fields are only used in stages I and IIA without extensive mediastinal involvement.

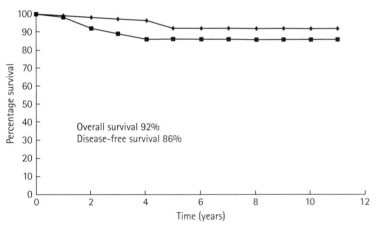

Figure 14.9 *Survival and disease-free survival for the 238 children included in the French study (personal communication).*

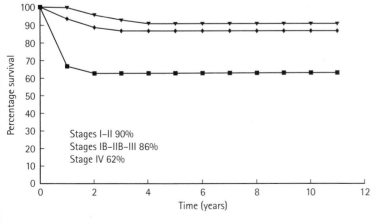

Figure 14.10 *Relapse-free survival according to stage for the 238 children involved in the French study (personal communication).*

Freedom from progression survival is 95 per cent at 7 years.[69]

In the German studies HD 82, HD 85 and HD 87, the radiation doses given were dependent on the duration of the preceding chemotherapy: 35 Gy in stages I–IIA after two cycles; 30 Gy in stages IIB–IIIA after four cycles; and 25 Gy after six cycles, with similar excellent results.[93] In HD 95 a response-adapted approach to chemotherapy determined the subsequent dose and volume of radiotherapy administered. This enabled a reduction in dosage for all patients achieving a good partial response, but also highlighted the need for radiotherapy in patients who had advanced disease. Many of these obtained a complete remission (CR), did not receive radiotherapy and subsequently relapsed.[94] The 5-year EFS for the whole group was maintained at 91 per cent, and OS at 98 per cent.

All these studies clearly demonstrate that low-dose radiotherapy can be safely used to cure patients after effective primary chemotherapy. The French study also gives a clear indication that chemotherapy can be limited to four cycles rather than six in an attempt to minimize the drug-related sequelae. In the same study, the response to primary chemotherapy appeared as a very strong prognostic indicator in terms of survival and DFS. The EFS of good responders (>70 per cent regression) was 89 per cent, whereas it was only 18 per cent for the poorly responding patients.[95] Stage IV patients have a lower DFS than those in the other stages. However, after adjustment for response to chemotherapy, extranodal involvement is not more predictive of outcome.

THE USE OF NON-TOXIC CHEMOTHERAPY

The next challenge in the treatment of children with Hodgkin's disease was to reduce exposure to MOPP, in order to minimize the late effects of sterility and acute leukaemias. The results reported initially in Milan have since been confirmed by many groups. The previously mentioned French study demonstrated, in a randomized trial, that four cycles of ABVD are equivalent to two of MOPP plus two of ABVD in localized stages.[95] The national Italian group and the Milan paediatric team confirmed the efficacy of ABVD in a non-randomized study.[69,96]

One of the aims of the German study, begun in 1985, was to eliminate procarbazine. One result was that the OPPA regimen became OPA, and methotrexate replaced the procarbazine in the COPP combination, resulting in the COMP regimen. Disease progression and relapse were significantly higher than in the preceding study (HD 82) in stages IE and IIE–IIIA, and the study was prematurely stopped, highlighting the need for an effective drug to replace procarbazine.[49]

Very few drugs are both non-toxic (or have acceptable toxicity) and active in Hodgkin's disease. Single-drug

phase II studies are difficult to carry out because of the small number of relapsing patients and the existing concept of giving combination chemotherapy as a salvage regimen. However, the French group has reported the use of a drug combination that is devoid of alkylating agents, vinblastine, bleomycin, etoposide (VP-16) and prednisolone (VBVP). Radiotherapy dosing was dependent on chemotherapy response, poor responders going on to receive OPPA. Radiotherapy doses were 20 Gy for good responders and 40 Gy for poor responders. The overall 5-year survival rate (mean ± SD) was 97.5 ± 2.1 per cent. These results suggest that most children with stage I and II Hodgkin's disease can be treated without alkylating agents and anthracyclines prior to low-dose radiotherapy.[21] An alternative UK regimen, VEEP (vincristine, epirubicin, etoposide, prednisolone), without routine radiotherapy appeared to be less effective than Chl VPP.[97]

THE OPTION OF USING CHEMOTHERAPY ALONE

The option of treating children without the use of radiotherapy has been taken up by some teams. In all these studies, patients are given six cycles of chemotherapy. In the Dutch study on a small group of patients, additional radiation therapy was given only to large lymph node tumours (>4 cm).[98,99] In the Australian study, no additional irradiation was used.[43] In the UK study, only patients with a large mediastinum received 35 Gy after the chemotherapy.[44] All these series are based on alkylating and procarbazine-containing chemotherapy, with its well known risks of late sterility and secondary leukaemia. Another question of concern about such strategies is the proportion of relapsing patients who will be cured after heavy salvage therapy and the sequelae of their whole treatment.

Treatment of advanced, resistant and relapsing cases

Stage IV disease patients have a poor prognosis according to many of the paediatric series published. DFS at 5 years ranges from 41 to 61 per cent in several studies.[44,91,95] The best paediatric results have been reported by the German study, in which 31 patients had an 81 per cent EFS.[99] A European cooperative study is being carried out by SIOP (International Society of Paediatric Oncology) to confirm these excellent results on a larger group of patients, limiting the radiation dose to 20 Gy for good responders.

Patients who fail to achieve CR or who relapse after an initial response to chemotherapy have a poor prognosis. The complete remission rate with further chemotherapy is around 50 per cent whatever the combination of non-cross-resistant drugs given. Various combinations of chemotherapy have been explored – including prednisolone, doxorubicin, bleomycin, vincristine and etoposide (PABIOE);[100,101] bleomycin, etoposide, adriamycin cyclophosphamide, vincristine, procarbazine and prednisolone (BEACOPP);[102] adriamycin, methylprednisolone, Ara-C and cisplatin (ASHAP);[103] etoposide, prednisolone and cisplatin (EPIC);[104] and mitoxantrone, fluoraline, cytarabine and cisplatin (MIFAP)[105] – in an attempt to achieve a CR prior to high-dose chemotherapy as the cure rate is low with conventional salvage therapy.

The therapeutic approach of high-dose chemotherapy with bone marrow rescue has shown good results in adults and initial results reported in a French paediatric study[106] were promising and have led to what is now accepted practice for patients with relapsed or refractory disease. In the adult population, the efficacy of an early high-dose chemotherapeutic approach for poor responders or relapsed disease has been confirmed.[107,108] Baker et al.[109] reported the outcome of 53 paediatric patients receiving high-dose chemotherapy who had a failure-free survival at 5 years of 31 per cent. Prognostic factors were a normal lactate dehydrogenase (LDH) prior to transplantation and disease sensitivity. The conditioning regimen used was cyclophosphamide, carmustine and etoposide.

CURRENT CONTROVERSIES

PROGNOSTIC FACTORS

Poor response to initial therapy and raised LDH are associated with a poor outcome. The former may be the best way to stratify patients. The use of PET imaging may lead to more accurate response definition.

WHAT IS THE OPTIMAL MANAGEMENT OF EARLY STAGE DISEASE?

One of the main therapeutic aims in childhood Hodgkin's disease is to minimize late toxicity without compromising the cure rate. What is optimal treatment for early stage disease in paediatric practice is a much debated topic, with some groups going as far as to adopt a wait-and-watch approach to totally excised stage I lymphocytic-predominant disease. In stage I disease, the current 5-year DFS is comparable for radiotherapy alone, combined radiotherapy/chemotherapy and chemotherapy ranging from 88 to 100 per cent.[110,111] The impact of age, histology and predictions of late effects have all been considered in the decision-making for this group.

Donaldson et al.[112] reviewed the treatment policies of two large centres comparing pathological staging and extended-field radiotherapy with clinical staging and involved-field radiotherapy. As one would predict, there was a higher relapse rate in stage I patients treated by clinical staging and involved-field radiotherapy; the critical

point, however, was that the OS of both groups was the same.

WHEN IS RADIOTHERAPY INDICATED?

The whole question of the necessity of radiotherapy in patients who achieve a CR after risk-adapted chemotherapy is under review. Nachman et al.[113] have reported no survival advantage for patients who receive low-dose involved-field radiotherapy when CR is attained following risk-adapted chemotherapy, although the follow-up time is short.

WHEN IS RADIOTHERAPY INDICATED IN SUPRADIAPHRAGMATIC STAGE II DISEASE?

It has been suggested that there is a good case for post-chemotherapy radiotherapy for patients presenting with large mediastinal masses.[114] Radiation portals of less than a full mantle may be advantageous,[115] but Ekert et al.[43] have produced good relapse-free survival data using chemotherapy alone in this situation. Moreover, omission of radiotherapy from a ChlVPP-based regimen in children with bulky mediastinal disease has no adverse effect on outcome (HD9201 and HD8201) (unpublished data). Increased use of FDG-PET scanning may help to refine exactly how much treatment is needed for mediastinal masses.

THE MOVE AGAINST ALKYLATING AGENT CHEMOTHERAPY

In a recent report from the United States Children's Cancer Study Group (USCCSG), 64 children with advanced Hodgkin's disease were treated with ABVD (12 courses) followed by low-dose regional radiotherapy. The EFS and OS were 87 per cent at 3 years.[116] The pulmonary toxicity rate of 9 per cent could be reduced by using less bleomycin. Why are the groups still studying a hybrid regimen of MOPP/ABVD when there are excellent results with a non-alkylating agent regimen? Is it the fear of late cardiotoxicity? Is it a fear that salvageability with MOPP after ABVD therapy may be less than expected?

Also relevant here is the use of etoposide in front-line Hodgkin's chemotherapy regimens. It is included in VEEP (vincristine, epirubicin, etoposide, prednisolone), which has been the first-line chemotherapy regimen of some UK and Australian groups.[97] A review of 54 children treated with VEEP has reported an OS and 5-year progression-free survival (PFS) for stage I–III patients of 93 and 82 per cent, respectively. However, for stage IV patients, OS and 5-year PFS were 44 and 50 per cent, respectively. Only 50 per cent of patients were salvageable by second-line therapy and this makes VEEP inadequate for stage IV patients.[117] In addition, there is the worrying aspect of reports of late acute myeloblastic leukaemia following etoposide therapy.

THE DOSE AND THE PLACE OF RADIOTHERAPY IN ADVANCED DISEASE

A radical dose of radiotherapy for childhood Hodgkin's disease would be 30 Gy over 3 weeks, conventionally fractionated to 35 Gy for bulk disease. There is, however, accumulating evidence that lower doses are effective when used after 'chemotherapeutic debulking'.[89] Whether such low-dose radiotherapy has a routine role in the management of patients presenting with advanced disease and bulky presentation sites is open to question, but some groups do this routinely.[116]

THE ROLE OF MEGATHERAPY AND BONE MARROW TRANSPLANTATION IN RELAPSE

Following relapse after primary chemotherapy where remission is achieved by further chemotherapy (chemosensitive disease) and in patients failing to achieve remission with primary chemotherapy (primarily chemorefractory disease), there is increasing evidence to support the use of megatherapy. However, the timing of such treatment and the ideal high-dose regimen still remain to be defined.

KEY POINTS

- The cure rate for Hodgkin's disease at 5 years is 95–100 per cent.
- Present treatment exposes patients to significant adverse late effects 10–20 years after treatment.
- Second malignancies are the most common adverse late effect, after infertility, with a cumulative risk of 6.5 per cent above the normal population at 20 years. These malignancies include breast, leukaemia, thyroid, bone/soft tissue, stomach and oesophagus, all of which are related to radiotherapy exposure.
- Optimum use of radiotherapy and chemotherapy needs further investigation
- Robust methods for assessing disease at diagnosis and response to treatment are needed.
- Biological prognostic indicators require further investigation
- Accurate patient grouping would allow the development of risk-adapted treatment strategies.

- Radiotherapy can be omitted in low-stage patients, with low-dose involved-field radiotherapy used to cure higher-stage patients.
- Appropriate chemotherapy regimens need to be developed alongside new radiotherapeutic strategies. Chemotherapy should exclude mechlorethamine, and procarbazine in boys, while limiting cumulative doses of alkylating agents, anthracyclines, etoposide and bleomycin.
- The ideal duration of chemotherapy has yet to be defined.
- An EFS >90 per cent should be the aim in view of the higher risk of second malignancies induced by salvage therapy.
- Combination low-dose involved-field radiotherapy with multiagent chemotherapy is the present mainstay of treatment for Hodgkin's disease.

REFERENCES

1. Dielh V, Von Kalle C, Fontash C et al. The cell of origin in Hodgkin's disease. Semin Oncol 1990; **17**: 660–72.
2. Alexander FE, Williams J, McKinney PA et al. A specialist leukaemia/lymphoma registry in the UK. Part 2: Clustering of Hodgkin's disease. Br J Cancer 1989; **60**: 948–52.
3. Guthenson N, Cole P. Childhood social environment and Hodgkin's disease. N Engl J Med 1981; **304**: 135–40.
4. Guthenson N, Cole P. Epidemiology of Hodgkin's disease. Semin Oncol 1980; **7**: 92–102.
5. Levine PH, Ablashi DV, Berard CW et al. Elevated antibody titers to Epstein Barr virus in Hodgkin's disease. Cancer 1971; **27**: 416–21.
6. Herbst H, Niedobitek G, Kneba M et al. High incidence of Epstein Barr virus genomes in Hodgkin's disease. Am J Pathol 1990; **137**: 13–18.
7. Jarrett R, Dones D, Gallagher A et al. Clonal EBV genomes are detectable in biopsy from the majority of older and paediatric Hodgkin's disease patients. J Pathol 1991; **163**: 169A.
8. Wright CF, Reid AH, Tsai MM et al. Detection of Epstein Barr virus sequences in Hodgkin's disease by the polymerase chain reaction. Am J Pathol 1991; **139**: 393–8.
9. Weinreb M, Dat PJR, Niggli F et al. The role of Epstein-Barr virus in Hodgkin's disease from different geographical areas. Arch Dis Child 1996; **74**: 27–31.
10. Glaser SL, Lin LJ, Stewart SL et al. Epstein-Barr virus associated Hodgkin's disease: epidemiologic characteristics in international data. Int J Cancer 1997; **70**: 375–82.
11. Mueller BU, Pizzo PA. Cancer in children with primary or secondary immunodeficiencies. J Pediatr 1995; **126**: 1–10.
12. Robinson LL, Stoker V, Frizzera G et al. Hodgkin's disease in pediatric patients with naturally occurring immunodeficiency. Am J Pediatr Hematol Oncol 1987; **9**: 189–92.
13. Svejgraad A, Platz P, Ryder LP et al. HLA and disease association. A survey. Transplant Rep 1975; **22**: 3–73.

14. Grufferman S, Cole P, Smith P, Lukes RJ. Hodgkin's disease in siblings. *N Engl J Med* 1979; **300**: 1006–11.

15. Swerdlow AJ, De Stavola B, Maconochie N et al. A population based study of cancer risk in twins: relationships to birth order and sexes of the twin pair. *Int J Cancer* 1996; **67**: 472–8.

16. Mack TM, Cozen W, Shibata DK et al. Concordance for Hodgkin's disease in identical twins suggesting genetic susceptibility to the young-adult form of the disease. *N Engl J Med* 1995; **332**: 413–18.

17. Parkin DM, Stiller CA, Draper GJ et al. *International Incidence of Childhood Cancer*. IARC Scientific Publications No 87. Lyon: IARC, 1988.

18. Stiller CA. What causes Hodgkin's disease in children? Review. *Eur J Cancer* 1998; **34**: 523–8.

19. Lukes RJ, Craver LF, Hall TC et al. Report of the nomenclature committee. *Cancer Res* 1966; **26**: 1311.

20. Shankar AG, Ashley S, Radford M et al. Does histology influence outcome in childhood Hodgkin's disease? Results from the United Kingdom Children's Cancer Study Group. *J Clin Oncol* 1997; **15**: 2622–30.

●21. Landman-Parker J, Pacquement H, Leblanc T et al. Localized childhood Hodgkin's disease: response-adapted chemotherapy with etoposide, bleomycin, vinblastine, and prednisolone before low-dose radiation therapy – results of the French Society of Pediatric Oncology Study MDH90. *J Clin Oncol* 2000; **18**: 1500–7.

22. Lukes RJ, Butler JJ. The pathology and nomenclature of Hodgkin's disease. *Cancer Res* 1966; **26**: 1063–81.

23. Trudel MA, Krikorian JG, Neiman RS. Lymphocytic predominance in Hodgkin's disease: a clinicopathologic reassessment. *Cancer* 1987; **59**: 99–106.

24. Thangavelu M, LeBeau MM. Chromosomal abnormalities in Hodgkin's disease. *Hematol Oncol Clin North Am* 1989; **3**: 221–36.

25. Fonatsch C, Gradel G, Rademacher J. Genetics of Hodgkin's lymphoma. In: Dielh V, Pfreundschuh M, Loeffler M, eds. *New Aspects in the Diagnosis and Treatment of Hodgkin's Disease*. Berlin: Springer, 1989; 35–9.

26. Bendini M, Zuiani C, Bazzocchi M et al. Magnetic resonance imaging and 67 Ga scan versus computed tomography in the staging and in the monitoring of mediastinal malignant lymphoma: a prospective pilot study. *MAGMA* 1996; **4**: 213–24.

27. Drossman SR, Schiff RG, Kronfeld GD et al. Lymphoma of the mediastinum and neck: evaluation with Ga-67 imaging and CT correlation. *Radiology* 1990; **174**: 171–5.

28. Devizzi L, Maffioli, L, Bonfante V et al. Comparison of gallium scan, computed tomography, and magnetic resonance in patients with mediastinal Hodgkin's disease. *Ann Oncol* 1997; **8**(Suppl. 1): 53–6.

29. Ha CS, Choe J, Kong JS et al. Agreement rates among single photon emission computed tomography using gallium-76, computed axial tomography and lymphangiography for Hodgkin Disease and correlation of image findings with clinical outcome. *Cancer* 2000; **89**: 1371–9.

30. De Wit M, Bohuslavizki KH, Buchert R et al. ¹⁸FDG-PET following treatment as valid predictor for disease-free survival in Hodgkin's lymphoma. *Ann Oncol* 2001; **12**: 29–37.

31. Weidmann E, Baican B, Hertel A et al. Positron emission tomography (PET) for staging and evaluation of response to treatment in patients with Hodgkin's Disease. *Leuk Lymphoma* 1999; **34**: 545–51.

32. Kostakoglu L, Leonard J, Kuji I et al. Comparison of fluorine-18 fluorodeoxyglucose positron emission tomography and Ga-67 scintigraphy in evaluation of lymphoma. *Cancer* 2002; **94**: 879–88.

33. Naumann R, Vaic A, Beuthien-Baumann B et al. Prognostic value of positron emission tomography in the evaluation of post-treatment residual mass in patients with Hodgkin's disease and non-Hodgkin's lymphoma. *Br J Haematol* 2001; **11**: 793–800.

34. Dunnick NR, Parker BR, Castellino RA. Pediatric lymphography: performance, interpretation and accuracy in 193 consecutive children. *AJR Am J Roentgenol* 1977; **129**: 639–45.

35. Andrieu JM, Asselain B, Bayle CH et al. La séquence polychimiothérapie MOPP-irradiation ganglionnaire sélective dans le traitement de la maladie de Hodgkin, stades cliniques IA-IIIB. *Bull Cancer* 1981; **68**: 190–9.

36. Russell KR, Donaldson SS, Cox RS, Kaplan HS. Childhood Hodgkin's disease: patterns of relapse. *J Clin Oncol* 1984; **2**: 80–7.

37. Jenkin RD, Berry MP. Hodgkin's disease in children. *Semin Oncol* 1980; **7**: 202–11.

38. Desser RK, Ultmann JE. Risk of severe infection in patients with Hodgkin's disease or lymphoma after diagnostic laparotomy and splenectomy. *Ann Intern Med* 1972; **77**: 143–6.

39. Rosenstock JG, D'Angio GJ, Kiesewetter WB. The incidence of complications following staging laparotomy for Hodgkin's disease in children. *Radiology* 1974; **120**: 531–5.

40. Chilcote RR, Baehner RL, Hammond D and Children's Cancer Study Group. Septicemia and meningitis in children splenectomized for Hodgkin's disease. *N Engl J Med* 1976; **295**: 798–800.

41. Donaldson SS, Glatestein E, Vosti KL. Bacterial infection in pediatric Hodgkin's disease: relationship to radiotherapy, chemotherapy and splenectomy. *Cancer* 1978; **41**: 1949–58.

42. Siber GR, Weitzman SA, Aisenberg AC et al. Impaired antibody response to pneumococcal vaccine after treatment for Hodgkin's disease. *N Engl J Med* 1978; **299**: 442–8.

43. Ekert H, Waters KD, Smith PJ et al. Treatment with MOPP or ChIVPP chemotherapy only for all stages of childhood Hodgkin's disease. *J Clin Oncol* 1988; **6**: 1845–50.

44. Martin J, Radford M. Current practice in Hodgkin's disease. The United Kingdom Children's Cancer Study Group. In: Kampo WA, Humphrey GB, Poppema S, eds. *Hodgkin's Disease in Children: Controversies and Current Practice*. Boston: Kluwer Academic, 1989; 263–75.

45. Loeffler M, Pfreundschuh M, Rühl U et al. Risk factor adapted treatment of Hodgkin's lymphoma: strategies and perspectives. In: Dielh V, Pfreundschuh M, Loeffler M, eds. *New Aspects in the Diagnosis and Treatment of Hodgkin's Disease*. Berlin: Springer, 1989; 142–62.

46. Oberlin O, Boilletot A, Leverger G et al. Clinical staging, primary chemotherapy and involved field radiotherapy in childhood Hodgkin's disease. *Eur Paediatr Hematol Oncol* 1985; **2**: 65–70.

47. Leverger G, Oberlin O, Quintana E et al. ABVD vs MOPP/ABVD before low-dose radiotherapy in CS IA–IIA childhood Hodgkin's disease: a prospective randomized trial from the French Society of Paediatric Oncology. Proc Am Soc Clin Oncol 1990; 9: 1060.

48. Vecchi V, Pileri S, Burnelli R et al. Treatment of pediatric Hodgkin disease tailored to stage, mediastinal mass, and age. An Italian (AIEOP) multicenter study on 215 patients. Cancer 1993; 72(6): 2049–57.

49. Brämswig JH, Hörnig-Franz I, Reipenhausen M, Schellong G. The challenge of pediatric Hodgkin's disease: where is the balance between cure and long-term toxicity? Leuk Lymphoma 1990; 3: 183–93.

50. Mefferd JM, Donaldson SS, Link MP. Pediatric HD. Pulmonary, cardiac and thyroid function following combined modality therapy. Int J Radiat Oncol Biol Phys 1989; 16: 679–85.

51. Schicha H, Franke M, Smolorz J et al. Diagnostic strategies and staging procedure for Hodgkin's lymphoma: bone marrow scintigraphy and magnetic resonance imaging. In: Dielh V, Pfreundschuh M, Loeffler M, eds. New Aspects in the Diagnosis and Treatment of Hodgkin's Disease. Berlin: Springer, 1989; 112–19.

52. Carbone PP, Kaplan HS, Musshof K et al. Report of the committee on Hodgkin's disease staging. Cancer Res 1971; 31: 1860–1.

53. Tubiana M, Henry-Amar M, Burgers MV et al. Prognostic significance of ESR in clinical stages I and II Hodgkin's disease. J Clin Oncol 1984; 2: 194–200.

54. Hrgovcic M, Tessmer CF, Thomas FB et al. Significance of serum copper in adult patients with Hodgkin's disease. Cancer 1973; 31: 1337–45.

55. Pui CH, Ip SH, Thompson E et al. Increased serum CD8 antigen level in childhood Hodgkin's disease relates to advanced stage and poor treatment outcome. Blood 1989; 73: 209–13.

56. Bohlen H, Kessler M, Sextro M et al. Poor clinical outcome of patients with Hodgkin's Disease and elevated interleukin-10 serum levels. Ann Hematol 2000; 79: 110–13.

57. Kaplan HS. On the natural history, treatment and prognosis of HD. Harvey Lectures, 1968–1969. New York: Academic Press, 1970; 251–9.

58. Donaldson S, Kleeberg P, Cox R. Growth abnormalities with radiation in children with HD. Proc Am Soc Clin Oncol 1988; 7: 864.

59. Sklar C, Whitton J, Mertens A et al. Abnormalities of the thyroid in survivors of Hodgkin's disease: Data from the childhood cancer survivor study. J Clin Endocrinol Metab 2000; 85: 3227–32.

60. Smith RE, Adler RA, Clark P et al. Thyroid function after mantle irradiation in HD. J Am Med Assoc 1981; 245: 46–9.

61. Green DM, Brecher ML, Yakar D et al. Thyroid function in pediatric patients after neck irradiation for HD. Med Pediatr Oncol 1984; 8: 127–36.

62. Meadows A, Obringer A, Marrero O et al. Second malignant neoplasms following childhood Hodgkin's disease: treatment and splenectomy as risk factors. Med Pediatr Oncol 1989; 17: 477–84.

63. Cosset JM, Henry-Amar M, Meerwaldt JH. Long-term toxicity of early stages of Hodgkin's disease therapy: the EORTC experience. EORTC Lymphoma Cooperative Group. Ann Oncol 1991; 2(suppl. 2): 77–82.

64. Green D, Gingell R, Pearce J et al. Evaluation of cardiac function in patients treated with mediastinal irradiation during childhood and adolescence for HD. Proc Am Soc Clin Oncol 1985; 4: C-818.

65. Carbone PP. The role of chemotherapy in the management of patients with Hodgkin's disease. Ann Intern Med 1967; 67: 433–7.

66. De Vita VT, Serpick A, Carbone PP. Combination chemotherapy in the treatment of advanced HD. Ann Intern Med 1970; 73: 881–95.

67. Radford M, Barrett A, Martin J, Cotterill S. Treatment of Hodgkin's disease in children. Study HDI. Med Pediatr Oncol 1991; 19: 400.

68. Schellong G. Pediatric Hodgkin's disease: treatment in the late 1990s. Ann Oncol 1998; 9(Suppl. 5): S115–19.

69. Bonadonna G, Valagussa P, Santoro A et al. Hodgkin's disease: the Milan experience with MOPP and AVBD. In: Dielh V, Pfreundschuh M, Loeffler M, eds. New Aspects in the Diagnosis and Treatment of Hodgkin's Disease. Berlin: Springer, 1989; 169–74.

●70. Van de Berg, Stuve W, Behrendt H. Treatment of Hodgkin's disease in children with alternating mechlorethamine, vincristine, procarbazine, and prednisolone (MOPP) and adriamycin, bleomycin, vinblastine, and dacarbazine (ABVD) courses without radiotherapy. Med Pediatr Oncol 1997; 29: 23–7.

71. Vecchi V, Pileri S, Burnelli R et al. Treatment of pediatric Hodgkin disease tailored to stage, mediastinal mass, and age. An Italian (AIEOP) multicenter study on 215 patients. Cancer 1993; 72: 2049–57.

72. Viviani S, Bonadonna G, Santoro A et al. Alternating versus hybrid MOPP and ABVD combination in advanced Hodgkin's disease: ten year results. J Clin Oncol 1996; 14: 1421–30.

73. Aubier F, Flamant F, Brauner R et al. Male gonadal function after chemotherapy for solid tumours in childhood. J Clin Oncol 1989; 7: 304–9.

●74. Schellong G, Pötter R, Brämswig J et al. High cure rates and reduced long-term toxicity in pediatric Hodgkin's Disease: The German-Austrian multicenter trial DAL-HD-90. J Clin Oncol 1999; 17: 3736–44.

75. Donaldson SS, Kaplan HS. Complications of treatment of Hodgkin's disease in children. Cancer Treat Rep 1982; 66: 977–89.

76. Pereyra Pacheco BP, Méndez Ribas JM, Milone G et al. Use of GnRH analogs for functional protection of the ovary and preservation of fertility during cancer treatment in adolescents: a preliminary report. Gynecol Oncol 2001; 81: 391–7.

77. Cosset JM, Henry-Amar M, Thomas J et al. Increased pulmonary toxicity in the ABVD arm of the EORTC H6-U Trial. Proc Am Soc Clin Oncol 1989; 8: 985.

78. Villani F, De Maria P, Bonfante V et al. Late pulmonary toxicity after treatment for Hodgkin's disease. Anticancer Res 1997; 17: 4739–42.

79. Bhatia S, Robison LI, Oberlin O et al. Breast cancer and other second neoplasms after childhood Hodgkin's disease. N Engl J Med 1996; 334: 745–51.

80. Walden SW, Lamborn KR, Cleary SF *et al.* Second cancers following pediatric Hodgkin's Disease. *J Clin Oncol* 1998; **16**: 536–44.

81. Green DM, Hyland A, Barcos MP *et al.* Second malignant neoplasms after treatment for Hodgkin's disease in childhood or adolescence. *J Clin Oncol* 2000; **18**: 1492–9.

82. Cutuli B, Borel C, Dhermain F *et al.* Breast cancer occurred after treatment for Hodgkin's disease: analysis of 133 cases. *Radiat Oncol* 2001; **59**: 247–55.

83. Hudson MM, Poquette CA, Lee J *et al.* Increased mortality after successful treatment for Hodgkin's disease. *J Clin Oncol* 1998; **16**: 3592–600.

♦84. Metayer C, Lynch FC, Clarke AE *et al.* Second cancers among long-term survivors of Hodgkin's Disease diagnosed in childhood and adolescence. *J Clin Oncol* 2000; **18**: 2435–43.

85. Bhatia S, Yasui Y, Robison LL *et al.* High risk of subsequent neoplasms continues with extended follow-up of childhood Hodgkin's disease: report from the Late Effects Study Group. *J Clin Oncol* 2003; **21**: 4386–94.

86. Valagussa P, Santora A, Foassati-Bellani F *et al.* Second acute leukaemia and other malignancies following treatment for Hodgkin's disease. *J Clin Oncol* 1986; **4**: 830–7.

87. Schellong G, Riepenhausen M, Creutig U *et al.* Low risk of secondary leukaemia after chemotherapy without mechlorethamine in childhood Hodgkin's disease. German-Austrian Pediatric Hodgkin's Disease Group. *J Clin Oncol* 1997; **15**: 2247–53.

♦88. Gehan EA, Sullivan MP, Fuller LM *et al.* The intergroup HD in children. A study of stages I and II. *Cancer* 1990; **65**: 1429–37.

●89. Donaldson SS, Link MP. Combined modality treatment with low dose radiation and MOPP chemotherapy for children with Hodgkin's disease. *J Clin Oncol* 1987; **5**: 742–9.

90. Jenkin RD, Chan H, Freeman M *et al.* Hodgkin's disease in children: treatment results with MOPP and low-dose, extended field irradiation. *Cancer Treat Rep* 1982; **66**: 949–59.

91. Hamilton VJ, Norris C, Bunin N *et al.* Cyclophosphamide-based, seven-drug hybrid and low-dose involved field radiation for the treatment of childhood and adolescent Hodgkin disease. *J Pediatr Hematol Oncol* 2001; **23**: 84–8.

92. Schellong G, Oberlin O, Riepenhausen M *et al.* Stage IV childhood Hodgkin's disease: updated results of the SIOP collaborative study. Abstr. 59. *Med Pediatr Oncol* 1997; **29**: 332.

93. Schellong G, Brämswig JH, Hörnig-Franz I. Treatment of children with Hodgkin's disease. Results of the German Pediatric Oncology Group. *Ann Oncol* 1992; **3**: S73–6.

●94. Rühl U, Albrecht M, Dieckmann K *et al.* Response-adapted radiotherapy in the treatment of pediatric Hodgkin's Disease: an interim report at 5 years of the German GPOH-HD 95 trial. *Int J Radiat Oncol Biol Phys* 2001; **52**: 1209–18.

95. Oberlin O, Leverger G, Paquement H *et al.* Low-dose radiation therapy and reduced chemotherapy in childhood Hodgkin's disease. The experience of the French Society of Paediatric Oncology. *J Clin Oncol* 1992; **10**: 1602–8.

96. Fossati-Bellani F, Gasparini M, Kenda A *et al.* Limited field and low-dose radiotherapy + ABVD chemotherapy for childhood Hodgkin's disease. Abstract. *Proceedings of the XVIIth SIOP meeting, Venice,* 1985; 323–4.

97. O'Brien MER, Pinkerton CR, Kingston J *et al.* VEEP in children with Hodgkin's disease. *Br J Cancer* 1992; **65**: 756–60.

98. Behrendt H, Van Bunningen, B, Van Leeuwen EF. Treatment of HD in children without radiotherapy. *Cancer* 1987; **59**: 1870–3.

99. Van den Berg H, Zsiros J, Behrendt H. Treatment of childhood Hodgkin's Disease without radiotherapy. *Ann Oncol* 1997; **8**(Suppl. 1): 515–17.

100. Schellong G, Oberlin O, Riepenhausen M *et al.* Stage IV childhood Hodgkin's disease: updated results of the SIOP collaborative study. *Med Pediatr Oncol* 1997; **29**: 332.

101. Hancock BW, Gregory WM, Cullen MH *et al.* ChlVPP alternating with PABlOE is superior to PABlOE alone in the initial treatment of advanced Hodgkin's disease: results of a British National Lymphoma Investigation/Central Lymphoma Group randomized controlled trial. *Br J Cancer* 2001; **84**: 1293–300.

●102. Engel C, Loeffler MS, Schmitz S *et al.* Acute hematologic toxicity and practicability of dose-intensified BEACOPP chemotherapy for advanced stage Hodgkin's Disease. *Ann Oncol* 2000; **11**: 1105–14.

103. Hänel M, Kröger N, Hoffknecht SO *et al.* ASHAP – an effective salvage therapy for recurrent and refractory malignant lymphomas. *Ann Hematol* 2000; **79**: 304–11.

104. Hickish T, Roldan A, Cunningham D *et al.* EPIC: an effective low toxicity regimen for relapsing lymphoma. *Br J Cancer* 1993; **68**: 599–604.

105. Hänel M, Kröger N, Kroschinsky F *et al.* Salvage chemotherapy with mitoxantrone, fludarabine, cytarabine, and cisplatin (MIFAP) in relapsing and refractory lymphoma. *J Cancer Res Clin Oncol* 2001; **127**: 386–95.

106. Bessa E, Pacquement H, Hartmann O *et al.* Long term survival of refractory or relapsed Hodgkin's disease treated by high dose chemotherapy with hematopoietic support. *Med Pediatr Oncol* 1993; **21**(8): 552.

107. Schimtz N, Pfistner B, Sextro M *et al.* Aggressive conventional chemotherapy compared with high-dose chemotherapy with autologous haemopoietic stem-cell transplantation for relapsed chemosensitive Hodgkin's disease: a randomised trial. *Lancet* 2002; **359**: 2065–71.

108. Ferme C, Mounier N, Divine M *et al.* Intensive salvage therapy with high-dose chemotherapy for patients with advanced Hodgkin's disease in relapse or failure after initial chemotherapy: results of the Groupe d'Etudes des Lymphomes de l'Adulte H89 Trial. *J Clin Oncol* 2002; **20**: 467–75.

109. Baker K, Gordon BG, Gross TG *et al.* Autologous hematopoietic stem-cell transplantation for relapsed or refractory Hodgkin's disease in children and adolescents. *J Clin Oncol* 1999; **17**: 825–31.

110. Hudson MM, Donaldson SS. Hodgkin's disease. *Pediatr Clin North Am* 1997; **44**: 891–906.

111. Raney BR. Hodgkin's disease in childhood: a review. *J Pediatr Hematol Oncol* 1998; **20**: 362–3.

112. Donaldson SS, Whitaker SJ, Plowman, PN *et al.* Stage I-II pediatric Hodgkin's disease: long term follow-up

demonstrates equivalent survival rates following different management schemes. *J Clin Oncol* 1990; **8**: 1128–37.

113. Nachman JB, Sposto R, Herzag P *et al.* Randomized comparison of low-dose involved-field radiotherapy and no radiation for children with Hodgkin's disease who achieve a complete response to chemotherapy. *J Clin Oncol* 2002; **20**: 3765–71.

114. Doreen MS, Wrigley PFM, Laidlow JM *et al.* The management of stage II supradiaphragmatic Hodgkin's disease at St Bartholomew's Hospital. *Cancer* 1984; **54**: 2882–8.

115. Glynne-Jones R, Whitaker SJ, Plowman PN. The 'urn' portal; an alternative to the 'mantle' portal in the chemoradiotherapy of paediatric Hodgkin's disease. *Clin Oncol* 1990; **2**: 235–40.

116. Fryer CJ, Hutchinson RJ, Krailo M *et al.* Efficacy and toxicity of 12 courses of ABVD chemotherapy followed by low dose regional radiation in advanced Hodgkin's disease in children: a report from the Children's Cancer Study Group. *J Clin Oncol* 1990; **8**: 1971–80.

117. Shankar A, Ashley S, Atra A *et al.* A limited role for VEEP (vincristine, etoposide, epirubicin, prednisolone) chemotherapy in childhood Hodgkin's disease. *Eur J Cancer* 1998; **34**: 2058–63.

118. Smith KL, Rivera G. Comparison of clinical course of Hodgkin's disease in children and adolescents. *Med Pediatr Oncol* 1976; **2**: 361–70.

119. Cavdar AO, Tacoy A, Babacan E *et al.* Hodgkin's disease in Turkish children: a clinical and histopathologic analysis. *J Natl Cancer Inst* 1977; **58**: 479–81.

120. Tan C, Jereb B, Chan KW *et al.* Hodgkin's disease in children. Results of management between 1970–82. *Cancer* 1983; **51**: 1720–5.

15

Tumours of the central nervous system*

DARREN R. HARGRAVE, BOO MESSAHEL & PIERS N. PLOWMAN

INTRODUCTION

Paediatric central nervous system (CNS) tumours are the commonest malignant solid tumours in childhood, representing 20 per cent of cancers in this age group.[1] They are the leading cause of cancer-related death under 15 years of age and the morbidity associated with CNS tumours is greater than any other tumour type.

Of all tumour types occurring in childhood, those located in the brain and spine best demonstrate the dilemma of seeking to improve survival whilst wishing to avoid or diminish toxicity (acute and late). The team required to care for children and adolescents with CNS tumours holistically has to be truly multidisciplinary, with input from multiple specialist doctors, nurses, therapists, psychologists, social care workers and educationalists.

An increased understanding of the biology of these tumours and the underlying normal nervous system will be central to the development of better and less toxic therapies for children and adolescents with CNS tumours.

CLASSIFICATION AND EPIDEMIOLOGY

The incidence of CNS tumours showed a rise during the late 1980s, but more recent data from the United States appear to show that rates are stabilizing.[2] It is thought that this rise may have been due to the increased use of magnetic resonance imaging (MRI) detecting low-grade tumours and also to changes in the histological classification of brain tumours. The centralization and development of specialized paediatric neurosurgical services may also have led to an increase in diagnosis and reporting of these tumours. The most accurate incidence rates should be those reported by population-based registries. The German Childhood Cancer Registry (GCCR) has reported data from over 5000 childhood CNS tumours from 1980 to 1999.[1] In the years 1990–1999 the incidence was estimated as 2.6 (2.8 males/2.4 females) per 100 000 children (<15 years old), as compared with other national registry estimates of 1.7 (Hong Kong), 2.7 (UK), 3.2 (USA) and 4.1 (Sweden). The calculated risk of a newborn German baby developing a CNS tumour in its first 15 years is 0.04 per cent (1 in 2500). Age-stratified incidence was shown as 2.7 (<1 year), 3.1 (1–4 years), 2.7 (5–9 years) and 2.0 (10–14 years) per 100 000 children. The relative frequency of individual tumour types as a percentage of all CNS tumours is indicated in Box 15.1.

*We would like to thank Dr Richard Grundy (Birmingham Children's Hospital) and Mr Conor Mallucci (Walton Centre for Neurology and Neurosurgery, Liverpool) for their contributions to the section on rare central nervous system tumours.

Box 15.1 *WHO classification and incidence of central nervous system tumours in children aged < 15 years (numbers in brackets refer to incidence as a percentage of CNS tumours in children < 15 years)*

Tumours of neuroepithelial tissue

Astrocytic tumours (37.1%)

Grade I	Pilocytic (14.8%) and subependymal giant-cell (0.4%) astrocytomas
Grade II	Diffuse astrocytomas – fibrillary (1.8%), protoplasmic (0.2%), gemistocytic (0.2%)
Grade III	Anaplastic astrocytoma (1.9%)
Grade IV	Glioblastoma (2.8%), gliosarcoma (0.1%)

Oligodendroglial tumours (1.4%)

Grade II	Oligodendroglioma (1.4%)
Grade III	Anaplastic oligodendroglioma (0.1%)

Mixed gliomas (0.6%)

Grade II	Oligoastrocytoma
Grade III	Anaplastic oligoastrocytoma

Ependymal tumours (8.5%)

Grade I	Myxopapillary ependymoma (0.3%) and subependymoma (0.1%)
Grade II	Ependymoma (5.2%)
Grade III	Anaplastic ependymoma (3.3%)

Embryonal tumours (25%)

Grade IV	Medulloblastoma (20.4%) – desmoplastic (0.9%), large cell, medullomyoblastoma
Grade IV	Supratentorial primitive neuroectodermal tumour (4.8%)
Grade IV	Medulloepithelioma and ependymoblastoma
Grade IV	Atypical teratoid/rhabdoid tumour

Other neuroepithelial tumours

Grade I	Choroid plexus papilloma (1.2%)
Grade I–III	Ganglioglioma (2.5%)
Grade II	Pineocytoma (0.4%)
Grade III	Choroid plexus carcinoma (0.6%)
Grade III	Gliomatosis cerebri (0.1%)
Grade IV	Pineoblastoma (0.6%)

Germ cell tumours (4.3%)

Germinoma (2.4%)

Embryonal carcinoma (0.2%), choriocarcinoma (0.4%), yolk sac tumour (0.5%)

Teratoma (1%) – mature (0.2%), immature (0.2%), with malignant transformation (0.1%)

Mixed germ cell tumours (0.1%)

Other tumours

Craniopharyngioma (4.7%), pituitary (0.4%), meningioma (0.7%)

In 2000 the World Health Organization (WHO) produced its revised classification of tumours of the nervous system.[3] Although there remains some debate, this is generally accepted as the standard classification system and is also outlined in Box 15.1. The system includes the WHO grading scale of malignancy, which can be interpreted as grades I–II representing benign tumours and grades III–IV malignant tumours. It is hoped that improving histopathological and molecular techniques may allow further refinement of the classification of CNS tumours, providing a closer correlation with the natural history and prognosis of these tumours in the future.

The aetiology of most cases of CNS tumours in childhood remains unknown, despite extensive epidemiological studies. However, there are a number of genetic disorders which can predispose to the development of a brain tumour, e.g. neurofibromatosis types (NF) 1 and 2, tuberous sclerosis, Gorlin's, Cowden's and Turcot's syndromes, and these will be discussed in greater detail in relation to the individual tumour types. The other proven risk factor of CNS malignancy is exposure of the brain to ionizing radiation, with cases of secondary brain tumours described following cranial radiotherapy for primary CNS tumours and treatment for leukaemia.

CLINICAL PRESENTATION AND DIAGNOSIS

Clinical features

Brain and spinal cord tumours have been found to have the greatest diagnostic delay of all childhood cancers.[4] This probably results from the often nonspecific nature and variability of symptoms arising from CNS tumours and the need for neuroimaging to confirm the diagnosis. The determinants of symptoms and signs include age, tumour type and, of course, anatomical site. The presentation may demonstrate features of raised intracranial pressure (ICP) or localizing neurological deficits.

Increased ICP can be due to direct tumour infiltration or compression of normal structures or may be secondary to obstruction of the cerebrospinal fluid (CSF). In older children this can present initially as mood/behavioural changes and declining school performance prior to development of the more classical features of headache, nausea and vomiting. Typically, headaches start as generalized and intermittent, and then increase in both intensity and frequency with time. The child may awake with headache at night, with the pain generally being worse in the morning and improving during the day with an upright posture. Nausea and vomiting may occur alone or with headache; again, this is often worse in the morning after being recumbent during sleep.

School-age children may also complain of visual disturbance with the development of cranial nerve palsies and papilloedema. False localizing signs related to raised ICP include a deficit of lateral gaze (VI nerve palsy) or a head tilt related to a IV nerve palsy. In infants and younger children, raised ICP is more insidious due to the plasticity of the developing skull and the inability to communicate symptoms easily. Infants may be irritable, with failure to thrive associated with anorexia and vomiting and possible regression of developmental milestones. Carers may notice increasing head circumference with widened sutures and a tense anterior fontanelle. In these late stages the 'sun-setting' sign may be noted due to paralysis of upward gaze (Parinaud's sign).

Focal neurological signs may help to localize a CNS tumour prior to imaging but are not always present. Box 15.2 demonstrates the typical distribution of anatomical sites in paediatric CNS tumours and the symptoms and signs associated with these sites. Specific tumours have characteristic presentations and will be discussed later. If the primary CNS tumour has spread, there may be associated signs and symptoms related to the sites of metastases although these are often asymptomatic at presentation.

Diagnostic management

In those patients who present with acute neurological deficit, the most urgent need is to stabilize their condition. In most cases this can be done with appropriate conservative measures to control pain, raised ICP, seizures and electrolyte abnormalities, allowing definitive surgery to be planned semi-electively. Occasionally, despite the use of high-dose corticosteroids, surgical CSF diversion is required urgently and this may involve external ventricular drainage, a III ventriculostomy or insertion of a ventriculoperitoneal shunt. During this initial period, the patient will obviously undergo full neurological examination (including ophthalmic assessment) and diagnostic investigations such as appropriate neuroimaging, serum and CSF tumour markers, CSF cytology and baseline endocrine testing.

Neuroimaging is essential in diagnosing a CNS tumour. Although computed tomography (CT) is still currently the most widely used initial imaging modality, magnetic resonance imaging (MRI) is in most cases a preferable and superior investigation. MRI with gadolinium contrast of both brain and spine ideally takes place prior to surgery, allowing better delineation of both local tumour extent and staging of any neuraxis metastases. Although paediatric CNS tumours have characteristic radiological appearances, in the majority of cases, conventional CT/MRI cannot replace a histological diagnosis. The exceptions to this are the typical diffuse intrinsic

Box 15.2 *Symptoms and signs according to anatomical site of central nervous system tumours (proportion of tumours at site)*

Supratentorial (30–40%)
- Cerebral hemisphere – hemiparesis, spasticity, seizures (focal or generalised)
- Para/suprasellar – endocrinopathy (growth failure, diabetes insipidus, pubertal abnormality)
- Hypothalamus – diencephalic syndrome (infants), developmental and behavioural abnormalities
- Optic pathway – visual field, acuity, colour vision deficits, optic atrophy, nystagmus, head tilt
- Pineal – Parinaud's syndrome, sleep abnormalities
- Thalamus, basal ganglia – pain, sensory loss, memory disturbance
- Intraventricular
- Meningeal

Infratentorial (60–70%)
- Posterior fossa – ataxia, nystagmus, dysmetria (presents as clumsiness or worse handwriting)
- Brainstem – multiple cranial nerve palsies, hemiparesis, spasticity, mood changes

Spinal (2–5%)
- Primary intramedullary – pain (local back and root pain), motor and sensory disturbance
- Spinal metastases – scoliosis, sphincter (bowel, bladder) disturbance, reflex changes

pontine glioma, optic pathway glioma in a child with NF-1 and secreting intracranial germ cell tumour. It has been hoped that more advanced imaging techniques may lead to better tumour preoperative characterization but this work is still ongoing. Promising newer modalities include magnetic resonance spectroscopy (MRS) and various nuclear medicine techniques, such as positron emission tomography (PET) and single photon emission computed tomography (SPECT); this area is described at the end of the chapter.

Neurosurgery is the principal modality in the management of the majority of CNS tumours and the extent varies from biopsy alone to attempting to remove the tumour completely. It is essential that children are referred to an experienced paediatric neurosurgical unit, as studies have suggested an improved resection rate with centralization of paediatric cases.[5] Difficult to access tumours may undergo CT/MRI stereotactic guided biopsies or, in the case of intraventricular tumours, endoscopic biopsy. But in most cases an open procedure is preferred and the degree of resection will be dictated by neuroanatomy, tumour invasion, histology (available intraoperatively by fresh frozen section) and haemostasis. The prognostic importance of the extent of surgical resection varies between tumour types and will be discussed individually. Accurate postoperative imaging is desirable as it serves to confirm the degree of surgical resection and acts as a baseline for future imaging. Again, MRI is preferable to CT, but either modality needs to be performed early after surgery to try to minimize the difficulties of distinguishing residual tumour from postsurgical changes such as blood and oedema. The United Kingdom Children's Cancer Study Group (UKCCSG) and the Society of French Paediatric Oncologists (SFOP) have jointly recommended preoperative MRI of brain and spine and a postoperative MRI within 72 hours.[6] The final histological diagnosis, along with the other staging investigations, will inform the need and type of any further adjuvant therapy.

ASTROCYTOMAS

Astrocytomas are the commonest childhood CNS tumour, representing approximately 40 per cent of the total. They are divided into low-grade (grade I and II of both the WHO and Kernohan systems) and high-grade (grade III and IV) tumours. Low-grade astrocytomas include the pilocytic variant which is generally confined to children or young adults and is the most common low-grade glioma. It is a well circumscribed, low-cellularity tumour which often exhibits Rosenthal fibres. Interestingly, this grade I benign tumour can demonstrate rare mitoses, occasional hyperchromatic nuclei and microvascular proliferation, but these are not a sign of malignancy in this slow-growing tumour. Grade II diffuse astrocytomas such as fibrillary, gemistocytic and protoplasmic astrocytomas are well differentiated, highly cellular tumours with diffuse infiltration of neighbouring tissues but without mitoses, necrosis or vascular proliferation. They tend to occur at an older age than the pilocytic variant. The pleomorphic xanthoastrocytoma is also more likely to occur at a younger age and is composed of fibrillary and giant multinucleated astrocytes with large xanthomatous cells. Although anaplasia is occasionally seen, these are generally benign grade II tumours.

High-grade astrocytomas are malignant tumours and consist of the grade III anaplastic astrocytoma and the grade IV glioblastoma and gliosarcoma. Anaplastic astrocytomas are diffusely infiltrating tumours with increased cellularity, distinct nuclear atypia and marked mitotic activity. Glioblastomas have the same features as anaplastic astrocytomas plus prominent microvascular proliferation and necrosis. The clinical behaviour of astrocytomas broadly corresponds to the histological grade, with low-grade gliomas being less aggressive and more responsive to treatment than high-grade gliomas, which relentlessly progress and respond poorly to adjuvant therapy. Proliferation indices as measured by Ki-67 and MIB-1 have both been shown to correlate with prognostic outcome in high-grade tumours,[7] but their prognostic use in low-grade astrocytomas is still unclear.[8,9] A new low-grade variant known as a pilomyxoid astrocytoma has been described as exhibiting a worse outcome than a typical pilocytic tumour.[10] Although malignant transformation of grade II tumours has been described in children, this is much less frequent than seen in the adult population. Astrocytomas can disseminate and seed to the CSF but this is the exception rather than the rule and has been described in both low- and high-grade lesions.

There are a number of genetic predisposition syndromes that can lead to astrocytoma development. The condition NF-1 is the most common and various series have described between 50 and 70 per cent of optic pathway tumours to be associated with the syndrome.[11,12] These tumours are usually pilocytic astrocytomas, with 15 per cent of NF-1 sufferers developing this variant;[13] however, other low- and high-grade astrocytomas at various sites have also been reported. Although mutation of the large NF-1 gene on the long arm of chromosome 17 is thought to act as a potential tumour suppressor, it has not been found to play a significant role in sporadic astrocytomas.[14] The rare subependymal giant-cell astrocytoma (SEGA) is almost exclusively reported in tuberous sclerosis, with 5–15 per cent of patients developing this tumour in their first two decades.[15,16] The familial cancer predisposition Li–Fraumeni syndrome also gives rise to an increase in astrocytoma development, presumably secondary to the initial germ-line p53 mutation and accumulation of subsequent oncogenic abnormalities.

The genetic abnormalities of sporadic astrocytomas are increasingly being defined, particularly in the adult population, but are less well known in childhood and low-grade tumours. The importance of abnormalities of the p53/MDM2/p21 pathway is well known in studies of adult high-grade gliomas and appears to be an early event and present in both de novo primary malignant gliomas and also secondary tumours that have transformed from low-grade lesions. Recent large multi-institutional studies have confirmed that p53 overexpression and mutation correlates independently with an adverse outcome.[17] Interestingly, p53 mutations in high-grade astrocytoma have also been shown to occur with increasing age in children; and indeed infants, who have a generally better outcome, have a low incidence of this mutation.[18] High-grade gliomas in adults are also known to demonstrate the following genetic abnormalities: amplification of the epidermal and platelet-derived growth factor receptors (EGFr/PDGFr), abnormalities of the p16/p15/CDK4/CDK6/RB pathway and deletion of the *PTEN* gene. The frequency and order of these accumulating changes remain to be fully elucidated, but available studies do suggest significant differences between paediatric and adult groups, with fewer genetic abnormalities being described in childhood tumours.[19–22] It is vital that this area is intensively investigated in paediatric astrocytomas, as abnormalities of these cell cycle pathways may provide new targets, and early clinical trials in adults are already using targeted novel therapies exploiting the above genetic changes.

Low-grade astrocytomas

The most common sites for low-grade (I–II) astrocytomas are the cerebellum (20 per cent of all CNS tumours), deep midline (15 per cent), cerebral hemispheres (10 per cent) and visual pathways (5 per cent), but they also arise in the brainstem and spinal cord.

CEREBELLAR ASTROCYTOMAS

The classic cerebellar astrocytoma occurs in the first decade of life, is slightly more common in boys and presents with midline cerebellar signs. The neuroradiological and operative findings are usually of a cystic tumour with a mural nodule (see Figure 15.1). In 15 per cent of tumours, the lesion is more solid and histologically it is a diffuse astrocytoma.

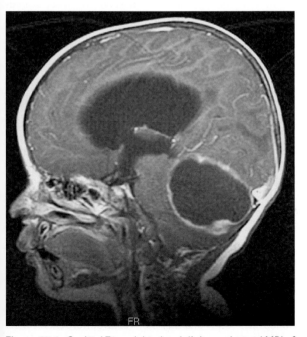

Figure 15.1 *Sagittal T1-weighted gadolinium enhanced MRI of a classical cerebellar pilocytic astrocytoma with hydrocephalus. Cystic tumour with enhancing cyst wall and mural nodule.*

Surgery is the principal therapeutic modality, aiming for maximal resection with minimal morbidity. Survival rates for greater than 90 per cent resection are in the order of 90 per cent at 10 years.[23,24] After surgery, the current recommendation is observation if the child is asymptomatic, as follow-up studies suggest that approximately 50 per cent of incompletely resected tumours will not progress over a period of 5 years and more.[23,25] If there is evidence of progression, further surgical resection should be undertaken followed by non-surgical treatment if the operation is incomplete. The choice between focal radiotherapy and chemotherapy is usually based on age and is primarily related to the risk of developing significant neurocognitive deficit following radiotherapy, which depends on the age of the child. The cut-off age for considering radiotherapy as first-line non-surgical therapy is around 8 years and the use of modern conformal CT/MRI planned radiotherapy minimizes the volume of normal brain irradiated in the treatment field. Chemotherapy comprising vincristine and carboplatin is used prior to radiotherapy in younger children.

VISUAL PATHWAY ASTROCYTOMAS

These tumours account for 5 per cent of all paediatric CNS tumours, with 50–70 per cent of tumours occurring in patients with NF-1.[12,13] The peak incidence is in the first 5 years of life, and 95 per cent have presented by 10 years of age. The tumour may involve only one optic nerve, usually within the orbit (intraorbital), and can present with proptosis (Figure 15.2). This pattern or bilateral isolated optic nerve involvement is more typical in NF-1, whereas sporadic tumours more often affect the optic chiasm. Extension can occur in the optic radiations and also superiorly to involve the hypothalamus. Presentation may be with visual disturbance of acuity and field loss or, in younger children, with strabismus, nystagmus and developmental difficulties. Tumours affecting the hypothalamus in infants may present with the diencephalic syndrome, manifested by failure to thrive despite apparent normal caloric intake in an apparently alert and cheerful child. Large tumours can cause neuroendocrine deficits and hydrocephalus. Dissemination of low-grade astrocytomas has been estimated to occur in about 2–5 per cent of cases and appears more likely in sporadic cases with a midline primary.

It is essential that neurocutaneous stigmata are searched for, as an optic pathway tumour may occur in a child with previously unrecognized NF-1. Full ophthalmological assessment is essential plus endocrine assessment if there are any concerns about growth, excessive fluid intake or diuresis. Imaging with modern spiral CT is acceptable but MRI is preferable. Figure 15.2 shows the difference in quality between the two modalities. In the unusual presence of back pain, bladder or bowel

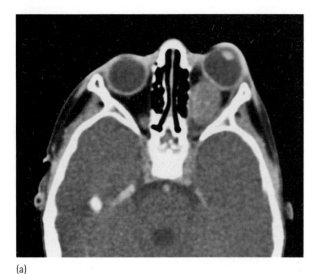

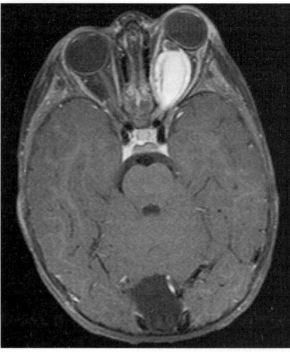

Figure 15.2 *(a) Axial non-contrast CT demonstrating a left-sided optic nerve glioma causing marked proptosis. (b) Axial T1-weighted gadolinium-enhanced MRI demonstrating large enhancing intraorbital left-sided optic nerve glioma with extension to chiasm and marked proptosis.*

symptoms, a spinal MRI should be included. The imaging is diagnostic in children with NF-1 and is likely to demonstrate other characteristic neuroradiological features such as hamartomas and 'unidentified bright objects' (UBOs).

The natural history of visual pathway tumours is very variable and, in patients with NF-1, may follow a very indolent course with more than 50 per cent not progressing.[26] In view of this, therapy should only be administered if there is definite evidence of symptoms from the tumour, impairment of visual function or neuroradiological evidence of progression.

Patients with optic pathway tumours should be observed and monitored intensively with the use of MRI scans and detailed serial opthalmic assessments including visual acuity, fields and colour vision, and the addition of visual evoked potentials (VEPs) in younger children. These investigations should be carried out at relatively short (3-monthly) intervals initially, until it is known whether the tumour is progressing or stable.

Surgery is curative in an isolated intraorbital optic nerve glioma where the tumour can be excised with clear margins anterior to the chiasm, but is reserved for those in whom there is no functional vision left in the affected eye. However, in most cases, it is reserved for debulking large exophytic/cystic chiasmatic-hypothalamic tumours that are causing hydrocephalus or for obtaining tissue to confirm the diagnosis in non-NF-1 patients.

As with other sites, the selection of non-surgical treatment is dependent on the child's age; for older children (8+ years) external beam radiotherapy is effective,

at least in preventing progression, in the majority of cases. Overall survival (OS) is usually reported as in excess of 90 per cent with progression-free survival (PFS) ranging from 60 to 85 per cent.[27–29] However, significant long-term effects are apparent, particularly in young children and those with NF-1. Due to the midline nature of these tumours, conventionally planned radiotherapy has resulted in young children with severe learning disabilities, vasculopathy, including 'moyamoya' syndrome, and neuroendocrine deficits.[27] Children with NF-1 have a fivefold increase in obstructive vasculopathy after irradiation[30,31] and may also have an increase in the rate of secondary tumour formation; it is therefore best avoided if possible in this group.[32,33] It is hoped, but as yet not proven, that stereotactic conformal radiotherapy and the use of radiotherapy at older ages will reduce these long-term side-effects.[34,35] Chemotherapy, with vincristine and carboplatin, is the treatment of choice for these tumours in young children (under 8 years of age) and those with NF-1. The response to chemotherapy with this regimen leads to an objective response with tumour shrinkage in approximately 60 per cent of cases, with a further 30 per cent achieving stable disease. The outcome as measured by visual function is more difficult to report due to inconsistency in ophthalmological examinations in multi-institutional studies. However, several small series report approximately 20 per cent improvement and 60–80 per cent stability of vision after chemotherapy.[36–38] The important prognostic variables for outcome are thought be age at diagnosis, with most recent reports suggesting those under 5 years have a worse outcome,[39–41] and NF-1 status, with improved outcome in those with the condition.[42,43]

LOW-GRADE ASTROCYTOMAS AT OTHER SITES

Low-grade tumours also occur in the supratentorial region in the cerebral hemispheres, deep midline structures such as the thalami, and the tectal plate. The same therapeutic approach is taken, with surgery needing to balance the benefit of near complete resection with morbidity, especially in deep tumours and those in eloquent areas of the cerebrum. The use of neuro-navigational techniques which register the position of the patient's brain with previous imaging via a computerized system in conjunction with functional imaging allows for previously unresectable tumours to be removed. Bithalamic tumours, even when low-grade on histology, have a poor prognosis despite adjuvant therapy,[44] whereas tectal plate gliomas are often very indolent and, after biopsy and CSF diversion, may remain stable without further therapy for many years.[45] Chemotherapy or radiotherapy are both used if progression occurs after surgery, again according to age.

Spinal cord astrocytomas are intramedullary tumours (see Figure 15.3), and surgical resection is the mainstay of treatment. Careful postoperative monitoring should be undertaken, with radiotherapy or chemotherapy given if there is progression.

CHEMOTHERAPY FOR LOW-GRADE ASTROCYTOMA

Historically, it was believed that chemotherapy would not be effective for these slow-growing tumours. However, following the demonstration of the activity of vincristine and actinomycin D,[46] numerous other reports and agents have been shown to have activity. The combination of vincristine and carboplatin in various schedules is now regarded as standard and was first described in the early 1990s.[47] This chemotherapy has been administered after an initial induction phase of 10 weeks for up to 12 months; in Europe the carboplatin has been given monthly at a dose of 500–560 mg/m^2, whereas elsewhere the dose is often fractionated to 175 mg/m^2 weekly for 4 weeks. Both regimens have demonstrated significant responses (objective + stable disease) of around 80–90 per cent, but it is not clear how response correlates with PFS. The PFS as reported by the American Children's Cancer Group (CCG)[48] was 68 per cent at 3 years, compared with that reported by the European consortium group of 48 per cent at 5 years' follow-up.[49] Both groups report a problem with carboplatin hypersensitivity, which can stop therapy due to severity and may occur in up to 30 per cent of patients. Other multiagent regimens have been reported, including a five-drug nitrosourea-based

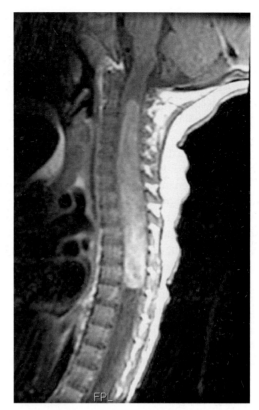

Figure 15.3 *Sagittal T1-weighted gadolinium-enhanced MRI of a cervical/thoracic low-grade astrocytoma.*

regimen, TPDCV (thioguanine, procarbazine, dibromodulcitol, vincristine), which originated in San Francisco[38] and showed good response rates (97 per cent objective response or stable disease) and OS of 75 per cent at 5 years.[40] This promising response rate has led to an American randomized study, CCG 9952, between standard vincristine/carboplatin and TPCV, and the results of this recently closed study are awaited. Multiple single agents have been shown to have activity, including cyclophosphamide, etoposide, ifosfamide, methotrexate, temozolomide, topotecan and vinblastine.[50–54] Response rates have ranged from 55 to 95 per cent and future multiagent studies may include some of these agents to try to improve both response and PFS rates. The next European consortium study will look at adding etoposide to vincristine and carboplatin in the induction phase followed by a prolonged maintenance phase of up to 18 months with vincristine and carboplatin.

High-grade astrocytomas

Malignant astrocytomas represent about 10–20 per cent of all paediatric CNS tumours if intrinsic brainstem gliomas are included. The most common sites are the supratentorial region and the brainstem, although they can occur in other sites in the brain and spine.

SUPRATENTORIAL TUMOURS

High-grade astrocytomas – anaplastic astrocytoma (AA) and glioblastoma multiforme (GBM) – are the most common supratentorial tumours. Conventional therapy with surgical resection followed by irradiation only very rarely results in survival in those with GBM[55] and in 20 per cent survival in those with AA.[56] This exceeds the survival rates seen in adults with similar histological tumours and, along with the differences emerging from molecular studies, suggests that there may be biological differences. Unlike the situation in adults, studies have demonstrated a prognostic benefit of near total resection (>90 per cent) in children.[57] However, the diffuse nature and location of these tumours in eloquent areas of the brain provide a considerable challenge for the neurosurgeon and, again, the use of sophisticated neuroimaging and neuro-navigation techniques can assist resection. The extent of local tumour invasion has been proven by stereotactic biopsies to extend beyond that shown by either contrast-enhanced CT, MRI or T2-weighted MRI. Typical radiological characteristics include marked heterogeneity on T2 with partial enhancement, with marked oedema and mass effect (see Figure 15.4). The selection of imaging for defining radiotherapy treatment volumes is a matter of debate due to the current inability of CT or MRI to delineate tumour invasion accurately. Originally, whole brain radiotherapy was used, but in order to avoid unnecessary normal brain being irradiated, limited fields are used with a margin added to the tumour volume according to either contrast-enhanced CT or T1-weighted MRI, although some use the T2-weighted signal. The other area of debate is the boosting of local tumour to obtain better local control and this is being investigated in current studies using stereotactic techniques.

In the late 1970s and early 1980s, there was a suggestion that nitrosoureas had some activity in high-grade astrocytomas.[58] In view of this, the first randomized phase II trial for children was undertaken by CCG in North America. CCG 943 entered only a relatively small number of children but a survival advantage was demonstrated for the use of adjuvant chemotherapy with lomustine (CCNU), vincristine and prednisone, in addition to irradiation compared with radiotherapy alone[55] (5-year PFS: 48 vs. 18 per cent). Subsequently, CCG 945 compared this regimen with the so-called 'eight drugs in 1 day' regimen (vincristine, CCNU, procarbazine, hydroxyurea, cisplatin, cytarabine, dacarbazine and methylprednisolone) which had shown activity in a previous pilot study. There was no significant difference in PFS between the two arms (26 and 33 per cent, respectively).[59] This study illustrated a number of important points, including the prognostic impact of

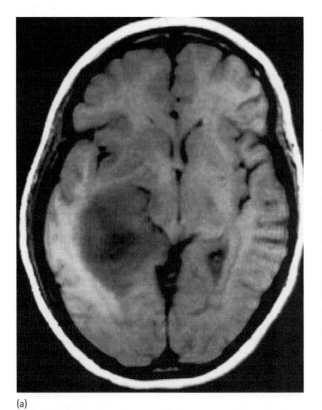

(a)

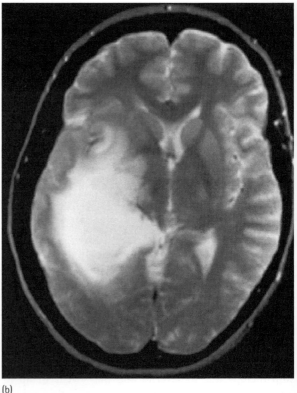

(b)

Figure 15.4 *Axial T1(a) and T2 (b) images of a right parietal glioblastoma. The T2 image shows marked peritumoral oedema.*

histology, 28 per cent PFS at 5 years for AA and 16 per cent for GBM and, as previously mentioned, the extent of surgical resection. Also, the fact that central histological review took place for the first time was important, as it demonstrated a discordant opinion in 51/172 tumours between central and local pathology review.[60] This is vital in that the inclusion of low-grade tumours in studies for high-grade gliomas or even the wrong classification of grade III or grade IV tumours may give misleading results. A more recent German randomized study looked at pre-irradiation chemotherapy (ifosfamide, etoposide, methotrexate, cisplatin and cytosine arabinoside) followed by radiotherapy vs. radiotherapy followed by so-called maintenance chemotherapy (lomustine, vincristine, and cisplatin).[61] This study again confirmed the benefit of a >90 per cent resection, with a median survival of 5.2 years compared with 1.3 years in those with <90 per cent resection. It also showed a benefit in those with >90 per cent resection in receiving the pre-irradiation chemotherapy compared with maintenance chemotherapy (median survival: 5.2 vs. 1.9 years). Although encouraging, there was no central pathological review presented and those that benefited were the better risk group who underwent macroscopic resection.

The major future therapeutic goal for high-grade astrocytomas is the identification of new active anti-cancer drugs. Platinum agents, etoposide, cyclophosphamide, ifosfamide as well as nitrosoureas and procarbazine have all shown some activity in phase II single-agent studies but have been disappointing as monotherapy. Newer agents such as the camptothecin derivatives topotecan and irinotecan have been studied, with disappointing results for the former[62,63] but encouraging response rates in phase II studies for irinotecan (45 per cent with two complete responses).[64] Topotecan is now being looked at as a potential radiosensitizer when given with irradiation. Irinotecan is of interest, as its relative lack of myelosuppression means its incorporation into multiagent regimens is feasible, and further studies are ongoing. The main interest has been focused on the drug temozolomide, which is already licensed in adult high-grade glioma therapy. Initial phase I studies of this oral alkylating agent, as conducted by both the UKCCSG[65] and the CCG,[66] were encouraging and determined a maximum tolerated dose (MTD) that was used for phase II studies. A dose of 200 mg/m^2 per day for 5 days was used by the UKCCSG with two arms for non-brainstem malignant glioma and brainstem glioma.[67] The response rate of 12 per cent in the non-brainstem arm was disappointing but the agent is still of interest in combination therapy and possibly given in a low-dose schedule concomitant with radiotherapy.[68] This latter regimen has shown some success in adult GBM and could theoretically help to reduce the activity of O^6-alkyl-transferase, an important resistance mechanism to this drug.[69]

High-dose myeloablative chemotherapy with stem cell rescue has been used with a number of agents (BCNU, carboplatin, cyclophosphamide, etoposide, thiotepa) with some significant responses but also with the expected toxicity of such high-dose regimens. An early example was the CCG 9922 trial of thiotepa/etoposide and BCNU of newly diagnosed high-grade gliomas, in which there was a high toxic deathd rate but a 42 per cent 2-year survival in those with GBM.[70] The later CCG 9883 study used carboplatin instead of BCNU and had a lower toxic mortality of 6 per cent with two out of nine high-grade gliomas having prolonged PFS at the time of reporting. More recent studies by the CCG (99702, 99703) are exploring sequential high-dose chemotherapy with stem cell support to explore this mode of therapy further.

Future targeted treatments may well be developed using the increasing knowledge of the abnormalities of the cell cycle as outlined earlier in this section and potential candidates are discussed at the end of the chapter.

BRAINSTEM GLIOMAS

Brainstem gliomas occur predominantly in children and young adults and compromise 15–20 per cent of paediatric CNS tumours. The sex incidence is equal and the most common presenting age is 5–10 years. Most brainstem gliomas arise in the pons and can extend into the medulla and midbrain. The majority are high-grade astrocytomas and usually present with a short history of cranial nerve palsies, ataxia and long tract signs. MRI scanning is the investigation of choice and the typical pontine glioma is a diffuse, poorly enhancing, hypointense on T1 or hyperintense on T2 lesion (see Figure 15.5). This characteristic appearance associated with the classical symptoms described above is now regarded as diagnostic and biopsy, which carries a risk of neurological morbidity, can be avoided. Focal tumours centred on the midbrain, medulla or tectal plate along with dorsally exophytic brainstem tumours often behave in a less aggressive manner (see Figure 15.6). Imaging consistent with one of these tumours should, where possible, lead to surgical biopsy or resection to confirm the probability of low-grade histology. Following surgery, low-grade lesions are treated with radiotherapy or vincristine and carboplatin as previously outlined.

The classical diffuse intrinsic pontine glioma has a dismal prognosis, with fewer than 5 per cent long-term survivors and a median survival of approximately 9 months. As surgery is not possible, conventional radiotherapy (50–54 Gy in 30 fractions) is the standard treatment and benefits up to 70 per cent of patients with regard to improving and palliating symptoms. Unfortunately this is not a durable response in the vast majority of patients, which led to extensive investigations involving increased

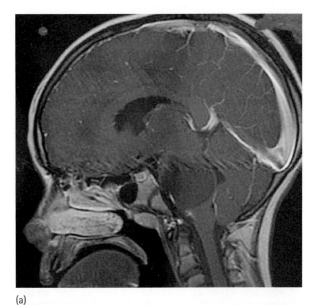

(a)

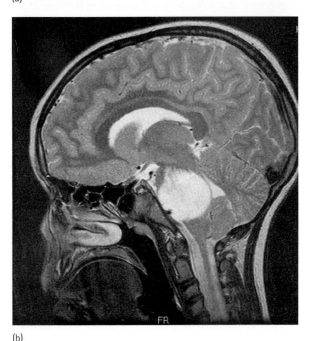

(b)

Figure 15.5 *Sagittal MRI, T1 (hypointense) (a) and T2 (hyperintense) (b) weighted images of a diffuse intrinsic pontine glioma.*

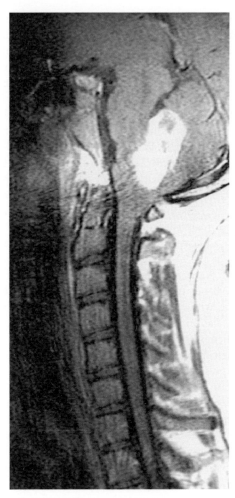

Figure 15.6 *Spinal MRI T1-weighted gadolinium-enhanced image of a dorsal exophytic cervicomedullary tumour prior to resection. Histology confirmed low-grade fibrillary astrocytoma.*

dose and scheduling of irradiation. Increasing the dose by hyperfractionation up to 78 Gy has not improved survival,[71,72] and a review of the very few long-term survivors demonstrated very significant late neurological toxicity.[73] More recently, efforts have concentrated on using concomitant drug administration to attempt to selectively sensitize glioma cells to irradiation; agents have included carboplatin, topotecan and gadolinium texaphyrin and the results are awaited.

To date, no chemotherapeutic agent has shown significant activity in high-grade brainstem gliomas. The following agents have been studied at the time of recurrent disease: AZQ, carboplatin, cisplatin, cyclophosphamide, etoposide, ifosfamide, iproplatin, BCNU, tamoxifen, temozolomide and topotecan.[74] Oral etoposide and temozolomide showed some initial promise in some patients with prolonged stable disease, but further studies have been disappointing.[65,67,75] The only randomized study between chemotherapy plus radiotherapy and irradiation alone found that adding vincristine, CCNU and prednisone to standard therapy made no significant difference.[76] Other multiagent schedules, including high-dose myeloablative chemotherapy with stem cell rescue, have not demonstrated any significant benefit either. Conventional MRI criteria for estimating response have not correlated with length of survival[77] and new imaging modalities are needed to assess response, especially for newer targeted therapies.

The reasons for the lack of progress in this most challenging tumour may include; relative inaccessibility leading to poor drug delivery, inherent aggressive biology and brainstem failure. Therefore new agents and techniques to improve drug delivery, target the underlying molecular defects and decrease the effects of brainstem failure are needed.

GLIOMATOSIS CEREBRI

Gliomatosis cerebri is characterized by a diffusely neoplastic proliferation of glial cells with the disease usually extensively involving both cerebral hemispheres and infratentorial structures. Clinically, the range of presentation is wide and the diagnosis often difficult to make due to the lack of early focal signs. The peak incidence is in middle age but has been reported in neonates. Diagnosis is by exclusion of other diffuse neurological processes but has been greatly aided by MRI imaging with diffuse high signal intensity seen on T2-weighted images. Biopsy is required to arrive at a diagnosis and surgery is usually restricted to this followed by radiotherapy. Whole-brain doses of 50 Gy appear to be of benefit and this is the therapy usually offered. Recently, temozolomide has demonstrated response and a survival advantage.[78]

SPINAL CORD TUMOURS

The therapeutic approach for high-grade astrocytomas of the spinal cord is very similar to that for other sites. Surgery is often restricted to biopsy only and radiotherapy is the standard treatment. Chemotherapy remains experimental and unproven.

PRIMITIVE NEUROECTODERMAL TUMOURS

Medulloblastoma is the most common malignant CNS tumour and accounts for 20 per cent of all childhood brain and spinal cord tumours and 40 per cent of those in the cerebellum. This is an embryonal tumour and considered a primitive neuroectodermal tumour (PNET) of the CNS. The term medulloblastoma is reserved for those PNETs arising in the posterior fossa, while those found in the pineal region are pineoblastomas and those in the cerebrum are called supratentorial primitive neuroectodermal tumours (SPNETs). Very rarely, they arise in the brainstem or the spinal cord. Histologically, PNETs are similar irrespective of location and comprise small round cells with disproportionately large hyperchromatic nuclei. These cells are clustered into rosettes. There has been quite extensive debate as to whether medulloblastomas and SPNETs arise from a common cell type in the subventricular germinal matrix or whether they are biologically distinct with medulloblastomas originating from the external cerebellar granule cells. Recent microarray gene expression profiling appears to confirm the latter hypothesis with a high correlation of several genes encoding transcription factors specific for cerebellar granule cells found only in medulloblastomas but not other CNS PNETs.[79] Morphologically, in addition to classical medulloblastoma there are a number of distinct subtypes: desmoplastic, large-cell anaplastic, medullomyoblastoma and melanotic medulloblastoma. It has been postulated that the large-cell anaplastic variant has an adverse prognosis, which has been confirmed recently by two large studies, and also that even in the absence of large-cell morphology, anaplasia imparts a worse prognosis compared with the classical histological type.[80,81]

A number of genetic conditions have been shown to predispose to medulloblastoma development. Gorlin's syndrome (naevoid basal cell carcinoma) is characterized by multiple basal cell carcinomas, jaw cysts, skeletal abnormalities, palmar pits and mental retardation. Approximately 5 per cent of sufferers develop medulloblastoma, usually during the first 3 years of life and of the desmoplastic variety. Gorlin's syndrome is autosomal dominant and 40 per cent are new mutations. The patched (PTCH) gene has been identified in a specific germ-line mutation and is located on chromosome 9q22.3. The gene product is known to act as a receptor for the sonic hedgehog family of proteins, which in turn act on the transcription factor Gli. Recently, germ-line mutations of another member of the sonic hedgehog pathway, SUFU, have been discovered and also predispose to desmoplastic medulloblastoma.[82] The gene is distinct from PTCH, located on chromosome 10q24.32, and confirms the importance of this pathway not only in normal cerebellar development but also in desmoplastic medulloblastoma. Further work is needed to investigate the relevance in sporadic tumours. Turcot's syndrome can predispose to both glioblastoma and medulloblastoma and actually comprises two distinct genetic conditions associated with familial adenomatous polyposis (FAP; mutation of the APC gene) and hereditary non-polyposis colorectal carcinoma syndrome (mutation in mismatch repair genes). The latter condition predisposes to medulloblastoma, usually in adolescence, whereas FAP predisposes to glioblastoma, also during late teenage years. Li–Fraumeni syndrome also predisposes to medulloblastoma, although less frequently than to astrocytic tumours.

In sporadic tumours, several genetic abnormalities have been noted, including deletions of the short arm of chromosome 17, most frequently as a component of an isochromosome in up to 50 per cent of tumours. This appears to be distinct from p53, which is only rarely mutated. Variable abnormalities of other chromosomal regions have been noted, including loss of 1q, 10q, 22 and gain of 7. Gene amplification of c-MYC (8q24) has been associated with aggressive disease and a poor outcome,[83] whilst high mRNA expression of the nerve growth factor receptor Trk C appears to correlate with a favourable prognosis.[84] The ErbB family of tyrosine kinases are important in cerebellar development, and high expression of ErbB-2 and ErbB-4 in medulloblastoma cells appears to result in a significantly worse prognosis.[85,86] Gene expression profiling has identified clusters of genes able to distinguish between good and poor outcome tumours,[79] and along with the other molecular prognostic factors described, could provide for more accurate stratification of patients at diagnosis. However, these new predictors of outcome need to be robustly trialed prospectively.

The classical paediatric cerebellar medulloblastoma is a midline vermis tumour, which has its peak incidence in 5-year-olds; 85 per cent of cases have presented by 15 years of age. There is a slight male predominance. In young adults, the tumour more often appears to arise in the cerebellar hemispheres and is histologically the desmoplastic type with prominent stroma. PNETs tend to invade locally, metastasize into the subarachnoid space and disseminate by CSF to other areas of the neuraxis. The incidence of CSF seeding at diagnosis ranges from 10 to 40 per cent in different reports, but the risk is always substantial and full MRI imaging of brain and spine is mandatory. Furthermore, medulloblastoma is the brain tumour *par excellence* for dissemination outside of the CNS (~5 per cent). Radiologically, sclerotic bone metastases are the most common metastatic site, but peritoneal seeding has been reported, presumably secondary to spread from ventriculoperitoneal shunts. Clinically, children with medulloblastoma more commonly present with features of raised ICP than with cerebellar signs due to compression of the IV ventricle.

Staging consists ideally of preoperative MRI of brain and spine, so avoiding the difficulties of interpreting post-surgical changes in the spine. If preoperative spinal imaging is not available, at least 14 days should elapse before imaging the spine to allow clearance of blood products. Imaging will usually demonstrate an iso/hyperintense well-defined lesion on CT, calcified in about 20 per cent of medulloblastomas and 40 per cent SPNETs. MRI characteristically shows a low T1/T2 signal, homogeneous enhancing mass in a medulloblastoma (see Figure 15.7), and a heterogeneous lesion, possibly with haemorrhage, necrosis and cysts, in SPNET. Spinal metastases show as either nodules or 'sugar-coating' on spinal MRI. The Chang staging system is used and measures the extent of primary tumour and metastases (M). However, only the M stage is of prognostic importance, as follows:

- M0 – localized disease with no evidence of metastasis
- M1 – microscopic tumour cells found in CSF
- M2 – nodular seeding intracranially
- M3 – nodular seeding on spinal cord
- M4 – extraneuraxial metastasis.

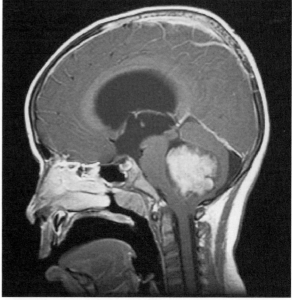

(a)

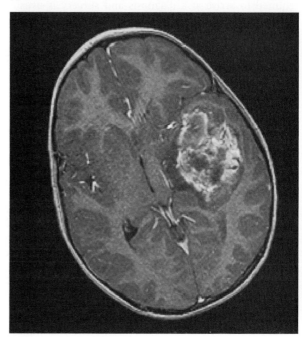

(b)

Figure 15.7 *(a) Sagittal T1-weighted enhanced MRI of posterior fossa medulloblastoma. (b) Axial T1-weighted MRI of left parietal supratentorial primitive neuroectodermal tumour (SPNET).*

The sampling of CSF is therefore of prognostic importance, as demonstrated in several multi-institutional studies.[87] The standard site of sampling is from lumbar puncture rather than ventricular CSF and should be performed preoperatively or, if this is not possible due to raised ICP, at least 14 days post-surgery.

Surgical resection is aimed to be maximal but avoiding significant morbidity, as studies have confirmed that in non-disseminated PNET a >90 per cent resection improves prognosis but this does not have to be complete. The CCG 921 study showed that a residuum of less than 1.5 cm^2 did not impart a significantly worse prognosis but that a larger residuum did in M0 patients.[87] This means that, to complete staging, a postoperative MRI/CT is required ideally within 72 hours of the operation. The combination of tumour residuum and Chang M stage leads to two risk groups:

- standard risk – residuum <1.5 cm^2 with localized disease (M0)
- high risk – either a tumour residuum >1.5 cm^2 or metastatic disease (M+).

Other prognostic factors indicating higher risk include anatomical site (SPNETs have a worse outcome than similar staged medulloblastomas) and young age (<36 months also results in a worse outcome as compared with the same stage in older children).

Resection usually establishes normal CSF flow, but in some cases a shunt may be required. Complications other than hydrocephalus after surgery include seizures, infections, pseudomeningocele and cerebellar mutism syndrome. This latter complication arises after posterior fossa craniotomy in about 8 per cent of cases and has been described in several tumour types but most commonly with medulloblastoma extending into the brainstem. Mutism occurs usually between 1 and 7 days after surgery and is associated with anorexia, behavioural abnormalities and decreased initiation of voluntary movements.[88,89] The deficits recover in the majority of cases but the syndrome may last for several months and mild speech abnormalities may persist.

It was noted over 70 years ago that surgery alone was insufficient to provide cure in medulloblastoma, and the addition of craniospinal radiotherapy has been the standard adjuvant therapy for decades. Craniospinal radiotherapy using a boosted dose of 54–55 Gy to the primary tumour and 34–36 Gy to the whole neuraxis has consistently resulted in a 5-year survival rate of 60–70 per cent. Due to the propensity of PNETs to disseminate in the neuraxis, irradiation of the whole brain and spine has been regarded as essential, but this leads to the risk of endocrine, growth and cognitive deficits. As previously described, the younger the age of the child and the greater the dose and volume of radiotherapy, the higher the risk. This has led to the desire to explore reducing the dose of craniospinal radiotherapy in standard-risk tumours and avoiding, delaying or reducing irradiation in infants. The American Pediatric Oncology Group (POG) 8631 study randomized standard-risk medulloblastoma patients to receive either standard-dose craniospinal radiotherapy (54 Gy posterior fossa, 36 Gy to whole brain and spine) or a reduced dose (54 and 23.4 Gy). There was an increased frequency of relapse in the reduced-dose arm, with event-free survival (EFS) at 8 years being 67 per cent in the standard arm and 52 per cent in the investigational arm.[90,91] Importantly, this study also included testing of cognitive functioning and demonstrated that children who received 23.4 Gy performed significantly better than those treated with a higher dose and also that older age at irradiation correlated with improved outcome.[92]

Many chemotherapy agents have been shown to have significant activity in PNET and there have now been several large multi-institution studies addressing the addition of chemotherapy to surgery and radiotherapy. The first two randomized studies from the International Society of Paediatric Oncology (SIOP) and the CCG compared surgery and radiotherapy with surgery, radiotherapy and chemotherapy. The SIOP I trial used vincristine and CCNU after standard-dose radiotherapy, and initial results at 2 years showed an EFS advantage for chemotherapy (71 vs. 53 per cent), but with further follow-up this advantage was lost (10-year EFS: 50 vs. 46 per cent).[93] However, subgroup analysis showed that those with high-risk disease continued to do better with additional chemotherapy. The CCG 942 study was similar in design but with prednisone added to the chemotherapy. The results showed no significant survival advantage at 5 years overall for chemotherapy but in high risk patients there was a 46 per cent EFS vs. 0 per cent in favour of chemotherapy.[94] Another randomized study by POG looked at the addition of MOPP (mustine, vincristine, procarbazine and prednisone) to radiotherapy and showed a marginal improvement versus radiotherapy alone (68 vs. 57 per cent at 5 years).[95]

A number of studies have looked at the feasibility of giving chemotherapy in the neoadjuvant setting after surgery but prior to radiotherapy. In theory, this may exploit the period in which the blood–brain barrier is maximally disrupted. The second SIOP study looked at both pre-radiotherapy 'sandwich' chemotherapy (procarbazine, vincristine and methotrexate) and dose reduction of craniospinal radiotherapy. A risk stratification (brainstem involvement, incomplete resection and metastasis) was used with low-risk patients randomized between reduced vs. standard-dose craniospinal radiotherapy as well as sandwich chemotherapy. High-risk patients received standard dose plus vincristine and CCNU post-radiotherapy. Sandwich chemotherapy did not benefit any group and there was concern that in low-risk patients it had a negative impact by the delay in radiotherapy.[96] Those receiving reduced vs. standard-dose radiotherapy fared less well, with 5-year EFS rates of 55 and 68 per cent, respectively. The CCG 921 study compared sandwich chemotherapy (eight drugs in 1 day regimen: vincristine, CCNU, procarbazine, hydroxyurea, cisplatin, cytarabine, dacarbazine and methylprednisolone) with post-radiotherapy vincristine, CCNU and prednisone. EFS at 5 years was 45 vs. 63 per cent, with the eight-in-1 regimen thought to be inferior due to delay in radiotherapy.[97] A German study, HIT 91, also looking at neoadjuvant (cisplatin, cytarabine, etoposide, ifosfamide and methotrexate) vs. post-radiotherapy chemotherapy (carboplatin, CCNU and vincristine), also raised concerns that chemotherapy given prior to radiotherapy may adversely affect survival by delaying onset of radiotherapy. However, SIOP recently reported the results of the PNET III study, which not only confirms in a randomized fashion the benefit of chemotherapy when added to radiotherapy, but also, for the first time, shows that neoadjuvant 'sandwich' chemotherapy can improve survival in standard non-metastatic risk medulloblastoma. The addition of four courses of chemotherapy (including carboplatin, cyclophosphamide, etoposide and vincristine) led to an EFS at 5 years of 74 per cent, compared with 60 per cent for radiotherapy alone.[98]

The advantage of chemotherapy in poor- or high-risk tumours was further documented by the Washington group using a combination of CCNU, cisplatin and vincristine,[99] and the results of a subsequent multi-institutional study confirmed these findings, with an EFS of 67 per cent at 5 years.[100] This same regimen was subsequently used in low/standard-risk medulloblastoma in combination with reduced-dose (23.4 Gy) craniospinal radiotherapy. The CCG 9892 non-randomized study reported a 5-year EFS of 79 per cent, at least comparable with historical controls using full-dose craniospinal radiotherapy.[101] However, 50 per cent of patients required dose modification of cisplatin due to significant ototoxicity with this regimen. For standard/low-risk medulloblastoma, the latest studies are looking at building on these results using reduced-dose craniospinal radiotherapy. Results are awaited from the CCG 9961 study, which randomized between two chemotherapy regimens following reduced-dose craniospinal radiotherapy; both contain vincristine and cisplatin, with cyclophosphamide and CCNU as the third agents in the differing arms. The next SIOP and German studies are investigating the use of differing schedules of radiotherapy in standard-risk medulloblastoma, randomizing between reduced-dose conventional once-daily craniospinal radiotherapy and a hyperfractionated (twice-daily) schedule. A pilot study with post-irradiation chemotherapy used a dose of 18 Gy for the neuraxis with a standard posterior fossa boost in standard-risk tumours, and showed a 70 per cent survival rate at 6 years; most interestingly, the IQ of the survivors was not altered from baseline.[102] This has prompted consideration for the next American study in younger children (3–8 years) to randomize between 23.4 and 18 Gy as the neuraxis dose and also to use conformal tumour volume-based boost rather than whole posterior fossa.

In high-risk tumours the main priority is not reduction of late effects as in standard-risk medulloblastoma but improvement of overall survival. Historically, high-risk PNETs (incompletely resected, metastatic medulloblastoma and SPNET) have had survival rates of between 30 and 50 per cent at 5 years in the early chemotherapy studies using high-dose radiotherapy. The best results reported so far are those using cisplatin, CCNU and vincristine, with a 67 per cent 5-year survival as previously described. In the PNET III study, pre-irradiation chemotherapy resulted in a 5-year EFS of 46 per cent, but pineal tumours had a better outcome than non-pineal sites (76 vs. 37 per cent).[103] Therapeutic strategies actively being explored in high-risk PNETs include hyperfractionated accelerated radiotherapy (HART; radiotherapy in a higher daily fraction in two doses) and high-dose chemotherapy with or without stem cell rescue and concomitant chemoradiotherapy. A combination of both intensive chemotherapy and HART has given encouraging preliminary results in an Italian group study, with a 3-year EFS of 78 per cent in metastatic medulloblastoma.[104] Combination of HART and chemotherapy with cisplatin, CCNU and vincristine is the basis of the next UKCCSG high-risk medulloblastoma and SPNET protocols. The POG 9631 trial is a phase II study of oral etoposide given concurrently with radiotherapy followed by dose-intensive adjuvant chemotherapy in high-risk PNETs and results are awaited. The CCG has two studies open for high-risk PNETs: CCG 99701 administers concurrent carboplatin and vincristine with radiotherapy followed by cisplatin, CCNU and vincristine, while CCG 99702 utilizes high-dose sequential chemotherapy (carboplatin, cyclophosphamide, thiotepa and vincristine) with stem cell rescue after radiotherapy.

The feasibility of this type of approach has been shown with a 2-year survival of 74 per cent in high-risk tumours.[105] Myeloablative chemotherapy has been used with limited success in relapsed PNETs using initial re-induction chemotherapy followed by high-dose consolidation chemotherapy in those proving to be chemosensitive.[106] Therefore this strategy is being used, with varying induction and consolidation regimens, up front in high-risk tumours with initial encouraging results.[107–109] Obviously, new anti-cancer agents are also being explored, with significant activity for irinotecan and temozolomide in phase I and II studies and interest in pre-clinical results for differentiating agents such as *cis*-retinoic acid.

EPENDYMOMAS

As expected from consideration of their cell of origin, ependymomas usually arise in paraventricular locations. They constitute 8 per cent of all paediatric brain tumours and 25 per cent of all spinal cord tumours. The maximum incidence of intracranial ependymomas is in the first decade of life, whereas spinal ependymomas tend to present a little later. Two-thirds of intracranial ependymomas occur in the posterior fossa. Ependymomas present as space-occupying lesions with clinical features appropriate for their site of origin (see Box 15.2). Obstructive hydrocephalus is common at presentation.

Ependymal tumours are graded according to the WHO criteria as follows:

- grade I – myxopapillary and subependymoma variants
- grade II – ependymoma (cellular, papillary, clear cell and tancytic)
- grade III – malignant anaplastic ependymoma.

Ependymomas are well delineated, moderately cellular gliomas with perivascular pseudo-rosettes and ependymal rosettes. Anaplastic features include brisk mitotic activity, associated microvascular proliferation and necrosis. There remains considerable variability between neuropathologists in assigning anaplastic grading, with the incidence varying between 7 and 89 per cent in reported series[110] and discordance rates of 69 per cent between local and central reviews.[111] This obviously means that histological grading is of limited prognostication without strict central review and agreement. In order to develop a more objective prognostic factor, Ki-67 and MIB-1 indices have been employed and shown to be of prognostic significance.[112–114] The genetics of ependymomas show some consistency with chromosomal deletions on 6q, 17 and 22 and gain of 1q;[115,116] however, the prognostic power of these abnormalities is complex.[117,118] As in medulloblastoma, ErB-B receptor signalling appears to promote aggressive behaviour in ependymoma and this pathway may be a potential therapeutic target.[119]

The natural history of ependymoma is one of local recurrence, often after many years. Overall, 10 per cent of tumours disseminate throughout the CNS and this appears more likely in high-grade and posterior fossa tumours. This means that both brain and spinal MRI imaging should be undertaken at diagnosis and possibly CSF cytology obtained if there is doubt. Ependymomas are usually iso/hypointense on T1-weighted MRI and hyperintense on T2 with enhancement on contrast (see Figure 15.8). Surgery alone can cure ependymoma if complete[120] and the extent of surgical resection has been demonstrated to be the most important prognostic factor in multiple studies, with a gross total (>90 per cent) resection imparting a better prognosis.[111,121,122] The site of origin of the tumour therefore is important as posterior fossa tumours often infiltrate the brainstem and wrap around cranial nerves and vessels, whereas supratentorial tumours may be more amenable to gross total resection. Due to the overriding importance of surgery to prognosis, more aggressive surgical approaches are being taken with the possibility of increased morbidity (e.g. bulbar palsy requiring tracheostomy/gastrostomy)

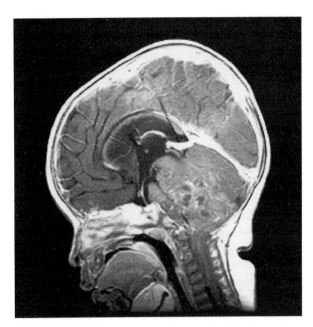

Figure 15.8 *Sagittal T1-weighted enhanced MRI of posterior fossa ependymoma.*

plus the concept of second look surgery after adjuvant chemotherapy/radiotherapy has emerged. Reduction in size or vascularization may allow the neurosurgeon to complete resection at a later point.[123]

Radiotherapy, except in very young children, has become the main adjuvant therapy to surgery despite the absence of any randomized studies confirming benefit. The 5-year EFS in completely resected tumours varies between 50 and 70 per cent, compared with 0–30 per cent in incompletely resected tumours. Historically, craniospinal radiotherapy was deemed necessary due to the possibility of spinal seeding, but several studies refute the need, as local failure is the main reason for relapse.[124,125] The dose of radiotherapy to the tumour bed is usually >50 Gy; various schedules and techniques have been used, including hyperfractionation, stereotactic and gamma knife radiosurgery, with varying results, and these still need to be further evaluated.[126,127]

Chemotherapeutic agents have been investigated in phase II studies, including AZQ, carboplatin, cisplatin, etoposide, idarubicin, ifosfamide, irinotecan, PCNU, temozolomide, thiotepa and topotecan.[128,129] Responses have been limited in these single-agent studies in relapsed patients and there is a continued need to identify anticancer drugs with activity, possibly in window phase II studies prior to second-look surgery. Combination therapy has also been limited in success; the CCG's first randomized study demonstrated no benefit of CCNU, prednisone and vincristine when added to craniospinal radiotherapy, with survival at 10 years of 37 per cent.[130] Other combinations include MOPP, vincristine/cyclophosphamide and eight-in-1-day, all with limited response. A regimen alternating vincristine/carboplatin with etoposide/ifosfamide after irradiation resulted in an EFS of 74 per cent at 5 years, which appeared to be an improvement compared with historical controls.[131] Baby brain protocols have demonstrated some efficacy and are described on page 305. High-dose chemotherapy with stem cell rescue has also been investigated with a number of agents, including busulphan/thiotepa, thiotepa/carboplatin/etoposide and cyclophosphamide/melphalan.[132–134] Although some objective responses have been documented, these are in relatively few tumours and most patients have relapsed despite high-dose chemotherapy suggesting inherent chemoresistance.[135,136] Ongoing studies by SIOP and the American cancer groups are looking at combination chemotherapy and the possibility of increasing the frequency of complete resection by second-look surgery.

The prognosis for spinal ependymomas is superior to that for intracranial tumours, although surgical resection may result in significant neurological deficit. Myxopapillary low-grade ependymoma often occurs in the lower cord or cauda equina and surgery may well be curative. Future directions in the treatment of ependymoma will require new active agents and continued improvements in neurosurgical and radiotherapy practice.

PINEAL TUMOURS

Tumours of different histology can arise in the pineal gland and account for 1–2 per cent of all CNS tumours. In a compilation of 278 histologically verified tumours collected from 12 series,[137] the calculated incidence of the various pineal tumour types was as follows:

- germinomas – 45 per cent
- astrocytomas – 17 per cent
- non-germinomatous germ cell tumours (NGGCTs), including teratomas – 16 per cent
- pineal parenchymal tumours (pineoblastoma and pineocytoma) – 15 per cent
- other – 7 per cent.

In Japan and the Far East, the incidence of germinoma is even higher, particularly in young men. A pineoblastoma may arise as part of the familial trilateral retinoblastoma syndrome.[138] This tumour is histologically identical to PNET at other sites and has a predisposition to disseminate to the neuraxis. Pineocytomas have larger cells which grow in sheets and are lower grade tumours.

Germ cell tumours (GCTs) arise in the pineal gland and other midline structures of the brain, including the third ventricle and suprasellar regions as well as the basal ganglia. Germinomas represent about two-thirds of all intracranial GCTs, the rest are NGGCTs and can be divided into secreting GCTs (embryonal carcinoma, yolk sac tumours and choriocarcinoma) and teratomas (mature and immature). There are also mixed GCTs. Germinomas are the most common pineal tumours, have a high incidence in young adult males and are fast-growing. Histologically they consist of uniform large cells with prominent nucleoli and glycogen-rich cytoplasm; there is often a lymphocytic infiltrate and they mark positive for placental alkaline phosphatase. They do not secrete alpha-fetoprotein (AFP), but low levels of beta-human chorionic gonadotrophin (β-hCG) can be detected if the tumour contains a few syncytiotrophoblasts and this does not preclude the diagnosis. Germinomas have a tendency to disseminate in the CSF in approximately 10–15 per cent of cases. NGGCTs are more likely to arise in the pineal region than the suprasellar area and their histological appearance is identical to extracranial tumours of the same type. A raised serum or CSF β-hCG is consistent with choriocarcinoma, whereas embryonal cell carcinomas, immature teratomas and yolk sac tumours secrete AFP.

Clinical presenting features are often due to hydrocephalus secondary to aqueductal obstruction. Pressure of a pineal tumour on the quadrigeminal plate gives rise to Parinaud's syndrome, consisting of paralysis of upward gaze, convergence retraction nystagmus, lid retraction and dissociation of the light and accommodation reflexes. GCTs arising anteriorly in the third ventricle may present with visual difficulties, precocious puberty and hypopituitarism. Diabetes insipidus is often an early presenting symptom from pineal germinomas and is due to the presence of microscopic seedling deposits. Secretion of high β-hCG levels can lead to pseudo-precocious puberty.

Due to the diversity of tumours that can arise in the pineal region, neuroimaging may help in the differential diagnosis but is not diagnostic. Germinomas are usually isointense on T1, hyperintense on T2 with homogeneous enhancement on MRI (see Figure 15.9). Pineal parenchymal tumours are hypointense on T1, hyperintense on T2 with variable enhancement and teratomas show heterogeneity in signal intensity with multi-loculated irregular enhancement (see Figure 15.10). Spinal preoperative imaging is indicated for a possible germinoma due to possible seedings. A secreting GCT with characteristic appearance on MRI with elevation of serum/CSF AFP or β-hCG (normalized for age) does not require histological confirmation. CSF cytology may be useful in staging, but timing in relation to surgery is important due to false positives from tumour spillage. However, biopsy may be possible via endoscopy, also allowing an endoscopic third ventriculostomy for CSF diversion. Alternatively, stereotactic biopsy can be performed but there is often concern over the possibility of injury to deep veins. Extensive resection is difficult to achieve in most pineal tumours and, due to the relative chemo/radiosensitivity, is not essential to successful management. Mature teratomas that are well encapsulated may be amenable to complete

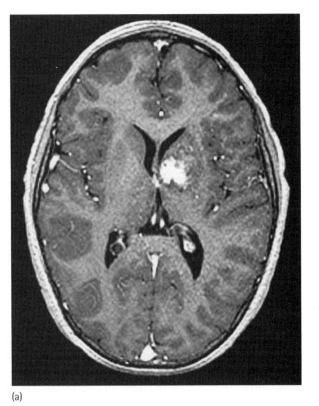

(a)

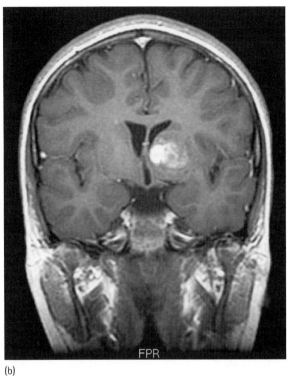

(b)

Figure 15.9 *Axial (a) and coronal (b) T1-weighted enhanced MRI of a basal ganglia germinoma.*

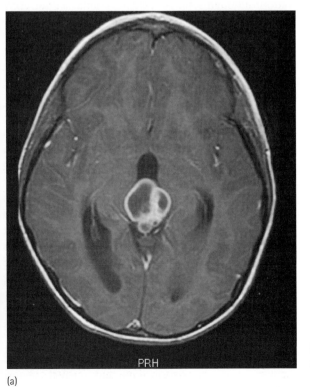

(a)

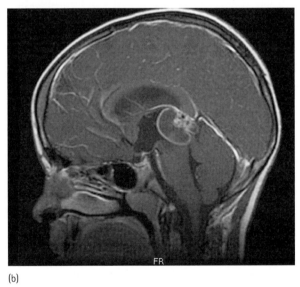

(b)

Figure 15.10 *Axial (a) and sagittal (b) T1-weighted enhanced MRI of a cystic heterogeneous pineal mature teratoma.*

resection. Therefore surgery is usually limited to biopsy and debulking to relieve hydrocephalus with the possibility of second-look surgery in those with significant residual disease.

Radiotherapy has traditionally been first-line adjuvant therapy and craniospinal with primary tumour boost was, for many years, standard. Pineoblastomas are usually treated as per other high-risk PNETs with craniospinal irradiation and chemotherapy. Pineocytoma, unless disseminated, can receive involved-field radiotherapy alone. Germinomas are extremely radiosensitive, with survival rates at 10 years in excess of 90 per cent after craniospinal radiotherapy.[139] As only 15 per cent of germinomas are disseminated at diagnosis and the majority of relapses occur locally, there has been a trend away from the routine use of craniospinal irradiation. Review of published studies has demonstrated that spinal recurrence is no more common in patients treated with whole-brain versus craniospinal radiotherapy.[140] Local-field radiotherapy in non-disseminated germinoma can considerably reduce long-term sequelae such as growth and neurocognitive deficits, particularly in younger children, and provides comparable 5-year EFS rates to craniospianal radiotherapy.[141] Whether to include the ventricular system in the field or to irradiate only the tumour bed is debatable. Several studies have shown local-field irradiation to be effective,[142,143] but results from the SIOP GCT study group suggest that focal irradiation of tumour plus margin, even with chemotherapy, led to more relapses in the ventricular system than previously encountered with extended-field irradiation.[144] This has led to a recommendation for the use of whole ventricular irradiation in non-metastatic germinoma in combination with chemotherapy. The dose of radiotherapy has been shown to be as effective in low-dose craniospinal (24 Gy + local boost to 45 Gy) as that previously used in several studies.[145,146]

Lower-dose focal radiotherapy of 40 Gy has also been shown not to affect survival adversely.[147] Although NGGCTs are generally less radiosensitive, the debate over field size is similar to germinoma but they generally require a higher dose in comparison.

As would be expected from the results in extracranial GCTs, they have been found to be highly chemosensitive tumours, and significant activity found with bleomycin, carboplatin, cisplatin, cyclophosphamide, etoposide, ifosfamide and vinca alkaloids. Chemotherapy has generally been used in germinoma to allow reduction of radiotherapy volume and dose, and in NGGCTs to try to improve the disappointing survival rates with surgery and radiotherapy alone (30–50 per cent OS). The French SFOP TC 90 study, used two courses of carboplatin, etoposide and ifosfamide with 40 Gy focal radiotherapy in localized germinomas and low-dose craniospinal irradiation in metastatic disease, with a 3-year EFS of 96.4 per cent.[148] The first international study for intracranial GCT used four cycles of carboplatin, etoposide and bleomycin in an attempt to avoid radiotherapy.[149] Those with a complete response received two further cycles; others received two cycles intensified by cyclophosphamide. The complete response rate was 84 per cent for germinomas and 78 per cent for NGGCTs. With a median follow-up duration of 31 months, 28 of 71 patients were alive without relapse or progression. Thirty-five showed tumour recurrence ($n = 28$) or progression ($n = 7$) at a median of 13 months. Twenty-six out of 28 patients (93 per cent) who recurred following remission underwent successful salvage therapy.

This approach has been modified and most current studies are investigating the combined use of chemotherapy with reduction in both dose and volume of radiotherapy in germinoma. As can be seen from this study, NGGCTs also respond to chemotherapy. The German and Italian cooperative group conducted a pilot study using four courses of PEI (cisplatin, etoposide, ifosfamide) prior to resection of residual tumour, if possible.[150] Following this, patients received craniospinal radiotherapy (30 Gy with 24 Gy tumour boost), which produced an impressive EFS of 86 per cent and was taken forward as the basis of the recent SIOP GCT 96 trial.

Prognostic factors for pineal tumours include histology (germinomas have a better outcome than NGGCTs and parenchymal pineal tumours), presence of metastases and grossly elevated tumour markers. In the case of relapse after radiotherapy, high-dose salvage chemotherapy has been successfully used in both germinomas and NGGCTs.[151–153] Mature and immature teratomas are the rarest CNS GCTs, and tumour markers may be slightly elevated. Therapy is surgical resection followed by observation, although subtotal resection confers a poor prognosis. Neither chemotherapy nor radiotherapy has been shown to be of significant benefit.

CRANIOPHARYNGIOMAS

Craniopharyngiomas account for about 8 per cent of all paediatric CNS tumours (2 per cent in adults), with a median age of 8 years at presentation. Usually occurring in the midline suprasellar region, they may also appear intrasellarly or, rarely, in adjacent locations. Derived from Rathke's pouch remnants, approximately 55 per cent of the tumours are entirely cystic, 15 per cent are almost entirely solid and the rest are mixed. The cyst content is usually thick cholesterol-laden fluid, escape into the CSF of which causes chemical meningitis. The surrounding tumour contains squamous epithelium. The capsule of the tumour adheres tightly to the adjacent brain tissue, making complete resection difficult and sometimes hazardous.

Clinical presentation varies but raised ICP, visual changes, pituitary dysfunction and mental abnormalities are common. Very young children tend to present with signs of hydrocephalus and older children with endocrinopathies, failure to thrive and diabetes insipidus. Adolescents and young adults more commonly have visual field deficits.

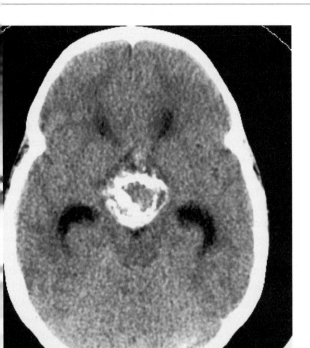

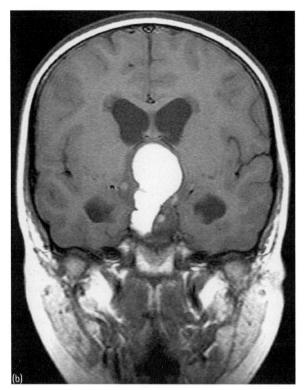

Figure 15.11 *(a) CT showing calcified craniopharyngioma. (b) T1-weighted coronal MRI of craniopharyngioma.*

Neuroimaging will generally distinguish these tumours from other parasellar tumours. CT demonstrates a low-density contrast-enhancing mass with calcification and erosion of the sella (see Figure 15.11). MRI delineates the surrounding anatomy well with a variable cystic/solid tumour with the cystic component enhancing readily with gadolinium enhancement.

A rigorous preoperative neuroendocrine and ophthalmic work-up is essential. Surgery is the most important initial therapy. The surgical technique is dependent on the exact anatomical site of the tumour and several radiological classification systems have been used, including those described by Hoffman[154] and Brunel *et al.*[155] Subfrontal, pterional, bifrontal interhemispheric, subtemporal, transcallosal and trans-sphenoidal approaches have all been used successfully with the aid of an operating microscope and are chosen according to site, size and operator experience. Trans-sphenoidal surgery is more common in adult craniopharyngioma due to location and also the fact that anatomically this technique is difficult in young children. The debate as to whether radical resection or subtotal resection with adjuvant radiotherapy should be attempted is still controversial. There is no doubt that complete compared with subtotal resection leads to a better PFS (60–90 vs. 30–50 per cent), but this comes at a cost in terms of increased neuroendocrine, neurocognitive, visual and marked behavioural deficits. However, the addition of adjuvant radiotherapy has been demonstrated

to improve PFS even in subtotal resections.[156,157] Some centres have preferentially performed subtotal resections with adjuvant radiotherapy and claim equivalent survival figures at a reduced morbidity. Both Great Ormond Street Hospital and St Jude Children's Research Hospital have presented patient series using limited surgery and radiotherapy and suggest fewer neuroendocrine deficits and neurocognitive changes, less postoperative morbid obesity and better quality of life scores.[158,159]

Patients who relapse after surgery and radiotherapy require individualized retreatment. In the case of cystic recurrence, this could include surgery, intracystic radioisotope installation or intracystic bleomycin. Radioisotopes used include yttrium-90[160] and phosphorus-32[161,162] and have been reported to have shown good control in those patients in whom further surgical intervention would have a high morbidity. Intracystic bleomycin has been used in cystic craniopharyngioma in childhood but significant side-effects have been described.[163–165] Systemic chemotherapy has had limited activity in this benign tumour.[166,167]

CENTRAL NERVOUS SYSTEM TUMOURS IN INFANTS

Central nervous system tumours in younger children warrant a separate discussion as they are often treated on specific 'infant' brain tumour protocols with a therapeutic approach different from that used in older children. The primary reason for this distinction has to do with therapy-related morbidity, particularly intellectual damage, which has been attributed to the effects of cranial irradiation at a young age. The definition of an infant, and the point at which therapy for a brain tumour changes, varies between different groups but generally 3 years of age is chosen. It has been shown that cranial irradiation has a more significant effect on the intellect of the developing brain; for example, a reduction in IQ of 40 has been found in children irradiated at under 12 months of age. The effect becomes less significant in children over the age of 3, but a reduction in IQ can still be observed in 7-year-olds.

Approximately 15 per cent of all paediatric CNS tumours occur in children less than 2 years of age and one-third in those below the age of 5 years. The distribution of histological tumour types shows some differences from that of older children. Astrocytomas are still the largest group, but the proportion of malignant gliomas (including brainstem gliomas) is reduced, with optic chiasm and hypothalamic sites representing more of the low-grade tumours. PNETs are the commonest malignant tumours and the incidence of ependymoma is slightly higher in children under the age of 3 years than in older children. Certain tumour types are much more common in infants, e.g. atypical teratoid/rhabdoid tumours, choroid plexus tumours and desmoplastic infantile ganglioglioma.

Infants often have different clinical presentation from that of older children, due to the compliance of their skull and their inability to report symptoms. Increasing head circumference may be noted as a first sign of a slow-growing tumour, whereas features of raised ICP (full bulging fontanelle, separation of sutures, irritability, vomiting) are the commonest presentation. Failure to thrive and poor feeding are also recognized associations, particularly with hypothalamic tumours. Localizing signs, seizures and visual disturbance are considerably less common in young children than in an older group.

The treatment of infants with malignant brain tumours presents a therapeutic dilemma between efficacy and trying to avoid unacceptable morbidity in survivors. Therefore, in the 1980s, 'baby brain' protocols were developed to try to delay, reduce or avoid radiotherapy in this vulnerable group. One of the first chemotherapy protocols described in infants was MOPP (mustine, vincristine, procarbazine, prednisone), which was used in 17 infants with mixed histology and resulted in 15 having a response (six with complete remission).[168] Radiotherapy was reserved for progressive disease or relapse, with four out of nine relapses being salvaged by irradiation/second-line chemotherapy. Those children who did not receive radiotherapy have IQ scores in the normal range.[169] The Pediatric Oncology Group study

POG 8633-34 used post-surgical chemotherapy comprising vincristine, cyclophosphamide, cisplatin and etoposide, initially aiming to delay radiotherapy (children aged <24 months received irradiation after 24 months' chemotherapy and those aged 24–36 months after 12 months' chemotherapy).[170] There was a 40 per cent PFS at 2 years. The protocol allowed delay of radiotherapy of 1–2 years in the majority of patients. At the same time, the CCG opened a study using the 'eight-in-1-day' regimen, previously described (p. 299). Infants were to receive either focal radiotherapy after two courses or craniospinal irradiation after 12 months of the regimen.[171] Interestingly, only nine of the 82 infants received radiotherapy prior to tumour progression due to investigator decision, and 24 children completed the full chemotherapy course, of whom 19 are event-free survivors, with only three being irradiated. This study suggested that a proportion of young children with malignant CNS tumours could be cured without recourse to radiotherapy, although the PFS remained poor (29 per cent at 3 years for localized disease and 11 per cent for metastatic disease). Survival rates in these two studies varied according to histology, with choroid plexus carcinoma, ependymoma, medulloblastoma and malignant glioma responding better to these regimens as compared with very poor results for brainstem glioma and other PNETs.[172–174] The results indicate that the chemosensitivity of infant tumours may be different from that seen in older children, reflecting possible different underlying biology.

Following on from these initial studies, several groups looked at dose intensification as a means of improving outcome in infants. A number of national study groups adopted protocols using multi-agent chemotherapy for a period of 12–18 months, with radiotherapy usually reserved for those with disseminated disease or salvage at progression or relapse. The drugs used and results are shown in Table 15.1.[175–181] These studies have shown some improvement from the original 'baby brain' protocols, mainly for those tumours that have been completely surgically resected and, interestingly, in children with ependymoma where there has been delayed radiotherapy that has been given as a salvage strategy.

The most recent generation of studies has developed further the idea of dose intensification, looking at the use of myeloablative chemotherapy with stem cell rescue. The French SFOP group used high-dose chemotherapy comprising busulphan and thiotepa plus focal radiotherapy in relapsed medulloblastoma after young children had progressed on their 'SFOP baby brain' protocol (see Table 15.1).[182] Among 16 of these patients with measurable disease, there was an overall response rate of 75 per cent. At a median follow-up of 31 months, the EFS was 50 per cent. Following on from these results, the French group have been investigating the use of high-dose chemotherapy with focal radiotherapy in high-risk

Table 15.1 *National 'baby brain' protocols for malignant infant CNS tumours*

National group	Chemotherapy (CT)	Duration	Radiotherapy	Results
POG 9233[175]	Dose intensive: Cyclo, VCR, CDDP, VP-16	72 weeks	Not if in CR	Improvement in PFS for EP but not MB over POG 8633
CCG 9921[180]	Randomized between: Cyclo, VCR, CDDP, VP-16 or Ifos, VP-16, Carbo, VCR	52 weeks	Delayed until either completed CT or 3 years	1-year PFS 48 vs. 30% for prior CCG study
UKCCSG[176]	VCR, Carbo, Cyclo, MTX, CDDP	52 weeks	Only if progression	Not published
SFOP[178,179]	Carbo, Proc, VP-16, CDDP, VCR, Cyclo	63 weeks	Only if progression	Low-risk MB: PFS 37%, 94% OS at 3 years EP: 22% PFS, 59% OS at 4 years
ANZCCSG[181]	VCR, VP-16, Cyclo, CDDP, Carbo (VETOPEC)	64 weeks	Progression or residual disease at 3 years	11% PFS, 34% OS at 3 years
German[177]	Cyclo, MTX, Carbo, VCR, VP-16, IT-(MTX)	24 weeks	Only if progression	52% PFS at 3 years

Carbo, carboplatin; CDDP, cisplatin; CR, complete response; CT, chemotherapy; Cyclo, cyclophosphamide; EP, ependymoma; Ifos, ifosfamide; IT-(MTX), intrathecal (methotrexate); MB, medulloblastoma; OS, overall survival; PFS, progression-free survival; Proc, procarbazine; VCR, vincristine; VP-16, etoposide.

metastatic medulloblastoma as well as relapses in children under the age of 3.

Similar results in relapsed CNS tumours in older patients were reported by a team in New York in collaboration with other institutions using high-dose thiotepa and etoposide with a response rate of 28 per cent and a PFS of 28 per cent at 3+ years.[183] A subsequent study by the same group in young children with recurrent CNS tumours was even more encouraging, with 50 per cent of patients alive and disease-free at a median follow-up of 39 months, including patients with high-grade glioma, medulloblastoma and SPNET.[184] This strategy was adapted to newly diagnosed CNS tumours in infants and young children less than 6 years of age with the addition of an induction regimen, 'Head Start I', consisting of five cycles of vincristine, cisplatin, cyclophosphamide and etoposide.[109] Irradiation was reserved for treatment of residual disease at consolidation or after progression or relapse and was administered to 19 out of 62 patients. Consolidation with thiotepa, carboplatin and etoposide occurred with stem cell rescue, and the 3-year PFS was 25 per cent and the OS was 40 per cent. An update of these results from the 'Head Start' series shows that results are improving due to a combination of lower treatment-related mortality and intensification of the induction regimen with high-dose methotrexate: OS rates at 3 years are 64 per cent for medulloblastoma, 43 per cent for SPNET, 66 per cent for ependymoma and 25 per cent for high-grade glioma.[185,186] The Italian group has also recently presented its data using myeloablative chemotherapy in infants. An initial induction regimen of vincristine, etoposide, high-dose methotrexate, cyclophosphamide and carboplatin was followed by sequential chemotherapy utilizing carboplatin and etoposide plus thiotepa and melphalan couplets with stem cell support. Those with residual tumour following chemotherapy or metastatic disease received radiotherapy. For high-risk medulloblastoma, 58 per cent of patients were alive and free of disease at

median follow-up of 20 months, with 50 per cent not receiving radiotherapy; results for other PNETs and malignant gliomas are also encouraging.[187]

Areas of active research in infant CNS tumours include the use of highly conformal radiotherapy in conjunction with chemotherapy and the possibility of new agents that may be used intrathecally either as treatment or as prophylaxis against disseminated disease in place of craniospinal radiotherapy. Increasingly, separate protocols for specific tumour types are being developed as in older children rather than one generic 'baby brain' protocol.

RARE PAEDIATRIC CNS TUMOURS

Tumours that occur in relatively small numbers present a difficult challenge when attempting to produce best evidence-based treatment plans. Collection of data from registries is essential and sharing of successful management is vital as an initial step to developing studies or guidelines for these infrequent tumours.

Atypical teratoid/rhabdoid tumour

This is a malignant embryonal CNS tumour consisting of rhabdoid cells but often resembling a classical PNET. It is histologically and genetically similar to the malignant rhabdoid tumour of the kidney (MRTK), and metachronous tumours of the CNS and kidney have been reported. The vast majority of tumours arise before the age of 5 years, but older cases have been confirmed, with peak incidence in the first 2 years of life. Over 60 per cent of tumours arise in the posterior fossa but most sites in the CNS have been reported for primary tumours. A third of patients present with disseminated disease from CSF spread. Presentation is dependent on site, with infants often showing lethargy, vomiting and failure to thrive. Head tilt and cranial nerve palsies may also be noted, with older children complaining of headache, motor weakness and ataxia. Unfortunately, neuroimaging is similar to that for medulloblastoma and PNET with high-density, non-uniform enhancement on CT and a hypointense enhancing lesion seen on T1-weighted MRI. The histology maybe a classical malignant rhabdoid tumour or may closely resemble PNET and classification can be difficult, but immunohistochemistry yields a unique pattern of expression positive for both epithelial membrane antigen (EMA) and vimentin on the rhabdoid cells. The majority (90 per cent) demonstrate monosomy deletion of chromosome 22. The gene involved is *hSNF5/INI1* located at 22q11.2, and germ-line mutations have been detected in patients with both CNS and renal lesions, one child with tumours of both organs.[188] Prognosis is poor compared with a similar stage PNET, with very few long-term survivors. Even with complete surgical resection and intensive multimodality therapy, little progress has been made in this aggressive tumour. Some reports have suggested that either high-dose chemotherapy or intensive chemotherapy as used in sarcoma protocols may lead to improved survival.[189,190]

Choroid plexus tumours

These usually occur in infants and represent between 1–4 per cent of paediatric CNS tumours. The choroid plexus papilloma is more common than carcinomas and classically is a frond-like mass arising in the ventricles and secreting CSF (see Figure 15.12). The infant usually presents with hydrocephalus and following diagnosis, complete excision is curative.

Choroid plexus carcinomas represent a considerable surgical challenge due to their high vascularity and in the past surgical mortality was high. With modern surgical techniques the majority of tumours can be fully excised but this may be in a two staged process after adjuvant chemotherapy has reduced the vascularity of the malignant tumour. Although complete resection is regarded as the goal of the neurosurgeon, survivors have been described with gross total resections without adjuvant therapy.[191] There is a debate over the role of adjuvant radiotherapy, although a review of the published literature suggested an advantage.[192] Chemotherapy has been shown to be effective both in producing a response and in allowing second-look surgery, but the most effective regimen is still to be developed. The most important positive prognostic factors are the absence of metastases and completeness of surgical resection.

Chordoma

Although they are presumed to arise from congenital notochordal remnants, it is rare for these tumours to present in childhood. They can arise anywhere within the

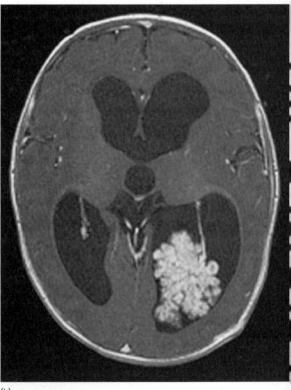

(a)

(b)

Figure 15.12 *Sagittal T1-weighted unenhanced (a) and axial T1 enhanced (b) MRIs of a choroid plexus papilloma in the lateral ventricle.*

axial skeleton but most frequently are found at the base of the skull or in the sacrococcygeal region. Compared with adults, paediatric lesions are more likely to follow an aggressive course and metastasize, which may include systemic lesions such as bone and lung, and skin lesions.[193]

Presentation is due to local invasion causing damage to neighbouring structures such as lower cranial nerve palsies, motor weakness, dysphagia and dysarthria in the case of a clival primary. Both CT and MRI are required to delineate disease and plan possible surgery (see Figure 15.13). Due to the location and invasion of chordomas, gross total resection with negative margins is rarely achieved and the incidence of local recurrence is high. The risks of functional, structural and cosmetic deficits limit the radiation dose using conventional radiation techniques, although this adjuvant therapy has been shown to improve survival. Therefore the use of conformal proton beam radiotherapy with its minimal exit beam allows safe dose escalation even in lesions close to vulnerable structures and is regarded as the gold standard in this condition.[194] Chemotherapy has been used with variable results and its position in the overall management of inoperable chordoma needs further evaluation.

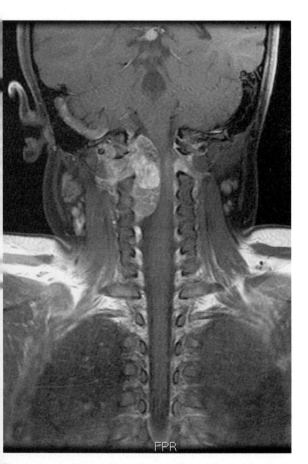

Figure 15.13 *Coronal T1-enhanced MRI of a cervical locally invasive chordoma.*

Dysembryoplastic neuroepithelial tumours

Dysembryoplastic neuroepithelial tumours (DNETs) are mixed neuronal and neuronoglial benign tumours and were only described in 1988.[195] They are slow-growing tumours that present with a chronic history of refractory seizures; rarely, there may be a history of headache. The most common location is the temporal lobe and a cortical lesion is classical, possibly extending subcortically. On neuroimaging, the lesion is well demarcated and hypodense on CT with a small degree of enhancement or calcification. MRI shows a hyperintense signal on T2. Surgical excision is curative and may improve seizures.

Ganglioglioma

These represent up to 4 per cent of paediatric CNS tumours and are more frequent in children than in adults. They are benign, slow-growing tumours composed of mature well-differentiated ganglion cells. The glial component demonstrates Rosenthal fibres and calcification. Anaplastic variants have been described but are very rare; there is also a tumour that occurs in infancy as a large supratentorial cystic mass with a desmoplastic matrix, which is known as a 'desmoplastic infantile ganglioglioma'. The clinical presentation is dependent on site, with half of patients developing seizures, usually associated with a supratentorial location such as the temporal lobe or another cortical site. Symptom history is usually long and may include headache, visual disturbance or spinal symptoms if a midline or spinal lesion is present. Imaging demonstrates a non-specific appearance on both CT and MRI, with diagnosis resting on histology. Treatment is with surgery, and gross total resection is attempted. Radiotherapy has been used in non-operable lesions or at recurrence, and the place of chemotherapy is debatable.[196]

Meningioma

The incidence of meningeal tumours is much lower in childhood than in adults, representing only 0.5–2 per cent of tumours. Histologically they are indistinguishable from the adult tumours and are classified into several variants that appear not to correlate with prognosis. Malignant meningiomas are thought to be more common in children but this reflects the inclusion of meningeal sarcomas which are not recognized as readily in adults. The main aetiological factors are the presence of neurofibromatosis types 1 and 2, with some series suggesting 25 per cent having these predisposing conditions and previous irradiation. The location varies in this age group compared with adults, with an increased incidence of non-dural-based, intraventricular and posterior fossa lesions. Therefore the presentation is often different, with more features of raised ICP. Imaging is interesting, with plain films able to demonstrate hyperostosis, calcification and bone erosion, although this is more commonly seen on CT. MRI provides excellent delineation of the anatomy with the characterization of the tapering enhancement along the periphery of the tumour, the so-called 'dural tail'. Angiography can be used if preoperative embolization is being considered and may demonstrate external carotid or cavernous sinus feeding vessels. Treatment options include surgery, which may be preceded by embolization. Radiotherapy can produce stabilization of disease and sometimes reduction in size; chemotherapy has no established role but hydroxyurea, interferon and anti-progesterones have all been used in adults. Prognosis is good but local recurrences do occur.

Neurocytoma

Predominately a tumour of young adults, central neurocytomas are usually found located in the septum pellucidum or the lateral ventricle wall but have been reported in a variety of other intra-, extra- and paraventricular sites. Most commonly the tumour presents with symptoms and signs of raised ICP. Imaging usually shows a tumour in the lateral ventricles but they can occur extraventricularly. Pathology demonstrates a typical honeycomb pattern resembling oligodendroglioma with uniform nuclei. The treatment of choice is gross total excision but the central location can limit resection. Prognosis is generally good but recurrence and dissemination have been reported. Radiotherapy has been suggested to be useful in those with a subtotal resection.

Oligodendroglioma

These tumours account for only 1 per cent of paediatric CNS tumours, being much more common in adults. They are well differentiated, diffusely infiltrating glial tumours that usually occur in the cerebral cortex, but they have been described throughout the neuraxis. Symptoms can occur over a long period, and seizures are the most common ones. Raised ICP can be a presenting feature of higher-grade faster-growing lesions. The most common sites are the frontal, temporal, parietal lobes followed by the hypothalamus and ventricles. Rarely, dissemination can occur. The histology is classical and described as having a 'fried egg' appearance with 'chicken wire' vasculature. The WHO system recognizes low-grade lesions and an anaplastic variant based on the presence of mitotic activity, microvascularization and necrosis but there has been a debate over the interobserver variability between

the classifications used. There is a high incidence of 19q and 1p chromosomal loss and also of *p53* mutations, P16/CDKN2A, 10q loss and overexpression of EGFr.[197] Treatment consists of surgery, with extent of resection correlating with survival. Interestingly, chemotherapy response in adult tumours correlates closely with the presence of 19q and 1p deletions, this group having up to a 70 per cent response rate to procarbazine, CCNU and vincristine (PCV) and more recently also to the alkylating agent temozolomide.[198–200] This has not as yet been established as being the same in the paediatric population. Radiotherapy is often used in anaplastic tumours as adjuvant therapy but its real benefit remains unclear.

Pleomorphic xanthoastrocytoma

This rare tumour is composed of mixed neuronal-glial cells that demonstrate glial fibrillary acidic protein (GFAP) positivity but have significant cellular atypia, pleomorphism and bizarre multinucleated giant cells. The intracellular lipid gives rise to the xanthomatous appearance and there is low mitotic activity, which is important as it can be mistaken for a more aggressive tumour. The majority of patients present in the second decade of life with seizures with an average duration of 2 years. Raised ICP signs and symptoms occur in a fifth of patients. It is located subcortically in the temporal lobe in over 75 per cent of cases and can be solid, cystic or have components of both. Treatment is by surgical excision and long-term survival is excellent. The presence of anaplasia and necrosis are poor prognostic features, and the benefit of radiotherapy and chemotherapy is as yet unproven.

Schwannomas and acoustic neuromas

These are rare benign tumours arising from the normal Schwann cells that wrap around peripheral nerves. They are most commonly associated with NF-2 but there are non-NF-2 affected patients. Acoustic neuromas arise from the sensory vestibular part of the VIIIth cranial nerve and, in the case of NF-2, usually bilaterally. The commonest symptoms are tinnitus and slow sensorineural hearing loss.[201] The next most common site is the Vth cranial nerve but they can also arise in the CNS parenchyma, ventricles and spinal cord. In children, symptoms may go unnoticed for some time and they may present late with cranial nerve palsies and raised ICP. Obviously, patients with NF-2 may have other signs and a family history, but this condition should be considered, and indeed screened for, if a Schwannoma is diagnosed. The surgical management is very specialized and aimed at conserving function of the VIIth and VIIIth nerves. Preoperative assessment is vital, as is intraoperative monitoring. Indications for surgery include rapid growth, brainstem compression, hydrocephalus and loss of hearing in the affected ear. Stereotactic radiotherapy is of interest and has shown good results in adult patients.[202,203]

CNS TREATMENT MORBIDITY

Damage can result to the CNS from several factors related to the development and subsequent treatment of tumours of the brain and spinal cord. The tumour itself can destroy neuronal tissue locally, and raised ICP can result in permanent damage. Surgical trauma and postoperative complications, such as infection, haemorrhage and ischaemia, can produce significant neurological sequelae. Chemotherapy can result in acute encephalopathy and cause haemorrhage and leucoencephalopathy. Radiotherapy can lead to microangiopathy, large-vessel stenosis such as moyamoya, neuroendocrinopathy and secondary brain tumours.

The neuropsychological sequelae of paediatric radiotherapy in children treated for both acute lymphoblastic leukaemia (ALL) and primary brain tumours have been extensively studied and reported. Initial studies on long-term survivors of ALL who were irradiated showed a significantly higher incidence of deficits than classmates, siblings and children with malignancy that had not received radiotherapy.[204,205] It became apparent that children who were irradiated at a younger age were more vulnerable to neuropsychological sequelae, and it is now clear that children under the age of 3–4 years are at most risk.[204,206,207] The dose of radiotherapy used in the cranial prophylaxis/ treatment of ALL has also been shown to correlate with the degree of neurocognitive deficit, with children treated with doses greater than 24 Gy (children retreated after CNS relapse) having significantly worse deficits.[208] The beneficial effect of reducing whole-brain radiotherapy to a dose of 18 Gy, compared with 24 Gy, has been more debatable but there is evidence that younger children in particular suffer fewer deficits.[209,210]

Studies on long-term survivors of primary brain tumours provide a number of interesting data that complement and augment the foregoing work. An early small case–control study of irradiated medulloblastoma survivors, none of whom had undergone chemotherapy, demonstrated a significant neurocognitive deficit compared with a sibling control group.[211] Another study, conducted at the same time, tested 10 children with posterior fossa tumours treated with radiation and chemotherapy.[212] Four children had undergone intelligence testing in school prior to treatment of their tumour. In each case, results following treatment revealed a deterioration of full-scale IQ of at least 25 points. Six children did not have prior testing; of these, two had IQs less than 20. Overall, 50 per cent of the patients had IQs of less than 80 and 20 per cent had IQs greater than 100. Furthermore, four children with normal intelligence (IQ > 80) had learning problems requiring special classes. The authors concluded that, of the 10 children evaluated, all had dementia, learning disabilities or evidence of intellectual retardation. Of concern is the fact that there appears to be a continuing decline in IQ of approximately 4 points per year after radiotherapy compared with their peer group.[213] The mechanism of this decline has been associated with loss of normal white matter on MRI[214,215] and this has been suggested to lead to decreased attentional abilities, and consequent declining IQ and academic achievement.[216] As would be expected, the volume of brain irradiated correlates with neurocognitive outcome, with whole-brain, supratentorial irradiation causing more deficit than posterior fossa fields, although the latter still results in measurable sequelae.[217,218] Focal radiotherapy results in significantly less decline in intellectual performance than craniospinal irradiation, as demonstrated by several studies comparing the two techniques.[219,220] The dose of radiotherapy also influences the neuropsychological sequelae, with recent studies looking at the de-escalation of the craniospinal therapy given to children with standard-risk medulloblastoma. A reduction in the dose of craniospinal irradiation from 36 to 24 Gy has been shown to preserve IQ by approximately 8 points,[92,220,221] but the continued decline previously described in neurocognition remains. A pilot study that further reduced the dose to 18 Gy demonstrated that low-dose craniospinal radiotherapy in conjunction with chemotherapy could prove effective in tumour control and lead to minimal intellectual decline.[102,222] Leading on from these observations, new protocols are aiming to explore reduction in both dose and volume of radiotherapy in combination with chemotherapy to try to reduce neurocognitive deficits. However, it must be remembered that intellectual decline is not only associated with irradiation but also with the effects of the tumour, as recently described in midline low-grade gliomas,[43] surgery and its complications,[219,223] and chemotherapy, with its potential detrimental effects on the brain.[224–226] As yet there is no evidence that intervention can reverse the actual biological deficits, but it is hoped that targeted educational/psychological input can maximize the child's academic and social skills. It is essential, therefore, that there is close cooperation between the neuro-oncology multidisciplinary team and the local educational authority and school.

Other CNS complications following treatment for brain tumours include neuroendocrine deficits. These can occur as a result of hypothalamic/pituitary damage directly from the tumour, as with craniopharyngioma or other midline tumours, or as a consequence of surgical damage to these sites.[36,43,159,227,228] Hypothalamic damage can cause major morbidity with regard to both behavioural problems and morbid obesity,[158,229] and multimodality therapy should aim to minimize this as far as possible. Endocrine deficiencies are common after treatment for CNS tumours, with 43 per cent of brain tumour survivors reporting one or more deficits;[230,231] a major risk factor is radiotherapy in which the field includes the hypothalamus or pituitary. Growth hormone secretion is the most vulnerable, but adrenocorticotrophic and thyroid-stimulating hormones can be affected, leading to the need for hydrocortisone and thyroid replacement, respectively. The latter hormone deficiencies can occur some time after treatment and lifelong monitoring is essential. Occasionally precocious puberty may also follow irradiation in young children. It is therefore essential that an experienced paediatric endocrinologist is part of the neuro-oncology team.

Growth may be affected not only by deficiency of growth hormone but also by the effects of spinal cord tumours and surgery plus irradiation to the spine. Scoliosis and kyphosis can result from spinal abnormalities, and growth and alignment of the spine must be continually monitored; neurosurgical/orthopaedic intervention may be required in severe cases.

Other deficits may include vascular complications, ranging from migraine-like headaches to stroke and vascular stenosis; NF and irradiation are particular risk factors.[30,31,231,232] Hearing impairment may result directly from the tumour or surgery but is also a complication of radiotherapy and platinum-based chemotherapy; it requires monitoring and appropriate dose adjustment during therapy as well as consideration of the use of conformal radiotherapy techniques to spare the cochlea.[101,233–236]

It can be appreciated that long-term follow-up is a vital role for any paediatric neuro-oncology team, not only to monitor for disease relapse but also to predict and monitor for the tumour/treatment-related morbidity. This will involve clinical examination, endocrine, psychometric and physiological testing (auxology, audiology, evoked potentials) and appropriate neuroimaging (MRI, spectroscopy, isotope studies), with arrangements made for a smooth transition to adult services when graduating from the paediatric/adolescent team.

CONCLUSIONS AND CURRENT CONTROVERSIES

Although considerable progress has been made in the management of CNS tumours of childhood, unfortunately in many tumour types this has not translated into significantly improved survival rates. It is hoped that advances in neuroradiology, neurosurgery, radiotherapy and the development of new anti-cancer agents will, in the near future, result in a better therapeutic/toxicity ratio, allowing not only an increase in the number of survivors but a parallel reduction in morbidity. It is also hoped that a better understanding of the molecular biology of CNS tumours will result in improved prognostic stratification and the evolution of targeted drug therapy aiming to exploit the knowledge of the oncogenic pathways of brain and spinal cord tumours.

Neuroradiology and neurosurgery

Neuroimaging is vital for the diagnosis, staging, therapeutic planning and monitoring of both treatment response and late effects. The evolution of MRI continues to have an impact on all of these areas, whilst novel nuclear medicine techniques may also contribute to neuro-oncology in the future.[237] Magnetic resonance spectroscopy (MRS) measures metabolites *in situ* and is therefore a useful tool that can potentially provide an *in vivo* method correlating with histology and treatment changes in CNS tumours.[238] Proton MRS principally measures the metabolites N-acetyl aspartate (NAA), creatine, choline, lactate and lipids. Whilst NAA is a neuronal marker and associated with normal intact brain, choline, lactate and lipids are at higher levels characteristic of malignant tumours. Several studies have confirmed that this spectral pattern is characteristic of malignant CNS tumours and even correlates with survival and histology in high-grade gliomas.[239–241] Spectroscopic techniques can also be used on frozen biopsy samples and, as the resolution is much higher than *in vivo* analysis, this may in future provide a link between histology and molecular changes and non-invasive imaging.[242,243] Previously, the use of MRS has been investigated as a potential marker of neurotoxicity with limited success, but new techniques such a two- or three-dimensional MRS may allow researchers to revisit this area.[244,245] Diffusion-weighted MRI techniques produce images whose signal is related to displacement of water, which allows an estimation of the direction of white matter tracts and possibly the cellularity (histological grade) of an individual tumour.[246,247] A particular type of imaging known as diffusion tensor imaging may provide valuable data in planning surgery in eloquent areas of the brain and may also be of interest in investigating neurotoxicity.[248,249] Neurosurgery is increasingly relying on advanced MRI techniques for neuro-navigation, such as those already described, and also the use of functional MRI to highlight eloquent areas.[250,251] The use of open magnet intraoperative MRI is already in practice in some centres and is currently being evaluated.[252,253] Nuclear medicine also has techniques that are being investigated in paediatric neuro-oncology, such as PET and SPECT imaging. The difficulty has been in the selection of isotopes that are suitable for neuro-oncology practice, i.e. that cross the blood–brain barrier (BBB), differentiate between tumour and normal brain and are stable. For PET, the use of the most common isotope, F-18 flourodeoxyglucose (FDG), has been restricted mainly to differentiating tumour from radiation-induced necrosis or as a marker in neuro-navigation by looking at function-specific metabolism.[254,255] The isotope C-11 methionine has been suggested to correlate with tumour proliferation and has been used as a way of guiding stereotactic biopsy, but it has a short half-life, which restricts its use.[256] Newer stable isotopes such as 18-flourothymidine and labelled annexin V may open up the possibility of measuring response for proliferation or degree of apoptosis induced by therapy.[257,258] SPECT imaging is more readily available and isotopes, including thallium-201 and Tc-99m MIBI, have been shown potentially to correlate with histological grade.[259–261] It is hoped that by combining these innovative neuroimaging modalities in the future, safer and more complete resections can be achieved and response to therapy and its side-effects more closely monitored.[262]

Molecular biology and tumour classification

In the post-human genome era, one may hope that the understanding of the inherent biology of paediatric CNS tumours will lead not only to improved therapies but also to safer treatments. This may occur in one of two ways:

- better classification/stratification and prognostication by use of molecular markers in association with conventional therapies
- definition of molecular targets for new anti-cancer treatments.

The former has already been developed in various settings in paediatric oncology, such as MYC-N status in neuroblastoma, allowing a more aggressive subset of tumours to be identified and treated more intensively. In childhood CNS tumours, medulloblastoma is following a similar path with myc, TRK-C, ErbB-2/4 and gene clusters from array analysis all being potential molecular prognostic markers in addition to conventional staging and histology.[79,83–86,263] In theory, this may allow a new subgroup of tumours to be identified, irrespective of conventional staging, which are either good-risk, allowing less intensive therapy (e.g. lower dose radiotherapy), or high-risk, needing consolidation therapy. Early studies have also suggested that ependymoma and oligodendroglioma may have their own molecular markers.[117,119,198,199] Further studies are needed in high-grade gliomas and also in infant tumours.

Targeted anti-cancer therapy

The idea of the 'magic bullet' has been with us for 100 years after first being used by the chemist Paul Ehrlich; however, in oncology for the first time we are now seeing therapies which are truly targeted. The development of the tyrosine kinase receptor (TKR) inhibitor STI571 (imatinib mesylate) which targets Bcr-Abl in chronic myeloid leukaemia (CML) has provided both encouragement and vital lessons.[264–266] Whilst developed specifically for the management of CML, it has also been shown to inhibit other TKRs, such as c-Kit, and prove useful in other malignancies such as gastrointestinal stromal tumours (GISTs).[267] In this latter condition, a specific activating mutation on exon 11 strongly predicts response to STI571, demonstrating the need to understand further the targets of this new class of drugs. Indeed, STI571 is now in clinical trials in paediatric CNS tumours where it is thought that both malignant gliomas and medulloblastoma may exhibit PGDFr, another class III TKR.[268,269] Other potential molecular targets include the family of ErbB receptors which have been shown to be overexpressed in malignant gliomas (ErbB-1 or EGFr),[270,271] ependymoma[199] and medulloblastoma (ErbB-2 and 4).[85,86,272] There are a number of agents on trial targeting these molecules, including small molecules (e.g. Iressa or erlotinib) or monoclonal antibodies such as cetuximab. It is likely, due to the problems of the blood–brain barrier, that small-molecule inhibitors will have more potential in CNS tumours. Other pathways that may be active targets, particularly in malignant gliomas, include the phosphoinositidine 3-kinase/Akt/mTOR pathway (e.g. inhibitor CCI-779, rapamycin analogue)[273,274] and the Ras pathway (e.g. R115777, farnesyl transferase inhibitor).[275] Future agents may include those targeting the cyclo-oxygenase pathway, proteasome inhibitors and integrin and endothelin receptor antagonists. Another area of active research in targeted therapy is focused on angiogenesis and the inhibition of neovascularization, which is thought to be vital to tumour growth.[271,276] Several specific compounds have been developed, including inhibitors of vascular endothelial growth factor (VEGF), such as PTK787 and semaxanib, and are in early clinical trials. Matrix metalloproteinase inhibitors stop the degradation of the extracellular matrix vital for tumour invasion and growth and a number of agents are on trial (e.g. marimastat, prinomastat).[277–280] Work is still needed in both adult and paediatric tumours to confirm these as important targets and, importantly, to define the interaction of these multiple pathways with each other and the effects of both single and multiple pathway inhibition.[281] If proven successful, the combination and scheduling of targeted therapies in relation to conventional therapies will need to be elucidated.

KEY POINTS

- Dedicated multidisciplinary paediatric neuro-oncology teams are essential for the management of these complex patients.
- CNS tumours are the most common solid tumours in childhood and the leading cause of cancer-related death.
- Survivors can face significant neurological and psychosocial morbidity and lifelong support is required.
- There have been improvements in both survival and decreased toxicity in the treatment of ependymoma, medulloblastoma and low-grade astrocytomas.
- Malignant gliomas, including pontine glioma, remain a very difficult challenge.
- Advances in neuroimaging may facilitate improved neurosurgical outcomes.
- Advances in the understanding of the molecular biology of paediatric CNS tumours may yield improved stratification for conventional therapeutic strategies.
- Molecularly targeted therapies hold potential for increased efficacy and diminished toxicity.

REFERENCES

1. Kaatsch P, Rickert CH, Kuhl J et al. Population-based epidemiologic data on brain tumors in German children. Cancer 2001; 92: 3155–64.
2. Legler JM, Ries LA, Smith MA et al. Cancer surveillance series [corrected]: brain and other central nervous system cancers: recent trends in incidence and mortality. J Natl Cancer Inst 1999; 91: 1382–90.
3. Kleihues P, Louis DN, Scheithauer BW et al. The WHO classification of tumors of the nervous system. J Neuropathol Exp Neurol 2002; 61: 215–25.
4. Saha V, Love S, Eden T et al. Determinants of symptom interval in childhood cancer. Arch Dis Child 1993; 68: 771–4.
5. Albright AL, Sposto R, Holmes E et al. Correlation of neurosurgical subspecialization with outcomes in children with malignant brain tumors. Neurosurgery 2000; 47: 879–85.
♦6. Griffiths PD. A protocol for imaging paediatric brain tumours. United Kingdom Children's Cancer Study Group and Societe Francaise d'Oncologie Pediatrique Panelists. Clin Radiol 1999; 54: 558–62.
7. Pollack IF, Hamilton RL, Burnham J et al. Impact of proliferation index on outcome in childhood malignant gliomas: results in a multi-institutional cohort. Neurosurgery 2002; 50: 1238–44.
8. Roessler K, Bertalanffy A, Jezan H et al. Proliferative activity as measured by MIB-1 labeling index and long-term

outcome of cerebellar juvenile pilocytic astrocytomas. J Neurooncol 2002; 58: 141–6.
9. Bowers DC, Gargan L, Kapur P et al. Study of the MIB-1 labeling index as a predictor of tumor progression in pilocytic astrocytomas in children and adolescents. J Clin Oncol 2003; 21: 2968–73.
10. Tihan T, Fisher PG, Kepner JL et al. Pediatric astrocytomas with monomorphous pilomyxoid features and a less favorable outcome. J Neuropathol Exp Neurol 1999; 58: 1061–8.
♦11. Listernick R, Louis DN, Packer RJ et al. Optic pathway gliomas in children with neurofibromatosis 1: consensus statement from the NF1 Optic Pathway Glioma Task Force. Ann Neurol 1997; 41: 143–9.
12. Sorensen SA, Mulvihill JJ, Nielsen A. Long-term follow-up of von Recklinghausen neurofibromatosis. Survival and malignant neoplasms. N Engl J Med 1986; 314: 1010–15.
13. Listernick R, Charrow J, Greenwald M et al. Natural history of optic pathway tumors in children with neurofibromatosis type 1: a longitudinal study. J Pediatr 1994; 125: 63–6.
14. Kluwe L, Hagel C, Tatagiba M et al. Loss of NF1 alleles distinguish sporadic from NF1-associated pilocytic astrocytomas. J Neuropathol Exp Neurol 2001; 60: 917–20.
15. Ahlsen G, Gillberg IC, Lindblom R et al. Tuberous sclerosis in Western Sweden. A population study of cases with early childhood onset. Arch Neurol 1994; 51: 76–81.
16. Shepherd CW, Scheithauer BW, Gomez MR et al. Subependymal giant cell astrocytoma: a clinical, pathological, and flow cytometric study. Neurosurgery 1991; 28: 864–8.
17. Pollack IF, Finkelstein SD, Woods J et al. Expression of p53 and prognosis in children with malignant gliomas. N Engl J Med 2002; 346: 420–7.
18. Pollack IF, Finkelstein SD, Burnham J et al. Age and TP53 mutation frequency in childhood malignant gliomas: results in a multi-institutional cohort. Cancer Res 2001; 61: 7404–7.
19. Louis DN, Rubio MP, Correa KM et al. Molecular genetics of pediatric brain stem gliomas. Application of PCR techniques to small and archival brain tumor specimens. J Neuropathol Exp Neurol 1993; 52: 507–15.
20. Cheng Y, Ng HK, Zhang SF et al. Genetic alterations in pediatric high-grade astrocytomas. Hum Pathol 1999; 30: 1284–90.
21. Newcomb EW, Alonso M, Sung T et al. Incidence of p14ARF gene deletion in high-grade adult and pediatric astrocytomas. Hum Pathol 2000; 31: 115–19.
22. Sung T, Miller DC, Hayes RL et al. Preferential inactivation of the p53 tumor suppressor pathway and lack of EGFR amplification distinguish de novo high grade pediatric astrocytomas from de novo adult astrocytomas. Brain Pathol 2000; 10: 249–59.
23. Wisoff JH, Sanford R, Holmes E et al. Impact of surgical resection on low grade gliomas of childhood: a report from the CCG 9891/POG 9130 low grade astrocytoma study. Neurooncology 2003; 5: 71.
24. Pollack IF, Claassen D, al Shboul Q et al. Low-grade gliomas of the cerebral hemispheres in children: an analysis of 71 cases. J Neurosurg 1995; 82: 536–47.
25. Fisher BJ, Leighton CC, Vujovic O et al. Results of a policy of surveillance alone after surgical management of pediatric low grade gliomas. Int J Radiat Oncol Biol Phys 2001; 51: 704–10.
26. Grill J, Laithier V, Rodriguez D et al. When do children with optic pathway tumours need treatment? An oncological

perspective in 106 patients treated in a single centre. *Eur J Pediatr* 2000; **159**: 692–6.

27. Cappelli C, Grill J, Raquin M *et al.* Long-term follow up of 69 patients treated for optic pathway tumours before the chemotherapy era. *Arch Dis Child* 1998; **79**: 334–8.

28. Horwich A, Bloom HJ. Optic gliomas: radiation therapy and prognosis. *Int J Radiat Oncol Biol Phys* 1985; **11**: 1067–79.

29. Jenkin D, Angyalfi S, Becker L *et al.* Optic glioma in children: surveillance, resection, or irradiation? *Int J Radiat Oncol Biol Phys* 1993; **25**: 215–25.

30. Kestle JR, Hoffman HJ, Mock AR. Moyamoya phenomenon after radiation for optic glioma. *J Neurosurg* 1993; **79**: 32–5.

31. Grill J, Couanet D, Cappelli C *et al.* Radiation-induced cerebral vasculopathy in children with neurofibromatosis and optic pathway glioma. *Ann Neurol* 1999; **45**: 393–6.

32. Kony SJ, de Vathaire F, Chompret A *et al.* Radiation and genetic factors in the risk of second malignant neoplasms after a first cancer in childhood. *Lancet* 1997; **350**: 91–5.

33. Little MP, de Vathaire F, Shamsaldin A *et al.* Risks of brain tumour following treatment for cancer in childhood: modification by genetic factors, radiotherapy and chemotherapy. *Int J Cancer* 1998; **78**: 269–75.

34. Saran FH, Baumert BG, Khoo VS *et al.* Stereotactically guided conformal radiotherapy for progressive low-grade gliomas of childhood. *Int J Radiat Oncol Biol Phys* 2002; **53**: 43–51.

35. Merchant TE, Zhu Y, Thompson SJ *et al.* Preliminary results from a phase II trail of conformal radiation therapy for pediatric patients with localized low-grade astrocytoma and ependymoma. *Int J Radiat Oncol Biol Phys* 2002; **52**: 325–32.

36. Janss AJ, Grundy R, Cnaan A *et al.* Optic pathway and hypothalamic/chiasmatic gliomas in children younger than age 5 years with a 6-year follow-up. *Cancer* 1995; **75**: 1051–9.

37. Mitchell AE, Elder JE, Mackey DA *et al.* Visual improvement despite radiologically stable disease after treatment with carboplatin in children with progressive low-grade optic/thalamic gliomas. *J Pediatr Hematol Oncol* 2001; **23**: 572–7.

38. Petronio J, Edwards MS, Prados M *et al.* Management of chiasmal and hypothalamic gliomas of infancy and childhood with chemotherapy. *J Neurosurg* 1991; **74**: 701–8.

●39. Laithier V, Raquin MA, Couanet D *et al.* Chemotherapy for children with optic pathway glioma: results of a prospective study by the French Society of Pediatric Oncology (SFOP) (meeting abstract). *Med Pediatr Oncol* 2000; **35**: 190.

40. Prados MD, Edwards MS, Rabbitt J *et al.* Treatment of pediatric low-grade gliomas with a nitrosourea-based multiagent chemotherapy regimen. *J Neurooncol* 1997; **32**: 235–41.

41. Gajjar A, Sanford RA, Heideman R *et al.* Low-grade astrocytoma: a decade of experience at St Jude Children's Research Hospital. *J Clin Oncol* 1997; **15**: 2792–9.

●42. Walker D, Gnekow AK, Perilongo G *et al.* Vincristine/carboplatin in hypothalamic-chiasmatic glioma: a report from the international consortium on low grade glioma. *Med Pediatr Oncol* 2003; **9**: 229.

43. Fouladi M, Wallace D, Langston JW *et al.* Survival and functional outcome of children with hypothalamic/chiasmatic tumors. *Cancer* 2003; **97**: 1084–92.

44. Reardon DA, Gajjar A, Sanford RA *et al.* Bithalamic involvement predicts poor outcome among children with thalamic glial tumors. *Pediatr Neurosurg* 1998; **29**: 29–35.

45. Bowers DC, Georgiades C, Aronson LJ *et al.* Tectal gliomas: natural history of an indolent lesion in pediatric patients. *Pediatr Neurosurg* 2000; **32**: 24–9.

46. Rosenstock JG, Packer RJ, Bilaniuk L *et al.* Chiasmatic optic glioma treated with chemotherapy. A preliminary report. *J Neurosurg* 1985; **63**: 862–6.

●47. Packer RJ, Lange B, Ater J *et al.* Carboplatin and vincristine for recurrent and newly diagnosed low-grade gliomas of childhood. *J Clin Oncol* 1993; **11**: 850–6.

●48. Packer RJ, Ater J, Allen J *et al.* Carboplatin and vincristine chemotherapy for children with newly diagnosed progressive low-grade gliomas. *J Neurosurg* 1997; **86**: 747–54.

49. Walker D, Gnekow AK, Perilongo G *et al.* Vincristine/carboplatin in hypothalamic-chiasmatic glioma: a report from the international consortium on low grade glioma. *Med Pediatr Oncol* 2003; **39**: 229.

50. Kadota RP, Kun LE, Langston JW *et al.* Cyclophosphamide for the treatment of progressive low-grade astrocytoma: a Pediatric Oncology Group phase II Study. *J Pediatr Hematol Oncol* 1999; **21**: 198–202.

51. Chamberlain MC, Grafe MR. Recurrent chiasmatic-hypothalamic glioma treated with oral etoposide. *J Clin Oncol* 1995; **13**: 2072–6.

52. Heideman RL, Douglass EC, Langston JA *et al.* A phase II study of every other day high-dose ifosfamide in pediatric brain tumors: a Pediatric Oncology Group Study. *J Neurooncol* 1995; **25**: 77–84.

53. Quinn JA, Reardon DA, Friedman AH *et al.* Phase II trial of temozolomide in patients with progressive low-grade glioma. *J Clin Oncol* 2003; **21**: 646–51.

54. Bouffet E, Hargrave D, Cairney E *et al.* Weekly vinblastine for recurrent/progressive low grade gliomas. *Med Pediatr Oncol* 2002; **39**: 229.

●55. Sposto R, Ertel IJ, Jenkin RD *et al.* The effectiveness of chemotherapy for treatment of high grade astrocytoma in children: results of a randomized trial. A report from the Children's Cancer Study Group. *J Neurooncol* 1989; **7**: 165–77.

56. Marchese MJ, Chang CH. Malignant astrocytic gliomas in children. *Cancer* 1990; **65**: 2771–8.

●57. Wisoff JH, Boyett JM, Berger MS *et al.* Current neurosurgical management and the impact of the extent of resection in the treatment of malignant gliomas of childhood: a report of the Children's Cancer Group trial no. CCG-945. *J Neurosurg* 1998; **89**: 52–9.

58. Walker MD, Alexander E Jr, Hunt WE *et al.* Evaluation of BCNU and/or radiotherapy in the treatment of anaplastic gliomas. A cooperative clinical trial. *J Neurosurg* 1978; **49**: 333–43.

●59. Finlay JL, Boyett JM, Yates AJ *et al.* Randomized phase III trial in childhood high-grade astrocytoma comparing vincristine, lomustine, and prednisone with the eight-drugs-in-1-day regimen. Children's Cancer Group. *J Clin Oncol* 1995; **13**: 112–23.

●60. Pollack IF, Boyett JM, Yates AJ *et al.* The influence of central review on outcome associations in childhood malignant gliomas: results from the CCG-945 experience. *Neurooncology* 2003; **5**: 197–207.

●61. Wolff JE, Gnekow AK, Kortmann RD *et al.* Preradiation chemotherapy for pediatric patients with high-grade glioma. *Cancer* 2002; **94**: 264–71.

62. Kadota RP, Stewart CF, Horn M *et al.* Topotecan for the treatment of recurrent or progressive central nervous system tumors – a pediatric oncology group phase II study. *J Neurooncol* 1999; **43**: 43–7.

63. Blaney SM, Phillips PC, Packer RJ *et al.* Phase II evaluation of topotecan for pediatric central nervous system tumors. *Cancer* 1996; **78**: 527–31.

64. Turner CD, Gururangan S, Eastwood J *et al.* Phase II study of irinotecan (CPT-11) in children with high-risk malignant brain tumors: the Duke experience. *Neurooncology* 2002; **4**: 102–8.

●65. Estlin EJ, Lashford L, Ablett S *et al.* Phase I study of temozolomide in paediatric patients with advanced cancer. United Kingdom Children's Cancer Study Group. *Br J Cancer* 1998; **78**: 652–61.

●66. Nicholson HS, Krailo M, Ames MM *et al.* Phase I study of temozolomide in children and adolescents with recurrent solid tumors: a report from the Children's Cancer Group. *J Clin Oncol* 1998; **16**: 3037–43.

●67. Lashford LS, Thiesse P, Jouvet A *et al.* Temozolomide in malignant gliomas of childhood: a United Kingdom Children's Cancer Study Group and French Society for Pediatric Oncology Intergroup Study. *J Clin Oncol* 2002; **20**: 4684–91.

68. Hargrave D, Stempak D, Coppes M *et al.* Phase I study of oral continuous administration of low dose temozolomide in paediatric brain tumours. *Neurooncology* 2003; **5**: 27.

●69. Stupp R, Dietrich PY, Ostermann KS *et al.* Promising survival for patients with newly diagnosed glioblastoma multiforme treated with concomitant radiation plus temozolomide followed by adjuvant temozolomide. *J Clin Oncol* 2002; **20**: 1375–82.

●70. Grovas AC, Boyett JM, Lindsley K *et al.* Regimen-related toxicity of myeloablative chemotherapy with BCNU, thiotepa, and etoposide followed by autologous stem cell rescue for children with newly diagnosed glioblastoma multiforme: report from the Children's Cancer Group. *Med Pediatr Oncol* 1999; **33**: 83–7.

●71. Packer RJ, Boyett JM, Zimmerman RA *et al.* Outcome of children with brain stem gliomas after treatment with 7800 cGy of hyperfractionated radiotherapy. A Children's Cancer Group Phase I/II Trial. *Cancer* 1994; **74**: 1827–34.

●72. Freeman CR, Krischer JP, Sanford RA *et al.* Final results of a study of escalating doses of hyperfractionated radiotherapy in brain stem tumors in children: a Pediatric Oncology Group study. *Int J Radiat Oncol Biol Phys* 1993; **27**: 197–206.

73. Freeman CR, Bourgouin PM, Sanford RA *et al.* Long term survivors of childhood brain stem gliomas treated with hyperfractionated radiotherapy. Clinical characteristics and treatment related toxicities. The Pediatric Oncology Group. *Cancer* 1996; **77**: 555–62.

74. Freeman CR, Perilongo G. Chemotherapy for brain stem gliomas. *Childs Nerv Syst* 1999; **15**: 545–53.

75. Chamberlain MC. Recurrent brainstem gliomas treated with oral VP-16. *J Neurooncol* 1993; **15**: 133–9.

●76. Jenkin RD, Boesel C, Ertel I *et al.* Brain-stem tumors in childhood: a prospective randomized trial of irradiation with and without adjuvant CCNU, VCR, and prednisone. A report of the Children's Cancer Study Group. *J Neurosurg* 1987; **66**: 227–33.

77. Hargrave D, Chaung N, Tariq N *et al.* Can radiological characteristics predict length of survival in pontine glioma? *Neurooncology* 2003; **5**: 43.

78. Benjelloun A, Delavelle J, Lazeyras F *et al.* Possible efficacy of temozolomide in a patient with gliomatosis cerebri. *Neurology* 2001; **57**: 1932–3.

79. Pomeroy SL, Tamayo P, Gaasenbeek M *et al.* Prediction of central nervous system embryonal tumour outcome based on gene expression. *Nature* 2002; **415**: 436–42.

80. McManamy CS, Lamont JM, Taylor RE *et al.* Morphophenotypic variation predicts clinical behavior in childhood non-desmoplastic medulloblastomas. *J Neuropathol Exp Neurol* 2003; **62**: 627–32.

81. Eberhart CG, Kepner JL, Goldthwaite PT *et al.* Histopathologic grading of medulloblastomas: a Pediatric Oncology Group study. *Cancer* 2002; **94**: 552–60.

82. Taylor MD, Liu L, Raffel C *et al.* Mutations in SUFU predispose to medulloblastoma. *Nat Genet* 2002; **31**: 306–10.

83. Grotzer MA, Hogarty MD, Janss AJ *et al.* MYC messenger RNA expression predicts survival outcome in childhood primitive neuroectodermal tumor/medulloblastoma. *Clin Cancer Res* 2001; **7**: 2425–33.

84. Grotzer MA, Janss AJ, Fung K *et al.* TrkC expression predicts good clinical outcome in primitive neuroectodermal brain tumors. *J Clin Oncol* 2000; **18**: 1027–35.

85. Gilbertson RJ, Pearson AD, Perry RH *et al.* Prognostic significance of the c-erbB-2 oncogene product in childhood medulloblastoma. *Br J Cancer* 1995; **71**: 473–7.

86. Gilbertson RJ, Perry RH, Kelly PJ *et al.* Prognostic significance of HER2 and HER4 coexpression in childhood medulloblastoma. *Cancer Res* 1997; **57**: 3272–80.

●87. Albright AL, Wisoff JH, Zeltzer PM *et al.* Effects of medulloblastoma resections on outcome in children: a report from the Children's Cancer Group. *Neurosurgery* 1996; **38**: 265–71.

88. Pollack IF, Polinko P, Albright AL *et al.* Mutism and pseudobulbar symptoms after resection of posterior fossa tumors in children: incidence and pathophysiology. *Neurosurgery* 1995; **37**: 885–93.

89. Doxey D, Bruce D, Sklar F *et al.* Posterior fossa syndrome: identifiable risk factors and irreversible complications. *Pediatr Neurosurg* 1999; **31**: 131–6.

●90. Deutsch M, Thomas PR, Krischer J *et al.* Results of a prospective randomized trial comparing standard dose neuraxis irradiation (3,600 cGy/20) with reduced neuraxis irradiation (2,340 cGy/13) in patients with low-stage medulloblastoma. A Combined Children's Cancer Group-Pediatric Oncology Group Study. *Pediatr Neurosurg* 1996; **24**: 167–76.

●91. Thomas PR, Deutsch M, Kepner JL *et al.* Low-stage medulloblastoma: final analysis of trial comparing standard-dose with reduced-dose neuraxis irradiation. *J Clin Oncol* 2000; **18**: 3004–11.

●92. Mulhern RK, Kepner JL, Thomas PR *et al.* Neuropsychologic functioning of survivors of childhood medulloblastoma randomized to receive conventional or reduced-dose craniospinal irradiation: a Pediatric Oncology Group study. *J Clin Oncol* 1998; **16**: 1723–28.

●93. Tait DM, Thornton-Jones H, Bloom HJ *et al.* Adjuvant chemotherapy for medulloblastoma: the first multi-centre control trial of the International Society of Paediatric Oncology (SIOP I). *Eur J Cancer* 1990; **26**: 464–9.

●94. Evans AE, Jenkin RD, Sposto R *et al.* The treatment of medulloblastoma. Results of a prospective randomized trial of radiation therapy with and without CCNU, vincristine, and prednisone. *J Neurosurg* 1990; **72**: 572–82.

●95. Krischer JP, Ragab AH, Kun L *et al.* Nitrogen mustard, vincristine, procarbazine, and prednisone as adjuvant chemotherapy in the treatment of medulloblastoma. A Pediatric Oncology Group study. *J Neurosurg* 1991; **74**: 905–9.

●96. Bailey CC, Gnekow A, Wellek S *et al.* Prospective randomised trial of chemotherapy given before radiotherapy in childhood medulloblastoma. International Society of Paediatric Oncology (SIOP) and the (German) Society of Paediatric Oncology (GPO): SIOP II. *Med Pediatr Oncol* 1995; **25**: 166–78.

●97. Zeltzer PM, Boyett JM, Finlay JL *et al.* Metastasis stage, adjuvant treatment, and residual tumor are prognostic factors for medulloblastoma in children: conclusions from the Children's Cancer Group 921 randomized phase III study. *J Clin Oncol* 1999; **17**: 832–45.

●98. Taylor RE, Bailey CC, Robinson K *et al.* Results of a randomized study of preradiation chemotherapy versus radiotherapy alone for nonmetastatic medulloblastoma: The International Society of Paediatric Oncology/United Kingdom Children's Cancer Study Group PNET-3 Study. *J Clin Oncol* 2003; **21**: 1581–91.

99. Packer RJ, Siegel KR, Sutton LN *et al.* Efficacy of adjuvant chemotherapy for patients with poor-risk medulloblastoma: a preliminary report. *Ann Neurol* 1988; **24**: 503–8.

●100. Packer RJ, Sutton LN, Elterman R *et al.* Outcome for children with medulloblastoma treated with radiation and cisplatin, CCNU, and vincristine chemotherapy. *J Neurosurg* 1994; **81**: 690–8.

●101. Packer RJ, Goldwein J, Nicholson HS *et al.* Treatment of children with medulloblastomas with reduced-dose craniospinal radiation therapy and adjuvant chemotherapy: A Children's Cancer Group Study. *J Clin Oncol* 1999; **17**: 2127–36.

●102. Goldwein JW, Radcliffe J, Johnson J *et al.* Updated results of a pilot study of low dose craniospinal irradiation plus chemotherapy for children under five with cerebellar primitive neuroectodermal tumors (medulloblastoma). *Int J Radiat Oncol Biol Phys* 1996; **34**: 899–904.

●103. Pizer BL, Taylor RE, Weston CL *et al.* Analysis of patients with supratentorial PNET entered in the SIOP PNET III trial. *Neurooncology* 2003; **5**: 57.

104. Gandola L, Cefalo G, Massimino M *et al.* Hyperfractionated accelerated radiotherapy (HART) for metastatic medulloblastoma. *Neurooncology* 2003; **5**: 39.

105. Strother D, Ashley D, Kellie SJ *et al.* Feasibility of four consecutive high-dose chemotherapy cycles with stem-cell rescue for patients with newly diagnosed medulloblastoma or supratentorial primitive neuroectodermal tumor after craniospinal radiotherapy: results of a collaborative study. *J Clin Oncol* 2001; **19**: 2696–704.

●106. Dunkel IJ, Boyett JM, Yates A *et al.* High-dose carboplatin, thiotepa, and etoposide with autologous stem-cell rescue for patients with recurrent medulloblastoma. Children's Cancer Group. *J Clin Oncol* 1998; **16**: 222–8.

107. Dhodapkar K, Dunkel IJ, Gardner S *et al.* Preliminary results of dose intensive pre-irradiation chemotherapy in patients older than 10 years of age with high risk medulloblastoma and supratentorial primitive neuroectodermal tumors. *Med Pediatr Oncol* 2002; **38**: 47–8.

108. Dunkel IJ, Finlay JL. High dose chemotherapy with autologous stem cell rescue for patients with medulloblastoma. *J Neurooncol* 1996; **29**: 69–74.

109. Mason WP, Grovas A, Halpern S *et al.* Intensive chemotherapy and bone marrow rescue for young children with newly diagnosed malignant brain tumors. *J Clin Oncol* 1998; **16**: 210–21.

♦110. Bouffet E, Perilongo G, Canete A *et al.* Intracranial ependymomas in children: a critical review of prognostic factors and a plea for cooperation. *Med Pediatr Oncol* 1998; **30**: 319–29.

●111. Robertson PL, Zeltzer PM, Boyett JM *et al.* Survival and prognostic factors following radiation therapy and chemotherapy for ependymomas in children: a report of the Children's Cancer Group. *J Neurosurg* 1998; **88**: 695–703.

112. Bennetto L, Foreman N, Harding B *et al.* Ki-67 immunolabelling index is a prognostic indicator in childhood posterior fossa ependymomas. *Neuropathol Appl Neurobiol* 1998; **24**: 434–40.

113. Ritter AM, Hess KR, McLendon RE *et al.* Ependymomas: MIB-1 proliferation index and survival. *J Neurooncol* 1998; **40**: 51–7.

114. Figarella-Branger D, Civatte M, Bouvier-Labit C *et al.* Prognostic factors in intracranial ependymomas in children. *J Neurosurg* 2000; **93**: 605–13.

115. Ward S, Harding B, Wilkins P *et al.* Gain of 1q and loss of 22 are the most common changes detected by comparative genomic hybridisation in paediatric ependymoma. *Genes Chromosomes Cancer* 2001; **32**: 59–66.

116. Reardon DA, Entrekin RE, Sublett J *et al.* Chromosome arm 6q loss is the most common recurrent autosomal alteration detected in primary pediatric ependymoma. *Genes Chromosomes Cancer* 1999; **24**: 230–7.

117. Carter M, Nicholson J, Ross F *et al.* Genetic abnormalities detected in ependymomas by comparative genomic hybridisation. *Br J Cancer* 2002; **86**: 929–39.

118. Dyer S, Prebble E, Davison V *et al.* Genomic imbalances in pediatric intracranial ependymomas define clinically relevant groups. *Am J Pathol* 2002; **161**: 2133–41.

119. Gilbertson RJ, Bentley L, Hernan R *et al.* ERBB receptor signaling promotes ependymoma cell proliferation and represents a potential novel therapeutic target for this disease. *Clin Cancer Res* 2002; **8**: 3054–64.

120. Awaad YM, Allen JC, Miller DC *et al.* Deferring adjuvant therapy for totally resected intracranial ependymoma. *Pediatr Neurol* 1996; **14**: 216–19.

121. Pollack IF, Gerszten PC, Martinez AJ *et al.* Intracranial ependymomas of childhood: long-term outcome and prognostic factors. *Neurosurgery* 1995; **37**: 655–66.

122. Horn B, Heideman R, Geyer R *et al.* A multi-institutional retrospective study of intracranial ependymoma in children: identification of risk factors. *J Pediatr Hematol Oncol* 1999; **21**: 203–11.

123. Foreman NK, Love S, Gill SS *et al.* Second-look surgery for incompletely resected fourth ventricle ependymomas: technical case report. *Neurosurgery* 1997; **40**: 856–60.

124. Goldwein JW, Corn BW, Finlay JL et al. Is craniospinal irradiation required to cure children with malignant (anaplastic) intracranial ependymomas? Cancer 1991; 67: 2766–71.

125. Vanuytsel L, Brada M. The role of prophylactic spinal irradiation in localized intracranial ependymoma. Int J Radiat Oncol Biol Phys 1991; 21: 825–30.

126. Hodgson DC, Goumnerova LC, Loeffler JS et al. Radiosurgery in the management of pediatric brain tumors. Int J Radiat Oncol Biol Phys 2001; 50: 929–35.

127. Aggarwal R, Yeung D, Kumar P et al. Efficacy and feasibility of stereotactic radiosurgery in the primary management of unfavorable pediatric ependymoma. Radiother Oncol 1997; 43: 269–73.

♦128. Bouffet E, Foreman N. Chemotherapy for intracranial ependymomas. Childs Nerv Syst 1999; 15: 563–70.

♦129. Grill J, Pascal C, Chantal K. Childhood ependymoma: a systematic review of treatment options and strategies. Paediatr Drugs 2003; 5: 533–43.

♦130. Evans AE, Anderson JR, Lefkowitz-Boudreaux IB et al. Adjuvant chemotherapy of childhood posterior fossa ependymoma: cranio-spinal irradiation with or without adjuvant CCNU, vincristine, and prednisone: a Children's Cancer Group study. Med Pediatr Oncol 1996; 27: 8–14.

131. Needle MN, Goldwein JW, Grass J et al. Adjuvant chemotherapy for the treatment of intracranial ependymoma of childhood. Cancer 1997; 80: 341–7.

●132. Mason WP, Goldman S, Yates AJ et al. Survival following intensive chemotherapy with bone marrow reconstitution for children with recurrent intracranial ependymoma – a report of the Children's Cancer Group. J Neurooncol 1998; 37: 135–43.

133. Grill J, Kalifa C, Doz F et al. A high-dose busulfan-thiotepa combination followed by autologous bone marrow transplantation in childhood recurrent ependymoma. A phase-II study. Pediatr Neurosurg 1996; 25: 7–12.

134. Mahoney DH Jr, Strother D, Camitta B et al. High-dose melphalan and cyclophosphamide with autologous bone marrow rescue for recurrent/progressive malignant brain tumors in children: a pilot pediatric oncology group study. J Clin Oncol 1996; 14: 382–8.

135. Grill J, Kalifa C. High dose chemotherapy for childhood ependymoma. J Neurooncology 1998; 40: 97.

♦136. Kalifa C, Valteau D, Pizer B et al. High-dose chemotherapy in childhood brain tumours. Childs Nerv Syst 1999; 15: 498–505.

137. Bloom HJ. Primary intracranial germ cell tumours. In: Clinics in Clinical Oncology. London: WB Saunders, 1983; 233–7.

138. Kingston JE, Plowman PN, Hungerford JL. Ectopic intracranial retinoblastoma in childhood. Br J Ophthalmol 1985; 69: 742–8.

♦139. Calaminus G, Bamberg M, Baranzelli MC et al. Intracranial germ cell tumors: a comprehensive update of the European data. Neuropediatrics 1994; 25: 26–32.

140. Brada M, Rajan B. Spinal seeding in cranial germinoma. Br J Cancer 1990; 61: 339–40.

141. Wolden SL, Wara WM, Larson DA et al. Radiation therapy for primary intracranial germ-cell tumors. Int J Radiat Oncol Biol Phys 1995; 32: 943–9.

142. Dattoli MJ, Newall J. Radiation therapy for intracranial germinoma: the case for limited volume treatment. Int J Radiat Oncol Biol Phys 1990; 19: 429–33.

143. Matsutani M, Sano K, Takakura K et al. Primary intracranial germ cell tumors: a clinical analysis of 153 histologically verified cases. J Neurosurg 1997; 86: 446–55.

●144. Alapetite C, Ricardi U, Saran FH et al. Whole ventricular irradiation in combination with chemotherapy in intracranial germinoma: the consensus of the SIOP CNS GCT study group. Med Pediatr Oncol 2002; 39: 248.

145. Hardenbergh PH, Golden J, Billet A et al. Intracranial germinoma: the case for lower dose radiation therapy. Int J Radiat Oncol Biol Phys 1997; 39: 419–26.

●146. Bamberg M, Kortmann RD, Calaminus G et al. Radiation therapy for intracranial germinoma: results of the German cooperative prospective trials MAKEI 83/86/89. J Clin Oncol 1999; 17: 2585–92.

147. Shibamoto Y, Takahashi M, Abe M. Reduction of the radiation dose for intracranial germinoma: a prospective study. Br J Cancer 1994; 70: 984–9.

●148. Bouffet E, Baranzelli MC, Patte C et al. Combined treatment modality for intracranial germinomas: results of a multicentre SFOP experience. Societe Francaise d'Oncologie Pediatrique. Br J Cancer 1999; 79: 1199–204.

●149. Balmaceda C, Heller G, Rosenblum M et al. Chemotherapy without irradiation – a novel approach for newly diagnosed CNS germ cell tumors: results of an international cooperative trial. The First International Central Nervous System Germ Cell Tumor Study. J Clin Oncol 1996; 14: 2908–15.

150. Calaminus G, Andreussi L, Garre ML et al. Secreting germ cell tumors of the central nervous system (CNS). First results of the cooperative German/Italian pilot study (CNS sGCT). Klin Padiatr 1997; 209: 222–7.

151. Tada T, Takizawa T, Nakazato F et al. Treatment of intracranial nongerminomatous germ-cell tumor by high-dose chemotherapy and autologous stem-cell rescue. J Neurooncol 1999; 44: 71–6.

152. Graham ML, Herndon JE, Casey JR et al. High-dose chemotherapy with autologous stem-cell rescue in patients with recurrent and high-risk pediatric brain tumors. J Clin Oncol 1997; 15: 1814–23.

153. Baranzelli MC, Patte C, Bouffet E et al. An attempt to treat pediatric intracranial alphaFP and betaHCG secreting germ cell tumors with chemotherapy alone. SFOP experience with 18 cases. Société Française d'Oncologie Pédiatrique. J Neurooncol 1998; 37: 229–39.

154. Hoffman HJ: Craniopharyngiomas. Can J Neurol Sci 1985; 12: 348–52.

155. Brunel H, Raybaud C, Peretti-Viton P et al. [Craniopharyngioma in children: MRI study of 43 cases]. Neurochirurgie 2002; 48: 309–18.

156. Sanford RA. Craniopharyngioma: results of survey of the American Society of Pediatric Neurosurgery. Pediatr Neurosurg 1994; 21(Suppl 1): 39–43.

157. Fischer EG, Welch K, Shillito J Jr et al. Craniopharyngiomas in children. Long-term effects of conservative surgical procedures combined with radiation therapy. J Neurosurg 1990; 73: 534–40.

158. Merchant TE, Kiehna EN, Sanford RA et al. Craniopharyngioma: the St Jude Children's Research Hospital experience 1984–2001. Int J Radiat Oncol Biol Phys 2002; 53: 533–42.

159. De Vile CJ, Grant DB, Kendall BE *et al.* Management of childhood craniopharyngioma: can the morbidity of radical surgery be predicted? *J Neurosurg* 1996; **85**: 73–81.

160. Blackburn TP, Doughty D, Plowman PN. Stereotactic intracavitary therapy of recurrent cystic craniopharyngioma by instillation of 90yttrium. *Br J Neurosurg* 1999; **13**: 359–65.

161. Pollock BE, Lunsford LD, Kondziolka D *et al.* Phosphorus-32 intracavitary irradiation of cystic craniopharyngiomas: current technique and long-term results. *Int J Radiat Oncol Biol Phys* 1995; **33**: 437–46.

162. Pollack IF, Lunsford LD, Slamovits TL *et al.* Stereotaxic intracavitary irradiation for cystic craniopharyngiomas. *J Neurosurg* 1988; **68**: 227–33.

163. Hader WJ, Steinbok P, Hukin J *et al.* Intratumoral therapy with bleomycin for cystic craniopharyngiomas in children. *Pediatr Neurosurg* 2000; **33**: 211–18.

164. Takahashi H, Nakazawa S, Shimura T. Evaluation of postoperative intratumoral injection of bleomycin for craniopharyngioma in children. *J Neurosurg* 1985; **62**: 120–7.

165. Savas A, Erdem A, Tun K *et al.* Fatal toxic effect of bleomycin on brain tissue after intracystic chemotherapy for a craniopharyngioma: case report. *Neurosurgery* 2000; **46**: 213–16.

166. Bremer AM, Nguyen TQ, Balsys R. Therapeutic benefits of combination chemotherapy with vincristine, BCNU, and procarbazine on recurrent cystic craniopharyngioma. A case report. *J Neurooncol* 1984; **2**: 47–51.

167. Lippens RJ, Rotteveel JJ, Otten BJ *et al.* Chemotherapy with adriamycin (doxorubicin) and CCNU (lomustine) in four children with recurrent craniopharyngioma. *Eur J Paediatr Neurol* 1998; **2**: 263–8.

●168. van Eys J, Cangir A, Coody D *et al.* MOPP regimen as primary chemotherapy for brain tumors in infants. *J Neurooncol* 1985; **3**: 237–43.

169. Ater JL, van Eys J, Woo SY *et al.* MOPP chemotherapy without irradiation as primary postsurgical therapy for brain tumors in infants and young children. *J Neurooncol* 1997; **32**: 243–52.

●170. Duffner PK, Horowitz ME, Krischer JP *et al.* Postoperative chemotherapy and delayed radiation in children less than three years of age with malignant brain tumors. *N Engl J Med* 1993; **328**: 1725–31.

●171. Geyer JR, Zeltzer PM, Boyett JM *et al.* Survival of infants with primitive neuroectodermal tumors or malignant ependymomas of the CNS treated with eight drugs in 1 day: a report from the Children's Cancer Group. *J Clin Oncol* 1994; **12**: 1607–15.

172. Duffner PK, Krischer JP, Burger PC *et al.* Treatment of infants with malignant gliomas: the Pediatric Oncology Group experience. *J Neurooncol* 1996; **28**: 245–56.

●173. Duffner PK, Cohen ME, Sanford RA *et al.* Lack of efficacy of postoperative chemotherapy and delayed radiation in very young children with pineoblastoma. Pediatric Oncology Group. *Med Pediatr Oncol* 1995; **25**: 38–44.

●174. Duffner PK, Kun LE, Burger PC *et al.* Postoperative chemotherapy and delayed radiation in infants and very young children with choroid plexus carcinomas. The Pediatric Oncology Group. *Pediatr Neurosurg* 1995; **22**: 189–96.

●175. Strother D, Kepner JL, Aronin P *et al.* Dose-Intensive (DI) chemotherapy (CT) prolongs event-free survival (EFS) for very young children with ependymoma (EP). Results of Pediatric Oncology Group (POG) Study 9233. *Proceedings of the 36th ASCO Annual Meeting.* 2000.

●176. Lashford LS, Campbell RH, Gattamaneni HR *et al.* An intensive multiagent chemotherapy regimen for brain tumours occurring in very young children. *Arch Dis Child* 1996; **74**: 219–23.

●177. Kuhl HJ, Berthold F, Bode U *et al.* Postoperative chemotherapy without radiation therapy in children less than three years of age with medulloblastoma: German pilot trial- HIT-SKK'92. *Proceedings of the 8th International Symposium on Pediatric Neuro-oncology.* San Francisco: ISPNO, 1998; 146.

●178. Kalifa C, Raquin M, Bouffet E *et al.* Chemotherapy without irradiation in medulloblastoma patients younger than three. *Proceedings of the 8th International Symposium on Pediatric Neuro-oncology.* San Francisco: ISPNO, 1998; 38.

●179. Grill J, Le Deley MC, Gambarelli D *et al.* Postoperative chemotherapy without irradiation for ependymoma in children under 5 years of age: a multicenter trial of the French Society of Pediatric Oncology. *J Clin Oncol* 2001; **19**: 1288–96.

●180. Geyer JR, Ater J, Axtell R *et al.* Multiagent chemotherapy and deferred radiotherapy in infants with malignant brain tumours. *Proceedings of the 8th International Symposium on Pediatric Neuro-oncology.* San Francisco: ISPNO, 1998; 41.

●181. White L, Kellie S, Gray E *et al.* Postoperative chemotherapy in children less than 4 years of age with malignant brain tumors: promising initial response to a VETOPEC-based regimen. A Study of the Australian and New Zealand Children's Cancer Study Group (ANZCCSG). *J Pediatr Hematol Oncol* 1998; **20**: 125–30.

182. Dupuis-Girod S, Hartmann O, Benhamou E *et al.* Will high dose chemotherapy followed by autologous bone marrow transplantation supplant cranio-spinal irradiation in young children treated for medulloblastoma? *J Neurooncol* 1996; **27**: 87–98.

●183. Finlay JL, Goldman S, Wong MC *et al.* Pilot study of high-dose thiotepa and etoposide with autologous bone marrow rescue in children and young adults with recurrent CNS tumors. The Children's Cancer Group. *J Clin Oncol* 1996; **14**: 2495–503.

184. Guruangan S, Dunkel IJ, Goldman S *et al.* Myeloablative chemotherapy with autologous bone marrow rescue in young children with recurrent malignant brain tumors. *J Clin Oncol* 1998; **16**: 2486–93.

♦185. Finlay J, Stephen D. Marrow ablative chemotherapeutic strategies in the treatment of high risk brain tumours of early childhood. *Neurooncology* 2003; **5**: 37.

186. Finlay J, Chi S, Gardner S *et al.* Newly diagnosed medulloblastoma with leptomeningeal dissemination in young children: Response to 'Head Start' induction chemotherapy intensified with high dose methotrexate. *Neurooncology* 2003; **5**: 37.

●187. Garre ML, Massimino M, Cefalo G *et al.* High risk malignant CNS tumours in infants: Standard versus myeloablative chemotherapy: The experience of the Italian co-operative study for children < 3 years of age. *Neurooncology* 2003; **5**: 40.

♦188. Biegel JA, Kalpana G, Knudsen ES *et al.* The role of INI1 and the SWI/SNF complex in the development of rhabdoid tumors: meeting summary from the workshop on childhood atypical teratoid/rhabdoid tumors. *Cancer Res* 2002; **62**: 323–8.

♦189. Hilden JM, Watterson J, Longee DC *et al.* Central nervous system atypical teratoid tumor/rhabdoid tumor: response to intensive therapy and review of the literature. *J Neurooncol* 1998; **40**: 265–75.

♦190. Packer RJ, Biegel JA, Blaney S *et al.* Atypical teratoid/rhabdoid tumor of the central nervous system: report on workshop. *J Pediatr Hematol Oncol* 2002; **24**: 337–42.

191. Fitzpatrick LK, Aronson LJ, Cohen KJ. Is there a requirement for adjuvant therapy for choroid plexus carcinoma that has been completely resected? *J Neurooncol* 2002; **57**: 123–6.

♦192. Wolff JE, Sajedi M, Brant R *et al.* Choroid plexus tumours. *Br J Cancer* 2002; **87**: 1086–91.

193. Borba LA, al Mefty O, Mrak RE *et al.* Cranial chordomas in children and adolescents. *J Neurosurg* 1996; **84**: 584–91.

194. Hug EB, Sweeney RA, Nurre PM *et al.* Proton radiotherapy in management of pediatric base of skull tumors. *Int J Radiat Oncol Biol Phys* 2002; **52**: 1017–24.

195. Daumas-Duport C, Scheithauer BW, Chodkiewicz JP *et al.* Dysembryoplastic neuroepithelial tumor: a surgically curable tumor of young patients with intractable partial seizures. Report of thirty-nine cases. *Neurosurgery* 1988; **23**: 545–56.

196. Johnson JH Jr, Hariharan S, Berman J *et al.* Clinical outcome of pediatric gangliogliomas: ninety-nine cases over 20 years. *Pediatr Neurosurg* 1997; **27**: 203–7.

197. Reifenberger G, Louis DN. Oligodendroglioma: toward molecular definitions in diagnostic neuro-oncology. *J Neuropathol Exp Neurol* 2003; **62**: 111–26.

198. Jenkins RB, Curran W, Scott CB *et al.* Pilot evaluation of 1p and 19q deletions in anaplastic oligodendrogliomas collected by a national cooperative cancer treatment group. *Am J Clin Oncol* 2001; **24**: 506–8.

199. Smith JS, Perry A, Borell TJ *et al.* Alterations of chromosome arms 1p and 19q as predictors of survival in oligodendrogliomas, astrocytomas, and mixed oligoastrocytomas. *J Clin Oncol* 2000; **18**: 636–45.

200. Chahlavi A, Kanner A, Peereboom D *et al.* Impact of chromosome 1p status in response of oligodendroglioma to temozolomide: preliminary results. *J Neurooncol* 2003; **61**: 267–73.

201. Pothula VB, Lesser T, Mallucci C *et al.* Vestibular schwannomas in children. *Otol Neurotol* 2001; **22**: 903–7.

202. Subach BR, Kondziolka D, Lunsford LD *et al.* Stereotactic radiosurgery in the management of acoustic neuromas associated with neurofibromatosis Type 2. *J Neurosurg* 1999; **90**: 815–22.

203. Wiet RJ, Mamikoglu B, Odom L *et al.* Long-term results of the first 500 cases of acoustic neuroma surgery. *Otolaryngol Head Neck Surg* 2001; **124**: 645–51.

204. Eiser C, Lansdown R: Retrospective study of intellectual development in children treated for acute lymphoblastic leukaemia. *Arch Dis Child* 1977; **52**: 525–9.

205. Meadows AT, Gordon J, Massari DJ *et al.* Declines in IQ scores and cognitive dysfunctions in children with acute lymphocytic leukaemia treated with cranial irradiation. *Lancet* 1981; **2**: 1015–18.

206. Jannoun L. Are cognitive and educational development affected by age at which prophylactic therapy is given in acute lymphoblastic leukaemia? *Arch Dis Child* 1983; **58**: 953–8.

207. Silber JH, Radcliffe J, Peckham V *et al.* Whole-brain irradiation and decline in intelligence: the influence of dose and age on IQ score. *J Clin Oncol* 1992; **10**: 1390–6.

208. Mulhern RK, Ochs J, Fairclough D *et al.* Intellectual and academic achievement status after CNS relapse: a retrospective analysis of 40 children treated for acute lymphoblastic leukemia. *J Clin Oncol* 1987; **5**: 933–40.

209. Harten G, Stephani U, Henze G *et al.* Slight impairment of psychomotor skills in children after treatment of acute lymphoblastic leukemia. *Eur J Pediatr* 1984; **142**: 189–97.

210. Trautman PD, Erickson C, Shaffer D *et al.* Prediction of intellectual deficits in children with acute lymphoblastic leukemia. *J Dev Behav Pediatr* 1988; **9**: 122–8.

211. Silverman CL, Palkes H, Talent B *et al.* Late effects of radiotherapy on patients with cerebellar medulloblastoma. *Cancer* 1984; **54**: 825–9.

212. Duffner PK, Cohen ME, Thomas P: Late effects of treatment on the intelligence of children with posterior fossa tumors. *Cancer* 1983; **51**: 233–7.

213. Walter AW, Mulhern RK, Gajjar A *et al.* Survival and neurodevelopmental outcome of young children with medulloblastoma at St Jude Children's Research Hospital. *J Clin Oncol* 1999; **17**: 3720–8.

214. Reddickaij WE, Russell JM, Glass JO *et al.* Subtle white matter volume differences in children treated for medulloblastoma with conventional or reduced dose craniospinal irradiation. *Magn Reson Imaging* 2000; **18**: 787–93.

215. Mulhern RK, Reddick WE, Palmer SL *et al.* Neurocognitive deficits in medulloblastoma survivors and white matter loss. *Ann Neurol* 1999; **46**: 834–41.

216. Reddick WE, White HA, Glass JO *et al.* Developmental model relating white matter volume to neurocognitive deficits in pediatric brain tumor survivors. *Cancer* 2003; **97**: 2512–19.

217. Duffner PK, Cohen ME, Thomas P. Late effects of treatment on the intelligence of children with posterior fossa tumors. *Cancer* 1983; **51**: 233–7.

218. Mulhern RK, Palmer SL, Reddick WE *et al.* Risks of young age for selected neurocognitive deficits in medulloblastoma are associated with white matter loss. *J Clin Oncol* 2001; **19**: 472–9.

219. Hoppe-Hirsch E, Brunet L, Laroussinie F *et al.* Intellectual outcome in children with malignant tumors of the posterior fossa: influence of the field of irradiation and quality of surgery. *Childs Nerv Syst* 1995; **11**: 340–5.

220. Grill J, Renaux VK, Bulteau C *et al.* Long-term intellectual outcome in children with posterior fossa tumors according to radiation doses and volumes. *Int J Radiat Oncol Biol Phys* 1999; **45**: 137–45.

●221. Ris MD, Packer R, Goldwein J *et al.* Intellectual outcome after reduced-dose radiation therapy plus adjuvant chemotherapy for medulloblastoma: a Children's Cancer Group study. *J Clin Oncol* 2001; **19**: 3470–6.

●222. Goldwein JW, Radcliffe J, Packer RJ *et al*. Results of a pilot study of low-dose craniospinal radiation therapy plus chemotherapy for children younger than 5 years with primitive neuroectodermal tumors. *Cancer* 1993; **71**: 2647–52.

223. Reimers TS, Ehrenfels S, Mortensen EL *et al*. Cognitive deficits in long-term survivors of childhood brain tumors: Identification of predictive factors. *Med Pediatr Oncol* 2003; **40**: 26–34.

224. Allen JC, Rosen G, Mehta BM *et al*. Leukoencephalopathy following high-dose iv methotrexate chemotherapy with leucovorin rescue. *Cancer Treat Rep* 1980; **64**: 1261–73.

225. Salloum E, Flamant F, Ghosn M *et al*. Irreversible encephalopathy with ifosfamide/mesna. *J Clin Oncol* 1987; **5**: 1303–4.

226. Glass JP, Lee YY, Bruner J *et al*. Treatment-related leukoencephalopathy. A study of three cases and literature review. *Medicine (Baltimore)* 1986; **65**: 154–62.

227. De Vile CJ, Grant DB, Hayward RD *et al*. Obesity in childhood craniopharyngioma: relation to post-operative hypothalamic damage shown by magnetic resonance imaging. *J Clin Endocrinol Metab* 1996; **81**: 2734–7.

228. Curtis J, Daneman D, Hoffman HJ *et al*. The endocrine outcome after surgical removal of craniopharyngiomas. *Pediatr Neurosurg* 1994; **21**(Suppl 1): 24–7.

229. Lustig RH, Post SR, Srivannaboon K *et al*. Risk factors for the development of obesity in children surviving brain tumors. *J Clin Endocrinol Metab* 2003; **88**: 611–16.

230. Duffner PK, Cohen ME, Anderson SW *et al*. Long-term effects of treatment on endocrine function in children with brain tumors. *Ann Neurol* 1983; **14**: 528–32.

231. Gurney JG, Kadan-Lottick NS, Packer RJ *et al*. Endocrine and cardiovascular late effects among adult survivors of childhood brain tumors: Childhood Cancer Survivor Study. *Cancer* 2003; **97**: 663–73.

232. Shuper A, Packer RJ, Vezina LG *et al*. 'Complicated migraine-like episodes' in children following cranial irradiation and chemotherapy. *Neurology* 1995; **45**: 1837–40.

●233. Packer RJ, Gurney JG, Punyko JA *et al*. Long-term neurologic and neurosensory sequelae in adult survivors of a childhood brain tumor: childhood cancer survivor study. *J Clin Oncol* 2003; **21**: 3255–61.

234. Walker DA, Pillow J, Waters KD *et al*. Enhanced cis-platinum ototoxicity in children with brain tumours who have received simultaneous or prior cranial irradiation. *Med Pediatr Oncol* 1989; **17**: 48–52.

235. Kirkbride P, Plowman PN. Platinum chemotherapy, radiotherapy and the inner ear: implications for 'standard' radiation portals. *Br J Radiol* 1989; **62**: 457–62.

236. Freilich RJ, Kraus DH, Budnick AS *et al*. Hearing loss in children with brain tumors treated with cisplatin and carboplatin-based high-dose chemotherapy with autologous bone marrow rescue. *Med Pediatr Oncol* 1996; **26**: 95–100.

237. Pomper MG, Port JD. New techniques in MR imaging of brain tumors. *Magn Reson Imaging Clin North Am* 2000; **8**: 691–713.

238. Howe FA, Barton SJ, Cudlip SA *et al*. Metabolic profiles of human brain tumors using quantitative in vivo 1H magnetic resonance spectroscopy. *Magn Reson Med* 2003; **49**: 223–32.

239. Curless RG, Bowen BC, Pattany PM *et al*. Magnetic resonance spectroscopy in childhood brainstem tumors. *Pediatr Neurol* 2002; **26**: 374–8.

240. Kuznetsov YE, Caramanos Z, Antel SB *et al*. Proton magnetic resonance spectroscopic imaging can predict length of survival in patients with supratentorial gliomas. *Neurosurgery* 2003; **53**: 565–74.

241. Nafe R, Herminghaus S, Raab P *et al*. Preoperative proton-MR spectroscopy of gliomas – correlation with quantitative nuclear morphology in surgical specimen. *J Neurooncol* 2003; **63**: 233–45.

242. Tzika AA, Cheng LL, Goumnerova L *et al*. Biochemical characterization of pediatric brain tumors by using in vivo and ex vivo magnetic resonance spectroscopy. *J Neurosurg* 2002; **96**: 1023–31.

243. Cheng LL, Chang IW, Louis DN *et al*. Correlation of high-resolution magic angle spinning proton magnetic resonance spectroscopy with histopathology of intact human brain tumor specimens. *Cancer Res* 1998; **58**: 1825–32.

244. Packer RJ, Zimmerman RA, Bilaniuk LT. Magnetic resonance imaging in the evaluation of treatment-related central nervous system damage. *Cancer* 1986; **58**: 635–40.

245. Davidson A, Tait DM, Payne GS *et al*. Magnetic resonance spectroscopy in the evaluation of neurotoxicity following cranial irradiation for childhood cancer. *Br J Radiol* 2000; **73**: 421–4.

246. Gauvain KM, McKinstry RC, Mukherjee P *et al*. Evaluating pediatric brain tumor cellularity with diffusion-tensor imaging. *AJR Am J Roentgenol* 2001; **177**: 449–54.

247. Tzika AA, Zarifi MK, Goumnerova L *et al*. Neuroimaging in pediatric brain tumors: Gd-DTPA-enhanced, hemodynamic, and diffusion MR imaging compared with MR spectroscopic imaging. AJNR *Am J Neuroradiol* 2002; **23**: 322–33.

248. Khong PL, Kwong DL, Chan GC *et al*. Diffusion-tensor imaging for the detection and quantification of treatment-induced white matter injury in children with medulloblastoma: a pilot study. *AJNR Am J Neuroradiol* 2003; **24**: 734–40.

249. Tummala RP, Chu RM, Liu H *et al*. Application of diffusion tensor imaging to magnetic-resonance-guided brain tumor resection. *Pediatr Neurosurg* 2003; **39**: 39–43.

250. Golder W. Functional magnetic resonance imaging – basics and applications in oncology. *Onkologie* 2002; **25**: 28–31.

251. Holodny AI, Schulder M, Liu WC *et al*. The effect of brain tumors on BOLD functional MR imaging activation in the adjacent motor cortex: implications for image-guided neurosurgery. *AJNR Am J Neuroradiol* 2000; **21**: 1415–22.

252. Schulder M, Carmel PW. Intraoperative magnetic resonance imaging: impact on brain tumor surgery. *Cancer Control* 2003; **10**: 115–24.

253. Hall WA, Kowalik K, Liu H *et al*. Costs and benefits of intraoperative MR-guided brain tumor resection. *Acta Neurochir Suppl* 2003; **85**: 137–42.

254. Roelcke U, Leenders KL. PET in neuro-oncology. *J Cancer Res Clin Oncol* 2001; **127**: 2–8.

255. Chao ST, Suh JH, Raja S *et al*. The sensitivity and specificity of FDG PET in distinguishing recurrent brain tumor from radionecrosis in patients treated with stereotactic radiosurgery. *Int J Cancer* 2001; **96**: 191–7.

256. Pirotte B, Goldman S, Salzberg S *et al.* Combined positron emission tomography and magnetic resonance imaging for the planning of stereotactic brain biopsies in children: experience in 9 cases. *Pediatr Neurosurg* 2003; **38**: 146–55.

257. Barthel H, Cleij MC, Collingridge DR *et al.* 3'-deoxy-3'-[18F]fluorothymidine as a new marker for monitoring tumor response to antiproliferative therapy in vivo with positron emission tomography. *Cancer Res* 2003; **63**: 3791–8.

258. Collingridge DR, Glaser M, Osman S *et al.* In vitro selectivity, in vivo biodistribution and tumour uptake of annexin V radiolabelled with a positron emitting radioisotope. *Br J Cancer* 2003; **89**: 1327–33.

259. Kirton A, Kloiber R, Rigel J *et al.* Evaluation of pediatric CNS malignancies with (99m)Tc-methoxyisobutylisonitrile SPECT. *J Nucl Med* 2002; **43**: 1438–43.

260. Ak I, Gulbas Z, Altinel F *et al.* Tc-99m MIBI uptake and its relation to the proliferative potential of brain tumors. *Clin Nucl Med* 2003; **28**: 29–33.

261. Sasaki M, Kuwabara Y, Yoshida T *et al.* A comparative study of thallium-201 SPET, carbon-11 methionine PET and fluorine-18 fluorodeoxyglucose PET for the differentiation of astrocytic tumours. *Eur J Nucl Med* 1998; **25**: 1261–9.

262. Tzika AA, Astrakas LG, Zarifi MK *et al.* Multiparametric MR assessment of pediatric brain tumors. *Neuroradiology* 2003; **45**: 1–10.

263. Grotzer MA, Janss AJ, Phillips PC *et al.* Neurotrophin receptor TrkC predicts good clinical outcome in medulloblastoma and other primitive neuroectodermal brain tumors. *Klin Padiatr* 2000; **212**: 196–9.

264. Capdeville R, Buchdunger E, Zimmermann J *et al.* Glivec (STI571, imatinib), a rationally developed, targeted anticancer drug. *Nat Rev Drug Discov* 2002; **1**: 493–502.

265. Fabbro D, Ruetz S, Buchdunger E *et al.* Protein kinases as targets for anticancer agents: from inhibitors to useful drugs. *Pharmacol Ther* 2002; **93**: 79–98.

266. Manley PW, Cowan-Jacob SW, Buchdunger E *et al.* Imatinib: a selective tyrosine kinase inhibitor. *Eur J Cancer* 2002; **38**(Suppl. 5): S19–27.

267. Verweij J, van Oosterom A, Blay JY *et al.* Imatinib mesylate (STI-571 Glivec, Gleevec) is an active agent for gastrointestinal stromal tumours, but does not yield responses in other soft-tissue sarcomas that are unselected for a molecular target. Results from an EORTC Soft Tissue and Bone Sarcoma Group phase II study. *Eur J Cancer* 2003; **39**: 2006–11.

268. McLaughlin ME, Robson CD, Kieran MW *et al.* Marked regression of metastatic pilocytic astrocytoma during treatment with imatinib mesylate (STI-571, Gleevec): a case report and laboratory investigation. *J Pediatr Hematol Oncol* 2003; **25**: 644–8.

269. Kilic T, Alberta JA, Zdunek PR *et al.* Intracranial inhibition of platelet-derived growth factor-mediated glioblastoma cell growth by an orally active kinase inhibitor of the 2-phenylaminopyrimidine class. *Cancer Res* 2000; **60**: 5143–50.

270. Muracciole X, Romain S, Dufour H *et al.* PAI-1 and EGFR expression in adult glioma tumors: toward a molecular prognostic classification. *Int J Radiat Oncol Biol Phys* 2002; **52**: 592–8.

271. Khatua S, Peterson KM, Brown KM *et al.* Overexpression of the EGFR/FKBP12/HIF-2alpha pathway identified in childhood astrocytomas by angiogenesis gene profiling. *Cancer Res* 2003; **63**: 1865–70.

272. Hernan R, Fasheh R, Calabrese C *et al.* ERBB2 up-regulates S100A4 and several other prometastatic genes in medulloblastoma. *Cancer Res* 2003; **63**: 140–8.

273. Schlegel J, Durchschlag G, Piontek G *et al.* Activation of the phosphatidylinositol-3'-kinase/protein kinase B-dependent antiapoptotic pathway plays an important role in the development of radioresistance of human glioma cells. *Ann NY Acad Sci* 2002; **973**: 224–7.

274. Maity A, Pore N, Lee J *et al.* Epidermal growth factor receptor transcriptionally up-regulates vascular endothelial growth factor expression in human glioblastoma cells via a pathway involving phosphatidylinositol 3'-kinase and distinct from that induced by hypoxia. *Cancer Res* 2000; **60**: 5879–86.

275. Sakata K, Kato S, Fox JC *et al.* Autocrine signaling through Ras regulates cell survival activity in human glioma cells: potential cross-talk between Ras and the phosphatidylinositol 3-kinase-Akt pathway. *J Neuropathol Exp Neurol* 2002; **61**: 975–83.

276. Huber H, Eggert A, Janss AJ *et al.* Angiogenic profile of childhood primitive neuroectodermal brain tumours/medulloblastomas. *Eur J Cancer* 2001; **37**: 2064–72.

277. Bodey B, Bodey B Jr, Siegel SE *et al.* Matrix metalloproteinase expression in childhood medulloblastomas/primitive neuroectodermal tumors. *In Vivo* 2000; **14**: 667–73.

278. Bodey B, Bodey B Jr, Siegel SE *et al.* Matrix metalloproteinase expression in childhood astrocytomas. *Anticancer Res* 2000; **20**: 3287–92.

279. Steward WP, Thomas AL. Marimastat: the clinical development of a matrix metalloproteinase inhibitor. *Expert Opin Invest Drugs* 2000; **9**: 2913–22.

280. VanMeter TE, Rooprai HK, Kibble MM *et al.* The role of matrix metalloproteinase genes in glioma invasion: co-dependent and interactive proteolysis. *J Neurooncol* 2001; **53**: 213–35.

281. Kapoor GS, O'Rourke DM. Receptor tyrosine kinase signaling in gliomagenesis: pathobiology and therapeutic approaches. *Cancer Biol Ther* 2003; **2**: 330–42.

16

Retinoblastoma

FRANÇOIS DOZ, H. BRISSE, D. STOPPA-LYONNET, X. SASTRE, JEAN-MICHEL ZUCKER & L. DESJARDINS

INTRODUCTION

Retinoblastoma is the most frequent eye tumour in children, with an incidence of 1 in 15 000–20 000 births.[1] About 60 per cent of cases correspond to unilateral involvement; the median age at diagnosis is 2 years and most of these unilateral forms are not hereditary. Retinoblastoma is bilateral in about 40 per cent of cases; the median age at diagnosis is 1 year. All bilateral forms and all multifocal unilateral forms are hereditary. The frequency of familial forms, defined by the presence of at least two cases in the same family, is increasing as a result of the improved efficacy of treatments. Hereditary retinoblastoma constitutes a cancer predisposition syndrome. A subject constitutionally carrying an *RB1* gene mutation has a greater than 90 per cent risk of developing retinoblastoma, but is also at increased risk of developing other types of cancer, usually secondary sarcomas.[2]

Management of patients with retinoblastoma must take into account the various aspects of the disease:

- the visual risk, which depends on whether the lesions are unilateral or bilateral, the topography of the tumours in the eye and the frequent need for enucleation
- the quite possibly hereditary nature of the disease (according to the clinical presentation and family history)
- the life-threatening risk – retinoblastoma itself is rarely fatal in industrialized countries, but patients may die from subsequent second

tumours in hereditary forms. In underdeveloped countries, retinoblastoma appears to be a more frequent form of cancer in children and is accompanied by a high mortality rate due to a frequently delayed diagnosis, at an advanced stage of the disease.[3]

DIAGNOSIS OF RETINOBLASTOMA

The most frequent presenting signs are leukocoria (white reflection in the pupil) (Figure 16.1) and strabismus. Leukocoria is often inconstant early in the disease, only visible at certain angles and under certain light conditions. It is particularly well demonstrated in flash photographs. Strabismus, when present, rapidly becomes constant, reflecting impaired vision. It must not be confused with physiological accommodation strabismus in infants. Both these signs are still neglected too frequently and justify ophthalmological consultation with fundoscopy. Presenting signs other than leukocoria and strabismus are observed more rarely (Box 16.1).

The diagnosis is usually established on fundoscopy under general anaesthesia, showing the characteristic appearance of a white tumour accompanied by angiomatous dilatation of the vessels. The diagnosis may be more difficult in the case of extensive unilateral forms when the tumour is atypical or poorly visualized. The main differential diagnoses are Coats' disease (unilateral retinal disease, more frequent in boys, with telangiectasia

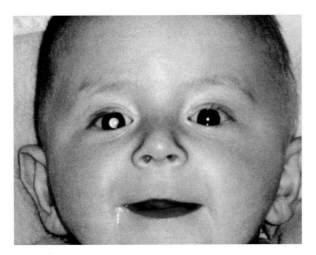

Figure 16.1 *Leukocoria.*

Box 16.1 *Main symptoms and circumstances for discovering retinoblastoma*

- Leukocoria
- Strabismus
- Iris rubeosis
- Hypopion
- Hyphaema
- Buphthalmia
- Orbital cellulitis, exophthalmia
- Screening (familial history, or dysmorphic syndrome with 13q14 deletion)

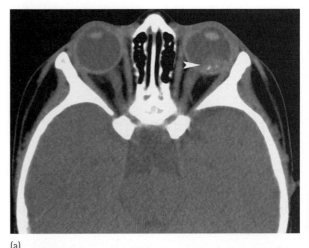

(a)

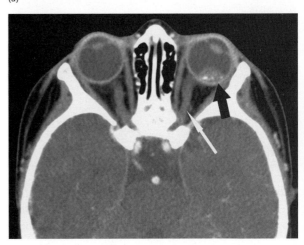

(b)

Figure 16.2 *Left unilateral retinoblastoma (CT scan): pre-contrast (a) and after iodinated contrast injection (b). Intraocular tumour with relative high density compared with the vitreous, containing calcifications (arrowhead, a), which are slightly enhanced after contrast injection. The sclera remains continuous (broad arrow, b), excluding extrascleral involvement. Normal size and density of the retrolaminar optic nerve (thin arrow, b).*

and subretinal exudates), *Toxocara canis* eye infection, persistence of the primitive vitreous and certain forms of uveitis. The most misleading forms of retinoblastoma are diffuse invasive forms, giving an appearance of pseudo-uveitis.

Several radiological examinations can contribute to the diagnosis:[4,5]

- Ultrasound performed during fundoscopy under general anaesthesia demonstrates a mass more echogenic than the vitreous, comprising highly hyperechoic zones with posterior acoustic shadow corresponding to calcifications, possibly associated with retinal detachment in the form of a fine echogenic border.
- Computed tomography (CT) typically demonstrates an intraocular mass with a higher density than the vitreous, calcified in 90 per cent of cases, and moderately enhanced after iodinated contrast agent injection (Figure 16.2).
- Magnetic resonance imaging (MRI) shows a mass with a signal equivalent to or slightly more

intense than that of the vitreous on T1-weighted sequences, with a relatively low-intensity signal on T2-weighted sequences, and variable enhancement on sequences after injection of gadolinium chelates (Figure 16.3). Fine calcifications are not visible on MRI.

The diagnosis is generally established on fundoscopy. Although not pathognomonic, the best diagnostic imaging criterion in favour of retinoblastoma is the presence of calcifications within the tumour, most reliably demonstrated by CT. In contrast, the rare, invasive, diffuse forms of retinoblastoma,[6] usually not calcified, are very difficult

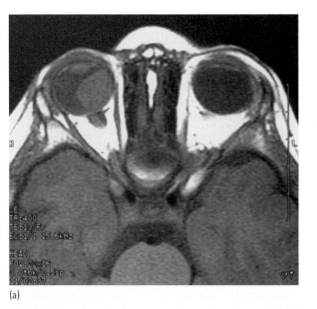

(a)

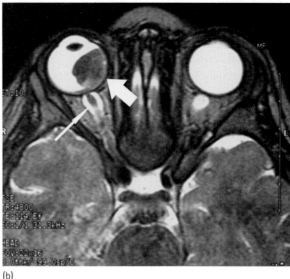

(b)

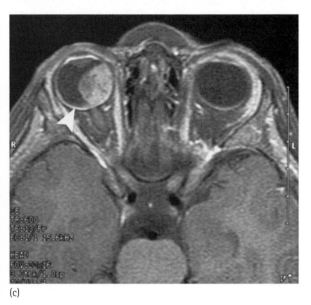

(c)

Figure 16.3 *Right unilateral retinoblastoma with prelaminar optic nerve involvement and massive choroidal invasion (MR scan). Pre-contrast T1-weighted (a), T2-weighted (b) and gadolinium-enhanced fat-saturated T1-weighted (c) images. Intraocular tumour with relatively high signal intensity compared with the vitreous on T1-weighted image, low signal intensity on T2-weighted image, and diffusely enhanced after gadolinium injection. The physiological choroidal enhancement can be seen (arrowhead, c), but choroidal invasion cannot be precisely assessed. The sclera remains continuous with physiologically low signal intensity on both T1- and T2-weighted images (broad arrow, b), excluding extrascleral involvement. Normal size and signal of the retrolaminar optic nerve (thin arrow, b).*

to diagnose due to their atypical clinical and radiological features, mimicking advanced forms of Coats' disease and toxocariasis,[7] and sometimes requiring the use of anterior chamber aspiration. However, the indications for diagnostic anterior chamber aspiration with assay of enolase (elevated in the case of retinoblastoma) and cytology must remain exceptional, as they increase the risk of orbital seeding to the conjunctiva along the needle track.

The diagnosis of retinoblastoma is sometimes made during routine fundoscopy in the context of a malformative syndrome with a known cytogenetic anomaly affecting the 13q14 region or during screening examination of a high-risk subject with a family history of retinoblastoma. These screening examinations are sometimes guided by molecular genetic analyses of the constitutional and tumour RB gene, performed in the subject and the family when they are available and informative.

STAGING

Intraocular staging

FUNDOSCOPY UNDER GENERAL ANAESTHESIA

Staging of the intraocular lesion must be performed by fundoscopy under general anaesthesia. This examination is ideally performed by indirect ophthalmoscopy using a Schepens ophthalmoscope and magnifying glass to visualize all of the retina from the posterior pole to the most anterior zone or ora serrata. Fundoscopy determines the unilateral or bilateral nature of the lesions, the number of tumours, their situation in the retina, their anatomical relations with the optic disc and macula, their dimensions (diameter and thickness), and the presence of invasion of the vitreous. Fundoscopy specifies the endophytic (arising

Box 16.2 *Reese–Ellsworth classification*[a]

Group I

a Solitary tumour, <4 disc diameters in size, at or behind the equator

b Multiple tumours, none >4 disc diameters in size, at or behind the equator

Group II

a Solitary tumour, 4–10 disc diameters in size, at or behind the equator

b Multiple tumours, 4–10 disc diameters in size, behind the equator

Group III

a Any lesion anterior to the equator

b Solitary tumour >10 disc diameters behind the equator

Group IV

a Multiple tumours, some >10 disc diameters

b Any lesion extending anteriorly to the ora serrata

Group V

a Massive tumours involving more than half the retina

b Vitreous seeding

---

[a] Reese grouping is the international reference for staging of intraocular tumours. It has been designed to predict the success of eye preservation after treatment with external beam radiotherapy. A new staging classification is presently being discussed in order to make it more relevant to the current practice of eye examination and the new conservative approaches

inside the vitreous cavity) and/or exophytic (associated with retinal detachment) nature of the tumour. When retinal detachment is complete, clinical measurement of the masses may be impossible. This assessment is currently completed in a specialized centre by a digital camera, allowing recording and follow-up of these clinical data. It is sometimes difficult to specify the number of tumours in extensive intraocular forms, as a very large solitary tumour cannot be distinguished from several confluent tumours. It is therefore impossible to determine whether the tumour is unifocal or multifocal in a large number of unilateral retinoblastomas. Precise staging of intraocular involvement must take into account the diameter of the tumour(s), the tumour topography and the presence or absence of invasion of the vitreous, specifying its extent (diffuse or localized vitreous invasion). The Reese classification, which defines five degrees of intraocular invasion (Box 16.2), remains the reference classification.[8] However, it is no longer perfectly adapted, as it was initially formulated in order to predict the probability of success of conservative management by external beam radiation at a time when indirect ophthalmoscopy was not available, making examination of the peripheral retina difficult. New international intraocular staging is now being validated, taking into account current practice of eye examination and conservative approaches.

OCULAR ULTRASOUND

Ocular ultrasound is often performed during the same general anaesthetic and also contributes to assessment of the lesions by measuring their diameter and especially their thickness.

Intraorbital staging

Intraorbital staging is based on CT or MRI imaging, which must be performed in almost all patients, except in the case of small unilateral or bilateral tumours, situated away from the optic disc, often diagnosed in a screening context. MRI is the most sensitive technique, but is less readily available and requires general anaesthesia to ensure complete immobility of the child. Cerebral imaging is systematically performed at the same time as orbital imaging.

Although now rarely observed, radiologically visible extension to the retrolaminar optic nerve must be carefully investigated, especially in the case of tumours involving the optic disc, as it determines the surgical approach for enucleation (prechiasmatic section via a subfrontal incision in the case of visible involvement of the optic nerve). Imaging may reveal extrascleral extension, but is unable to predict choroidal invasion.[4]

Distant staging

The other staging investigations depend on the clinical features (Figure 16.4).[9–13] A staging assessment looking for metastasis is useless in most cases of retinoblastoma and must be reserved for forms with extraretinal involvement documented by histological examination of the enucleation specimen or forms with primary orbital or extraocular involvement that have now become exceptional in industrialized countries.

TREATMENT OF LOCALIZED FORMS OF RETINOBLASTOMA

Management of extensive unilateral retinoblastoma

Most unilateral forms of retinoblastoma correspond to extensive intraocular lesions (Reese group V) with invasion of the great majority of the retina, frequently associated with complete retinal detachment and vitreous invasion.

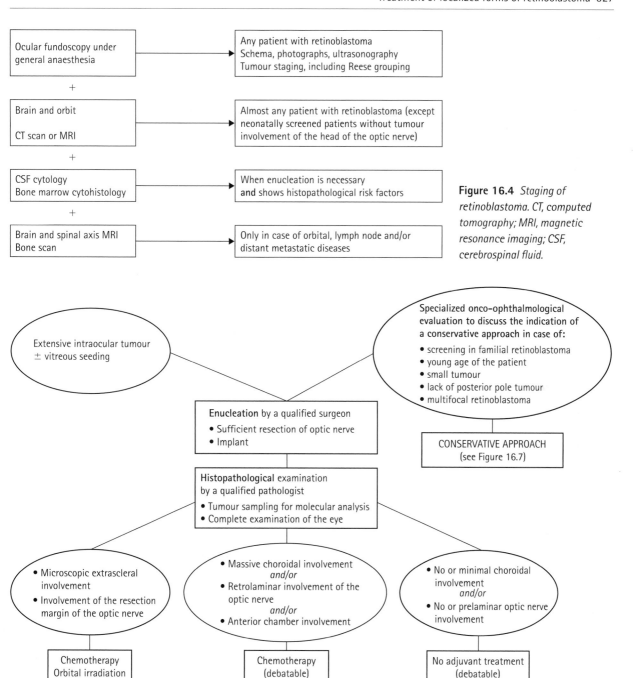

Figure 16.4 *Staging of retinoblastoma. CT, computed tomography; MRI, magnetic resonance imaging; CSF, cerebrospinal fluid.*

Figure 16.5 *Unilateral retinoblastoma treatment algorithm.*

Under these conditions, conservative management is impossible and enucleation remains mandatory (see Figure 16.5).

ENUCLEATION

The conditions of enucleation must strictly comply with the following criteria: section of the optic nerve as posteriorly as possible inside the orbit, avoiding effraction of the eyeball; placement of an orbital implant, preferably a coral implant,[14] to limit the risks of rejection of the implant and allow better subsequent mobility of the

prosthesis; and, finally, collection of tumour samples for genetic studies, in collaboration with the pathologist.

HISTOLOGICAL RISK CRITERIA

Histological examination must also be performed by a pathologist experienced in this field, on the basis of the following criteria:

- examination of the whole eyeball, taking into account artefacts induced by tumour aspiration for genetic studies

- identification of the endophytic and/or exophytic nature of the tumour
- examination of all of the available optic nerve with particular attention to the prelaminar and retrolaminar segments, the optic nerve resection margins and its meningeal sheaths
- search for minimal or massive choroidal involvement, scleral involvement or a microscopic extrascleral lesion
- search for invasion of the ciliary body and anterior segment of the eye.

Histological examination therefore defines risk groups, guiding the indications for adjuvant therapy, as follows:

- High-risk group in the case of microscopically incomplete resection – invasion of the optic nerve resection margin or meningeal sheaths, extrascleral invasion.
- Low-risk group – no invasion of the optic nerve or limited to its prelaminar segment, minimal or no choroidal invasion. Definition of minimal choroidal invasion remains complex, as quantification may be unreliable.[15] Based on our experience, we have defined minimal choroidal invasion as the presence of localized superficial involvement of the choroid with less than three clumps of tumour cells.[16]
- Intermediate-risk group – retrolaminar invasion of the optic nerve (Plate 18), massive choroidal invasion (Plate 19), invasion of the anterior segment. Quantification of choroidal invasion is also difficult in this situation; in our experience, any choroidal invasion that cannot be considered to be minimal according to the above definition must be considered to be massive.

INDICATION FOR ADJUVANT THERAPY

A general consensus has been reached concerning the indication for adjuvant therapy in the presence of invasion of the optic nerve resection margins (or its meningeal sheaths) and microscopic extrascleral invasion.[16,17] This treatment generally comprises irradiation of the orbital cavity and conventional chemotherapy. The value of intensive chemotherapy with haemopoietic stem cell support in these high-risk forms has not been clearly established.[18]

However, the indications are much more controversial in the case of choroidal invasion, even when massive, and in the case of retrolaminar optic nerve invasion.[19] Various authors, usually on the basis of single-centre retrospective series, have either recommended or contraindicated adjuvant therapy in these intermediate-risk forms.[20] Only one single-centre prospective study has recently been published and this did not conclude in favour of adjuvant therapy.[17] The Institut Curie experience

argues in favour of adjuvant chemotherapy in these intermediate-risk cases,[16] but no randomized trials are available on this subject.

In low-risk cases (minimal choroidal invasion and/or invasion of the prelaminar segment of the optic nerve), most authors agree that adjuvant therapy is not indicated. However, in view of the difficulty of reliably quantifying choroidal invasion, some authors recommend chemotherapy regardless of the degree of the apparent choroidal invasion, minimal or massive.[15]

Research is underway to try to define new risk criteria, based on the study of tumour gene anomalies distinct from alterations of the *RB1* gene.[21,22]

MODALITIES OF ADJUVANT THERAPY

Combination chemotherapy

The cytotoxic drugs used in the adjuvant setting after enucleation in retinoblastoma are mainly alkylating agents, e.g. platinum derivatives, etoposide, vincristine and doxorubicin. The drug combinations used are those with a demonstrated efficacy in extraocular forms of retinoblastoma.[23] Historically, these drug combinations were also determined by analogy with those used in the treatment of neuroblastoma. Among the various platinum derivatives, carboplatin is now preferred to cisplatin because of the lower auditory risk in these children who already have a compromised sensory prognosis and its good cerebromeningeal penetration. The combinations most frequently used are etoposide-carboplatin[23] and vincristine-cyclophosphamide-doxorubicin.

Orbital irradiation

Orbital irradiation after enucleation is now rarely performed, as it is only indicated in the case of microscopically incomplete resection. Some authors have proposed more extensive external beam radiation along the optic tracts, or even including the brain in the presence of invasion of the resection margins, but such indications are limited by the neuroendocrine and neurocognitive sequelae of extensive irradiation in children with a median age of 2 years at diagnosis. External beam radiation of the orbital cavity after enucleation is usually performed via an anterior approach, with a high risk of sequelae affecting orbitopalpebral development and major implant fitting difficulties. An orbital cavity irradiation technique using interstitial brachytherapy has been developed in South Africa, and appears to give much better cosmetic results.[24]

UNILATERAL RETINOBLASTOMA AND CONSERVATIVE TREATMENTS

In a few rare cases of unilateral retinoblastoma, conservative treatment may be indicated after a specialist onco-ophthalmological assessment, as follows:

- diagnosis of unilateral retinoblastoma in the context of screening of high-risk subjects – the tumour is generally very small and accessible to conservative treatments and there is a high risk of 'metachronous' bilateral retinoblastoma[25,26]
- young age at diagnosis – even in the absence of a family history, a young age at diagnosis is suggestive of a hereditary form with, once again, a risk of secondary bilateral involvement
- tumour-sparing vital visual structures (macula, optic disc), with a possibility of preservation of vision in the case of ocular conservation
- small tumour, accessible to the available conservative treatments without external beam radiation – could allow ocular preservation, possibly even without useful vision or with only peripheral vision.

Management of bilateral retinoblastoma

The indication for conservative management, at least on one side, is systematically considered in cases of bilateral retinoblastoma (Figure 16.6). These indications depend on the number of tumours, their situation in relation to the macula and optic disc, the presence of partial or total retinal detachment, the presence of invasion of the vitreous and preretinal space, the age at diagnosis and the presence of a family history of retinoblastoma. The indications, practical modalities, assessment and follow-up of these conservative treatments require management in a specialized ophthalmological cancer centre.

CONSERVATIVE TREATMENT MODALITIES

Up until recently, the reference conservative treatment was external beam radiation, which guaranteed a high ocular preservation rate.[27–33] However, alternative solutions are being developed in view of the numerous adverse effects of external beam radiation in these patients. These adverse effects comprise:

- cosmetic sequelae – temporal depression, enophthalmos, loss of eyelashes and eyebrows
- ophthalmological sequelae – risk of retinopathy, maculopathy, radiation optic neuropathy, cataract, dry eye, keratitis;[34,35] irradiation techniques, generally performed under general anaesthesia, designed to spare the lens, have been developed[36,37]
- endocrine sequelae, especially decreased growth hormone secretion[38]
- cognitive sequelae have been rarely described, depending on irradiation techniques and fields

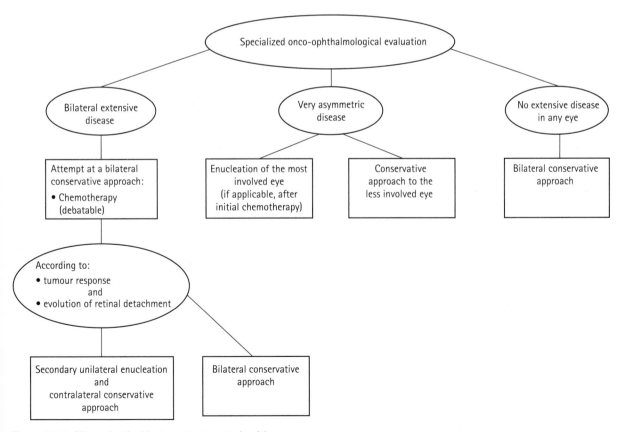

Figure 16.6 *Bilateral retinoblastoma treatment algorithm.*

- potentiation of the risk of life-threatening secondary sarcoma in the irradiation field.

The first alternatives to external beam radiation were developed for tumours situated away from the macula and optic disc, anterior to the equator of the eye. The first technique consists of cryotherapy, which can be used to treat tumours 2–3 mm in diameter and thickness, with no localized vitreous invasion.[39] Larger tumours (up to 15 mm in diameter) with localized vitreous invasion or refractory to cryotherapy may be suitable for interstitial brachytherapy[32,40–42] by iodine, ruthenium or radium plaques. The first interstitial radiotherapy treatments using cobalt plaques were abandoned because, like external beam radiation, they also induced irradiation of orbital bone and muscle, which is no longer the case with the isotopes used at the present time.

Another technique has recently been developed for tumours situated posteriorly to the equator of the eye, combining the synergistic effects of tumour hyperthermia and carboplatin. This technique, called thermochemotherapy, is based on experimental data and was introduced into the treatment of human retinoblastoma in 1994 by A.L. Murphree.[43] It is able to control tumours up to 10 mm in diameter without vitreous invasion. The intravenous infusion of carboplatin is performed 2 hours before laser treatment under general anaesthesia. The laser spot dimensions, power and exposure time are adjusted to the tumour diameter and degree of local involvement during administration of treatment (Plate 20). A second laser session is generally performed on day 8, without chemotherapy, and the following sequence is performed 3 weeks later. The current tendency is to omit the second session of laser only for small tumours. Argon laser photocoagulation, which acts by tumour devascularization, is only used for tumours less than 2 mm in diameter, situated in the posterior pole.[44,45] Its indications are actually very limited, often confined to tumours detected in a screening context, provided there is no risk of macular damage. Overall, the recently introduced modality of thermochemotherapy is the first conservative treatment for posterior pole tumours that eliminates the need for external beam radiation[46–48] with promising functional results.[49]

Other types of laser treatment associated with chemotherapy are also used.[50] All these local treatments can be administered after a phase of neoadjuvant chemotherapy. The objectives of neoadjuvant chemotherapy are as follows:[46,47,51–54]

- to make ocular tumours accessible to conservative management
- to allow conservative management other than external beam radiation
- to improve the visual prognosis by promoting retinal reapplication and by decreasing or eliminating macular invasion

- to allow creation of a healthy retinal space between the tumour and the optic disc.

The neoadjuvant chemotherapy most frequently used in recent years in the treatment of intraocular retinoblastoma comprises etoposide and carboplatin,[46,55] based on the marked efficacy of this combination in phase II trials in retinoblastomas with orbital or metastatic extraocular involvement.[23] These two drugs have also been combined with vincristine.[51,54,56] Recently published results of the use of carboplatin combined with vincristine are encouraging.[56a] Local administration of carboplatin by subconjunctival injection has recently been reported[57,58] and appears to be able to control intravitreous disease. However, the follow-up is not yet sufficient to confirm the long-term efficacy of chemotherapy alone, even topical chemotherapy, and, in the vast majority of cases, neoadjuvant chemotherapy must be combined with local conservative treatments. However, primary chemotherapy alone has been used successfully in selected patients.[59] Neoadjuvant chemotherapy provides a clear advantage when it allows ocular preservation by avoiding external beam radiation, by making tumours accessible to other conservative treatments. However, the advantage of this modality is less certain when conservative treatment requires external beam radiation in extensive intraocular tumours. In these cases, neoadjuvant chemotherapy may have an advantage in terms of the visual prognosis by providing a larger area of healthy retina prior to external beam radiation. It may also allow a reduction of the doses of external irradiation, but this has not yet been confirmed. However, the drugs used are potentially mutagenic[60] and neoadjuvant chemotherapy in combination with external beam radiation could therefore potentiate the risk of second tumours in the irradiation field.

INDICATIONS FOR CONSERVATIVE TREATMENTS

The indications for neoadjuvant chemotherapy and the place of the various conservative treatment modalities are complex issues and require diagnostic assessment, follow-up of the efficacy of treatment, and post-treatment follow-up in a specialized ophthalmological cancer centre. The indications for conservative management in unilateral and bilateral retinoblastoma are summarized in Figures 16.5 and 16.6, while Figure 16.7 summarizes the place of the various conservative treatment modalities currently available according to the size of the tumours, their anatomical relationships and the presence of vitreous invasion.

Follow-up and therapeutic results of localized forms of retinoblastoma

Ophthalmological follow-up comprises fundoscopy, performed at gradually increasing intervals after the end of

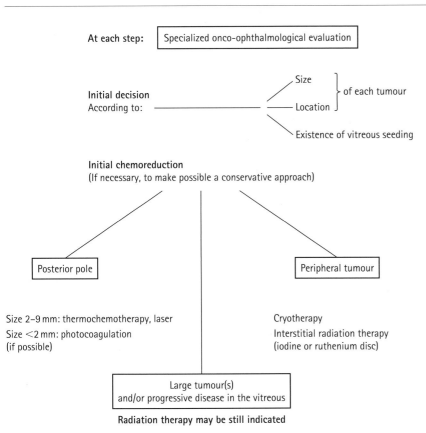

At each step: | Specialized onco-ophthalmological evaluation

Initial decision
According to: ——————— Size ⎤ of each tumour
Location ⎦
Existence of vitreous seeding

Initial chemoreduction
(If necessary, to make possible a conservative approach)

Posterior pole   Peripheral tumour

Size 2–9 mm: thermochemotherapy, laser   Cryotherapy
Size <2 mm: photocoagulation   Interstitial radiation therapy
(if possible)   (iodine or ruthenium disc)

Large tumour(s)
and/or progressive disease in the vitreous
Radiation therapy may be still indicated

Figure 16.7 *Conservative treatment approaches in retinoblastoma.*

treatment, while maintaining an examination every 3 months, and is recommended even in unilateral forms because of the rare, but significant, risk of late bilateral involvement.[25,26] The ophthalmologist must assess the retinal scars, looking for vitreous changes and the appearance of new tumours, often situated peripherally when they occur later.[61] The examination must also look for any ocular complications induced by treatment, affecting the retina, optic disc, macula and anterior segment of the eye. Clinical follow-up by an ophthalmological oncologist is usually sufficient. Ultrasound and MRI are only indicated in the case of vitreous haemorrhage due to rupture of vitreoretinal adhesions to ensure the absence of tumour progression, before performing vitrectomy. Similarly, in the case of radiation-induced cataract making fundoscopy impossible, surgery with insertion of an intraocular lens is currently recommended. Ophthalmological follow-up also comprises complete follow-up of visual functions, especially visual acuity, and correction of any disorders of refraction. Ophthalmological follow-up is generally performed under general anaesthesia until the age of 4–5 years, and then usually in the office in older children. Secondary disease progression and/or severe ocular complications may require secondary enucleation. Ophthalmological examination after enucleation must also include assessment of the orbital cavity. Follow-up by orbital imaging after enucleation is useless, as an orbital recurrence would very rapidly result in expulsion of the implant.

Paediatric follow-up is complementary to ophthalmological follow-up. The risk of extraocular involvement has become very low in industrialized countries as a result of earlier diagnosis and the strategy of adjuvant therapy adapted to histological risk criteria. Follow-up of the sequelae of treatment is obviously a priority in coordination with teams managing the child's visual handicap. A psychomotor assessment is recommended even in the case of unilateral normal vision, as it may sometimes reveal the need for further management.

The vital prognosis, related to retinoblastoma itself, is now barely threatened in patients with unilateral or bilateral retinoblastoma in industrialized countries. The visual prognosis depends on ocular preservation, the initial tumour volume, the anatomical relationships of the tumours with the macula and optic disc, and the adverse effects of treatments. The long-term visual prognosis of new conservative treatment strategies appears to be encouraging compared with that of patients classically treated with external beam radiation.[48] The long-term survival in hereditary forms is threatened by the development of other cancers. However, the current reduction in the indications for external beam radiation should result in a reduction in the incidence of second tumours, the most frequent being sarcomas arising in the irradiation field. Nevertheless, the long-term follow-up of these patients and the information given to families and the patients themselves, when they are old enough to understand, are essential to ensure early diagnosis of these second tumours. This is particularly important in that the spontaneous incidence of these tumours could also be increased by the use of neoadjuvant chemotherapy or thermochemotherapy.

RETINOBLASTOMAS WITH EXTRAOCULAR INVOLVEMENT

The sites of extraocular involvement of retinoblastoma include:

- soft tissues of the orbit[62]
- pretragal and cervical lymph nodes
- metastases, primarily affecting bone, bone marrow and central nervous system (meningeal lesions, along the optic tracts or cerebral lesions).

These extraocular forms have become exceptional in industrialized countries, but remain the most frequent presenting forms of the disease in poor countries.[3]

Considerable progress in the treatment of extraocular forms of retinoblastoma not involving the central nervous system (CNS) has been achieved by intensification of chemotherapy.[17,18,23,63] Preoperative chemotherapy is also an interesting approach in the case of extensive unilateral retinoblastoma, preceding a combined neurosurgical and ophthalmological approach for the prechiasmatic section of the optic nerve.[64] Numerous publications have reported tumour control in forms with orbital soft tissue involvement[62,65,66] and/or pretragal and cervical lymph node involvement, even with conventional chemotherapy alone.[17] Several cases of cure have also been reported after bone or bone marrow recurrence in chemosensitive forms, after high-dose chemotherapy with haemopoietic stem cell support.[18,67] On the other hand, CNS involvement has a persistently poor prognosis despite various attempts at treatment intensification.[18,65]

SECOND TUMOURS

The reported incidence of these second tumours varies considerably from one series to another, ranging from 8.4 per cent of cases at 18 years[68] to 50 per cent of cases at 20 years of follow-up.[69] The relative risk of developing a second cancer in patients with hereditary forms of retinoblastoma has been estimated to be 13 at the age of 35 years.[2] The most frequent and earliest second tumours are sarcomas, especially osteosarcomas, but also soft tissue sarcomas, which are often difficult to type precisely. The other types of cancer most frequently reported are malignant melanomas, generally occurring later than sarcomas, and malignant gliomas.[2] Some patients can present several successive second tumours. The predisposing factors for these second tumours, apart from the constitutional predisposition related to anomalies of the *RB1* gene, are essentially treatment-related. Second sarcomas are usually situated in irradiation fields,[69–71] although the incidence of osteosarcomas of the extremities is also higher in patients with hereditary forms of retinoblastoma than in the general population.[2,72,73] Alkylating chemotherapy has also been demonstrated to increase the risk of second tumours.[68] Second tumours after retinoblastoma have a poor prognosis,[74,75] because of their limited chemosensitivity and poor operability, especially when the facial bones are involved.

A special type of second cancer corresponds to the increased incidence of pineal tumours, such as pinealoblastoma, in patients followed for hereditary retinoblastoma.[76,77] This tumour usually occurs during the first 5 years of life. It is a non-metastasizing embryonic tumour, whose development could be favoured by photon beam external radiation. According to some authors, pinealoblastoma has become the leading cause of death after retinoblastoma.[78] In the Institut Curie experience, the incidence of pinealoblastoma is low, possibly partly due to the use of electron beam external radiation. Like all forms of CNS involvement related to retinoblastoma, the prognosis is very poor: no cases of cure of histologically documented pinealoblastoma have been reported in patients followed for hereditary retinoblastoma. In addition to the pineal lesion, these so-called 'trilateral' forms of retinoblastoma may also comprise suprasellar involvement.

GENETIC COUNSELLING FOR FAMILIES AND PATIENTS

The genetic counselling visit is designed to answer questions raised by patients treated during childhood, or by the patient's parents when the patient is still a young child, concerning the risk of transmission of a predisposition to retinoblastoma, the risk of having an affected child, the risk for a couple of having another child with retinoblastoma and the risk of second cancers. The follow-up of high-risk children is guided by the detection of a high cancer risk. The genetic counselling visit is conducted by a geneticist in close collaboration with the ophthalmology, paediatric oncology and radiotherapy teams looking after the child. The geneticist's tools include an analysis of the child's personal and family history, and direct and indirect molecular studies.

Analysis of the child's personal and family history

The unilateral or bilateral, unifocal or multifocal nature of the tumour, the age at diagnosis, and the presence of psychomotor retardation, or even a malformative syndrome, are crucial elements. The systematic search for a family history of retinoblastoma, and fundoscopy of the parents and siblings, looking for retinomas, tumours that have spontaneously involuted, also help to guide the analysis. The mode of transmission dominating predisposition to retinoblastoma is characterized by distribution of cases in only one parental branch.

Young age at diagnosis (less than 24 months), multifocal nature (bilateral or unilateral multifocal), presence of a family history of retinoblastoma and retinoma are arguments in favour of an underlying genetic predisposition. The affected child carries a constitutional mutation of the *RB1* gene and has one chance in two of transmitting it to each of his or her children (dominant transmission). The risk of retinoblastoma in the patient's children presenting this mutation is about 90 per cent.

Multifocal forms of retinoblastoma without a family history are mostly related to a neo-mutation in the gametes of one of the two parents. The risk of predisposition of the affected child's brothers and sisters is low (<5 per cent). These less frequent cases are due to the low penetrance of the mutations or germ-line mosaics in one of the two parents (generally the father). Inversely, the unilateral nature of the tumour, an older age at diagnosis and the absence of a family history argue in favour of the absence of predisposition. Note, however, that this interpretation is not unequivocal, as an estimated 5–10 per cent of these unilateral cases are associated with a constitutional alteration of the *RB1* gene. The risk of predisposition of the siblings of a subject with unilateral retinoblastoma is very low, of the order of 0.5 per cent.

Molecular tests

The *RB1* gene, the first tumour suppressor gene suspected,[79] and subsequently identified,[80] is situated on the long arm of chromosome 13 (segment 13q14) and possesses 27 exons, which makes an exhaustive study of this gene complex and expensive.

Development of a retinoblastoma is related to the necessary (but probably not sufficient) inactivation of the two alleles of the *RB1* gene. In predisposed children, one of the two alleles is constitutionally altered (all cells of the body carry the mutant allele); the mutation responsible is demonstrated by analysis of DNA extracted from a blood sample. The second alteration is acquired and is only present in tumour cells. Inactivation of the second allele is very frequently (65 per cent of cases) due to loss of all of the chromosomal region flanking the *RB1* gene. This allele loss is demonstrated indirectly by looking for loss of heterozygosity in the tumour. Briefly, this consists of identifying intragenic or *RB1* gene flanking genetic markers which are constitutionally heterozygous (presence of two different alleles for a given marker locus) and comparing them with the tumour DNA to detect any loss of one of the two alleles. The remaining allele is the one potentially carrying the constitutional mutation.

Molecular tests allowing the most precise genetic analysis in affected children are:

- direct search for a constitutional mutation of the *RB1* gene performed on the constitutional DNA[81–85]
- indirect demonstration of the allele carrying the mutation (in familial forms)
- study of tumour loss of heterozygosity.

DIRECT SEARCH FOR A CONSTITUTIONAL MUTATION OF THE *RB1* GENE

The complex structure of the *RB1* gene and the diversity of the mutations, generally different from one family to another, are the limiting factors of this study. In familial forms of retinoblastoma, the maximum mutation detection rate is about 85 per cent of cases.[85] These mutations are usually point mutations or small mutations leading to a truncated RB1 protein. The sensitivity of detection of *RB1* gene mutations is far from complete, even in clearly hereditary forms. This is due to the frequency of germ-line mosaicism,[86,87] the poor understanding of the role of intronic mutations and methodological limitations of detection techniques, some of which are now more clearly understood.[88] The mutations sometimes consist of deletions or duplications of part of the gene or even the whole gene, corresponding to deletions or complex chromosomal rearrangements of the long arm of chromosome 13, associated with psychomotor and growth retardation or even a malformative syndrome. Chromosomal rearrangements can be identified by high-resolution karyotyping.[89,90]

INDIRECT DEMONSTRATION OF THE ALLELE CARRYING THE MUTATION

In familial forms of retinoblastoma, indirect demonstration of the allele carrying the mutation is essential and easy to perform. Briefly, as for loss of heterozygosity in the tumour, this test consists of identifying intragenic or *RB1* gene flanking markers common to all affected members of the family (generally a parent and a child). In order to reconstitute the phase of markers (haplotype), it is often useful to also study the non-affected parent and the siblings.

STUDY OF TUMOUR LOSS OF HETEROZYGOSITY

This study depends on the availability of tumour material, which is increasingly rare due to the increasing use of conservative treatments. In the context of a family history and when only one affected subject is available, this approach can detect the mutant allele in 65 per cent of cases (when loss of the second allele has occurred in this way). In the absence of a family history, this study is able to detect a high-risk allele (i.e. 'potentially carrying the predisposition') in an average of one case in four.[91]

Test procedure and significance according to family history

RISK OF A CHILD WITH ONE PARENT PRESENTING A HISTORY OF RETINOBLASTOMA

- In a parent (or future parent) with a history of retinoblastoma in childhood and a family history of retinoblastoma, indirect study of constitutional DNA can reveal a high-risk *RB1* allele in the majority of cases, leading to proposal of antenatal or postnatal diagnosis (depending on the availability of samples from at least two affected members of the family), which is positive in 50 per cent of cases.
- In the case of bilateral retinoblastoma with no family history, the indirect approach based on tumour DNA, whenever tumour material is available, can detect the high-risk allele in an average of one out of four cases. In the other cases, only demonstration of a constitutional mutation of the *RB1* gene by the direct approach justifies proposal of a diagnostic test for predisposition, which will be positive in 50 per cent of cases. When the diagnosis of predisposition is confirmed, or when the study of the index case is not informative, ophthalmological surveillance right from the neonatal period is essential.
- In the case of unilateral retinoblastoma with no family history, the indirect approach based on tumour DNA may detect the allele at potential risk. Note that, although this examination avoids the need for surveillance in about one case in four, it does not eliminate the need for surveillance in three out of four cases, but this surveillance is only positive in less than 10 per cent of cases. In isolated unilateral forms, the probability of constitutional mutation of the affected parent is less than 10 per cent. Ideally, a systematic search for *RB1* gene mutations with no false-negative results (100 per cent detection of existing mutations) would be able to reassure these affected parents.

RISK FOR A CHILD WITH A BROTHER OR SISTER WITH RETINOBLASTOMA

- In the case of family history comprising at least two cases, the risk of predisposition of younger brothers and sisters is 50 per cent. As indicated in the previous section, constitutional and tumour indirect approaches are generally able to detect the high-risk allele.
- In the absence of a family history, but in the presence of bilateral or multifocal retinoblastoma, the risk for young brothers and sisters is low (>5 per cent). Once again, the indirect approach may eliminate the need for surveillance if children do not present any alleles in common with their affected sibling or if they do not carry the allele lost in the tumour. If, in contrast, a child shares an allele in common with an affected sibling, only demonstration of a constitutional mutation in the index case can lead to proposal of a diagnosis of predisposition, which will give a clearly interpretable result: carrier or non-carrier.
- In the presence of unilateral, unifocal retinoblastoma, with no family history, the risk of predisposition of younger brothers and sisters is very low (<1 per cent). Constitutional and tumour indirect approaches can eliminate the need for surveillance in the situations described above, but once again, in the majority of cases, surveillance will be continued uselessly. Only detection and identification of an *RB1* gene mutation can allow a diagnosis of predisposition with an unequivocal interpretation.
- Classification into the stereotyped situations described above is obviously somewhat artificial: the unifocal or multifocal nature of the tumours in a unilateral form can be difficult to determine, as the tumours are often extensive and possibly confluent. Some non-hereditary unilateral forms can also be diagnosed early, while, conversely, a unilateral retinoblastoma, even diagnosed at the age of 2 years or later, can actually be hereditary.[92,93] The precautions of ophthalmological surveillance are therefore the same as above; non-informative laboratory analyses are obviously more frequent in these unilateral forms.

Risk of second cancers

No laboratory parameters are currently available to predict the increased risk of second tumours. Although certain *RB1* gene mutations appear to have a low phenotypic expression or even a low penetrance in terms of retinoblastoma *per se*,[94] there is no evidence, at the present time, that a particular anomaly of the *RB1* gene is associated with a higher risk of second cancer.

CONCLUSION

Retinoblastoma is a disease whose various aspects require integrated multidisciplinary management. This malignant tumour, although very often curable, is associated with a risk of mutilation (ranging from enucleation to facial sequelae of conservative management by external beam radiation), unilateral or bilateral visual handicap and a risk of second tumours in hereditary forms.

The increasingly frequent use of new conservative treatments avoiding external beam radiation can only be achieved in the greatest number of cases when the symptoms (leukocoria and strabismus) are rapidly recognized and managed.[95] A reduction in the mortality related to retinoblastoma in poor countries also depends on early recognition of the first signs. However, the risks of treatment and the constitutional predisposition to the development of a second tumour cannot be completely eliminated in hereditary forms of retinoblastoma.

KEY POINTS

- Early diagnosis may save vision, eye and life:
  - one should listen to the parents describing a leukocoria
  - strabismus in a young child should not be considered as a banal symptom and requires ophthalmological examination with ocular fundoscopy
  - genetic counselling should be proposed to any patient who was treated for retinoblastoma during childhood, including late and unilateral cases; appropriate molecular and clinical screening should be the rule.
- All bilateral, unilateral and clearly plurifocal retinoblastoma cases, as well as familial cases, are hereditary; only 10 per cent of unilateral retinoblastoma is hereditary.
- Although retinoblastoma is highly curable, children still die of the disease in economically disadvantaged countries, often because of late referral and parental refusal of enucleation.
- The diagnosis is mainly clinical: ocular fundoscopy under general anaesthesia by an experienced ophthalmologist; the presence of calcification (ultrasound, CT) is a strong positive argument.
- The best neuroradiological examination for initial staging and diagnosis is CT scan (small calcification may be seen) or MRI (no radiation, better optic nerve imaging).
- Therapeutic management aims to offer:
  - the most efficient treatment with fewer sequelae
  - the taking into account of the risk of second cancer in patients with genetic predisposition.
- Adjuvant therapy after enucleation:
  - there is a consensus in favour of chemotherapy and radiotherapy in cases of microscopically incomplete surgery (extrascleral disease, invasion of resection margin or subarachnoid space of optic nerve)
  - debatable in case of retrolaminar invasion of optic nerve and/or so-called 'massive choroidal invasion'.
- Conservative approaches:
  - therapeutic indication and procedures as well as follow-up should be performed by specialized ophthalmologists and paediatric oncologists
  - tumours anterior to the equator of the eye: cryotherapy (inefficient in the case of localized vitreous seeding); brachytherapy
  - tumours posterior to the equator of the eye: laser; thermochemotherapy
  - external beam radiotherapy is still indicated in large bilateral tumours and diffuse vitreous seeding
  - chemoreduction helps to achieve a condition that allows less aggressive local treatments; thus, this treatment is often, but not always, useful before or during local treatment (the type and duration of chemotherapy are debated).

REFERENCES

1. Desjardins L, Doz F, Schlienger P *et al.* Le rétinoblastome. *Ann Pediatr* 1996; **43**: 359–71.
2. Moll AC, Imhof SM, Bouter LX *et al.* Second primary tumors in patients with hereditary retinoblastoma: a register-based follow-up study 1945–1994. *Int J Cancer* 1996; **67**: 515–19.
3. Chantada G, Fandino A, Manzitti J *et al.* Late diagnosis of retinoblastoma in a developing country. *Arch Dis Child* 1999; **80**: 171–4.
4. Barkhof F, Smeets M, Van Der Valk P *et al.* MR imaging in retinoblastoma. *Eur Radiol* 1997; **7**: 726–31.
5. Smirniotopoulos JG, Bargallo N, Mafee MF. Differential diagnosis of leukokoria: radiologic-pathologic correlation. *Radiographics* 1994; **14**: 1059–79.
6. Brisse HJ, Lumbroso L, Freneaux PC *et al.* Sonographic, CT, and MR imaging findings in diffuse infiltrative retinoblastoma: report of two cases with histologic comparison. *AJNR Am J Neuroradiol* 2001; **22**: 499–504.
7. Kaufman LM, Mafee MF, Song CD. Retinoblastoma and simulating lesions. Role of CT, MR imaging and use of Gd-DTPA contrast enhancement. *Radiol Clin North Am* 1998; **36**: 1101–17.
8. Reese AB, Ellsworth RM. The evaluation and current concept of retinoblastoma treatment. *Trans Am Acad Ophthalmol* 1963; **67**: 164–72.
9. Karcioglu ZA, Al-Mesfer SA, Abboud E *et al.* Workup for metastatic retinoblastoma. A review of 261 patients. *Ophthalmology* 1997; **104**: 307–12.

10. Mohney BG, Robertson DM. Ancillary testing for metastasis in patients with newly diagnosed retinoblastoma. *Am J Ophthalmol* 1994; **118**: 707–11.

11. Moscinski LC, Pendergrass TW, Weiss A *et al.* Recommendations for the use of routine bone marrow aspiration and lumbar punctures in the follow-up of patients with retinoblastoma. *J Pediatr Hematol* 1996; **18**: 130–4.

12. Pratt CB, Meyer D, Chenaille P, Crom DB. The use of bone marrow aspirations and lumbar punctures at the time of diagnosis of retinoblastoma. *J Clin Oncol* 1989; **7**: 140–3.

13. Pratt CB, Crom DB, Magill L *et al.* Skeletal scintigraphy in patients with bilateral retinoblastoma. *Cancer* 1990; **65**: 26–8.

14. Jordan DR, Allen LH, Ells A *et al.* The use of Vicryl mesh (polyglactin 910) for implantation of hydroxyapatite orbital implants. *Ophthal Plast Reconstr Surg* 1995; **11**: 95–9.

15. Shields CL, Shields JA, Baez K *et al.* Choroidal invasion of retinoblastoma: metastatic potential and clinical risk factors. *Br J Ophthalmol* 1993; **77**: 544–8.

16. Khelfaoui F, Validire P, Auperin A *et al.* Histopathological risk factors in retinoblastoma. A retrospective study of 172 patients treated in a single institution. *Cancer* 1996; **77**: 1206–13.

17. Schwartzman E, Chantada G, Fandino A *et al.* Results of a stage-based protocol for the treatment of retinoblastoma. *J Clin Oncol* 1996; **14**: 1532–6.

18. Namouni F, Doz F, Tanguy ML *et al.* High dose chemotherapy with carboplatin, etoposide and cyclophosphamide followed by hematopoietic stem cell rescue in patients with high risk retinoblastoma: a SFOP and SFGM study. *Eur J Cancer* 1997; **33**: 2368–75.

19. Shields CL, Shields JA, Baez K *et al.* Optic nerve invasion of retinoblastoma. Metastatic potential and clinical risk factors. *Cancer* 1994; **73**: 692–8.

20. Kopelman JE, Mc Lean IW, Rosenberg H. Multivariate analysis of risk factors in retinoblastoma treated by enucleation. *Ophthalmology* 1987; **94**: 371–7.

21. Doz F, Peter M, Schleiermacher G *et al.* Nmyc amplification loss of heterozygosity on the short arm of chromosome 1 and DNA ploidy in retinoblastoma. *Eur J Cancer* 1996; **32A**: 645–9.

22. Mairal A, Pinglier E, Gilbert E *et al.* Detection of chromosome imbalances in retinoblastoma by parallel karyotype and CGH analyses. *Genes Chromosomes Cancer* 2000; **28**: 370–9.

23. Doz F, Neuenschwander S, Plantaz D *et al.* Etoposide and carboplatin in extraocular retinoblastoma: a study by the Société Française d'Oncologie Pédaitrique. *J Clin Oncol* 1995; **13**: 902–9.

24. Sealy R, Stannard C, Shackleton D. Improved cosmesis in retinoblastoma patients treated with iodine-125 orbital irradiation. *Ophthalmic Pediatr Genet* 1987; **8**: 95–9.

25. Fontanesi J, Pratt C, Meyer D *et al.* Asynchronous bilateral retinoblastoma: the St Jude Children's Research Hospital experience. *Ophthalmic Genet* 1995; **16**: 109–12.

26. Poncet P, Lévy C, Doz F *et al.* Rétinoblastomes unilatéraux avec bilatéralisation tardive. A propos de 3 cas. *J Fr Ophtalmol* 1998; **21**: 223–6.

27. Abramson DH, Ellsworth RM, Tretter P *et al.* Simultaneous bilateral irradiation for advanced bilateral retinoblastoma. *Arch Ophthalmol* 1981; **99**: 1763–6.

28. Abramson DH, Ellsworth RM, Tretter P *et al.* Treatment of bilateral groups I through III retinoblastoma with bilateral radiation. *Arch Ophthalmol* 1981; **99**: 1761–2.

29. Fontanesi J, Pratt CB, Kun LE *et al.* Treatment outcome and dose response relationship in infants younger than 1 year treated for retinoblastoma with primary irradiation. *Med Pediatr Oncol* 1996; **26**: 297–304.

30. Fontanesi J, Pratt CB, Hustu HO *et al.* Use of irradiation for therapy of retinoblastoma in children more than 1 year old: The St Jude Children's Hospital experience and review of literature. *Med Pediatr Oncol* 1995; **24**: 321–6.

31. Haye C, Schlienger P, Calle R *et al.* Conservative treatment of tumors of the retina at the Curie Institut. 5 year ophthalmologic results of 129 cases treated with the Stallard disc and electrons. *Bull Cancer* 1986; **73**: 260–70.

32. Hernandez JC, Brady LW, Shields JA, DePotter P. Conservative treatment of retinoblastoma. The use of plaque brachytherapy. *Am J Clin Oncol* 1993; **16**: 397–401.

33. Hernandez JC, Brady LW, Shields JA *et al.* External beam radiation for retinoblastoma: results, patterns of failure, and a proposal for treatment guidelines. *Int J Radiat Oncol Biol Phys* 1996; **35**: 125–32.

34. Coucke PA, Schmid C, Balmer A *et al.* Hypofractionation in retinoblastoma: an increased risk of retinopathy. *Radiother Oncol* 1993; **28**: 157–61.

35. Imhof SM, Hofman P, Tan K. Quantification of lacrimal function after D-shaped field irradiation for retinoblastoma. *Br J Ophthalmol* 1993; **77**: 482–4.

36. Griem ML, Ernest JT, Rozenfeld ML *et al.* Eye lens protection in the treatment of retinoblastoma with high-energy electrons. *Radiology* 1987; **90**: 351–2.

37. McCormick B, Ellsworth R, Abramson D *et al.* Radiation therapy for retinoblastoma: comparison of results with lens-sparing versus lateral beam techniques. *Int J Radiat Oncol Biol Phys* 1988; **16**: 733–61.

38. Pomarede R, Czernichow P, Zucker JM *et al.* Incidence of anterior pituitary deficiency after radiotherapy at an early age: study in retinoblastoma. *Act Paediatr Scand* 1984; **73**: 115–19.

39. Shields JA, Parsons H, Shields CL *et al.* The role of cryotherapy in the management of retinoblastoma. *Am J Ophthalmol* 1989; **108**: 260–4.

40. Desjardins L, Levy C, Labib A. An experience of the use of radioactive plaques after failure of external beam radiation in the treatment of retinoblastoma. *Ophthalmic Paediatr Genet* 1993; **14**: 39–42.

41. Shields JA, Giblin ME, Shields CL *et al.* Episcleral plaque radiotherapy for retinoblastoma. *Ophthalmology* 1989; **96**: 530–7.

42. Shields CL, Shields JA, Minelli S *et al.* Regression of retinoblastoma after plaque radiotherapy. *Am J Ophthalmol* 1993; **115**: 181–7.

43. Murphree AL, Villablanca JG, Deegan WF *et al.* Chemotherapy plus local treatment in the management of intraocular retinoblastoma. *Arch Ophthalmol* 1996; **114**: 1348–56.

44. Augsburger JJ, Faulkner CB. Indirect ophthalmoscope Argon laser treatment of retinoblastoma. *Ophthalm Surg* 1992; **23**: 591–3.

45. Shields JA, Shields CL, Parson H. The role of photocoagulation in the management of retinoblastoma. *Am J Ophthalmol* 1989; **108**: 205–8.

46. Levy C, Doz F, Quintana E *et al*. The role of chemotherapy alone or in combination with hyperthermia in the primary treatment of intraocular retinoblastoma: preliminary results in 30 patients treated at Institut Curie. *Br J Ophthalmol* 1998; **82**: 1154–8.

47. Shields CL, Shields JA, Needle M *et al*. Combined chemoreduction and adjuvant therapy for intraocular retinoblastoma. *Ophthalmology* 1997; **104**: 2101–11.

48. Lumbroso L, Doz F, Urbieta M *et al*. Chemothermotherapy in the management of retinoblastoma. *Ophthalmology* 2002; **109**: 1130–6.

49. Desjardins L, Charif Chefchaouni M, Lumbroso L *et al*. Functional results after treatment of retinoblastoma. *J Am Assoc Pediatr Ophthalmol Strabismus* 2002; **6**(2): 108–11.

50. Gallie BL, Budning A, DeBoer G *et al*. Chemotherapy with focal therapy can cure intraocular retinoblastoma without radiotherapy. *Arch Ophthalmol* 1996; **114**: 1321–8.

51. Friedman DL, Himelstein B, Shields CL *et al*. Chemoreduction and local ophthalmic therapy for intraocular retinoblastoma. *J Clin Oncol* 2000; **18**: 12–17.

52. Gallie B, Budning A, Deboer G *et al*. Chemotherapy with focal therapy can cure intraocular retinoblastoma without radiotherapy. *Arch Ophthalmol* 1996; **114**: 1321–8.

53. Greenwald MJ, Strauss LC. Treatment of intraocular retinoblastoma with carboplatin and etoposide chemotherapy. *Ophthalmology* 1996; **103**: 1989–97.

54. Kingston J, Hungerford JL, Madreperla SA, Plowman PN. Results of combined chemotherapy and radiotherapy for advanced intraocular retinoblastoma. *Arch Ophthalmol* 1996; **114**: 1339–43.

55. Beck MN, Balmer A, Dessing C *et al*. First-line chemotherapy with local treatment can prevent external-beam irradiation and enucleation in low-stage intraocular retinoblastoma. *J Clin Oncol* 2000; **18**: 2881–7.

56. Shields CL, Meadows AT, Shields JA *et al*. Chemoreduction for retinoblastoma may prevent intracranial neuroblastic malignancy (trilateral retinoblastoma). *Arch Ophthalmol* 2001; **119**: 1269–72.

56a. Rodriguez-Galindo C, Wilson MW, Haik BG *et al*. Treatment of intraocular retinoblastoma with vincristine and carboplatin. *J Clin Oncol* 2003; **21**: 2019–25.

57. Abramson DH, Franck CM, Dunkel IJ. A phase I/II study of subconjunctival carboplatin for intraocular retinoblastoma. *Ophthalmology* 1999; **106**: 1947–50.

58. Seregard S, Kock E, Af Trampe E. Intravitreal chemotherapy for recurrent retinoblastoma in an only eye. *Br J Ophthalmol* 1995; **79**: 194–5.

59. Gombos DS, Kelly A, Coen PG *et al*. Retinoblastoma treated with primary chemotherapy alone: the significance of tumour size, location and age. *Br J Ophthalmol* 2002; **86**: 80–3.

60. Winick NJ, Mc Kenna RW, Shuster JJ. Secondary acute myeloid leukemia in children treated for acute lymphoblastic leukemia with etoposide. *J Clin Oncol* 1993; **11**: 209–17.

61. Munier FL, Balmer A, van Melle G, Gailloud C. Radial asymmetry in the topography of retinoblastoma. Clues to the cell of origin. *Ophthalmic Genet* 1994; **15**: 101–6.

62. Goble RR, McKenzie J, Kingston JE *et al*. Orbital recurrence of retinoblastoma successfully treated by combined therapy. *B J Ophthalmol* 1990; **74**: 97–8.

63. Chantada G, Fandino A, Mato G *et al*. Phase II window of idarubicin in children with extraocular retinoblastoma. *J Clin Oncol* 1999; **17**: 1847–50.

64. Bellaton E, Bertozzi AI, Behar C *et al*. Neoadjuvant chemotherapy for extensive unilateral retinoblastoma. *Br J Ophthalmol* 2003; **87**: 327–9.

65. Doz F, Khelfaoui F, Mosseri V *et al*. The role of chemotherapy in orbital involvement of retinoblastoma: the experience of a single institution in 33 patients. *Cancer* 1994; **74**: 722–32.

66. Kiratli H, Bilgiç S, Ozerdem U. Management of massive orbital involvement of intraocular retinoblastoma. *Ophthalmology* 1998; **105**: 322–6.

67. Dunkel IJ, Aledo A, Kernan NA *et al*. Successful treatment of metastatic retinoblastoma. *Cancer* 2000; **89**: 2117–21.

68. Draper GJ, Sanders BM, Kingston JE. Second primary neoplasms in patients with retinoblastoma. *Br J Cancer* 1986; **53**: 661–71.

69. Abramson DH, Ellsworth RM, Kitchin FD *et al*. Second non ocular tumors in retinoblastoma survivors: are they radiation-induced? *Ophthalmology* 1984; **91**: 1351–5.

70. Desjardins L, Haye C, Schlienger P *et al*. Second non-ocular tumours in survivors of bilateral retinoblastoma. A 30-year follow-up. *Ophthalmic Paediatr Genet* 1992; **12**: 145–8.

71. Winter J, Olsen JH, De Nully Brown P. Risk of nonocular cancer among retinoblastoma patients and their parents. A population based study in Denmark 1943–1984. *Cancer* 1988; **62**: 1458–62.

72. Abramson DH, Ronner HJ, Ellsworth RM. Second tumors in nonirradiated bilateral retinoblastoma. *Am J Ophthalmol* 1979; **87**: 624–7.

73. Roarty JD, Mac Lean IW, Zimmerman LE. Incidence of second neoplasm in patients with bilateral retinoblastoma. *Ophthalmology* 1988; **95**: 1583–7.

74. Dunkel IJ, Gerald WL, Rosenfield NS *et al*. Outcome of patients with a history of bilateral retinoblastoma treated for a second malignancy: the Memorial Sloan-Kettering experience. *Med Pediatr Oncol* 1998; **30**: 515–19.

75. Eng C, Li FP, Abramson DH *et al*. Mortality from second tumors among long term survivors of retinoblastoma. *J Natl Cancer Inst* 1993; **85**: 1121–8.

76. Kingston JE, Plowman PN, Hungerford JL. Ectopic intracranial retinoblastoma in childhood. *Br J Ophthalmol* 1985; **69**: 742–8.

77. Kivelä T. Trilateral retinoblastoma: a meta-analysis of hereditary retinoblastoma associated with primary ectopic intracranial retinoblastoma. *J Clin Oncol* 1999; **17**: 1829–37.

78. Blach LE, McCormick B, Abramson DH. External beam radiation therapy and retinoblastoma: long-term results in the comparison of two techniques. *Int J Radiat Oncol Biol Phys* 1996; **35**: 45–51.

79. Knudson AG. Mutation and cancer: statistical study of retinoblastoma. *Proc Natl Acad Sci USA* 1971; **68**: 820–3.

80. Friend SH, Bernards R, Rogelj S *et al*. A human DNA segment with properties of the gene that predisposes to retinoblastoma and osteosarcoma. *Nature* 1986; **22**: 643–6.

81. Blanquet V, Turleau C, Gross-Moran MS *et al*. Spectrum of germline mutations in the RB1 gene: a study of 232 patients with hereditary and non-hereditary retinoblastoma. *Hum Mol Genet* 1995; **4**: 383–8.

82. Cavanee WK, Murphree AL, Shull MM *et al.* Prediction of familial predisposition to retinoblastoma. *N Engl J Med* 1986; **314**: 1201–7.

83. Harbour JW. Overview of RB gene mutations in patients with retinoblastoma. Implications for clinical genetic screening. *Ophthalmology* 1998; **105**: 1442–7.

84. Lohman DR, Brandt B, Höpping W *et al.* The spectrum of RB1 germ line mutations in hereditary retinoblastoma. *Am J Hum Genet* 1996; **58**: 940–9.

85. Lohmann DR. RB1 gene mutations in retinoblastoma. *Hum Mutat* 1999; **14**: 283–8.

86. Munier FL, Thonney F, Girardet A *et al.* Evidence of somatic and germinal mosaicism in pseudo-low-penetrant hereditary retinoblastoma, by constitutional and single-sperm mutation analysis. *Am J Hum Genet* 1998; **63**: 1903–8.

87. Sippel KC, Fraioli RE, Smith GD *et al.* Frequency of somatic and germ-line mosaicism in retinoblastoma: implications for genetic counseling. *Am J Hum Genet* 1998; **62**: 610–19.

88. Otterson GA, Modi S, Nguyen K *et al.* Temperature-sensitive RB mutations linked to incomplete penetrance of familial retinoblastoma in 12 families. *Am J Hum Genet* 1999; **65**: 1040–6.

89. Baud O, Cormier-Daire V, Turleau C *et al.* Dysmorphic phenotype and neurological impairment in 22 retinoblastoma patients with constitutional cytogenetic 13-q deletion. *Clin Genet* 1999; **55**: 478–82.

90. Pratt CB, Raimondi SC, Kaste SC *et al.* Outcome for patients with constitutional 13q chromosomal abnormalities and retinoblastoma. *Pediatr Hematol Oncol* 1994; **11**: 541–7.

91. Hagstrom SA, Dryja TP. Mitotic recombination map of 13cen-13q14 derived from an investigation of loss of heterozygosity in retinoblastoma. *Proc Natl Acad Sci USA* 1999; **96**: 2952–7.

92. Lohmann DR, Gerick M, Brandt B *et al.* Constitutional RB1-gene mutations in patients with isolated unilateral retinoblastoma. *Am J Hum Genet* 1997; **61**: 282–94.

93. Lohmann DR, Horsthemke B. No association between the presence of a constitutional RB1 gene mutation and age in 68 patients with isolated unilateral retinoblastoma. *Eur J Cancer* 1999; **35**: 1035–6.

94. Bremner R, Chan Du D, Connolly-Wilson MJ *et al.* Deletion of RB exons 24 and 25 causes low-penetrance retinoblastoma. *Am J Hum Genet* 1997; **61**: 556–70.

95. Canzano JC, Handa JT. Utility of pupillary dilation for detecting leukocoria in patients with retinoblastoma. *Pediatrics* 1999; **104**: e44.

17

Soft tissue sarcomas

MODESTO CARLI, GIOVANNI CECCHETTO, GUIDO SOTTI, RITA ALAGGIO & MICHAEL C. G. STEVENS

INTRODUCTION

Soft tissue sarcomas (STSs) are a heterogeneous group of neoplasms showing different lines of differentiation according to the putative tissues of origin. These mainly include contractile, connective and supportive tissues, vascular tissue, adipose tissue and, arguably, some derived from the neural crest. STSs constitute approximately 6.5 per cent of all the childhood cancers.

In the USA the annual incidence of STS has been estimated to be 10.0 per million white children under 15 years of age.[1] The figures are similar in Europe: data obtained from several cancer registries indicate that the incidence of STS ranges from 6.2 to 12.2 per million children.[2] The incidence of STSs is fairly constant among adolescents aged 15–19 years, although the relative frequencies of histological subtypes vary with age.[3] Rhabdomyosarcoma (RMS) is the most common STS in children and young adults under the age of 21, accounting for approximately half of all sarcomas in this age group. Fibrosarcoma, synovial sarcoma, neurogenic sarcoma, extraskeletal Ewing's sarcoma, haemangiosarcoma, haemangiopericytoma, alveolar soft part sarcoma and peripheral primitive neuroectodermal tumours (pPNETs) occur less frequently. For this reason, RMS has been the object of multi-institutional clinical trials organized on a national or multinational basis in both Europe and the USA, and the management of this tumour has become the model for managing practically all other types of STS in childhood.

AETIOLOGY AND GENETICS

The aetiology of childhood RMS is still unknown. Data derived from epidemiological studies indicate that genetic factors may play an important role in the aetiology of at least some childhood sarcomas.

An increased incidence of congenital anomalies, mostly involving the genitourinary and central nervous systems, has been associated with RMS. In particular, the incidence of genitourinary anomalies is comparable to that found in patients with Wilms' tumour.[4] RMS has also been associated with several congenital disorders, including neurofibromatosis,[5] Gorlin's naevoid basal cell carcinoma syndrome[6] and fetal alcohol syndrome.[7] Furthermore, STSs in children and young adults have been associated with an excess incidence of breast cancer in the mothers and other close relatives, as well as an excess of cancers (breast carcinoma, gliomas) in the siblings.[8,9,10] According to Birch et al.,[10] this pattern of cancers is consistent with the well known Li–Fraumeni cancer family syndrome. Among the 24 families originally studied by Li et al.,[11] bone and soft tissue sarcomas and breast cancer were the most frequent cancers, but brain tumours, leukaemias and adrenocortical carcinomas had also occurred to excess in those below the age of 45 years.

Birch et al.[10] analysed 754 first-degree relatives of a population-based series of 177 children with STS. They were able to identify the following factors in the index children associated with high cancer risk in relatives:

- age at diagnosis <24 months
- histological type such as embryonal RMS or other unspecified STS
- male sex.

Such findings have important implications in the identification of a group of patients at high cancer risk who may benefit from genetic counselling and screening.

Developments in molecular genetic and biological methods in the past few years have made possible the identification of characteristic chromosomal abnormalities in several varieties of malignant STS.

In RMS, two characteristic reciprocal chromosomal translocations, either t(2;13)(q35;q14) or t(1;13) (p36;q14), are found in the majority of tumours with the alveolar subtype.[12] The more frequent t(2;13)(q35;q14) involves the *PAX3* gene on chromosome 2 and the *FKHR* gene on chromosome 13, while the t(1;13)(p36;q14) translocation involves the *PAX7* gene on chromosome 1 and the *FKHR* gene.

PAX-FKHR chimeric mRNA can be detected by reverse-transcriptase polymerase chain reaction (RT-PCR) even when these are translocations not detected by standard cytogenetic techniques. This represents a useful tool for diagnosis as well as providing a method to ascertain the presence of minimal residual disease (MRD).

Among RMSs identified as alveolar by histological classification, RT-PCR will detect t(2;13)(q35;q14) (*PAX3-FKHR*) fusion product in 50–70 per cent of cases and t(1;13)(p36;q14) (*PAX7-FKHR*) in 10–20 per cent of cases. No fusion product is identified in 10–30 per cent of cases but there is evidence that the two translocations occur in different subsets of patients and that those with t(1;13) may have a better outcome.[13] The t(2;13) and t(1;13) translocations have not been associated with any other tumour and appear to be specific markers for alveolar RMS (ARMS).

No karyotype abnormalities have so far been identified in the more common embryonal histological subtype. However, loss of constitutional heterozygosity at the 11p15 locus has been detected in embryonal RMS (ERMS)[14] and this genotype change, which seems to distinguish between the embryonal and alveolar subtypes, suggests that a gene, or genes, on 11p may be involved in malignant transformation. It is worth noting that partial loss of chromosome 11 involves the *IGF-II* gene, the product of which has been shown to stimulate the growth of RMS cells *in vitro*.[15]

Other specific cytogenetic abnormalities in STS include the translocations t(11;22)(q24;q12) or t(21;22)(q22;q12) which are present in 90–95 and 5–10 per cent, respectively, of Ewing's sarcomas and pPNETs.[16,17] These translocations involve the *EWS* gene (22q12) and partner genes, most often *FLI1* (11q24) or *ERG* (21q12). It is possible to identify the chimeric message derived from the reciprocal translocations by RT-PCR.[18] This is used for the primary diagnosis of Ewing's sarcoma and pPNET and for the detection of metastatic or residual disease. More than 10 different transcripts have been identified so far. Patients with tumour expressing a type 1 *EWS-FLI1* transcript appear to have a better prognosis.[19,20] Less frequently additional genetic changes have been described, including gains of chromosome 8 and a non-reciprocal translocation der(16)t(1;16)(q11;q11).[21] Other cytogenetic findings include the translocation (X;18)(p11.2;q11.2) in synovial sarcoma,[22] the recurrent translocation t(11;22)(p13;q12) associated with desmoplastic small round-cell tumour,[23] and the recurrent reciprocal translocation t(12;16) (q13;p11) in myxoid liposarcomas.[24] A novel t(12;15) (p13;q25) translocation was recently identified in infantile fibrosarcoma but it has not been found in either adult-type fibrosarcoma or infantile fibromatosis.[25] Other abnormalities associated with congenital infantile fibrosarcomas include gains of chromosomes 8, 11, 17 and 20.[26]

RHABDOMYOSARCOMA

Rhabdomyosarcoma is a highly malignant tumour and is thought to arise from primitive mesenchymal cells committed to develop into striated muscles. It can be found virtually anywhere in the body, including those sites where striated muscles are not normally found.

RMS has an annual incidence of 5.3 per million Caucasians under the age of 15. Of these, 70 per cent of cases occur before the age of 10 years. It shows two peaks of incidence, the first and most important being in children aged 2–5 years, and the second being during adolescence. A slight male predominance (1.4–1.7:1) is generally reported.

Classification and histological subtypes

Since the first report,[27] four types of RMS have been described on the basis of their cytoarchitectural features.

- embryonal
- botryoid
- alveolar
- pleomorphic.

Initially no prognostic distinctions were made between these different histotypes, but with the introduction of multimodality therapy, it was found that some RMSs responded better to treatment than others.[28] Several classifications were proposed for RMS in an attempt to correlate the morphological appearance of the tumour with the prognosis. All these schemes claimed a good prognostic significance and an International Study Committee was formed to look at the different classifications with a view

Box 17.1 *International classification for childhood rhabdomyosarcoma (RMS) (Newton et al.[30])*

> 1) Superior prognosis
>   a) Botryoid RMS
>   b) Spindle cell RMS
> 2) Intermediate prognosis
>   a) Embryonal RMS
> 3) Poor prognosis
>   a) Alveolar RMS

to working out a standardized scheme.[29] A new prognostically significant classification was published in 1995 whereby RMS can be divided into three main classes (Box 17.1). This classification system does not include the pleomorphic category, as this is very rarely observed in children.[30]

SUPERIOR PROGNOSIS

This category consists of two special variants: botryoid RMS and spindle cell or leiomyomatous RMS.

Botryoid RMS

This is observed in hollow organs, such as the vagina, nasal sinuses and bladder. Histologically, this variant is defined by the presence of a discrete submucosal hypercellular zone called the 'cambium layer' and an abundant oedematous myxoid stroma, occasionally mimicking a myxoma.

Spindle cell RMS

This is almost exclusively composed of short or long fascicles of eosinophilic spindle cells, sometimes intersecting at right angles, and the appearances may be confused with leiomyosarcoma, although scattered cytoplasmic cross-striations can be detected in the majority of cases.[31,32] An analysis of 21 cases from the German-Italian Soft Tissue Study showed that this variant occurred chiefly at paratesticular sites (12 cases) and head and neck sites (five cases) and with clear male predominance. Sufficient follow-up information was available in 17 cases, of whom 15 patients were alive and well 24–89 months after diagnosis. Based on these findings, this tumour seems to represent a very well differentiated variant of RMS, characterized by a low malignant potential and an excellent prognosis.

INTERMEDIATE PROGNOSIS

Embryonal RMS is characterized by a loose myxoid stroma and a proliferation of undifferentiated stellate mesenchymal cells that tend to differentiate into muscle cells. A wide spectrum of cellular differentiation is consequently observed. The cells have round or oval eccentric hyperchromatic nuclei with uniformly distributed chromatin and small or absent nucleoli. The eosinophilic cytoplasm at times shows typical cross-striations (strap cell) or has the characteristic angular irregular shape. Intermediate-sized cells with eccentric nuclei and elongated eosinophilic 'comma'-shaped cytoplasm (tadpole cells), as well as occasional large polygonal cells, are usually scattered in the stroma. Pleomorphic cells are occasionally observed in classic ERMS. Although worrisome, these cells show the same nuclear characteristics described above, and their presence does not affect the final prognosis.

POOR PROGNOSIS

This category consists of ARMS and solid variants. Microscopically, classical ARMS is characterized by the presence of alveolar spaces, usually lined with a single row of small or intermediate-sized cells with dark hyperchromatic nuclei, evident nucleolus and eosinophilic cytoplasm. Multinucleated giant cells are commonly observed.

The term mixed-type RMS was advanced for cases in which areas of embryonal or pleomorphic RMSs were present within the alveolar tumour.[33] Subsequently, it was proposed that only tumours consisting of 70 per cent alveolar spaces should be classified as ARMS,[34] but in the proposed new international classification, those RMSs in which even a single alveolar space is present are to be classified as ARMS. In fact, no difference has been found in biological behaviour between tumours with 70 per cent of alveolar spaces and those with only a small percentage. At the periphery of ARMS, solid areas of closely packed round cells may be present, as originally observed by Riopelle and Theriault.[35] More recently, Tsokos et al.[36] proposed that tumours consisting almost entirely of these solid areas should be considered to be a solid variant of ARMS. Microscopically, this variant presents a compact proliferation of round cells with hyperchromatic nuclei, evident nucleolus and scarce cytoplasm; any factors indicating a rhabdomyoblastic differentiation are rare or absent. Cross-striations are invariably absent, whereas atypical mitoses as well as single cell necrosis and nuclear pyknosis are frequently observed. No stroma is interspersed between the tumour cells, and a vague alveolar pattern is occasionally present. Cytologically, the cells are identical to those lining the alveolar spaces and show the same degree of cellular pleomorphism present in classical ARMS. The solid areas occasionally consist of sheets of small round monomorphous cells with the typical nuclear features already described. This variety, named monomorphous RMS by Palmer and Foulkes,[37] must be considered within the spectrum of morphological variations of the solid variant of RMS, and shows a very aggressive clinical course.

Primary sites (Figures 17.1 and 17.2)

Rhabdomyosarcoma may arise anywhere in the body. In order to reduce the differences of categorization of primary sites between different institutional and cooperative cancer clinical trial groups, a common classification of primary sites was adopted by European and US clinical investigators. The international definition of anatomical sites, adopted since 1986 in the workshop organized by the International Society of Pediatric Oncology (SIOP), is as follows:

- orbit
- parameningeal (PM) head-neck
- head-neck non-PM
- genitourinary tract
  - bladder and prostate (BP)
  - vagina, vulva, uterus, paratesticular (non-BP)
- extremities
- others.

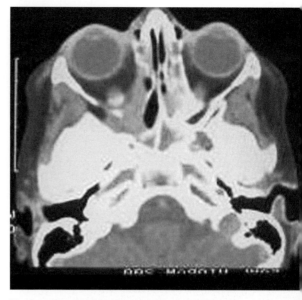

Figure 17.1 *CT scan of orbital rhabdomyosarcoma.*

The latter group includes the wall of the trunk and intrathoracic, intra-abdominal, pelvic, perineal and paravertebral regions. Due to the fact that in some cases the determination of origin is uncertain, it is usual to describe the tumour by its assumed origin and its possible secondary extension according to the topographical coding system described by Donaldson *et al.*[38]

The relative frequency of occurrence at primary sites based on 907 RMS cases enrolled in four European studies (SIOP 1984–88; CWS 81 and 86; ICG RMS 79–86) is given in Table 17.1.

Pattern of spread

Rhabdomyosarcoma is a very aggressive tumour that tends to infiltrate along fascial planes and into surrounding tissue as well as disseminating along both lymphatic and haematogenous routes. About 20 per cent of patients present with distant metastatic disease at diagnosis, the most common sites of metastases being lung, lymph nodes, bone and bone marrow (Figure 17.3). More rarely, metastases can occur in the liver, brain and breast.

The frequency of regional lymph node involvement is still not precisely defined due to the fact that lymph node sampling is not always routinely performed. Among 592 children with localized RMS enrolled in the first two Intergroup Rhabdomyosarcoma Studies (IRS), who had systematic regional lymph node sampling, 14 per cent had lymphatic spread at presentation. The incidence by primary site was 0 per cent for orbital, 8 per cent for non-orbital head and neck, 12 per cent for extremity, 24 per cent for genitourinary tract, 3 per cent for trunk, and 23 per cent for pelvis-retroperitoneum.[39] The high incidence of retroperitoneal lymph node involvement previously

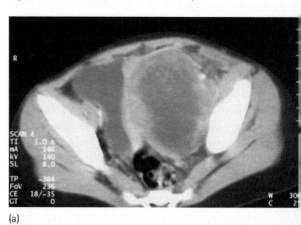

(a)

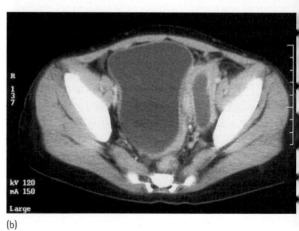

(b)

Figure 17.2 *Pelvic rhabdomyosarcoma on CT scan before (a) and after (b) chemotherapy.*

reported in the paratesticular RMS[40] was not subsequently confirmed.[39,41,42] It should be noted that these data may reflect a bias since some sites are much more easily and frequently sampled than others and pathological evaluation

Table 17.1 *Rhabdomyosarcoma: distribution of primary site[a]*

	n	Relative frequency (%)
Orbit	95	10.5
Parameningeal head-neck	190	21
Head-neck non-parameningeal	83	9.5
Genitourinary	211	23
Bladder and prostate (BP)	89	10
Non-BP	122	13
Extremity	124	14
Others	204	22

[a] Data based on 907 cases enrolled in the following studies: International Society of Pediatric Oncology (SIOP) MMT-84; German Soft Tissue Sarcoma Study CWS-81 and CWS-86; Italian Rhabdomyosarcoma Study RMS-79.

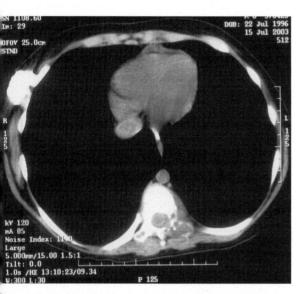

Figure 17.3 *Spinal bone metastasis presenting with back pain.*

is, in most instances, limited to the confirmation of clinically suspected lymph nodes. Thus the figure reported here is only indicative of real differences in the incidence of lymphatic spread within these broad anatomical categories.

Clinically involved lymph nodes documented by physical and imaging investigations were found in 10 and 13 per cent of cases with localized RMS enrolled in the SIOP MMT 89 and the ICS RMS-88, respectively. These data indicate that, when lymph nodes are clinically positive, the clinical and pathological findings correlate quite closely with each other. The results of the histological examination of clinically negative lymph nodes remain to be investigated.

Clinical manifestation and staging systems

The initial signs and symptoms depend on the site of origin and on the extension of the tumour to contiguous organs

Box 17.2 *Presenting signs and symptoms by primary site*

- Head-neck – asymptomatic mass
- Orbit – proptosis, chemosis, ocular paralysis, eyelid mass
- Nasopharynx – airway obstruction, nasal voice, epistaxis, local pain, dysphagia, cranial nerve palsies
- Paranasal sinuses – swelling, pain, sinusitis, obstruction, epistaxis, cranial nerve curve palsies
- Neck – hoarseness, dysphagia
- Middle ear – polypoid mass, chronic otitis media, haemorrhagic discharge, cranial nerve palsies
- Larynx – hoarseness, irritating cough
- Genitourinary tract – haematuria, urinary retention, polypoid vaginal extrusion of mucosanguineous tissue, vulval nodule or painless scrotal mass
- Trunk – asymptomatic mass (usually)
- Retroperitoneum – painless mass, ascites, gastrointestinal or urinary tract obstruction
- Extremity – painless mass (may be associated with bruising)

or tissues or the presence of metastases. The most important signs and symptoms are summarized in Box 17.2.

Several peculiarities should be noted: tumours arising in parameningeal sites (nasopharynx, nasal cavity, paranasal sinuses, pterygoid-infratemporal fossae and middle ear mastoid) are associated with a high risk of spreading to the meninges by contiguous bony destruction. Thus, they may present with isolated or multiple cranial nerve palsies, sometimes with meningeal or increased intracranial pressure symptoms. This subtle presentation is a reason for these patients to have advanced stage at diagnosis.

Bladder tumours are most frequently observed in young boys; they originate from the neck or trigone and tend to proliferate intraluminally and to remain localized. In contrast, prostatic lesions are more aggressive and infiltrate the bladder neck and urethra and tend to metastasize earlier, mostly to the lungs. However, it is often difficult to define clinically whether a tumour is arising primarily in the bladder or in the prostate, unless the lesion is very small.

Extremity lesions have a high propensity for involving the regional lymph nodes as well as for early dissemination to distant lymph nodes, lung, bone marrow, bone and central nervous system (CNS).

Tumours of the trunk generally present as asymptomatic masses, but dyspnoea and thoracic pain associated with pleural effusion may also be present, depending on the extension of the disease. Particular attention should be paid to the neurological signs, due to the possibility of involvement of the thoracolumbar spine.

Rare primary sites for RMS include the biliary tract. These lesions may present a clinical picture of asymptomatic jaundice or even as symptoms of acute cholecystitis.

Unusual forms of the disease are represented by clinical symptoms characteristic of leukaemic patients, e.g. fever, bone pain, anaemia and pancytopenia. The primary tumour is often so small that it may at first go unnoticed. The differential diagnosis often requires special immunocytochemistry stains to reveal the nature of the non-haemopoietic bone marrow infiltrate. In these cases, cytogenetic studies showing the translocation t(2:13) (q37;q14) may substantiate the diagnosis of ARMS.[43]

Staging investigations

A precise definition of locoregional extension of disease and a detailed investigation of the potential metastatic sites are mandatory before planning therapy. For histological diagnosis, an incisional biopsy is necessary. This approach generally gives sufficient material to avoid any difficulty in histopathological interpretation and allows the clinician to perform a wide variety of ancillary techniques, such as cytogenetic or molecular biological studies, that could be helpful in differential diagnosis.

Pretreatment evaluation may vary depending on the anatomical sites affected and clinical presentation, but it should include the following for all patients:

- Complete physical examination, with a precise definition of tumour site and size, and a careful regional lymph nodes assessment
- Laboratory studies – complete blood count, liver and renal function tests, serum electrolytes plus calcium, phosphorus and magnesium, uric acid and coagulation parameters
- Magnetic resonance imaging (MRI) and/or computed tomography (CT) scan of the primary lesion, with three-dimensional measurement if possible. Ultrasonography is also important, particularly in the assessment of pelvic tumours; it avoids radiation and may be easily repeated in evaluating tumour volume reduction
- Bone marrow aspiration plus two trephine biopsies for patients with evidence of node or distant metastases and all those with alveolar histology
- Technetium bone scan, with plain X-rays of abnormal sites
- Chest X-ray and CT scan
- Biopsy of any clinically suspicious regional lymph nodes.

Other complementary investigations appropriate to the primary site include the following:

- Parameningeal head and neck – brain MRI and/or CT scan and cerebrospinal fluid (CSF) cytology

- Genitourinary – CT scan or MRI with or without ultrasound of retroperitoneum; cystourethroscopy with biopsy for bladder prostate lesions
- Extremity – CT scan with or without ultrasound of regional lymph nodes and retroperitoneum for lower extremity; brain CT scan should be considered as brain metastases seem more commonly associated with extremity primaries; regional lymph node biopsy is highly recommended
- Trunk – spinal MRI or myelography if neurological signs of medullary compression are present
- Intra-abdominal – CT scan with or without ultrasound of the liver.

In defining soft tissue tumours and intracranial extension, MRI appears to be superior to the CT scan. In addition, MRI has the ability to define vascular involvement without contrast enhancement as well as the ability to perform sagittal and coronal scans. Bone destruction, however, is more accurately defined on CT scan. Ultrasonography is also a useful, easily repeated diagnostic technique for measuring therapy response. In summary, these examinations are often complementary and it is recommended that the same imaging procedure for response evaluation be used throughout management.

Staging systems

The primary purpose of staging is to classify tumours into categories from which treatment can be planned and prognosis predicted. It is also an essential way of defining similar groups of patients so that outcome can be compared between different approaches to treatment. The characteristics of the disease selected for use within a staging system must not only take into account the extent of the disease at first presentation but should also reflect the impact of any initial surgery and the amount of residual disease before starting chemotherapy, i.e. a consideration of both pre- and post-surgical influences on potential outcome.

Historically, two main approaches have been used in the staging of rhabdomyosarcoma, both of which have been applied more generally to all STSs in childhood: the post-surgical clinical grouping system developed by the North American Intergroup Rhabdomyosarcoma Study Group (IRSG – now the Soft Tissue Sarcoma Committee of the Children's Oncology Group) and a TNM system used by the SIOP MMT committee (Boxes 17.3–17.5). There have been attempts by the major collaborative treatment groups to compare and standardize the systems used in clinical trials,[44] but until recently both have been in use.

Prior to the availability of effective multiagent chemotherapy, there was a much greater emphasis on

Box 17.3 *Intergroup Rhabdomyosarcoma Studies (IRS) clinical grouping system*

Group I

Localized disease, completely resected, confined to organ or muscle of origin, infiltration outside organ or muscle of origin. Regional nodes not involved

Group II

Compromised or regional resection of three types:

- Grossly resected tumours with microscopic residual, no evidence of regional lymph node involvement
- Regional disease, completely resected, in which nodes may be involved, and/or extension of tumour into an adjacent organ but with no microscopic residual
- Regional disease with involved nodes, grossly resected, but with evidence of microscopic residual

Group III

Incomplete resection or biopsy only with gross (macroscopic) residual disease

Group IV

Distant metastases present at diagnosis

Box 17.4 *International Society of Paediatric Oncology (SIOP) presurgical clinical staging – TNM characteristics*

Stage I	T1a, T1b	N0, NX	M0
Stage II	T2a, T2b	N0, NX	M0
Stage III	Any T	N1	M0
Stage IV	Any T	Any N	M1

T = Primary tumour

T0 No evidence of primary tumour

T1 Tumour confined to the organ or tissue of origin

T1a Tumour 5 cm or less in its greatest dimension

T1b Tumour more than 5 cm in its greatest dimension

T2 Tumours involving one or more contiguous organs or tissues or with adjacent malignant effusion, or multiple tumours in the same organ

T2a Tumour 5 cm or less in its greatest dimension

T2b Tumour more than 5 cm in its greatest dimension

N = Regional lymph nodes

N0 No evidence of regional lymph node involvement

N1 Evidence of regional lymph node involvement

NX Lymph node status uncertain

M 5 Distant metastases

M0 No evidence of distant metastases

M1 Evidence of distant metastases

radical primary surgery, but the value of chemotherapy and the possibility of delaying surgery (when feasible) until later in the course of treatment have reduced the number of patients in which primary tumour resection is attempted. Now the great majority of patients (approximately 75 per cent) have macroscopic residual disease at the primary site (IRS Group III or post-surgical pT3bc in the SIOP TNM staging system) at the start of chemotherapy, whether or not they also have node or distant metastases. It has become necessary, therefore, to identify ways to subdivide this large group of patients so as to provide better discrimination between subgroups with different prognoses. Apart from the adverse impact of regional node and distant metastatic disease, one of the most important and consistent additional prognostic factors is the site of the primary tumour.[45] Neither of the previous systems considered this, but in 1997 IRSG introduced a new staging system which integrates primary site with TNM stage[46] (Table 17.2). The IRS-IV study treatment stratification has been based on a system of risk categories utilizing both IRS stage and IRS group. Plans for a new European collaborative study for RMS are likely to include a system for treatment stratification based on similar criteria.

Both European and North American data identify pathological subtype as an important prognostic

influence for RMS and use it as another determinant of treatment intensity.

Children with other forms of STS are usually staged according to the systems devised for RMS. There is no evidence that this is inappropriate, although for those tumours with limited chemosensitivity, the adequacy of surgical resection is of overriding prognostic importance.[47]

Prognostic factors

Several prognostic factors have so far been identified through different cooperative studies conducted in Europe and the USA.

Univariate analysis for a study performed on 951 children with non-metastatic RMS enrolled in four European and US cooperative studies[45] identified the following variables as favourable prognostic factors:

- tumour invasiveness T1
- tumour size ≤ 5 cm

Box 17.5 *International Society of Paediatric Oncology (SIOP) post-surgical clinicopathological (pTNM) classification*

---

pT = Primary tumour

pT0 No evidence of tumour found on histological examination of specimen

pT1 Tumour limited to organ or tissue of origin
Excision complete and margins histologically free

pT2 Tumour with invasion beyond the organ or tissue of origin
Excision complete and margins histologically free

pT3 Tumour with or without invasion beyond the organ or tissue of origin
Excision incomplete

    pT3a Evidence of microscopic residual tumour

    pT3b Evidence of macroscopic residual tumour or biopsy only

    pT3c Adjacent malignant effusion regardless of the size

pN = Regional lymph nodes

pN0 No evidence of tumour found on histological examination of regional lymph nodes

pN1 Evidence of invasion of regional lymph nodes

    pN1a Evidence of invasion of regional lymph nodes
Involved nodes considered to be completely resected

    pN1b Evidence of invasion of regional lymph nodes
Involved nodes considered to be incompletely resected

- negative regional lymph nodes
- primary site in orbit and genitourinary (GU) non-bladder prostate (BP) sites.

Multivariate Cox regression analysis of the pooled data identified tumour invasiveness, primary site and the interaction between tumour invasiveness and primary site as significant independently predictive factors for survival, while lymph node involvement was no longer predictive. In particular, the prognosis of orbital tumours was consistently favourable, whereas the prognosis of 'other sites' was consistently unfavourable regardless of T status.

In addition, T status appeared to determine the relative risk of treatment failure for primary sites in the GU, head and neck, parameningeal and extremity sites. The risk was low for T1 tumour in GU non-BP, head and neck, and GU-BP, and high for patients with T2 tumours in extremity and parameningeal primary sites. In this study, tumour size was not considered for the multivariate Cox regression analysis since it was not available for all centres. Tumour size was, however, confirmed as a strong factor in predicting survival[48,49] and is utilized in defining risk group in the IRS-V and in the new European collaborative RMS studies.

All studies to date have also demonstrated the crucial role of disease extent, as defined by the post-surgical clinical groups or the pre-surgical TNM system, in predicting survival: survival decreases from approximately 80 per cent in stage I patients to approximately 20 per cent in stage IV patients.[48–52]

Histological type is now also recognized as an important variable. Practically all reports indicate that patients with ARMS fare worse than those with the embryonal subtype.[30,49,50,53–56] This finding was not confirmed in the IRS-III study, where the more intensive therapy used for groups I and II ARMS may have reduced the adverse

Table 17.2 *North American Intergroup Rhabdomyosarcoma Study Group pretreatment staging system*

Stage	Site	T stage	Size	Node	Metastases
1	Orbit Non-parameningeal head and neck GU, non-bladder/prostate	T1 or T2	a or b	N0 or N1	M0
2	Bladder/prostate Limb Parameningeal Other (trunk, retroperitoneum)	T1 or T2	a	N0 or NX	M0
3	Bladder/prostate Limb	T1 or T2	a	N1	M0
	Parameningeal Other (trunk, retroperitoneum)		b	N0 or N1	
4	All	T1 or T2	a or b	N0 or N1	M1

GU, genitourinary.

impact of the alveolar subtype on the clinical outcome (5-year survival rate of 80 per cent).[51]

The most recent studies demonstrated that age at diagnosis is also an important predictor of survival with the best outcome in patients aged 1–9 years.[55,56]

Response to treatment is another important variable and this must be taken into account. Speed of response to chemotherapy has only been evaluated in a German Co-operative Soft Tissue Sarcoma Study (CWS), which found a strong correlation between the degree of tumour reduction in response to induction chemotherapy and the relapse-free survival in clinical group III patients.[57]

Biological factors may emerge that affect prognosis. The prognostic value of DNA ploidy in RMS is still a matter of controversy. Several studies have shown that DNA ploidy and proliferative status (S-phase) are important prognostic indicators of tumour behaviour; non-hyperdiploidy (DI < 1.1 and > 1.8) and a high rate of proliferative activity (S-phase > 14 per cent) were associated with a poor prognosis.[58–60] A recent study, however, showed that DNA ploidy was not an independent risk factor to predict outcome in such tumours despite the prognostic relationship in univariate analysis.[61]

TREATMENT MODALITIES FOR RMS

Multimodality therapy involving surgery, chemotherapy and radiotherapy is necessary in childhood RMS. The optimal timing and intensity of these three treatment modalities must be planned with regard to the primary tumour, site, extent of disease, histology and late effects of treatment.

Surgery

Surgical management of RMS is less aggressive in children than the approach usually taken towards STS in adults. Primary excision should be attempted only when the surgeon thinks it is possible to achieve a complete but non-mutilating procedure. Primary surgery should otherwise be limited to biopsy alone and the child should undergo a secondary excision, if this becomes feasible, after chemotherapy ± radiotherapy. Not only does the surgical choice depend on the location, size and extent of the tumour and on the study design, but it is also influenced by the surgeon's own judgment and experience.[61a,61b]

DIAGNOSTIC BIOPSY

The surgeon must carry out at least an initial diagnostic biopsy to identify the histological nature of the tumour. Needle cores or aspirates can establish malignancy,[62] but they are not always able to identify the subtypes of sarcoma, and in many cases they are not able to supply the tissue required for biological investigation and research. Surgical biopsies are usually incisional. If the surgeon has carried out an excisional biopsy that indicates a sarcoma, this cannot be considered to be a radical excision. It should instead be considered as an excision where there is likely to be at least microscopic residual tumour. Frozen sections prepared in the operating room can be sufficient for a generic diagnosis of sarcoma, making immediate definitive surgical excision possible in some cases.

PRIMARY EXCISION

The goal in these cases is the complete removal of the tumour by a non-mutilating procedure. Mutilating procedures are those that result in major functional or cosmetic impairment, such as orbital exenteration, head and neck dissection, total cystectomy or vaginectomy, pneumonectomy, permanent urinary or intestinal diversion, limb amputation or local excision with significant functional limb impairment. Non-mutilating operations are pulmonary lobectomy, partial intestinal or liver resection, nephrectomy, partial cystectomy, unilateral orchidectomy or ovariectomy, or finger amputation. Excision is complete (radical) when no microscopic residue of the tumour remains. It is generally believed that an initial excision that leaves macroscopic residual disease does not offer any advantage over a biopsy and should therefore be discouraged. Opinions differ as far as initial excision with microscopic residue is concerned. If the tumour can be grossly resected, many surgeons prefer to undertake primary excision even when it is unlikely that a specimen with free microscopic margins can be obtained. However, microscopic residual disease receives local irradiation, while the alternative of initial chemotherapy and secondary surgery would allow complete excision, making it possible to avoid radiotherapy at least in selected cases. For these reasons, we recommend primary excision only if there is a reasonable probability of removing the tumour without microscopic residues; otherwise biopsy is preferred.[63] Other authors have discussed the possibility to avoid radiotherapy in young patients with microscopic residue of ERMS.[64]

The local microscopic spread of many sarcomas goes far beyond the macroscopic limits of the tumour. To obtain a specimen with free microscopic margins, it is obviously necessary to resect the tumour together with some surrounding normal tissue (wide excision). There are, however, no rules on how much apparently normal tissue should be resected to guarantee the absence of microscopic residual tumour. An adequate histological study is therefore necessary in order to decide whether the excision has been radical. Apart from the microscopic examination of the specimen margins, it is important that the surgeon performs many biopsies around the margins of the excision, especially in doubtful areas. In this way the risk of an incorrect evaluation of adequate surgery is minimized. After an initial excision, if margins or biopsies are found to be positive for microscopic disease, or there are insufficient data on its completeness, but complete surgical excision is possible by a non-mutilating procedure, a wider local re-excision should be undertaken before any further therapy.[65] The aim of this primary re-excision is to avoid local irradiation; it is usually most effective in RMSs smaller than 5 cm and in limb, trunk and paratesticular sites.[66]

Adopting these criteria, initial surgery should be limited to biopsy for all parameningeal sarcomas, for the majority of orbital and other head and neck sarcomas, and for vulvovaginal and uterine tumours. In order to preserve the urinary bladder, endoscopic biopsy alone is the initial procedure of choice for bladder and prostate sarcomas. Primary excision is nearly always indicated in paratesticular sarcomas and consists of inguinal orchidectomy without trans-scrotal biopsy to avoid scrotal contamination. Complete non-mutilating excision should also be feasible in most limb and trunk sarcomas. The choice between excision and biopsy for pelvic, retroperitoneal and intrathoracic tumours requires great surgical experience; these tumours often cannot be completely resected and the operation is limited to biopsy.

An important aspect of all initial surgery relates to the indications and techniques for regional lymph node exploration. In limb sarcomas, regional lymph nodes should always be explored. Preoperative lymphoscintigraphy, using technetium-labelled sulphur colloid, has been proposed to address the correct lymph node sampling of paediatric limb sarcomas.[67] In other sites, it is common practice to explore lymph nodes at diagnosis if clinically or radiologically enlarged. In paratesticular sarcomas, surgical sampling of retroperitoneal lymph nodes is currently required in patients over 10 years of age by the IRS-V Study. In European protocols the evaluation is based on clinical (thin-cut CT scans) data, reserving the surgical assessment for patients with enlarged or suspected nodes.[68] Radical lymph node dissections are discouraged. However, when nodes are clearly metastatic and the primary tumour has been radically removed, the surgeon should also remove all enlarged nodes, if possible.

SECONDARY SURGERY

When the initial surgical approach has been a biopsy or an excision with macroscopic residue, the tumour mass may become surgically resectable after chemotherapy ± radiotherapy. The feasibility of secondary surgery depends on the tumour location and the clinical response to therapy. However, the response evaluated by physical and imaging data often differs from the pathological findings during surgical exploration. In IRS-III, 46 per cent of group III patients achieving a clinical partial remission (PR) were found to have no evidence of tumour, i.e. complete remission (CR) at surgical exploration, and another 28 per cent were converted to CR by excision of tumour residue. The most surprising fact was that 30 per cent of group III patients with no clinical response were shown to be in CR at surgical exploration, and another 43 per cent could be converted to CR (i.e. completely resected) by the surgeon.[69] These data underline the importance of secondary surgery in cases of residual mass, even when a poor clinical response to chemotherapy has been obtained. The value of histological verification of the complete clinical remission is uncertain. The European groups recommend avoiding surgical exploration when no tumour mass is detectable by imaging investigations, as this may make no difference to outcome. For example, in the SIOP MMT 84 study, the relapse rates in histologically and clinically proven complete remission were, respectively, 51 and 48 per cent.[70]

The timing of secondary surgery depends on the study design and the response to therapy. Surgical excision is carried out after chemotherapy or after chemotherapy plus radiotherapy. The goal of surgical exploration after chemotherapy alone is to avoid radiotherapy or to utilize reduced doses. Mutilating excisions at this time are discouraged. Generally, repeated surgical explorations may be planned, if feasible, in patients with persistent and residual disease, in order to achieve local control of the disease.

Tumours that are unresectable or incompletely resected after initial chemotherapy can be removed after further chemotherapy plus radiotherapy. At this point, the aim is the complete excision of residual disease, and any surgical procedure, mutilating or non-mutilating, is acceptable if technically feasible.

Radiotherapy

The role of radiotherapy in the management of childhood RMS is well known. High doses (60–65 Gy) of irradiation have been demonstrated to achieve local control in 90 per cent of orbital tumours[71] but with subsequent severe long-term morbidity. Several studies conducted in the USA and Europe since this study have answered important clinical and biological questions about the behaviour of RMS; the role of radiotherapy, too, has undergone change. In IRS-I, patients in group I (completely resected tumours) were randomized to receive post-operative chemotherapy with or without radiation. No significant advantage was apparent with the addition of radiotherapy to chemotherapy after surgery, and it was concluded that group I patients do not require irradiation. Subsequently, patients in group I with unfavourable histology and/or extremity primary tumour treated without irradiation in IRS-II, Italian RMS-79 and German CWS-81 studies showed an unexpectedly high local regional relapse rate. In the German CWS-81 study, patients with RMS of the extremities (stages I–III) who received radiotherapy had a significantly better disease-free survival (DFS) than patients who were not irradiated (60 vs. 12 per cent).[72]

More recently a report from the IRS-I to III has evaluated the outcome of 439 group I disease patients. The conclusion was that patients with group I ERMS have an excellent prognosis when treated with chemotherapy without irradiation. Patients with ARMS or undifferentiated sarcoma fare worse, but failure-free survival (FFS) and overall survival (OS) are substantially improved when radiotherapy is added to chemotherapy. The best results occurred in IRS-III, when radiotherapy was used in conjunction with intensified chemotherapy.[73] For this reason, radiation therapy is now widely used for patients with unfavourable histology, even if the tumour has been completely resected at primary surgery.

Patients with parameningeal tumours who were enrolled in the IRS-I protocol had a lower relapse-free survival (46 per cent) than those with other head and neck primaries. The reason for treatment failure in 35 per cent of these patients was tumour invasion into the CNS and almost all patients died as a consequence. The introduction of CNS-directed therapy with whole-brain irradiation in IRS-II increased the 5-year survival to 65 per cent, compared with 45 per cent in IRS-I. However, in IRS-I, 42 per cent of relapsed patients received a radiation dose to the tumour of below 4000 cGy, and in 58 per cent of cases the irradiated tumour volume was too small. These findings suggest that the delivered dose or the irradiated volume, or both, might have influenced the clinical course.[74] Currently, it is recommended that the target volume is limited to the site of the tumour plus a margin that includes the local meninges. This modification of the target volume resulted in local tumour control and survival comparable to that seen when whole-brain irradiation was used.[51] Several other factors may have contributed to this improved outcome. Early introduction of radiation therapy may contribute to better outcome. In IRS-I, radiation therapy for patients with group III disease was withheld until week 6 to allow for assessment of response to chemotherapy. With the high incidence of meningeal relapse and mortality, it was felt that delaying the start of radiation therapy might reduce the chance of tumour control. Subsequently, in RMS studies, it was recommended that radiation therapy should begin as soon as possible in all patients with high-risk meningeal features[75]. It is also important to acknowledge other reasons for better results following the first IRS study, such as the

availability of better diagnostic imaging studies and increasingly sophisticated irradiation techniques. Several studies have compared classic radiotherapy with modern techniques, such as stereotactic, intensity-modulated or proton beam radiation therapy, in order to optimize radiotherapy. Intensity-modulated proton or X-ray beams may succeed in reducing severe toxicity, while optimally covering the target volume in any site.[76]

The IRS-I study was unable to show an overall dose–response relationship but reported that doses of 40 Gy might be sufficient for treatment of sub-clinical disease in patients with completely resected tumours.[71] Subsequent studies demonstrated that radiation doses of 40 Gy delivered to adequate volumes allowed a local control of about 90 per cent in patients with microscopic post-surgical residual disease (group II). Moreover, the same low-dose irradiation permitted quite good local control in group III patients left with apparent microscopic disease after prior chemotherapy with or without delayed surgery. In a paper by Regine et al.,[77] a local control rate of 79 per cent was reported in highly selected IRS group III patients using a similar irradiation approach. All local failures occurred in patients with unfavourable site disease. These patients, together with those with gross residual disease after initial chemotherapy, showed an unacceptable local failure rate ranging from 30 to 70 per cent when doses of 40–50 Gy were administered. Despite a much better knowledge of risk factors and the improvement of multiagent chemotherapy, the lack of local control still represents the greatest problem in the treatment of RMS. Higher radiation doses are found to be associated with unacceptable late effects.

In an attempt to improve therapeutic effectiveness, maintaining a safety margin for late effects, the division of the daily dose into two or more small fractions (hyperfractionation) has been the subject of intense interest. Several clinical studies on head and neck tumours in adults have confirmed that a daily dose of 200–250 cGy can be fractionated into two smaller fractions of 100–125 cGy, increasing the tolerance dose for late-responding tissues and allowing an increase in total dose. Through a greater capacity for repair of sublethal injury, slow-responding tissues are spared more by reducing dose per fraction than are tumours. In addition, studies conducted in weanling rats indicated that significant sparing of radiation-induced epiphyseal growth arrest may be achieved using hyperfractionation, demonstrating that a proportion of the epiphyseal damage caused by ionizing radiation is recoverable during the 6-hour interval between the two fractions.[78] These data are very important since damage to growing bone is a major dose-limiting factor in the radiotherapeutic management of childhood cancer.

A small study of hyperfractionated radiation therapy (HFRT) at 1.1-Gy fractions twice daily to a total dose of 59.4–63 Gy was published by the St Jude Children's Research Hospital.[79] HFRT was tested in patients with gross residual disease after induction chemotherapy. In 14 selected patients, the 2-year local tumour control rate was 75 per cent. St Jude's previously reported experience, using conventional fractionated irradiation (50 Gy, 1.8 Gy daily fraction) in 50 patients with gross residual disease following chemotherapy, showed a local tumour control rate of only 40 per cent.[80] HFRT was associated with the expected enhancement of acute reactions, all resolving with conservative medical management. Long-term outcome and late effects continue to be monitored in these patients. A disadvantage of this strategy is the very high number of fractions and its overall length, which may decrease the treatment compliance.

In an attempt to improve local control, but keeping the late effects of therapy comparable to those achieved when 5040 cGy are given, a HFRT programme has been tested in 459 children enrolled in the IRS-IV. This was designed as a prospective randomized trial to test the value of HFRT versus conventionally fractionated radiation therapy (CFRT), with 5040 cGy in 28 daily fractions, in children with group III RMS. HFRT consisted of 110-cGy fractions given twice daily, at an interfractional interval of 6 hours, for a total tumour dose of 5940 cGy. Using the linear quadratic formula,[81] this would provide an increase of 10 per cent in tumour response and similar late effects as in a standard schedule of 5040 cGy in 28 fractions of 180 cGy. However, HFRT as given in this study did not improve local/regional control, FFS or overall survival. As a result, the standard irradiation technique for group III RMS continues to be CFRT.[82]

It is possible to look for an improvement in radiotherapeutic regimens by combining a decrease in dose per fraction with a reduction in the overall duration of treatment; this is called hyperfractionated accelerated radiotherapy (HART). An example of HART would be to give a fraction size greater than 125 cGy and less than 180 cGy twice daily. In this way, one might expect a decrease in late effects and an improvement in tumour control by hindering cell proliferation during treatment.[83] The limitation of HART is acute toxicity, which may necessitate a rest period during the treatment. In order to maintain the advantage of acceleration, these pauses must be as short as possible. A HART regimen was adopted in a pilot study conducted at the Memorial Sloan-Kettering Cancer Center from 1984 to 1986 on 12 children with gross residual disease. Radiotherapy was delivered at two daily fractions of 150 cGy to a total dose of 5400 cGy in two courses of 3000 and 2400 cGy, respectively, alternating with intensive chemotherapy.[84] Despite a rest period of 4 weeks between the two courses, losing some of the benefits expected from hyperfractionation, the study proved to be beneficial for local control (83 per cent at 21 years) and well tolerated.

The German CWS-86 study was the first to introduce a HART regimen given simultaneously with chemotherapy. Two daily fractions of 160 cGy were delivered to a total dose of 3200 cGy in patients who were good responders to chemotherapy (PR > 2/3). Poor responders received 5400 cGy in two courses of HART with a rest period of 9 days. The published data show that reduction in tumour volume after preoperative chemotherapy combined with tumour size in patients with residual disease can be used as a basis for risk-adapted radiotherapy and suggest that early HART given simultaneously with chemotherapy improved local tumour control in patients with a good response after preoperative chemotherapy. This study also suggested that a radiation dose of 32 Gy, when hyperfractionated and accelerated, given simultaneously with chemotherapy, is adequate for local tumour control in patients who show a good response to preoperative chemotherapy.[49] The same hyperfractionated accelerated schedule was utilized in the Italian cooperative study RMS-88. Here, 160 cGy were given twice daily, with concomitant chemotherapy beginning at week 11. Patients with microscopic residual disease after surgery or good responders to chemotherapy received a total dose of 4000 cGy in 2.5 weeks. Gross residual tumour received a boost of 1440 cGy (total dose 5440 cGy) after 10 days of rest accompanied by the following cycle of chemotherapy. Sixty-five (65 per cent) patients enrolled in the ICS-RMS 88 received 40 Gy of HART concomitantly with chemotherapy according to the protocol, 30 (35 per cent) had 54 Gy, and local control in the irradiated group was 77 per cent. Nine (13 per cent) patients had to stop the treatment because of acute toxicity. The most important factor influencing acute toxicity was the site of irradiation: all nine of these patients had abdominal or pelvic tumours.[85] The efficacy of HART was also explored in the MMT 89 SIOP study. No difference was apparent in terms of local control achieved with this strategy, although acute toxicity (cutaneous and mucosal) may have been greater than with conventional fractionation. In the Italian cooperative study RMS-96, 128 patients (57 per cent) have received radiotherapy as part of initial treatment: 24 had 32 Gy and 79 had 44.8 Gy, while 25 were boosted up to a total dose of 54 Gy. Preliminary data show an encouraging local control of 85 per cent (G. Sotti, unpublished data, 2002).

Apart from dose and fractionation, another important radiotherapeutic issue in the management of RMS is the treatment volume. Locoregional invasiveness is a relevant feature in STS. Even if a pseudocapsule gives an impression that it confines the tumour, it is by no means an effective barrier, and tumour extensions are typically identified far beyond it. In the IRS-I, no significant difference was found in terms of local control between patients who received irradiation of the entire muscle and those in whom it was limited to the tumour bed or residual tumour, with at least a 5 cm margin in all directions.[71] In most current protocols, the volume of irradiation is based on the dimension of the tumour before chemotherapy, including a margin of 2 cm. The possibility of targeting irradiation to the residual tumour volume after completion of chemotherapy is currently being explored by SIOP in some favourable circumstances. Moreover, SIOP and IRSG are both trying to avoid radiation therapy in special sites when chemotherapy achieves complete remission. For instance, in female genital tract tumours, SIOP uses chemotherapy irrespective of histology, reserving local therapy for patients who do not achieve complete remission or experience local relapse. The IRS group uses delayed radiotherapy in a very selected group of patients who do not achieve complete remission after chemotherapy or who do not have clear margins after resection.[86]

As a rule, 'prophylactic' irradiation of adjacent lymph nodes is not recommended. Regional nodes are only irradiated when they are clinically, radiologically or histologically involved. Usually the treatment volume should be gauged to encompass the level of the affected lymph node plus the adjacent one.

In certain instances, brachytherapy should be considered, particularly when the tumour is clinically accessible and limited in volume. This approach is recommended in the SIOP study in patients with incompletely resected tumour of the perineum, bladder, prostate and genital tract. Late complications of brachytherapy appear to be fewer than those caused by external radiotherapy. This is due to the small size of the target volume and also probably to a better tolerance by normal tissues of a continuous low-dose rate (LDR) irradiation compared with standard fractionated radiotherapy.[87] However, the radiation hazard associated with LDR brachytherapy is of particular concern when treating children since they require constant attention from parents and care-givers. More recently, high-dose rate (HDR) brachytherapy has been proposed in the treatment of childhood sarcomas.[88] Even if there is no consensus in the brachytherapy community regarding the total dose or total number of HDR fractions, it may be possible to substitute HDR brachytherapy for LDR brachytherapy without affecting tumour control. HDR brachytherapy provides the benefits of radiation protection, outpatient treatment, shortened overall treatment time, cost reduction, increased patient tolerance and improved nursing care.

HDR brachytherapy uses a computer-controlled machine with a high-intensity radioactive source to administer irradiation inside a shielded room through catheters previously placed in the patient. The treatment can be administered in minutes, obviating the need for prolonged sedation and immobilization. In the study by Nag et al.,[88] these catheters were left in place for 8–14 days until the treatment was concluded. The minimum peripheral dose was 36 Gy in 12 fractions, 3 Gy each fraction given twice daily, 6 hours apart, over a period of 8 days.

Nine of the 11 patients in first remission had no recurrences. Although the outcome appeared satisfactory, the authors conclude that HDR brachytherapy in young children should be restricted until long-term morbidity and efficacy results are obtained from pilot studies.[88a] A new Children's Cancer Group protocol for HDR (CCG-6005) will continue to investigate the toxicity and local control rate in a multi-institutional trial in children with STS.

Recently the American Brachytherapy Society[89] recommended that, due to the complexities involved, paediatric brachytherapy should be limited to centres that have extensive implant experience in children.

Chemotherapy

Childhood RMS is a chemosensitive tumour. In the 1960s and 1970s, phase II single-agent studies were used to identify the most effective agents. High tumour responses were reported mainly with vincristine (VCR) (59 per cent), cyclophosphamide (CYC) (54 per cent), adriamycin (ADR) (31 per cent), actinomycin D (AMD) (24 per cent) and DTIC (11 per cent).[90] Subsequently, other drugs have been included in the list of effective agents, e.g. cisplatin (CDDP),[91] etoposide (VP-16),[92] ifosfamide (IFO),[93] high-dose methotrexate[94,95] and melphalan, used in conventional doses[96] or, in association with bone marrow rescue, in high doses.[97] More recently, the camptothecin derivatives, topotecan and irinotecan, topoisomerase I inhibitors, have been identified as promising new agents.[98] In particular, the response rate of 46 per cent achieved in a phase II window trial of topotecan alone in previously untreated patients with metastatic RMS indicates that topotecan is very effective against RMS, particularly active in patients with alveolar histological subtype[99] (although response rates in conventional phase II evaluation of relapsed patients are relatively disappointing).[100] Finally, vinorelbine, a semisynthetic vinca alkaloid, has been described as having a favourable toxicity profile with evidence of activity in already heavily pretreated paediatric sarcomas. The 50 per cent response rate recently observed in patients with RMS (six cases of PR out of 12 RMS patients) seems very promising.[101]

The combination most commonly utilized so far has been the association of VCR, AMD, CYC and ADR in two- three- and four-drug combinations (Box 17.6).

In the early 1970s, large cooperative national and international study groups focusing on childhood RMS were started. The IRS has played a pivotal role in designing prospective randomized clinical trials. Patients were usually stratified according to the extent of the initial surgery. The first two studies[102,103] showed that a two-drug regimen with VCR and AMD (without local radiotherapy) was effective in achieving local tumour control in the majority of children with a group I (microscopically

Box 17.6 *Combination chemotherapy for RMS*

VA

VCR	1.5 mg/m^2 (max. 2 mg)/week × 4 weeks
AMD	1.5 mg/m^2 (max. 2 mg) weeks 1 and 4

or

VCR	1.5 mg/m^2/week × 6 weeks
AMD	0.015 mg/kg/day × 5 days

PulseVAC

VCR	1.5 mg/m^2(max. 2 mg)
AMD	0.015 mg/kg/day × 5 days
CYC	10 mg/kg/day × 3 days

or

VCR	1.5 mg/m^2 (max. 2 mg)
AMD	1.5 mg/m^2 (max. 2 mg)
CYC	250 mg/m^2/day × 5–7 days

Intensive pulse VAC (IRS-IV)

VCR	1.5 mg/m^2 (max. 2 mg)/week × 9 or × 6
AMD	0.015 mg/m^2 (max. 0.5 mg)/day × 5 days, q3 weeks × 3 or × 2
CYC	2.2 g/m^2, q3 weeks × 3 or × 2

VADRC

VCR	2 mg/m^2 (max. 2 mg)
ADR	30 mg/m^2/day × 2 days
CYC	10 mg/kg/day × 3 days

VACA

VCR	1.5 mg/m^2/week, weeks 1–4
ADR	30 mg/m^2 × 2, weeks 1 and 7
CYC	1200 mg/m^2, weeks 1, 4 and 7
AMD	0.05 mg/m^2/day × 3, week 4

ADR, adriamycin; AMD, actinomycin D; CYC, cyclophosphamide; VCR, vincristine.

Box 17.7 *Ifosfamide-containing regimens*

IVA (SIOP MMT-89)

IFO	3 g/m^2/day × 3 days
VCR	1.5 mg/m^2 (max. 2 mg)
AMD	1.5 mg/m^2 (max. 2 mg)

IVA (SIOP MMT-95)

IFO	3 g/m^2/day × 2 days
VCR	1.5 mg/m^2 (max. 2 mg)
AMD	1.5 mg/m^2 (max. 2 mg)

VAIA (ICS RMS-88)

IFO	2 g/m^2/day × 5 days, weeks 1, 4 and 7
AMD	1.5 mg/m^2 (max. 2 mg), weeks 1 and 7
VCR	1.5 mg/m^2 (max. 2 mg), weeks 1, 2, 3, 4 and 7
ADR	40 mg/m^2/day × 2, week 4

VAIA (CWS-86)

IFO	3 g/m^2/day × 2 days, weeks 1, 4 and 7
AMD	0.5 mg/m^2/day (max. 0.5 mg) × 3 days, weeks 1 and 7
VCR	1.5 mg/m^2 (max. 2 mg), weeks 1, 2, 3, 4 and 7
ADR	40 mg/m^2/day × 2, week 4

EVAIA (CWS-91)

IFO	2 g/m^2/day × 3 days, weeks 1, 4, 7 and 10
VP-16	150 mg/m^2/day × 3 days, weeks 1, 4, 7 and 10
ADR	20 mg/m^2/day × 3 days, weeks 1 and 7
AMD	0.5 mg/m^2/day × 3 days, weeks 4 and 10
VCR	1.5 mg/m^2/day × 1 day, weeks 1, 4, 7 and 10

CEVAIE

CARBO	500 mg/m^2, week 1
EPI	150 mg/m^2, week 1
IFO	3 g/m^2/day × 3 days, weeks 4 and 7
AMD	1.5 mg/m^2/day (max. 2 mg), week 4
VP-16	200 mg/m^2/day × 3, week 7
VCR	1.5 mg/m^2 (max. 2 mg), weeks 1, 2, 3, 4, 5, 7 and 8

ADR, adriamycin; AMD, actinomycin D; CARBO, carboplatin; EPI, epirubicin; IFO, ifosfamide; VCR, vincristine; VP-16, etoposide.

complete resection) non-ARMS. The same regimen, in association with local radiotherapy, was as effective in maintaining local tumour control in group II RMS as a three-drug regimen including CYC (VAC). The addition of ADR to pulse VAC (VADRC-VAC regimen) did not significantly improve survival for patients with group III or IV disease. The rate of complete clinical remission after 6–8 weeks of chemotherapy of VAC ± ADR in patients with measurable tumour was approximately 30 per cent.[102–105] The need to improve the tumour response fostered research for new active agents and for more effective drug combinations. Encouraging results with IFO-containing regimens (Box 17.7) were reported mainly in Europe in the late 1980s. The German CWS obtained a higher response rate in their CWS-86 protocol (CR + tumour reduction ≥ 2/3 = 71 per cent) than in the previous study (CWS-81, 55 per cent). This result

was attributed to substitution of IFO for CYC.[106] Otten et al.[107] reported the highest CR rate so far documented (59 per cent within 1 year) with an IVA regimen as the sole treatment in RMS patients in the SIOP-84 study. IFO in combination with VP-16 was employed by Miser et al.[108] in patients with recurrent sarcoma of soft tissue and bone. A very favourable response rate of 69 per cent was obtained for nine out of 13 patients with RMS. The combination IFO + doxorubicin was evaluated as a phase 'window' therapy in newly diagnosed metastatic rhabdomyosarcoma. The 63 per cent response rate (CR + PR at week 12) has identified this drug pair as highly active against both alveolar and embryonal subtypes of RMS.[109]

CDDP-based combination regimes, such as CDDP/VP-16[110] and CDDP/ADR,[111] have also been shown to be effective, with response rates of 33 and 40 per cent, respectively, in children with advanced RMS. The second-generation compounds carboplatin and epirubicin have also been shown to be effective in chemosensitive childhood STS. A combination of carboplatin and high-dose epirubicin has been utilized in newly diagnosed children with metastatic STS as front-line therapy in the European Intergroup Study MMT-4. With this combination, a 53 per cent response rate[112] has been achieved.

The newer agent topotecan was evaluated in combination with CYC in a phase II Pediatric Oncology Group (POG) study in heavily pretreated patients who had previously received CYC or IFO. Ten out of 15 patients with RMS achieved a good response (CR + PR), with substantial activity for both alveolar and embryonal RMS.[113] In contrast, topotecan alone showed no activity in 22 patients with relapsed RMS.[100] Topotecan is also utilized in association with VCR. In fact, topoisomerase I inhibitors have demonstrated enhanced activity when administered in combination with VCR or alkylating agents in the xenograft model.[98,114,115]

Intrathecal (IT) chemotherapy including methotrexate (MTX) or the combination of MTX + cytosine arabinoside (Ara-C) + hydrocortisone has been utilized in association with whole-brain irradiation to prevent the development of occult meningeal deposits in patients with parameningeal primary tumour and signs of extension to meningeal spaces such as erosion of the bones at the skull base, presence of cranial nerve palsy and intracranial extension of the tumour.[103] However, the role of IT chemotherapy in the marked improvement in survival observed in this group of patients is not clear and there has been some concern about cumulative toxicity in the presence of radiotherapy.[116]

Although great advances have been made in the treatment of RMS, progress is still needed, particularly for patients with locally advanced and metastatic disease. With this objective, more aggressive treatment must be utilized, with the goal of rapidly eliminating as many tumour cells as possible and preventing the development of drug resistance. Increased toxicity is likely to be expected, but the achievement of complete remission is of critical importance.

A recent observation pointed to the importance of dose intensity to achieve a maximal therapeutic effect.[117] This concept could have an impact on the treatment of RMS, and strategies for improving chemotherapy effectiveness in RMS must include:

- the incorporation of as many active agents as possible to try to overcome drug resistance[118]

- the use of chemotherapeutic regimens with higher dose intensity, which may result in a higher CR rate.

Based on these concepts, intensive chemotherapy is being increasingly utilized as an initial therapy with the aim of using less aggressive methods of local treatment. In all European studies, primary chemotherapy (IVA, or VAIA or CEVAIE) is given, unless complete non-mutilating excision of the primary tumour is considered feasible.

The major difference between the German, the Italian and the IRS studies in comparison to the SIOP trial is the timing of local therapy, which may include surgery and/or radiotherapy, according to the degree of tumour shrinkage after primary chemotherapy and tumour resectability. At present, within a common framework, two parallel trials are running in Europe, one by SIOP and the other by the combined Italian and German study groups. These two groups launched a randomized study for 'high risk' RMS, sharing a chemotherapy arm represented by the six-drug combination (CEVAIE) adopted in the European Intergroup Study (EIS) for stage IV STSs. This arm is compared with IVA in the SIOP study, while the comparison will be with VAIA in the combined Italian-German trial. The two studies differ in their timing of delivery of local therapy, which will be within the ninth week of therapy for the latter group and later, after week 17, for the former. In this way the possible prognostic impact of these two different strategies can be compared.

The treatment guidelines utilized by the Italian and German groups for localized RMS, extraosseous Ewing's sarcoma, pPNET, undifferentiated sarcoma and synovial sarcoma are shown in Figure 17.4. The intensity, the duration and the type of chemotherapy are stratified according to risk groups defined on the basis of histology, site and TNM status. An effort is currently being made to plan a new European collaborative study for STS since differences in treatment philosophy mostly related to local therapy between the European Groups have begun to converge and the treatment concepts are very similar.

The IRS-III study utilized a combination of two to seven drugs (VCR, ADM, CYC, ADR, CDDP, VP-16 and DTIC). Irradiation was delivered in all but group I favourable histology patients. Second- and third-look operations, to document tumour response and to excise residual tumour, were also recommended. Treatment duration (1–2 years) and intensity of chemotherapy were related to initial clinical group and histology. The results of this study showed that the addition of CDDP and VP-16 in the front-line therapy of selected patients did not appear to improve the complete response rate or FFS, while the role of ADR remains controversial.[51]

Intensive, multimodal therapy was also adopted by the IRS-IV protocol in a randomized three-arm study. The principal aim was to compare the intensive pulse VAC regimen with IVA (IFO is substituted for CYC) and

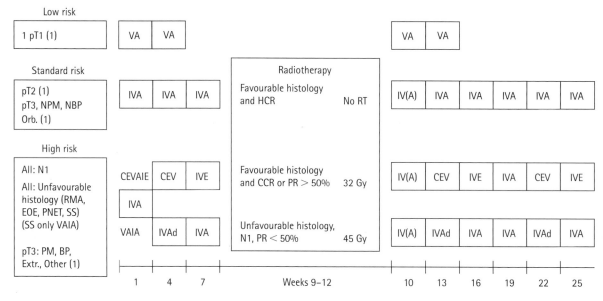

Low risk

| 1 pT1 (1) | | VA | VA | | | | VA | VA | | | | |

Standard risk

pT2 (1)
pT3, NPM, NBP
Orb. (1)

| IVA | IVA | IVA | | IV(A) | IVA | IVA | IVA | IVA | IVA |

Radiotherapy

Favourable histology and HCR	No RT
Favourable histology and CCR or PR > 50%	32 Gy
Unfavourable histology, N1, PR < 50%	45 Gy

High risk

All: N1
All: Unfavourable histology (RMA, EOE, PNET, SS)
(SS only VAIA)

pT3: PM, BP, Extr., Other (1)

CEVAIE	CEV	IVE		IV(A)	CEV	IVE	IVA	CEV	IVE
IVA			
VAIA	IVAd	IVA		IV(A)	IVAd	IVA	IVA	IVAd	IVA

Weeks: 1 4 7   Weeks 9–12   10 13 16 19 22 25

(1) Favourable (favourable histology: RME) and N0.

Figure 17.4 *Treatment overview ICS-CWS-96 for localized rhabdomyosarcoma (RMS), Ewing's sarcoma (EOE), peripheral primitive neuroectodermal tumour (pPNET) and synovial sarcoma (SS). A, actinomycin D; Ad, adriamycin; C, carboplatin; CCR, clinical complete remission; E, etoposide; HCR, histological complete remission; I, ifosfamide; PR, partial remission; RMA, alveolar rhabdomyosarcoma; RME, embryonal rhabdomyosarcoma; RT, radiation therapy; V, vincristine.*

VIE (IFO + VP-16 are substituted for AMD + CYC). In addition, CFRT was randomized against HFRT in patients with gross residual disease after initial surgery in an attempt to verify whether hyperfractionated radiotherapy improved local control rate. The major finding of this study, whose 3-year FFS was the same as that of IRS-III (about 76 per cent in both studies), was that patients with embryonal histology fared significantly better than similar patients treated in IRS-III (3-year FFS rates, 83 vs. 74 per cent). Much of the improvement, however, occurred in patients in groups I and II who, in comparison to those treated on IRS-III, received the additional alkylating agent. No differences in either FFS or OS were observed between the three chemotherapy treatment regimens in an analysis of patients with embryonal or with alveolar and undifferentiated RMS. Finally, the use of HFRT did not appear to offer any advantage over CFRT.[55]

The current IRS-V study allocates treatment according to the risk categories defined by tumour histology, group and stage. Three groups are identified – low, intermediate and high risk – which, according to the IRS-III and IV data, are expected to achieve 3-year FFS rates of 88, 55–76 per cent and <30 per cent, respectively.

Patients at 'intermediate risk', who account for about 55 per cent of the total, are those with group III ERMS at unfavourable sites (stages 2 and 3), group I–III ARMS at all sites (stages 1–3) and ERMS stage 4 patients aged < 10 years. For these patients, the protocol is testing the potential therapeutic value of intensive VAC (Box 17.6) alternating with VCR, topotecan and CYC compared with intensive VAC which, according to the results of IRS-IV, is considered the 'gold standard' therapy for these patients. Both groups receive CFRT.

Patients at 'low risk' are those with group I-III ERMS at favourable sites (stage 1) or group I–II ERMS at unfavourable sites (stages 2 and 3). These patients are divided into two subgroups: they receive chemotherapy with VA (Box 17.6) (subgroup A) or VAC (subgroup B) and CFRT to any residual tumour.

Patients at 'high risk' (stage 4 ARMS or stage 4 ERMS patients >10 years old) are being evaluated in an upfront window with irinotecan followed-up by VAC and CFRT.[119]

In all studies, second-line chemotherapeutic regimens together with radical surgery, if feasible, and/or radical wide field radiotherapy are considered for all patients who have tumour progression or stable residual disease after first-line chemotherapy. The optimum duration of adjuvant chemotherapy for patients who attain complete response is still unknown. The current tendency is to shorten treatment programmes utilizing intensive multiagent chemotherapeutic regimens to a duration of 6–12 months.

High-dose chemotherapy (HDCT) followed by haemopoietic stem cell rescue (HSCR) has been an attractive strategy for selected very high-risk patients, mostly those with metastatic or recurrent RMS. In particular, HDCT with HSCR has been investigated in patients with metastatic disease as a means of eliminating microresidual disease in patients in complete remission after intensive conventional chemotherapy. However, the results of the EIS MMT4-91, which evaluated the potential role of high-dose melphalan as consolidation therapy for newly diagnosed children with metastatic disease in first complete remission, showed that high-dose melphalan did not improve the overall survival of these patients.[120] Similar results have been obtained by other investigators who utilized more intensive myeloablative regimens such as rapid VAC and melphalan,[121] or a combination of melphalan, carboplatin and VP-16 (MEC regimen),[122,123] thiothepa, CYC and carboplatin,[124] or melphalan and VP-16.[125] The event-free survival at 2–3 years in such studies ranged from 19 to 44 per cent.

A new strategy, which utilizes repetitive courses of HDCT with HSRC earlier in the treatment, in an attempt to avoid drug resistance, is at present being evaluated in two studies, one conducted by the SIOP group, the other by the Italian group. These are still in progress and it is not yet clear if this novel approach could be of some benefit for metastatic patients.

Combined modality therapy for special sites

ORBIT

Chemotherapy [VA (Box 17.6) or IVA (Box 17.7)] in conjunction with radiotherapy is the preferred treatment in almost all cases. The surgical approach is usually limited to biopsy, and routine regional lymph node sampling is not justified. As tumours at this site have an excellent prognosis, major efforts are now being made to limit the late effects of treatment by trying to reduce the radiotherapy dose or even to avoid radiation altogether. The results of an International Workshop on orbital RMS suggest that a subset of patients can be cured without systemic local therapy, although the total burden of treatment (primary therapy and treatment for relapse) must be taken into account when assessing the implications for late effects.[126]

PARAMENINGEAL HEAD–NECK

Primary excision is never indicated here and in only a few cases does secondary excision become feasible. Radiotherapy should begin as soon as possible in all patients with a high risk of meningeal extension or by week 10 provided that chemotherapy is effective. Whole-brain irradiation is now limited to cases with intracranial tumour extension. In all other cases the radiotherapy field will include the skull base and the volume of the tumour with 2–3 cm margins. SIOP studies, MMT-84 and MMT-89, attempted to avoid radiotherapy in children under 3 years of age by evaluating prospects for local control with more intensive chemotherapeutic regimens. However, the incidence of local recurrence was high and few children with tumours at this site are ultimately cured without radiotherapy.[53] Intrathecal chemotherapy is no longer routinely required for parameningeal sarcoma with meningeal impingement.[119]

BLADDER–PROSTATE

All therapeutic efforts are directed towards avoiding cystectomy and to limiting pelvic radiotherapy. The tumour response to primary chemotherapy determines subsequent therapy. Patients who obtain a complete response with chemotherapy + conservative surgery can continue with chemotherapy alone, while a reduced dose of radiotherapy (32 Gy is delivered in the current Italian and German study) is suggested for those achieving complete clinical remission with chemotherapy alone. Conventional dose but limited field radiotherapy or brachytherapy should be given when there is micro- or macroresidual disease after initial chemotherapy and limited surgery. The timing of delivery of irradiation may vary depending on treatment policy. Second-line chemotherapy might be employed in poorly responding patients before proceeding to radical surgery (cystectomy).

PARATESTICULAR

Paratesticular tumours have a very favourable prognosis. Inguinal orchidectomy is the primary therapeutic approach. The value of retroperitoneal surgical lymph node sampling, as part of staging procedures, is still a matter of controversy. In contrast to earlier IRS group studies, European protocols reserve laparotomy for regional lymph node sampling only when imaging findings are doubtful. Less favourable results observed in boys > 10 years of age in the IRS-IV study, where this procedure was not required, prompted US investigators to reintroduce surgical sampling of retroperitoneal lymph nodes for such patients in the IRS-V study. The majority of patients with paratesticular tumours have favourable prognostic features (group I, pT1 ERMS) and have an excellent outcome with limited chemotherapy utilizing a regimen of VCR and AMD.[68,68a]

Treatment results

The use of a multimodal approach resulted in a dramatic improvement in the cure rate of childhood RMS; this has risen from less than 20 per cent in historical series[127] to 50–70 per cent in the more recent reports.[48,49,51,53,102,103] The major improvement has been observed in patients with localized tumours of embryonal histology (5-year OS, 70–85 per cent).[49,53,55,56] By contrast no improvement was noted for patients with metastatic RMS, whose 5-year OS remains disappointing at 20–30 per cent.[51,57,109,110] The OS rate according to the extent of disease for non-metastatic patients in four representative cooperative studies is shown in Table 17.3 (note that these data are reported separately for studies utilizing IRS group and TNM stage). Overall survival is strongly influenced by the primary site, as demonstrated by the results achieved in different series of patients (Table 17.4).

ARMS is consistently associated with poor prognosis, as indicated by the 5-year survival rate of 53 per cent, compared with 95 per cent for botryoid, 88 per cent for spindle cell, and 64 per cent for embryonal subtypes.[30] Even with more modern and intensive chemotherapy no significant overall improvement has occurred for children with ARMS.[55] The patients who have benefited most from an intensified treatment programme are those with extremity and parameningeal primary sites and those with group I or II alveolar tumours.[51,103]

A conservative approach in relation to organ preservation is feasible. This approach, already achieved in orbit and extremity tumours, has also been confirmed for bladder-prostate tumours, as shown by the 65 per cent bladder salvage rate[128] achieved in surviving patients

treated with intensive chemotherapeutic regimens with or without radiotherapy.

Age less than 1 year may be associated with a less favourable outcome.[55,56] Whether the drug dose reduction recommended for infants and the limited use of radiotherapy in this group of patients are relevant factors remains to be ascertained.

Local relapse is the main cause of treatment failure. A review of relapse patterns in RMS patients[129] demonstrated that the first recurrence took the form of an isolated local or regional relapse in 50–60 per cent of cases. Distant metastases occurred in 30 per cent of cases, while a combined distant and local relapse affected the remaining 10–20 per cent. Specific patterns of tumour progression were also associated with certain histological subtypes or primary tumour locations. The DFS curve for childhood RMS seems to plateau at six years.[102]

NON–RHABDO SOFT TISSUE SARCOMAS

Non-rhabdo soft tissue sarcomas (NRSTSs) are a heterogeneous group of tumours of different origins and distinctive histological characteristics that are much more common in adults than in children. In the paediatric age group, NRSTSs have two peaks of incidence, the first under the age of 5 years and the second in early adolescence. The prevalent entities are:[130]

- pPNET
- extraosseous Ewing's sarcoma (EOE)
- malignant peripheral nerve sheath tumour (MPNST)
- fibrosarcoma
- synovial sarcoma (SS).

Less common types include undifferentiated sarcoma, haemangiosarcoma, haemangiopericytoma, epithelioid sarcoma and alveolar soft part sarcoma. Any histological subtype of STS can, however, be found in children and adolescents: even sporadic cases of liposarcoma, malignant

Table 17.3 *Rhabdomyosarcoma: 5-year survival rate according to extent of disease for non-metastatic patients in four representative cooperative studies*

Studies	Clinical group		
	I	II	III
IRS-I	83	70	52
IRS-II	81	80	65
IRS-III	93	81	73
IRS-IV (3-year EFS)	83	86	73
ICS RMS-79	83	68	55
ICS RMS-88	93	76	70
CWS-81	93	85	61
CWS-86 (5-year FFS)	83	67	62
	TNM stage		
SIOP-84	89	63	42
SIOP-89	80	66	60

EFS, event-free survival; FFS, failure-free survival; IRS, Intergroup Study; ICS, Italian Co-operative Study; CWS, German Co-operative Study; SIOP, International Society of Pediatric Oncology.

Table 17.4 *Rhabdomyosarcoma: 5-year survival according to primary site*

Primary site	IRS-III		SIOP-84		CWS-86 (5-year EFS)		ICS-88	
	n	Alive (%)	n	Alive (%)	n	Alive (%)	n	Alive (%)
Orbit	107	95	19	88	36	71	23	74
Head-neck	106	78	17	77	28	51	29	79
Parameningeal	134	74	41	58	55	60	43	74
GU bladder/prostate	104	81	14	79	30	70	26	88
GU non-bladder/prostate	158	89	35	88	38	89	29	97
Extremity	156	74	23	65	25	56	18	56
Other	147	67	37	45	39	58	50	59

EFS, event-free survival; GU, genitourinary.
IRS-III, Intergroup RMS Study III; SIOP-84, International Society of Pediatric Oncology RMS-84 study; CWS-86, German Co-operative Soft Tissue Sarcoma Study 86; ICS-88, Italian Co-operative Study RMS-88.

fibrous histiocytoma and leiomyosarcoma are described in the literature. Recently, other histological types occurring in the paediatric age group have been described. Some of them have a tendency to relapse locally, such as giant cell fibroblastoma, fibrous plexiform histiocytoma, fibrous angiomatoid histiocytoma; others show aggressive biological behaviour with metastatic capacity and poor prognosis, e.g. extrarenal rhabdoid tumour and intra-abdominal desmoplastic small-cell tumour. The incidence of different NRSTSs registered by the Italian cooperative studies is shown in Figure 17.5.

NRSTSs can be found anywhere in the body, but the most common sites are the extremities, the wall of the trunk and the retroperitoneum. The most important symptom is a painless mass that usually grows rapidly; indirect signs of vascular or peripheral nerve compression may be present. When the mass is retroperitoneal, intestinal obstruction is possible. Involvement of regional lymph nodes is less frequent than that observed in RMS (10 per cent), and distant metastases are present at diagnosis in about 10–12 per cent of cases.

Since these tumours are rare and include different histological types, the diagnostic work-up and the staging systems are the same as those adopted for RMS. The definitive diagnosis is obtained by an incisional biopsy; fine-needle biopsy does not yet provide sufficient accuracy.[131]

Chemotherapy responsiveness is one of the main therapeutic problems and our knowledge in this field is incomplete, particularly for the less common entities. Responsiveness depends on the histological type, but it is generally lower than that observed in RMS. Furthermore, not all the authors agree on the indications and on the use of chemotherapy. The experience of the recent international cooperative studies indicates that three different therapeutic groups of NRSTS exist:

- Group A – tumours with proven chemosensitivity, which should be treated as RMS; these are pPNET, EOE and undifferentiated sarcoma
- Group B – tumours with possible chemosensitivity, e.g. SS, malignant fibrous histiocytoma, liposarcoma and congenital-infantile fibrosarcoma; this category should be stratified according to post-surgical stage and grading; adjuvant chemotherapy is given unless there is no response to primary (neoadjuvant) chemotherapy
- Group C – tumours with unproven chemosensitivity (juvenile or 'adult type' fibrosarcoma and MPNST) for which surgery is the mainstay of treatment; if complete excision cannot be obtained, a trial of chemotherapy may be justified.

In the Italian studies, pPNET and EOE have demonstrated a 60 per cent good-response rate to primary chemotherapy, SS a 50 per cent good-response rate, while fibrosarcoma and MPNST were less sensitive to chemotherapy regimens.

Excluding pPNET and EOE, NRSTSs have a higher tendency than RMS to relapse locally. For this reason, it is generally agreed that local treatment should be more aggressive for these tumours. A wide, non-mutilating

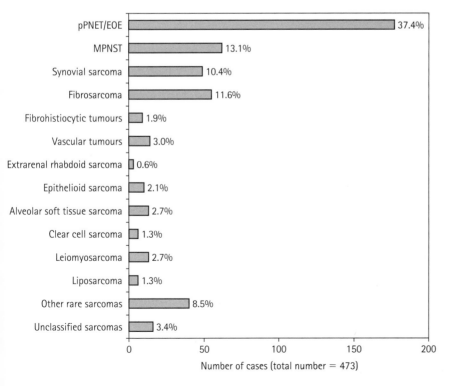

Figure 17.5 *Incidence of different non-rhabdo soft tissue sarcomas (NRSTSs) in childhood (data from the Italian cooperative studies). EOE, extraosseous Ewing's sarcoma; MPNST, malignant peripheral nerve sheath tumour; pPNET, peripheral primitive neuroectodermal tumour.*

surgical resection, performed at diagnosis and completed by exploration of regional lymph nodes, is recommended, if feasible. This is particularly important for NRSTS with unproven chemosensitivity, such as adult-type fibrosarcomas and MPNST; otherwise a trial of presurgical chemotherapy is preferred. Response to chemotherapy should predict the need for, and timing of, local treatment according to the schema for the individual treatment strategies. Radiotherapy can help in achieving local control of the disease in patients with minimal residual disease; doses of at least 40–50 Gy on the tumour bed are indicated. Low-dose brachytherapy can be used in place of external radiotherapy for superficial NRSTS. Postoperative radiotherapy is no longer utilized when a radical excision, histologically confirmed, is carried out.

Prognostic factors are as follows:

- Extension of the disease at diagnosis – survival varies from 85 per cent in patients with localized tumours to 7–10 per cent in children with disseminated disease[132]
- Quality of initial surgery for localized disease (IRS group)
- Size and site of the tumour – local control of the disease can be obtained with greater difficulty in patients with tumours > 5 cm in size and at thoracic/abdominal sites
- Histological type and consequent different response rates to combined treatments
- Grading has been advocated as a means of standardizing therapy for NRSTS. The POG schema indicates that patients may be assigned to grade 1, 2 or 3 according to the histological type, the number of mitoses and amount of necrosis, the degree of nuclear atypia and the degree of cellularity[133]
- Younger patients have a more favourable behaviour, although this may reflect histological type.

The clinical features and treatment of the most common NRSTSs are described in Table 17.5. The principal diagnostic morphological features of NRSTSs are listed in Table 17.6.

Peripheral primitive neuroectodermal tumours and extraosseous Ewing's sarcoma

Since the clinical behaviour, the cytogenetic alterations and probably the histogenesis of these tumours are similar, they are generally considered in the same family of tumours (Ewing's sarcoma family tumours).

pPNETs make up a controversial and poorly defined class of extracranial and extraspinal small round-cell malignant tumours with 'neural' characteristics supposedly of neuroectodermal origin.[134] Microscopically, pPNET is composed of a uniform population of round cells arranged in lobular or diffuse patterns, with small nucleoli and numerous mitoses; Homer-Wright or Flexner rosettes are frequently seen. Undifferentiated areas with Ewing's-like appearance are occasionally observed, and PAS-positive, diastase-sensitive material (glycogen) has been found in 40 per cent of cases.[135] The identification of neural characteristics (neurosecretory granules) sometimes requires the use of electron microscopy and immunocytochemical analyses (presence of neuron-specific enolase (NSE), S-100 protein, and synaptophysin). pPNET occurs in children and young adults with a median age of around 12–15 years; it is a very aggressive tumour most commonly found on the chest wall and extremities, and has the tendency to metastasize to regional lymph nodes, lungs and bone.

EOE appears to be a very primitive member of the same neuroectodermal family on the basis of several common features.[136] Two specific cytogenetic abnormalities, the translocations t(11;22)(q24;q12) and t(21;22)(q22;q12), are present in 90–95 and 5–10 per cent, respectively, of tumours within the Ewing's sarcoma family.[16,17] These findings confirm a close histogenetic relationship between EOE and pPNET. Therefore, it seems convenient to use the term Ewing's sarcoma for undifferentiated blastematous soft tissue small round-cell tumours that, unlike pPNET, lack any morphological or immunohistochemical evidence of neural differentiation.

Up to now, in most parts of Europe, EOE and pPNET of soft tissue have been included in RMS protocols and treated according to the guidelines for unfavourable histology RMS. Combinations of VAIA, CEVAIE (Box 17.7), VAC ± ADR (Box 17.6) have been adopted in the various European and IRS studies, and high-dose chemotherapy with HSCR has been investigated in metastatic patients. The most important unfavourable prognostic factor is the presence of metastases at diagnosis, and survival in such cases is <30 per cent.[137] Among patients with localized disease, the most important variables are the tumour size and the site (pelvis being the least favourable and the distal extremities the most favourable). EOE and pPNET are frequently present as large masses which may involve the contiguous bone; the resection of the tumours of the chest may require reconstructive procedures adopting muscular flaps or grafts, while the removal of the masses arising in the extremities needs the evaluation of experienced orthopaedic specialists. Treatment results achieved in a series of 130 patients with EOE are similar to those obtained in RMS patients; in fact, the overall survival varies from 61 per cent (IRS-I) to 77 per cent (IRS-III). No benefit to survival was demonstrated from the addition of adriamycin to a VAC combination in IRS grade III patients.[138] The results of

Table 17.5 *Clinical features and treatment in paediatric non-rhabdo soft tissue sarcomas*

	Age	Site	Treatment/prognosis
pPNET and EOE	Adolescence	Chest wall, head, extremities	Aggressive multimodal therapy Stage-related prognosis
Infantile fibrosarcoma	<2 year	Extremities (distal)	Excellent prognosis with complete surgery alone
Adolescent fibrosarcoma	10–15 years	Extremities (proximal)	Aggressive excision Poor response to chemotherapy/radiotherapy/unfavourable prognosis
MPNST	Child, adolescent (20% associated with von Recklinghausen's disease)	Extremities, retroperitoneum	Aggressive surgical treatment Poor response to chemotherapy/radiotherapy
Synovial sarcoma	Young adults	Legs (knee, foot)	Resection Doubtful response to chemotherapy Stage-related prognosis
Haemangiosarcoma	Rare in children	Liver, head-neck	Multimodal treatment High malignancy Unfavourable prognosis
Childhood haemangiopericytoma	<1 year	Chest wall, head, neck	Excellent prognosis with complete excision
Haemangiopericytoma in young adult	15–20 years	Retroperitoneum, legs	Multimodal treatment Stage-related prognosis
Epithelioid sarcoma	Rare in children	Extremities (distal)	Radical excision and radiotherapy Good prognosis if complete excision
Alveolar rhabdoid tumour	Children	Deep soft tissue	Multimodal treatment Unfavourable prognosis
Intra-abdominal desmoplastic small cell tumour	Adolescents/young adults	Abdomen	Multimodal treatment Unfavourable prognosis

EOE, extraosseous Ewing's sarcoma; MPNST, malignant peripheral nerve sheath tumour; pPNET, peripheral primitive neuroectodermal tumour.

Table 17.6 *The principal diagnostic morphological features of non-rhabdo soft tissue sarcomas*

Tumour	Morphology		Immunocytochemistry							
	Pattern of growth	Nuclear shape	S-100	NSE	Keratin	EMA	Desmin	Vimentin	Factor VIII	CD99
pPNET	Lobular or diffuse	Oval-round	+	++	−	−	−	+	−	+
Fibrosarcoma	Herringbone	Sharp-pointed	−	−	−	−	−	+	−	−
Synovial sarcoma	Nodular and/or biphasic	Spindle and/or roundish	−	−	++	+	−	−	−	+
MPNST	Whorls	Comma	++	+	±	−	−	+	−	−
Haemangiosarcoma	Lobular	Roundish and/or spindle	−	−	+[a]	−	−	+	+	−
Epithelioid sarcoma	Multinodular	Polygonal	−[b]	−	+	+	−	+	−	−
Alveolar soft tissue sarcoma	Alveolar	Large round	±	−	−	−	±	+	−	−

pPNET, peripheral primitive neuroectodermal tumour; MPNST, malignant peripheral nerve sheath tumour; NSE, neuron-specific enolase; EMA, epithelial membrane antigen.
[a]In epithelioid variant.
[b]Occasionally positive.

the CWS-86 study on pPNET and EOE showed that the EFS was slightly worse than that of RMS (47 ± 7 vs. 60 ± 3 per cent).[49] The same less favourable outcome of patients with EOE/pPNET was confirmed by the SIOP-MMT89 study; the most common cause of failure was metastatic relapse.[139] The results of the European MMT4-89 and MMT4-91 studies demonstrated that the survival of patients with metastatic disease has not been improved despite the high CR rate achieved with intensive chemotherapy with or without high-dose melphalan.[140]

Fibrosarcoma

Two forms of fibrosarcoma with different peaks of age incidence are recognized: the first occurs in children under 2 years of age (congenital-infantile fibrosarcoma), and the second in patients aged between 10 and 15 years (juvenile or 'adult type' fibrosarcoma).[140,141] The two forms of fibrosarcoma are histologically identical, consisting of small round or spindle-shaped fibroblasts exhibiting variable collagen production and showing no evidence of other differentiation. Histological grading, which is a predictor of tumour aggressiveness in adults, has not been proved to be an indicative factor for the infantile form. A recurring t(12;15)(q22;q13) translocation has recently been documented in congenital-infantile fibrosarcoma; this abnormality may help to differentiate infantile myofibromatosis from adult-type fibrosarcoma.[25] Translocations (2,5) and (7,22) have also been described in adult-type fibrosarcoma.[142]

In adolescents, fibrosarcoma has clinical features similar to those found in adults. The most frequent sites are proximal regions of the extremities and deep trunk, where the tumour is most aggressive. This form has an unfavourable prognosis and the survival rate is less than 60 per cent. The most effective treatment is radical surgery. If a wide excision can be achieved, no further treatment is required. Improved local control may be obtained with the use of radiotherapy in patients with minimal residual disease. Brachytherapy, which may be employed in adults with residual disease, may also be a useful alternative in the paediatric age group. The role of chemotherapy remains uncertain, in both unresectable and disseminated fibrosarcomas.

Congenital-infantile fibrosarcomas are usually located in the distal region of the extremities and present as a fast-growing masses. Some authors believe that this should be considered an intermediate form of disease between fibromatosis and adult fibrosarcoma.[141] Surgery alone is generally able to cure the disease. Even if these tumours have a tendency to relapse locally (30–40 per cent), metastases are extremely rare and the overall survival is about 85–90 per cent.[143,144] Recent reports have demonstrated a good response to primary chemotherapy in patients with inoperable infantile fibrosarcoma: vincristine and dactinomycin are the recommended drugs, in some cases associated with ifosfamide or cyclophosphamide.[145,146]

Other fibrous proliferations of infancy and childhood are the so-called fibromatoses. Because of their unusual histological features, they pose special diagnostic problems. Exuberant cellular proliferation, high mitotic index and infiltrative growth pattern do not necessarily indicate aggressive clinical behaviour. On the other hand, innocent-looking fibrous proliferation may relapse repeatedly. After the original series published by Stout[147] on 'juvenile fibromatosis', many other entities have been recognized and categorized.[141,148] Of all the forms, infantile fibromatosis, desmoid-type, is the most controversial and difficult to delineate with precision.[149] In fact, it displays a considerable histological variability, from immature mesenchymal lesions to mature fibroblastic proliferations with abundant collagen production that closely resemble adult musculoaponeurotic fibromatosis. In the more cellular variant of infantile fibromatosis, differential diagnosis from fibrosarcoma is sometimes very difficult. Such difficulty in diagnosis is emphasized by the great variety of terms used in the past (e.g. aggressive fibromatosis, differentiated fibrosarcoma, fibrosarcoma grade I desmoid type). In our experience, high mitotic rate, minor collagen production and destructive growth generally favour a diagnosis of infantile fibrosarcoma over fibromatosis. Fibromatosis does not usually metastasize but has high local aggressiveness; it requires complete surgical excision and must be distinguished from other NRSTSs by a precise histological examination. Again, low-dose VA or VAC as well as the combination of methotrexate and vinblastine may be effective if the tumour is unresectable.[150] Responses have been reported in adults using antioestrogen hormone therapy (tamoxifen). Regional perfusion systems have occasionally been employed in adolescents with desmoid-type fibromatosis of the extremities.

Other myofibroblastic lesions with locally invasive behaviour are mesenchymal hamartoma, giant-cell fibroblastoma and nodular fasciitis.[141] They are superficially located and sometimes underestimated at clinical evaluation. Complete surgical excision is the only treatment.

Synovial sarcoma

Synovial sarcoma is one of the most common NRSTSs in adolescents and young adults. It is mostly characterized by two histological subtypes, biphasic and monophasic, the biphasic subtype being the most common, accounting for 60 per cent of cases. It is characterized by an epithelial–glandular component and a spindle cell–fibrous component. SS shows a characteristic t(X;18)(p11;q11) translocation[22] and fresh tissue should always be submitted for cytogenetic analysis.[149] SS occurs most often in the region of a large joint; the lower extremity, particularly the knee, is the most common site (80 per cent). Many prognostic factors have been defined. Those so far identified as favourable are IRS group, tumour invasiveness, tumour size < 5 cm,[149–156] and distal site.[157] The prognostic value of histological subtype is still debated. The best outcome seems to be linked to biphasic subtype,[158,159] particularly in those tumours in which a high percentage of glandular tissue and a low mitotic activity are evident.

A wide excision of the primary mass offers the best chance of a favourable outcome in localized forms; controversy still exists as to whether adjuvant radiotherapy and chemotherapy are useful after complete excision. Radiotherapy is indicated in the treatment of microscopic residual disease. In inoperable SS, chemotherapy should be given with the aim of improving local treatment with surgery and radiotherapy. IFO or CYC and ADR-based regimens are the most commonly used. In the German CWS-81 study, a chemotherapy response rate of 77 per cent (VACA combination: Box 17.6) was recorded for stage III and IV patients[155] and 5-year EFS rates of 84 and 85 per cent were achieved with a mulitmodality therapy in the CWS-81 and CWS-86 studies, respectively.[160] In one large retrospective analysis of 220 children and adolescents treated in different centres between 1966 and 1999, the overall survival at 5 years after diagnosis was 88 ± 4 per cent for patients with tumours that were grossly resected at diagnosis (IRS groups I and II) and 75 ± 7 per cent for patients with localized unresectable tumour (IRS group III). Patients with distant metastases fared poorly. The results of this study suggest that neoadjuvant chemotherapy should be utilized to facilitate delayed surgery, whereas group I and II patients do not seem to benefit from adjuvant chemotherapy.[157]

Malignant peripheral nerve sheath tumour (malignant schwannoma)

These tumours originate from the peripheral nerve sheaths. About 20 per cent of MPNSTs occur in association with neurofibromatosis type I.[162] The most common sites are the extremities and the trunk. This tumour has a poor response to chemotherapy and radiotherapy, and surgical excision is the optimal treatment and the most important prognostic factor. In a review of 24 patients, Raney et al.[163] found that 9/12 patients with MPNST who had undergone a complete excision were alive without disease, whereas none of the 12 who had residual disease had a favourable outcome. In the Italian and German studies, local control was the major cause of treatment failure for MPNST, although distant metastases can also occur. Radiotherapy appears to improve the local control in patients with minimal residual disease, but the role of chemotherapy in curing these patients is not well established, although a 45 per cent response rate (CR and PR) was achieved with different drug combinations, particularly the VAIA or CEVAIE regimens; in some cases it allowed delayed complete surgical excision. Low IRS group, extremity site, T1 status and absence of neurofibromatosis type 1 (NF1) have been identified in multivariate analysis as significant factors influencing overall survival.[164]

Other non-rhabdo soft tissue sarcomas

Other rare histological types do not have specific therapeutic strategies and follow the treatment guidelines of NRSTS. The experience of the Italian and German Soft Tissue Sarcoma Group on leiomyosarcoma,[165] alveolar soft part sarcoma[166] and haemangiopericytoma shows that complete surgical resection is the mainstay of treatment and that the tumour size is the most significant prognostic factor. In infants, haemangiopericytoma exhibits more favourable behaviour, sharing clinical features with infantile myofibroblastic lesions.[167] The outcome of angiosarcomas remains dismal (OS < 30 per cent at 5 years); complete surgical excision is the main therapy but is probably sufficient in only a minority of cases, while the role of chemotherapy is uncertain.[168] The experience of the Italian and German group on clear cell sarcoma of tendons and aponeuroses indicates the aggressive behaviour of this entity. Complete surgery is curative for cases with small tumours, radiotherapy may control microscopic residues, while chemotherapy is ineffective in cases with unresectable tumours.[169] Desmoplastic small round-cell tumour is a highly aggressive neoplasm, typically presenting as a large abdominal mass; survival rates remain disappointing despite aggressive multimodality therapy. Surgery and radiotherapy play a crucial role when the disease is localized. The best chemotherapeutic treatment has yet to be established, although some evidence points towards an intensive use of alkylating agents.[170]

LATE EFFECTS

The importance of an accurate prognostic assessment at diagnosis is as much to ensure that patients with a good prognosis are not overtreated as to identify those with a poorer prognosis who require more intensive therapy. Much concern has been focused on the late sequelae of local treatment for RMS, particularly after radiotherapy and after the types of aggressive surgery which may result in significant functional or cosmetic problems (e.g. procedures such as orbital exenteration, total cystoprostatectomy and bilateral retroperitoneal lymph node dissection).

The majority of children with RMS are very young and 40 per cent of tumours occur in the region of the head and neck where the need for radiotherapy as part of optimal treatment, particularly for those with parameningeal tumours, creates especial concern.[171] Exenteration rates for children with RMS of the orbit are, fortunately, very low and this procedure is usually performed only when disease recurs after previous radiotherapy. Nevertheless, the majority of children with orbital tumours who receive radiotherapy experience important late sequelae, including cataract, dry eye, orbital hypoplasia and pituitary insufficiency.[172] Only approximately 50 per cent of children with bladder-prostate RMS retain their bladder after successful treatment and a significant minority of these have a degree of bladder dysfunction.[173] There has been particular controversy about the value of retroperitoneal lymph node dissection as part of staging procedures for paratesticular RMS. Clinicians in Europe have tended to consider this unnecessary,[174] particularly as bilateral sampling may cause intestinal obstruction, loss of ejaculatory function and lymphoedema of the leg.[175] The policy of the IRS group (COG) studies has varied in recent years with omission of this procedure in IRS-IV. However, concern about less favourable results in this group of patients, who otherwise have an excellent prognosis, has stimulated its reintroduction, albeit on a more selective basis.[176]

Chemotherapy is also associated with significant sequelae in some patients and the concept that more intensive chemotherapy may reduce the use of local treatment must be balanced against the additional toxicity this may bring. The use of agents such as alkylating agents and anthracycline drugs is of particular concern in relation to the risks of gonadal toxicity, cardiotoxicity and second malignancy.

The use of ifosfamide as the alkylating agent component of chemotherapy for RMS in Europe is well established but remains controversial. Historical evaluation of its efficacy against earlier studies that used lower doses of cyclophosphamide will not have provided an equivalent biological comparison. Data from IRS-IV[55] showed no apparent advantage of combination chemotherapy utilizing ifosfamide at a dose of $9 \, \text{g/m}^2$ per course compared with cyclophosphamide at a dose of $2.2 \, \text{g/m}^2$ per course. Furthermore, there is concern about the renal toxicity profile of ifosfamide, although the incidence of significant nephrotoxicity is very low when the cumulative dose is less than approximately $60 \, \text{g/m}^2$.[177] Data are not yet available to determine whether ifosfamide is less damaging to gonadal function than cyclophosphamide and this requires prospective evaluation, particularly as the majority of children are exposed to treatment that includes alkylating agents.

Other chemotherapy-induced late effects depend on specific drug exposures, but reports have included evidence of significant pulmonary toxicity in patients exposed to chemotherapy combinations including bleomycin and BCNU,[178] and a high risk of neurotoxicity when intrathecal chemotherapy was delivered in conjunction with cranial radiotherapy for parameningeal tumours.[116]

All survivors of cancer in childhood are at risk of second malignancy. The reported cumulative incidence in survivors of RMS is reassuringly low, estimated at less than 2 per cent at 10 years in one series.[179] Although radiotherapy is the dominant risk factor, there is a compound effect from concurrent exposure to chemotherapy, particularly alkylating agents,[180] and there must be at least theoretical concern that rates may increase in those treated with more recent, higher-dose multiagent chemotherapy schedules.[181]

Long-term follow-up and prospective evaluation of all survivors is required in order to document the frequency and functional significance of the sequelae of all types of therapy.

CURRENT CONTROVERSIES

Comparing results of different approaches to treatment

Many clinicians find protocols for treatment of RMS confusing and difficult to implement. This is partly due to the use of different staging systems and partly because the complexity of prognostic variables often results in a relatively large number of possible treatment assignments. Moreover, when reading the literature it is often hard to separately identify similar groups of patients in different studies, preventing easy comparison of the outcome with different approaches to treatment. There is, however, increasing collaboration between the major international study groups working in this field. A series of international workshops have been held at which specific subtypes of RMS have been explored,[125,182] and there is an expectation that staging systems and definition of factors used to determine treatment allocation will become more consistent in the future.

Perhaps the most important difficulty in evaluating current literature lies in understanding the form in which results are reported and outcome is defined. This relates to philosophical differences in the approach to therapy, particularly towards the method and timing of local treatment, and, most specifically, to the place of radiotherapy in guaranteeing local control for patients who may achieve complete remission with chemotherapy, with or without significant surgery. This represents an important philosophical difference between the SIOP MMT studies and those of the IRS group and, to some extent, those of the CWS and ICS cooperative groups. Local relapse rates are generally higher in the SIOP studies than those experienced elsewhere, although the SIOP experience has also made it clear that a significant number of patients who relapse may be cured with alternative treatment.[53] In the context of such differences, OS rather than DFS or progression-free survival (PFS) becomes the most important criteria for measuring outcome. Ultimately, there should also be some measure of the 'cost' of survival, which takes into account the total burden of therapy experienced by an individual patient and the predicted late sequelae that may result.[183]

OPTIMAL USE OF RADIOTHERAPY?

Radiotherapy has been a standard component of therapy for the majority of patients since the outset of IRS group studies. Randomized studies within IRS-I to III established that radiotherapy is unnecessary for group I (completely resected) patients with embryonal histology, although analyses from the same studies suggest that it offers improved FFS in patients with completely resected alveolar RMS. Studies from the European groups have attempted to relate the use of radiotherapy to response to initial chemotherapy, the most radical approach being by the SIOP group who have tried to withhold radiotherapy in patients with group III (pT3b) disease if CR is achieved with initial chemotherapy with or without conservative second surgery. This approach has produced evidence that it is possible to delay or even avoid local therapy in some children who would otherwise receive radiotherapy, but there is a need to try to define such favourable patients at the outset so as to reduce the risk of relapse in those for whom this strategy would not be suitable.

Doses of radiotherapy have, somewhat pragmatically, been tailored to age, with reduced doses in younger children, although there is no defined threshold below which late effects can be avoided and yet tumour control can still be achieved. In IRS-IV, a pilot study established the feasibility of hyperfractionated (twice daily) radiotherapy treatment (an approach also explored by the European groups), but the data from this study showed no difference between those who received conventional radiotherapy at a dose of 50.4 Gy and HFRT at a dose of 59.4 Gy.[184] The German (CWS) group has explored the use of reduced radiation dose in children who demonstrate better response to chemotherapy (32 vs. 54 Gy) but also delivered treatment using a twice-daily hyperfractionation schedule prior to second surgery. Although there was no significant difference in local relapse rate between those who received standard therapy and those who had a reduced dose, it is difficult to interpret the results in the presence of the other variables, but the possibility of reducing radiation dose must remain a target for future investigation.

OPTIMAL CHEMOTHERAPY FOR RMS

Based on the results of the IRS group studies, many clinicians assert that the VAC (vincristine, actinomycin D and cyclophosphamide) combination remains the 'gold standard' for the treatment of RMS. There have been changes in this regimen over time. For example, cyclophosphamide doses have been increased with the use of granulocyte colony-stimulating factor (G-CSF) support, and whilst actinomycin D was originally given in a fractionated schedule, subsequent experience showed no advantage in terms of outcome and even suggested that fractionation may increase toxicity; single dose scheduling is now standard across all studies. There have never been any results that challenge the use of these drugs as first-line therapy, and the results of all randomized studies that compare alternatives with VAC have failed to show significant advantage. This includes experience with ifosfamide, which has assumed greater importance in Europe as the alkylating agent of choice, although a comparison of outcome between ifosfamide and cyclophosphamide in the IRS-IV study showed no significant difference between combinations using these two agents.[55] It is likely that toxicity profile, ease of administration, the need for G-CSF support and long-term sequelae will ultimately be the criteria that distinguish between them.

Alternative agents of particular interest include doxorubicin, which has been evaluated in a number of IRS group studies. A total of 1431 patients with group III and IV disease were randomized to receive or not receive doxorubicin in addition to VAC during studies in IRS-I to IRS-III. The results did not indicate any significant advantage for those who received doxorubicin. Furthermore, also in IRS-III, patients with group II (microscopic residual) tumours were randomized between VA alone and VA + doxorubicin without any significant difference in survival.[119] Despite these results, and the lack of historical phase II data for the use of doxorubicin in RMS, many paediatric oncologists continue to consider the value of anthracycline in the treatment of RMS. Recent data from an 'up front' window study of doxorubicin in newly diagnosed patients with high-risk metastatic RMS performed in France has confirmed response rates in excess of 70 per cent (C. Bergeron, personal communication) and current European studies (MMT 95 and CWS-ICG 96) include randomizations between their ifosfamide-based standard chemotherapy options and an intensified six-drug combination which includes epirubicin (with carboplatin and etoposide). The first study from the European Soft Tissue Sarcoma Study Group (ESSG RMS 2004) will address the value of adding doxorubicin to IVA in high-risk patients.

Experience of the value of other drugs in IRS group studies has been relatively limited. IRS-III included the addition of cisplatin and etoposide in a three-way randomization between VAC, VAC + doxorubicin and cisplatin, and VAC + doxorubicin, cisplatin and etoposide. No advantage was seen in selected group III and all group IV patients, and there were concerns about additive toxicity.[51] IRS-IV (and an earlier IRS-IV pilot) explored the value of melphalan in a three-way randomization which compared initial treatment for metastatic (group IV) patients with vincristine/melphalan (VM), ifosfamide/ etoposide (IE) and ifosfamide/doxorubicin (ID). Patients who received IE did best and those who received VM did worst. This was almost certainly due to enhanced myelotoxicity, which reduced tolerance of subsequent treatment, but there was the additional anxiety that this combination also produced the highest rate of second malignancy (7.2 per cent at 5 years).[119]

More recent new drugs evaluated in RMS include topotecan which, although showing high activity in a window study with newly diagnosed high-risk patients, showed a disappointingly poor response rate in conventional phase II evaluation.[115] This drug was first identified as a potentially active agent in a xenograft model system, as was irinotecan,[98] which shows promise in current phase II trials. These drugs may be more effective in combination with vincristine.[114] Few other new conventional chemotherapy agents are under evaluation. Two particular areas of controversy are:

- trying to assess the clinical relevance of the results of xenograft experiments
- comparing the data derived from conventional phase II studies with those from window studies in naïve patients.

WHAT IS THE VALUE OF 'MEGATHERAPY' (HIGH-DOSE CHEMOTHERAPY WITH HAEMOPOIETIC STEM CELL SUPPORT)?

The place of high-dose chemotherapy strategies necessitating autologous bone marrow or peripheral blood stem cell support remains unclear. Some experience has been gained in individual institutions using a variety of chemotherapy schedules and, predominantly, in the treatment of patients with relapsed disease. More recently, the European collaborative groups shared a strategy for the treatment of newly diagnosed patients with metastatic disease. The results suggest that there is no overall survival advantage from consolidation chemotherapy with melphalan for patients who achieve CR with conventional therapy.[120] On the basis of current knowledge, it would be difficult to justify the use of high-dose chemotherapy outside the framework of a clinical trial.

MOLECULAR CHARACTERIZATION AND NEW TUMOUR TARGETS

Basic cancer treatment is changing as a result of the development of agents targeted to molecular characteristics of individual tumour types. Thus far, there are limited data in a paediatric setting, although sarcoma is an area that has attracted attention in adult practice and there is interest from *in vivo* data in agents such as Iressa (an epidermal growth factor receptor TK inhibitor) and TRAIL (tumour necrosis factor alpha-related apoptosis-inducing ligand) as candidates for evaluation in RMS. It is becoming increasingly important that all patients with relapsed tumours are systematically considered for new drug studies in order to adequately address the potential of such new agents in a timely manner.

SHOULD NRSTS BE TREATED LIKE RMS?

There is a clear challenge to be faced in the management of non-RMS soft tissue sarcoma in childhood. With a few notable exceptions (e.g. infantile fibrosarcoma and haemangiopericytoma) there is little evidence that the biological characteristics of tumours more frequently encountered in adult practice are significantly different when diagnosed in childhood. Strategies for the management of such tumours in children generally derive from experience with RMS. Patients with unresectable tumours are often offered a trial of chemotherapy on a neoadjuvant basis whilst the management of the same pathology seen in an adult emphasizes local control (surgery and radiotherapy) with more selective use of chemotherapy (usually doxorubicin ± ifosfamide).[182] There is evidence for the chemosensitivity of many non-RMS malignant mesenchymal tumours, but it is not clear whether this translates into a survival advantage.[185] There is an urgent need for randomized studies to address this question, and further work will be needed to elucidate prognostic variables to aid treatment stratification. One particular area that merits attention is the evaluation of the prognostic value of pathological grading, as used in adult sarcoma practice, to these tumours in childhood. Drugs such as ET-743, gemcitabine and STI571 (Glivec) have all attracted interest in adult sarcoma[186] and need to be evaluated in similar paediatric tumours, particularly if the appropriate molecular targets are shown to be present.

KEY POINTS

- Although overall survival rates for children with STS have improved, progress for some subgroups of patients has been less encouraging than might be expected.
- Increasing international collaboration should improve standardization of approach to staging and treatment stratification and help to eliminate some of the difficulties encountered in comparing results of different approaches to treatment.
- Priorities for the future include the better identification of patients who can be cured with minimal therapy and the development of better treatment for those who have a poor outcome with current therapy.
- Improved understanding of the biology of this heterogeneous group of tumours is slowly being accrued, which may provide opportunities to capitalize on novel forms of therapy aimed at molecular targets.
- Although considerable amounts of valuable clinical data have been acquired through clinical trials in patients with RMS, further efforts to systematically explore therapy in children with non-RMS soft tissue sarcoma are now required.

REFERENCES

1. Ries LAG, Hankey BF, Percy CL *et al.* United States of America, SEER Program, 1983–1992 In: Parkin DM, Kramàrovà E, Draper GJ *et al.*, eds. *International Incidence of Childhood Cancer.* IARC Scientific Publication No. 144. Lyon: IARC, 1998; 131–44.

2. Parkin DM, Kramàrovà E, Draper GJ *et al.*, eds. *International Incidence of Childhood Cancer.* IARC Scientific Publication No. 144, Vol. II. Lyon IARC, 1998.

3. Stiller C. Epidemiology of cancer in adolescents. *Med Pediatr Oncol* 2002; **39**: 149–55.

4. Ruymann FB, Maddux HR, Ragab A *et al.* Congenital anomalies associated with rhabdomyosarcoma: an autopsy study of 115 cases. A report from the Intergroup Rhabdomyosarcoma Study Committee. *Med Pediatr Oncol* 1988; **16**: 33–9.

5. Mckeen EA, Bodurtha J, Meadows AT *et al.* Rhabdomyosarcoma complicating multiple neurofibromatosis. *J Pediatr* 1978; **93**: 992–3.

6. Becker H, Zaunschirm A, Muntean W, Domej W. Alkoholembryopathie und maligner tumor. *Wien Klin Wochenschr* 1982; **94**: 364.

7. Beddis IR, Mott MG, Bullimore J. Case report: nasopharyngeal rhabdomyosarcoma and Grolin's nevoid basal cell carcinoma syndrome. *Med Ped Oncol* 1983; **11**: 178–9.

8. Li FP, Fraumeni JR. Jr. Rhabdomyosarcoma in children: epidemiologic study and identification of a family cancer syndrome. *J Natl Cancer Inst* 1969; **43**: 1365–73.

9. Pastore G, Mosso ML, Carli M *et al.* Cancer mortality among relatives of children with soft tissue sarcoma: a national survey in Italy. *Cancer Lett* 1987; **37**: 17–24.

10. Birch JM, Hartley AL, Blair V *et al.* Cancer in the families of children with soft tissue sarcoma. *Cancer* 1990; **66**: 2239–48.

11. Li FP, Fraumeni JR Jr, Mulvihill JT *et al.* A cancer family syndrome in twenty-four kindreds. *Cancer Res* 1988; **48**: 5358–62.

♦12. Barr FG. Molecular genetics and pathogenesis of rhabdomyosarcoma. *J Pediatr Hematol Oncol* 1997; **19**: 483–91.

13. Kelly KM, Worner RB, Sorensen PHB *et al.* Common and variant gene fusions predict distinct clinical phenotypes in rhabdomyosarcoma. *J Clin Oncol* 1997; **15**: 1831–6.

14. Scrable H, Witte D, Shimada H *et al.* Molecular differential pathology of rhabdomyosarcoma. *Genes Chromosomes Cancer* 1989; **1**: 23–35.

15. El-Badry OM, Minniti C, Kohn EC *et al.* Insulin-like growth factor II acts as an autocrine growth and motility factor in human rhabdomyosarcoma tumors. *Cell Growth Differ* 1990; **1**: 325–31.

16. Whang-Peng, J, Triche TJ, Krusten T *et al.* Chromosomal translocation in peripheral neuroepithelioma. *N Engl J Med* 1985; **311**: 584–5.

17. Turc-Carel C, Aurias A, Mugneret F *et al.* Chromosomes in Ewing' s sarcoma. An evaluation of 85 cases and remarkable consistency of t(11;22)(q24;q12). *Cancer Genet Cytogenet* 1988; **32**: 229–38.

♦18. Delattre O, Zucman J, Melot T *et al.* The Ewing family of tumors: a subgroup of small-round-cell tumors defined by specific chimeric transcripts. *N Engl J Med* 1995; **331**: 294–9.

●19. Zubek A, Dockhorn-Dworniczak B, Delattre O *et al.* Does expression of different EWS chimeric transcripts define clinically distinct risk groups of Ewing tumour patients? *J Clin Oncol* 1996; **14**: 1245–51.

●20. De Avala E, Kawai A, Healey JH *et al.* EWS-FLI 1 fusion transcript structure is an independent determinant of prognosis in Ewing's sarcoma. *J Clin Oncol* 1998; **4**:1248–55.

21. Mugnaret F, Lizard S, Aurias A, Turc-Carel C. Chromosomes in Ewing's sarcoma. Non random additional changes, trisomy 8 and (16) t(1;16). *Cancer Genet Cytogenet* 1988; **32**: 239–45.

22. Turc-Carel C, Dal Cin P, Limon J *et al.* Involvement of chromosome X in primary cytogenetic change in human neoplasia: non random translocation in synovial sarcoma. *Proc Natl Acad Sci USA* 1987; **84**: 1981–5.

23. Gerald WL, Roasi J, Ladanyi M. Characterization of the genomic breakpoint and chimeric transcript in the EWS-WT1 gene fusion of desmoplastic small round cell tumour. *Med Sci* 1995; **92**: 1028–32.

24. Turc-Carel C, Lienon T, Dal Cin P *et al.* Cytogenetic studies of adipose tissue tumors. II Recurrent reciprocal translocation t(12;16) (q13;p11) in myxoid liposarcomas. *Cancer Genet Cytogenet* 1986; **23**: 291–9.

25. Bourgeios JM, Knezevich SR, Mathers JA, Sorensen PHB. Molecular detection of the ETV6-NTRK3 gene fusion differentiates congenital fibrosarcoma from other childhood spindle cell tumors. *Am J Surg Pathol* 2000; **24**: 937–46.

26. Mandahl N, Heim S, Rydholm A *et al.* Non random numerical chromosome aberrations (+8, +11, +17, +20) in infantile fibrosarcoma. *Cancer Genet Cytogenet* 1989; **37**: 139–40.

27. Horn RC, Enterline H. Rhabdomyosarcoma: a clinico-pathological study and classification of 39 cases. *Cancer* 1958; **11**: 181–99.

28. Hays DM, Newton WA, Soule EH *et al.* Mortality among children with rhabdomyosarcoma of the alveolar histological subtype. *J Pediatr Surg* 1983; **18**: 412.

29. Asmar L, Gehan EM, Newton WA Jr *et al.* Agreement among and within groups of pathologists in the classification of rhabdomyosarcoma and related childhood sarcomas: report of an international study of four pathology classifications. *Cancer* 1994; **74**: 2579–88.

♦30. Newton WA, Gehan EA, Webber BL *et al.* Classification of rhabdomyosarcomas and related sarcomas: pathologic aspects and proposal for a new classification – an Intergroup Rhabdomyosarcoma Study. *Cancer* 1995; **76**: 1073–85.

31. Cavazzana AO, Schmidt D, Ninfo V *et al.* Spindle cell rhabdomyosarcoma: a prognostically favorable variant of rhabdomyosarcoma. *Am J Pathol* 1992; **16**: 229–35.

32. Leuschener J, Newton WA, Schmidt D *et al.* Spindle cell variants of embryonal rhabdomyosarcoma in the paratesticular region: a report of the Intergroup Rhabdomyosarcoma study. *Am J Surg Pathol* 1993; **17**: 221–30.

33. Gonzalez-Crussi F, Black-Shaffer S. Rhabdomyosarcoma of infancy and childhood. Problems of morphologic classi-fication. *Am J Surg Pathol* 1979; **3**: 157–71.

34. Bale PM, Parson RE, Stevens MM. Pathology and behavior of juvenile rhabdomyosarcoma. In: Finegold M, ed. *Pathology of Neoplasia in Children and Adolescents.* Philadelphia: WB Saunders, 1986; 196–222.

35. Riopelle JL, Theriault JP. Sur une forme meconnue de sarcome des parties molles: le rhabdomyosarcome alveolaire. *Ann Pathol* 1956; **1**: 88–111.

36. Tsokos M, Webber BL, Parham DM *et al*. Rhabdomyosarcoma; a new classification scheme related to prognosis. *Arch Pathol Lab Med* 1992; **116**: 847.

37. Palmer NF, Foulkes M. Histopathology and prognosis in the second Intergroup Rhabdomyosarcoma Study (IRS II). *Proc Am Soc Clin Oncol* 1983; **3**: 229.

38. Donaldson SS, Draper GJ, Flamant F *et al*. Topography of childhood tumours: Pediatric Coding System. *Pediatr Hematol Oncol* 1986; **3**: 249–58.

39. Lawrence W Jr, Hays DM, Heyn R *et al*. Lymphatic metastases with childhood rhabdomyosarcoma. A report from the Intergroup Rhabdomyosarcoma Study. *Cancer* 1987; **60**: 910–15.

40. Raney RB Jr, Hays DM, Lawrence W Jr *et al*. Paratesticular rhabdomyosarcomas in childhood. *Cancer* 1978; **42**: 729–36.

41. Olive D, Flamant F, Zucker JM *et al*. Paraaortic lymphade-nectomy is not necessary in the treatment of localized paratesticular rhabdomyosarcoma. *Cancer* 1984; **54**: 1283–7.

42. Cecchetto G, Grotto P, De Bemardi B *et al*. Paratesticular rhabdomyosarcoma in childhood: experience of the Italian Cooperative Study. *Tumori* 1988; **74**: 645–7.

43. Engel R, Ritterbach J, Shwabe D *et al*. Chromosome translocation (2;13)(q37;q1) in a disseminated alveolar sarcoma. *Eur J Pediatr* 1988; **18**: 69–71.

●44. Rodary C, Flamant F, Donaldson SS (for the SIOP-IRS Committee). An attempt to use a common staging system in rhabdomyosarcoma: a report of an International Workshop initiated by the International Society of Pediatric Oncology (SIOP). *Med Pediatr Oncol* 1989; **17**: 210–15.

●45. Rodary C, Gehan E, Flamant F *et al*. Prognostic factors in 951 nonmetastatic rhabdomyosarcoma in children: a report from the International Rhabdomyosarcoma Workshop. *Med Pediatr Oncol* 1991; **19**: 89–95.

46. Lawrence W, Anderson JR, Gehan EA *et al*. Pre-treatment TNM staging of childhood rhabdomyosarcoma. A report of the Intergroup Rhabdomyosarcoma Study Group. *Cancer* 1997; **80**: 1165–70.

47. Pratt CB, Maurer HM, Gieser P *et al*. Treatment of unresectable or metastatic pediatric soft tissue sarcomas with surgery, irradiation and chemotherapy: a Pediatric Oncology Group study. *Med Pediatr Oncol* 1998; **30**: 201–9.

48. Carli M, Guglielmi M, Sotti G *et al*. Prognostic factors in children with rhabdomyosarcoma. Results of the Italian Cooperative Study RMS-79. *Med Pediatr Oncol* 1991; **19**: 398.

●49. Koscielniak E, Harms D, Henze G *et al*. Results of treatment for soft tissue sarcomas in childhood and adolescence: a final report of the German Cooperative Soft Tissue Sarcoma Study CWS-86. *J Clin Oncol* 1999; **17**: 3706–19.

50. Crist WM, Garnsey L, Beltangady M *et al*. Prognosis in children with rhabdomyosarcoma: a report of the Intergroup Rhabdomyosarcoma Studies I and II. *J Clin Oncol* 1990; **8**: 443–52.

●51. Crist W, Geham EA, Ragab AH *et al*. The third Intergroup Rhabdomyosarcoma Study. *J Clin Oncol* 1995; **13**: 610–30.

●52. Koscielniak E, Rodary C, Flamant F *et al*. Metastatic rhabdomyosarcoma and histologically similar tumors in childhood. A retrospective European multicenter analysis. *Med Pediatr Oncol* 1992; **20**: 209–15.

●53. Flamant F, Rodary C, Rey A *et al*. Treatment of non-metastatic rhabdomyosarcomas in childhood and adolescence. Results of the second study of the International Society of Pediatric Oncology: MMT84. *Eur J Cancer* 1998; **34**: 1050–62.

54. Carli M, Grotto P, Cavazzana A *et al*. Prognostic significance of histology in childhood rhabdomyosarcoma: improved survival with a new histologic 'leiomyomatous' subtype. *Proc Am Soc Clin Oncol* 1990; **9**: 297.

●55. Crist WM, Anderson JR, Meza JL *et al*. Intergroup Rhabdomyosarcoma Study-IV: results for patients with nonmetastatic disease. *J Clin Oncol* 2001; **19**: 3091–102.

56. Ferrari A, Casanova M, Bisogno G *et al*. Rhabdomyosarcoma in infants younger than one year old: a report from the Italian Cooperative Group. *Cancer* 2003; **97**: 2597–604.

57. Treuner J, Suder J, Keim M *et al*. The predictive value of initial cytostatic response in primary unresectable rhabdomyosarcoma in children. *Acta Oncol* 1989; **28**: 67.

58. Pappo AS, Crist WM, Kuttesch J *et al*. Tumor-cell DNA content predicts outcome in children and adolescents with clinical group III embryonal rhabdomyosarcoma: the Intergroup Rhabdomyosarcoma Study Committee of the Children's Cancer Group and the Pediatric Oncology Group. *J Clin Oncol* 1993; **11**: 1901–5.

59. Niggli FK, Powell JE, Parkes SE *et al*. DNA ploidy and proliferative activity (S-phase) in childhood soft-tissue sarcomas: their value as prognostic indicators. *Br J Cancer* 1994; **69**: 1106–10.

60. De Zen L, Sommaggio A, D'Amore ESG *et al*. Clinical relevance of DNA ploidy and proliferative activity in childhood rhabdomyosarcoma: a retrospective analysis of patients enrolled onto the Italian Cooperative Rhabdomyosarcoma Study RMS88. *J Clin Oncol* 1997; **15**: 1198–205.

61. Niggli FK, Mathien MC, Chassevent A *et al*. Prognostic value of flow cytometric DNA ploidy in childhood rhabdomyo-sarcomas enrolled in SIOP-MMT 89 study. *Med Pediatr Oncol* 2001; **37**: 222.

61a. Cecchetto G, Bisogno G, Treuner J *et al*. Role of surgery for nonmetastatic abdominal rhabdomyosarcomas: a report from the Italian and German Soft Tissue Cooperative Groups Studies. *Cancer* 2003; **97**: 1974–80.

61b. Blakely ML, Andrassy RJ, Raney RB *et al*. Prognostic factors and surgical treatment guidelines for children with rhabdomyosarcoma of the perineum or anus: a report of Intergroup Rhabdomyosarcoma Studies I through IV, 1972 through 1997. *J Pediatr Surg* 2003; **38**: 347–53.

62. Pohar-Marinsek Z, Anzic J, Jereb B. Value of fine needle aspiration biopsy in childhood rhabdomyosarcoma: twenty-six years of experience in Slovenia. *Med Pediatr Oncol* 2002; **38**: 416–20.

63. Cecchetto G, Carli M, Sotti G *et al*. Importance of local treatment in pediatric soft tissue sarcomas with microscopic residual after primary surgery: results of the Italian Cooperative Study RMS-88. *Med Pediatr Oncol* 2000; **34**: 97–101.

64. Flamant F, Rodary C, Praquin MT *et al*. Treatment of non-metastatic rhabdomyosarcomas in childhood and adolescence. Results of the second study of the International Society of Paediatric Oncology: MMT84. *Eur J Cancer* 1998; **34**: 1050–62.

65. Hays DM, Lawrence W Jr *et al*. Primary re-excision for patients with 'microscopic residual' tumor following initial

excision of sarcomas of trunk and extremity sites. *J Pediatr Surg* 1989; **24**: 5–10.

66. Cecchetto G, Guglielmi M, Inserra A *et al.* Primary re-excision: the Italian experience in patients with localized soft tissue sarcomas. *Pediatr Surg Int* 2001; **17**: 532–4.

67. Neville HL, Andrassy RJ, Lally KP *et al.* Lymphatic mapping with sentinel node biopsy in pediatric patients. *J Pediatr Surg* 2000; **35**: 961–4.

●68. Ferrari A, Bisogno G, Casanova M *et al.* Paratesticular rhabdomyosarcoma: report from the Italian and German Cooperative Group. *J Clin Oncol* 2002; **20**: 449–55.

68a. Stewart RJ, Martelli H, Oberlin O *et al.* Treatment of children with nonmetastatic paratesticular rhabdomyosarcoma: results of the Malignant Mesenchymal Tumors studies (MMT 84 and MMT 89) of the International Society of Pediatric Oncology. *J Clin Oncol* 2003; **21**: 793–8.

69. Wiener E, Lawrence W, Hays DM *et al.* Complete response or not complete response? Second look operations are the answer in children with rhabdomyosarcoma. *Proc Am Soc Clin Oncol* 1991; **10**: 316.

70. Godzinski J, Flamant F, Rey A *et al.* Value of post-chemotherapy bioptical verification of complete clinical remission in previously incompletely resected (St I and IIpT3) malignant mesenchymal tumors in children: SIOP MMT 84. *Med Pediatr Oncol* 1994; **22**: 22–6.

71. Tefft M,Lindberg RD, Gehan A. Radiation therapy combined with systemic chemotherapy of rhabdomyosarcoma in children: local control in patients enrolled in the Intergroup Rhabdomyosarcoma Study. *NCI Monogr* 1981; **56**: 75–81.

72. Koscielniak E, Jurgens H, Winkler K *et al.* Treatment of soft tissue sarcoma in childhood and adolescence. *Cancer* 1992; **70**: 2557–67.

73. Wolden SL, Anderson JR, Crist WM *et al.* Indications for radiotherapy and chemotherapy after complete resection in rhabdomyosarcoma: a report from the Intergroup Rhabdomyosarcoma Studies I to III. *J Clin Oncol* 1999; **17**: 3468–75.

●74. Raney B, Tefft M, Newton WA *et al.* Improved prognosis with intensive treatment of children with cranial soft tissue sarcomas arising in nonorbital parameningeal sites. *Cancer* 1987; **59**: 147–55.

●75. Raney RB, Meza J, Anderson IR *et al.* Treatment of children and adolescents with localized parameningeal sarcoma: experience of the Intergroup Rhabdomyosarcoma Study Group protocols IRS-II through-IV, 1978–1997. *Med Pediatr Oncol* 2002; **38**: 22–32.

76. Miralbell R, Cella L, Weber D, Lomax A. Optimizing radiotherapy of orbital and paraorbital tumors: intensity modulated X ray beams vs intensity modulated proton beams. *Int J Radiat Oncol Biol Phys* 2000; **47**: 1111–19.

77. Regine WF, Fontanesi J, Kumar P *et al.* A phase II trial evaluating selective use of altered radiation dose and fractionation in patients with unresectable rhabdomyosarcoma. *Int J Radiat Oncol Biol Phys* 1995; **31**: 779–805.

78. Eifel PJ. Decreased bone growth arrest in weanling rats with multiple radiation fractions per day. *Int J Radiat Oncol Biol Phys* 1988; **15**: 141–5.

79. Regine WF, Fontanesi J, Kumar P *et al.* Local tumor control in rhabdomyosarcoma following low-dose irradiation: comparison of group II and select group III patients. *Int J Radiat Oncol Biol Phys* 1995; **31**: 485–91.

80. Kun L, Etcubanas E, Pratt C *et al.* Treatment factors affecting local control in childhood rhabdomyosarcoma. *Proc Am Soc Clin Oncol* 1986; **5**: 207.

81. Fowler JF. The linear-quadratic formula and progress in fractionated radiotherapy. *Br J Radiol* 1989; **62**: 679–94.

●82. Donaldson SS, Meza J, Breneman JC *et al.* Results from the IRS-IV randomized trial of hyperfractionated radiotherapy in children with rhabdomyosarcoma – A report from the IRSG. *Int J Radiat Oncol Biol Phys* 2001; **51**: 718–28.

83. Saunders MI, Dische S, Hong A *et al.* Continuous hyperfractionated accelerated radiotherapy in locally advanced carcinoma of the head and neck region. *Int J Radiat Oncol Biol Phys* 1989; **17**: 1287–93.

84. Mandell LR, Ghavimi F, Exelby P *et al.* Preliminary results of alternating combination chemotherapy and hyperfractionated radiotherapy in advanced rhabdomyosarcoma. *Int J Radiat Oncol Biol Phys* 1988; **15**: 197–203.

85. Sotti G, Scarzello G, Bisogno G *et al.* Combined hyperfractionated-accelerated radiation therapy and chemotherapy related toxicity in the Italian Cooperative Study RMS-88. *Med Pediatr Oncol* 1994; **25**: 273.

86. Arndt C, Donaldson S, Anderson J *et al.* What constitutes optimal therapy for patients with rhabdomyosarcoma of the female genital tract. *Cancer* 2001; **91**: 2454–68.

87. Gerbaulet A, Panis X, Flamant F *et al.* Iridium afterloading curietherapy in the treatment of pediatric malignancies. The Institute Gustave Roussy Experience. *Cancer* 1985; **56**: 1274–9.

88. Nag S, Grecula J, Ruymann F. Aggressive chemotherapy, organ preserving surgery and high-dose rate remote brachytherapy in the treatment of rhabdomyosarcoma in infants and young children. *Cancer* 1993; **72**: 2769–76.

88a. Nag S, Tippin D, Ruymann FB. Long-term morbidity in children treated with fractionated high-dose-rate brachytherapy for soft tissue sarcomas. *J Pediatr Hematol Oncol* 2003; **25**: 448–52.

♦89. Nag S, Shasha D, Janjan N *et al.* The American Brachytherapy Society recommendations for brachytherapy of soft tissue sarcomas. *Int J Radiat Oncol Biol Phys* 2001; **49**: 1033–43.

●90. Green DM, Jaffe N. Progress and controversy in the treatment of childhood rhabdomyosarcoma. *Cancer Treat Rev* 1978; **5**: 7–27.

91. Baum ES, Gaynon P, Greenberg L *et al.* Phase II trial of cisplatin in refractory childhood cancer: Children's Cancer Study Group report. *Cancer Treat Rep* 1981; **65**: 815–22.

92. Schniall H. Review of etoposide single agent activity. *Cancer Treat Rev* 1982; **9**: 21–30.

93. Carli M, Passone E, Perilongo G *et al.* Ifosfamide in pediatric solid tumors. *Oncology* 2003; **65**(Suppl. 2): 99–104.

94. Bode V. Methotrexate as relapse therapy for rhabdomyosarcoma. *Am J Pediatr Hematol Oncol* 1986; **8**: 70–2.

95. Pappo AB, Bowman LC, Furman WL *et al.* A phase II trial of high-dose methotrexate in previously untreated children and adolescents with high-risk unresectable or metastatic rhabdomyosarcoma. *J Pediatr Hematol Oncol* 1997; **19**: 438–42.

96. Horowitz ME, Etcubanas E, Christensen NL *et al.* Phase II testing of melphalan in children with newly diagnosed rhabdomyosarcoma: a model for anticancer drug development. *J Clin Oncol* 1988; **6**: 308–14.

97. Bagnulo S, Perez DJ, Barrett A et al. High dose melphalan and autologous bone marrow transplantation for solid tumors of childhood. Eur Paediatr Haematol Oncol 1985; 1: 129.

98. Houghton PJ, Cheshire PJ, Hallman JD et al. Efficacy of topoisomerase 1 inhibitors, topotecan and irinotecan, administered at low dose levels in protracted schedules to mice bearing xenografts of human tumors. Cancer Chemother Pharmacol 1995; 36: 393–403.

99. Pappo AS, Lyden E, Breneman J et al. Up-front window trial of topotecan in previously untreated children and adolescents with metastatic rhabdomyosarcoma: an intergroup rhabdomyosarcoma study. J Clin Oncol 2001; 19: 213–19.

100. Nitschker R, Parkhurst J, Sullivan J et al. Topotecan in pediatric patients with recurrent and progressive solid tumors: a Pediatric Oncology Group phase II study. J Pediatr Hematol Oncol 1998; 20: 315–18.

● 101. Casanova M, Ferrari A, Spreafico F et al. Vinorelbine in previously treated advanced childhood sarcomas: evidence of activity in rhabdomyosarcoma. Cancer 2002; 94: 3263–8.

● 102. Maurer HM, Beltangady M, Gehan EA et al. The Intergroup Rhabdomyosarcoma Study-I. A final report. Cancer 1988; 1: 209–20.

103. Maurer HM, Gehan EA, Beltangady M et al. The Intergroup Rhabdomyosarcoma Study-II. Cancer 1993; 71: 1904–22.

104. Flamant F, Rodary F, Voute PA et al. Primary chemotherapy in the treatment of rhabdomyosarcoma in children: Trial of the International Society of Pediatric Oncology (SIOP). Preliminary results. Radiat Oncol 1985; 3: 227–36.

105. Carli M, Pastore G, Perilongo G et al. Tumor response and toxicity after single high-dose versus standard five-day divided-dose dactinomycin in childhood rhabdomyosarcoma. J Clin Oncol 1988; 6: 654–8.

106. Treuner J, Koscielniak E, Keim M. Comparison of the rates of response to ifosfamide and cyclophosphamide in primary unresectable rhabdomyosarcoma. Cancer Chemother Pharmacol 1989; 24: 48–50.

107. Otten J, Flamant F, Rodary C et al. Treatment of rhabdomyosarcoma and other malignant mesenchymal tumors of childhood with ifosfamide + vincristine + dactinomycin (IVA) as front-line therapy. Cancer Chemother Pharmacol 1989; 24: 30.

● 108. Miser JS, Kinsella TJ, Triche TJ et al. Ifosfamide with mesna uroprotection and etoposide: an effective regimen in the treatment of recurrent sarcomas and other tumors of children and young adults. J Clin Oncol 1987; 5: 191–8.

109. Sandler E, Lyden E, Ruymn F et al. Efficacy of ifosfamide and doxorubicin given as a phase II 'window' in children with newly diagnosed metastatic rhabdomyosarcoma: a report from the Intergroup Rhabdomyosarcoma Study Group. Med Pediatr Oncol 2001; 37: 442–8.

110. Carli M, Perilongo G, Cordero di Montezemolo L et al. Phase II trial of cisplatin and etoposide in children with advanced soft tissue sarcoma: a report from the Italian Cooperative Rhabdomyosarcoma Group. Cancer Treat Rep 1987; 71: 525–7.

111. Schimitt C, Flamant F, Rodary C. Efficacy of cisplatin-adriamycin in combination in children with rhabdomyo-sarcoma. Proc Am Soc Clin Oncol 1989; 9: 306.

112. Frascella E, Pritchard-Jones K, Modak S et al. Response of previously untreated metastatic rhabdomyosarcoma to combination chemotherapy with carboplatin, epirubicin and vincristine. Eur J Cancer 1996; 32: 821–5.

113. Sailors RL, Stine KC, Sullivan J et al. Cyclophosphamide plus topotecan in children with recurrent or refractory solid tumors: a Pediatric Oncology Group Phase II Study. J Clin Oncol 2001; 19: 3463–9.

114. Thompson J, George EO, Poquette CA et al. Synergy of topotecan in combination with vincristine for treatment of pediatric solid tumor xenografts. Clin Cancer Res 1999; 5: 3617–31.

115. Coggins CA, Elion GB, Houghton PJ et al. Enhancement of irinotecan (CPT-11) activity against central nervous system tumor xenografts by alkylating agents. Cancer Chemother Pharmacol 1998; 41: 485–90.

116. Raney B, Tefft M, Heyn R et al. Ascending myelitis after intensive chemotherapy and radiation therapy in children with cranial parameningeal sarcoma. Cancer 1992; 69: 1498–506.

117. De Vita VT. Dose-response is alive and well. J Clin Oncol 1986; 4: 1157–9.

♦ 118. Goldie JH, Coldman AJ. The genetic origin of drug resistance in neoplasms: implications for systemic therapy. Cancer Res 1984; 44: 3643–53.

● 119. Raney RB, Anderson JR, Barr FG et al. Rhabdomyosarcoma and undifferentiated sarcoma in the first two decades of life: a selective review of Intergroup Rhabdomyosarcoma Study group experience and rationale for Intergroup Rhabdomyosarcoma Study V. J Pediatr Hematol Oncol 2001; 23:215–20.

120. Carli M, Colombatti O, Oberlin O et al. High dose melphalan with autologous stem cell rescue in metastatic rhabdomyosarcoma. J Clin Oncol 1999; 17: 2796–803.

● 121. Pinkerton CR, Groot-Loonen J, Barrett A et al. Rapid VAC high dose melphalan regimen, a novel chemotherapy approach in childhood soft tissue sarcomas. Br J Cancer 1991; 64: 381–5.

122. Koscelniak E, Klingebiel TH, Peters C et al. Do patients with metastatic and recurrent rhabdomyosarcoma benefit from high-dose therapy with hematopoietic rescue? Report of the German/Austrian Pediatric Bone Marrow Transplant Group. Bone Marrow Transplant 1997; 19: 227–31.

123. Malogolowkin MH, Sposto R, Grovas L et al. Lack of improvement in survival of children with metastatic rhabdomyosarcoma treated with intensive therapy followed by stem cell transplant for control of minimal residual disease. Proc Am Soc Clin Oncol 1999; 18: 555a.

● 124. Walterhouse DO, Hoover ML, Marymont MAH et al. High-dose chemotherapy followed by peripheral blood stem cell rescue for metastatic rhabdomyosarcoma: the experience at Chicago Children's Memorial Hospital. Med Pediatr Oncol 1999; 32: 88–92.

● 125. Boulad F, Kernan NA, LaQuaglia MP et al. High-dose induction chemotherapy followed by peripheral blood stem cell rescue for metastatic rhabdomyosarcoma: the experience at Chicago Children's Memorial Hospital. J Clin Oncol 1998; 16: 1697–706.

126. Oberlin O, Rey A, Anderson J et al. Treatment of orbital rhabdomyosarcoma: survival and late effects of treatment. Results of an international workshop. *J Clin Oncol* 2001; **19**: 197–204.

127. Sutow W, Sullivan MP, Ried HL et al. Prognosis in childhood rhabdomyosarcoma. *Cancer* 1979; **25:** 1384–91.

128. Anderson J, Carli M, Oberlin O et al. International study of characteristics and outcome of patients with primary rhabdomyosarcoma of the bladder/prostate. *Med Pediatr Oncol* 2001; **37**: 181.

129. Carli M, Perilongo G. Pattern of treatment failure and the meaning of complete response in rhabdomyosarcoma. In: Murer HM, Ruymann F, Pochedly C, eds. *Rhabdomyosarcoma and Related Tumours in Childhood and Adolescence.* Boca Raton, FL: CRC Press, 1991; 261–71.

130. Dehner LP. Soft tissue sarcomas. In: Dehner LP, ed. *Pediatric Surgical Pathology,* 2nd edn. Baltimore: Williams and Wilkins, 1987: 869.

●131. Hays D. New approaches to the surgical management of rhabdomyosarcoma in childhood. *Chir Pediatr* 1990; **31**: 197–201.

132. Horowitz ME, Pratt CB, Webber L et al. Therapy for childhood soft-tissue sarcomas other than rhabdomyosarcoma: a review of 62 cases. *J Clin Oncol* 1986; **4**: 559–64.

133. Parham DM, Webber BL, Jenkins JJ III et al. Nonrhabdomyosarcomatous soft tissue sarcomas of childhood: formulation of a simplified system for grading. *Mod Pathol* 1995; **8**: 705–10.

134. Dehner LP. Peripheral and central primitive neuroectodermal tumors. A nosologic concept seeking a consensus. *Arch Pathol Lab Med* 1986; **110**: 997–1005.

135. Cavazzana A, Ninfo V, Roberts J. Peripheral neuroepithelioma: a light microscopy, immunocytochemical and ultrastructural study. *Mod Pathol* 1992; **5**: 71–8.

●136. Cavazzana AO, Miser JS, Jefferson J et al. Experimental evidence for a neural origin of Ewing's sarcoma of bone. *Am J Pathol* 1987; **127:** 507–18.

137. Raney RB, Asmar L, Newton WA et al. Ewing sarcoma of soft tissue in childhood: a report from the Intergroup Rhabdomyosarcoma Study, 1972 to 1991. *J Clin Oncol* 1999; **15**: 574–82.

138. Niggli FK, Scopinaro M, Rey A et al. Treatment of non metastatic peripheral primitive neuroectodermal tumor (PNET) extraosseous Ewing's sarcoma (EOES): experience in the SIOP-MMT 89 Study. *Med Pediatr Oncol* 2001; **37**: 188.

●139. Bisogno G, Carli M, Stevens M et al. Intensive chemotherapy for children and young adults with metastatic primitive neuroectodermal tumors of the soft tissue. *Bone Marrow Transplant* 2002; **30**: 297–302.

140. Chung EB, Enzinger FM. Infantile fibrosarcoma. *Cancer* 1976; **38**: 729–39.

141. Coffin CM. Congenital-infantile fibrosarcoma: a comparison with adult-type fibrosarcoma. In: Coffin CM, Dehner LP, O'Shea PA, eds. *Pediatric Soft Tissue Tumors. A Clinical, Pathological and Therapeutic Approach.* Baltimore: Lippincott 1997; 164–70.

●142. Fisher C. Fibromatosis and fibrosarcoma in infancy and childhood. *Eur J Cancer* 1996; **32A**: 2094–100.

143. Soule EH, Pritchard DJ. Fibrosarcoma in infants and children. A review of 110 cases. *Cancer* 1977; **40**: 1711–21.

144. Cecchetto G, Carli M, Alaggio R et al. Fibrosarcoma in pediatric patients: results of the Italian Cooperative Group Studies (1979–1995). *J Surg Oncol* 2001; **78**: 225–31.

145. Ninane J. Chemotherapy for infantile fibrosarcoma. *Med Pediatr Oncol* 1991; **19**: 209.

146. Shetty AK, Yu LC, Gardner RV et al. Role of chemotherapy in the treatment of infantile fibrosarcoma. *Med Pediatr Oncol* 1999; **33**: 425–7.

147. Stout AP. Juvenile fibromatoses. *Cancer* 1954; **7**: 953–78.

148. Chung EB. Pitfalls in diagnosis of benign soft tissue tumours in infancy and childhood. *Pathol Annu* 1985; **20**: 323–86.

●149. Ayala AG, Ro JY, Goepfert H et al. Desmoid fibromatosis: a clinicopathologic study of 25 children. *Semin Diagn Pathol* 1986; **3**: 138–50.

150. Shapek SX, Hawk BJ, Hoffer FA et al. Combination chemotherapy using vinblastine and methotrexate for the treatment of progressive desmoid tumor in children. *J Clin Oncol* 1998; **16**: 3021–7.

151. Schmidt D, Thum P, Harms D et al. Synovial sarcoma in children and adolescents. A report from the Kiel Pediatric Tumor Registry. *Cancer* 1991; **67**: 1667–72.

152. Pilz T, Ganz C, Knietig R et al. Synovial sarcoma in childhood and adolescence in CWS 81–96 Trials. *Med Pediatr Oncol* 2000; **35**: 179.

153. Ladenstein R, Treuner J, Koscielniak E et al. Synovial sarcoma of childhood and adolescence. Report of the German CWS-81 study. *Cancer* 1993; **71**: 3647–55.

154. Pappo AS, Fontanesi J, Luo X et al. Synovial sarcoma in children and adolescents: the St Jude Children's Research Hospital experience. *J Clin Oncol* 1994; **12**: 2360–6.

155. Ferrari A, Casanova M, Massimino M et al. Synovial sarcoma: report of a series of 25 consecutive children from a single institution. *Med Pediatr Oncol* 1999; **32**: 32–7.

156. Okcu MF, Despa S, Choroszy M et al. Synovial sarcoma in children and adolescents: thirty three years of experience with multimodal therapy. *Med Pediatr Oncol* 2001; **37**: 90–6.

157. Okcu MF, Munsell M, Treuner J et al. Synovial sarcoma of childhood and adolescence: a multicenter, multivariate analysis of outcome. *J Clin Oncol* 2003; **21**: 1602–11.

158. Cagle LA, Mirra JM, Storm FK. Histologic features relating to prognosis in synovial sarcoma. *Cancer* 1987; **59**: 1810–14.

159. Flamant F. Tumours mesenchymateuse malignes en dehors du rhabdomyosarcoma. In: Lemerle J, ed. *F. Cancer de l'Enfant Encyclopedie des Cancers.* Paris: Flammarion, 1989; 446–56.

160. Ladenstein R, Treuner J, Koscielniak E et al. Synovial sarcoma of childhood and adolescence. Report of the German CWS-81 study. *Cancer* 1993; **71**: 3647–55.

162. Meis JM, Enzinger FM, Martz KL, Neal JA. Malignant peripheral nerve sheath tumors (malignant Schwannomas) in children. *Am J Surg Pathol* 1992; **16**: 694–707.

163. Raney B, Schnauffer L, Ziegler M et al. Treatment of children with neurogenic sarcoma. Experience at the Children's Hospital of Philadelphia 1958–1984. *Cancer* 1987; **59**: 1–5.

●164. Carli M, Bisogno G, Matte AC et al. Malignant peripheral nerve sheath tumors in childhood (MPNST). A combined experience of the Italian and German co-operative study groups (ICG and CWS). Med Pediatr Oncol 2001; 37: 184.

●165. Ferrari A, Bisogno G, Casanova M et al. Childhood leiomyosarcoma: a report from the Soft Tissue Sarcoma Italian Cooperative Group. Ann Oncol 2001; 12: 1163–8.

●166. Casanova M, Ferrari A, Bisogno G et al. Alveolar soft part sarcoma in children and adolescents: a report from the Soft Tissue Sarcoma Italian Cooperative Group. Ann Oncol 2000; 11: 1445–9.

●167. Ferrari A, Casanova M, Bisogno G et al. Hemangiopericytoma in pediatric ages. A report from the Italian and German Soft Tissue Sarcoma Cooperative Group. Cancer 2001; 92: 2692–8.

●168. Ferrari A, Casanova M, Bisogno G et al. Malignant vascular tumours in children and adolescents: a report from the Italian and German Soft Tissue Sarcoma Cooperative Group. Med Pediatr Oncol 2002; 39: 109–14.

169. Ferrari A, Casanova M, Bisogno G et al. Clear cell sarcoma of tendons and aponeuroses in pediatric patients. A report from the Italian and German Soft Tissue Sarcoma Cooperative Group. Cancer 2002; 94: 3269–76.

●170. Bisogno G, Roganovich J, Sotti G et al. Desmoplastic small round cell tumour in children and adolescents. Med Pediatr Oncol 2000; 34: 338–42.

●171. Raney RB, Asmar L, Vassilopoulou-Sellin R et al. Late complications of therapy in 213 children with localised, non orbital soft tissue sarcoma of the head and neck: a descriptive report from the Intergroup Rhabdomyosarcoma Studies (IRS) II and III. Med Pediatr Oncol 1999; 33: 362–71.

●172. Raney RB, Anderson JR, Kollath J et al. Late effects of therapy in 94 patients with localised rhabdomyosarcoma of the orbit: report from the Intergroup Rhabdomyosarcoma Study (IRS)-III, 1984–1991. Med Pediatr Oncol 2000; 34: 413–20.

173. Raney RB, Heyn R, Hays D et al. Sequelae of treatment in 109 patients followed for five to fifteen years after diagnosis of sarcoma of the bladder and prostate: a report from the Intergroup Rhabdomyosarcoma Committee. Cancer 1993; 71: 2387–94.

174. Gamba PG, Cecchetto G, Katende M et al. Paratesticular rhabdomyosarcoma (RMS) and paraaortic lymphadenectomy. Eur J Pediatr Surg 1994; 4: 158–60.

175. Hughes LL, Baruzzi MJ, Ribeiro RC et al. Paratesticular rhabdomyosarcoma: delayed effects of multimodality therapy and implications for current management. Cancer 1994; 73: 467–82.

176. Weiner ES, Anderson JR, Ojimba JI et al. Controversies in the management of paratesticular rhabdomyosarcomas: is staging retro peritoneal lymph node dissection necessary for adolescents with resected paratesticular rhabdomyosarcoma? Semin Pediatr Surg 2001; 10: 146–52.

177. Skinner R, Cotterill SJ, Stevens MCG. Risk factors for nephrotoxicity after ifosfamide treatment in children: a UKCCSG Late Effects Group Study. Br J Cancer 2000; 82: 1636–45.

178. Kaplan E, Sklar C, Wilmott R, Michaels S, Ghavimi F. Pulmonary function in children treated for rhabdomyosarcoma. Med Pediatr Oncol 1996; 27: 79–84.

179. Heyn R, Haeberlen V, Newton WA et al. Second malignant neoplasms in children treated for rhabdomyosarcoma. J Clin Oncol 1993; 11: 262–70.

180. Hawkins MM, Kinnier Wilson LM, Burton HS et al. Radiotherapy, alkylating agents and the risk of bone cancer after childhood cancer. J Natl Cancer Inst 1996; 88: 270–8.

●181. Scaradavou A, Heller G, Sklar C, Ren L, Ghavimi F. Second malignant neoplasms in long term survivors of childhood rhabdomyosarcoma. Cancer 1995, 76: 1860–7.

182. Benk V, Rodary C, Flamant F et al. Parameningeal rhabdomyosarcoma. Results of an international workshop. Int J Radiat Oncol Biol Phys 1996; 36: 534–40.

183. Stevens MCG. The treatment of soft tissue sarcoma, the philosophy of treatment and the concept of the 'total burden of therapy'. Med Pediatr Oncol 2001; 37: 196.

184. Bramwell VH. Adjuvant chemotherapy for adult soft tissue sarcoma: Is there a standard of care? J Clin Oncol 2001; 19: 1235–7.

●185. Pratt CB, Maurer HM, Gieser P et al. Treatment of unresectable or metastatic pediatric soft tissue sarcoma with surgery, irradiation and chemotherapy. A Pediatric Oncology Group Study. Med Pediatr Oncol 1998; 30: 201–9.

186. Meco D, Colombo T, Ubezio P et al. Effective combination of ET-743 and doxorubicin in sarcoma: preclinical studies. Cancer Chemother Pharmacol 2003; 52: 131–8.

18

Bone tumours

JEREMY WHELAN & BRUCE MORLAND

INTRODUCTION

Primary tumours of bone are generally uncommon but have a well recognized peak incidence between 10 and 20 years of age. The second commonest solid malignancy in this age group, these diseases provide distinct challenges to both patient and carer alike. In particular, the adverse functional consequences of reconstructive surgery can be especially burdensome in addition to the side-effects of intensive chemotherapy. Most importantly, recent survival trends have been disappointing after the initial dramatic improvements recognized when effective chemotherapy was first introduced 20 years ago. The commonest primary bone cancers, osteosarcoma and Ewing's family of tumours (EFT), remain biological puzzles, the unravelling of which may hold the key to further improvements in survival.

AETIOLOGY AND EPIDEMIOLOGY

Osteosarcoma and Ewing's sarcoma account for over 90 per cent of primary bone tumours occurring in children and adolescents. While the biological relationship of these diseases seems very distant, there are distinct clinical characteristics suggesting aetiological similarities. Both diseases occur in children and young adults, principally in teenagers, and commonly coincide with maximum linear bone growth, both in tumour location and age of incidence. However, in a paper by Buckley et al.[1] investigating epidemiological factors in 305 cases of bone tumour in children, no consistent differences between controls and cases were identified.

Genetic factors associated with both diseases are shown in Table 18.1. Sarcomas of all types occur as a feature of Li–Fraumeni syndrome. Osteosarcoma is one of the

Table 18.1 *Aetiological factors in the development of osteosarcoma and Ewing's tumours*

	Osteosarcoma	Ewing's family of tumours
Retinoblastoma	Common second malignancy after inherited retinoblastoma. Alterations in *Rb* common in sporadic osteosarcoma	Exceptionally uncommon after retinoblastoma
Li–Fraumeni	Common association but *p53* mutations account for very small proportion of sporadic osteosarcoma	No clear association
Racial	No clear racial differences	Uncommon in some races
Radiation	Common second malignancy after radiation	No clear association
Prior alkylator therapy	Associated with osteosarcoma as second malignancy	No clear association
Skeletal growth	Clear but unexplained association with rapid bone growth	Clear but unexplained association with rapid bone growth

commoner associated tumours, but in contrast EFT have no clear association. Survivors of retinoblastoma have an excess risk of osteosarcoma occurring both within and without an irradiated area. The additional risk that therapeutic radiation poses for the development of osteosarcoma is well documented but principally accounts for tumours occurring in adults rather than in children.[2]

Ewing's sarcomas are approximately half as common as osteosarcomas in the paediatric population, accounting for approximately 30 per cent of all bone tumours seen in this age group. This translates into an estimate of 0.18 cases per 100 000 of the population under 14 years of age.[1,3] There is a slight male predominance, tumours are most commonly seen in the second decade of life and there are clear racial differences: EFT are unusual in black and oriental populations.[4]

OSTEOSARCOMA

Clinical presentation and diagnosis

The initial clinical features of osteosarcoma are rarely so characteristic as to indicate the diagnosis. The most common complaint is pain. When examined, early signs may be few. Thus pain is often ascribed to trauma or, worse, 'growing pains' and the underlying cause may remain unrecognized until the pain is intolerable or other features, most often swelling, become obvious. If the primary site is in the pelvis or other axial skeleton site, diagnosis may be very delayed. Too often the significance of persistent pain, especially pain which disturbs the sleep of adolescents, is ignored.

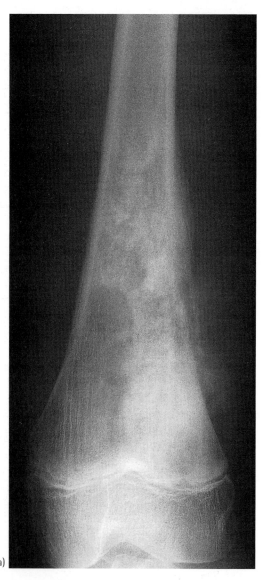

(a)

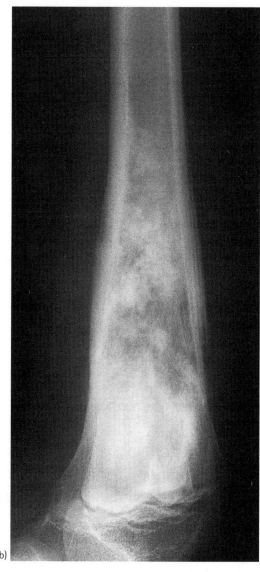

(b)

Figure 18.1 *Plain radiograph of osteosarcoma of distal femur showing chaotic new bone formation, cortical destruction and cortical elevation ('Codman's triangle').*

Although 10–15 per cent of patients will be found to have metastases when staged, indicative symptoms such as cough or shortness of breath are rare. Systemic symptoms such as weight loss or fever are very uncommon and may indicate unusually aggressive and extensive disease.

Plain radiography is a crucial investigation, as characteristic radiological features of osteosarcoma may be present (Figure 18.1). Further three-dimensional imaging with magnetic resonance (MRI) should then be undertaken before proceeding to biopsy. MRI will identify both the intraosseous and extraosseous extents of tumour, and show its relationship to the neurovascular bundle and to the epiphysis, all of which are important factors for the planning of surgery (Figure 18.2).

Biopsy should be carried out with meticulous care. In the past an open procedure was carried out with a carefully planned longitudinal incision, the track of which is excised at the time of definitive tumour resection. This has been replaced in most specialist centres by core needle biopsy. In acknowledgement of the histological heterogeneity of osteosarcoma, diagnostic yield is ensured by correlation of the area biopsied with imaging. Additionally, the biopsy is placed to allow subsequent excision of the track. Needle biopsy is quicker and carries lower morbidity. Multiple cores can be taken to provide additional information for ancillary diagnostics or for biological studies.

Staging for newly diagnosed osteosarcoma is completed by an isotope bone scan and thoracic computed tomography (CT) scan (Figures 18.3 and 18.4). The most important route of spread is in the bloodstream, principally to the lungs. Continuing improvements in the sensitivity of imaging techniques are leading to a greater proportion of patients identified as having metastatic disease at presentation, probably between 15 and 20 per cent, in contrast to the previous figure of 10 per cent. Bone metastases are less common. 'Skip' metastases are those identified proximally in the same bone as the primary. More distant metastases may be suggested by the isotope scan but are always confirmed by additional MRI. Biopsy of suspected metastatic lesions is occasionally indicated when the radiology is equivocal and when the information thus gained will alter management.

Another investigation that may be helpful in certain situations to aid diagnosis or treatment planning is additional imaging of the primary with high-resolution CT, which may highlight bone cortex and arteriography. Positron emission tomography (PET) scanning has as yet not been clearly identified as adding valuable discriminatory information to standard staging investigations.[5,6] Serum alkaline phosphatase provides prognostic information, although this is uncommonly independent in multivariate analyses.

Histology

The histological classification of bone tumours is shown in Box 18.1. Diagnosis may be made rapidly by examination of cytological imprint impressions of a core biopsy. Morphology supplemented by staining for cytoplasmic

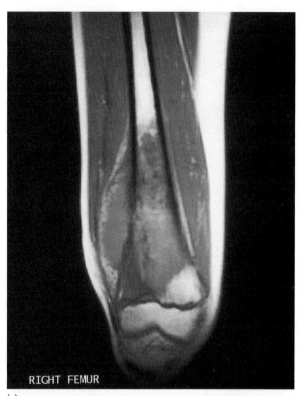

RIGHT FEMUR

(a)

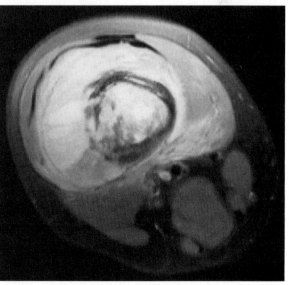

(b)

Figure 18.2 *(a, b) Magnetic resonance scan of tumour shown in Figure 18.1. The intramedullary and extraosseous extents are clearly seen. The relationship to the neurovascular bundle is evident on the transverse image (b).*

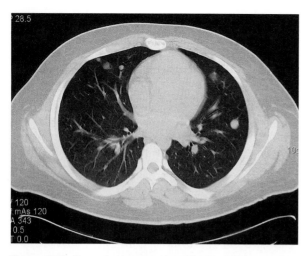

Figure 18.3 *Computed tomography of thorax showing characteristic appearance of pulmonary metastases.*

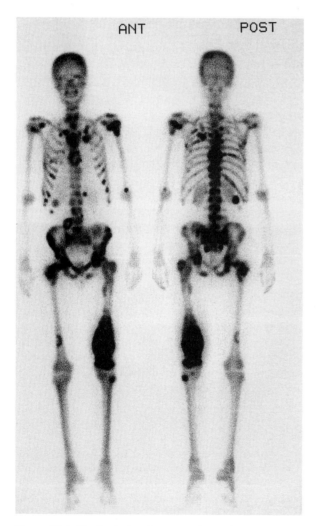

Figure 18.4 *Staging isotope bone scan demonstrating extensive skeletal metastases from an osteoblastic osteosarcoma.*

Box 18.1 *Histological classification of bone tumours*

> A Osteosarcoma
>   1 High-grade central:
>   mixed, fibroblastic, osteoblastic,
>   chondroblastic, osteoclast-rich, small cell
>   2 Low-grade central
>   3 Surface
>   4 High-grade surface, periosteal, parosteal
> B Ewing's family of tumours
> C Chondrosarcoma
>   1 Chondrosarcoma (grades 1–3)
>   2 Dedifferentiated chondrosarcoma
>   3 Mesenchymal chondrosarcoma
> D Malignant fibrous histiocytoma of bone
> E Other spindle cell tumours of bone:
>   fibrosarcoma, leiomyosarcoma,
>   liposarcoma, haemangiopericytoma,
>   haemangioendothelioma
> F Primary bone lymphoma
> G Post-radiation sarcoma
> H Paget's sarcoma

expression of alkaline phosphatase is the main diagnostic technique, with immunocytochemistry usually adding little further information.

The majority of osteosarcomas are high-grade intramedullary lesions. The morphological appearances may be quite varied depending on the dominant cell type and the amount of osteoid (abnormal disorganized new bone formation) being produced by the tumour. The majority of high-grade lesions contain an admix of malignant cells, while in others, dominant components are evident, reflected in the nomenclature as chondroblastic and osteoblastic types. The significance of subtype is unclear, as in large series the number of the less common subtypes is small.[7] Telangiectatic osteosarcoma may be suspected by a very lytic radiographic appearance and biopsy may be very bloody, reflecting the blood-filled spaces that characterize this tumour. There is some evidence that the outcome of such tumours may be relatively favourable. Osteoclast-rich tumours may also be predominantly lytic and contain large numbers of osteoclasts, sometimes leading to a mistaken diagnosis of giant cell tumour.

Low-grade intramedullary and surface tumours are very uncommon. It is particularly important to recognize the latter, correlation between radiology and biopsy being essential. While some high-grade lesions arise on the cortical surface of the bone, other types, periosteal and parosteal osteosarcomas, have a lower propensity to metastasize. Chemotherapy is not indicated for the latter while its role in the management of periosteal osteosarcoma is unclear.

A key role for the pathologist in the management of osteosarcoma is the examination of the resected primary tumour after preoperative chemotherapy. As well as establishing the completeness of excision, the extent of chemotherapy-induced necrosis provides prognostic information as discussed below. This is laborious as the entire tumour must be mapped, and blocks taken from selected areas and then examined for the extent of viable tumour. Scoring systems are then applied which reflect the degree of non-viable tumour as a percentage.

Treatment

Like many other cancers occurring in the young, significant improvements in the outcome of treatment have occurred since the introduction of combined modality therapies and the greater acceptance that treatment should be given within well designed clinical trials. Concentration of expertise in specialist centres, particularly for complex reconstructive surgery, seems especially desirable, and additional consideration should be given to the particular needs of teenagers in whom such tumours have their peak incidence.

Sufficient information exists to inform us of the poor outcome of osteosarcoma treated by surgery alone, as this, in the form of amputation, remained the standard care until the 1970s. Until then, survival rarely exceeded 15–20 per cent, with most patients rapidly succumbing to lung metastases. During the 1970s, developments such as the identification of active chemotherapy agents against advanced disease, limb reconstruction methods that avoided amputation and, finally, an aggressive approach to the surgical excision of lung metastases all led to the now accepted approach to treatment of this disease, i.e. preoperative ('neoadjuvant') chemotherapy followed by limb-salvage surgery and further chemotherapy. This strategy results in more that half of all patients with extremity tumours being cured.

LOCAL THERAPY

Complete surgical excision is a prerequisite for cure of osteosarcoma.[8] In contrast to EFT, radiotherapy does not provide a satisfactory alternative as the dose required to give any expectation of local control would be associated with unacceptable morbidity. Thus, experienced surgical evaluation is an essential part of initial assessment and should continue through the period of preoperative chemotherapy.

Most osteosarcomas arise in the extremity, especially around the knee and shoulder girdle. Surgery must achieve complete excision of the tumour at the least subsequent cost to limb function. While amputation is associated with very low local recurrence rates, it is less acceptable to patients and there are significant lifelong 'maintenance' costs of the prosthetic limb.[9] Limb salvage involves excision of the affected segment of bone and its replacement either with a metallic endoprosthesis or so-called biological reconstructions in which harvested host bone such as the fibula or bone allograft, or a combination, is used. Functional consequences of such surgery principally relate to the need for joint excision and replacement or the need to replace a segment of a growing limb. A variety of 'growing' prostheses may be used for the latter but often involve numerous 'lengthening' operations until maximum height is gained. Preservation of joints can more often be achieved with biological reconstruction, but rehabilitation may be prolonged and failure through either poor incorporation or infection is not uncommon (Figure 18.5).

An alternative to such techniques is the van Ness rotationplasty which may be appropriate for young children with tumours around the knee. The distal limb is re-implanted after excision of distal femur and proximal tibia. The foot is rotated 180° and the ankle provides an effective joint over which a special prosthesis can be secured. The function achieved by such surgery can be excellent, exceeding that of amputation and the other methods of reconstruction described above. However, the technique has not been widely adopted, as there are significant issues about patient acceptability that can only be addressed in centres undertaking rotationplasty regularly and that have in place the necessary support for patients and families.[10,10a]

When osteosarcoma arises in the pelvis or vertebrae, the surgical challenges may be extreme. Pelvic tumours that do not involve the acetabulum or cross the sacroiliac joint can often be excised with acceptable morbidity and functional outcome, but more often hindquarter amputation is required, after which rehabilitation with a prosthesis is only achieved by a few.

Choice of surgery and reconstructive approach must come through a dialogue between patient and surgeon, preferably after consideration in a multidisciplinary forum. Comparison between approaches is assisted by several scoring systems for functional outcome, but we remain relatively poorly informed as to ascertaining the best approaches in individual patients.[11]

SYSTEMIC THERAPY

The introduction of chemotherapy has transformed the outlook for osteosarcoma. However, both short- and long-term toxicities of current schedules are unacceptably high. Furthermore, for those with metastatic disease at presentation, axial tumours or those who relapse, current treatment outcomes remain disappointing.

As indicated above, investigation of new approaches to the management of osteosarcoma during the 1970s and

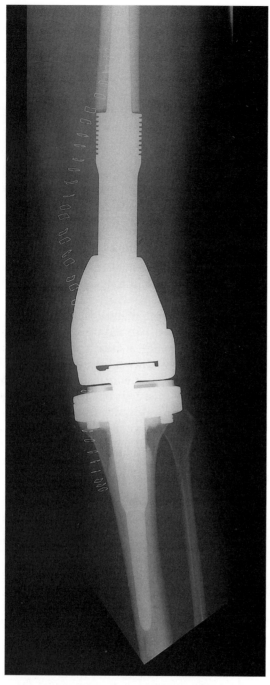

Figure 18.5 *Postoperative radiograph of endoprosthetic replacement after resection of a distal femoral osteosarcoma.*

early 1980s led to several crucial observations that have subsequently stood the test of time and remain enshrined in current treatment schedules. Of particular importance was that the pioneers of preoperative chemotherapy identified that examination of the resected tumour specimen to assess the extent of chemotherapy-induced necrosis could be correlated with prognosis. It is now known that patients who achieve a good histological response to

preoperative chemotherapy, most often defined as <1 per cent residual viable tumour, experience considerabl[y] better survival than those who have a poor respons[e] (≥10 per cent viable tumour). Five-year survival for goo[d] responders is in the region of 75–80 per cent, compare[d] with 45–55 per cent for poor responders.[8,12]

The cytotoxic agents identified in early studies as bein[g] most active against osteosarcoma were doxorubicin, cis[-] platin and methotrexate. These three drugs remain centra[l] to most current first-line schedules. More recently, ifos[-] famide, sometimes in combination with etoposide, ha[s] been demonstrated to have efficacy.[13] It is not yet clea[r] which is the most effective first-line combination, as to[o] few studies have been carried out in which a randomize[d] comparison has been made of different regimens.

The European Osteosarcoma Intergroup has under[-] taken two large randomized trials comparing first-lin[e] neoadjuvant regimens in localized extremity osteosar[-] coma. The first compared the combination of cisplati[n] and methotrexate with or without high doses o[f] methotrexate (the doses of methotrexate used in osteosar[-] coma have traditionally been 8–12 g/m^2). This study faile[d] to identify any advantage for three drugs over two and ha[s] been frequently cited, along with the second Europea[n] Osteosarcoma Intergroup (EOI) study, as evidence agains[t] the inclusion of methotrexate.[14] However, the trial desig[n] was flawed and did not make a true comparison, as th[e] total dose and dose intensity of doxorubicin and cisplati[n] in the methotrexate-containing arm were significantl[y] lower. A subsequent study then compared these two drug[s] with a more complex and prolonged multidrug regime[n] the T10 schedule, which was widely used as a standard reg[-] imen in the United States and parts of Europe. There wa[s] no overall survival difference between the two treatment[s] (55 per cent at 5 years) but this was notably inferior to tha[t] being reported from many single centres and non-ran[-] domized studies from specialist study groups.[15]

One such, the Cooperative Osteosarcoma Study Grou[p] (COSS), consisting of centres in Germany, Austria an[d] Switzerland, has reported a 10-year survival of 71 per cen[t] with the use of methotrexate, cisplatin, doxorubicin an[d] ifosfamide.[16] This trial also evaluated the use of intra[-] arterial cisplatin and found no benefit compared wit[h] intravenous administration.[17]

Similarly, Italian investigators have reported a series o[f] open studies and small randomized trials from the Rizzoll[i] Institute. More recent results using four drugs for mos[t] patients report a 5-year event-free survival (EFS) an[d] overall survival of 56 and 71 per cent, respectively.[18]

The North American Children's Oncology Grou[p] (COG) has reported the results of INT 0133, a 2 × 2 fac[-] torial trial examining the addition of ifosfamide an[d] muramyl tripeptide (MTP), a biological agent, to a contro[l] regimen of MAP (methotrexate, doxorubicin, cisplatin[:] Figure 18.6).[19] Preliminary results of INT 0133 have

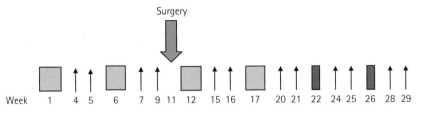

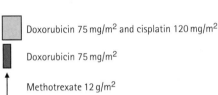

Doxorubicin 75 mg/m^2 and cisplatin 120 mg/m^2

Doxorubicin 75 mg/m^2

Methotrexate 12 g/m^2

Figure 18.6 *Chemotherapy schedule for osteosarcoma based on a three-drug standard regimen used in the Children's Oncology Group randomized clinical trial, INT 0133.*

indicated that although neither treatment tested offers an EFS benefit when added to MAP individually, there may be an unexpected synergistic effect when ifosfamide and MTP are administered together. Because of the conflicting information from this study, the results require reproduction in a further study. Unfortunately, MTP is no longer available, so such a study is unlikely to be undertaken in the foreseeable future.

Considerable consistency has emerged from the groups above regarding prognostic factors for osteosarcoma.[8,20] Certainly, surgical respectability of the primary tumour is critical, as radiotherapy is largely ineffective at rescuing unresectable axial tumours. Patients in whom metastases are present at diagnosis have an inferior survival, with mature results rarely exceeding 20 per cent survival at 5 years. Histological response to preoperative chemotherapy is assessed by careful analysis of the entire resected tumour. Grading systems can be applied to categorize the extent of necrosis. A cut-off of more or less than 90 per cent tumour necrosis is most often used and can separate a group with survival in excess of 70 per cent from those with less than 40 per cent survival. Discussion continues as to the value of division by smaller differences in percentage necrosis, assessment of which has a potentially significant element of subjectivity.

Adjustment of postoperative chemotherapy on the basis of histological response is widely practised but evidence to support this is very limited.[17] Due to the small number of active agents, treatment options in these circumstances are limited and determined by the constituents of preoperative chemotherapy. The use of high doses of ifosfamide has attracted attention as there is some evidence of a dose response, but the ceiling beyond which any further dose escalation is ineffective is unknown.[13,21] Toxicity may be substantial. Further studies are certainly indicated.

More valuable prognostic information should emerge from a greater understanding of the biology of osteosarcoma.[21a,21b] Frequent alterations have been identified in *Rb*,[22,23] *p53* and p-glycoprotein[24,25] and Her 2/neu,[26,27] but there have been inconsistencies in these observations and

so far no factor has been prospectively studied and shown to provide unambiguous prognostic, and thus therapeutically influential, information. It is hoped that further studies using cDNA microarrays may provide more reliable information.[28]

Thus, although significant improvements in survival have been achieved since the widespread use of chemotherapy for osteosarcoma, recent progress has been very limited. While important questions regarding the most effective delivery of the available active agents remain outstanding, it is unlikely that further manipulation of these same drugs will be good enough for those with adverse disease features. New directions are therefore required.

METASTATIC DISEASE AND MANAGEMENT OF RECURRENCE

Between 10 and 15 per cent of patients will have evidence of metastatic disease at presentation, mostly to the lungs and to other bones.[28a] A further 20–50 per cent with initially localized disease will relapse, generally with distant disease, some 10 per cent having a local recurrence. Surgical resectability of metastatic disease should always be considered, as some patients, particularly those with disease confined to the lung, will be cured. Any further role for chemotherapy is determined by the previous treatment received, with responses to previously used drugs rarely occurring. For those with unresectable disease, further chemotherapy will occasionally prolong survival.[29–31]

Future directions

The introduction of innovative new therapies in osteosarcoma is urgently needed. Testing of new cytotoxic agents has been disappointing, as has the application of other techniques which have shown value in other treatments such as high-dose therapy with stem cell support.[32,33] Bone-seeking radioisotopes provide a potentially attractive technique to deliver radiation therapy more effectively but they are still in the early phases of evaluation.[34,35]

It is hoped that insights provided by a greater understanding of the biology of osteosarcoma will lead to better treatments.

EWING'S FAMILY OF TUMOURS

James Ewing first described the tumour that now bears his name over 75 years ago.[36] His original description identified two issues which are still of relevance today:

- the difficulty at times of differentiating the tumour from osteomyelitis
- the radiosensitivity of the tumour.

Despite the fact that the tumour has been recognized for such a period of time, one mystery remains – the identity of the cell of origin of Ewing's sarcoma.

Clinical presentation and diagnosis

Most patients with Ewing's sarcoma present with pain followed by swelling of the overlying affected bone. The duration from the onset of first symptoms to diagnosis is often many months, reflecting the population of patients commonly seen with these tumours who, in the main, are active adolescents and young adults. Thus, symptoms are frequently explained away as being a result of minor trauma or 'growing pains'.

Persistent pain following minor trauma should warrant further investigation as this may reveal an underlying bony tumour such as osteosarcoma or Ewing's sarcoma. The presence of systemic symptoms such as fever are, however, much more likely to be seen in Ewing's sarcoma. In addition, because of the large soft tissue mass commonly associated with Ewing's sarcoma, the presence of nerve root pain or neuropathies from nerve compression may also be a presenting symptom, especially in vertebral/paravertebral and pelvic tumours.

Almost half of Ewing's tumours will present in the femur or pelvis, with other long bones (tibia, fibula, humerus), ribs and vertebrae making up the majority of other primary sites (Figure 18.7). Metastatic disease is present in approximately one-quarter of patients, with half of all metastatic patients having solely lung metastases.[37]

It is not possible to make an accurate diagnosis of bone tumour without a surgical biopsy even if 'classical' radiological features are present. Plain radiographs of Ewing's sarcoma often demonstrate a degree of bone destruction with periosteal changes and a 'moth-eaten' appearance of the underlying bone. New bone formation, unlike in osteosarcoma, is rare, but its absence is not pathognomonic of Ewing's sarcoma. The soft tissue component associated with Ewing's tumours is often seen even on plain radiographs (Figure 18.8).

MRI scanning is the imaging modality of choice for the primary tumour. It is often not possible to define the limits of the soft tissue component of the tumour accurately without MRI. MRI also has the added benefit of demonstrating intramedullary tumour spread and/or metastases. All patients should have a plain chest radiograph, but this should be supported by a chest CT scan if the diagnosis is confirmed. Technetium-labelled bone scanning will normally demonstrate uptake in the primary tumour but is also helpful in delineating areas of bony metastatic disease. MRI scanning of these bony sites is often useful in addition, particularly to assess response to treatment since the technetium labelled bone scan often remains abnormal for some time even after the tumour has been eradicated, due to new bone formation/remodelling.

A number of haematological and biochemical parameters are often abnormal in patients with Ewing's sarcoma, but none is specific and they are commonly seen in other malignancies. Raised erythrocyte sedimentation rate,

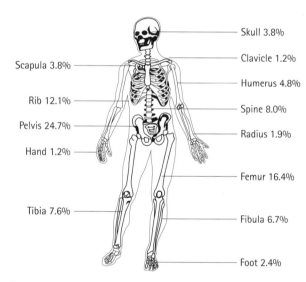

Figure 18.7 *Distribution of primary site of Ewing's tumours.*

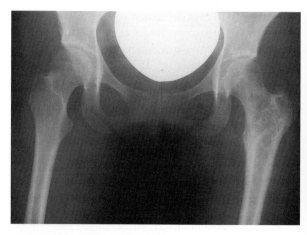

Figure 18.8 *Plain radiograph of Ewing's tumour of proximal femur. Features include infiltrative destruction, cortical thickening and a soft tissue mass.*

anaemia, raised lactate dehydrogenase and neuron-specific enolase (NSE) have all been reported and some linked with prognosis.[38,39] However, it is important for all patients with Ewing's sarcoma to have bone marrow aspirates and trephines prior to commencing chemotherapy in order to detect the bone marrow disease present in around 10 per cent of patients. Detection of subclinical bone marrow disease based on reverse transcriptase polymerase chain reaction (RT-PCR) of the i.e. *EWS-Fli1* gene product is currently under investigation as a further diagnostic and prognostic tool.[40–42]

Ultimately the diagnosis of Ewing's sarcoma is based on histopathology linked with immunohistochemical and, increasingly, molecular genetic characteristics. The planning of a surgical biopsy should therefore be made by an experienced team involved in the management of bone tumours in a facility having access to the full complement of diagnostic and molecular tests required. The site of any biopsy must be planned in the knowledge of the need for future local therapy (surgery and/or radiotherapy) and tissue samples must be handled and prepared appropriately.

Histology

Ewing's sarcoma is one of the 'small blue cell tumours of childhood'. This describes the microscopic features of these tumours which comprise uniform tightly packed round cells with rounded nuclei and pale, indistinct cytoplasm. In many cases, positive staining with periodic acid–Schiff (PAS) can be demonstrated, indicating the presence of glycogen.[43] Historically the presence of PAS-positive small blue cell tumours was deemed diagnostic of Ewing's sarcoma; however, cross-reactivity with other tumour types (rhabdomyosarcoma, neuroblastoma and lymphoma) makes this unreliable. Newer techniques such as immuno-histochemisty and molecular biology must be relied upon to make the diagnosis of Ewing's sarcoma reliably.

Neuroepithelial differentiation is commonly seen in Ewing's sarcoma with staining positivity for, among others, NSE and S100.[44] The addition of electron microscopy may reveal the presence of neurosecretory granules, but the degree of neuroepithelial differentiation does not appear to be of prognostic significance.[45]

The most useful immunohistochemical marker for the differential diagnosis of Ewing's sarcoma is the surface membrane protein expression of the MIC2 gene product (CD99).[46,47] However, there is clearly considerable overlap between classical Ewing's sarcoma and peripheral primitive neuroectodermal tumours (pPNETs), and histologically and immunohistochemically, they are impossible to differentiate accurately, such that most histopathologists these days seldom bother to do so. Instead, the differential between Ewing's sarcoma and pPNET depends much more on the clinical and radiological findings of these tumours. To add further to the confusion, pPNETs may be termed extraosseous Ewing's sarcoma (EOE) when they occur as isolated soft tissue tumours with no bone involvement. It is probably safest to regard classical Ewing's sarcoma, EOE and pPNET as biologically identical tumours; despite this, the choice of treatment for these tumour types remains controversial.

Molecular pathology

Cytogenetic abnormalities in Ewing's sarcoma have been recognized for many years. With the explosion in technology around the investigation of cytogenetic abnormality at the molecular level, a great deal more is known about the gene products of cytogenetic variables. The 'classic' chromosomal abnormality seen in around 85 per cent of cases of Ewing's sarcoma is the t(11;22)(q24;q12). At a molecular level this translocation juxtaposes the N-terminal segment of the *EWS* gene located at 22q12, with the C-terminal part of the *Fli1* gene located at 11q24.[48,49] The resulting *EWS-Fli1* transcript appears to provide the oncogenic stimulus for Ewing's sarcoma as suggested by reversal of tumorigenesis in models where the fusion transcript is antagonized by antisense oligonucleotides.[50,51] The breakpoint on each of the *EWS* and *Fli1* exons can vary, with the commonest variant (type 1 transcript) joining exon 7 of *EWS* with exon 6 of *Fli1*. There is a suggestion that the type 1 variant may confer improved prognosis compared with other breakpoint variants.[52]

Other *EWS* fusion transcripts have also been described, of which the *EWS-ERG* fusion resulting from the translocation t(21;22)(q22;q12) accounts for a further 10 per cent of reported abnormalities. Additional, rare translocations also include t(7;22)(p22;q12) (*EWS-ETV1*), t(17;22) (q12;q12) (*EWS-E1AF*) and t(2;22)(q33;q12) (*EWS-FEV*).[49,53] There does not appear to be any difference in outcome between patients with the two most common transcripts, *EWS-Fli1* and *EWS-ERG*.[54,55] Ultimately it may be possible to manipulate *EWS* fusion products using gene therapy as a therapeutic tool in the management of Ewing's sarcoma.[56,57]

Staging and stratification according to risk factors

In deciding the clinical management of patients with Ewing's sarcoma, a number of prognostic features should be taken into account. The most important of these is the presence or absence of metastatic disease. It is possible to identify three groups of patients based on the distribution of metastatic disease:

- patients without metastases who are currently experiencing 5-year survival rates in the order of 50–70 per cent

- those with isolated pulmonary metastases with around 30 per cent survival
- a very poor risk group with pulmonary and/or bone/bone marrow disease with <20 per cent survival.[58–64]

Tumour volume has also been demonstrated to be of prognostic significance, with larger tumours having poorer outcome.[65,66] Tumour volume (in mL) can be calculated using the formula $a \times b \times c \times F$ where a, b and c represent the maximum tumour dimensions (in cm) and $F = 0.52(\pi/6)$ for spherical tumours and $F = 0.785(\pi/4)$ for cylindrical tumours. Both the metastatic status and tumour volume are the basis for treatment stratification/randomization within the current European Ewing Tumour Working Initiative of National Groups (EURO-EWING) clinical trial (EE99).

Table 18.2 summarizes a number of prognostic factors that influence outcome in Ewing's sarcoma. In three of the series, and in other reports, a very strong correlation exists between histological response to chemotherapy and outcome in patients in whom surgery is the local therapy undertaken.[67–72] This again forms part of the randomization in the EE99 trial in which patients with poor histological response (>10 per cent viable tumour) after induction chemotherapy are treated with standard ifosfamide, vincristine, actinomycin (IVA) chemotherapy or intensive therapy with busulphan and melphalan followed by peripheral stem cell transplantation.

Treatment

James Ewing noted the fact that Ewing's sarcoma is sensitive to radiotherapy in the original report in 1921. However Ewing's sarcoma must be regarded as a systemic disease and prior to the introduction of multiagent chemotherapy the vast majority of patients died from progressive disease, usually lung metastases.

SYSTEMIC THERAPY

Developments in the use of chemotherapy in the 1970s alongside the increasing use of limb-salvage surgery have resulted in the cornerstones of modern therapeutic strategies for Ewing's sarcoma. Some of the first experiences with multiagent chemotherapy came from the reports of superior activity of 'VAC' chemotherapy (vincristine, actinomycin D and cyclophosphamide) compared with single-drug therapy.[73] Subsequent addition of doxorubicin demonstrated further improvement in results and formed the basis of the first Intergroup Ewing's Sarcoma Study (IESS-I) in the United States.[74–76] The IESS-I study confirmed the superiority of the doxorubicin-containing arm of the trial with a 20 per cent improvement in disease-free survival compared with VAC chemotherapy.

The next major development in chemotherapy was the introduction of ifosfamide to replace some of the cyclophosphamide within the 'standard' VACA four-drug chemotherapy regimen (vincristine, actinomycin D, cyclophosphamide, doxorubicin). Ifosfamide had been demonstrated to be effective in children with relapsed sarcomas and there was hope that the incidence of haemorrhagic cystitis would be reduced compared with cyclophosphamide with mesna protection.[77,78] In addition, the fact that, on a gram for gram basis, six times more ifosfamide could safely be given compared with cyclophosphamide led to high hopes that significant benefits could be gained. Thus the IESS-II in the USA, CESS-86 in Germany and ET-1 studies in the UK all introduced ifosfamide into the chemotherapy schedule.[58,69,79]

Whilst survival rates continued to be encouraging with these regimens, without any data from randomized trials there was no convincing evidence for superiority of ifosfamide over cyclophosphamide. Indeed, the comparison to historic treatment regimens is problematic because we now appreciate that the dose intensity of cyclophosphamide was limited by lack of bladder protection from

Table 18.2 *Statistical significance of prognostic factors influencing outcome in Ewing's sarcoma patients*

	References			
	Bacci *et al.*[67]	Cotterill *et al.*[39]	Paulussen *et al.*[37]	Oberlin *et al.*[68]
Age	$P < 0.001$m	$P < 0.0001$m	NSm	NSu
Sex	$P < 0.04$m	$P < 0.001$u	NSm	NSu
Fever	$P < 0.0002$m			
Anaemia	$P < 0.02$m			
LDH	$P < 0.0003$m	$P = 0.03$m		NSu
Tumour site	$P < 0.02$m	$P < 0.03$m	$P = 0.0157$u	NSu
Volume	NS	$P = 0.001$m	$P = 0.0008$m	$P = 0.006$u
Presence of metastases		$P < 0.0001$u		
Histological response	$P < 0.001$m		$P = 0.0206$m	$P \leq 0.0001$m

LDH, lactate dehydrogenase; NS, not significant; u, univariate analysis; m, multivariate analysis.

the routine use of mesna and growth factors such as granulocyte colony-stimulating factor. Modern scheduling of cyclophosphamide we now know can deliver doses of cyclophosphamide similar to that of ifosfamide ($6\,g/m^2$). Response rates in relapsed and high-risk solid tumour patients with high-dose cyclophosphamide-containing regimens are similar to those of ifosfamide.[80,81]

Compelling data exist for the use of ifosfamide,[82–84] supported by the increased efficacy of higher doses of ifosfamide in the ET-2 trial in the UK, in which EFS in localized tumours increased from 44 to 62 per cent with $6\,g/m^2$ ifosfamide vs. $9\,g/m^2$.[85] However, other groups have been unable to demonstrate the benefits of ifosfamide.[85–87] In an attempt to answer this question in a randomized setting, the combined forces of the German/Austrian (GPOH) and United Kingdom (UKCCSG) study groups formed the European Intergroup Cooperative Ewing's Sarcoma Study (EICESS 92). In this study, standard-risk patients (non-metastatic with tumour volume less than $100\,mL$) were randomized between VACA and VAIA chemotherapy (ifosfamide substituted for cyclophosphamide). Only preliminary results of this study are currently available.[88]

The most recent introduction to the chemotherapy schedules in Ewing's sarcoma has been etoposide. Encouraging results of combined ifosfamide and etoposide schedules in sarcoma patients have led to its incorporation into many front-line strategies.[83,89] The use of etoposide was tested in a randomized setting in the EICESS 92 study when high-risk non-metastatic patients (tumour volume > $100\,mL$) were randomized between standard VAIA chemotherapy and the addition of etoposide (EVAIA).[88] In the current EE99 study, both doxorubicin and etoposide are administered in a dose-intensive fashion with ifosfamide to all patients during induction (vincristine $1.5\,mg/m^2$, ifosfamide $9\,g/m^2$, doxorubicin $60\,mg/m^2$ and etoposide $450\,mg/m^2$ per course; Figure 18.9).

LOCAL THERAPY

Whilst chemotherapy is an important therapeutic modality for the control of systemic disease in Ewing's sarcoma, the management of the primary tumour itself must also be considered. Technological advances in the surgical management of patients with bone tumours and the tendency towards limb-salvage procedures alongside the desire to reduce the toxicity and long-term sequelae of radiotherapy have all had an influence on the evolving picture of local tumour management. However, in common with many of the decisions surrounding choice of chemotherapy, modality of local tumour control has not been subjected to any randomized comparisons. Whatever the choice of treatment, local control rates in Ewing's sarcoma are high (>95 per cent in larger published series).[90,90a]

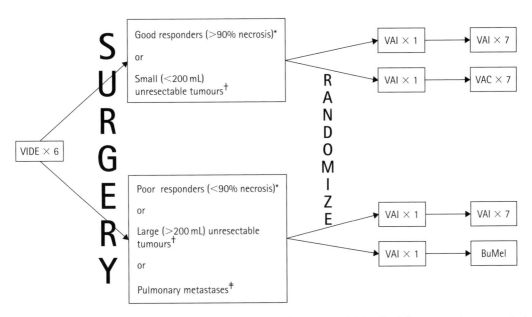

Figure 18.9 *Schematic representation of the EURO-EWING 99 protocol for patients with localized disease ± pulmonary metastases. VIDE = vincristine 1.5 mg/m², ifosfamide 9 g/m², doxorubicin 60 mg/m², etoposide 450 mg/m² per course. VAI = vincristine 1.5 mg/m², actinomycin D 1.5 mg/m², ifosfamide 6 g/m² per course. VAC = vincristine 1.5 mg/m², actinomycin D 1.5 mg/m², ifosfamide 6 g/m² per course. BuMel = busulphan 600 mg/m², melphalan 140 mg/m² followed by peripheral blood stem cell rescue. *Tumour necrosis on resected specimen when no irradiation prior to surgery; †unresectable tumours receive radiotherapy concurrently with randomized VAI or VAC chemotherapy, or following recovery from BuMel; ‡patients with pulmonary metastases receive pulmonary radiation if randomized to VAI. Local therapy may be surgery or radiotherapy (central axis tumours needing irradiation to primary electively treated with VAI).*

The completeness of surgical excision of the primary tumour was emphasized before the routine use of multiagent chemotherapy, whilst early studies such as IESS-I emphasized the poorer outcome of pelvic primary tumours and failed to demonstrate a clear difference between survival after either surgery or radiotherapy.[91,92] IESS-I and IESS-II set the standard for multimodality therapy in the 1970s and 1980s. The CESS 81 study highlighted the need for stringent attention to planning of radiotherapy when an attempt to reduce the dose resulted in poor outcomes for patients treated with radiotherapy alone (28 per cent 5-year overall survival). However, protocol deviations had occurred in 17/19 patients who relapsed following radiotherapy.[93] CESS 86 investigated the use of hyperfractionated radiotherapy, but no significant difference was observed between these patients and those receiving conventional radiotherapy.[94]

The publication of the combined follow-up data of 975 patients treated in the European Intergroup Cooperative Ewing's Sarcoma Study Group[39] allows us some insight into the role of local therapy in a large cohort of patients with long follow-up duration (median 6.6 years). Whilst local relapse rates for both axial and non-axial tumours fell during the study period (from 24 to 4 per cent for axial, and 31 to 15 per cent for non-axial), the suggestion that surgery or surgery plus radiotherapy seemed superior to radiotherapy alone was made. It was also emphasized, however, that other compounding influences are likely to impact on this analysis, e.g. the fact that axial tumours are likely to be of a larger volume and have increased metastatic disease. Clearly, without a randomized trial of local therapy, it will be impossible for us to distinguish between the success of radiother-apy and surgery. However, the following principles of local therapy should be adopted based on available evidence:

- Incomplete surgery should be avoided.
- Contaminated margins at the site of surgical excision should be irradiated.
- There is no proven role for preoperative radiotherapy to facilitate surgical excision.
- Postoperative radiotherapy should deliver a compartmental dose in the region of 45 Gy and a tumour boost to >50 Gy.

Future directions

The definition of first-line therapy for EFT remains the subject of clinical trials, as does the value of high-dose chemotherapy. Those with metastatic disease beyond the lungs or recurrent disease[95] still have exceptionally poor survival in spite of intensification of chemotherapy and investigational programmes can continue to be appropriately developed for this group.

OTHER BONE TUMOURS

Other primary bone tumours may occur in children and adolescents but all are exceptionally uncommon and information about treatment is sporadic. In some instances, a close histological relationship exists, e.g. between osteosar-coma and malignant fibrous histiocytoma of bone (MFH-B). The principles of staging and treatment for osteosarcoma can be appropriately applied to MFH-B.[96] With the exception of primary bone lymphoma, the value of chemotherapy in other tumours has been less clearly defined.

KEY POINTS

- Osteosarcoma and Ewing's tumour are the commonest bone tumours affecting children and adolescents.
- Aetiological links include genetic factors such as abnormalities of *Rb* and *p53* genes and therapeutic radiation.
- The key clinical symptom is pain. Plain radiographic appearances may be diagnostic.
- Between 50 and 70 per cent of patients may be cured with neoadjuvant chemotherapy and surgical resection of the primary tumour.
- An adverse prognosis is associated with the presence of metastases, large tumours and poor histological response to preoperative chemotherapy.
- Management should be undertaken at specialist centres with patients entered in multicentre clinical trials.
- New therapeutic approaches are needed for patients with adverse prognostic features.

REFERENCES

1. Buckley JD, Pendergrass TW, Buckley CM *et al.* Epidemiology of osteosarcoma and Ewing's sarcoma in childhood: a study of 305 cases by the Children's Cancer Group. *Cancer* 1998; **83**(7): 1440–8.
2. Hawkins MM, Wilson LM, Burton HS *et al.* Radiotherapy, alkylating agents, and risk of bone cancer after childhood cancer. *J Natl Cancer Inst* 1996; **88**(5): 270–8.
3. Cotterill SJ, Parker L, Malcolm AJ *et al.* Incidence and survival for cancer in children and young adults in the North of England, 1968–1995: a report from the Northern Region Young Persons' Malignant Disease Registry. *Br J Cancer* 2000; **83**(3): 397–403.
4. Fraumeni JF Jr, Glass AG. Rarity of Ewing's sarcoma among US Negro children. *Lancet* 1970; **1**(7642): 366–7.

5. Franzius C, Daldrup-Link HE, Sciuk J et al. FDG-PET for detection of pulmonary metastases from malignant primary bone tumors: comparison with spiral CT. Ann Oncol 2001; 12(4): 479–86.

6. Franzius C, Daldrup-Link HE, Wagner-Bohn A et al. FDG-PET for detection of recurrences from malignant primary bone tumors: comparison with conventional imaging. Ann Oncol 2002; 13(1): 157–60.

7. Hauben EI, Weeden S, Pringle J et al. Does the histological subtype of high-grade central osteosarcoma influence the response to treatment with chemotherapy and does it affect overall survival? A study on 570 patients of two consecutive trials of the European Osteosarcoma Intergroup. Eur J Cancer 2002; 38(9): 1218–25.

8. Bielack SS, Kempf-Bielack B, Delling G et al. Prognostic factors in high-grade osteosarcoma of the extremities or trunk: an analysis of 1702 patients treated on neoadjuvant cooperative osteosarcoma study group protocols. J Clin Oncol 2002; 20(3): 776–90.

9. Grimer RJ, Carter SR, Pynsent PB. The cost-effectiveness of limb salvage for bone tumours. J Bone Joint Surg Br 1997; 79(4): 558–61.

10. Nagarajan R, Neglia JP, Clohisy DR et al. Limb salvage and amputation in survivors of pediatric lower-extremity bone tumors: what are the long-term implications? J Clin Oncol 2002; 20(22): 4493–501.

10a. Ozaki T, Flege S, Kevric M et al. Osteosarcoma of the pelvis: experience of the Cooperative Osteosarcoma Study Group. J Clin Oncol 2003; 21: 334–41.

11. Davis AM, Devlin M, Griffin AM et al. Functional outcome in amputation versus limb sparing of patients with lower extremity sarcoma: a matched case-control study. Arch Phys Med Rehabil 1999; 80(6): 615–18.

12. Whelan JS, Weeden S, Uscinska B, McTiernan A. Localised extremity osteosarcoma: mature survival data from two European Osteosarcoma Intergroup randomised clinical trials. Proc ASCO 2000; 19: 552.

13. Goorin AM, Harris MB, Bernstein M et al. Phase II/III trial of etoposide and high-dose ifosfamide in newly diagnosed metastatic osteosarcoma: a pediatric oncology group trial. J Clin Oncol 2002; 20(2): 426–33.

14. Bramwell VHC, Burgess M, Sneath R et al. A comparison of two short intensive adjuvant chemotherapy regimens in operable osteosarcoma of limbs in children and young adults: the first study of the European Osteosarcoma Intergroup. J Clin Oncol 1992; 10: 1579–91.

15. Souhami RL, Craft AW, Van der Eijken JW et al. Randomised trial of two regimens of chemotherapy in operable osteosarcoma: a study of the European Osteosarcoma Intergroup. Lancet 1997; 350(9082): 911–17.

16. Fuchs N, Bielack SS, Epler D et al. Long-term results of the co-operative German-Austrian-Swiss osteosarcoma study group's protocol COSS-86 of intensive multidrug chemotherapy and surgery for osteosarcoma of the limbs. Ann Oncol 1998; 9(8): 893–9.

17. Winkler K, Beron G, Delling G et al. Neoadjuvant chemotherapy of osteosarcoma: results of a randomized cooperative trial (COSS-82) with salvage chemotherapy based on histological tumor response. J Clin Oncol 1988; 6(2): 329–37.

18. Bacci G, Briccoli A, Ferrari S et al. Neoadjuvant chemotherapy for osteosarcoma of the extremity: long-term results of the Rizzoli's 4th protocol. Eur J Cancer 2001; 37(16): 2030–9.

19. Meyers P, Schwartz CL, Bernstein M et al. Addition of ifosfamide and muramyl tripeptide to cisplatin, doxorubicin, and high-dose methotrexate improves event-free survival (EFS) in localised osteosarcoma (OS). Proc ASCO 2001; 20: 1483a.

20. Davis AM, Bell RS, Goodwin PJ. Prognostic factors in osteosarcoma: a critical review. J Clin Oncol 1994; 12(2): 423–31.

21. Bacci G, Picci P, Ferrari S et al. Primary chemotherapy and delayed surgery for nonmetastatic osteosarcoma of the extremities. Results in 164 patients preoperatively treated with high doses of methotrexate followed by cisplatin and doxorubicin. Cancer 1993; 72(11): 3227–38.

21a. Ozaki T, Neumann T, Wai D et al. Chromosomal alterations in osteosarcoma cell lines revealed by comparative genomic hybridization and multicolor karyotyping. Cancer Genet Cytogenet 2003; 140: 145–52.

21b. Ulaner GA, Huang HY, Otero J et al. Absence of a telomere maintenance mechanism as a favorable prognostic factor in patients with osteosarcoma. Cancer Res 2003; 63: 1759–63.

22. Feugeas O, Guriec N, Babin-Boilletot A et al. Loss of heterozygosity of the RB gene is a poor prognostic factor in patients with osteosarcoma. J Clin Oncol 1996; 14(2): 467–72.

23. Miller CW, Aslo A, Won A et al. Alterations of the p53, Rb and MDM2 genes in osteosarcoma. J Cancer Res Clin Oncol 1996; 122(9): 559–65.

24. Gokgoz N, Wunder JS, Mousses S et al. Comparison of p53 mutations in patients with localized osteosarcoma and metastatic osteosarcoma. Cancer 2001; 92(8): 2181–9.

25. Serra M, Scotlandi K, Reverter-Branchat G et al. Value of P-glycoprotein and clinicopathologic factors as the basis for new treatment strategies in high-grade osteosarcoma of the extremities. J Clin Oncol 2003; 21(3): 536–42.

26. Thomas DG, Giordano TJ, Sanders D et al. Absence of HER2/neu gene expression in osteosarcoma and skeletal Ewing's sarcoma. Clin Cancer Res 2002; 8(3): 788–93.

27. Zhou H, Randall RL, Brothman AR et al. Her-2/neu expression in osteosarcoma increases risk of lung metastasis and can be associated with gene amplification. J Pediatr Hematol Oncol 2003; 25(1): 27–32.

28. Wolf M, El-Rifai W, Tarkkanen M et al. Novel findings in gene expression detected in human osteosarcoma by cDNA microarray. Cancer Genet Cytogenet 2000; 123(2): 128–32.

28a. Kager L, Zoubek A, Potschger U et al. Primary metastatic osteosarcoma: presentation and outcome of patients treated on neoadjuvant Cooperative Osteosarcoma Study Group protocols. J Clin Oncol 2003; 21: 2011–18.

29. Saeter G, Hoie J, Stenwig AE et al. Systemic relapse of patients with osteogenic sarcoma. Prognostic factors for long term survival. Cancer 1995; 75(5): 1084–93.

30. Aung L, Gorlick R, Healey JH et al. Metachronous skeletal osteosarcoma in patients treated with adjuvant and neoadjuvant chemotherapy for nonmetastatic osteosarcoma. J Clin Oncol 2003; 21(2): 342–8.

31. Ferrari S, Briccoli A, Mercuri M et al. Postrelapse survival in osteosarcoma of the extremities: prognostic factors for long-term survival. J Clin Oncol 2003; 21(4): 710–15.

32. Sauerbrey A, Bielack S, Kempf-Bielack B et al. High-dose chemotherapy (HDC) and autologous hematopoietic stem cell transplantation (ASCT) as salvage therapy for relapsed osteosarcoma. Bone Marrow Transplant 2001; 27(9): 933–7.

33. Janinis J, McTiernan A, Driver D et al. A pilot study of short-course intensive multiagent chemotherapy in metastatic and axial skeletal osteosarcoma. Ann Oncol 2002; 13(12): 1935–44.

34. Anderson PM, Wiseman GA, Dispenzieri A et al. High-dose samarium-153 ethylene diamine tetramethylene phosphonate: low toxicity of skeletal irradiation in patients with osteosarcoma and bone metastases. J Clin Oncol 2002; 20(1): 189–96.

35. Franzius C, Schuck A, Bielack SS. High-dose samarium-153 ethylene diamine tetramethylene phosphonate: low toxicity of skeletal irradiation in patients with osteosarcoma and bone metastases. J Clin Oncol 2002; 20(7): 1953–4.

36. Ewing J. Diffuse endothelioma of bone. Proc NY Pathol Soc 1921; 21: 17–24.

37. Paulussen M, Frohlich B, Juergens H. Ewing tumour. Incidence, prognosis and treatment options. Paediatric Drugs 2001; 3: 899–913.

38. Bacci G, Ferrari S, Longhi A et al. Prognostic significance of serum LDH in Ewing's sarcoma of bone. Oncol Rep 1999; 6(4): 807–11.

39. Cotterill SJ, Ahrens S, Paulussen M et al. Prognostic factors in Ewing's tumor of bone: analysis of 975 patients from the European Intergroup Cooperative Ewing's Sarcoma Study Group. J Clin Oncol 2000; 18(17): 3108–14.

40. Fischmeister G, Zoubek A, Jugovic D et al. Low incidence of molecular evidence for tumour in PBPC harvests from patients with high risk Ewing tumours. Bone Marrow Transplant 1999; 24(4): 405–9.

41. Merino ME, Navid F, Christensen BL et al. Immunomagnetic purging of Ewing's sarcoma from blood and bone marrow: quantitation by real-time polymerase chain reaction. J Clin Oncol 2001; 19(16): 3649–59.

42. Leung W, Chen AR, Klann RC et al. Frequent detection of tumor cells in hematopoietic grafts in neuroblastoma and Ewing's sarcoma. Bone Marrow Transplant 1998; 22(10): 971–9.

43. Schajowicz F. Ewing's sarcoma and reticulum cell sarcoma of bone. With special reference to the histochemical demonstration of glycogen as an aid to differential diagnosis. J Bone Joint Surg 1959; 41: 349–356.

44. Schmidt D, Harms D, Pilon VA. Small-cell pediatric tumors: histology, immunohistochemistry, and electron microscopy. Clin Lab Med 1987; 7(1): 63–89.

45. Parham DM, Hijazi Y, Steinberg SM et al. Neuroectodermal differentiation in Ewing's sarcoma family of tumors does not predict tumor behavior. Hum Pathol 1999; 30(8): 911–18.

46. Ambros IM, Ambros PF, Strehl S et al. MIC2 is a specific marker for Ewing's sarcoma and peripheral primitive neuroectodermal tumours. Cancer 1991; 67: 1886–93.

47. Perlman EJ, Dickman PS, Askin FB et al. Ewing's sarcoma – routine diagnostic utilization of MIC2 analysis: a Pediatric Oncology Group/Children's Cancer Group Intergroup Study. Hum Pathol 1994; 25(3): 304–7.

48. Delattre O, Zucman J, Melot T et al. The Ewing family of tumors – a subgroup of small-round-cell tumors defined by specific chimeric transcripts. N Engl J Med 1994; 331(5): 294–9.

49. Denny CT. Gene rearrangements in Ewing's sarcoma. Cancer Invest 1996; 14(1): 83–8.

50. Ouchida M, Ohno T, Fujimura Y et al. Loss of tumorigenicity of Ewing's sarcoma cells expressing antisense RNA to EWS-fusion transcripts. Oncogene 1995; 11(6): 1049–54.

51. Tanaka K, Iwakuma T, Harimaya K et al. EWS-Fli1 antisense oligodeoxynucleotide inhibits proliferation of human Ewing's sarcoma and primitive neuroectodermal tumor cells. J Clin Invest 1997; 99(2): 239–47.

52. de Alava E, Kawai A, Healey JH et al. EWS-FLI1 fusion transcript structure is an independent determinant of prognosis in Ewing's sarcoma. J Clin Oncol 1998; 16(4): 1248–55.

53. Urano F, Umezawa A, Yabe H et al. Molecular analysis of Ewing's sarcoma: another fusion gene, EWS-E1AF, available for diagnosis. Jpn J Cancer Res 1998; 89(7): 703–11.

54. Ginsberg JP, de Alava E, Ladanyi M et al. EWS-FLI1 and EWS-ERG gene fusions are associated with similar clinical phenotypes in Ewing's sarcoma. J Clin Oncol 1999; 17(6): 1809–14.

55. Zoubek A, Dockhorn DB, Delattre O et al. Does expression of different EWS chimeric transcripts define clinically distinct risk groups of Ewing tumor patients? J Clin Oncol 1996; 14(4): 1245–51.

56. Lambert G, Bertrand JR, Fattal E et al. EWS fli-1 antisense nanocapsules inhibit Ewing sarcoma-related tumor in mice. Biochem Biophys Res Commun 2000; 279(2): 401–6.

57. Maruyama-Tabata H, Harada Y, Matsumura T et al. Effective suicide gene therapy in vivo by EBV-based plasmid vector coupled with polyamidoamine dendrimer. Gene Ther 2000; 7(1): 53–60.

58. Burgert EJ, Nesbit ME, Garnsey LA et al. Multimodal therapy for the management of nonpelvic, localized Ewing's sarcoma of bone: intergroup study IESS-II [see comments]. J Clin Oncol 1990; 8(9): 1514–24.

59. Craft A, Cotterill S, Malcolm A et al. Ifosfamide-containing chemotherapy in Ewing's sarcoma: The Second United Kingdom Children's Cancer Study Group and the Medical Research Council Ewing's Tumor Study. J Clin Oncol 1998; 16(11): 3628–33.

60. Elomaa I, Blomqvist CP, Saeter G et al. Five-year results in Ewing's sarcoma. The Scandinavian Sarcoma Group experience with the SSG IX protocol. Eur J Cancer 2000; 36(7): 875–80.

61. Rosito P, Mancini AF, Rondelli R et al. Italian Cooperative Study for the treatment of children and young adults with localized Ewing sarcoma of bone: a preliminary report of 6 years of experience. Cancer 1999; 86(3): 421–8.

62. Cangir A, Vietti TJ, Gehan EA et al. Ewing's sarcoma metastatic at diagnosis. Results and comparisons of two intergroup Ewing's sarcoma studies. Cancer 1990; 66(5): 887–93.

63. Paulussen M, Ahrens S, Craft AW et al. Ewing's tumors with primary lung metastases: survival analysis of 114 (European Intergroup) Cooperative Ewing's Sarcoma Studies patients. J Clin Oncol 1998; 16(9): 3044–52.

64. Paulussen M, Ahrens S, Burdach S et al. Primary metastatic (stage IV) Ewing tumor: survival analysis of 171 patients from the EICESS studies. European Intergroup Cooperative Ewing Sarcoma Studies. Ann Oncol 1998; 9(3): 275–81.

65. Gobel V, Jurgens H, Etspuler G et al. Prognostic significance of tumor volume in localised Ewing's sarcoma of bone in children and adolescents. J Cancer Res Clin Oncol 1987; 113: 187–91.

66. Hayes FA, Thompson EI, Meyer WH et al. Therapy for localized Ewing's sarcoma of bone. J Clin Oncol 1989; 7(2): 208–13.

67. Bacci G, Ferrari S, Bertoni F et al. Prognostic factors in nonmetastatic Ewing's sarcoma of bone treated with

adjuvant chemotherapy: analysis of 359 patients at the Istituto Ortopedico Rizzoli. *J Clin Oncol* 2000; **18**(1): 4–11.

68. Oberlin O, Deley MC, Bui BN *et al*. Prognostic factors in localized Ewing's tumours and peripheral neuroectodermal tumours: the third study of the French Society of Paediatric Oncology (EW88 study). *Br J Cancer* 2001; **85**(11): 1646–54.

69. Paulussen M, Ahrens S, Dunst J *et al*. Localized Ewing tumor of bone: final results of the cooperative Ewing's Sarcoma Study CESS 86. *J Clin Oncol* 2001; **19**(6): 1818–29.

70. Wunder JS, Paulian G, Huvos AG *et al*. The histological response to chemotherapy as a predictor of the oncological outcome of operative treatment of Ewing sarcoma. *J Bone Joint Surg Am* 1998; **80**(7): 1020–33.

71. Donaldson SS, Torrey M, Link MP *et al*. A multidisciplinary study investigating radiotherapy in Ewing's sarcoma: end results of POG #8346. Pediatric Oncology Group. *Int J Radiat Oncol Biol Phys* 1998; **42**(1): 125–35.

72. Picci P, Rougraff BT, Bacci G *et al*. Prognostic significance of histopathologic response to chemotherapy in nonmetastatic Ewing's sarcoma of the extremities. *J Clin Oncol* 1993; **11**(9): 1763–9.

73. Jaffe N, Paed D, Traggis D *et al*. Improved outlook for Ewing's sarcoma with combination chemotherapy (vincristine, actinomycin D and cyclophosphamide) and radiation therapy. *Cancer* 1976; **38**(5): 1925–30.

74. Cangir A, Morgan SK, Land VJ *et al*. Combination chemotherapy with adriamycin (NSC-123127) and dimethyl triazeno imidazole carboxamide (DTIC) (NSC-45388) in children with metastatic solid tumors. *Med Pediatr Oncol* 1976; **2**(2): 183–90.

75. Pomeroy TC, Johnson RE. Combined modality therapy of Ewing's sarcoma. *Cancer* 1975; **35**(1): 36–47.

76. Nesbit MJ, Gehan EA, Burgert EJ *et al*. Multimodal therapy for the management of primary, nonmetastatic Ewing's sarcoma of bone: a long-term follow-up of the First Intergroup study. *J Clin Oncol* 1990; **8**(10): 1664–74.

77. Pinkerton CR, Rogers H, James C *et al*. A phase II study of ifosfamide in children with recurrent solid tumours. *Cancer Chemother Pharmacol* 1985; **15**(3): 258–62.

78. Bryant BM, Jarman M, Ford HT, Smith IE. Prevention of isophosphamide-induced urothelial toxicity with 2-mercaptoethane sulphonate sodium (mesnum) in patients with advanced carcinoma. *Lancet* 1980; **2**(8196): 657–9.

79. Craft AW, Cotterill SJ, Bullimore JA, Pearson D. Long-term results from the first UKCCSG Ewing's Tumour Study (ET-1). United Kingdom Children's Cancer Study Group (UKCCSG) and the Medical Research Council Bone Sarcoma Working Party. *Eur J Cancer* 1997; **33**(7): 1061–9.

80. Zoubek A, Holzinger B, Mann G *et al*. High-dose cyclophosphamide, adriamycin, and vincristine (HD-CAV) in children with recurrent solid tumor. *Pediatr Hematol Oncol* 1994; **11**(6): 613–23.

81. Kushner BH, Meyers PA, Gerald WL *et al*. Very-high-dose short-term chemotherapy for poor-risk peripheral primitive neuroectodermal tumors, including Ewing's sarcoma, in children and young adults. *J Clin Oncol* 1995; **13**(11): 2796–804.

82. Wexler LH, DeLaney TF, Tsokos M *et al*. Ifosfamide and etoposide plus vincristine, doxorubicin, and cyclophosphamide for newly diagnosed Ewing's sarcoma family of tumors. *Cancer* 1996; **78**(4): 901–11.

83. Meyer WH, Kun L, Marina N *et al*. Ifosfamide plus etoposide in newly diagnosed Ewing's sarcoma of bone. *J Clin Oncol* 1992; **10**(11): 1737–42.

84. Grier HE, Krailo MD, Tarbell NJ *et al*. Addition of ifosfamide and etoposide to standard chemotherapy for Ewing's sarcoma and primitive neuroectodermal tumor of bone. *N Engl J Med* 2003; **348**(8): 694–701.

85. Bacci G, Toni A, Avella M *et al*. Long term results in 144 Ewing's sarcoma patients treated with combined therapy. *Cancer* 1989; **63**: 1477–86.

86. Oberlin O, Habrand JL, Zucker JM *et al*. No benefit of ifosfamide in Ewing's sarcoma: a nonrandomized study of the French Society of Pediatric Oncology. *J Clin Oncol* 1992; **10**(9): 1407–12.

87. Bacci G, Picci P, Ferrari S *et al*. Neoadjuvant chemotherapy for Ewing's sarcoma of bone: no benefit observed after adding ifosfamide and etoposide to vincristine, actinomycin, cyclophosphamide, and doxorubicin in the maintenance phase – results of two sequential studies. *Cancer* 1998; **82**(6): 1174–83.

88. Paulussen M, Craft A, Lewis I *et al*. Ewing tumor of bone – updated report of the European Intergroup Cooperative Ewing's Sarcoma Study EICESS 92. *Proc ASCO* 2002:1568.

89. Miser JS, Kinsella TJ, Triche TJ *et al*. Ifosfamide with mesna uroprotection and etoposide: an effective regimen in the treatment of recurrent sarcomas and other tumors of children and young adults. *J Clin Oncol* 1987; **5**: 1191–8.

90. Dunst J, Sauer R, Burgers JM *et al*. Radiation therapy as local treatment in Ewing's sarcoma. Results of the Cooperative Ewing's Sarcoma Studies CESS 81 and CESS 86. *Cancer* 1991; **67**(11): 2818–25.

90a. Shankar AG, Pinkerton CR, Atra A *et al*. Local therapy and other factors influencing site of relapse in patients with localised Ewing's sarcoma. United Kingdom Children's Cancer Study Group (UKCCSG). *Eur J Cancer* 1999; **35**: 1698–704.

91. Pritchard DJ, Dahlin DC, Dauphine RT *et al*. Ewing's sarcoma. A clinicopathological and statistical analysis of patients surviving five years or longer. *J Bone Joint Surg Am* 1975; **57**(1): 10–16.

92. Pritchard DJ. Surgical experience in the management of Ewing's sarcoma of bone. *Natl Cancer Inst Monogr* 1981; **56**:169–71.

93. Sauer R, Jurgens H, Burgers JM *et al*. Prognostic factors in the treatment of Ewing's sarcoma. The Ewing's Sarcoma Study Group of the German Society of Paediatric Oncology CESS 81. *Radiother Oncol* 1987;**10**(2): 101–10.

94. Dunst J, Jurgens H, Sauer R *et al*. Radiation therapy in Ewing's sarcoma: an update of the CESS 86 trial. *Int J Radiat Oncol Biol Phys* 1995; **32**(4): 919–30.

95. Shankar AG, Ashley S, Craft AW, Pinkerton CR. Outcome after relapse in an unselected cohort of children and adolescents with Ewing sarcoma. *Med Pediatr Oncol* 2003; **40**: 141–7.

96. Bramwell VH, Steward WP, Nooij M *et al*. Neoadjuvant chemotherapy with doxorubicin and cisplatin in malignant fibrous histiocytoma of bone: a European Osteosarcoma Intergroup study. *J Clin Oncol* 1999; **17**(10): 3260–9.

19

Neuroblastoma

ANDREW D. J. PEARSON & ROSS PINKERTON

INTRODUCTION

Neuroblastoma is a malignant tumour derived from the sympathetic nervous system. It is the most frequent extracranial solid tumour occurring in children. Up to the 1980s it was almost invariably fatal for children over 1 year of age with metastatic disease. The short-term prognosis has steadily improved over the past two decades due to a combination of better understanding of the natural history of the disease, more sophisticated investigation methods and new therapeutic approaches. This chapter focuses on the clinical characteristics of neuroblastoma and treatment strategies for the various stages of disease. Further details of pathology, diagnostic markers and the role of very high-dose therapy with stem cell rescue are provided in Chapters 3, 9 and 26 respectively.

EPIDEMIOLOGY

Neuroblastoma accounts for approximately 10 per cent of all the solid malignancies encountered in paediatric practice. Its annual incidence is between six and eight per million children under 15 years of age. The median age of onset is 2 years, making neuroblastoma the most frequent malignant tumour of early childhood. Moreover, age is an independent prognostic factor – the onset is usually inversely proportional to the survival rate. The existence of less advanced stages in younger patients only partly explains the correlation with prognosis.

Table 19.1 and Figure 19.1 present 1310 cases of neuroblastoma taken from seven early clinical studies of more than 100 cases each. The most frequent anatomical sites of the primary tumours are, in decreasing order of frequency, the adrenal gland, the paravertebral

Table 19.1 *Primary sites of neuroblastoma*

References	Adrenal		Abdomen		Pelvis		Thorax		Neck		Other		Total (*n*)
	n	%	*n*	%	*n*	%	*n*	%	*n*	%	*n*	%	
Gross et al.[1]	89	41	28	13	12	6	25	12	4	2	59	27	217
Bodian[2]	48	37	41	32	10	8	14	11	7	5	9	7	129
Fortner et al.[3]	67	50	25	19	5	4	11	8	3	2	22	17	133
Stella et al.[4]	42	29	62	43	5	3	24	17	4	3	6	4	143
Wilson and Draper[5]	112	23	155	32	32	7	80	16	0	0	108	22	487
Total	358	32	311	28	64	6	154	14	18	2	204	18	1109

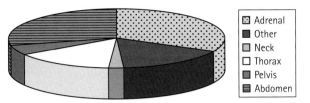

Figure 19.1 *Primary sites of neuroblastoma (n = 1310).*

retroperitoneum, the posterior mediastinum, the pelvis and the cervical area.

As for other malignant tumours, neuroblastoma tends to metastasize to specific sites, i.e. bones, bone marrow and lymph nodes. Liver and skin are less frequent sites of metastasis, while lungs and brain are only exceptionally affected.[6]

CLINICAL PRESENTATION

The initial symptoms of neuroblastoma are frequently non-specific and may mimic a wide variety of more common paediatric conditions. This is due to the numerous possible sites of both the primary tumour and metastases, and to some symptoms that can be attributed to the associated metabolic disturbances. A growing infiltrative tumour in the neck, thorax, abdomen or pelvis may invade and compress surrounding structures. In the head and neck region, a palpable mass and Horner's syndrome (Figure 19.2) can be the first symptoms. In the chest, the tumour can cause respiratory distress, dysphagia and venous compression. A palpable mass, with or without abdominal pain, is usually the sign of an abdominal tumour, whereas pelvic tumours may be revealed by problems with defaecation and voiding urine. Tumours growing through the intravertebral foramina and compressing the spinal cord ('dumb-bell' neuroblastoma) may present with neurological symptoms such as flaccid paralysis of the legs and/or urinary dysfunction with distension of the bladder.

The clinical symptoms due to metastases also vary widely. In infants, the first sign is usually a rapidly enlarging liver, sometimes accompanied by skin nodules with a bluish colour and bone marrow involvement. Older children show a different pattern of metastatic spread. Symptoms due to metastases in older children include bone pain, frequently manifesting as a limp, and lymph node enlargement. Signs and symptoms can sometimes be confused with those of leukaemia, consisting of anaemia and mucosal or skin haemorrhage due to pancytopenia caused by bone marrow infiltration by neuroblastoma cells (Figure 19.3).

The metabolic effects of the tumour can also cause systemic symptoms. The high level of catecholamines and sometimes vasoactive intestinal peptides (VIPs) produced by neuroblastoma cells can result in bouts of sweating

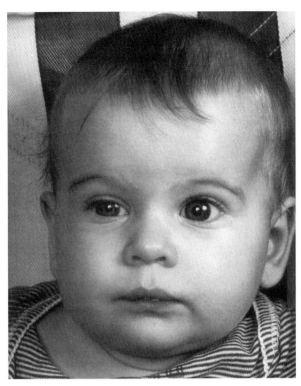

Figure 19.2 *Horner's syndrome: miosis, ptosis and enophthalmia in a 9-month-old girl with a neuroblastoma of the right cervical sympathetic side-chain.*

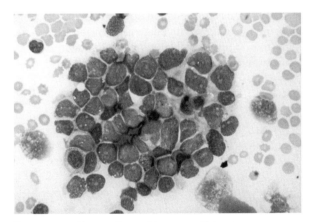

Figure 19.3 *Cluster of neuroblastoma cells in a bone marrow smear (H&E stain).*

and pallor associated with watery diarrhoea and hypertension. These symptoms are probably unrelated to the site and size of the tumour and regress following successful therapy. Finally the tumour may be disclosed by a routine clinical examination.

STAGING SYSTEMS FOR NEUROBLASTOMA

Until 1988, three major staging systems for neuroblastoma were used throughout the world, making

Box 19.1 *International Staging System for neuroblastoma (INSS)[12]*

Stage 1

Localized tumour with complete gross excision, with or without microscopic residual disease; representative ipsilateral and contralateral lymph nodes negative for tumour microscopically (nodes attached to and removed with the primary tumour may be positive)[a]

Stage 2a

Localized tumour with incomplete gross excision; representative ipsilateral and non-adherent lymph nodes negative for tumour microscopically

Stage 2b

Localized tumour with complete or incomplete gross excision; with ipsilateral non-adherent lymph nodes positive for tumour. Enlarged contralateral lymph nodes must be negative microscopically

Stage 3

Unresectable unilateral tumour infiltrating across the midline[b] with or without regional lymph node involvement; **or** localized unilateral tumour with contralateral regional lymph node involvement; **or** midline tumour with bilateral extension by infiltration (unresectable) or by lymph node involvement

Stage 4

Any primary tumour with dissemination to distant lymph nodes, bone, bone marrow, liver, skin and/or other organs (except as defined in stage 4S)

Stage 4S

Localized primary tumour (as defined for stage 1, 2a or 2b) with dissemination limited to skin, liver and/or bone marrow[c] (limited to infants younger than 1 year old).

---

[a] Multifocal primary tumours (e.g. adrenal primary tumours) should be staged according to the greatest extent of the disease, as defined above, and followed by $_m$, e.g. 3_m.

[b] The midline is defined as the vertebral column. Tumours originating on one side and 'crossing the midline' must infiltrate to or beyond the opposite side of the vertebral column.

[c] Marrow involvement of stage 4S should be minimal, i.e. fewer than 10 per cent of total nucleated cells identified as malignant on bone marrow biopsy or on marrow aspirates. More extensive marrow involvement will be considered to be stage 4. The *m*IBG scan (if done) should be negative in marrow.

---

communication between clinicians and researchers very difficult:

- the system used by the Children's Cancer Group (CCG) in the USA as well as many others[7]
- the system utilized by St Jude Children's Research Hospital (SJCRH) and the Pediatric Oncology Group (POG)[8]
- the TNM system proposed by the International Union Against Cancer.[9]

In general, the various staging systems gave comparable results in distinguishing low-stage, good-prognosis patients from high-stage, poor-prognosis patients. However, some of the differences between these staging systems are substantial, particularly when applied to individual patients. The results of clinical trials or studies performed by different groups cannot therefore be readily compared. Points of disagreement included the prognostic importance of tumours crossing the midline; the prognostic importance of ipsilateral and/or contralateral lymph node involvement;[10] and the importance of resectability of the primary tumour.

Agreement on the definition of stage with regard to these and other issues was achieved in 1988.[11] This has substantially facilitated the comparison of different studies. This staging system, known as INSS (International Neuroblastoma Staging System), was modified in 1993[12] and is now internationally accepted. It is a postsurgical staging system with substantial dependence on the assessment of resectability and surgical examination of lymph node involvement. The modified INSS is shown in Box 19.1, and incidence and survival by stage are shown in Table 19.2.

In 1993, the definition of stage 4S was brought into line with that initially intended by Evans *et al.*[7] In stage 4S, there is localized primary tumour; metastases are limited to the liver, skin and bone marrow but not bone; bone marrow involvement is minimal and the entity occurs only in children under 1 year of age. Prognosis for these children without therapy is very good, the majority regressing spontaneously.

Table 19.2 *Incidence and survival by International Neuroblastoma Staging System (INSS) stage*

Stage	Incidence (%)	Five-year survival (%)
1	5	≥90
2a + 2b	10	70–80
3	20	40–70
4	60	60 if age <1 year
		20 if age >1 year
4S	5	>80

TUMOUR MARKERS

Five circulating markers, detectable in patient's blood or urine, are discussed below: catecholamines, neuron-specific enolase (NSE), ferritin, lactate dehydrogenase (LDH) and gangliosides (see also Chapter 9).

Catecholamines

In 1959, excessive secretion of vanillylmandelic acid (VMA) was noticed in children with ganglioneuroma and ganglioneuroblastoma. Today, the fact that neuroblastoma cells secrete large amounts of one or more catecholamines, in addition to their metabolites, is well documented. Despite the fact that VMA and homovanillic acid (HVA) are relatively easy to measure and are usually raised in neuroblastoma patients, there are 'non-secreting' tumours for which less frequently measured metabolites may be useful, e.g. dopamine. A good understanding of the synthesis and metabolism of catecholamines is therefore useful, although for practical clinical reasons, HVA and VMA are the most widely used in diagnosis and follow-up (Figure 19.4).

During the past 20 years, the measurement of urinary VMA and HVA has become a routine test for diagnosis and follow-up of patients with neuroblastoma.[13] It is now accepted that random urinary HVA and VMA levels are adequate not only for diagnosis but also for follow-up, and that 24-hour collections are not necessary.[14,15] Urinary catecholamine values are presented as ratios to urinary creatinine. Although HVA and VMA levels in the pretreatment urine of children with neuroblastoma were initially believed to be of prognostic value, it is now generally agreed that there is no correlation between these values

and outcome.[16,17] Plasma HVA and VMA concentrations parallel urinary levels and can be used for monitoring. Furthermore, in some children, elevated plasma levels are found while urine levels are normal.[18,19] Dopamine in urine or plasma is a particularly sensitive marker.[20]

Neuron-specific enolase

Enolase is a glycolytic enzyme: brain and neuroendocrine tissues contain two forms of enolase, denoted $\alpha\alpha$ and $\gamma\gamma$ to indicate that they are dimers of biochemically and immunologically distinct subunits. A hybrid form ($\alpha\gamma$) is also present in these tissues. The γ-enolase is found in neurons and has therefore been called neuron-specific enolase (NSE). In children, although high serum NSE levels are suggestive of neuroblastoma, increased levels have been reported in other malignancies such as Wilms' tumour, Ewing's sarcoma, non-Hodgkin's lymphoma, soft tissue sarcoma and acute leukaemias.[21] Caution should thus be exercised in using NSE as a diagnostic test in children with a malignant disease. Furthermore, the test is not particularly sensitive since raised serum NSE levels have been described in all stages of neuroblastoma at diagnosis. In general, a low level predicts a good prognosis and a high level a poor outcome, this being mainly due to the fact that children with advanced disease present high serum NSE levels.[22] It is interesting to observe that patients with 4S neuroblastoma, who generally present with a large tumour burden but have a good prognosis, usually have lower NSE levels than children with stage 4 disease of equivalent tumour bulk. In summary, NSE is a 'marker' of neuroblastoma but not a very good one since it lacks both good specificity and good sensitivity; it is nevertheless of prognostic importance.

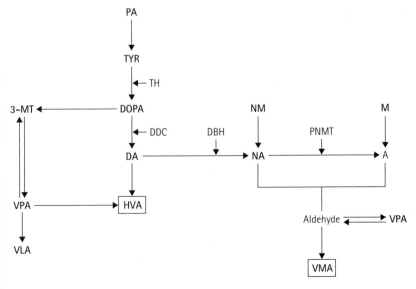

Figure 19.4 *Synthesis of homovanillic acid (HVA) and vanillylmandelic acid (VMA). Enzymes – DBH, dopamine-β-hydroxylase; DDC, dopa-decarboxylase; PNMT, phenylethanolamine-N-methyl transferase; TH, tyrosine hydroxylase. Catecholamines, metabolites and precursors – A, adrenaline; DA, dopamine; DOPA, 3,4-dihydroxylphenylalanine; M, metanephrine; NA, noradrenaline; NM, normetanephrine, 3-MT, 3-methoxytyramine; PA, phenylalanine; TYR, tyrosine; VLA, vanillactic acid; VPA, vanilpuric acid.*

Ferritin

Children with advanced neuroblastoma frequently present with an increased level of ferritin; the levels usually decrease during treatment and may reach normal when the patients are in clinical remission. The increase in serum ferritin levels in patients with neuroblastoma is due to augmented synthesis of ferritin by the tumour cells and subsequent secretion in plasma.[23]

Ferritin is not frequently elevated in serum from children with stage 1 and 2 disease, but is abnormally raised in some patients with stage 3 and 4 disease.[24] In one study on prognostic factors in neuroblastoma, it was possible to define three groups of children with different prognoses:[25]

- good – normal ferritin, aged under 2 years, 2-year survival 93 per cent
- intermediate – normal ferritin, aged 2 years or older, 2-year survival 58 per cent
- poor – raised ferritin, 2-year survival 19 per cent.

More recent analyses have confirmed that the serum ferritin concentration is a powerful prognostic indicator.[26,27]

Lactate dehydrogenase

Serum lactate dehydrogenase (LDH) concentrations are elevated in patients with advanced disease. Following the initial recognition of the prognostic significance of serum LDH levels, by the German group, this has been confirmed by other investigators.[27,28]

Gangliosides

Gangliosides, sialic acid-containing glycosphyngolipids, are mainly detected in the cell surface membrane. These membrane-bound glycolipids are shed or released *in vitro* by a variety of cells, particularly tumours cells. It now appears that these markers are present in both tumours and the plasma of most children with neuroblastoma. Concentrations of disialoganglioside G_{D2} elevated to more than 50 times the normal value have been demonstrated in the plasma of children with active neuroblastoma. Sequential determination of circulating G_{D2} has revealed that plasma levels decreased in children responding to treatment and reappeared in patients in relapse. In contrast, raised circulating G_{D2} has not been demonstrated in the plasma of children with ganglioneuroblastoma or ganglioneuroma.[29] There is a relationship between the ganglioside composition of neuroblastoma tumours and outcome, with the lack of G_{T1b} indicating a poor outlook. In particular, thoracic neuroblastomas, which are associated with a favourable outcome, contain more complex gangliosides of the b series (G_{D1b} and G_{T1b}) and few monosialogangliosides, suggesting a more differentiated cellular composition.[30]

In summary, the ideal neuroblastoma marker has yet to be found. It is a molecule of neuroblastoma cell origin, released in the circulation and/or in the urine in amounts that are easily detectable and proportional to the stage of the disease. This molecule should disappear when the child is in remission and reappear in advance of clinical evidence of relapse. Not all of the above criteria for an ideal neuroblastoma marker are met by catecholamines, NSE, ferritin, LDH or gangliosides when taken individually.

In conclusion, only catecholamine concentrations are valuable in the diagnosis and monitoring of response to treatment of neuroblastomas. Serum ferritin and LDH concentrations are powerful prognostic indicators, while the importance of the other markers mentioned above has not been borne out in studies of a large number of patients.

PATHOLOGY

Current nomenclature generally classifies three types of tumour:

- undifferentiated neuroblastoma
- ganglioneuroblastoma – a tumour with both maturing or mature ganglion cells together with neuroblasts
- ganglioneuroma – the most mature end of the spectrum.

The microscopic appearance of undifferentiated neuroblastoma (Figure 19.5) is that of diffusely arranged sheets of cells showing some focal evidence of aggregation. Differentiating neuroblastomas (Figure 19.6) show definite evidence of neurofibril formation: neurofibrils may be arranged at the centre of 'pseudorosettes'. Ganglioneuroblastoma contains both neuroblasts and ganglion cells in two histological patterns: complex

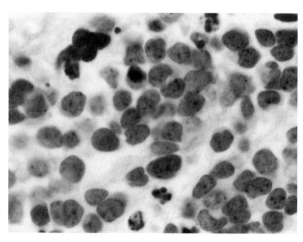

Figure 19.5 *Undifferentiated neuroblastoma (H&E).*

ganglioneuroblastoma (Figure 19.7), in which the tumour has a lobular arrangement, and undifferentiated neuroblasts are intermixed with ganglion cells and intermediate forms, all within any lobule; and composite ganglioneuroblastoma, in which undifferentiated neuroblasts and mature ganglion cells are located in different parts of the tumour.

Ganglioneuroblastoma (Figure 19.8) consists of mature ganglion cells lying against a background of neurofibrous tissue. Although it is clear that the prognosis for ganglioneuroma is extremely good, and that for ganglioneuroblastoma is considerably better than for neuroblastoma, it is not always easy to demonstrate prognostic correlations within the neuroblastoma subtypes. Systems for histological grading must take account of varying degrees of differentiation from field to field within a tumour since the potential for metastasis is probably determined, at least in part, by the most undifferentiated component. In general, there is a correlation between more neural differentiation and better prognosis.[31,32]

The Shimada system[33] is an age-related classification based on the amount of stroma and tumour cell differentiation, and an index of mitosis and karyorrhexis in the tumour. With the classification, neuroblastomas are categorized into two groups: stromal-rich and stromal-poor. Each group is then divided into those with favourable or unfavourable histological features. Using the system, a correlation was demonstrated between histology and survival, the better prognosis being achieved within the favourable stromal group, with more than 80 per cent survival at 2 years from diagnosis.

In 1992, Joshi et al.[34] modified the Shimada classification and recommended the terms neuroblastoma and ganglioneuroblastoma rather than stroma poor and stroma rich, and identified both undifferentiated and poorly differentiated neuroblastoma. In a ganglioneuroblastoma there should be a predominant ganglioneuromatous component with a minor neuroblastomic component. Using this classification system, tumours could be grouped according to prognosis. The system is easier to employ than the Shimada system and does not include age.

In 1995, the International Neuroblastoma Pathology Committee (INPC) further modified this classification to include various histological features (Table 19.3):

- degree of differentiation towards ganglion cells
- amount of Schwann cell stroma present
- whether the tumour is nodular, noting particularly macronodules (which tend to be associated with a poor prognosis compared with intermixed nodules)
- degree of calcification
- mitotic–karyorrhexis index.

The main aim of this classification is to differentiate those neuroblastomas that are embryonic and will regress from those that are neoplastic. The INPC proposes comparing the pathology, particularly the nuclear morphology of neuroblastomas that are known to express TRKA and those that do not. The aim is to relate histological

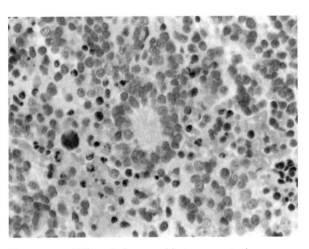

Figure 19.6 *Differentiating neuroblastoma – note the pseudorosettes (H&E).*

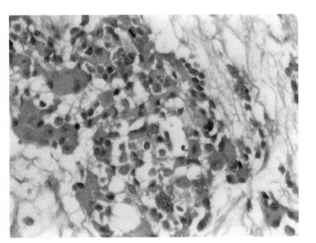

Figure 19.7 *Complex ganglioneuroblastoma with both mature and undifferentiated tumour cells (H&E).*

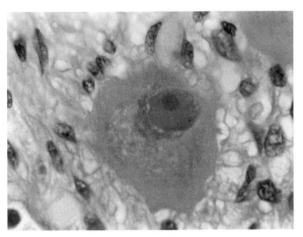

Figure 19.8 *Ganglioneuroma (H&E).*

Table 19.3 *International Neuroblastoma Pathology Committee classification*

INPC classification	Age (years)	Mitosis karyorrhexis index	Prognosis
Neuroblastoma			
Undifferentiated			Unfavourable
Poorly differentiated	<1.5	Low or intermediate	Favourable
	>1.5	Any	
Differentiating	1.5–5.0	Low	Favourable
	<1.5	Low or intermediate	Favourable
	>1.5	Low, intermediate or high	Unfavourable
Ganglioneuroblastoma			
Intermixed			Favourable
Nodular			Unfavourable
Ganglioneuroma			
Maturing			Favourable
Mature			Favourable

appearances to molecular pathological features and outcome.

All three of these histopathological classifications are valid only with adequate histopathological material and not if needle biopsy material alone is available. Similarly, these classifications are only applicable to tumours examined before any therapy. Previously treated primary tumours may have different appearances.

MOLECULAR PATHOLOGY OF NEUROBLASTOMA

It has become apparent that neuroblastoma is at least two, or perhaps three, distinct entities. The clinical behaviour or neuroblastoma varies greatly and includes tumours that regress spontaneously, by either apoptosis or differentiation into ganglioneuroblastoma, and those that are chemosensitive, chemocurable and chemoresistant malignancies. Spontaneous regression is very obvious in patients with stage 4S neuroblastoma, although some patients with stage 1, 2 and 3 tumours, and possibly infants with stage 4 disease, may be long-term survivors without therapy. Not all the tumours that do not require therapy can be identified at present. Treatment is sometimes required to induce 'regression' in children who have life-threatening symptoms. Some long-term survivors of stage 2 neuroblastoma have received chemotherapy and have late sequelae without any therapeutic benefit. Recently, patients with stage 3 neuroblastoma who are long-term survivors treated with chemotherapy or irradiation have been reported.[35] Was even surgery necessary in these patients?

Such cases are in marked contrast to patients with poor-prognosis neuroblastoma who, despite intensive chemoradiotherapy, often consolidated by high-dose chemotherapy with autologous bone marrow rescue, relapse and die. Commonly, these tumours are initially chemosensitive but are chemoresistant at relapse. This pattern is particularly seen with *MYCN* amplified tumours. Neuroblastomas that are chemoresistant at presentation are less frequent.

There is a great deal known about the molecular pathology of neuroblastoma, and this can now be linked to variations in clinical behaviour.[36] Major attempts are being made internationally to develop a classification system for neuroblastoma based on this knowledge.[37,38]

Cytogenetic studies identified the first abnormalities which have subsequently been investigated extensively.[39] Chromosome 1 was noted to be most frequently involved in structural and numerical abnormalities. These include deletions or rearrangements leading to the loss of material from the short arm (1p) and additional long arm segments (1q). Chromosome 17 has also been reported to be frequently involved. Other cytogenetic findings include homogeneously staining regions (HSRs) and double minutes (DMs). The HSR is a chromosome segment that is usually longer than a single band in the standard karyotype, staining with intermediate density over its length and not showing the alternating pattern of dark and light bands characteristic of a normal karyotype. DMs, which are paired chromosome bodies lacking centromeres, have the same staining pattern. Both HSRs and DMs have been shown to be the site of gene amplification.

Non-random genetic losses

Non-random genetic abnormalities in neuroblastoma can either be losses (1p, 4p, 11q and 14q) or amplification/gains (*MYCN*, 17q) of genetic material (Table 19.4). Genetic losses indicate the loss of function of some as yet unknown tumour suppressor genes. Allelic loss of chromosome 1p in neuroblastoma has been shown, to date, to have greater importance in terms of effects on clinical outcome. Deletions of 1p were first detected from cytogenetic studies;[39] more recently, Southern blot analysis with

Table 19.4 *Non-random genetic alterations and altered gene expression in neuroblastoma*

	Feature	Approximate incidence (%)	Adverse prognostic factor	Relative importance
Genetic gains	*MYCN* amplification	20	Amplification gain	+++
	17q gain	42		++
Gene expression	CD44		Lack of expression	++++?
	TRKA		Lack of expression	++
	MRP		Expression	++++?
Genetic loss	1p	33	Loss	+++++
	4p	23	–	–
	11q	21	–	–
	14q	21	–	–
DNA ploidy			Diploidy	++

DNA hybridization has been employed.[40–42] Allelic loss of 1p occurs in approximately 33 per cent of neuroblastomas.[43–47] Its presence does not appear to be related to the clinical features of age and stage,[47] but is associated with elevations of serum concentrations of LDH and ferritin. Of great importance is the relationship between *MYCN* amplification and allelic loss of 1p. *MYCN* amplification does not occur without 1p loss, i.e. 20 per cent of neuroblastomas have *MYCN* amplification and 1p loss, and 14 per cent have 1p loss alone; no tumours have *MYCN* amplification with no loss of 1p.[47] 1p loss is also associated with gains of genetic material on 17q and DNA diploidy.[47]

An association between poor outcome and allelic loss of 1p has been documented for a number of years in studies of limited numbers of patients where only one genetic feature has been examined.[40–42] However, more recent studies are documenting the relevant prognostic value of 1p loss in larger series when a number of features are considered.[43,44,47–49]

Caron *et al.*[47] suggested that allelic loss of 1p may be a better prognostic indicator than *MYCN*, as 1p deletion identifies more patients with adverse outcome than *MYCN*. Also, all patients with *MYCN* amplification have 1p loss. However, as with *MYCN* the relationship with prognosis is not absolute as there are some long-term survivors whose tumours have allelic loss of 1p. Similarly, in multivariate analysis the most powerful indicators of prognosis were stage, serum ferritin concentrations and 1p loss when age, serum concentrations of LDH, gain of 17q and DNA ploidy were also considered.[47] The prognostic value of 1p is perhaps strongest in patients with stage 1, 2 and 4S neuroblastoma in which patients who have no deletion of 1p all survive. Conversely, in patients with advanced stage neuroblastoma (stage 3 and 4), all of those with 1p deletion succumb to their disease. Patients with stage 1, 2 and 4S neuroblastoma with 1p deletion, and those with advanced stage neuroblastoma with no abnormalities of 1p, have an intermediate prognosis (between 35 and 50 per cent).[47] Interpretation of 1p data is made more complex as, although with localized disease the recurrence rate is higher, high salvage rates with second-line therapy may reduce any adverse impact on survival.

Initial molecular studies suggested that the deletion on chromosome 1 encompassed a single region in the 1p 36.2-3 subband.[50,51] Subsequent studies have indicated that there are at least two genes that can be lost on chromosome 1p: a distal gene in the region of 1p 36.2-3 that is associated with a single copy *MYCN*; and a more proximal gene in the region of 1p 35-36.1, which is associated with *MYCN* amplification.[45,46,52] There has been some suggestion that these different genes are associated with different prognoses and clinical behaviours, but these observations must be confirmed by larger studies. The possibility of other genes mapped to the 1p 35-36 region playing a role in neuroblastoma genesis has been suggested.[53] There is a gene at 1p 36.2 identified from studies in a constitutional balanced translocation in a patient with neuroblastoma and a gene at 1p 35-36 involved in modification of methylation. 17q gain is the commonest abnormality and is usually associated with advanced disease and age >1 year.[54] A large European collaborative study[55] demonstrated 17q gain in 54 per cent of 313 tumours. *MYCN* amplification was not seen in the absence of 1p deletion or 17q gain. In multivariate analysis, the latter was the most significant independent adverse prognostic factor.

MYCN oncogene

The oncogene *MYCN* is located on chromosome 2p at 2p 23-24.[56] Early reports described increased numbers of over 100 copies in approximately 25–30 per cent of neuroblastomas.[57,58] The amplification of the gene most commonly occurred in DMs in primary tumours, while amplification occurs in cell lines in HSRs. A relationship between higher tumour stage and rapid disease progression with *MYCN* copy number was first documented by Seeger *et al.*,[58] and the independent prognostic value of

MYCN amplification was established subsequently. For example, with stage 3 disease, the 3-year event-free survival (EFS) for patients with a single copy of *MYCN* is 80 per cent, and for those with *MYCN* amplification it is 20 per cent. Similar results have been seen for stage 4 disease under the age of 1 year, and stage 4S. However, in patients with stage 4 disease over the age of 1 year, *MYCN* does not have such discriminatory value,[59] especially following high-dose chemotherapy with autologous bone marrow rescue (ABMR).[60] It is becoming increasingly apparent from recent observations that not all tumours with *MYCN* amplification fare poorly.

MYCN gene copy number appears to be constant in a tumour throughout its natural history, i.e. the time of initial presentation and relapse and between primary tumours and metastases.[61] A definite relationship between *MYCN* expression, either at the mRNA or protein level, and survival has not been established.[62]

Recently, it has been observed that another gene, a DEAD-box protein gene (*DDX1*), is coamplified with *MYCN* in about one-third of patients. The coamplification of *DDX1* and *MYCN* is associated with a shorter disease-free interval than amplification of *MYCN* alone.[63] *Mdm2* has also been shown to be amplified in a small proportion of neuroblastomas.[64]

DNA ploidy

The majority of neuroblastoma tumours are diploid and have 46 chromosomes, but tumours are frequently hyperdiploid or near triploid. These occur most often in infants and are associated with few, if any, structural rearrangements and a very good outcome.[65,66] The combination of hyperdiploidy without amplification of *MYCN* in an infant indicates an excellent prognosis.[67] In contrast, triploid tumours tend to have structural rearrangements, e.g. deletions, translocation and marker chromosomes, and are associated with a poor prognosis.[68]

Nerve growth factor receptors

Neurotrophins are related molecules that promote neuron survival and differentiation in the nervous system. These include nerve growth factor (NGF), brain-derived neurotrophic factor (BDNF) and neurotrophin 3 (NT3). These are ligands for high-affinity tyrosine kinase receptors TRKA, TRKB and TRKC, respectively, which appear to be of prognostic importance in neuroblastoma.[69–71]

TRKA has been shown to be expressed at the mRNA level in 91 per cent of neuroblastomas and at a high level in 82 per cent.[72] A high level of TRKA expression is associated with *MYCN* single-copy, low-stage tumours and a good prognosis; the 5-year survival in patients with tumours expressing TRKA is 86 per cent, in contrast to 14 per cent in patients with tumours with low expression. Combining TRKA expression with *MYCN* gene copy number produced accurate survival information. Patients with a single copy of *MYCN* whose tumours express TRKA have 87 per cent 5-year survival, in contrast to those with *MYCN* amplification and no expression of TRKA, who have a very poor survival. Patients with tumours with a single copy of *MYCN* but with a low expression of TRKA have an intermediate survival. Long-term survival of stage 4 neuroblastoma over the age of 1 year (a very poor prognosis group) has been reported with tumours expressing high levels of TRKA.[73–75] The favourable effect of TRKA may be associated with a reduction in angiogenesis factors and less tumour vascularization.[76]

In contrast, expression of full-length TRKB occurs in association with *MYCN* amplified tumours and is associated with a poor prognosis.[77] Expression of truncated TRKB, i.e. lacking the tyrosine receptor, occurs in mature neuroblastomas.[77] TRKB transfection in cell lines induces chemotherapy resistance to cisplatin, doxorubicin and etoposide. This is reversed by CEP-2563, a TRKB-specific inhibitor.[78]

As well as providing important prognostic information, the expression of TRKA and its interaction with NGF may provide information about its role in the biology of the spontaneous regression and differentiation of neuroblastoma.[79–81] TRKC mRNA expression is associated with normal *MYCN* and low-stage disease.[62,82]

Cell surface glycoprotein CD44 expression

The cell surface glycoprotein CD44 is a polymorphic molecule. The most prevalent form is an 80–90 kDa molecule, CD44 H. CD44 molecules act as the principal receptor for hyaluronate and are involved in cell–cell or cell–extracellular matrix interactions, lymphocyte activation and the homing process. In the majority of tumours in which expression of CD44 has been examined, overexpression of large alternately spliced molecular variants have been associated with metastatic behaviour. However, expression of CD44 in neuroblastoma occurs in good-prognosis tumours.[59,83,84] Expression of CD44 correlates with low tumour stages, a favourable histology, young age and a single copy of *MYCN*. CD44 expression is a very powerful indicator of a favourable outcome, with a 3-year survival rate of 81 per cent in patients with tumour expressing CD44, compared with 7 per cent for associated tumours with-out expression. CD44 expression appears to be more discriminatory than *MYCN*, as patients over the age of 1 year with stage 4 neuroblastoma can be identified who have better prognosis (3-year EFS of 35 vs. 7 per cent). In multivariate analysis, CD44 expression and tumour stage were the only independent prognostic factors when *MYCN*, patient age and histology were also examined.[59]

As CD44 is expressed on non-neuronal derivatives of the neural crest, its expression in neuroblastoma may be related to differentiation, maturation and spontaneous regression. It is unknown whether the very strong interaction between *MYCN* amplification and lack of expression of CD44 is casual.

Multiple drug-resistant proteins, multidrug resistance–associated protein and P-glycoprotein

Various studies have addressed the prognostic importance of the different mechanisms involved in multidrug resistance in neuroblastoma. P-glycoprotein, which is encoded by the *MDR-1* gene, mediates drug resistance by facilitating the efflux of anticancer agents from the cell. Investigations relating to the *MDR-1* gene have resulted in very controversial findings.[85–89] PgP expression is detectable in about 20 per cent of neuroblastomas, but its chemical significance is unclear.[90] Expression at the mRNA level of the multidrug-resistance-associated protein (MRP) gene has, in one study, yielded more clear associations with outcome. The *MRP* gene is located in chromosome 16p 13.1 and encodes a 190-kDa membrane-bound glycoprotein that is associated with efflux of a number of anticancer agents (vinca alkaloids, anthracyclines and epipodophyllotoxins) and glutathione S conjugates.[91] Cisplatin and cyclophosphamide, both important drugs in the therapy of neuroblastoma, undergo glutathione S conjugation but are not substrates for P-glycoprotein.

The level of *MRP* expression has been shown to be greater in neuroblastoma cell lines with *MYCN* amplification and to be reduced when there is differentiation.[92] The level of *MRP* expression also appears to be an independent prognostic indicator in neuroblastoma, as shown in a multivariate analysis when only *MRP* was of independent prognostic significance when *MYCN* gene copy number, age, TRKA expression and tumour stage were also examined. *MRP* expression has prognostic importance to the subgroups of patients with neuroblastoma with *MYCN* amplification, and in stage 1, 2 and 3 tumours.[93] Future studies will determine whether *MRP* expression is causally linked to poor prognosis through efflux of anticancer agents or their glutathione conjugates.

Telomerase

The telomerase is a nucleotide sequence at the tip of the eukaryotic chromosomes and its loss with repeated cell division is responsible for cell senescence. Telomerase is responsible for maintaining telomere length and high levels in cancer cells may reflect tumour aggressiveness.[94–96] In one study, 24 per cent of neuroblastomas contained full-length telomerase catalytic subunit hTERT, which was associated with *MYCN* amplification and poor outcome.[97]

Conclusion

The third meeting of the INSS attempted to carry out a recursive partition analysis of data from over 2800 patients to identify the most powerful prognostic feature. A definitive conclusion was not possible, however, because of insufficient data. Nevertheless, based on published information, three priority levels for 'biological' features of prognostic value were determined:

- First priority:
  – histopathology
  – *MYCN*
  – 1p deletion
  – serum ferritin
  – serum LDH
- Second priority:
  – ploidy
- Third priority:
  – CD44
  – TRKA
  – *MRP*
  – platelet count.

The aim is that prospective collection of these factors in all patients with neuroblastoma will permit a definitive analysis and identify conclusively the most discriminatory molecular pathological features.

In the future, gene expression profiling and proteomics will inevitably play an important role in diagnosis and classification.[98,99]

ASSESSMENT OF MOLECULAR PATHOLOGICAL FEATURES

The ultimate goal is a therapeutic classification based upon clinical features, probably age and stage, together with the most discriminatory molecular pathological feature. In addition, the molecular pathological feature needs to be reproducible and easily assessed and measured. The established technique for determining *MYCN* gene copy number is by Southern blotting, although this does require relatively large amounts of DNA. False-negative results may occur in tumours where there is a high proportion of normal cells (fibroblasts, Schwann cells and lymphocytes) with only a small number of neuroblastoma cells with *MYCN* amplification. Techniques employing the polymerase chain reaction (PCR) have been reported but have not yet been widely used. Fluorescent *in-situ* hybridization (FISH) is a technique that has recently been developed using *MYCN* probes, which enables individual tumours cells to be examined. A very small number of cells is required, especially if tumour imprints are used.[100] False-negative results are less likely, as only tumour cells are examined. There is usually a marked heterogeneity in the number of copies of the *MYCN* gene in different cells in amplified tumours.

The standard technique for determining deletion of chromosome 1p has been Southern analysis with DNA hybridization to investigate loss of heterozygosity (LOH). However, more recently FISH techniques have been further developed.[101] A centromere probe for chromosome 1 is hybridized to the tumour imprint together with a distal probe for chromosome 1p. In a normal diploid cell, four signals should be detected (two centromere and two distal 1p), whereas in a diploid tumour with 1p deletion, only three signals will be seen. Multiplex PCR techniques have been developed to identify the extent and position of 1p deletions.[102] It has been suggested that the examination of tumour samples for allelic loss of 1p should optimally include both FISH and LOH. FISH allows individual tumour cells to be examined and provides information about the number of chromosomes, with LOH defining the position and extent of the deletion.

Flow cytometric analysis is the standard technique for estimating DNA ploidy. FISH techniques can be used to determine the number of individual chromosomes. However, the results obtained by FISH and those by cytometry may not be equivalent.

The expression of CD44 is demonstrated by immunohistology using a monoclonal antibody (J173) in frozen material.[59] In addition, CD44 expression is relatively simply determined on marrow or tumour aspirates. The technique is sensitive, rapid, requires minimum amounts of tissue and can be easily standardized for laboratory use.

The prognostic significance of both TRKA and *MRP* expression has been established examining mRNA levels using rapidly frozen material and Northern analysis or a reverse transcriptase PCR (RT-PCR) technique. Monoclonal antibodies have been used to detect TRKA protein expression.[73,103]

Whatever methods are used for molecular pathological stratification in clinical trials, quality control is essential. This will involve one or several reference laboratories to ensure standardization.[104]

Therapeutic classification system for neuroblastoma

A therapeutic classification system for neuroblastoma using molecular pathological features is the ultimate aim of the INSS. This classification would identify 'risk groups'. Tumours in each group would require different therapy so that patients could be long-term survivors with the least possible treatment. These 'risk groups' would define tumours that require:

- no therapy
- surgery alone
- conventional/minimal chemotherapy
- intensive chemotherapy
- novel approaches.

Patients can be categorized according to age, tumour stage, pathology or biology (Table 19.5).

MYCN amplification has already made an impact on the classification of stage 3 tumours, with those tumours with *MYCN* amplification being treated in a similar manner to stage 4 disease in children over the age of 1 year.

This classification system is imprecise. Some patients with stage 2 tumour succumb to their disease, while there are some survivors of stage 4 disease over the age of 1 year. The inclusion of molecular pathological features will hopefully provide more accurate prognostic groupings. A potential future classification is shown in Table 19.6.

CLINICAL EVALUATION

The diagnostic methods are numerous and include a range of imaging techniques, bone marrow biopsies and trephines, blood sampling and urine collection for the search for tumour markers, and open or closed biopsy of the primary tumour for histological grading and biological studies.

Locoregional involvement

A computed tomography (CT) scan or magnetic resonance imaging (MRI) should be carried out to localize the mass accurately, provide measurements and give anatomical information, particularly about both intra- and extraperitoneal structures in the case of an abdominal mass (Figure 19.9). A CT scan will differentiate cystic from solid tumours and define the extent of a primary tumour as well as its relationship with other structures. It will also detect small calcifications in a neuroblastoma that cannot be demonstrated with standard radiological studies.

The evaluation of metastases

To detect bone marrow metastases, bone marrow aspiration and trephine biopsies are required from two different sites; the two posterior iliac spines are currently recommended. For the assessment to be evaluable, it is important that at least 1 cm of bone marrow is obtained and not cartilage. Often, after chemotherapy, detectable tumour may be eradicated from the bone marrow but

Table 19.5 *Risk group classification based on stage, pathology and biology*

Risk group	Treatment
Low risk	
Stage 1	
Stage 2	
Favourable biology	Surgery
Non-amplified *MYCN*	
Stage 4S	Observe ± minimal chemotherapy
Non-amplified *MYCN*	
Intermediate risk	
Stage 3	
<1 year, non-amplified *MYCN*	
>1 year, non-amplified *MYCN* and	Surgery + ? chemotherapy
favourable histology	
Stage 4	
<1 year, non-amplified *MYCN*	Standard chemotherapy
Stage 4S	
Unfavourable histology	Observe ± chemotherapy
High risk	
Stage 2	
Amplified *MYCN*, unfavourable histology	
Stage 3	Intensive chemotherapy
<1 year, amplified *MYCN*, unfavourable	Surgery
histology	Radiotherapy
>1 year, unfavourable histology	High-dose therapy
Stage 4	Retinoic acid
<1 year, amplified *MYCN*	? Novel therapy
All >1 year	
Stage 4S	
Amplified *MYCN*	

Table 19.6 *Potential future therapeutic classification*

Group	Tumour stage	Patient age	*MYCN* amplification[a]	1p deletion[b]	Triploid DNA[c]	Therapy
1	1, 2, 4S	Any	−	−	+	Biopsy
2	3	Any	−	−	+	Surgery + ? chemotherapy
3	4	<1	−	−	+	Standard chemotherapy
4	4	>1	−	−	−	⎧ Intensive chemotherapy
	4S	>1	+	+	−	⎨ Surgery, high dose
						⎩ chemotherapy ± radiotherapy
5	3, 4	>1	+	+	−	New approaches

[a] −, no amplification; +, amplified >4 copies.
[b] −, intact chromosome 1p; +, allelic loss 1p.
[c] +, triploid DNA; −, diploid or tetraploid.

fibrosis may persist. The prognostic significance of fibrosis is uncertain, although a prospective study is evaluating the long-term implications of bone marrow appearances. If there is no morphological evidence of infiltration of bone marrow with neuroblastoma cells, examination by immunocytochemistry using antibody for neuroectodermal antigens may be of value.

Neuroblastoma has a predilection for metastasizing widely to the skeletal system. Radiographic bone changes on skeletal X-ray survey can occur very rapidly. Skeletal metastases are generally more frequent in children aged 2 years or older. The frequency of detecting skeletal metastases with standard radiography at the time of the initial diagnosis is approximately 50–60 per cent. With the introduction of ^{99m}Tc methylene diphosphate for bone imaging, the accuracy of detecting metastatic bone disease in children has improved dramatically to 80 per cent. *m*IBG, a guanethidine analogue labelled with iodine-123 (^{123}I), is now routinely used for the diagnosis and follow-up of children with neuroblastoma. ^{123}I-*m*IBG scintigraphy correctly demonstrates primary, residual and recurrent tumour masses, as well as diffuse bone marrow infiltration

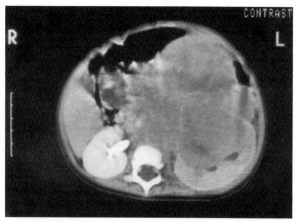

(a)

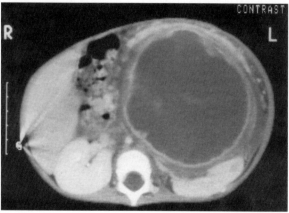

(b)

Figure 19.9 *An 18-month-old girl with stage 3 neuroblastoma of the left adrenal gland: (a) pretreatment CT scan; (b) preoperative CT scan following four courses of chemotherapy. Note that the entire tumour looks 'necrotic', showing a good response to chemotherapy.*

Box 19.2 *Recommended tests (according to site) to be used in assessing extent of disease (INSS)*

Primary tumour

CT and/or MRI scan[a] with 3D measurements; *m*IBG scan (if available)[b]

Metastatic sites[b]

Bone marrow

Bilateral posterior iliac crest marrow aspirates and trephine (core) bone marrow biopsies required to exclude marrow involvement; a single positive site documents marrow involvement; core biopsies must contain at least 1 cm of marrow (excluding cartilage) to be considered adequate

Bone

*m*IBG scan; ^{99}Tc scan is required if *m*IBG scan is negative or unavailable; plain radiographs of positive lesions are recommended

Lymph nodes

Clinical examination (palpable nodes), confirmed histologically; CT scan for non-palpable nodes (3D measurements)

Abdomen/liver

CT and/or MRI scan[a] with 3D measurements

Chest

Anteroposterior and lateral chest radiographs; CT/MRI is necessary if chest radiograph is positive or if abdominal mass/nodes extend into chest

---

[a] Ultrasound considered suboptimal for accurate 3D measurements.
[b] The *m*IBG scan is applicable to all sites of disease.

---

and skeletal, lymph node and soft tissue metastases.[105] The current INSS recommendations are that [123]I-*m*IBG scintigraphy should be carried out at every assessment, both at initial presentation and following therapy.

MRI can detect focal marrow and bone abnormalities in neuroblastoma.[106] However, the technique is not recommended as routine at the present time and its role in the follow-up of children with neuroblastoma requires evaluation.[107,108] More recently, fluorodeoxyglucose positron emission tomography (FDG-PET) scanning has been studied at diagnosis and following treatment.[109] This was highly effective at detecting tumours in soft tissue and the extracranial skeleton. Physiological uptake in brain precluded skull vault evaluation. It was suggested that PET plus normal examination was at least as good as *m*IBG to detect disease at follow-up.

The current recommendations of the INSS for disease evaluation are shown in Box 19.2.

In conclusion, during the past 10 years, the development of CT, MRI and radionuclide imaging has improved the accuracy of diagnosis, staging and follow-up of children with neuroblastoma. These technical advances and the need for cost containment place new responsibilities on the paediatric oncologist to consult the surgeon and the radiologist in selecting the most appropriate diagnostic modalities: the temptation to test excessively must be resisted.

Evaluation of response to treatment

The INSS recommends that the response to treatment is assessed at regular intervals, i.e. after about 10 weeks, the end of induction chemotherapy, after surgery and at the end of therapy. On each occasion the primary tumour should be evaluated and maximal dimensions measured, the extent of bone marrow metastases should be assessed, bone marrow involvement ascertained, and the

Table 19.7 *International Neuroblastoma Staging System (INSS) response to treatment criteria*

Response	Primary tumour[a]	Metastatic sites[a,b]
CR	No tumour	No tumour; catecholamines normal
VGPR	Decreased by 90–99%	No tumour; catecholamines normal; residual ^{99}Tc bone changes allowed
PR	Decreased by >50%	All measurable sites decreased by >50%; bones and bone marrow: number of positive bone sites decreased by >50%; no more than one positive bone marrow site allowed[b]
MR	No new lesions; >50% reduction of any measurable lesion (primary or metastases) with <50% reduction in any other; <25% increase in any existing lesion	
NR	No new lesions; <50% reduction but >25% increase in any existing lesion	
PD	Any new lesion; increase of any measurable lesion by >25%; previous negative marrow positive for tumour	

CR, complete response; MR, minimal response; NR, no response; PD, progressive disease; PR, partial response; VGPR, very good partial response.
[a] Evaluation of primary and metastatic disease.
[b] One positive marrow aspirate or biopsy allowed for PR if this represents a decrease from the number of positive sites at diagnosis.

concentrations of the urinary catecholamines measured. Based upon this information, responses at individual sites and an overall response can be calculated. Table 19.7 shows the INSS response criteria. Different therapeutic approaches can thus be compared on a national and international basis.

TREATMENT STRATEGY

Surgery

The diagnosis of some localized tumours may be suspected preoperatively by elevated urinary catecholamine concentrations. Surgery is the initial and only therapy for non-metastatic resectable tumours (stage 1 and 2). Surgery should include the examination of regional lymph nodes according to the INSS. It is particularly important that the procedure is associated with no, or very low, morbidity.

Most stage 3 tumours are deemed unresectable before or during operation. At presentation, usually only biopsy is possible, although there are some initial complete resections. The conventional approach is delayed surgical resection following a course of chemotherapy that causes tumour shrinkage. As the degree of resection is of prognostic importance, complete excision is the aim. An alternative approach is surgical excision alone for stage 3 tumours without *MYCN* amplification or 1p deletion.[110]

As the diagnosis for most stage 4 neuroblastomas is obtained by elevation of urinary catecholamine concentrations and bone marrow involvement, in the past surgery has not been considered at presentation. However, in view of the increasing importance of the molecular pathology, biopsy of the primary tumour for biological studies at the time of diagnosis is strongly recommended by the INSS. Biopsy should be associated with minimal morbidity and is often undertaken at the time of other procedures that require general anaesthetic, such as insertion of central venous catheters. Multiple needle biopsies may give adequate information on the molecular pathological features. If there is concern about the child's general condition or the primary tumour is very small, where the marrow is heavily infiltrated molecular studies can be done on marrow samples.

In stage 4 disease, the standard approach is to attempt surgical resection of the primary tumour after there has been a response to chemotherapy at the metastatic sites, particularly the bone marrow. In view of recent data relating surgical excision to survival, the aim should be complete resection. In one retrospective review,[111–116] the impact of complete resection in stage 4 disease seems less with the recent use of more aggressive chemotherapy. There remains, however, significant benefit for *MYCN* amplified tumours.[111]

The traditional practice of resecting the primary tumour in stage 4S disease after regression of metastatic disease is now questioned.

Chemotherapy

SINGLE AGENTS

At conventional doses, a number of drugs have shown definite activity when used as monotherapy in children with neuroblastoma,[117–119] including vincristine, cyclophosphamide, ifosfamide, dacarbazine, cisplatin, carboplatin, doxorubicin, epipodophyllotoxins (etoposide/teniposide), peptichemio and melphalan. Although ifosfamide is active in neuroblastoma, there is no convincing evidence to suggest that it is superior to high-dose cyclophosphamide.[120] There has been a suggestion that there is lack of cross-resistance between cisplatin and carboplatin,[120] but there has been no direct comparison of the two agents and it is not known if they are equally effective when given at the appropriate dose.

COMBINATION CHEMOTHERAPY

Initial multiagent schedules utilized vincristine, cyclophosphamide and dacarbazine or doxorubicin.[121,122] Unfortunately, combination therapy with these drugs resulted in a survival rate of 10 per cent or less for children with metastatic disease over the age of 1 year. The addition of cisplatin and epipodophyllotoxins significantly increased initial response rates but produced a minimal increase in overall survival rates.[123,124] These regimens had a more substantial effect on survival in stage 3 disease and in infants with metastatic disease.

HIGH–DOSE CHEMOTHERAPY AS INITIAL THERAPY

Based on the steep dose–response relationship for chemotherapy, high doses of active agents have been administered as initial chemotherapy. High-dose cisplatin ($200 \, mg/m^2$), ifosfamide ($9 \, g/m^2$), cyclophosphamide and carboplatin have been used. Higher response rates were reported than with conventional doses. A review of several different induction regimens using a wide range of doses failed to show any real evidence of an advantage.[125–128] Unfortunately, no randomized studies have been carried out to confirm the therapeutic benefit of escalating the dose.

RAPID SCHEDULE CHEMOTHERAPY

A review of the literature showed a correlation between dose intensity and response, median survival and median progression-free survival in metastatic neuroblastoma.[129] This was the most significant with cisplatin and etoposide.

Previous chemotherapeutic regimens have adhered to the convention that the bone marrow must be allowed to recover between courses to avoid morbidity. This has led to a gap of 3 weeks or longer between courses of chemotherapy, during which drug-resistant cell clones may develop. Rapid administration of the maximally tolerated dose of drugs could potentially lead to more rapid cell kill with a reduced chance of the emergence of resistance. In order to achieve the target of rapid administration, it is inevitable that some drugs will need to be given when the bone marrow has been suppressed by previous chemotherapy, or growth factors will have to be employed. An intensive chemotherapy protocol has been developed. Chemotherapy was administered with 10-day intervals between treatment. Relatively non-myelotoxic drugs (vincristine and cisplatin) were alternated with myelotoxic drugs. Ifosfamide and doxorubicin could not be used in this approach because of their prohibitive toxicity.[130]

However, the combinations of high-dose cisplatin and etoposide, and cyclophosphamide and etoposide, were used as the myelotoxic modules. This schedule produced rapid responses and its toxicity was manageable.[131] The major non-haemopoietic toxicity, renal dysfunction, hypertension, convulsions and persistent nausea were presumed to be caused by cisplatin. Carboplatin was therefore substituted for cisplatin in the first myelotoxic module. A randomized study is in progress (ENSG 5) in which the same drugs (carboplatin, cisplatin, etoposide, cyclophosphamide and vincristine) in the same total dose are administered in both arms, with the only variable being dose intensity. Patients are randomized to receive either the high-dose rapid COJEC schedule (eight courses of chemotherapy administered at 10-day intervals regardless of myelosuppression) or the conventional OPEC/OJEC schedule (seven courses of chemotherapy, given when there is haemopoietic recovery, at 21-day intervals). Dose intensity is 1.8 times higher in the COJEC than in the OPEC/OJEC schedule. This trial will determine whether increasing dose intensity and drug scheduling will improve response rates and overall survival in children over the age of 1 year with stage 4 neuroblastoma.[132]

HIGH–DOSE THERAPY WITH AUTOLOGOUS STEM CELL RESCUE

Based on the steep dose–response relationship between alkylating agents and malignant cells, the concept of high-dose chemotherapy followed by autologous bone marrow (ABM) and subsequently peripheral blood progenitor cell (PBPC) rescue was first suggested for neuroblastoma in the 1970s. Melphalan was initially chosen, as the drug's main toxicity was myelosuppression at conventional doses and this could be overcome by ABMR. The efficacy of melphalan in neuroblastoma was demonstrated in relapsed patients, and following this the agent was used as consolidation therapy prior to progression. In order to investigate whether high-dose melphalan improved overall survival in patients with advanced (stages 3 and 4) neuroblastoma, a randomized study, ENSG1, was carried out.[133,134] Patients who responded to induction chemotherapy – vincristine, cisplatin, teniposide and cyclophosphamide – had surgical removal of the primary tumour attempted and were then randomized to receive high-dose melphalan with ABMR. With a follow-up of 10 years, there is a survival advantage for patients receiving high-dose melphalan.

Encouraged by the response to high-dose melphalan, combinations of agents have been used. These include total body irradiation (TBI);[135] vincristine, melphalan and TBI;[136] teniposide, carmustine and melphalan;[137] teniposide, doxorubicin, melphalan, cisplatin and TBI;[138] cisplatin, etoposide, melphalan and TBI;[139] vincristine, cisplatin, etoposide and melphalan or thiotepa;[140] and vincristine, melphalan, etoposide and carboplatin.[141,142]

The Children's Oncology Group (COG) confirmed the benefit of high-dose therapy in a trial comparing TBI/melphalan-etoposide-carboplatin with standard therapy (see Chapter 26 for a detailed review of high-dose therapy).

Radiotherapy

EXTERNAL BEAM RADIOTHERAPY

In vitro data suggest that neuroblastoma is a radiosensitive tumour with a low capacity for repair of radiation damage.[143] This is confirmed by clinical response to radiation, with the suggestion that tumours arising in children under 2 years of age respond better to radiation than those in older children.[144]

Despite the acknowledged radiosensitivity of neuroblastoma, the role of radiation therapy in the disease remains unclear at present. Moreover, the introduction of more sophisticated techniques such as conformal and intraoperative radiotherapy may alter its role.[145,146] There are five situations where radiation therapy is of value or is being investigated, as discussed below.

Stage 3 neuroblastoma

From histological series, the addition of local radiation therapy appears to improve survival in these patients. The randomized trial by the Pediatric Oncology Group (POG) of North America indicated that local radiotherapy improved event-free and overall survival in patients who received surgery plus low-dose cyclophosphamide and doxorubicin.[147] The benefit of local radiotherapy may disappear when more intensive chemotherapy is used and is also probably unnecessary in good histology tumours where residual disease is of uncertain significance. In most current protocols, local irradiation is not given or is restricted to significant residual disease.[148]

Stage 4 disease

The value of radiotherapy to the primary tumour or areas of persistent metastatic disease at the end of induction chemotherapy has been a contentious issue. Non-randomized data have recently suggested that doses around 20 Gy reduce local failure rate in the setting of intensive chemotherapy. Moreover, an analysis of the COG3891 trial has shown that TBI added to 10 Gy local dose reduced local failure from 52 to 22 per cent, suggesting a dose–response relationship.[149] The potential beneficial effect of the high-dose chemotherapy combined with TBI on local control is a complicating factor.

Radiation therapy as a component of high–dose chemoradiotherapy

Total body irradiation is a component of a number of high-dose regimens used as consolidation therapy with ABMR. The benefit of including TBI and the conditioning regimen has not been proven in a randomized study.

The use of radiotherapy to relieve serious symptoms in stage 2 and 4S neuroblastoma

Radiotherapy is effective in producing decompression in patients with stage 2 neuroblastoma in whom there is spinal cord compression, and in patients with stage 4S neuroblastoma who have life-threatening symptoms from a large tumour burden, particularly in the liver. However, the consensus is that chemotherapy is probably more appropriate and effective in stage 4S disease.

Control of pain and symptoms in palliative care

Radiotherapy has a major role to play in the control of bone metastases in patients with relapsed neuroblastoma undergoing palliative care. In view of the radiosensitivity of neuroblastoma, good pain control can be achieved after one fraction of radiotherapy. Symptoms due to disease at other sites can similarly be relieved.

TARGETED RADIOTHERAPY

*m*IBG is structurally related to the adrenergic blocking antihypertensive drugs and functionally related to noradrenaline. *m*IBG is actively concentrated in tumours derived from the sympathetic nervous system. When labelled with ^{131}I or ^{123}I, this internally administered radiopharmaceutical targets radiation into neuroblastoma tissue. Accumulation of *m*IBG may be predictable by the measurement of noradrenaline transporter genes.[150,151] Studies in patients with relapsed neuroblastoma have demonstrated the activity of ^{131}I-*m*IBG.[152] Phase I and II studies indicate a response rate in the region of 30–40 per cent.[105,153,154] Following the demonstration of its activity as a single agent, ^{131}I-*m*IBG has been combined with high-dose chemotherapy and TBI and used as a consolidation regimen with ABMR, or in patients who have resistant or relapsed disease.[155,156] The toxicity of ^{131}I-*m*IBG when administered as a single or multiple agent is predominately thrombocytopenia, and it was initially suggested that this adverse effect was more severe if there was bone marrow infiltration, prior myelosuppressive chemotherapy and impairment of renal function. However, recent data suggest that bone marrow infiltration may not have a significant effect.

Currently, ^{131}I-*m*IBG is undergoing investigation when administered in four situations:

- *As consolidation therapy either alone or in combination with chemotherapy with or without total body irradiation.* Addition of high-dose chemotherapy followed by PBPC rescue is feasible and does not result in prohibitive toxicity. However, the preliminary results have not yet shown an increase in efficacy.[155–159]
- *As initial single agent therapy.* This approach, in which repeated therapy with ^{131}I-*m*IBG is administered until the primary tumour is deemed resectable, has been pioneered by the Amsterdam group. The toxicity is minimal and there is limited

thrombocytopenia.[160] Long-term evaluation of the efficacy of this approach is required. The benefit of *m*IBG therapy in non-metastatic disease must be set against the risk of secondary malignancies.[161,162]

- *Concomitant administration of chemotherapy and ^{131}I-mIBG at initial presentation.* This approach is based on the different and cross-resistant effects of [131]I-*m*IBG-delivered radiation and chemotherapy and the potential lack of cross-resistance between the modalities. Preliminary reports suggest no increase in toxicity.[163] One study combined [131]I-*m*IBG with vincristine, cisplatin, etoposide and cyclophosphamide. As irradiation from [131]I-*m*IBG is delivered at low dose rates, it is effectively fractionated and there is therefore no additional benefit to administering [131]I-*m*IBG in multiple doses. A single administration is therefore given with potentially maximum efficacy. Furthermore, the microdosimetry of β particle irradiation suggests that very small tumours would be ineffectively treated using *m*IBG because they are too small to absorb β energy efficiently. Mathematical modelling suggests that [131]I-*m*IBG is therefore likely to be most effective when given at presentation, when tumour masses are at their largest. Hyperbaric oxygen has been used to try to enhance efficacy although its value is unproven.[164] Recent work has focused on improving dosimetry to optimize dose delivery.[165–167]
- *Palliation.* Effective pain control may be obtained with minimal morbidity but significant thrombocytopenia limits the use of *m*IBG. This strategy may be appropriate for multifocal bone disease.[168,169]

Differentiation therapy

The retinoids 13-*cis*- and all-*trans*-retinoic acid cause decreased proliferation, morphological differentiation, decreased expression of *MYCN* and increased expression of retinoic acid receptors in neuroblastoma cells *in vitro*.[170] These changes have been observed in neuroblastoma cell lines resistant to cytotoxic drugs, suggesting that treatment with retinoids may be an alternative and complementary therapeutic strategy to chemotherapy. 13-*cis*-retinoic acid was chosen for clinical study in view of its lower toxicity and more favourable pharmacokinetics, as plasma concentrations of *trans*-retinoic acid fall during therapy. This decrease in concentration may be due to induction of drug metabolism by a cytochrome P450 system and/or increased expression of the cellular retinoic acid binding proteins (CRABP).

In the first clinical trial, 13-*cis*-retinoic acid was administered at a dose of 100 mg/m² per day on a continuous schedule.[171] There was little efficacy against advanced recurrent disease, with only 9 per cent of patients responding.

However, a phase I study of 13-*cis*-retinoic acid using an intermittent schedule with two equally divided doses being given daily for 2 weeks followed by a 2-week rest period, reported responses in patients with resistant disease in the bone marrow.[172] This suggested that 13-*cis*-retinoic acid had a greater potential for therapy when there was minimal residual disease than at the time of recurrence or initial presentation. With this schedule, the maximal dosage was 60 mg/m² per day with the major toxicities being hypercalcaemia and rash.

Two phase III studies have examined the therapeutic benefit of 13-*cis*-retinoic acid. In both these studies, 13-*cis*-retinoic acid was administered after completion of therapy, i.e. after high-dose therapy with ABMR. Different schedules were employed. In the CCG study, retinoic acid was given intermittently for 2 out of every 4 weeks at a higher dose of 60 mg/m² compared with continuous oral administration of 0.75 mg/kg in the ENSG study. The ENSG study failed to show any benefit in terms of relapse-free or overall survival.[173,174] In contrast, the CCG trial, which included 258 children, showed a significant advantage, the relapse-free survival being 46 per cent at 3 years from randomization in those receiving retinoic acid compared with 29 per cent in the control arm.

13-*cis*-Retinoic acid does not bind to either retinoic acid receptors or retinoid X receptors, which are thought to be responsible for the mechanism of retinoid action. 13-*cis*-Retinoic acid *in vivo* isomerizes to all-*trans*- and 9-*cis*-retinoic acid. 9-*cis*-Retinoic acid binds with high affinity to both retinoic acid and retinoid X receptors, and *in vitro* shows greater therapeutic potential.[175–177] Xenograft studies have, however, shown disappointing *in vivo* activity.[178]

Fenretinide, a synthetic retinoid (N-4-hydroxyphenyl reinamide), has the ability to induce apoptosis in neuroblastoma cell lines.[179] The compound has entered phase I trial in a 4 weeks on, 1 week off schedule. Night blindness and skin toxicity were the main side-effects.[180] One xenograft study has failed to confirm *in vitro* activity.[181]

Appropriate therapy for different groups

STAGE 1 AND 2 TUMOURS

The present international consensus is that surgery alone is required for the majority of these tumours.[35,182,183] It is important that surgery should not be associated with significant mortality or morbidity. Additional chemotherapy or radiotherapy has not been shown to be of value.[184]

There are two groups of patients in whom the situation is more controversial: stage 1 and 2 neuroblastoma with *MYCN* amplification and stage 2b neuroblastoma.

Stage 1 and 2 neuroblastoma with *MYCN* amplification

These patients have a worse prognosis than those with other low-stage tumours. Some groups therefore suggest that these patients require very intensive chemotherapy, including high-dose regimens. However, 50 per cent of these patients will be cured without any additional treatment to surgery.[185] There is no evidence that intensive treatment at presentation is of benefit compared with treatment at the time of relapse. Furthermore, it appears that conventional chemotherapy will not improve the prognosis of these tumours.[184,186] If treatment is given, intensive chemotherapy, with its attendant morbidity and mortality, is therefore required. The current policy in the European Collaborative Group is to use surgery alone for stage 1 *MYCN* amplified and to use the current high-risk protocol with very intensive therapy for stage 2 *MYCN* amplified (as for stage 4).

Stage 2b neuroblastoma

Early studies indicated that these tumours have a worse prognosis.[8,10] However, only a minority progress, and as there is no compelling evidence that treatment at progression is inferior to therapy at initial presentation, the consensus in a number of groups is that tumours should be treated similarly to stage 2a disease, i.e. surgery alone if good histology.

STAGE 3 NEUROBLASTOMA

The standard treatment for this group of patients is initial surgery, usually biopsy, followed by conventional chemotherapy and then delayed surgical excision. Five-year survival rates of approximately 65 per cent are expected. As complete excision of the primary, particularly if confirmed by histological examination, confers a survival advantage, complete surgical resection should be attempted after initial chemotherapy.[112,187,188] The better prognosis observed in patients in whom there is no microscopic residual tumour present after surgery may simply be a reflection of the degree of chemosensitivity of the tumour and not primarily due to the surgical procedure.

There are two specific questions related to these patients, which are discussed below.

The role of radiotherapy

A randomized study carried out by POG showed a survival advantage for local radiotherapy in addition to chemotherapy with cyclophosphamide and doxorubicin.[147] However, the chemotherapy employed was not intensive and it has been suggested that radiotherapy may not be of benefit when a cisplatin-based chemotherapy regimen is used. Although never clearly demonstrated, it seems likely that only bad biology tumours have a high risk of recurrence and, as these are now treated on high-risk regimens, low-morbidity chemotherapy and surgery are appropriate for the rest of stage 3 tumours. It has even been suggested that after initial incomplete surgery, no additional therapy is needed for good biology tumours, i.e. treat like stage 2. This philosophy requires prospective evaluation.[189]

Treatment for stage 3 neuroblastoma with *MYCN* amplification

It is generally agreed that these patients have a worse prognosis; they should be treated by the protocol used for stage 4 disease over the age of 1 year. High-dose therapy with ABMR and local radiotherapy are given in addition to conventional chemotherapy. Loss of chromosome 1p has also been shown to influence outcome.[190]

STAGE 4 DISEASE OVER THE AGE OF 1 YEAR

The treatment currently used by most cooperative groups comprises initial chemotherapy followed by attempted surgical resection of the primary tumour and then high-dose chemotherapy with PBPC rescue.[191] With this approach there has been a steady improvement in outcome with survival in unrelated series of 30–40 per cent.[192–195]

A number of different types of initial chemotherapy have been given. Combinations of cyclophosphamide (occasionally ifosfamide), cisplatin or carboplatin, and etoposide are the most frequent. Doxorubicin, vincristine or peptichemio are given in some protocols. Different doses and schedules of these drugs have been used. A review of the induction regimen has shown that there is little, if any, difference in the complete response (CR) or very good partial response (VGPR) rates with the various protocols[196] and the well tolerated OPEC/OJEC remains a standard regimen.[197] In one study, an attempt to intensify therapy appeared to worsen outcome.[193]

ENSG 5 is one of the few randomized studies of induction chemotherapy in neuroblastoma. The results of this study should determine whether increasing dose intensity really improves survival.

Local irradiation follows high-dose therapy and *cis*-retinoic acid is then given for a 6-month period. The current European high-risk study compares two high-dose regimens, busulphan/melphalan and melphalan, etoposide, carboplatin. The role of anti-GD2 antibody is also planned to be evaluated. In the COG trial, the role of peripheral blood stem cell (PBSC) purging and of anti-GD2 combined with granulocyte/monocyte colony-stimulating factor (GM-CSF) are studied.

INFANTS WITH STAGE 4 NEUROBLASTOMA

For a considerable time it has been recognized that infants have a better prognosis than older children. Five-year

EFS rates have ranged from 50 to 75 per cent when multiagent chemotherapy has been used. In some early studies with a very good survival rate, patients with 4S disease may have been included. The degree of marrow involvement influences outcome.[198] Various multiagent chemotherapy regimens have been utilized followed by surgical resection of the primary tumour. High-dose chemotherapy with ABMR is not recommended for infants with stage 4 disease in view of the high morbidity of the procedure and the high survival rates when conventional chemotherapy is used. Although infants with bone metastases tend to have a worse outcome, this is not a very powerful prognostic feature. *MYCN* amplification may be a better feature for identifying patients who require more intensive treatment. In contrast, infants with diploid tumours without allelic loss of 1p or *MYCN* amplification have an excellent prognosis. Thus two groups of infants with disseminated neuroblastoma may be emerging. The poor prognosis patients require intensive therapy, perhaps including innovative treatment modalities. Due to late sequelae, irradiation is used sparingly in this age group. Sophisticated planning and intensity-modulated radiotherapy (IMRT) may facilitate administration where there is a strong indication.[199]

STAGE 4S NEUROBLASTOMA

The overall prognosis for these patients is very good, with an EFS rate of about 85 per cent. However, the behaviour of 4S neuroblastoma varies and includes:

- spontaneous regression without symptoms
- progression with life-threatening symptoms but response to therapy
- progression unresponsive to therapy
- regression with recurrence in stage 4 disease with bone involvement.

With the exception of *MYCN* amplification, the behaviour of the tumour cannot currently be predicted at presentation.[48,200,201] Therapy should only be administered for life-threatening symptoms. The Philadelphia scoring system is a useful guide and may be used to choose treatment strategy. Radiotherapy or single or multiple agent chemotherapy has been given. The overall consensus is that chemotherapy is probably the most efficient modality. A single course of combination chemotherapy, such as carboplatin and etoposide is advocated. If there is response to this no further treatment is given. If not, more intensive chemotherapy is used. With this approach, overall survival should approach 90 per cent.[202,203] Considerable attention is now paid to identifying more clearly what biological features predict behaviour, including novel chromosome changes and telomerase activity.[204–206]

NEUROBLASTOMA PRESENTING WITH SPINAL CORD COMPRESSION

Spinal cord compression can occur with stage 2, 3 or 4 neuroblastoma. The goals of therapy differ with stage 2 disease where the major objective is relief of the spinal cord compression in the expectation that the tumour will regress spontaneously. Surgery (laminectomy or laminotomy), radiotherapy and chemotherapy have been employed. The optimal method of spinal cord decompression is the one associated with the least acute or long-term toxicity. In the past, laminectomy was associated with late scoliosis. However, the newer techniques of laminotomy should not be associated with this problem. Recent preliminary reports express some concern regarding laminotomy in the cervical region. Radiotherapy has little acute toxicity and small doses should not have long-term sequelae. Two courses of chemotherapy with carboplatin/etoposide are associated with few long-term side-effects, although there is a risk of myelosuppression and infection in the short term. If chemotherapy is employed, only one or two courses of treatment are necessary to cause regression. An objective response will take a number of weeks to become apparent and it is therefore important that dexamethasone is continued for 3–4 weeks or until there is definite neuroradiological evidence of regression. The best method of treatment of spinal cord compression in patients with neuroblastoma is uncertain. Large cooperative groups need to present their results with different modalities in order that results can be compared.

In the case of spinal cord compression in stage 4 disease, decompression by chemotherapy should be attempted, as systemic chemotherapy is required for overall treatment. If this fails, surgical decompression should be undertaken.

SCREENING FOR NEUROBLASTOMA

Neuroblastoma appeared to be the ideal candidate for a tumour screening programme. There were a number of features that supported the concept of screening:

- The prognosis for infants presenting before their first birthday is superior to that of older children.
- Localized disease has a better outcome than disseminated disease.
- Metastatic neuroblastoma was a major cause of death from childhood cancer in the 1990s.
- Neuroblastoma can be detected by the elevation of urinary catecholamines.

Screening for neuroblastoma began in Japan in the early 1970s, and initial results were encouraging.[207] However, the incidence of neuroblastoma doubled from 8.2 to 20.1 per million children and the majority of the tumours detected were of low stage and had good biological features (triploid tumours with neither amplification of *MYCN* nor allelic loss of 1p).[208,209] Furthermore, there was no reduction in either the death rate from neuroblastoma or the incidence of metastatic disease in older children.[210] Studies were subsequently undertaken in the north of England, France, Stuttgart and Hamburg, and Quebec, Canada.

In the German study 2.5 million children were screened and compared with 2.1 million controls. This was based on geographical location. The incidence of stage 4 disease was the same in both groups.[211] In the Canadian study almost half a million were screened at 3 weeks and 6 months of age. Compared with a control group in Florida there was no benefit in terms of death from neuroblastoma.[212]

It is therefore concluded that it is possible to detect asymptomatic cases of neuroblastoma by screening, resulting in an overdiagnosis. These children are exposed to therapy that is not required and carries potential morbidity and mortality consequences.

These investigations do not support the concept that poor-prognosis metastatic neuroblastoma evolves from localized disease, but rather confirm that there are two distinct entities of good- and poor-prognosis disease. The consensus is therefore that screening infants under 1 year is highly unlikely to reduce mortality from neuroblastoma. Whether screening for neuroblastoma at the age of 12 months would be of therapeutic benefit has been considered, but this would be an enormous undertaking, requiring the screening of 1.25–2 million children, together with a control group of equal size.[213]

CONCLUSIONS AND CURRENT CONTROVERSIES

Neuroblastoma has the greatest diversity in clinical behaviour of any tumour, and it is the malignancy in which there is the greatest knowledge of molecular pathology. The prognostic importance of many biological features has already allowed therapy to be altered according to molecular pathological features. There are great expectations that a therapeutic classification can be developed in the future. Despite this and the fact that neuroblastoma is one of the commonest childhood malignancies, there are still many questions about the optimal therapy of neuroblastoma and the role of the different therapeutic modalities. These questions can only be answered through large randomized, probably international, studies. Research into the genetics and cellular behaviour of this tumour will soon identify new targets for treatment.

Further significant progress in the treatment of neuroblastoma demands both international randomized studies of new therapeutic modalities and close collaboration between basic scientists and clinicians.

HOW CAN THE THERAPEUTIC CLASSIFICATION OF NEUROBLASTOMA BE IMPROVED?

It is anticipated that, through the INSS and the International Neuroblastoma Risk Groups (INRG) working group, a more precise therapeutic classification for neuroblastoma can be achieved by the inclusion of molecular pathological features as well as tumour stage and patient age. There are now a large number of molecular pathological variables that have been shown to be of prognostic importance. Further progress must depend on the analysis of a large number of patients in whom the important molecular pathological and clinical features and outcome are known. Such analysis has to be on an international basis.[214] Only one or two molecular pathological features should be included. Simple, reliable, reproducible techniques to assess these features on small quantities are mandatory for the success of this approach.

To date, *MYCN* amplification in stage 3 neuroblastoma has probably had the greatest impact on therapy. In the future, similar changes to treatment may be made in infants with stage 4 and 4S neuroblastoma who also have *MYCN* amplification. Not only can therapy be intensified in lower stage patients, but it can also be reduced in very good prognosis patients detected by molecular pathology, e.g. stage 1, 2 and 3 tumours that are triploid, have no *MYCN* amplification, and no allelic loss of 1p. Despite the recent publication of new molecular pathological features, *MYCN* gene copy number, allelic loss of 1p and DNA ploidy appear to be the most important factors on which to base therapy. Attempts to identify at presentation those patients over the age of 1 year with stage 4 disease who will be long-term survivors have not yet been very fruitful. Of particular interest are features that influence outcome independent of *MYCN*.[205]

The reproducibility of accurate surgical staging, particularly the detection of lymph node metastases, appears to be a difficult goal on an international basis. It is anticipated that future staging systems will not require this degree of detail.

IN WHICH NEUROBLASTOMAS CAN THERAPY BE REDUCED?

A relatively easy realizable goal is the reduction of therapy in some patients with neuroblastoma who are long-term survivors with current therapy. The ongoing European Neuroblastoma Study of surgery alone for stage 1 and 2 tumours without *MYCN* amplification is a major step forward. A decade ago many of these patients would have received chemotherapy and radiation. In future, surgery may be the only therapy for some groups of infants and patients with stage 3 neuroblastoma.

WHAT IS THE ROLE OF SURGERY IN NEUROBLASTOMA?

This question cannot be answered accurately at present because the current therapeutic grouping of neuroblastoma is imprecise. Surgery may not be necessary in some stage 1, 2 and even 3 tumours. In contrast, recent studies indicate that complete surgical resection of stage 3 and 4 neuroblastomas is a good prognostic factor. Maximal surgical resection of stage 3 and 4 disease should therefore be the aim at present. It is possible that resectability is a surrogate for a good prognostic molecular pathological feature and that these tumours would be associated with a favourable outcome regardless of the degree of surgery. Only a study in which the degree of surgical resection is randomized will answer this question.

IS THERE A ROLE FOR RADIOTHERAPY IN STAGE 3 AND 4 DISEASE?

The contribution of irradiation treatment to macroscopic or microscopic disease in stage 2 patients has been shown to be insignificant. Although one randomized study in stage 3 patients indicated that it may be beneficial, the value of radiotherapy in stage 3 disease without *MYCN* amplification when current chemotherapy protocols are used needs to be established.

Whether local radiotherapy to sites of disease in patients with stage 4 neuroblastoma prior to high-dose therapy is of benefit is uncertain. As local radiotherapy in stage 4 disease is favoured in North America, and has now been included in European protocols, a randomized study investigating this question is unlikely.

WHAT IS THE ROLE OF *m*IBG THERAPY?

Although targeted irradiation with ^{131}I*m*-IBG is active in neuroblastoma, there have not yet been any convincing studies to demonstrate that its inclusion in therapeutic regimens will improve overall survival in any group of patients. ^{131}I*m*-IBG appears not to add benefit to TBI and chemotherapy as consolidation treatment in neuroblastoma. The use of *m*IBG as the only initial therapy has been pioneered by the Amsterdam group. Although this approach results in significant response rates with little toxicity, a substantial number of patients with stage 4 disease still die. The concurrent use of *m*IBG and chemotherapy at presentation is an interesting approach as both modalities have different mechanisms of cell death in neuroblastoma. A pilot/feasibility study by the UKCCSG investigating a combination of *m*IBG and topotecan is underway.

WHAT IS THE ROLE FOR DIFFERENTIATION THERAPY INCLUDING THE RETINOIDS?

cis-Retinoic acid has been shown to produce ganglionic differentiation in undifferentiated neuroblastoma cell lines. Responses have been observed in patients with persistent disease when treated with 13-*cis*-retinoic acid. The results of the CCG randomized studies carried out investigating the role of 13-*cis*-retinoic acid when administered after chemotherapy showed clear benefit. Future studies need to address the clinical benefit of the newer retinoids and to determine the optimal time for administration.

HOW SHOULD RESPONSE BE ASSESSED?

Completeness of response is an important prediction of subsequent outcome, but the ideal methods of assessment remain unclear. In one study, plasma (but not urinary catecholamines) and marrow aspirates (but not *m*IBG) were predictive.[215]

In another study, *m*IBG added to the sensitivity of assessment, decreasing CR rate from 85 to 78 per cent.[216] An *m*IBG scoring system may improve patient stratification. One divides the skeleton into nine segments and each segment is scored 1–3. In this system, early response after four courses of chemotherapy appeared to predict outcome better than prior to high-dose therapy.[217]

Early response may be assessed by molecular methods such as RT-PCR for tyrosine hydroxylase and GD2[218–221] and perhaps by non-invasive imaging with magnetic resonance spectroscopy.[222,223]

MANAGEMENT OF UNUSUAL SITES/BEHAVIOUR

- Opsoclonus-myoclonus is generally associated with localized good biology tumours.[224] Although the symptoms often respond to steroid or immune globulin there is significant risk of neurological morbidity.[225] The role of low-dose chemotherapy to reduce this risk is under study.
- Central nervous system disease may rarely be present at diagnosis, in some cases as an isolated tumour. With better survival in stage 4 disease, it is now more common to see CNS disease at relapse.[226,227] Similarly, lung disease, rare at diagnosis,[228] may occur at relapse after intensive first-line therapy.
- 'Chronic' smouldering metastatic disease is now also seen more frequently. This is often in older children and may respond to repeated courses of standard or investigational therapy.[229]
- Neonatal tumours may be detected antenatally and are invariably of good biology and similar to screened tumours. Detailed staging with marrow, *m*IBG etc. is not necessary. Almost all tumours resolve on ultrasound follow-up. Raised catecholamines without biopsy or resection confirm the diagnosis.

HOW SHOULD PATIENTS BE FOLLOWED UP?

Close surveillance of localized disease may be appropriate if further treatment options are available. Late relapses beyond 5 years are seen.[230] With initial stage 4 disease, the chance of cure after relapse is remote and, moreover, surveillance imaging is not particularly effective in detecting disease prior to symptoms.[231] Clinical follow-up is more related to late effects in the survivors than salvage therapy.

WHAT ARE THE NEW TREATMENT APPROACHES?

- *Chemotherapy.* The role of newer drugs such as topotecan and irinotecan remain to be clarified and novel individualized pharmacokinetic guided approaches may hold promise.[232–235] Prodrug strategies include the use of a tyrosine hydroxylase-activated etoposide derivative[236] and VDEPT (virus-detected enzyme prodrug therapy), used to activate CPT11 at a cellular level.[237]
- *Molecular targets.* A number of the neuroblastoma-specific alterations, including *MYCN*, 17q gain and TRKB, are under evaluation using antisense and small molecules.[238–241]
- *Immunotherapy.* Antibody approaches with anti-GD2 +/− GM-CSF are currently under randomized trial.[242,243] Post-transcriptionally modified DNA vaccine is effective in the murine model[244] and vaccine therapy using allogeneic tumour cells transduced to secrete lymphotoctin and IL-2 is in clinical trial.[245]

KEY POINTS

- The clinical behaviour of neuroblastoma in children under the age of one year is significantly different from older children and their prognosis is superior.
- The genetic feature of the tumour, *MYCN* amplification, is currently being used to stratify therapy for children with localized disease and those under the age of one year.
- Patients with neuroblastoma are currently being grouped into those with a low, medium or high risk of recurrence.
- It has recently become appreciated that the group of children with metastatic neuroblastoma under the age of one year whose tumours will regress spontaneously and who do not need treatment (previously stage 4S) can be widened.
- High-risk disease is stage 4 disease over the age of one year, *MYCN* amplified localized or *MYCN* amplified infant disease.
- The internationally recognized therapy for high-risk disease is initial chemotherapy followed by surgical resection of the primary tumour, consolidation with myleoablative therapy with haemopoietic stem cell support, followed by radiation therapy to the site of the primary tumour and differentiation therapy with 13-*cis* retinoic acid.

REFERENCES

1. Gross RE, Farber S, Martin LW. Neuroblastoma sympatheticum: a study and report of 217 cases. *Pediatrics* 1959; **23**: 1179–91.
2. Bodian M. Neuroblastoma. *Pediatr Clin North Am* 1959; **6**: 449–518.
3. Fortner H, Nicastri A, Murphy ML. Neuroblastoma: natural history and results of treating 133 cases. *Ann Surg* 1968; **167**: 132–42.
4. Stella JG, Scheisguth O, Schlienger M. Neuroblastoma: a study of 144 cases treated in the Institute Gustave Roussy over a period of 7 years. *Am J Roentgenol* 1970; **108**: 325–32.
5. Wilson LMK, Draper GJ. Neuroblastoma: its natural history and prognosis – a study of 487 cases. *Br Med J* 1974; **3**: 301–7.
6. de la Monte SM, Moore GW, Hutchins GM. Non random distribution of metastases in neuroblastic tumors. *Cancer* 1983; **52**: 915–20.
7. Evans AE, D'Angio GJ, Randolph J. A proposed staging for children with neuroblastoma. Children's Cancer Study Group A. *Cancer* 1971; **27**: 374–8.
8. Hayes F, Green A, Hutsu O et al. Surgicopathologic staging of neuroblastoma: prognostic significance of regional lymph node metastases. *J Pediatr* 1983; **102**: 59–62.
9. UICC-TNM. *Classification of Malignant Tumours*, 4th edn. Berlin: Springer-Verlag, 1987.
10. Ninane J, Pritchard J, Morris Jones PH et al. Stage II neuroblastoma. Adverse prognostic significance of lymph node involvement. *Arch Dis Child* 1982; **57**: 438–42.
11. Brodeur GM, Seeger RC, Barrett A et al. International criteria for diagnosis, staging and response to treatment in patients with neuroblastoma. *J Clin Oncol* 1998; **6**: 1874–81.
12. Brodeur GM, Pritchard J, Berthold F et al. Revisions of international criteria for neuroblastoma diagnosis, staging and response to treatment. *J Clin Oncol* 1993; **11**: 1466–77.
13. Monsaingeon M, Perel Y, Simonnet G, Corcuff JB. Comparative values of catecholamines and metabolites for the diagnosis of neuroblastoma. *Eur J Pediatr* 2003; **162**: 397–402.
14. Tuchman M, Ramnaraine M, Woods W, Krivit W. Three years of experience with random urinary homovanillic and vanillylmandelic acid levels in the diagnosis of neuroblastoma. *Pediatrics* 1987; **79**: 203–5.
15. Tuchman M, Morros L, Ramnaraine M et al. Value of random unrinary homovanillic and vanillylmandelic acid levels in the diagnosis and management of patients with neuroblastoma: comparison with 24-hour urine collections *Pediatrics* 1985; **75**: 324–8.
16. Siegel SE, Laug WE, Harlow PJ et al. Effects of retinoic acid (RA) on the growth and phenotypic expression of several human neuroblastoma cell lines. *Exp Cell Res* 1983; **148**: 21–30.
17. Ninane J, Vangyseghem S, Andre F et al. Long term survivors of advanced neuroblastoma: factors affecting prognosis. An ENSG study. Abstract. International Society of Paediatric Oncology, XIII Meeting, Belgrade, Yugoslavia, 15–20 September 1986.
18. Krivit W, Mirkin BL, Freier E et al. Serum catecholamine metabolites in stage IV neuroblastoma. In: Evans AE, ed. *Advances in Neuroblastoma Research*. New York: Raven Press, 1980; 33–42.
19. Gahr M, Hunneman DH. The value of determination of homovanillic and vanillylmandelic acids in plasma for the

diagnosis and follow-up of neuroblastoma in children. *Eur J Pediatr* 1987; **146**: 489–93.

20. Eldrup E, Clausen N, Scherling B, Schmiegelow K. Evaluation of plasma 3,4-dihydroxyphenylacetic acid (DOPAC) and plasma 3,4-dihydroxyphenylalanine (DOPA) as tumor markers in children with neuroblastoma. *Scand J Clin Lab Invest* 2001; **61**: 479–90.

21. Cooper EH, Pritchard J, Bailey C, Ninane J. Serum neurone-specific enolase in children's cancer. *Br J Cancer* 1987; **56**: 65–7.

22. Zeltzer PM, Marangos PJ, Evans AE *et al*. Serum neuron-specific enolase in children with neuroblastoma. Relationship to stage and disease course. *Cancer* 1986; **57**: 1230–4.

23. Hann HL, Stahlut MW, Evans AE. Source of increased ferritin in neuroblastoma: studies with cancanavilin A-sepharose binding. *J Natl Cancer Inst* 1986; **76**: 1031–3.

24. Hann HL, Evans AE, Siegal SE *et al*. Prognostic importance of serum ferritin in patients with stage III and IV neuroblastoma: the Children's Cancer Study Group experience. *Cancer Res* 1985; **45**: 2843–8.

25. Evans AE, D'Angio GJ, Propert K *et al*. Prognostic factors in neuroblastoma. *Cancer* 1987; **59**: 1853–9.

26. Silber JH, Evans AE, Fridman M. Models to predict outcome from childhood neuroblastoma: the role of serum ferritin and tumor histology. *Cancer Res* 1991; **51**: 1426–33.

27. Berthold F, Trechow R, Utsch S *et al*. Prognostic factors in metastatic neuroblastoma: a multivariate analysis of 182 cases. *Am J Pediatr Hematol Oncol* 1992; **14**: 207–15.

28. Shuster JJ, McWilliams NB, Castleberry R *et al*. Serum lactate dehydrogenase in childhood neuroblastoma: a Pediatric Oncology Group recursive partitioning study. *Am J Clin Oncol* 1992; **15**: 295–303.

29. Ladisch S, Wu ZL. Shedding of G_{D2} ganglioside by human neuroblastoma. *Int J Cancer* 1985; **39**: 73–6.

30. Schochat S, Corbelletta N, Repman M, Schengrund CL. A biochemical analysis of thoracic neuroblastomas: a Pediatric Oncology Group study. *J Pediatr Surg* 1987; **22**: 660–4.

31. Beckwith JB, Martin RF. Observations on the histopathology of neuroblastomas. *J Pediatr Surg* 1968; **3**: 106–10.

32. Hugues M, Marsden HB, Palmer MK. Histologic patterns of neuroblastoma related to prognosis and clinical staging. *Cancer* 1974; **34**: 1706–11.

33. Shimada H, Chatten J, Newton WA *et al*. Histopathologic prognostic factors in neuroblastomic tumours. Definition of subtypes of ganglioneuroblastoma and an age-linked classification of neuroblastomas. *J Natl Cancer Inst* 1984; **73**: 405–9.

34. Joshi VV, Cantor AB, Altshuler G *et al*. Age-linked prognostic categorisation based on a new histologic grading system for neuroblastoma: a clinicopathologic study of 211 cases from the Pediatric Oncology Group. *Cancer* 1992; **69**: 2197–211.

35. Kushner BH, Cheung N-KV, LaQuaglia MP *et al*. Survival from locally invasive or widespread neuroblastoma without cytotoxic therapy. *J Clin Oncol* 1996; **14**: 373–81.

36. Schwab M, Westermann F, Hero B, Berthold F. Neuroblastoma: biology and molecular chromosomal pathology. *Lancet* 2003; **4**: 472–80.

37. Brodeur GM. Neuroblastoma: biological insights into a clinical enigma. *Nat Rev Cancer* 2003; **3**: 203–16.

38. George RE, Variend S, Cullinane C *et al*. Relationship between histopathological features, MYCN amplification, and prognosis: a UKCCSG study. United Kingdom Children's Cancer Study Group. *Med Pediatr Oncol* 2001; **36**: 169–76.

39. Brodeur GM, Sekhon GS, Goldstein MN. Chromosomal aberrations in human neuroblastomas. *Cancer* 1977; **40**: 2256–63.

40. Christiansen H, Lampert F. Tumour karyotype discriminates between good and bad prognostic outcome in neuroblastoma. *Br J Cancer* 1988; **57**: 121–6.

41. Christiansen H, Schestag J, Christiansen NM *et al*. Clinical impact of chromosome 1 aberrations in neuroblastoma: a metaphase and interphase cytogenetic study. *Genes Chromosomes Cancer* 1992; **5**: 141–9.

42. Hayashi Y, Kanada N, Inaba T *et al*. Cytogenetic findings and prognosis in neuroblastoma with emphasis on marker chromosome 1. *Cancer* 1989; **63**: 126–32.

43. Fong CT, White PS, Peterson K *et al*. Loss of heterozygosity for chromosomes 1 or 14 defines subsets of advanced neuroblastomas. *Cancer Res* 1992; **52**: 1780–5.

44. Caron HN, Van Sluis P, van oeve M *et al*. Allelic loss of chromosome 1p36 in neuroblastoma is of preferential origin and correlates with N-myc amplification. *Nat Genet* 1993; **4**: 187–90. (Erratum: *Nat Genet* 1993; **4**: 431.)

45. Schleiermacher G, Peter M, Michon J *et al*. Two distinct deleted regions on the short arm of chromosome 1 in neuroblastoma. *Genes Chromosomes Cancer* 1994; **10**: 275–81.

46. Takeda O, Homma C, Maseki N *et al*. There may be two tumour suppressor genes on chromosome arm 19 closely associated with biologically distinct subtypes of neuroblastoma. *Genes Chromosomes Cancer* 1994; **10**: 30–9.

47. Caron H, Van Sluis PD, de Kraker J *et al*. Allelic loss of chromosome 1p as a predictor of unfavourable outcome in patients with neuroblastoma. *N Engl J Med* 1996; **334**: 225–30.

48. Ambros PF, Ambros IM, Strehl S *et al*. Regression and progression in neuroblastoma: does genetics predict tumour behaviour? *Eur J Cancer* 1995; **31A**: 510–16.

49. Caron HN. Allelic loss of chromosome 1 and additional chromosome 17 material are both unfavourable prognostic markers in neuroblastoma. *Med Pediatr Oncol* 1995; **24**: 215–21.

50. Fong CT, Dracopoli NC, White PS *et al*. Loss of heterozygosity for the short arm chromosome 1 in human neuroblastomas: correlation with N-myc amplification. *Proc Natl Acad Sci USA* 1989; **86**: 3753–7.

51. Weith A, Martinsson T, Cziepluch C *et al*. Neuroblastoma consensus deletion maps to 1p36.1–2. *Genes Chromosomes Cancer* 1989; **1**: 159–66.

52. Cheng NC, Van Roy N, Chan A *et al*. Deletion mapping in neuroblastoma cell lines suggests two distinct tumour suppressor genes in the 1p35–36 region, only one of which is associated with *n-myc* amplification. *Oncogene* 1995; **10**: 291–7.

53. Versteeg R, Caron H, Cheng NC *et al*. 1p36: Every subband a suppressor? *Eur J Cancer* 1995; **31A**: 541–4.

54. Bown N, Lastowska M, Cotterill S *et al*. 17q gain in neuroblastoma predicts adverse clinical outcome. UK Cancer Cytogenetics Group and the UK Children's Cancer Study Group. *Med Pediatr Oncol* 2001; **36**: 14–19.

55. Bown N, Cotterill S, Lastowska M *et al*. Gain of chromosome arm 17q and adverse outcome in patients with neuroblastomas. *N Engl J Med* 1999; **340**: 1954–61.

56. Schwab M, Alitalo K, Klempnauer KH *et al*. Amplified DNA with limited homology to myc cellular oncogene is shared by human neuroblastoma cell lines and a neuroblastoma tumour. *Nature* 1983; **305**: 245–8.

57. Brodeur GM, Seeger RC, Schwab M et al. Amplification of MYCN in untreated human neuroblastoma correlates with advanced disease. Science 1984; 224: 1121–4.

58. Seeger RC, Brodeur GM, Sathe H et al. Association of multiple copies of the N-myc oncogene with rapid progression of neuroblastomas. N Engl J Med 1985; 313: 1111–16.

59. Combaret V, Gross N, Lasset C et al. Clinical relevance of CD44 cell-surface expression and n-myc gene amplification in a multicentric analysis of 121 pediatric neuroblastomas. J Clin Oncol 1996; 14: 25–34.

60. Matthay KK, O'Leary MC, Ramsey NK et al. Role of myeloablative therapy in improved outcome for high risk neuroblastoma: reviews of recent Children's Cancer Group results. Eur J Cancer 1995; 31A: 572–5.

61. Brodeur GM, Hayes FA, Green AA et al. Consistent N-myc copy number in simultaneous or consecutive neuroblastoma samples from sixty individual patients. Cancer Res 1987; 47: 4248–53.

62. Brodeur GM. Molecular basis for heterogeneity in human neuroblastomas. Eur J Cancer 1995; 31A: 505–10.

63. George RE, Kenyon R, McGuckin AG et al. Investigation of co-amplification of the candidate genes ornthine decarboxylase, ribonucleotide reductase, syndecan 1 and a DEAD box gene, DDX1 in primary neuroblastoma tumours. Oncogene 1996; 12: 1583–7.

64. Corvi R, Savelyeva L, Breit S et al. Non-syntenic amplification of MDM2 and MYCN in human neuroblastoma. Oncogene 1995; 10: 1081–6.

65. Look AT, Hayes FA, Nitschke R et al. Cellular DNA content as predictor of response to chemotherapy in infants with unresectable neuroblastoma. N Engl J Med 1984; 311: 231–5.

66. Gansler T, Chatten J, Varello M et al. Flow cytometric DNA analysis of neuroblastomas. Correlation with histology and clinical outcome. Cancer 1986; 58: 2453–8.

67. Look AT, Hayes FA, Schuster JJ et al. Clinical relevance of tumour cell ploidy and Nmyc gene amplification in childhood neuroblastoma. J Clin Oncol 1991; 9: 581–91.

68. Oppedal BR, Storm-Mathisen I, Lie SO et al. Prognostic factors in neuroblastoma. Clinical, histopathologic and immunohistochemical features and DNA ploidy in relation to prognosis. Cancer 1988; 62: 772–80.

69. Brodeur GM, Nakagawara A, Yamashiro DJ et al. Expression of TrkA, TrkB and TrkC in human neuroblastoma. J Neurooncol 1997; 31: 49–55.

70. Hempstead BL, Martin-Zanca D, Kaplan DR et al. High-affinity NGF binding requires coexpression of the trk proto-oncogene and the low-affinity NGF receptor. Nature 1991; 350: 678–83.

71. Glass DJ, Yancopoulos GD. The neurotrophins and their receptors. Trends Cell Biol 1993; 3: 262–8.

72. Nakagawara A, Arima M, Azar CG et al. Inverse relationship between trk expression and N-myc amplification in human neuroblastomas. Cancer Res 1992; 52: 1364–8.

73. Kramer K, Gerald W, Lesauteur L et al. Prognostic value of TrkA protein detection by monoclonal antibody 5C3 in neuroblastoma. Clin Cancer Res 1996; 2: 1361–7.

74. Kogner P, Barbany G, Dominici C et al. Coexpression of messenger RNA for TRK protocogene and low-affinity nerve growth factor receptor in neuroblastoma with favourable prognosis. Cancer Res 1993; 53: 2044–50.

75. Nakagawara A, Arima-Nakagawara M, Scarvarda NJ et al. Association between high levels of expression of the TRK gene and favorable outcome in human neuroblastoma. N Engl J Med 1993; 328: 847–54.

76. Eggert A, Grotzer MA, Ikegaki N et al. Expression of neutrotrophin receptor TrkA inhibits angiogenesis in neuroblastoma. Med Pediatr Oncol 2000; 35: 569–72.

77. Nakagawara A, Azar CG, Scarvarda NJ et al. Expression and function of TRK-B and BDNF in human neuroblastomas. Mol Cell Biol 1994; 14: 759–67.

78. Ho R, Eggert A, Hishiki T et al. Resistance to chemotherapy mediated by TrkB in neuroblastomas. Cancer Res 2002; 62: 6462–6.

79. Eggert A, Ho R, Ikegaki N et al. Different effects of TrkA expression in neuroblastoma cell lines with or without MYCN amplification. Med Pediatr Oncol 2000; 35: 623–7.

80. Eggert A, Ikegaki N, Liu XG et al. TrkA signal transduction pathways in neuroblastoma. Med Pediatr Oncol 2001; 36: 108–10.

81. Tanaka T, Sugimoto T, Sawada T. Prognostic discrimination among neuroblastomas according to Ha-ras/trk A gene expression: a comparison of the profiles of neuroblastomas detected clinically and those detected through mass screening. Cancer 1998; 83: 1626–33.

82. Yamashiro DJ, Nakagawara A, Ikegaki N et al. Expression of TrkC in favorable human neuroblastomas. Oncogene 1996; 12: 37–41.

83. Favrot MC, Lasset C, Combaret V. CD44: a new prognostic marker for neuroblastoma. N Engl J Med 1993; 329: 1965.

84. Gross N, Beretta C, Peruisseau G et al. CD44H expression by human neuroblastoma cells: relation to MYCN amplification and lineage differentiation. Cancer Res 1994; 54: 4238–42.

85. Bourhis J, Bernard J, Hartmann O et al. Correlation of MDRI gene expression with chemotherapy in neuroblastoma. J Natl Cancer Inst 1989; 81: 1401–5.

86. Goldstein LJ, Fojo AT, Ueda K et al. Expression of the multidrug resistence, MDRI, gene in neuroblastoma. J Clin Oncol 1990; 8: 128–36.

87. Nakagawara A, Kadomatsu K, Sato S et al. Inverse correlation between expression of multidrug resistance gene and N-myc oncogene in human neuroblastomas. Cancer Res 1990; 50: 3043–7.

88. Chan HSL, Haddad G, Thorner PS et al. P-glycoprotein expression as a predictor of the outcome of therapy for neuroblastoma. N Engl J Med 1991; 325: 1608–14.

89. Favrot M, Combaret V, Goillot E et al. Expression of P-glycoprotein restricted to normal cells in neuroblastoma biopsies. Br J Cancer 1991; 64: 233–8.

90. Kurowski C, Berthold F. Presence of classical multidrug resistance and P-glycoprotein expression in human neuroblastoma cells. Ann Oncol 1998; 9: 1009–14.

91. Zaman GJR, Flens MJ, van Leusden MR et al. The human multidrug resistant-associated protein MRP is a plasma membrane drug-efflux pump. Proc Natl Acad Sci USA 1994; 91: 8822–6.

92. Bordow SB, Haber M, Madafiglio J et al. Expression of the multidrug resistance-associated protein (MRP) gene correlates with amplification and overexpression of the N-myc oncogene in childhood neuroblastoma. Cancer Res 1994; 54: 5036–40.

93. Norris MD, Bordow SB, Marshall GM *et al.* Expression of the gene for multidrug-resistance-associated protein and outcome in patients with neuroblastoma. *N Engl J Med* 1996; **334**: 231–8.

94. Poremba C, Hero B, Heine B *et al.* Telomerase is a strong indicator for assessing proneness to progression in neuroblastoma. *Med Pediatr Oncol* 2000; **35**: 651–5.

95. Poremba C, Willenbring H, Hero B *et al.* Telomerase activity distinguishes between neuroblastoma with good and poor prognosis. *Ann Oncol* 1999; **10**: 715–21.

96. Hiyama E, Hiyama K, Yokoyama T *et al.* Correlating telomerase activity levels with human neuroblastoma outcomes. *Nat Med* 1995; **1**: 249–55.

97. Krams M, Hero B, Berthold F *et al.* Full-length telomerase reverse transcriptase messenger RNA: an independent prognostic factor in neuroblastoma. *Am J Pathol* 2003; **162**: 1019–26.

98. Khan J, Wei JS, Ringner M *et al.* Classification and diagnostic prediction of cancer using genetic expression profiling and artificial neural networks. *Nat Med* 2001; **7**: 673–9.

99. Gilbert J, Haber M, Bordow SB *et al.* Use of tumor-specific gene expression for the differential diagnosis of neuroblastoma from other paediatric small round cell malignancies. *Am J Pathol* 1999; **155**: 17–21.

100. Taylor CPF, McGurckin AG, Brown NP *et al.* Rapid detection of prognostic biological factors in neuroblastoma using fluorescence *in situ* hybridisation on tumour imprints and bone marrow smears. *Br J Cancer* 1994; **69**: 445–56.

101. Spitz R, Hero B, Ernestus K, Berthold F. FISH analysis for alterations in chromosomes 1, 2, 3 and 11 define high-risk groups in neuroblastomas. *Med Pediatr Oncol* 2003; **41**: 30–5.

102. Schleiermacher G, Peter M, Michon J *et al.* A multiplex PCR assay for routine evaluation of deletion of the short arm of chromosome 1 in neuroblastoma. *Eur J Cancer* 1995; **31A**: 535–8.

103. Dominici C, Nicotra MR, Digiesi G *et al.* Immunohistochemical detection of high affinity nerve growth factor receptor in neuroblastoma. *Eur J Cancer* 1995; **31A**: 444–6.

104. Ambros IM, Benard J, Boavida M *et al.* Quality assessment of genetic markers used for therapy stratification. *J Clin Oncol* 2003; **21**: 2077–84.

105. Hoefnagel CA, Vooute PA, de Kraker J *et al.* [131I] metaiodobenzylguanidine therapy after conventional therapy for neuroblastoma. *J Nucl Biol Med* 1991; **35**: 202–6.

106. Cohen MD, Klatte EC, Baehner R *et al.* Magnetic resonance imaging of bone marrow disease in children. *Radiology* 1984; **151**: 715–18.

107. Leonidas JC. MR imaging in the assessment of staging neuroblastoma. *Radiology* 2003; **226**: 285.

108. Cheung NK, Kushner BH. Should we replace bone scintigraphy plus CT with MR imaging for staging of neuroblastoma? *Radiology* 2003; **226**: 286–7.

109. Kushner BH, Yeung HW, Larson SM *et al.* Extending positron emission tomography scan utility to high risk neuroblastoma: fluorine-18 fluorodeoxyglucose: positron emission tomography as sole imaging modality in follow-up patients. *J Clin Oncol* 2001; **15**: 3397–405.

110. Kushner BH, Cheung NK, LaQuaglia MP *et al.* International neuroblastoma staging system stage 1 neuroblastoma: a prospective study and literature review. *J Clin Oncol* 1996; **14**: 2174–80.

111. von Schweinitz D, Hero B, Berthold F. The impact of surgical radicality on outcome in childhood neuroblastoma. *Eur J Pediatr Surg* 2002; **12**: 402–9.

112. Haase GM, O'Leary MC, Ramsey NK *et al.* Aggressive surgery combined with intensive chemotherapy improves survival in poor-risk neuroblastoma. *J Pediatr Surg* 1991; **26**: 1119–23.

113. Haase GM, Atkinson JB, Stram DO *et al.* Surgical management and outcome of locoregional neuroblastoma: comparison of the Children's Cancer Group and the international staging systems. *J Pediatr Surg* 1995; **30**: 289–94.

114. Strother D, van Hoff J, Rao PV *et al.* Event free survival of children with biologically favourable neuroblastoma based on the degree of initial tumour resection: results from the Pediatric Oncology Group. *Eur J Cancer* 1997; **33**: 2121–5.

115. La Quaglia MP, Kushner BH, Heller G *et al.* Stage 4 neuroblastoma diagnosed at more than one year of age – gross total resection and clinical outcome. *J Pediatr Surg* 1994; **29**: 1162–5.

116. Castel V, Tovar JA, Costa E *et al.* The role of surgery in stage IV neuroblastoma. *J Pediatr Oncol* 2002; **37**: 1574–8.

117. Carli M, Green AA, Hayes FA *et al.* Therapeutic efficacy of single drugs for childhood neuroblastoma: a review. In: Raybaud E, Clement R, Lebreuil G, Bernard JL, eds. *Pediatric Oncology.* Amsterdam: Exerpta Medica, 1982; 141–50.

118. de Kraker J, Pritchard J, Hartmann O, Ninane J. Single agent ifosfamide in patients with recurrent neuroblastoma. (ENSG Study 2). *Pediatr Hematol Oncol* 1987; **4**: 101–4.

119. Pinkerton CR, Lewis IJ, Pearson ADJ *et al.* Carboplatin or cisplatin? *Lancet* 1989; **ii**: 161 (letter).

120. Pearson ADJ. Use of ifosfamide in neuroblastoma and medulloblastoma. *Am J Pediatr Hematol Oncol* 1993; **15**(suppl): S62–6.

121. Finklestein JZ, Klemperer MR, Evans AE *et al.* Multiagent chemotherapy for children with metastatic neuroblastoma: a report from children's cancer study group. *Med Pediatr Oncol* 1979; **6**: 179–88.

122. Ninane J, Pritchard J, Malpas JS. Chemotherapy of advanced neuroblastoma: does adriamycin contribute? *Arch Dis Child* 1981; **56**: 544–8.

123. Shafford EA, Roger DW, Pritchard J. Advanced neuroblastoma: improved response-rate using a multiagent regimen (OPC) including sequential *cis*platinum and VM26. *J Clin Oncol* 1984; **5**: 1952–9.

124. Bernard JL, Philip T, Zucker JM *et al.* Sequential cisplatin/VM26 and vincristine/cyclophosphamide/doxorubicin in metastatic neuroblastoma: an effective alternating non-cross resistant regimen? *J Clin Oncol* 1987; **5**: 1952–9.

125. Hartmann O, Pinkerton CR, Philip T *et al.* (for ENSG). Very high dose cisplatin and etoposide in children with untreated advanced neuroblastoma. *J Clin Oncol* 1988; **2**: 742–6.

126. Pinkerton CR, Zucker JM, Hartmann O *et al.* Short duration, high dose, alternating chemotherapy in metastatic neuroblastoma (ENSG 3C induction regimen). *Br J Cancer* 1990; **62**: 319–23.

127. Cheung NK, Kushner BH, LaQuaglia M *et al.* N7: a novel multi-modality therapy of high risk neuroblastoma (NB) in children diagnosed over 1 year of age. *Med Pediatr Oncol* 2001; **36**: 227–30.

128. Frappaz D, Michon J, Coze C *et al.* LMCE3 treatment strategy: results in 99 consecutively diagnosed stage 4 neuroblastomas

in children older than 1 year at diagnosis. *J Clin Oncol* 2000; **18**: 468–76.

129. Cheung NKV, Heller G. Chemotherapy dose intensity correlates strongly with response, median survival and median progression-free survival in metastatic neuroblastoma. *J Clin Oncol* 1991; **9**: 1050–8.

130. Lowis SP, Pearson ADJ, Reid MM *et al*. Prohibitive toxicity of a dose-intense regime for metastatic neuroblastoma containing ifosfamide, doxorubicin and cisplatin. *Cancer Chemother Pharmacol* 1993; **31**: 415–8.

131. Pearson ADJ, Craft AW, Pinkerton CR *et al*. High dose rapid schedule chemotherapy for disseminated neuroblastoma. *Eur J Cancer* 1992; **28A**: 1654–9.

132. Pearson ADJ, Pinkerton CR, Lewis IJ. European Neuroblastoma Group fifth study (ENSG 5). A randomised study of dose intensity in stage 4 neuroblastoma over the age of one. In: Evans AE, Biedler JL, Brodeur GM *et al*., eds. *Advances in Neuroblastoma Research*, 4th edn. New York: Wiley-Liss, 1994: 444.

133. Pritchard J, Germond FN, Jones D. Is high dose melphalan (HDM) of value in treatment of advanced neuroblastoma (AN)? Preliminary review results of a randomized trial by the European Neuroblastoma Study Group (ENSG). Proceedings ASCO. *J Clin Oncol* 1986; **5**: 205.

134. Pinkerton CR, Pritchard J, de Kraker J *et al*. ENSG 1– a randomised study of high dose melphalan in neuroblastoma. In: Dicke KA, Spitzer G, Jagonnoth S, eds. *Autologous Bone Marrow Transplantation*. Texas: University of Texas Press, 1987; 401–5.

135. Pole JG, Casper J, Elfrenbein G *et al*. High dose chemoradiotherapy supported by marrow infusions for advanced neuroblastoma: a pediatric oncology group study. *J Clin Oncol* 1991; **9**: 152–8.

136. Philip T, Bernard JL, Zucker JM *et al*. High dose chemo-radiotherapy with bone marrow transplantation as consolidation treatment in neuroblastoma: an unselected group of stage IV patients over 1 year of age. *J Clin Oncol* 1987; **5**: 266–72.

137. Hartmann O, Benhaumou E, Beaujean F *et al*. Repeated high dose chemotherapy followed by purged autologous bone marrow transplantation as consolidation therapy in metastatic neuroblastoma. *J Clin Oncol* 1987; **5**: 1205–11.

138. Seeger RC, Moss TJ, Feig SA *et al*. Bone marrow transplantation for poor prognosis neuroblastoma. In: Evans AE, D'Angio GJ, Knudson AG, Seeger RC, eds. *Advances in Neuroblastoma Research*, 2nd edn. New York: Wiley-Liss, 1988; 203–13.

139. Matthay KK, O'Leary MC, Ramsay NK *et al*. Role of myeloablative therapy in improved outcome for high risk neuroblastoma: reviews of recent Children's Cancer Group results. *Eur J Cancer* 1995; **31A**(4): 572–5.

140. Kushner BH, O'Reily RJ, Mandell LR *et al*. Myeloablative combination without total body irradiation for neuroblastoma. *J Clin Oncol* 1991; **9**: 274–9.

141. Corbett R, Pinkerton CR, Pritchard J *et al*. Pilot study of high dose vincristine, etoposide, carboplatin and melphalan with autologous bone marrow rescue in advanced neuroblastoma. *Eur J Cancer* 1992; **28A**: 1324–8.

142. Gordon SJ, Pearson ADJ, Reid MM *et al*. Toxicity of single-day high-dose vincristine, melphalan, etoposide and carboplatin consolidation with autologous bone marrow rescue in advanced neuroblastoma. *Eur J Cancer* 1992; **28A**: 1319–23.

143. Deacon JM, Wilson PA, Peckham MJ. The radiobiology of human neuroblastomas. *Radiother Oncol* 1985; **3**: 210–19.

144. Jacobson GM, Sause WI, O'Brien RT. Dose response analysis of pediatric neuroblastoma to megavoltage radiation. *Am J Clin Oncol* 1984; **7**: 693.

145. Hug EB, Nevinny-Stickel M, Fuss M *et al*. Conformal proton radiation treatment for retroperitoneal neuroblastoma: introduction of a novel technique. *Med Pediatr Oncol* 2001; **37**: 36–41.

146. Tacharious Z, Sievrts H, Eble MJM. IORT (intraoperative radiotherapy) in neuroblastoma: Experience and first results. *J Pediatr Surg* 2003; **38**: 992.

147. Castleberry L, Kun J, Shuster G *et al*. Radiotherapy (RT) improves the outlook for children older than 1 year with POG stage C neuroblastoma (NB). *Clin Oncol* 1991; **9**: 789–95.

148. Rubie H, Michon J, Plantaz D *et al*. Unresectable localised neuroblastoma: improved survival after primary chemotherapy including carboplatin-etoposide. Neuroblastoma Study Group of the Société Française d'Oncologie Pédiatrique (SFOP). *Br J Cancer* 1998; **77**: 2310–17.

149. Haas-Kogan DA, Swift PS, Selch M *et al*. Impact of radiotherapy for high-risk neuroblastoma: a Children's Cancer Group study. *Int J Radiat Oncol Biol Phys* 2003; **56**: 28–39.

150. Mairs RJ, Livingstone A, Gaze MN *et al*. Prediction of accumulation of ^{131}I-labelled meta-iodobenzylguanidine in neuroblastoma cell lines by means of reverse transcription and polymerase chain reaction. *Br J Cancer* 1994; **70**: 97–101.

151. Lode HN, Bruchelt G, Seitz G *et al*. Reverse transcriptase-polymerase chain reaction (RT-PCR) analysis of monoamine transporters in neuroblastoma cell lines: correlations to meta-iodobenzylguanidine (MIBG) uptake and tyrosine hydroxylase gene expression. *Eur J Cancer* 1995; **31A**: 586–90.

152. Mastrangelo R, Voute PA. Session on the treatment of neuroblastoma with radio-iodinated metaiodobenzylguanidine. *J Nucl Med Biol* 1991; **35**: 260–2.

153. Klingebiel T, Berthold F, Treunder J *et al*. Metaiodobenzylguanidine (mIBG) in the treatment of 47 patients with neuroblastoma: results of the German Neuroblastoma Trial. *Med Pediatr Oncol* 1991; **19**: 84–8.

154. Lashford LS, Lewis IJ, Fielding SL *et al*. A phase I/II study of ^{131}I-mIBG in chemo-resistant neuroblastoma. *J Clin Oncol* 1992; **10**: 1889–96.

155. Corbett R, Pinkerton R, Tait D, Meller S. [^{131}I] metaiodobenzylguanidine and high dose chemotherapy with bone marrow rescue in advanced neuroblastoma. *J Nucl Biol Med* 1991; **35**: 228–31.

156. Gaze MN, Wheldon TE, O'Donoghue JA *et al*. Multimodality megatherapy with ^{131}Imetaiodobenzylguanidine, high-dose melphalan and total body irradiation with bone marrow rescue: feasibility study of a new strategy for advanced neuroblastoma. *Eur J Cancer* 1995; **31A**: 252–6.

157. Mairs RJ. Neuroblastoma therapy using radiolabelled [^{131}I]meta-iodobenzylguanidine ([131I]MIBG) in combination with other agents. *Eur J Cancer* 1999; **35**: 1171–3.

158. Miano M, Garaventa A, Pizzitola MR *et al*. Megatherapy combining I(131) metaiodobenzylguanidine and high dose chemotherapy with haematopoietic progenitor cell rescue for neuroblastoma. *Bone Marrow Transplant* 2001; **27**: 571–4.

159. Yanik GA, Levine JE, Matthay KK *et al*. Pilot study of iodine-131-metaiodobenzylguanidinie in combination with myeloablative chemotherapy and autologous stem cell support for the treatment of neuroblastoma. *J Clin Oncol* 2002; **20**: 2142–9.

160. de Kraker J, Hoefnagel CA, Caron H *et al*. First line targeted radiotherapy, a new concept in the treatment of advanced stage neuroblastoma. *Eur J Cancer* 1995; **31A**: 600–2.

161. Garaventa A, Gambini C, Villavecchia G *et al*. Second malignancies in children with neuroblastoma after combined treatment with ^{131}I-metaiodobenzylguanidine. *Cancer* 2003; **97**: 1332–8.

162. Weiss B, Vora A, Huberty J *et al*. Secondary myelodysplastic syndrome and leukemia following ^{131}I-metaiodobenzyl-guanidine therapy for relapsed neuroblastoma. *J Pediatr Hematol Oncol* 2003; **25**: 543–7.

163. Mastrangelo R, Tornesello A, Riccardi R *et al*. A new approach in the treatment of stage 4 neuroblastoma using a combination of (^{131}I) meta-iodobenzylguanidine (MIBG) and cisplatin. *Eur J Cancer* 1995; **31A**(4): 606–11.

164. Voute PA, van der Kleij AJ, de Kraker J *et al*. Clinical experience with radiation enhancement by hyperbaric oxygen in children with recurrent neuroblastoma stage IV. *Eur J Cancer* 1995; **31A**: 596–600.

165. Flux GD, Guy MJ, Papavasileiou P *et al*. Absorbed dose ratios for repeated therapy of neuroblastoma with I-131 mIBG. *Cancer Biother Radiopharm* 2003; **18**: 81–7.

166. Monsieurs M, Brans B, Bacher K *et al*. Patient dosimetry for (131)I-MIBG therapy for neuroendocrine tumours based on (123)I-MIBG scans. *Eur J Nucl Med Mol Imaging* 2002; **29**: 1581–7.

167. Matthay KK, Panina C, Huberty J *et al*. Correlation of tumor and whole-body dosimetry with tumor response and toxicity in refractory neuroblastoma treated with (131)I-MIBG. *J Nucl Med* 2001; **42**: 1713–21.

168. Westlin JE, Letocha H, Jakobson A *et al*. Rapid, reproducible pain relief with ^{131}I]iodine-meta-iodobenzylguanidine in a body with disseminated neuroblastoma. *Pain* 1995; **60**: 111–14.

169. Castellani MR, Rottoli L, Maffioli L *et al*. Experience with palliative ^{131}I]metaiodobenzylguanidine therapy in advanced neuroblastoma. *J Nucl Biol Med* 1991; **35**: 241–3.

170. Reynolds CP. Differentiating agents in pediatric malignancies: retinoids in neuroblastoma. *Curr Oncol Rep* 2000; **2**: 511–18.

171. Finklestein JZ, Krailo MD, Lenarsky C *et al*. 13-cis-retinoic acid (NSC 122758) in the treatment of children with metastatic neuroblastoma unresponsive to conventional chemotherapy: report from the children's cancer study group. *Med Pediatr Oncol* 1992; **20**: 307–11.

172. Villablanca JG, Khan AA, Avramis VI *et al*. Phase I trial of 13-cis retinoic acid in children with neuroblastoma following bone marrow transplantation. *J Clin Oncol* 1995; **13**: 894–901.

173. Kohler JA, Imeson J, Ellershaw C, Lie SO. A randomized trial of 13-cis retinoic acid in children with advanced neuroblastoma after high-dose therapy. *Br J Cancer* 2000; **83**: 1124–7.

174. Matthay KK, Villablanca JG, Seeger RC *et al*. Treatment of high-risk neuroblastoma with intensive chemotherapy, radiotherapy, autologous bone marrow transplantation, and 13-cis-retinoic acid. Children's Cancer Group. *N Engl J Med* 1999; **341**: 1165–73.

175. Redfern CPF, Lovat PE, Malcolm AJ, Pearson AD. Gene expression and neuroblastoma cell differentiation in response to retinoic acid: differential effects of 9-cis and all trans retinoic acid. *Eur J Cancer* 1995; **31A**: 486–94.

176. Lovat PE, Irving H, Annicchiarico-Petruzzelli M *et al*. Apoptosis of N-type neuroblastoma cells after differentiation with 9-cis-retinoic acid and subsequent washout. *J Natl Cancer Inst* 1997; **89**: 446–52.

177. Hewson QC, Lovat PE, Pearson AD, Redfern CP. Retinoid signalling and gene expression in neuroblastoma cells: RXR agonist and antagonist effects on CRABP-II and RARbeta expression. *J Cell Biochem* 2002; **87**: 284–91.

178. Ponthan F, Kogner P, Bjellerup P *et al*. Bioavailability and dose-dependent anti-tumour effects of 9-cis-retinoic acid on human neuroblastoma xenografts in rat. *Br J Cancer* 2001; **85**: 2004–9.

179. Lovat PE, Ranalli M, Corazzari M *et al*. Mechanisms of free-radical induction in relation to fenretinide-induced apoptosis of neuroblastomas. *J Cell Biochem* 2003; **89**: 698–708.

180. Garaventa A, Luksch R, Piccolo MS *et al*. Phase I trial and pharmacokinetics of fenretinide in children with neuroblastoma. *Clin Cancer Res* 2003; **9**: 2032–9.

181. Ponthan F, Lindskog M, Karnehed N *et al*. Evaluation of anti-tumour effects of oral fenretinide (4-HPR) in rats with human neuroblastoma xenografts. *Oncol Rep* 2003; **10**: 1587–92.

182. Rubie H, Plantaz D, Coze C *et al*. Localised and unresectable neuroblastoma in infants: excellent outcome with primary chemotherapy. Neuroblastoma Study Group, Société Française d'Oncologie Pédiatrique. *Med Pediatr Oncol* 2001; **36**: 247–50.

183. Evans AE, Sillber JH, Shpilsky A, D'Angio GJ. Successful management of low-stage neuroblastoma without adjuvant therapies: a comparision of two decades, 1972 through 1981 and 1982 through 1992, in a single institution. *J Clin Oncol* 1996; **14**: 2504–10.

184. Matthay KK, Sather HN, Seeger RC *et al*. Excellent outcome of stage II neuroblastoma is independent of residual disease and radiation therapy. *J Clin Oncol* 1989; **7**: 236–44.

185. DeBernardi B, Conte M, Mancini A *et al*. Localised resectable neuroblastoma: results of the second study of the Italian Cooperative Group for Neuroblastoma. *J Clin Oncol* 1995; **13**: 884–93.

186. Lockwood L, Lewis J, Pritchard J *et al*. Stage 1 and 2 neuroblastoma. Results of the ENSG survey. *Med Pediatr Oncol* 1990; **18**: 363.

187. Tsuchida Y, Yokoyama J, Kaneko M *et al*. Therapeutic significance of surgery in advanced neuroblastoma: a report from the study group of Japan. *J Pediatr Surg* 1992; **27**: 616–22.

188. Powis MR, Imeson JD, Holmes SJ. The effect of complete excision on stage III neuroblastoma: report of the European Neuroblastoma Study Group. *J Pediatr Surg* 1996; **31**: 516–19.

189. Kushner NH, LaQuaglia MP, Cheung NK. Rethinking management of localised neuroblastoma. *J Clin Oncol* 1993; **36**: 1832–4.

190. Rubie H, Delattre O, Hartmann O *et al*. Loss of chromosome 1p may have a prognostic value in local neuroblastoma: results of the French NBL 90 study. Neuroblastoma Study Group of the Société Française d'Oncologie Pédiatrique (SFOP). *Eur J Cancer* 1997; **33**: 1917–22.

191. Ladenstein R, Philip T, Lasset C et al. Mutlivariate analysis of risk factors in stage 4 neuroblastoma patients over the age of one year treated with megatherapy stem cell transplantation: a report from the European Bone Marrow Transplantation Solid Tumour Registry. J Clin Oncol 1998; **16**: 953–65.

192. De Bernardi B, Nicolas B, Boni L et al. Disseminated neuroblastoma in children older than one year at diagnosis: comparable results with three consecutive high-dose protocols adopted by the Italian Cooperative Group for Neuroblastoma. J Clin Oncol 2003; **21**: 1592–601.

193. Frappaz D, Perol D, Michon J et al. The LMCE5 unselected cohort of 25 children consecutively diagnosed with untreated stage 4 neuroblastoma over 1 year at diagnosis. Br J Cancer 2002; **18**: 1197–203.

194. Berthold F, Hero B. Neuroblastoma: current drug therapy recommendations as of the total treatment approach. Drugs 2000; **59**: 1261–77.

195. Castel V, Canete A, Navarro S et al. Outcome of high-risk neuroblastoma using a dose intensity approach: improvement in initial but not long term results. Med Pediatr Oncol 2001; **37**: 537–42.

196. Pinkerton CR, Blanc Vincent MP et al. Induction chemotherapy in metastatic neuroblastoma – does dose influence response? A critical review of published data; standards, options and recommendations (SOR) project of the National Federation of French Cancer Centres (FNCLCC). Eur J Cancer 2000; **36**: 1808–15.

197. Tweddle DA, Pinkerton CR, Lewis IJ et al. OPEC/OJEC for stage 4 neuroblastoma in children over one year of age. Med Pediatr Oncol 2001; **36**: 239–42.

198. Hero B, Simon T, Horz S, Berthold F. Metastatic neuroblastoma in infancy: what does the pattern of metastases contribute to prognosis? Med Pediatr Oncol 2000; **35**: 683–7.

199. Paulino AC, Mayr NA, Simon JH, Buatti JM. Locoregional control in infants with neuroblastoma: role of radiation therapy and late toxicity. Int J Radiat Oncol Biol Phys 2002; **52**: 1025–31.

200. Matthay KK. Stage 4S neuroblastoma: what makes it special? J Clin Oncol 1998; **16**: 2003–6.

201. Pritchard J, Hickman JA. Why does stage 4s neuroblastoma regress spontaneously? Lancet 1994; **344**: 869–70.

202. Schleiermacher G, Rubie H, Hartmann O et al. Treatment of stage 4s neuroblastoma – report of 10 years' experience of the French Society of Paediatric Oncology (SFOP). Br J Cancer 2003; **89**: 470–6.

203. Nickerson HJ, Matthay KK, Seeger RC et al. Favorable biology and outcome of stage IV-S neuroblastoma with supportive care or minimal therapy: a Children's Cancer Group study. J Clin Oncol 2000; **18**: 477–86.

204. Brinkschmidt C, Poremba C, Christiansen H et al. Comparative genomic hybridisation and telomerase activity analysis identify two biologically different groups of 4s neuroblastomas. Br J Cancer 1998; **77**: 2223–9.

205. Spitz R, Hero B, Ernestus K, Berthold F. Deletions in chromosome arms 3p and 11q are new prognostic markers in localized and 4s neuroblastoma. Clin Cancer Res 2003; **9**: 52–8.

206. Noguera R, Canete A, Pellin A et al. MYCN gain and MYCN amplification in a stage 4s neuroblastoma. Cancer Genet Cytogenet 2003; **140**: 157–61.

207. Sawada T, Nakata T, Takasugi N et al. Mass screening for neuroblastoma in infants in Japan. Interim report of a Mass Screening Study Group. Lancet 1984; **ii**: 271–3.

208. Kaneko Y, Kanda N, Maseki N et al. Current urinary mass screening for catecholamine metabolites at 6 months of age may be detecting only a small proportion of high-risk neuroblastomas: a chromosome and N-myc amplification study. J Clin Oncol 1990; **8**: 2005–13.

209. Hayashi Y, Hananda R, Yamamoto K. Biology of neuroblastomas in Japan found by screening. Am J Pediatr Hematol Oncol 1992; **14**: 343–7.

210. Yamamoto K, Hayashi Y, Handada R et al. Mass screening and age-specific incidence of neuroblastoma in Saitama Prefecture, Japan. J Clin Oncol 1995; **13**: 2033–8.

211. Schilling FH, Spix C, Berthold F et al. Neuroblastoma screening at one year of age. N Engl J Med 2002; **346**: 1047–53.

212. Woods WG, Gao RN, Shuster JJ et al. Screening of infants and mortality due to neuroblastoma. N Engl J Med 2002; **346**: 1041–6.

213. Treuner I, Schilling FH. Neuroblastoma mass screening: the arguments for and against. Eur J Cancer 1995; **31A**: 565–8.

214. Cotterill SJ, Pearson AD, Pritchard J et al. Clinical prognostic factors in 1277 patients with neuroblastoma: results of the European Neuroblastoma Study Group 'Survey' 1982–1992. Eur J Cancer 2000; **36**: 901–8.

215. Hero B, Hunneman DH, Gahr M, Berthold F. Evaluation of catecholamine metabolites, mIBG scan and bone marrow cytology as response markers in stage 4 neuroblastoma. Med Pediatr Oncol 2001; **36**: 220–3.

216. Kushner BH, Yeh SD, Kramer J et al. Impact of metaiodobenzylguanidine scintigraphy on assessing response of high-dose neuroblastoma to dose-intensive induction chemotherapy. J Clin Oncol 2003; **21**: 1082–6.

217. Matthay KK, Edeline V, Lumbroso J et al. Correlation of early metastatic response by ^{123}I-metaiodobenzylguanidine scintigraphy with overall response and event-free survival in stage IV neuroblastoma. J Clin Oncol 2003; **21**: 2486–91.

218. Cheung IY, Cheung NK. Detection of microscopic disease: comparing histology, immunocytology, and RT-PCR of tyrosine hydroxylase GAGE and MAGE. Med Pediatr Oncol 2001; **36**: 210–2.

219. Cheung IY, Cheung NK. Quantitation of marrow disease in neuroblastoma by real-time reverse transcription-PCR. Clin Cancer Res 2001; **7**: 1698–705.

220. Träger C, Kogner P, Lindskog M et al. Quantitative analysis of tyrosine hydroxylase mRNA for sensitive detection of neuroblastoma cells in blood and bone marrow. Clin Chem 2003; **49**: 104–12.

221. Burchill SA, Lewis IJ, Abrams KR et al. Circulating neuroblastoma cells detected by reverse transcriptase polymerase chain reaction for tyrosine hydroxylase mRNA are an independent poor prognostic indicator in stage 4 neuroblastoma in children over 1 year. J Clin Oncol 2001; **19**: 1795–801.

222. Vaidya SJ, Payne GS, Leach MO, Pinkerton CR. Potential role of magnetic resonance spectroscopy in assessment of tumour response in childhood cancer. Eur J Cancer 2003; **39**: 728–35.

223. Lindskog M, Kogner P, Ponthan F et al. Noninvasive estimation of tumour viability in a xenograft model of human

neuroblastoma with proton magnetic resonance spectroscopy (1H MRS). *Br J Cancer* 2003; **88**: 478–85.

224. Gambini C, Conte M, Bernini G *et al.* Neuroblastic tumors associated with opsoclonus-myoclonus syndrome: histological, immunohistochemical and molecular features of 15 Italian cases. *Virchows Arch* 2003; **442**: 555–62.

225. Cooper R, Khakoo Y, Matthay KK *et al.* Opsoclonus-myoclonus-ataxia syndrome in neuroblastoma: histopathological features – a report from the Children's Cancer Group. *Med Pediatr Oncol* 2001; **36**: 623–9.

226. Kramer K, Kushner B, Heller G, Cheung NK. Neuroblastoma metastatic to the central nervous system. The Memorial Sloan-Kettering Cancer Center experience and a literature review. *Cancer* 2001; **91**: 1510–19.

227. Matthay KK, Brisse H, Couanet D *et al.* Central nervous system metastases in neuroblastoma: radiologic, clinical and biologic features in 23 patients. *Cancer* 2003; **98**: 155–65.

228. Baka M, Pourtsidis A, Bouhoutsou D *et al.* Neuroblastoma metastatic to the lungs at diagnosis. *Med Pediatr Oncol* 2003; **41**: 147–9.

229. Kushner BH, Kramer K, Cheung NK. Chronic neuroblastoma. *Cancer* 2002; **95**: 1366–75.

230. Cotterill SJ, Pearson AD, Pritchard J *et al.* Late relapse and prognosis for neuroblastoma patients surviving 5 years or more: a report from the European Neuroblastoma Study Group 'Survey'. *Med Pediatr Oncol* 2001; **36**: 235–8.

231. Bruggers CS, Bolinger C. Efficacy of surveillance radiographic imaging in detecting progressive disease in children with advanced stage neuroblastoma. *J Pediatr Hematol Oncol* 1998; **20**: 104–7.

232. Langler A, Christaras A, Abshagen K *et al.* Topotecan in the treatment of refractory neuroblastoma and other malignant tumors in childhood – a phase II study. *Klin Padiatr* 2002; **214**: 153–6.

233. Kushner BH, Cheung NK, Kramer K *et al.* Topotecan combined with myeloablative doses of thiotepa and carboplatin for neuroblastoma, brain tumours and other poor-risk solid tumours in children and young adults. *Bone Marrow Transplant* 2001; **28**: 551–6.

234. Shitara T, Shimada A, Tsuchida Y *et al.* Successful clinical response to irinotecan in relapsed neuroblastoma. *Med Pediatr Oncol* 2003; **40**: 126–8.

235. Surico G, Muggeo P, De Leonardis F, Rigillo N. New paclitaxel-cisplatin based chemotherapy regimen for advanced stage, recurrent, or refractory neuroblastoma: preliminary report. *Med Pediatr Oncol* 2003; **40**: 130–2.

236. Jikai J, Shamis M, Huebener N *et al.* Neuroblastoma directed therapy to be a rational prodrug design of etoposide as a substrate for tyrosine hydroxylase. *Cancer Lett* 2003; **197**: 219–24.

237. Wagner LM, Guichard SM, Burger RA *et al.* Efficacy and toxicity of a virus-detected enzyme prodrug therapy purging method: preclinical assessment and application to bone marrow samples from neuroblastoma patients. *Cancer Res* 2002; **62**: 5001–7.

238. Lu X, Pearson A, Lunec J. The MYCN oncoprotein as a drug development target. *Cancer Lett* 2003; **197**: 125–30.

239. Saito-Ohara F, Imoto I, Inoue J *et al.* PPM1D is a potential target for 17q gain in neuroblastoma. *Cancer Res* 2003; **63**: 1876–83.

240. Evans AF, Kisselbach KD, Yamashiro DJ *et al.* Antitumor activity of CEP-751 (KT-6587) on human neuroblastoma and medulloblastoma xenografts. *Clin Cancer Res* 1999; **5**: 3594–602.

241. Brignole C, Pagnan G, Marimpietri D *et al.* Targeted delivery system for antisense oligonucleotides: a new experimental strategy for neuroblastoma treatment. *Cancer Lett* 2003; **197**: 231–5.

242. Cheung NK, Kushner BH, Cheung IY *et al.* Anti-G(D2) antibody treatment of minimal residual stage 4 neuroblastoma diagnosed at more than 1 year of age. *J Clin Oncol* 1998; **16**: 3053–60.

243. Kushner BH, Kramer K, Cheung NK. Phase II trial of the anti-G(D2) monoclonal antibody 3F8 and granulocyte-macrophage colony-stimulating factor for neuroblastoma. *J Clin Oncol* 2001; **19**: 4189–94.

244. Pertl U, Woodrich H, Ruehlmann JM *et al.* Immunotherapy with a posttranscriptionally modified DNA vaccine induces complete protection against metastatic neuroblastoma. *Blood* 2003; **101**: 649–54.

245. Rousseau RF, Haight AE, Hirschmann-Jax C *et al.* Local and systemic effects of an allogenic tumor cell vaccine combining transgenic human lymphotactin with interleukin-2 in patients with advanced or refractory neuroblastoma. *Blood* 2003; **101**: 1718–26.

20

Wilms' tumour

CHRISTOPHER D. MITCHELL

INTRODUCTION AND DEFINITION

Wilms' tumour (WT)[1] is the most common genitourinary malignancy of childhood, and is a triphasic embryonal neoplasm consisting of varying proportions of blastema, stroma and epithelium. Although this specific histological appearance was described by Max Wilms in 1899, the eponym is now loosely applied to virtually any malignant tumour arising in the kidney in childhood, some of which are pathologically, clinically and probably genetically distinct.

The development of WT treatment is often cited as a paradigm for the multicentre cooperative clinical trial in cancer. The period from 1969 to 1985 saw an impressive improvement in outcome, so that by the end of this era the great majority of patients were cured with relatively simple management strategies. The emphasis of subsequent trials was therapy reduction for this majority group of patients. However, there remains a small but stubborn group of patients for whom current strategies are not successful; additionally, the chances of retrieval following relapse are still poor. Thus, although new trials continue to focus on refinement of therapy, the real challenges now lie in identifying, at the time of diagnosis, those patients likely to fail therapy; developing successful therapies for this small group of patients with biologically aggressive disease; and improving relapse strategies.

EPIDEMIOLOGY, GENETICS AND PREDISPOSING CONDITIONS

The annual incidence of WT is around eight per million children under the age of 15 years. There are both racial and regional variations in incidence, so that the previously held view that the incidence was constant throughout the world (the 'index' tumour) is not correct.[2] The risk of developing WT is approximately 1 in 10 000 live births. The tumour accounts for about 8 per cent of childhood malignancies and so, in incidence, ranks fifth among the solid tumours of childhood, after tumours of the central nervous system (CNS), lymphoma, neuroblastoma and soft tissue sarcoma. The tumour occurs with equal frequency in boys and girls, with a peak incidence in the third year. Although very rare in the neonatal period,[3] over 75 per cent of children affected are under 4 years of age and at least 90 per cent under 7 years at diagnosis. Only a very few cases are diagnosed after the age of 11 years (see Figure 20.1).

The molecular genetics of WT and predisposing conditions are discussed in Chapter 2.

CLINICAL FEATURES AND INVESTIGATIONS

Most children with WT are well and present only because they have an abdominal mass detected by a parent or by

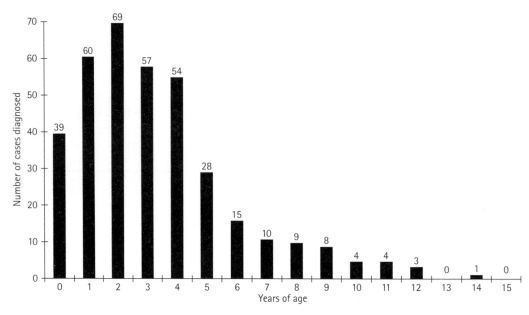

Figure 20.1 *Number of Wilms' tumour cases diagnosed per year of life (United Kingdom Children's Cancer Study Group data – 361 cases; absolute numbers of cases for each year are given at the top of each bar).*

someone else. Symptoms such as abdominal pain, haematuria and fever may occur,[4] but generally the contrast with the clinical picture of abdominal neuroblastoma, the major differential diagnosis, is marked. The frequency of presenting symptoms (from the first UK Wilms' tumour study) is as follows:

- abdominal mass – 74 per cent
- fever – 1 per cent
- pain – 44 per cent.

Physical examination should include a search for the stigmata of the various associated conditions, such as hemihypertrophy, Beckwith–Wiedemann syndrome, genital abnormalities and aniridia (see 'Follow-up and screening investigations'. Hypertension, which may arise from excessive renin production, vascular compression by the tumour or as part of pre-existing renal disease, occurs in a few patients and may be sufficiently severe to require treatment. The blood pressure must therefore be measured. Abdominal examination reveals a smooth, rounded or lobulated mass arising in the loin, which is usually ballotable and does not move with respiration, thus allowing distinction from liver or spleen. The previously held view that abdominal examination should not be repeated for fear of tumour rupture or tumour emboli is unfounded. Any metastases present at diagnosis, which are usually pulmonary, will only rarely be detected by clinical examination.

The objectives of investigation are to confirm the diagnosis, delineate the extent of the tumour, determine that the contralateral kidney is functional, discover any metastases, and ensure that the child is fit enough to undergo anaesthesia and surgery.

A blood count may detect anaemia resulting from haemorrhage into the tumour; there may also be thrombocytosis in response to haemorrhage. A few patients develop a bleeding diathesis secondary to an acquired form of von Willebrand's disease. An incidence of 8 per cent was noted in one study,[5] and so the prothrombin and partial thromboplastin times should be estimated. Further investigations of coagulation may be necessary either because of these results or because of the clinical state of the patient. Urinalysis, particularly for protein, and measurement of serum electrolytes, urea and creatinine will detect any gross abnormalities of renal function. Measurement of urinary catecholamines is essential to exclude neuroblastoma, especially in hypertensive children, if immediate surgery is contemplated. No imaging technique can exclude neuroblastoma, some of which are intrarenal, with complete accuracy. There are two reasons for taking care to exclude the diagnosis of neuroblastoma: first, immediate surgery may then not be appropriate; and second, catecholamine-secreting tumours pose particular anaesthetic problems, which should be recognized preoperatively. Catecholamine secretion is now usually measured by a chromatographic method, which removes the need for 24-hour collections of urine or the use of special diets, and renders the previous 'spot' method obsolete.

An abdominal ultrasound scan is usually the first investigation for determining the organ of origin, the extent of any spread within the abdomen, and the patency of the inferior vena cava, and also for detecting any involved lymph nodes. Most centres would subsequently perform computed tomography (CT) or magnetic resonance imaging (MRI) to define further the anatomy of

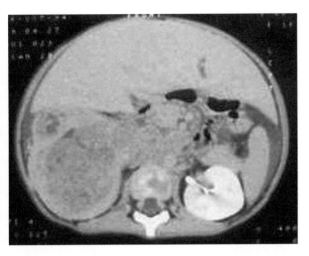

Figure 20.2 *Large Wilms' tumour with nodal involvement on computed tomography (CT) scan.*

the tumour and as an aid to assessing subsequent response to preoperative therapy (Figure 20.2). Paediatric radiologists prefer the latter as it keeps radiation exposure to a minimum.

It is important to know that the contralateral kidney is functioning adequately before surgery. Some radiologists and urologists hold the view that normal renal size and indices of renal function are sufficient to exclude a non-functioning contralateral kidney. The excretion of contrast at the end of computed axial tomography of the chest will provide an indication of function of the contralateral kidney. A DMSA scan is an alternative investigation that is also invaluable in planning surgery for patients with bilateral tumours or single functioning kidneys.

Posteroanterior and lateral chest radiographs are essential to exclude pulmonary metastases. CT is more sensitive in the detection of pulmonary metastases in WT, but its role in management is not yet established. A report by the United Kingdom Children's Cancer Study Group (UKCCSG) identified 31 patients with metastases detected by CT that were not found by conventional radiography of 142 patients. Seven of these patients relapsed. However, relapses were more common in patients who were otherwise stage I than in those who were stages II–V. Overall, four of the seven patients were salvaged by second-line treatment (including two of three stage I patients).[6] These data suggest that the majority of higher-stage patients will have their pulmonary disease adequately treated by their stage-appropriate chemotherapy. Wilimas *et al.*[7] found pulmonary disease by scanning, but not by conventional radiography, in 11 out of 124 children. There was no significant difference in the relapse rate between that small group and the larger number of patients whose lung lesions could be seen on ordinary radiography. The third National Wilms' Tumor Study (NWTS 3) identified 32 patients with CT-positive,

X-ray-negative pulmonary disease, of whom 18 were treated as stage IV and nine as stage III on the basis of their locoregional disease. There was no difference in the 4-year event-free survival (EFS) or overall survival (OS) between the two groups.[8] Thus, the place of CT scanning of the chest should still be assessed prospectively and not be considered part of routine staging.

Postoperatively, other imaging investigations may be indicated by specific histological findings. A technetium-99 bone scan is indicated after the diagnosis of the so-called bone-metastasizing renal tumour (also called clear-cell sarcoma. A radiological survey of the skeleton is unnecessary. In malignant rhabdoid tumour of the kidney the presence of an intracranial second tumour should be excluded with CT or MRI.[9]

PROGNOSTIC FEATURES

Prognostic factors arise because of the variable efficacy of treatment regimens in different patient groups. In WT, the policy of directing intensive treatment to patients with 'bad risk' disease and the refinement or reduction of treatment for patients with 'good risk' disease is based on a number of factors, the most important of which are histological appearance and stage.[10–12] The recent trend towards preoperative chemotherapy with delayed surgical resection has added response to treatment to the factors to be considered in overall management. Cytogenetic and molecular biological factors promise further refinement and are now under assessment.[12a]

PATHOLOGY

In patients who have immediate surgery, as pioneered by the North American National Wilms' Tumor Studies, two broad groups of tumours may be recognized by their histological appearances; by far the larger group has 'favourable' appearances (see Beckwith[13] for a review). The SIOP group, however, have explored the use of preoperative chemotherapy, which has provided an opportunity to study the association of pathological appearance in response to therapy and its effect on prognosis. However, it is easier to consider first the pathological appearances seen in patients having immediate nephrectomy.

Favourable histology

The major proportion of the favourable group consists of classical triphasic tumours, in which epithelial, blastemal and stromal elements are all present. Some triphasic tumours may have rhabdomyoblastic differentiation, such that the cells resemble fetal rhabdomyoblasts, often with cross-striations. This appearance is not unfavourable but it must not be confused with the 'malignant rhabdoid tumour of the kidney', which is a variant with poor prognosis (see below).

The monomorphic epithelial variant, usually found in children less than 1 year old, is easily recognized, as it appears to consist entirely of primitive tubules. This appearance has a very favourable prognosis, as do stage I tumours weighing less than 550 g in patients under 2 years of age.[14] Both of these subtypes are effectively treated by nephrectomy only.

Unfavourable histology

Anaplasia is an unfavourable feature occasionally observed in triphasic tumours. It is characterized by large (greater than four times normal) hyperchromatic nuclei, an increased nuclear:cytoplasmic ratio, and abnormal (e.g. tripolar) mitoses. Anaplasia in WT is often a patchy, focal change, which may escape notice unless a deliberate search is made, including widespread sampling with blocks cut every centimetre across the widest diameter of the tumour. The appearances are often best recognized by scanning the slide at low power.

The major unfavourable histological types are pathologically and genetically distinct tumours, rather than true variants of WT. The bone-metastasizing renal tumour of childhood was first reported by Kidd,[15] and later identified by Marsden and Lawler[16] in the UK, and Beckwith and Palmer[17] in the USA; they all describe a distinctive neoplasm with a propensity for skeletal metastasis and aggressive clinical behaviour. The incidence of reported bone metastases was 76 per cent of 38 cases in the British series and 17 per cent of 75 cases in the American series.

In NWTS 3, the bone-metastasizing tumour represented nearly 6 per cent of cases, making it the most frequent form of 'unfavourable' histology. Its age distribution is similar to that of WT. There appears to be a distinct male preponderance for this type in both American and British series, although not as great as originally suggested. There have been no reports of bone-metastasizing renal tumours in patients with WT-associated conditions such as sporadic aniridia.

The other unfavourable type is the malignant rhabdoid tumour of the kidney, described in the first National Wilms' Tumor Study.[18] It is the least common of the unfavourable entities and was found in only 2 per cent of patients entered in the national (American) studies. The age distribution is markedly different from that of WT, with nearly half the patients being diagnosed in the first year of life. It is also associated with second primary tumours of various types (usually primitive neuroectodermal tumours) arising in the midline of the posterior intracranial fossa.[9] The intracranial tumour may precede or follow

the renal tumour. Hypercalcaemia has been reported in a number of cases of malignant rhabdoid tumour,[19,20] and may also occur in congenital mesoblastic nephroma.

Benign variants

Two further distinct low-risk entities have been described. The first is congenital mesoblastic nephroma (CMN), which is a rare, distinctive tumour of the infantile kidney, usually regarded as a benign tumour. However, there have been a number of reports of metastasis or recurrence. Beckwith has described a pathological spectrum, with unequivocally malignant spindle cell sarcoma at one extreme, through a 'grey zone or cellular variant', to typical CMN at the other.[21] In a presentation in 1998, he redefined CMN and cellular CMN as infantile renal fibromatosis and infantile renal fibrosarcoma, respectively, according to their histological patterns.[22] Moreover, cytogenetic studies have shown that cellular CMN and congenital fibrosarcoma (CFS) share similar polysomies of chromosomes 8, 11, 17 and 21. They have also both been shown to contain a novel t(12;15)(p13;q25) translocation resulting in *ETV6-NTRK3* gene fusion.[23] Cellular CMN and CFS therefore share histological and cytogenetic features, which may be relevant in the management of patients with apparent recurrence or metastasis of CMN.[24]

The other low-risk entity is cystic partly differentiated nephroblastoma (CPDN), which is usually seen in children under the age of 2 years.[25] The tumour is composed entirely of cysts and their thin walls, with the septa forming the only 'solid' component of the tumour. The cysts are lined by cuboidal epithelium and the septa contain blastema together with stroma or epithelium. The tumour forms a discrete mass, well demarcated from the non-cystic renal parenchyma. Surgery alone is usually adequate therapy for both of these tumours.

Response to therapy

In the SIOP risk assessment system,[26] use is made of the response to chemotherapy, which now consists of four doses of vincristine at weekly intervals and actinomycin D at weeks 1 and 3. Low-risk tumours, as noted above, include mesoblastic nephroma and CPDN. In addition, completely necrotic nephroblastoma is also recognized as a low-risk entity, with 100 per cent survival regardless of stage and hence with no further therapy necessary after resection. The histological criteria for making this diagnosis are the absence of any viable tumour tissue on gross or microscopic examination of multiple blocks and the presence of regressive or necrotic changes caused by the chemotherapy.

The criteria for histological subtyping of WT established by Beckwith and Palmer[27] state that one component of the tumour must comprise at least 66 per cent of the tumour mass before a subclassification may be assigned. Preoperative chemotherapy may alter the original appearances and often results in the appearance of areas of regression or necrosis. In consequence, the criteria used in subclassification of immediately resected tumours must be adapted to take the chemotherapy-induced changes into account. It has been demonstrated that chemotherapy-induced changes are prognostically favourable.[28,29] Conversely, the persistence of blastema after chemotherapy indicates chemoresistance and has been shown to be associated with a poor outcome.[30] Designating intermediate-risk tumours involves first assessing the percentage of necrosis or regression that is present. If these changes are present in more than 66 per cent of the tumour, it may then be designated as being of regressive subtype. If the degree of change is less than 66 per cent, the tumour may be subtyped according to the predominant histological component, or designated as mixed if there is no predominance. Five entities may be recognized – epithelial, stromal, mixed, regressive or with focal anaplasia. Each of these entities is of intermediate prognosis.

The high-risk entities include, as noted above, tumours with persistence of blastema, together with diffuse anaplasia, clear-cell sarcoma of the kidney (CCSK) and malignant rhabdoid tumour of the kidney. In order to make a diagnosis of blastemal-type nephroblastoma, the viable component must be more than 33 per cent of the tumour mass and at least 66 per cent of the viable areas must be blastema. Other components may also be present in varying amounts.

STAGING SYSTEMS

Several staging systems have been used for WT, evolving as successive studies have redefined the criteria for each stage. The major contribution to these systems has been from the North American national studies. The current system, in use since the third national study, makes use of the data accumulated in NWTS 1 and 2[31–33] to define five stages, summarized in Box 20.1. This staging system has

Box 20.1 *National Wilms' Tumor Study 3, staging system*

Stage I	Tumour within renal capsule, completely excised
Stage II	Extension outside the renal capsule
Stage III	Extension outside renal capsule, with incomplete surgical excision or locoregional lymph node involvement
Stage IV	Metastatic spread to lungs, liver, bones, brain
Stage V	Bilateral tumours

Box 20.2 *International Society of Pediatric Oncology (SIOP) staging system*

Stage I
a) The tumour is limited to kidney or surrounded with a fibrous pseudocapsule if outside of the normal contours of the kidney. The renal capsule or pseudocapsule may be infiltrated with the tumour but it does not reach the outer surface, and it is completely resected (resection margins 'clear')
b) The tumour may be protruding ('bulging') into the pelvic system and 'dipping' into the ureter (but it is not infiltrating their walls)
c) The vessels of the renal sinus are not involved
d) Intrarenal vessel involvement may be present

Stage II
a) The tumour extends beyond kidney or penetrates through the renal capsule and/or fibrous pseudocapsule into perirenal fat but is completely resected (resection margins 'clear')
b) Tumour infiltrates the renal sinus and/or invades blood and lymphatic vessels outside the renal parenchyma but is completely resected
c) Tumour infiltrates adjacent organs or vena cava but is completely resected

Stage III
a) Incomplete excision of the tumour which extends beyond resection margins (gross or microscopic tumour remains postoperatively)
b) Any abdominal lymph nodes are involved
c) Tumour rupture pre- or intraoperatively (irrespective of other criteria for staging)
d) The tumour has penetrated through the peritoneal surface
e) Tumour implants are found on the peritoneal surface
f) The tumour thrombi present at resection margins of vessels or ureter are transected or removed piecemeal by surgeon
g) The tumour has been surgically biopsied (wedge biopsy) prior to preoperative chemotherapy or surgery

Stage IV
Haematogeneous metastases (lung, liver, bone, brain, etc.) or lymph node metastases outside the abdominopelvic region

Stage V
Bilateral renal tumours at diagnosis

Box 20.3 *International Society of Pediatric Oncology (SIOP) histological risk assignment*

Delayed nephrectomy cases

Low-risk tumours
- Mesoblastic nephroma
- Cystic partially differentiated nephroblastoma
- Completely necrotic nephroblastoma

Intermediate-risk tumours
- Nephroblastoma – epithelial type
- Nephroblastoma – stromal type
- Nephroblastoma – mixed type
- Nephroblastoma – regressive type
- Nephroblastoma – focal anaplasia

High-risk tumours
- Nephroblastoma – blastemal type
- Nephroblastoma – diffuse anaplasia
- Clear-cell sarcoma of the kidney
- Rhabdoid tumour of the kidney

Immediate nephrectomy cases

Low-risk tumours
- Mesoblastic nephroma
- Cystic partially differentiated nephroblastoma

Intermediate-risk tumours
- Non-anaplastic nephroblastoma and its variants
- Nephroblastoma – focal anaplasia

High-risk tumours
- Nephroblastoma – diffuse anaplasia
- Clear-cell sarcoma of the kidney
- Rhabdoid tumour of the kidney

---

been used subsequently in NWTS studies 4 and 5 and also in the UKCCSG (UKW) series of studies 1–3.

The use of preoperative chemotherapy has a major impact on the validity of the NWTS staging system. As a consequence, the SIOP group have refined their system, by using a combination of NWTS staging and pathological appearances, which take account of the implications of early disease response to chemotherapy, in order to categorize patients into risk groups (see Boxes 20.2 and 20.3).

MOLECULAR GENETIC PROGNOSTIC FACTORS

Consistent genetic changes have been identified in WT at chromosome regions 11p13, 11p15, 16q and 1p. Genes in these regions may be involved in processes such as proliferation, differentiation or localization, which might affect the behaviour of a tumour. A study of 232 patients registered in NWTS 3 and 4 found that those with loss of heterozygosity (LOH) of markers on 16q, found in 17.2 per cent of patients with favourable histology or anaplasia, had a significantly lower relapse-free and overall survival, even after allowing for stage or histology.[34] LOH for markers at region 1p was found in 11 per cent of the samples, and again was associated with poorer relapse-free and overall survival. LOH at 11p or duplication of 1q were not associated with any difference in outcome.

These early results are now being studied in a prospective fashion in the NWTS 5 and SIOP WT2001 trials; if confirmed, these features might be a useful way of further stratifying therapy.

TREATMENT

Place of treatment

There is overwhelming evidence that WT ought only to be treated in recognized paediatric oncology centres and that there is no place for the casual therapist. Early studies indicated that there was a survival advantage for children treated within a trial or at a specialist centre.[35,36] A more recent study has not shown any such advantage,[37] reflecting the high survival rate obtainable with WT when surgery is accompanied by adjuvant chemotherapy and radiotherapy and the difficulty of detecting differences in outcome when only small numbers of patients are involved. Subsequently, it has been shown that patients not included in a recognized trial, or not treated at a recognized centre, are overtreated by comparison with current recommendations, being more likely to receive radiotherapy.[38] Surgeons, radiotherapists, paediatricians or nephrologists not working in a centre with paediatric oncological expertise, who find themselves unexpectedly dealing with a child with WT, should make an urgent referral to an appropriate unit immediately.

Surgery

THE ROLE OF BIOPSY AND THE TIMING OF DEFINITIVE SURGERY

Despite advances in chemotherapy, surgical extirpation is, and will almost certainly remain, fundamental treatment for WT. Nevertheless, there is now considerable debate about the timing of surgical intervention, the place of percutaneous needle biopsy and the use of preoperative chemotherapy. North American practice remains steadfastly in favour of immediate surgery followed by adjuvant therapy dictated by the surgical stage. In contrast, the SIOP group in Europe has conducted a series of trials

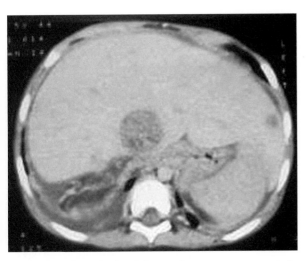

Figure 20.3 *Extensive involvement of vena cava on computed tomography (CT) scan.*

based on the use of preoperative therapy. While it remains to be proven that the latter approach is superior, there is increasing recognition that preoperative treatment may be of benefit in some circumstances. In an attempt to resolve the issues posed by the findings from these two groups, the UKCCSG has conducted a prospective randomized trial comparing immediate surgery with 6 weeks of chemotherapy and delayed surgery (UKW3). Preliminary analysis of the results shows that the preoperatively treated arm has an over-representation of stage I cases and a deficit of stage II cases compared with the immediate surgery arm.[39]

There are no generally accepted absolute contraindications to immediate surgery, but there are circumstances in which many surgeons would deem immediate operative intervention less appropriate. The presence of major tumour thrombus in the inferior vena cava will make an operation considerably more risky, and may well necessitate the use of cardiac bypass if the thrombus is to be removed (Figure 20.3). It seems illogical to subject a child with disseminated disease to immediate surgery for removal of the primary tumour until control of the metastases has been established. Very large tumours may pose considerable surgical problems, particularly if the tumour is found to be invading other organs, such as liver, spleen or bowel. It is abundantly clear that the vast majority of WTs will respond readily to treatment with vincristine and actinomycin D, and in the circumstances outlined above it may well be beneficial to use preoperative chemotherapy to shrink the tumour so as to facilitate the resection.

Accepting that, in some cases, immediate definitive surgery may be inappropriate, the choice facing the clinician will be either to proceed with therapy based solely on the clinicoradiological data or to subject the patient to a biopsy. Many paediatric oncologists and surgeons feel that a biopsy is unnecessary. However, an analysis of

biopsies in UKW3 from 297 patients thought on clinicoradiological grounds to have WT confirmed the diagnosis in 266 cases.[40] Twenty-two patients (7 per cent) were considered not to have WT by the local pathologist and a further nine cases (making a total of 10 per cent) were found on central review to have either unfavourable histology (four cases) or other diagnoses (five cases). Some of these diagnoses have been of less common renal tumours such as mesoblastic nephroma or renal cell carcinoma, but others have been of non-renal tumours, such as neuroblastoma, which may be radiologically difficult to distinguish. In the SIOP I trial,[41] 21 of 169 randomized patients – and in SIOP V,[42] 10 of 164 randomized patients – were found to have diagnoses other than WT. Thus, with reliance solely on clinicoradiological features yielding an error rate of around 8–10 per cent, pretreatment histological confirmation seems essential.

Typically, biopsy in these circumstances will be a closed procedure using a 'Trucut' or similar needle. There are two major concerns about the use of such a procedure:

- Needle biopsy may not provide a representative sample of the tumour and may fail to reveal unfavourable features such as anaplasia. Preoperative treatment may then mask the unfavourable features in the eventually resected specimen, and result in undertreatment. Review of 266 confirmed WT cases, with no evidence of anaplasia in the biopsy specimen, revealed anaplasia in the nephrectomy specimen in 25 cases. In 10 per cent of cases confirmed as WT, anaplasia could still be detected in the nephrectomy specimen after the preoperative chemotherapy.
- Does the process of biopsy in itself render the patients more likely to suffer a subsequent local recurrence? Since a needle biopsy must interrupt the integrity of the renal capsule, there is at least a theoretical concern that the procedure might result in local spillage of the tumour along the biopsy track. In the series of patients reported above, no patient suffered such a complication. In the current UKCCSG UKW3 trial, only one patient randomized to biopsy so far has had a biopsy track recurrence, out of a total of 297 procedures. These data suggest that the risk of recurrence posed to the patient is probably very minimal.

In the past it has been usual to regard patients with 'unresectable' tumours who have undergone a biopsy, whether open or closed, as having stage III tumours, for which they must then receive three-drug chemotherapy and flank irradiation. Whether such radical therapy is, in fact, necessary, is one of the outcomes awaited from the UKW3 trial.

In the NWTS 3, 131 children were judged to have primarily unresectable disease. The patients were assigned a pretreatment stage on clinicoradiological grounds and then treated accordingly. The 4-year survival for this group of patients was only 74 per cent, compared with 88 per cent for those patients having immediate surgery,[43] but because of patient selection, these data cannot be used as evidence that the preoperative treatment approach is flawed. In the first UKCCSG Wilms' Tumour Study (UKW1), 23 patients (6 per cent of the total number studied) had initially unresectable disease. Instead of being assigned a pretreatment stage, all were treated as stage III patients with four-drug chemotherapy and, in those patients with local residual disease after delayed surgery, 30 Gy flank or whole abdominal irradiation.[44] Unfortunately, the outcome for this small group of patients is not analysed separately from other stage III patients, but the EFS at 6 years for all stage III patients with favourable histology was 82 per cent (106 patients), and for those patients with unfavourable histology it was 50 per cent (18 patients).

It is essential that surgery for WT should start with a generous transverse abdominal incision, so that examination of the abdominal cavity can be thorough, and to ease the manipulation of the tumour during its removal. Review of the practice of mobilizing and inspecting the contralateral kidney has shown that no abnormalities are found surgically if preoperative imaging (e.g. by CT or MRI) was normal. Thus, the contralateral kidney need not be mobilized and inspected provided preoperative imaging has not revealed any abnormalities. The remainder of the abdominal cavity must then be examined. Once the surgeon is satisfied about the resectability of the tumour, the operation then proceeds with the mobilization of surrounding structures, at this stage disturbing the tumour as little as possible. The ureter is dissected free, transected, and a plane of cleavage developed towards the renal pelvis and its associated vessels. The vein, which lies anterior to the artery, is mobilized so that the artery can be tied first. The vein is then tied and the tumour mobilized. Finally, the tumour, with associated tissue, is removed *en bloc*, with care to avoid rupture and contamination of the abdominal cavity. Para-aortic lymph nodes should then be biopsied, especially if they are enlarged.

Chemotherapy

Stratification of therapy, based on the extent of the primary tumour, presence of involved lymph nodes or metastases, and the extent of any tumour spillage at operation, is the key to rational use of chemotherapy. Reduction in therapy for 'good risk' patients and more intensive therapy for 'bad risk' patients result in fewer adverse effects of treatment in the former group, and good survival in the latter.

The first NWTS study in North America was the first concerted, systematic attempt to analyse postoperative chemotherapy and radiotherapy.[31] That study and its

Box 20.4 *Main findings in National Wilms' Tumor Studies (NWTS) 1–3*

NWTS1	
Group I	Patients under 2 years of age do not all need radiotherapy
Group II/III	AMD plus VCR is better than either alone
Group IV	Preoperative VCR is of no benefit
Other findings	Unfavourable histology and lymph node involvement are adverse features
NWTS 2	
Stage I	No patients benefit from radiotherapy, regardless of age. Six months of VCR and AMD is as good as 15 months
Stages II–IV	Addition of doxo to VCR and AMD improves survival
Other findings	Stages II and III have the same survival. Local spillage and invasion of the renal vein do not affect outcome
NWTS 3	
Stage I	10 weeks' therapy with VCR/AMD is as effective as 6 months
Stage II	Intensive VCR/AMD is as effective as three drugs. Addition of radiotherapy does not affect survival
Stage III	Intensive VCR/AMD is as effective as three drugs. 10 Gy flank irradiation is as effective as 20 Gy
Other findings	Addition of cyclophosphamide to VCR/AMD/doxo does not improve survival

AMD, Actinomycin D; doxo, doxorubicin; VCR, vincristine.

successors[32,33,45] have been instrumental in devising prognostic stages and revising them, as has already been noted. Equally important has been the steady progress in delineating optimal treatment within the various disease stages. The major findings in the national series are summarized in Box 20.4. The fourth national study ran from 1986 to 1994; a major objective of this study, apart from the usual questions of efficacy and toxicity, was the cost of treatment. In total, 905 children were randomized to study the duration of therapy and/or to study single- vs. divided-dose drug administration. Short courses of therapy (6 months) were as effective as long (15 month) ones, and single-dose administration of actinomycin D was no more toxic than fractionated dosing, thus confirming the previous finding of a large Brazilian study.[46] Thus, treatment costs can be substantially reduced.

At the end of the fourth national study, therapy had been significantly reduced compared with the first study and vincristine, actinomycin D and doxorubicin were confirmed as very effective drugs for adjuvant treatment. Thus, stage I patients needed only 10 weeks of adjuvant chemotherapy and no radiotherapy. In stage II patients, by using a more intensive regimen of vincristine and actinomycin D, neither doxorubicin, with its associated cardiotoxicity, nor radiotherapy were required. For stage III disease the intensive two-drug regimen was as effective as the three-drug one, and it had been possible to reduce radiotherapy from 20 to 10 Gy. The use of doxorubicin appeared specifically to improve the outlook for patients with bone-metastasizing renal tumour, but the addition of cyclophosphamide to doxorubicin, actinomycin D, and vincristine did not enhance survival of stage IV or 'unfavourable histology' patients.

The UKCCSG has built its study in part on the results of these American national studies and also on those of United Kingdom Medical Research Council (MRC) trials.[47,48] In the UKW1 trial, stage I patients treated with 10 weeks of vincristine at weekly intervals, followed by five 3-weekly doses, had 98 per cent survival at 2 years, suggesting that actinomycin D can be avoided in these patients.[44] In the second Wilms' trial, this treatment was reduced still further to 10 weeks of vincristine at weekly intervals only, without diminution of relapse-free survival.[49] Analysis of this approach in WT2 and WT3 has shown older age to influence outcome adversely.[49a] As with the American national studies, the recognition of unfavourable histology and of the adverse impact of lymph node metastases has led to the use of more aggressive therapy for these patients. Their overall survival improved, so that the current 2-year disease-free survival of patients with unfavourable histology, stages I–III, is around 50 per cent. Results for the first and second United Kingdom studies are given in Box 20.5.

Unlike the American or British studies, the cooperative European studies run by SIOP have concentrated on the use of preoperative therapies in an effort to reduce surgical morbidity, particularly tumour rupture. In the first SIOP study, patients were randomized either to immediate surgery or to preoperative radiotherapy (20 Gy).[41] The frequency of tumour spillage at operation was significantly reduced by radiotherapy. Although there was no difference in the OS, recurrence-free survival was better in the rupture-free group. The second SIOP study was non-randomized and observational. Some patients had immediate surgery at the discretion of the investigator, usually because the tumour was thought to be suitable for primary resection; others received preoperative radiation (20 Gy) and five doses of actinomycin D. Again,

Box 20.5 *Main findings in United Kingdom Children's Cancer Study Group trials UKW1 and UKW2*

- Vincristine alone is as effective for stage I tumours as two-drug regimens
- Fractionation of actinomycin D is unnecessary
- Prognosis for clear-cell sarcoma is as good as classic favourable histology

a reduced incidence of tumour rupture was found with preoperative treatment. The fifth SIOP study[42] compared preoperative chemoradiotherapy, as used in the second, with preoperative chemotherapy, consisting in this instance of two 5-day courses of actinomycin D and four weekly doses of vincristine. There were no significant differences in recurrence or OS, or in the frequency of tumour spillage, indicating the equal efficacy of the chemotherapy and the chemoradiotherapy.

When the chemotherapy of the fifth SIOP study is compared with the immediate surgery of the first, the skewing of stages towards the more favourable ones is clearly seen. Thus, the proportion of stage I patients is increased from 22 to 48 per cent, with a concomitant reduction in the proportion with stage II node-negative tumours (45 to 32 per cent) and stage II node-positive or stage III tumours (33 to 19 per cent). In the sixth SIOP study,[50] all patients received preoperative chemotherapy. Seventeen weeks of therapy in total were as effective as 38 weeks in the treatment of stage I tumours; stage II node-negative tumours did not benefit from postoperative radiotherapy; and stage II node-positive and stage III patients benefited from the addition of doxorubicin.[51]

In addition to the obvious benefits of reducing the risk of tumour rupture, a possible further benefit of preoperative treatment might be a reduction in the total amount of treatment given. The use of preoperative chemotherapy would permit the selection of 'good responders' who might be cured with less treatment compared with 'bad responders'. An inkling of this possibility is gained by studying the distribution of patients according to their postoperative stages. The data for SIOP 1, SIOP 5, UKW1 and NWTS 3 are shown in Table 20.1. Comparison of SIOP 1 and SIOP 5 data shows that the introduction of preoperative chemotherapy is associated with a shift of patients out of stage II node-positive/stage III and into stage I. This shift in distribution would lead to a major reduction in the total doses of chemotherapy and radiotherapy delivered. The SIOP 5 distribution, however, approximates to the distributions seen in the UK and NWT studies where immediate surgery has been the rule, indicating the interaction of factors other than just the presence or absence of preoperative treatment. One important difference is the centralization of paediatric oncology care in the US and UK, whereas many of

Table 20.1 *Comparison of percentage stage distribution in International Society of Paediatric Oncology trials SIOP 1[a] and SIOP 5[a], the United Kingdom Children's Cancer Study Group trial UKW1 and the third National Wilms' Tumor Study, NWTS 3*

Stage	SIOP 1	SIOP 5	UKW 2	NWTS 3
I	22	48	47	53
II N0	45	32	18	24
II N+/III	33	19	34	24

[a] Immediate surgery arms of SIOP 1, chemotherapy arm of SIOP 5; N0, node-negative; N+, node-positive.

Table 20.2 *Outcome for patients in the International Society of Paediatric Oncology trial SIOP 9: 3-year estimates of overall survival (OS) and event-free survival (EFS) for 360 trial patients (stages I–III) and 83 stage IV patients*

Stage	Number	EFS (%)	OS (%)
I	229	89	95
II, N0	84	74	87
II, N+/III	47	73	91
IV	83	66	77

N0, node-negative; N+, node-positive.

the SIOP patients are treated in hospitals that only occasionally see children with WT.

SIOP 9 examined the question of duration of preoperative chemotherapy and showed that 4 weeks was as good as 8 weeks in terms of proportion of stage I patients, intraoperative rupture rate, 2-year EFS and 5-year OS.[52] The most recent study, SIOP 93-01, examined the duration of postoperative chemotherapy in stage I tumours with intermediate-risk histology or anaplasia and showed that 4 weeks of postoperative therapy was as good as 18 weeks for stage I patients with intermediate-risk histology. There appeared to be no benefit to prolonged postoperative treatment. Results from SIOP 9 are summarized in Table 20.2.

By extrapolation from these findings it would appear that with the SIOP approach, and a survival rate of 88–92 per cent, only about 20 per cent of patients need flank irradiation; in the third American National study, with similar survival rates, 30 per cent of patients with favourable histology, non-metastatic tumours required flank irradiation.[53]

The third UK Wilms' study examined, in a randomized way, the question of whether preoperative chemotherapy improved staging and thereby led to a reduction in treatment, in effect by early identification of patients with responsive tumours, without any diminution in outcome. Patients deemed at the time of diagnosis to have 'resectable' and localized (i.e. no evidence of metastatic tumours) tumours were randomly assigned to either immediate surgery or 6 weeks of chemotherapy with vincristine and

actinomycin D. In the latter group, surgery was then carried out at about week 6–7, and in both groups the postoperative treatment was based on the NWTS 3 stage at the time of surgery. The study proved very difficult to conduct with a very low randomization rate, but over a 10-year period, just over 200 patients were randomized. Interim analyses confirmed that histological confirmation of diagnosis was essential, and that there were fewer surgical complications in the preoperatively treated group. It also became clear that vincristine monotherapy was not adequate for stage I patients unless the chest CT was normal at the time of diagnosis. Preliminary analyses of the staging distribution show that the preoperatively treated group has an excess of stage I and II patients, with a reduction in the proportion of stage III patients, as compared with the immediate surgery group. Overall there is no suggestion of a deterioration in outcome. Thus, adoption of this approach will result in an overall reduction in the amount of therapy needed.[39]

UNFAVOURABLE HISTOLOGY TUMOURS

It will be clear from the previous discussions of pathology and treatment that it is questionable whether the bone-metastasizing and malignant rhabdoid variants should continue to be included under the heading of Wilms' tumour. The Wilms'-based strategy works well for patients with the bone-metastasizing variant, with outcomes little different to those of favourable histology patients. The outlook for patients with malignant rhabdoid tumour is rather different. Extrarenal rhabdoid tumours are well described and are often treated as malignant mesenchymal tumours with alkylating agents such as ifosfamide or cyclophosphamide rather than doxorubicin. While this change in emphasis may be rational, it must be said that the results are still poor and there is the additional problem of using ifosfamide, which is very nephrotoxic, in uninephric patients. Until better therapy is available, the distinction between Wilms'- and sarcoma-based strategies, for this subgroup of patients, will remain academic.

Radiotherapy

Radiotherapy is now used less, and in lower doses, in the treatment of WT because of its local deleterious effects on growing tissues. The general trend has been to reduce the dose delivered, as successive trials have indicated that dose reduction does not compromise cure rates. It should be noted, however, that doxorubicin has generally been used to supplant radiation. However, there is increasing evidence that this drug, in addition to its short-term effects, may cause a significant long-term incidence of cardiac dysfunction. It may well be that the relative demerits of these two forms of treatment will, in due course, necessitate a reappraisal of their places in the treatment of WT.

In the first NWTS trial, for patients in groups I and II, the irradiation portal covered the kidney and the associated tumour. The other border came across the midline to encompass the whole of the vertebral bodies but not the contralateral normal kidney. Group III patients, and those patients in groups I and II with intraoperative tumour spillage, were treated with whole-abdominal radiation from the domes of the diaphragm to the pelvic floor and to the lateral reflections of the peritoneum. The results of this trial suggested that whole-abdominal radiation was not necessary if tumour spillage was restricted to the flank.[54,55] The second national study showed that omission of radiotherapy in all stage I patients was safe.[32] Data from the third study suggest that reduction of dosage from 20 to 10 Gy in stage III patients is acceptable, particularly if three-drug chemotherapy is used.[33]

Pulmonary metastases

The outlook for patients with pulmonary disease at diagnosis, if they have favourable histology, is excellent, with more than 75 per cent of patients still alive 4 years later (NWTS 3, UKW2). However, the treatment used in these trials comprised both doxorubicin and pulmonary radiotherapy. Both are associated with potentially significant long-term side-effects, however, and a worthwhile objective would be the removal of one or both from current treatment regimens. Appraisal of the preceding trials suggests that a substantial proportion of cases are cured without the use of one or both of these agents. In UKW1, 50 per cent of stage IV cases were cured without radiotherapy, while in NWTS 1 around the same proportion were cured without the use of doxorubicin.

No randomized prospective study has yet examined the need for pulmonary irradiation in patients with pulmonary metastases at the time of diagnosis, and no study has systematically examined the role of speed of response of metastases to chemotherapy in determining outcome. However, comparison of the regimens used by the various study groups provides some information.

NWTS 3 employed 12 Gy of whole-lung irradiation for stage IV patients, in addition to three- or four-drug chemotherapy given for 15 months. The EFS and OS for these patients were 75 and 82 per cent, respectively, 4 years from diagnosis. The contemporary UKW1 employed three-drug chemotherapy for 12 months and recommended radiotherapy only if pulmonary metastases had not resolved after 12 weeks of chemotherapy – thus only 4/40 patients were irradiated. The outcomes of 50 per cent (EFS) and 65 per cent (OS) at 6 years are clearly inferior. In the subsequent UKW2, with the same chemotherapy as UKW1, pulmonary radiotherapy was recommended for all patients with pulmonary disease at diagnosis and the outcomes improved to 70 per cent (EFS)

and 75 per cent (OS) at 4 years, figures more in line with the NWTS data. However, of the 59 patients with stage IV disease at diagnosis, only 37 actually received the radiotherapy. The chemotherapy regimens are very similar, although marginally shorter in UKW1 and 2 (12 vs. 15 months' duration), which suggests that the improvement must have been due to the greater use of radiotherapy.

The SIOP group has adopted a different approach. All stage IV patients have preoperative chemotherapy with vincristine, actinomycin D and doxorubicin for 6 weeks followed by nephrectomy. Subsequent treatment is determined on the basis of response to this initial treatment, assessed by chest radiography. If pulmonary metastases are still visible on a plain chest X-ray after 6 weeks of treatment, and are deemed resectable, then the metastases are surgically excised. If the metastases are deemed unresectable, or if surgical excision is incomplete on a postoperative X-ray, radiotherapy (15 Gy in 10 fractions) is given. Thus, if patients are in complete remission following preoperative chemotherapy, with or without surgical excision of metastatic disease, no pulmonary radiotherapy is given. Using this approach, only nine out of 36 patients had detectable metastases after preoperative chemotherapy. Five of the nine underwent surgical excision and subsequently remained free of disease. Four were judged to have unresectable disease, of whom one died of disease. Twenty-seven patients received chemotherapy only, one of whom was subsequently irradiated, and the relapse-free survival for the whole group was 83 per cent at 5 years.[56] There remains, however, a major disparity with the UK data. Apart from the use of preoperative therapy by SIOP, the chemotherapy is little different, yet even without the use of surgery, 75 per cent of the SIOP patients were long-term disease-free survivors, compared with only 50 per cent of the UK patients. This discrepancy most likely reflects the small number of patients in each study.

Thus, a significant number of patients – at least 50 per cent – with pulmonary metastases at the time of diagnosis, can be cured without radiotherapy, and possibly even more with the aggressive use of surgery. Identification of these patients remains problematic. It is possible that early complete response is sufficient in the majority of cases, but it could be argued that this group as a whole might benefit even more from the use of radiotherapy. It could also be argued that the long-term effects of 15 Gy of whole-lung radiotherapy will be less deleterious than those of 200–250 mg/m^2 of doxorubicin and that a more rational aim might be to explore the avoidance of this agent. It is unlikely that any individual cooperative group will be able to identify the best strategy for dealing with pulmonary stage IV disease because of the already very good prognosis, the number of patients needed to identify significant changes in outcome associated with changes in treatment, and the very long-term follow-up needed to identify the adverse consequences of particular treatment modalities.

Bilateral tumours

Bilateral tumours provide a particular challenge, and here the key is 'conservation of nephrons'. Initial surgery in these circumstances is limited to establishing the histological diagnosis, either by open or closed (Trucut) biopsy from both kidneys, because the histology can differ between them. Chemotherapy is then instituted. Once a maximal response has been obtained, the operation is usually bilateral partial nephrectomy. If these procedures will not clear the residual tumour and preserve adequate renal function, then 'bench surgery' has been advocated. Here, the kidney is removed and residual tumour resected; the kidney is then reimplanted. In the presence of extensive nephroblastomatosis, where there could be a subsequent metachronous tumour, it has been suggested that surgery should be conservative.[57] Approaches similar to those outlined for bilateral tumours may be useful in these patients.

Data from SIOP studies[58] show that the highest local stage is important in determining prognosis, and that children with synchronous tumours do better than those with metachronous tumours. In addition, children with metachronous tumours tend to be younger at diagnosis than those with synchronous tumours (mean age 13.2 vs. 32.1 months).

Resection of bilateral tumours with preservation of renal function may be impossible in a few children. It may be necessary to remove both kidneys, with renal transplantation after a period of dialysis. This strategy, though, is one of last resort, and should not be contemplated until conventional therapies have clearly failed.

WT in patients with a single kidney

Very occasionally, WT will be found in a patient with a single functioning kidney. Management should follow the guidelines for patients with bilateral tumours, as preservation of normal, functioning renal tissue is critical. Thus, initial chemotherapy with careful monitoring of response and timing of definitive surgery will provide the most favourable result. Immediate nephrectomy followed by dialysis, chemotherapy and then transplantation would be an option, but one with many additional problems so that it is best avoided if at all possible.

WT in patients with pre-existing renal disease

In these patients, the type and prognosis of the pre-existing disease will dictate variations in management.

Where there is likely to be inexorable progression to end-stage renal failure there seems little virtue in delaying surgical removal of the tumour and associated kidney. If necessary, dialysis can be instituted to supplement residual renal function. The timing of transplantation is more difficult, but to avoid the complexity of simultaneous cancer chemotherapy and transplantation immunosuppression, it seems better to delay transplantation until chemotherapy has been completed and enough time has elapsed for the recurrence of malignancy to be unlikely. In practice, this period would be about 2 years from completion of chemotherapy.

RELAPSE

With the refinement of initial treatment and the excellent disease-free survival, the treatment of relapse has assumed greater importance. The most frequent site of relapse overall is the lungs. In the fifth SIOP study, 54 per cent of all relapses were isolated pulmonary events, the remainder being in other or multiple sites.[42] Sixteen per cent of all relapses involved the abdomen, but only in association with other sites. In the second and third American National Wilms' Tumor Studies, the lungs accounted for 58 per cent of all relapses, whilst abdominal relapse accounted for a further 29 per cent.[59] Isolated pulmonary relapse accounted for 41 per cent of all relapses in the first UK study, with abdominal relapses accounting for 24 per cent, and the remaining 35 per cent being patients with multiple simultaneous sites of relapse.[60]

Both American and British studies[59,60] have identified factors that indicate an increased likelihood of salvaging patients with relapsed tumours. These factors include tumours with favourable histology that recurred only in the lungs; relapse in the abdomen where radiotherapy had not been included in the primary treatment; and relapse that occurred more than 12 months from diagnosis. Each category was associated with a more favourable outcome. Patients with relapsed, 'unfavourable histology' tumours had poor survival regardless of the site or timing of relapse. Nevertheless, the overall survival following relapse was only 24 and 30 per cent in the UK and US series, respectively, and only 50 and 40 per cent, respectively, in the 'better' risk patients. Both studies showed that a variety of retrieval strategies were being used, in part dictated by the previous therapy. Subsequently both groups have introduced standard relapse regimens to provide consistent data on response rates to the agents employed.

Support for the use of multiagent regimens containing drugs to which the patient has not previously been exposed is provided by a report from St Jude Hospital.[61] The introduction of more modern, effective, drugs for relapsed WT in this report has been associated with a significant improvement in both EFS and OS (35 and 65 per cent, respectively). This improvement in survival after relapse occurred concurrently with a decrease in the primary relapse rate, further emphasizing the improvement in relapse therapy. Apart from the three standard agents – vincristine, actinomycin D and doxorubicin – other agents useful in relapse include ifosfamide[62] or cyclophosphamide, carboplatin[63] and etoposide.[64] The best reported results for relapsed and refractory WT come from the SFOP group. Using a combination of carboplatin and etoposide, response rates of 73 per cent and a survival rate of 33 per cent at 3 years have been obtained.[65] All patients with anaplasia responded to this combination. A Children's Cancer Group (CCG) study suggests that ifosfamide and etoposide may be a more potent combination for the treatment of bone-metastasizing renal tumours.[66]

One might ask why at least some of these drugs are not incorporated into the initial regimens so as to improve the initial relapse-free survival, and how it is that, for example, cyclophosphamide can be useful in relapse but not be shown to confer any advantage when prospectively assessed in poor-risk tumours in prospective trials. Presumably, overall, vincristine, actinomycin D and doxorubicin are so successful for the great majority of patients that the addition of a drug that benefits only a minority of patients who cannot be identified before initiation of treatment has only a trivial impact on relapse-free and overall survival.

Initial surgery may not be necessary for non-irradiated abdominal recurrences of tumours with favourable histology, when radiotherapy and further chemotherapy can be given – an important consideration if the tumour appears not to be resectable. If not previously used, radiotherapy is indicated for multiple pulmonary relapses and is used in conjunction with salvage chemotherapy. A small number of children with tumours of favourable histology who developed solitary lung metastases after treatment in NWTS 1, 2 or 3 had a poor outcome with surgery and chemotherapy alone. The group of patients who received radiotherapy as part of their relapse regimen did not have their outcome improved further by the addition of surgery,[67] implying that surgery is unnecessary. The St Jude group has also identified radiation as an important part of relapse therapy.[61]

There has been enthusiasm for the adoption of high-dose chemotherapy regimens, particularly for patients deemed to be at high risk of further relapse following retreatment. A total of 51 children with recurrent or chemoresistant WT who have had high-dose chemotherapy with autologous marrow or peripheral blood stem cell reconstitution have been registered with the European Bone Marrow Transplantation Solid Tumour Registry. Forty-three children underwent the procedure after at least one relapse, or without ever entering a remission. Although a variety of chemotherapy regimens were used, the commonest was melphalan, either alone or in combination (with vincristine or BCNU), which was received by 40 patients. Twenty-one patients died after the procedure from progressive disease, and three died of respiratory complications. Nineteen patients survived disease-free 2–10 years after the procedure, two are alive with progressive disease, and no follow-up data are available on six.[68] The variety of approaches to the treatment of relapsed WT make it impossible to reach firm conclusions about the indications for, and best method of, administering high-dose therapy, but these data suggest that high-dose chemotherapy may offer some chance of cure in patients who are resistant to conventional chemotherapy. Two prospective studies with conditioning regimens containing carboplatin/etoposide/melphalan and thioTEPA/etoposide/cyclophosphamide show encouraging results.[69,70] It is worth noting, however, that the results obtained after such an intensive procedure are no better than those obtained by the St Jude group for high-risk patients using modern era chemotherapy.[61]

FOLLOW-UP AND SCREENING INVESTIGATIONS

The place of repeated 'screening' investigations in patients with conditions associated with, or predisposing to, WT has not been established. Often the physicians taking care of such patients are not primarily oncologists, and may not recognize all of the issues involved when making a decision to start screening. Some physicians propose that repeated screening permits earlier detection of clinically occult tumours and leads to an improvement in outcome. Others note that tumours may be clinically detectable only a few weeks after apparently normal (usually ultrasonographic) screening.

There are two separate issues to consider. First, what is the evidence that screening of presymptomatic, predisposed children will lead to earlier detection of tumours? Second, will detection of presymptomatic tumours result in fewer deaths or less treatment-related morbidity (as less therapy would be necessary for lower-stage disease)? Palmer and Evans[71] reviewed nine patients with WT, known to have aniridia, who had been screened routinely by intravenous urography in an attempt to diagnose their tumours presymptomatically; an unsuspected tumour was detected in only one patient. Green et al.[72] reviewed data from 3675 patients registered with the National Wilms' Tumor Study and identified 24 WT patients with aniridia, 19 with Beckwith–Wiedemann syndrome, and 96 with hemihypertrophy. Screening examinations were associated with lower stage at diagnosis in aniridia, but not in the other two conditions. Craft *et al.*[73] reviewed 1622 WT patients in the United Kingdom Children's Cancer Registry and found 16 with aniridia, 18 with Beckwith–Wiedemann syndrome, and 18 with hemihypertrophy. There were no significant differences in stage distribution or outcome for any of the three predisposing conditions whether they were not screened, had a tumour detected by screening or had an interval diagnosis of tumour. At present, therefore, the utility of presymptomatic screening is not proven. Any randomized trial attempting to address this question will require an impracticably long accrual period because of the rarity of the predisposing conditions and the very high cure rates for WT.

During and after treatment, investigation is aimed at detecting early local or distant relapses. Generally, local relapses are less frequent than pulmonary relapse. Chest radiographs (posteroanterior and lateral) should be obtained regularly during treatment, and then continued over the time when relapse is most likely to occur. Pulmonary relapse may be clinically undetectable until quite advanced, whereas local (abdominal) relapses are usually more overt. Typically, therefore, chest radiographs should be obtained every 9 weeks during treatment, every 2 months for the first year and every 3 months for the second year after completion of treatment. Stage IV patients should continue to have chest radiographs at 3-monthly intervals for a further year. Screening for local relapse need not be so frequent, and abdominal ultrasonography at completion of treatment and then 6-monthly for 2 years is enough. Other sites of relapse are rare, even (despite its name) in bone-metastasizing renal tumour, in which pulmonary metastases are most common. Thus, patients with this tumour need radionuclide bone scans, if at all, only at 6-monthly intervals for 2 years.

PROGNOSIS

With the use of modern anaesthetic and surgical techniques and the rational application of combination chemotherapy, the majority of patients with WT will be cured. In part, this is because most patients will present with histologically favourable, low-stage disease, but there have also been genuine advances in chemotherapy. Results for the better arm of treatment for each stage of the third American national study and those from the second UK study are shown in Tables 20.3 and 20.4. The overall survival from the fifth SIOP trial was 86 per cent at 3 years, with a relapse-free survival of 71 per cent. Thus, the vast majority of WT patients are cured of their disease, many with minimal short- or long-term morbidity.

Stage V patients are often treated in a very 'individualized' fashion, and so the available findings are usually

Table 20.3 *Percentage outcome for patients in the third National Wilms' Tumor Study, NWTS 3*

	2-year RFS	2-year OS	Treatment
Stage I	92	97	10 weeks vincristine + actinomycin D
Stage II/III	87	91	15 months vincristine + actinomycin D + doxorubicin
Stage III	78	86	10 Gy + vincristine + actinomycin D ± doxorubicin
Stage IV + UH	72	81	

OS, overall survival; RFS, relapse-free survival; UH, unfavourable histology.

Table 20.4 *Percentage outcome for patients in the United Kingdom Children's Cancer Study Group trial UKW1*

Stage	3-year EFS	3-year OS	6-year EFS	6-year OS
I	90	96	89	96
II	85	94	85	93
III	82	83	82	83
IV	58	65	50	65

EFS, event-free survival; OS, overall survival.

those of single centres. Data collected from 22 SIOP centres indicate an overall survival of 64 per cent with a follow-up of 6 years.

TOXICITY OF TREATMENT

The majority of short-term toxicity caused by the treatment of WT is predictable according to the various modalities that are used. Thus neurotoxicity from vincristine, and myelosuppression from doxorubicin are both well known and well documented. Seven per cent (27/384) of patients in UKW1 developed clinically significant neurotoxicity secondary to treatment with vincristine. In eight cases the principal feature was paralytic ileus, and in the other 19 cases, it was peripheral neuropathy varying in severity from mild ptosis to severe foot drop. All patients regained their neurological function. There were 421 episodes of hospitalization necessitated by myelosuppression. In 29 instances the episode was fever in association with neutropenia, and in 13 it was bleeding secondary to thrombocytopenia.[44]

Actinomycin D, which in the past was often given fractionated over a 5-day period, is now more usually given as a single fraction.[45,46,74] This change has led to the emergence of an associated hepatopathy characterized by deranged liver function tests and thrombocytopenia.

The phenomenon is of variable severity, ranging from a mild elevation in aminotransferase activities and bilirubin, and a mild concurrent fall in platelet count, to a severe disorder with liver failure and disseminated intravascular coagulation, which may result in death. It is important to monitor for the occurrence of this condition as it may recur with subsequent courses of actinomycin D. Normally, dose reduction or readopting a fractionated schedule is sufficient to prevent recurrence.[75,76]

Concern about the possible long-term cardiotoxicity of anthracyclines was heightened by the detection of abnormalities of cardiac function in children who had received only low or moderate doses of anthracyclines[77] for the treatment of leukaemia. Although only a minority of patients with WT receive anthracyclines, many will also have received radiation with fields that may encompass part or all of the heart. Twenty-five per cent of 97 patients previously treated for WT, with a mean cumulative anthracycline dose of 303 mg/m^2, had abnormalities of cardiac function compared with a control group of patients with WT who had not received anthracyclines.[78] This incidence of abnormalities is disconcertingly high, but the full relevance of the findings remains unclear, and careful long-term evaluation remains essential. Patients with increased left ventricular wall stress should probably be advised to avoid extremely strenuous exercise and be monitored carefully during pregnancy.

It is often assumed that unilateral nephrectomy has only minimal, if any, long-term morbidity. An evaluation of renal function in a group of long-term WT survivors (more than 13 years of treatment) has shown some evidence of dysfunction of the remaining kidney in 32 per cent. Nineteen per cent had chrome EDTA glomerular filtration rates of less than 80 mL/min/1.73 m^2, 11 per cent had hypertension, and 9 per cent had increased urinary albumin excretion. Only 55 per cent of patients had undergone significant compensatory contralateral renal hypertrophy. Children of less than 24 months at the time of diagnosis and those children who had received radiation doses of greater than 1200 cGy to the remaining kidney were most at risk of dysfunction.[79] A similar study in adults who had undergone unilateral nephrectomy for a renal malignancy concluded that there was an increased risk of proteinuria, glomerulopathy and progressive renal failure.[80] Thus, there is a clear case for continuing follow-up with measurements of blood pressure and checks for proteinuria.

The major long-term side-effect of radiotherapy for WT is disturbance of growth. As the radiation field in virtually all children irradiated for this condition is the hemiabdomen, the most obvious disturbance is asymmetrical growth of soft tissue. As the field includes the full width of the vertebral bodies, there is also a loss in final height. The younger the patient at the time of irradiation, the more severe is the restriction and the more disproportionate they become as adults. The loss in potential height ranges from 10 cm at the age of 1 year to 7 cm at 5 years.[81]

FUTURE PROSPECTS

The two continuing clinical challenges in WT are to continue refining therapy in patients with good prognosis, so as to minimize treatment-related morbidity, and to improve therapy for poor prognosis and relapsing patients, so that their survival improves. Advances in the understanding of the genetic basis of WT may help to define more precisely patients with good and poor prognosis than the clinical staging currently in use. Patients with stage I tumours with favourable histology already receive minimal treatment, but the recognition of highly favourable histological or genetic patterns may define a group that needs no adjuvant chemotherapy. Preoperative chemotherapy may provide a route to overall reduction of chemotherapy and obviation of radiotherapy. Improvement in the treatment of cases with unfavourable histology awaits the development of novel strategies.

KEY POINTS

- Overall, the chances of cure are excellent.
- Novel therapies are needed, especially for malignant rhabdoid tumour.
- Preoperative chemotherapy is increasingly favoured.
- Both surgery and radiotherapy may have important roles in the treatment of pulmonary metastases.

REFERENCES

1. Wilms M. *Die Mischgeschwulste der Nieren*. Leipzig: Arthur Georgi, 1899; 1–90.
2. Parkin DM, Stiller CA, Draper GJ. The international incidence of childhood cancer. *Int J Cancer* 1988; **42**: 511–20.
3. Hrabovsky EE, Othrsen HB, de Lorimier A *et al*. Wilms' tumor in the neonate: a report from the National Wilms' Tumor Study. *J Pediatr Surg* 1986; **21**: 385–7.
4. Ledlie EM, Mynors LS, Draper GJ, Gorbach PD. Natural history and treatment of Wilms' tumour: an analysis of 335 cases occurring in England and Wales, 1962–1966. *Br Med J* 1970; **4**: 195–200.
5. Coppes MJ, Zandvoort SW, Sparling CR *et al*. Acquired von Willebrand disease in Wilms' tumour patients. *J Clin Oncol* 1992; **10**: 422–7.

6. Owens CM, Veys PA, Pritchard J *et al.* Role of chest computed tomography at diagnosis in the management of Wilms' tumor: a study by the United Kingdom Children's Cancer Study Group. *J Clin Oncol* 2002; **20**: 2768–73.

7. Wilimas JA, Douglass EC, Magill HL *et al.* Significance of pulmonary computed tomography at diagnosis in Wilms' tumour. *J Clin Oncol* 1988; **6**: 1144–6.

8. Green DM, Fernbach DJ, Norkool P *et al.* The treatment of Wilms' tumor patients with pulmonary metastases detected only with computed tomography: a report from the National Wilms' Tumor Study. *J Clin Oncol* 1991; **9**: 1776–81.

9. Bonnin JM, Rubinstein LJ, Palmer NF, Beckwith JB. The association of embryonal tumours originating in the kidney and in the brain. A report of seven cases. *Cancer* 1984; **54**: 2137–6.

10. Breslow NE *et al.* Wilms' tumor: prognostic factors for patients without metastases at diagnosis: results of the National Wilms' Tumor Study. *Cancer* 1978; **41**: 1577–89.

11. Breslow NE, Palmer NF, Hill LR *et al.* Prognostic factors for Wilms' tumor patients with non-metastatic disease at diagnosis. Results of the second National Wilms' tumor study. *J Clin Oncol* 1985; **3**: 521–31.

12. Breslow NE, Churchill G, Nesmith B *et al.* Clinicopathologic features and prognosis for Wilms' tumor patients with metastases at diagnosis. *Cancer* 1986; **58**: 2501–11.

12a. Bown N, Cotterill SJ, Roberts P *et al.* Cytogenetic abnormalities and clinical outcome in Wilms tumor: a study from the UK Cancer Cytogenetics Group and the UK Children's Cancer Study Group. *Med Pediatr Oncol* 2002; **38**: 11–21.

♦13. Beckwith JB. Wilms' tumor and other renal tumors of childhood. In: Finegold MWB, ed. *Pathology of Neoplasia in Children and Adolescents.* Philadelphia: Saunders, 1986; 313–32.

14. Green DM, Beckwith JB, Weeks NM *et al.* The relationship between microstaging variables, age at diagnosis, and tumor weight of children with stage I/favorable histology Wilms' tumor. *Cancer* 1994; **74**: 1817–20.

15. Kidd JM. Exclusion of certain renal neoplasms from the category of Wilms' tumour. *Am J Pathol* 1970; **59**: 16a.

16. Marsden HB, Lawler W. Bone-metastasising renal tumour of childhood. *Br J Cancer* 1978; **38**: 437–41.

17. Beckwith JB, Palmer NF. Histopathology and prognosis of Wilms' tumor: results from the first National Wilms' Tumor Study. *Cancer* 1978; **41**: 1937–48.

18. Weeks DA, Beckwith JB, Merau GW, Luckey DW. Rhabdoid tumor of the kidney. A report of 111 cases from the National Wilms' Tumor Study center. *Am J Surg Pathol* 1989; **13**: 439–58.

19. Rousseau-Merck MF, Boccon-Gibod L, Nogues C *et al.* An original hypercalcemic infantile renal tumor without bone metastasis: heterotransplantation to nude mice. *Cancer* 1982; **50**: 85–93.

20. Mitchell CD, Harvey W, Gordon D *et al.* Rhabdoid Wilms' tumour and prostaglandin-mediated hypercalcaemia. *Eur Paediatr Haematol Oncol* 1985; **2**: 153–7.

21. Beckwith JB. Mesenchymal renal neoplasms of infancy revisited. *J Pediatr Surg* 1974; **9**: 803–5.

22. Beckwith JB, Storkel S. Tumours of the kidney in adults and children. *Presented at the 22nd International Congress of the International Academy of Pathology and 13th World Congress of Academic and Environmental Pathology.* October, 1998 Nice, France.

23. Rubin BP, Chen CJ, Morgan TW *et al.* Congenital mesoblastic nephroma t(12;15) is associated with ETV6-NTRK3 gene fusion: cytogenetic and molecular relationships to congenital (infantile) fibrosarcoma. *Am J Pathol* 1998; **153**(5): 1451–8.

24. Patel Y, Mitchell CD, Hitchcock RJ. Use of sarcoma based chemotherapy in a case of congenital mesoblastic nephroma with liver metastases. *Urology* 2003; **61**: 1260.

25. Argani P, Beckwith JB. Metanephric stromal tumor: report of 31 cases of a distinctive pediatric renal neoplasm. *Am J Surg Pathol* 2000; **24**: 917–26.

26. Vujanic GM, Delemarre JFM, Sandstedt B *et al.* The new SIOP (Stockholm) working classification of renal tumours of childhood. *Med Pediatr Oncol* 1996; **26**: 145–6.

27. Beckwith JB, Palmer NF. Histopathology and prognosis of Wilms' tumour: results from the first National Wilms' Tumor Study. *Cancer* 1978; **41**: 1937–48.

28. Zuppan CW, Beckwith JB, Weeks DA *et al.* The effects of preoperative chemotherapy on the histologic features of Wilms' tumor. An analysis of cases from the third National Wilms' Tumor Study. *Cancer* 1991; **68**: 385–94.

29. Boccon-Gibod L, Rey A, Sandstedt B *et al.* Complete necrosis induced by preoperative chemotherapy in Wilms' tumor as an indicator of low risk: Report of the International Society of Paediatric Oncology (SIOP) Nephroblastoma Trial and Study 9. *Med Pediatr Oncol* 2000; **34**: 193–200.

30. Weirich A, Leuschner I, Harms D *et al.* Clinical impact of histologic subtypes in localised non anaplastic nephroblastoma treated according to trial and study SIOP9/GPOH. *Ann Oncol* 2001; **12**: 311–19.

●31. D'Angio GJ, Evans AE, Breslow N *et al.* The treatment of Wilms' tumor: results of the National Wilms' Tumor Study. *Cancer* 1976; **38**: 633–46.

●32. D'Angio GJ, Evans AE, Breslow N *et al.* The treatment of Wilms' tumour: results of the second National Wilms' Tumor Study. *Cancer* 1981; **47**: 2302–11.

●33. D'Angio GJ, Breslow N, Beckwith JB *et al.* The treatment of Wilms' tumor. Results of the third National Wilms' Tumor Study. *Cancer* 1989; **64**: 349–60.

34. Grundy PE, Telzerow PE, Breslow N *et al.* Loss of heterozygosity for chromosomes 16q and 1p in Wilms' tumors predicts an adverse outcome. *Cancer Res* 1994; **54**: 2331–3.

35. Griffel M. Wilms' tumour in New York State: epidemiology and survivorship. *Cancer* 1977; **40**: 3140–5.

36. Lennox EL, Stiller CA, Morris-Jones PH, Kinnier-Wilson LM. Nephroblastoma: treatment during 1970–73 and the effect on survival of inclusion in the first MRC trial. *Br Med J* 1979; **2**: 567–9.

37. Stiller CA. Centralisation of treatment and survival rates for cancer. *Arch Dis Child* 1988; **63**: 23–30.

38. Pritchard J, Stiller CA, Lennox EL. Over-treatment of children with Wilms' tumour outside paediatric oncology centres. *Br Med J* 1989; **299**: 835–6.

●39. Mitchell CD, Shannon R, Imeson J *et al.* The treatment of Wilms' tumour: results of the third United Kingdom Children's Cancer Research Group (UKCCSG) Wilms' Tumour Study (UKW3). *N Engl J Med* 2004, submitted.

40. Vujanic GM, Kelsey A, Mitchell CD et al. The role of biopsy in the diagnosis of renal tumors of childhood: results of the UKCCSG Wilms' Tumor Study 3. Med Pediatr Oncol 2003; 40: 18–22.

●41. Lemerle J, Voute PA, Tournade MF et al. Preoperative versus post-operative radiotherapy, single versus multiple courses of actinomycin D in the treatment of Wilms' tumours. Preliminary results of a controlled clinical trial conducted by the International Society of Pediatric Oncology (SIOP). Cancer 1976; 38: 647–54.

●42. Lemerle J, Voute PA, Tournade MF et al. Effectiveness of preoperative chemotherapy in Wilms' tumor: results of an International Society of Pediatric Oncology (SIOP) clinical trial. J Clin Oncol 1983; 1: 604–9.

43. Ritchey ML, Pringle KC, Breslow NE et al. Management and outcome of inoperable Wilms' Tumor. A report of the National Wilms' Tumor Study 3. Ann Surg 1994; 220: 683–90.

●44. Pritchard J, Imeson J, Barnes J et al. Results of the United Kingdom Children's Cancer Study Group (UKCCSG) first Wilms' Tumor Study (UKW-1). J Clin Oncol 1995; 13: 124–33.

●45. Green DM, Breslow NE, Beckwith JB et al. Comparison between single-dose and divided-dose administration of dactinomycin and doxorubicin for patients with Wilms' tumor: a report from the National Wilms' Tumor Study group. J Clin Oncol 1998; 16: 237–45.

●46. de Camargo B, Franco EL. A randomized clinical trial of single-dose versus fractionated-dose dactinomycin in the treatment of Wilms' tumor. Cancer 1993; 73: 3081–6.

47. Medical Research Council's Working Party on Embryonal Tumours in Childhood. Management of nephroblastoma in childhood. Clinical study of two forms of maintenance chemotherapy. Arch Dis Child 1978; 53: 112–19.

48. Morris-Jones P, Marsden HB, Pearson D, Barnes J. MRC second nephroblastoma trial, 1974–78: long-term results. SIOP Proceedings, abstract 121. Jerusalem: SIOP, 1987.

●49. Mitchell CD, Morris-Jones P, Kelsey A et al. The treatment of Wilms' tumour: results of the UKCCSG second Wilms' Tumour Study. Br J Cancer 2000; 83: 602–8.

49a. Pritchard-Jones K, Kelsey A, Vujanic G et al. Older age is an adverse prognostic factor in stage I, favorable histology Wilms' tumor treated with vincristine monochemotherapy: a study by the United Kingdom Children's Cancer Study Group, Wilms' Tumor Working Group. J Clin Oncol 2003; 21: 3269–75.

●50. Tournade MF, Com-Nougue C, Voute PA et al. Results of the International Society of Paediatric Oncology 6 Wilms' tumor trial and study; a risk adapted therapeutic approach in Wilms' tumor. J Clin Oncol 1993; 11: 1014–23.

●51. Voute PA, Lemerle J, de Kraker J et al. Preoperative chemotherapy (CT) as first treatment in children with Wilms' tumour. Results of the SIOP nephroblastoma trials and studies. SIOP Proceedings, abstract. 123. Jerusalem: SIOP, 1987.

●52. Tournade MF, Com-Nougue C, De Kraker J et al. Optimal duration of therapy in unilateral and non-metastatic Wilms' tumor in children older than 6 month; Results of the ninth International Society of Pediatric Oncology Wilms' tumor trial and study. J Clin Oncol 2001; 19: 488–500.

53. D'Angio GJ. SIOP and the management of Wilms' tumour. J Clin Oncol 1983; 1: 595–6.

54. Tefft M, D'Angio GJ, Grant W. Post-operative radiation therapy for residual Wilms' tumor. Review of group III patients in the National Wilms' Tumor Study. Cancer 1976; 37: 2768–72.

55. D'Angio GJ, Tefft M, Breslow N, Meyer JA. Radiation therapy of Wilms' tumor: results according to dose, field, post-operative timing and histology. Int J Radiat Oncol Biol Phys 1979; 4: 769–80.

56. de Kraker J, Lemerle J, Voute PA et al. Wilms' tumour with pulmonary metastases at diagnosis: the significance of primary chemotherapy. J Clin Oncol 1990; 8: 1187–90.

57. Heidemann RL, Haase GM, Foley CL et al. Nephro-blastomatosis and Wilms' tumour: clinical experience and management of seven patients. Cancer 1985; 555: 1446–51.

58. Coppes MJ, de Kraker J, van Dijken PJ et al. Bilateral Wilms' tumor: long-term survival and some epidemiological features. J Clin Oncol 1989; 7: 310–15.

59. Grundy P, Breslow N, Green DM et al. Prognostic factors for children with recurrent Wilms' tumor: results from the second and third National Wilms' Tumor Study. J Clin Oncol 1989; 7: 638–47.

60. Groot-Loonen JJ, Pinkerton CR, Morris-Jones PH, Pritchard J. How curable is relapsed Wilms' tumour? The United Kingdom Children's Cancer Study Group. Arch Dis Child 1990; 65: 968–70.

61. Dome JS, Liu T, Krasin M et al. Improved survival for patients with recurrent Wilms' tumour: the experience at St Jude Children's Research Hospital. J Pediatr Hematol Oncol 2002; 24: 192–8.

62. Tournade MF, Lemerle J, Brunat-Mentigny M et al. Ifosphamide is an active drug in Wilms' tumour: a phase II study by the French Society of Paediatric Oncology. J Clin Oncol 1988; 6: 793–6.

63. de Camargo B, Melaragno R, Saba e Silva N et al. Phase II study of carboplatin as a single drug for relapsed Wilms' tumour: experience of the Brazilian Wilms' Tumour Study Group. Med Pediatr Oncol 1994; 22, 258–60.

64. Pein F, Pinkerton CR, Tournade MF et al. Etoposide in relapsed or refractory Wilms' tumour: a phase II study by SFOP and UKCCSG. J Clin Oncol 1993; 11: 1478–81.

65. Pein F, Tournade MF, Zucker JM et al. Etoposide and carboplatin: a highly effective combination in relapsed or refractory Wilms' tumour – a phase II study by SFOP. J Clin Oncol 1994; 12, 931–6.

66. Miser J, Krailo M, Hammond GD et al. The combination of ifosfamide, etoposide and mesna: a very active regimen in the treatment of recurrent Wilms' tumour (abstract). Proc Am Soc Clin Oncol 1993; 12: 417.

67. Green DM, Breslow NE, Ii Y et al. The role of surgical excision in the management of relapsed Wilms' tumor patients with pulmonary metastases: a report from the National Wilms' Tumor Study. J Pediatr Surg 1991; 26: 728–33.

68. Garaventa A, Hartmann O, Bernard JL et al. Autologous bone marrow transplantation for pediatric Wilms' tumor: the experience of the European Bone Marrow Transplantation Solid Tumor Registry. Med Pediatr Oncol 1994; 22: 11–14.

69. Pein F, Michon J, Valteau-Couanet D et al. High-dose melphalan, etoposide and carboplatin with bone marrow

transplantation as consolidation therapy in high risk Wilms' tumour. A prospective study by SFOP. *Proc Am Soc Clin Oncol* 1995; **14**: 455.

70. Warkentin PI, Brochstein JA, Strandjord SE *et al.* High-dose chemotherapy followed by autologous stem cell rescue for recurrent Wilms' tumor. *Proc Am Soc Oncol* 1993; **12**: 414.

71. Palmer N, Evans AE. The association of aniridia and Wilms' tumour: methods of surveillance and diagnosis. *Med Pediatr Oncol* 1983; **11**: 73–5.

72. Green DM, Breslow NE, Beckwith JB, Norkool P. Screening of children with hemihypertrophy, aniridia and Beckwith–Wiedemann syndrome in patients with Wilms' tumor. *Med Pediatr Oncol* 1993; **21**: 188–92.

73. Craft AW, Parker L, Stiller C, Cole M. Screening for Wilms' tumour in patients with aniridia, Beckwith syndrome or hemihypertrophy. *Med Pediatr Oncol* 1995; **24**: 231–4.

74. Green DM, Breslow NE, Evans I *et al.* Relationship between dose schedule and charges for treatment on National Wilms' Tumor Study 4. A report from the National Wilms' Tumor Study Group. *J Natl Cancer Inst Mongr* 1995; **19**: 21–5.

75. Green DM, Finklestein JZ, Norkool P *et al.* Severe hepatic toxicity after treatment with single-dose dactinomycin and vincristine. *Cancer* 1988; **62**: 270–3.

76. Raine J, Bowman A, Wallendszus K *et al.* Hepatopathy-thrombocytopenia syndrome. A complication of actinomycin-D therapy for Wilms' tumour. *J Clin Oncol* 1991; **9**: 268–73.

77. Lipshultz SE, Colan SD, Gelber RD *et al.* Late cardiac effects of doxorubicin therapy for acute lymphoblastic leukaemia in children. *N Engl J Med* 1991; **324**: 808–15.

78. Sorensen K, Levitt G, Sebag-Montefiore D *et al.* Cardiac function in Wilms' tumour survivors. *J Clin Oncol* 1995; **13**: 1546–56.

79. Levitt GA, Yeomans E, Dicks-Mireaux C *et al.* Renal size and function after cure of Wilms' tumour. *Br J Cancer* 1992; **66**: 877–82.

80. Novick C, Gephardt MD, Guz B *et al.* Long-term follow-up after partial removal of a solitary kidney. *N Engl J Med* 1991; **325**: 1058–62.

81. Wallace WHB, Shalet SM, Morris-Jones PH *et al.* The effect of abdominal irradiation on growth in boys treated for a Wilms' tumor. *Med Pediatr Oncol* 1990; **8**(6): 441–6.

21

Germm cell tumours

JILLIAN R. MANN

PATHOGENESIS

In the human embryo, the first germ cells can be identified in the extraembryonal yolk sac at 4 weeks. From here they migrate through the middle and dorsal mesentery, reaching the germinal epithelium of the gonadal ridge at 6 weeks where they populate the developing testis or ovary (Figure 21.1).

The commonest sites of extragonadal germ cell tumours, namely, the sacrococcygeal area, retroperitoneum, mediastinum, neck and pineal area of the brain, can be explained by aberrant migration along the gonadal ridge which lies adjacent to the vertebral column from the cervical to the lower lumbar region.

The morphological subtype reflects the pathway of differentiation to which the cell is committed prior to malignant transformation. The cell line may remain in the germinal state as a dysgerminoma or seminoma, or the transforming event may occur in a population that differentiates towards either embryonal or extraembryonal cell types (Figure 21.2). The degree of differentiation will range from benign, fully differentiated teratoma to completely undifferentiated embryonal carcinoma. Mature or immature teratomas may include somatic tissues from the three basic embryonal layers – mesoderm, ectoderm and endoderm. A number of classifications have been used, such as those by Dehner[1] and Ablin and Isaacs[2] (Box 21.1). The UK has recently adopted a classification agreed by an international working group (Box 21.2).

In the case of tumour developing in cells destined to form extraembryonal tissues, differentiation is towards either the yolk sac or placenta. This produces either

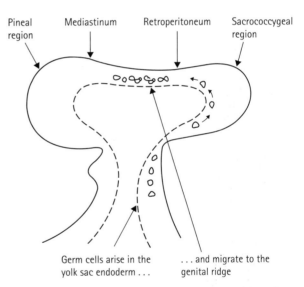

Pineal region   Mediastinum   Retroperitoneum   Sacrococcygeal region

Germ cells arise in the yolk sac endoderm . . .   . . . and migrate to the genital ridge

Figure 21.1 *Diagrammatic representation of the origin and migration of germ cells from yolk sac to gonadal ridge, showing possible aberrant sites of migration.*

malignant yolk sac tumour (endodermal sinus tumour) or choriocarcinoma.

Germ cell tumours (GCTs) account for approximately 3 per cent of childhood malignancies. The true incidence is difficult to ascertain, as many of the benign GCTs will not be registered with central cancer registries. However, the incidence of malignant GCTs in British children is rising.[3] In 1981–90 the age-standardized rates of germ cell and gonadal neoplasms were 4.2 per million per year for England and Wales and 4.8 for Scotland.[4] Two-thirds of GCTs in children occur in extragonadal sites and the

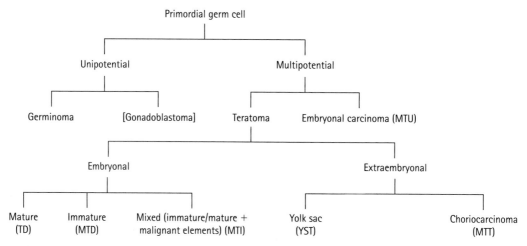

Figure 21.2 *Schema of differentiation pathway for germ cell tumours. MTD, malignant teratoma differentiated; MTI, malignant teratoma intermediate; MTU, malignant teratoma undifferentiated; MTT, malignant teratoma trophoblastic; TD, teratoma differentiated; YST, yolk sac tumour.*

Box 21.1 *Classification of germ cell tumours in childhood[2]*

> I   Teratoma
>   A   Mature = TD
>   B   Immature = MTD
>   C   With malignant germ cell tumour component(s) = MTI
> II   Germinoma
> III Embryonal carcinoma = MTU
> IV   Yolk sac tumour (endodermal sinus) = YST
> V   Choriocarcinoma = MTT
> VI   Gonadoblastoma
> VII Polyembryoma
>
> ---
>
> MTD, malignant teratoma differentiated; MTI, malignant teratoma intermediate; MTU, malignant teratoma undifferentiated; MTT, malignant teratoma trophoblastic; TD, teratoma differentiated; YST, yolk sac tumour.

Box 21.2 *International working classification of germ cell tumours in childhood*

> I   Germinoma
>   A   Intratubular germ cell neoplasia
>   B   Invasive (dysgerminoma, germinoma)
> II   Teratoma
>   A   Mature
>   B   Immature
>   Grade 1 immature tissue, <1 low power field (LPF) (4 × objective) per slide
>   Grade 2 immature tissue, 1–4 LPF/slide
>   Grade 3 immature tissue, >3 LPF/slide
>   Microfoci of probable yolk sac tumour (Heifetz lesions) may be present
>   C   Malignant teratoma (teratoma with non-germ cell malignant component)
> III Embryonal carcinoma (adult type)
> IV   Yolk sac tumour (endodermal sinus tumour)
> V   Choriocarcinoma
> VI   Gonadoblastoma
> VII Mixed malignant germ cell tumour (each component to be listed)

incidence of the commonest GCT, sacrococcygeal teratoma, is 1 in 40 000 live births. Epidemiological studies have shown a bimodal age distribution with one peak in children under 3 years of age and a second peak after 12 years of age. The early peak reflects the incidence of sacrococcygeal tumours and yolk sac tumour of the testis, the latter GCTs of the ovary, testis and intracranial sites.[4] It is of interest that the sacrococcygeal teratomas are commonly found in females, whereas those in the gastric, mediastinal and central nervous systems more often affect males.

Black children have low mortality rates from testicular tumours, whereas pineal teratomas are more common in Japan than in western countries.[5,6] GCTs of the gonads, pineal and sacrococcygeal regions may be familial and/or associated with a variety of malformations.[7,8] For example, sacrococcygeal teratoma may occur with sacral agenesis, meningocele or anomalies of the genitourinary tract and hind gut. Gonadoblastoma and malignant GCTs occur in

the gonads of individuals with intersex states, especially gonadal dysgenesis and a Y chromosome or 46XY/45XO mosaicism.[9–11] Boys with undescended testes have an increased risk of testicular cancer[5] and mediastinal tumours occur in Klinefelter's syndrome.

The karyotypes of mature teratomas are diploid, as are some yolk sac tumours of boys aged less than 2 years.[12–14] However, aneuploidy is found in high-grade immature and malignant GCTs, a variety of non-random gains and losses of chromosomes or parts of chromosomes having been described.[12–14] Isochromosome 12p is the most frequent chromosome anomaly in malignant GCTs of adults,[15–17] with over-representation of 12p being found in i(12p)-negative cases.[15,18] In malignant tumours of pre-pubertal children, i(12p) is rare, although gains of 12p are often present, especially in gonadal tumours.[19,20] On the other hand, deletions of 1p are common in paediatric malignant GCTs,[19,21] but not in benign teratomas. Carcinoma-*in-situ* is almost invariably present adjacent to testicular GCTs of adults, but is not usually associated with paediatric tumours.[22,23]

TUMOUR MARKERS

Because the majority of malignant GCTs in childhood involve extraembryonal differentiation, i.e. have at least some component of yolk sac tumour or choriocarcinoma, serum markers are of great value in both diagnosis and management. Alpha-1-globulin alpha-fetoprotein (AFP) is produced in the fetal yolk sac and later in embryonal hepatocytes and the gastrointestinal tract.

Synthesis of AFP peaks around the 13th week of gestation when serum levels of 3–4 mg/mL (approximately 3×10^6 IU/mL) are found.[24] The level decreases to approximately 50 000 ng/mL (42 000 IU/mL) at birth and continues to fall, reaching adult levels of less than 12 ng/mL (10 IU/mL) during the second 6 months of life. There is a wide range of normal levels in infancy and levels are higher in premature babies.[25–27] In adults and children, the half-life of AFP is approximately 5 days, and successful treatment of AFP-producing tumours is reflected by a similar fall in AFP.[28] In infants the half life is longer because the liver continues to produce some AFP during the first months of life.[25–27] These facts must be taken into account when using serial serum AFP levels to monitor the success of treatment of GCTs. Also, AFP levels may be raised in children with hepatomas, hepatitis, tyrosinosis, ataxia-telangiectasia, Indian childhood cirrhosis and other disorders.[29]

The beta subunit of human chorionic gonadotrophin (β-hCG) is produced by placental cells. Any tumour with trophoblastic elements, i.e. choriocarcinoma, will produce β-hCG. Its half-life is about 24 hours and its value in diagnosis and follow-up of gestational and non-gestational GCTs is well established.[30] Over 90 per cent of children with malignant GCTs have elevated serum AFP, whereas β-hCG is raised in fewer than 25 per cent.[31]

Further details of serum markers and their role in patient management are described in Chapter 9. They are important both in diagnosis and in evaluating response to therapy. They may be the most sensitive indicators of residual or recurrent tumour and the need to change treatment. For example, boys with testicular yolk sac tumour and apparent complete resection, but with rising AFP, may have no imageable disease but achieve normal AFP decline and cure after chemotherapy.[28] Conversely, a rapid fall in a tumour marker, even in the absence of change in bulk disease, may reflect a good response in the malignant component of the tumour and only benign differentiated teratoma may remain. In this context, surgery may be more appropriate than a change in chemotherapy.

MORPHOLOGICAL CATEGORIES

Box 21.1 shows the paediatric classification suggested by Albin and Isaacs,[2] with British Testicular Tumour Panel definitions added for clarity as these terms are in common usage in adults.[32] The more recent international working classification for children is shown in Box 21.2. The following discussion will describe pathological subtypes in order of the degree of differentiation as indicated in Figure 21.2. The clinical features and common anatomical sites of the different histological subtypes are listed in Box 21.3.

Germinoma

Germinoma develops in the undifferentiated germ cell and does not show features of differentiation towards embryonal or extraembryonal tissue. In the testis, this tumour is called a seminoma, in the ovary it is called a dysgerminoma, and in extragonadal sites, simply germinoma. This histological subtype is often found combined with others rather than in the pure form. In children the pure form occurs mainly in ovarian tumours in adolescent females and in the pineal gland/third ventricle in teenage males. It may also occasionally be found in the anterior mediastinum or testis. In the adult testis, the pre-invasive stage is called intratubular germ cell neoplasm or carcinoma-*in-situ*. Germinoma is the commonest malignant GCT to occur in the dysgenetic gonad or undescended testis.[1]

Histologically, the tumour contains a monotonous infiltrate of large mononuclear cells which, when occurring as a mediastinal mass, must be distinguished from non-Hodgkin's lymphoma. The microscopic pattern may be of fibrous septae and lymphoid infiltrate, with necrosis and granulomatous reactions. The latter may be very prominent. Rarely, germinomas may contain syn cytiotrophoblasts which produce β-hCG. This accounts for the raised levels of this marker in serum and cerebrospinal fluid (CSF) in some patients with pineal tumours.

Teratoma

It is within this subgroup that most terminological confusion arises. Three main subgroups should be considered (see Box 21.2):

- mature
- immature
- tumour with non-germ cell malignant component.

Box 21.3 *Sites of different histological subtypes*

Germinoma
- Ovary
- Pineal
- Mediastinum
- Testis

Teratoma
- Sacrococcyx
- Ovary
- Head and neck
- Abdomen/pelvis
- Retroperitoneum
- Stomach
- Liver
- Vagina

Embryonal carcinoma
- Usually mixed with yolk sac or choriocarcinoma

Yolk sac tumour
- Ovary
- Sacrococcyx
- Testis
- Pineal
- Mediastinum
- Vagina
- Uterus
- Abdomen
- Retroperitoneum

Choriocarcinoma
- Pineal
- Third ventricle
- Mediastinum
- Ovary
- Testis

The mature teratoma (the monodermal variant is called dermoid cyst) is a benign, highly differentiated tumour, composed of tissue derived from ectoderm, endoderm or mesoderm, often predominantly cystic with mucoid or keratinous content. Histologically, there may be mature neuroglia, bone, hair, cartilage, glandular structures resembling pancreas, cysts with retinal differentiation, hepatocytes, smooth muscle, etc. By definition, the mature teratoma should not contain any evidence of extraembryonal tumour or embryonal carcinoma. Mature teratomas occur most commonly in the sacrococcygeal area and ovary, and may also arise in the abdomen/pelvis, stomach, liver, vagina, and pineal and suprasellar areas.

The immature teratoma has a similar anatomical distribution and should not be regarded as a 'malignant' teratoma, as in childhood its natural history is benign, although local recurrences may present a problem. Mature glial implants on the peritoneum or omentum (gliomatosis peritonei) occur in about 25 per cent of girls with ovarian immature teratomas, with or without glial implants in lymph nodes. While they may demand additional surgery, they do not adversely affect the overall outcome.[33] Immature teratomas contain some fully mature tissue but also immature epithelial (neural or blastemal) or immature stromal tissue. Immature neural tissue consists of primitive neural tubes and immature rosettes, which resemble neuroblastoma, primitive neuroectodermal tumour or peripheral neuroepithelioma.[1,34,35] Microfoci of yolk sac tumour (or, more rarely, embryonal carcinoma, choriocarcinoma or germinoma) may be found,[33,36] probably only in immature teratomas arising in children. The presence of Heifetz (yolk sac tumour microfoci) lesions increases the risk of recurrence,[33] but even so, the majority of such patients will be cured by complete surgical resection.[37] The risk of recurrence is also related to resectability, histological grade and site, with incomplete resection, higher grade and sacrococcygeal site carrying greater risk of recurrence.[36] A recurrence may consist of immature teratoma or may be malignant, the latter nearly always being yolk sac tumour, presumably arising from a Heifetz lesion.

The third very rare group, malignant teratoma, consists of immature teratoma with a non-germ cell malignant component, e.g. sarcoma. Treatment consists of complete surgical resection, if feasible, and further therapy as appropriate to the malignant component.

Confusingly, in earlier classifications the term malignant teratoma described tumours containing mature/immature teratoma and one or more malignant germ cell elements (germinoma, embryonal carcinoma, yolk sac tumour, choriocarcinoma).[1,2] In the current international working classification, these are now called mixed malignant GCTs. In some cases, elevated serum markers may be the only clue to the presence of malignancy and treatment should be directed to the most malignant element.

Embryonal carcinoma

Embryonal carcinoma has been divided into adult and infantile types based on histological differences. The infantile type is essentially a yolk sac tumour and should be classified as such. Cellular anaplasia, mitotic activity, embryoid bodies, necrosis and haemorrhage are indicative of the 'adult' embryonal carcinoma. Pure embryonal carcinoma is one of the commoner types of germ cell neoplasm in the testis of young adults and occasionally is seen in the ovary. It is rarely seen in children. By definition, pure carcinoma will not produce AFP or β-hCG.[38]

Table 21.1 *Relative incidence according to age, site and pathological subtype*[1,43,48]

Site	Relative incidence (%)	Commonest age	Pathology
Sacrococcyx	41	Neonate	Mature 60%, immature 10%, malignant 30%
Ovary	28	Early teens	Mature 65%, immature 5%, malignant 30%
Testis	7	Infant and adolescent	Mature 20%, malignant 80% – yolk sac 90% – germinoma 10% – embryonal carcinoma <1%
Central nervous system	6	Child, adolescent	Germinoma, yolk sac, choriocarcinoma, embryonal carcinoma, mature/immature
Mediastinum	6	Adolescent	Mature/immature, mixed, germinoma, embryonal carcinoma
Head/neck	6	Infant and neonate	Usually mature, immature – rarely malignant
Retroperitoneum	4	Infant, child <2 years	Usually mature, immature – rarely malignant
Vagina/uterus	<1	Infant, child <3 years	Usually yolk sac
Other sites	1		

Mature = teratoma undifferentiated; yolk sac = yolk sac tumour (endodermal sinus).

Yolk sac tumour

This is also known as an endodermal sinus tumour because of its structural similarity to the mouse endodermal sinus. Like the term 'yolk sac carcinoma', this term is unhelpful. It is the commonest type of malignant GCT in children and is found in 10–20 per cent of sacrococcygeal tumours. Other common sites are the ovary and testis. Less commonly, the pineal region, mediastinum, vagina and retroperitoneum may be involved. Four histological patterns have been described – pseudopapillary, reticular, polyvesicular vitelline and solid – the pseudopapillary type being the commonest. Papillary projections associated with characteristic perivascular sheets of cells give rise to the term endodermal sinus and are also known as Schiller–Duval bodies. In most cases, there are intracellular and extracellular hyaline droplets which are periodic acid–Schiff (PAS) and AFP-positive. AFP is clearly demonstrable using immunohistochemical techniques.

Choriocarcinoma

Pure choriocarcinoma is rare in children and more commonly is a feature of mixed histological subtypes. Pure tumour may, however, be found in the pineal region, mediastinum, ovary and testis. In the neonate, multiple visceral metastases from gestational placental neoplasms have been reported. Tumours in the posterior aspect of the third ventricle occur almost exclusively in young males. Anterior lesions may occur in females. Mediastinal choriocarcinoma is more common in young adults.[39]

Microscopically, choriocarcinoma consists of two components: syncytiotrophoblasts and cytotrophoblasts. The former form syncytial knots and contain abundant vacuoles containing β-hCG. Considerable haemorrhage and necrosis may be seen.

Gonadoblastoma

The gonadoblastoma is a rare intratubular neoplasm occurring in dysgenetic gonads, usually in patients under the age of 20 years. The karyotype of the patient is generally 46XY (male pseudohermaphroditism, usually with a female phenotype) or 46XY/45XO (mosaicism). This tumour is often found by chance on examination of a dysgenetic gonad at the time of surgery for other reasons, and generally it behaves in a benign fashion. In about 20 per cent of patients, the tumour may contain malignant components and prophylactic gonadectomy is advocated in patients with XY karyotypes and gonadal dysgenesis.[11] Microscopically, the tumour is composed of ovoid or irregular cell nests separated by connective tissue. Primordial germ cells and stromal cells resembling Sertoli cells are seen. Smaller stromal cells resembling Call–Extner bodies of the granulosa cell tumour are occasionally found.[40,41]

CLINICAL CHARACTERISTICS AND MANAGEMENT

The relative incidence, age and pathological subtypes of tumours at different sites are shown in Table 21.1, and the overall management strategy for extracranial

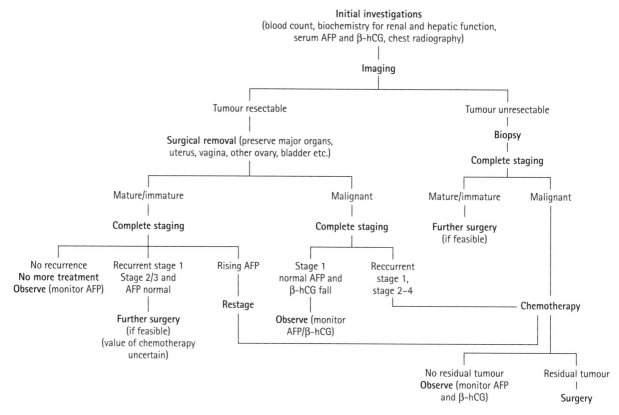

Figure 21.3 *Management strategy for extracranial germ cell tumours.*

tumours in Figure 21.3. When, following initial examination and investigations, a GCT is suspected, appropriate imaging is undertaken and complete excision is performed, if this is possible without major morbidity. Otherwise biopsy is performed. Mutilating surgery, such as hysterectomy, should be avoided and ovarian tissue, the vagina and uterus should be preserved even if adherent to the tumour.

Further treatment depends upon histology, resectability, site and stage. Serum AFP and β-hCG should be measured at diagnosis in all cases. Many different staging systems have been used in the past,[42] but for current and future protocols the TNM system is now recommended (Table 21.2).

For benign (mature and immature) teratomas, after appropriate imaging, surgery alone is suggested, with careful follow-up, and in infants AFP monitoring, to permit early detection of yolk sac tumour recurrence, which takes place in some 12 per cent of cases.[36] For recurrent mature and immature teratomas, the value of chemotherapy is doubtful, so further surgery is preferred when clinically necessary. Some 10–30 per cent of children with mature and immature teratomas have somewhat elevated AFP (presumably due to immature liver or intestine within the tumour or foci of yolk sac tumour). The AFP level is generally less than 1000 IU/mL and returns to normal after successful treatment. More rarely β-hCG may be a little

elevated.[38,43] Rising or markedly elevated markers indicate malignant GCT and, after investigations to confirm this and to restage the disease, treatment is with chemotherapy.

For malignant tumours, computed tomography (CT) or magnetic resonance imaging (MRI) scans of the primary, its lymphatic drainage and the liver, chest X-ray or CT scan of the lungs and bone scan are required, and also bone marrow aspirate when other metastatic disease is present. A 'watch and wait' strategy with AFP/β-hCG monitoring is recommended for stage I completely resected (pT1) tumours: about two-thirds of testicular and a smaller proportion of ovarian tumours can be managed in this way, but very few non-gonadal tumours are completely resectable. Chemotherapy is highly effective for patients with unresectable disease and the watch-and-wait group who relapse. Patients with distant metastases, usually involving lung, bone or bone marrow, are best treated by chemotherapy after biopsy, any further surgery being delayed to deal with tumour residuum. Residual tumour after completion of chemotherapy should be resected if feasible without causing disability. Follow-up is by clinical and AFP/β-hCG monitoring.

Chemoresistant disease should be treated by alternative chemotherapy regimens with or without 'megatherapy' and stem cell rescue. Radiotherapy has little role in children except in palliative therapy and in intracranial GCTs (see 'Intracranial tumours').

Table 21.2 *TNM classification*

		Clinical				Post-surgical		
T: Primary tumour	T0	No primary tumour				pT0	No tumour on histological examination	
	T1	Localized T < 5 cm				pT1	Complete resection of a localized tumour	
	T2	Localized T > 5 cm and < 10 cm				pT2	Complete resection of a T4 tumour	
	T3	Localized T > 10 cm				pT3	Residual tumour	
	T4	T of any size with locoregional extension					pT3a Microscopic	
	T5	Bilateral T					pT3b Macroscopic	
	Tx	Unknown					pT3c Biopsy alone	
						pTx	Unknown	
N: Regional lymph node	N0	No lymph node involvement				pN0	No regional lymph nodes	
	N1	Lymph node involvement at clinical examination or on imaging				pN1	Involvement of regional lymph nodes	
							pN1a Completely removed	
	Nx	Unknown					pN1b Not completely removed	
						pNx	Unknown	
M: Metastasis	M0	No metastasis						
	M1	Metastasis						
	Mx	Unknown						

Stages

CSI	T1	N0Nx	M0	pSI	pT1	pN0 pNx	pM0
CSII	T2T3	N0Nx	M0	pSII	pT1pT2	pN1a	pM0
					pT2	pN0 pNx pN1a	pM0
CSIIIA	T1T2T3	N1	M0	pSIIIa	pT3a	pN0 pN1a pNx	pM0
CSIIIB	T4	N0N1Nx	M0	pSIIIb	pT2	pN1b	pM0
					pT3bpT3c	All pN	pM0
CSIV	T1T2T3T4	N0N1Nx	M1	pSIV	All PT	All pN	pM1

Classification

Stage 1	Tumour <5 cm, no adenopathy, no metastasis	pSI	Tumour without locoregional extension, completely removed, with no metastasis
Stage 2	Tumour ≥5 cm, no adenopathy, no metastasis	pSII	Tumour with locoregional extension, with or without lymph node involvement, completely removed, with no metastasis
Stage 3a or 3b	Tumour of any size, locoregional extension and/or lymph node involvement, no metastasis	pSIII	Tumour with locoregional extension, with no metastasis, incompletely removed
			pSIIIa Microscopic residue
			pSIIIb Macroscopic residue
Stage 4	Metastatic tumour, including distant lymph nodes (lumbar aortic are locoregional for testicular tumour)	pSIV	Tumour with distant metastases

Sacrococcygeal tumours

Of all GCTs, 40 per cent (malignant and benign) are found in the sacrococcygeal region. Half are present at birth, mainly in girls, and may be diagnosed by antenatal ultrasound. A classification based on the anatomical location of sacrococcygeal tumours has been devised by Altman *et al*:[44]

- type I (47 per cent) – predominantly external and least likely to be malignant
- type II (34 per cent) – both external and intrapelvic
- type III (9 per cent) – external, pelvic and abdominal
- type IV (10 per cent) – entirely presacral.

Types I, II and III are easily diagnosed clinically because of the visible mass, but type IV may be missed until it causes symptoms such as constipation or urinary symptoms or extends through the sciatic notch into the buttock. Other diagnoses to be considered are listed in Box 21.4. Neurological problems due to extension into the spinal canal or involvement of the lumbosacral plexus may occur especially when the tumour is malignant. Rectal examination reveals a presacral mass. Plain X-rays, ultrasound and CT scans or MRI (Figure 21.4) will help to define the extent of the tumour. When neurological signs are present, MRI may be better for showing intraspinal extension; such symptoms suggest malignancy, as benign tumours are generally asymptomatic.[45,46]

The majority of congenital tumours are benign mature or immature teratomas and are cured by surgical resection, which may be difficult, sometimes necessitating a

Box 21.4 *Differential diagnosis of sacrococcygeal, testicular and anterior mediastinal and intracranial masses*

Sacrococcygeal
- Meningomyelocele
- Imperforate anus
- Pilonidal cyst
- Abscess
- Lipoma
- Lymphangioma
- Chondroma
- Giant cell tumour
- Neurogenic tumour
- Soft tissue sarcoma

Testicular
- Torsion
- Infarct
- Epididymo-orchitis
- Haematoma
- Hernia
- Hydrocele
- Leukaemia/lymphoma
- Paratesticular rhabdomyosarcoma

Anterior mediastinum
- Thymus
- Bronchogenic cyst
- Goitre
- Enteric cyst
- Lipoma
- Lymphangioma
- Thymoma
- T-cell lymphoma

Pineal/suprasellar
- Astrocytoma
- Ependymoma
- Pinealoma
- Ganglioneuroma

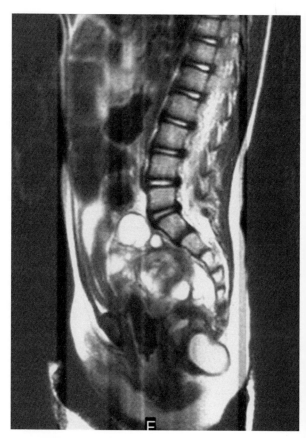

Figure 21.4 *Sacrococcygeal teratoma with large intra-abdominal component on MRI scan.*

combined abdominal and sacrococcygeal approach, and must include removal of the coccyx but avoid damage to the lumbosacral plexus. Microfoci of yolk sac tumour may be present within them and when resection is incomplete, local recurrence is likely and may be malignant, usually a yolk sac tumour.[36]

Delay in removing a congenital teratoma and initial presentation after the neonatal period are associated with a greater risk of malignancy.[44] Complete excision of malignant sacrococcygeal teratomas is usually impossible. Therefore, while surgical excision is required for benign teratomas, malignant teratomas, once confirmed by radiology, markers and biopsy, are generally better managed by chemotherapy and delayed tumour resection.[47] Modern chemotherapy is highly effective, and at delayed surgery after completion of chemotherapy any residual tumour usually consists of necrotic or fibrotic material or mature/immature teratoma.[48]

To facilitate early diagnosis of malignant recurrence of neonatal tumours, and thereby perhaps to reduce the risk of neurological complications, regular serum AFP monitoring for 2–3 years is recommended after resection of all sacrococcygeal teratomas, whether diagnosed as mature or immature. This is because these tumours are often very large and small areas of immature teratoma or Heifetz lesions can be missed.

Other extracranial non-gonadal tumours

Abdominal tumours are found in the retroperitoneum, stomach, liver, abdominal wall, umbilical cord and almost any other organ, and may present with abdominal pain or symptoms due to compression on the bowel or urinary tract. They are mostly present in the neonatal period, in infancy or early childhood. Usually they are mature or immature teratomas or, if malignant, are of yolk sac tumour histology. Hepatic teratoma must be distinguished by biopsy from the more common hepatoblastoma and hepatocellular carcinoma, as all these tumours may produce elevated AFP. For the mature and immature teratomas the treatment is surgical resection, while the malignant cases are highly curable with chemotherapy.

VAGINAL/UTERINE/BLADDER/PROSTATE TUMOURS

These tumours resemble botryoid rhabdomyosarcoma with a polypoid friable mass and are generally of yolk sac histology. After biopsy to confirm the diagnosis, chemotherapy is generally curative, and normal genital structure and function should be preserved. The very rare mature/immature teratomas are treated surgically.

HEAD AND NECK TERATOMAS

Head and neck teratomas occur in the nasopharynx, orbit, cervical region and thyroid and are generally present at birth and of benign mature or immature histology. They present with extensive solid and cystic masses, which may result in respiratory or oral obstruction and lead to major management problems. Surgical excision is the only real option as the tumour is chemoresistant, except in the very rare case of mixed histology (generally immature teratoma and yolk sac tumour).

THORACIC AND MEDIASTINAL TUMOURS

These types of tumour, while investigated and treated following the general strategy shown in Figure 21.3, present particular problems. Firstly, anterior mediastinal tumours (the commonest site) must be distinguished from a number of other conditions (Box 21.4). Secondly, they are usually asymptomatic until they reach a considerable size and produce tracheal or bronchial compression. Coughing, wheezing or chest pain may result and haemoptysis has been described. Unusual presentations include hypoglycaemia and precocious puberty due to ectopic production of insulin or sex hormones.

In adolescents, most teratomas in females are mature, cystic and benign, but in males there is a higher incidence of mixed malignant teratoma, germinoma and embryonal carcinoma. In younger children, mature, immature and malignant (usually mixed or yolk sac) tumours occur very rarely.

Investigation and treatment may be hazardous if there is respiratory compromise or superior vena caval obstruction, but imaging is helpful. For example, on plain X-ray in a mature teratoma a dense rounded opacity with calcification may be seen, and perhaps teeth. CT or MRI provides further detail. Urgent measurement of serum markers may show elevated AFP or β-hCG, which provides sufficient evidence of the diagnosis to commence chemotherapy without the hazards of biopsy. Attempts at radical surgery, if serum markers are elevated or biopsy shows malignant tumour, are unnecessary and dangerous; chemotherapy followed by removal of any residual tumour is preferred. If the patient has respiratory compromise and may require oxygen, bleomycin should not be given; another drug such as vincristine may be used instead as part of combination chemotherapy.

Gonadal tumours

TESTICULAR TUMOURS

Testicular tumours represent only about 10 per cent of paediatric GCTs but about a third of all the malignant GCTs of childhood.[1,48] Thus, about 20 per cent are mature (rarely immature) benign teratomas and about 80 per cent are malignant, mostly yolk sac tumours in boys aged less than 4 years. About 5 per cent of cases (often presenting during adolescence) have seminoma (germinoma) or embryonal carcinoma. Testicular tumours are very rarely seen between the ages of 5 and 10 years. In childhood, testicular tumours are almost always unilateral.

The differential diagnosis is shown in Box 21.4. Benign teratomas are usually multicystic and partially solid and may contain bone or cartilage. Yolk sac tumour is solid but has often been mistaken for hydrocele. Malignant tumours spread to the retroperitoneal, thoracic and cervical nodes and to the lungs, bone and bone marrow. Scrotal ultrasound and serum AFP and β-hCG are helpful in diagnosis, but retroperitoneal node sampling or lymphadenectomy generally have no place in paediatric practice. This is because CT or MRI should detect significant nodal involvement, and, as nearly all paediatric malignant GCTs produce AFP, marker monitoring after orchidectomy provides a sensitive method for detection of recurrent or residual disease,[28] for which chemotherapy is almost always curative. Retroperitoneal node biopsy is only necessary if there are enlarged nodes on imaging and serum markers are normal.

Resection of testicular tumour should be by inguinal orchidectomy, with high ligation of the spermatic cord. To avoid skin contamination with tumour, trans-scrotal biopsy is contraindicated. Orchidectomy alone cures patients with benign teratoma and about two-thirds of boys with malignant tumours. Thus, after non-invasive staging, all boys with stage I malignant disease are managed by a 'watch and wait' strategy, i.e. clinical and AFP monitoring, and the 15–20 per cent who develop clinical or marker evidence of residual disease or relapse are given chemotherapy.

OVARIAN TUMOURS

Ovarian tumours account for about one-third of paediatric GCTs. The peak incidence is in early adolescence and 70 per cent are benign, mature cystic teratomas. A cystic mass replaces all or part of the ovary and the tumour may be bilateral in about 10 per cent. It is often asymptomatic until it reaches a large size or may present with torsion, infarction or rupture. Occasionally, chronic abdominal pain or an acute abdomen resembling appendicitis may occur.

Detailed histological examination of any solid elements is essential to detect a malignant component. It should be noted that peritoneal 'spread' with mature glial tissue (gliomatosis peritonei) does not influence prognosis (although additional surgery may be needed) and neither systemic chemotherapy nor radiotherapy is required. The pattern of spread of immature teratomas or tumours with malignant components is usually that of ascites, peritoneal implants and distant metastasis to lymph nodes, liver and lung. Tumours with trophoblastic elements produce β-hCG, which may lead to premature breast enlargement, pubic hair or menarche. Serum AFP is elevated when there is a yolk sac component.

Plain abdominal X-rays often show calcification particularly in benign tumours. There may be urinary tract obstruction due to pressure or infiltration of the ureters, so ultrasound scan is useful, Further staging procedures should be done, as outlined in 'Sacrococcygeal tumours', but also, if ascites is present at laparotomy, this should be sent for cytological examination. If the other ovary appears abnormal, this should be biopsied as should any peritoneal or omental nodule or enlarged para-aortic node. Constitutional chromosome analysis should be done, too, to exclude XY gonadal dysgenesis and other intersex conditions. If the patient is already known to have XY gonadal dysgenesis, bilateral oophorectomy (gonadectomy) should be performed.

The overall treatment strategy is as in Figure 21.3. Patients with mature and immature teratomas are generally cured by surgical excision, although further surgery may be needed for intraperitoneal recurrences of immature teratoma. Chemotherapy is needed for the majority of girls with malignant GCTs apart from those with completely resected (pT1) tumours who can be managed by a watch-and-wait regimen as for testicular pT1 cases. Girls with clinically very advanced ovarian tumours are likely to benefit from biopsy, chemotherapy and delayed surgery (or even be treated on the basis of radiology and markers if they are unfit for biopsy). Bilateral malignant tumours should be treated avoiding bilateral oophorectomy if possible, chemotherapy often allowing preservation of ovarian tissue and preservation of fertility. There is no place, now that chemotherapy is so effective, for extensive surgery and hysterectomy.

Intracranial tumours

About 1 per cent of all primary intracranial neoplasms are GCTs, occurring mostly in the pineal or suprasellar areas, or sometimes in both. The majority are pure germinomas

(albeit some produce small amounts of β-hCG, serum or CSF levels being <50 IU/L). The remainder are mostly mixed malignant GCTs, which may include mature/immature teratoma as well as malignant elements – embryonal carcinoma, yolk sac tumour, choriocarcinoma – and most produce AFP and/or β-hCG and so are often referred to as 'secreting' tumours. They are seen predominantly in children and adolescents, and characteristic symptoms include third ventricular obstruction with hydrocephalus, visual symptoms, diabetes insipidus, hypopituitarism, precocious puberty and Parinaud's syndrome. Other diagnoses to be considered are shown in Box 21.4.

CT or MRI scan shows a mass which enhances after contrast and may be cystic or calcified. 'Secreting' tumours are confirmed by imaging and elevated serum and/or CSF markers – CSF should also be obtained for cytology, as GCTs metastasize via the CSF, but caution must be exercised over performing lumbar puncture, so that when there is raised intracranial pressure CSF may be obtained during a shunt procedure. Urgent management of hydrocephalus may be required. Biopsy of the tumour is unnecessary and is contraindicated in 'secreting' tumours because of the surgical hazards. However, biopsy, preferably open because of the risks of haemorrhage, is necessary to confirm the diagnosis of pure germinoma, but complete resection need not be attempted as the tumour is highly radio- and chemosensitive. Patients also require full evaluation of their endocrine status, visual fields and acuity.

Conventional treatment for pure germinoma has been craniospinal irradiation, with almost 100 per cent cure rates,[49] but to spare the patient's cerebral cortex and spine, platinum-based chemotherapy with focal irradiation has been used successfully for localized tumours.[50] The two approaches, conventional craniospinal radiotherapy and chemotherapy with focal irradiation, are being compared for localized disease in the SIOP CNS Germ Cell Tumour 1996 Study; for metastatic tumours additional radiotherapy and chemotherapy may be given. The prognosis for 'secreting' tumours before the introduction of chemotherapy was very poor.[51] Platinum-based chemotherapy, followed (if needed) by surgery to the residuum and either craniospinal or focal radiotherapy, has yielded cure rates of some 60–80 per cent.[52] In the SIOP CNS 96 protocol all patients are given chemotherapy, with local irradiation for non-metastatic disease or craniospinal irradiation for metastatic disease.

CHEMOTHERAPY

Extracranial tumours

The treatment of mature and immature teratomas is by surgical excision, there being no proven benefit from chemotherapy, except for tumours that also contain malignant germ cell elements (mixed malignant GCTs).

Before effective chemotherapy was available, while about two-thirds of boys with malignant testicular GCTs were cured by surgery alone, cures of metastatic disease were rare,[53] the results of treating malignant ovarian tumours were poor[53] and malignant sacrococcygeal teratomas were nearly always fatal.[54] Combination chemotherapy based on vincristine, actinomycin and cyclophosphamide (VAC), sometimes with doxorubicin, methotrexate or radiotherapy, was introduced during the 1970s and improved the results, but was more effective in limited than in advanced disease.[55–59] Following the successful use of cisplatin, vinblastine and bleomycin (PVB) for disseminated testicular cancer in adults,[60] cisplatin-containing regimens were introduced in children.[61] Survival rates from 75 per cent to over 90 per cent with cisplatin-based regimens have since been reported from the United States,[62–65] France[66] and Germany.[47,67,68] Children with gonadal tumours generally fare better than those with non-gonadal primary tumours.

However, there has been concern about both acute and long-term toxicities of these treatments. Bleomycin-induced lung damage caused fatalities in children treated with either PVB or BEP (bleomycin, etoposide and cis-platin) in the first germ cell study of the UK Children's Cancer Study Group (UKCCSG), until bleomycin was reduced from three doses per cycle to one. Moreover, although the 5-year survival rate was 85 per cent following BEP, some degree of renal impairment was present in about 40 per cent of survivors, and deafness in about 10 per cent, while one child died of leukaemia during the chemotherapy.[31] Cisplatin was considered to be responsible for the renal toxicity and ototoxicity, and therefore in a pilot study carboplatin was substituted with promising results.[69] Thus carboplatin, etoposide and bleomycin (JEB) was the combination used in the UKCCSG's second study, with good results and acceptable toxicity.[48] JEB consists of etoposide $120 \, mg/m^2$ intravenously daily on days 1–3, carboplatin on day 2 (dose calculated using a formula to give an AUC of $7.9 \, mg \cdot min/mL$, or, if glomerular filtration rate cannot be measured, $600 \, mg/m^2$) and bleomycin $15 \, mg/m^2$ on day 3. Courses were given every 3–4 weeks until remission was achieved, followed, if possible, by two further courses. Overall 5-year survival for 184 patients was 93 per cent, of whom 47 were cured by surgery alone. For the 137 patients requiring JEB, 5-year survival was 91 per cent and event-free survival (EFS) 88 per cent. Non-fatal haematological toxicity was common, but deafness and pulmonary and renal toxicities were rare. JEB remains the chemotherapy regimen in UKCCSG's third study, but to reduce toxicity further, except in high-risk cases, a maximum of four cycles are being given. For patients with recurrence after JEB, VIP (vinblastine $3 \, mg/m^2$ on days 1 and 2, ifosfamide $1.5 \, g/m^2$ daily on days 1–5, and cisplatin $20 \, mg/m^2$ daily on days 1–5) is now recommended. There are also a number of high-dose regimens that can be used with stem cell rescue in refractory disease.

Intracranial tumours

For germinoma, the French used alternating courses of carboplatin with etoposide and etoposide with ifosfamide, four courses in total, with 40 Gy local irradiation,[50] and this protocol was adopted for one arm of SIOP CNS GCT 96. Patients in the other arm received craniospinal irradiation without chemotherapy.

For 'secreting' tumours the Germans use PEI (cisplatin, etoposide and ifosfamide) and craniospinal irradiation (30 Gy, with 24 Gy tumour boost).[70] In SIOP CNS GCT 96, four cycles of PEI are followed by surgery if there is a significant residuum and then local irradiation (54 Gy) for non-metastatic disease, or by craniospinal irradiation as above for metastatic disease.

Follow-up must include endocrine surveillance, as all patients receive pituitary irradiation and some have diabetes insipidus.

CURRENT CONTROVERSIES

ARE THERE DIFFERENCES BETWEEN GCTs IN CHILDREN AND ADULTS THAT MAY AFFECT APPROACHES TO TREATMENT?

While the same ranges of histological subtypes are seen in children and adults, yolk sac tumour is the predominant malignant subtype in children, followed by mixed malignant GCTs, whereas in adults germinoma, embryonal carcinoma and mixed tumours are more common. In children, non-gonadal tumours are more frequent than gonadal tumours but testicular tumours predominate in adults, in whom ovarian and non-gonadal GCTs are rare. There are also biological differences; for example, isochromosome 12p, which characterizes most testicular tumours in adults, is hardly ever seen in prepubertal children.

Paediatric and adult malignant GCTs respond to the same range of drugs, but the randomized trials comparing different treatments have been performed almost entirely in adults with testicular tumours. The small numbers of patients, the high cure rates and the diversity of their tumours make it difficult to conduct randomized trials in children; therefore treatment modifications to improve cure rates and reduce toxicities have mostly been compared with historical series. Thus, international collaboration is needed for future trials, together with comprehensive data collection to include primary site, stage, histology (unless pre-chemotherapy biopsy is hazardous), serum markers and tumour biology as well as acute and long-term toxicities.

CAN CURE RATES BE IMPROVED FURTHER?

Most groups now achieve overall cure rates of greater than 90 per cent, but additional children might be cured with more intensive initial chemotherapy for the high-risk patients and/or better 'salvage' therapy after relapse. Primary site, stage, histology and chemotherapy efficacy have long been recognized to be relevant, leading to treatment stratification by several groups according to perceived risk. Recently, both the French and British have undertaken multivariate analyses and confirmed the importance of these factors and also that AFP levels above 10 000 kU/L confer a poorer prognosis.[48,71] However, the highest risk group that could be defined in the British series (in which JEB was used) had a 5-year EFS of 73 per cent and overall survival of 85 per cent. In adults with testicular tumours, cisplatin-based combinations have been shown to be more effective than those containing carboplatin (albeit in lower doses than in the UKCCSG JEB protocol).[72,73] The results of the French TGM 90 study, which incorporated carboplatin (also in a lower dose than JEB), were inferior to its predecessor, which contained cisplatin.[31] Nevertheless, in view of the renal toxicity and ototoxicity of cisplatin in children, the UKCCSG has decided to continue using JEB, but to try to rescue more of those who relapse, using an intensive VIP protocol and, if necessary, megatherapy with stem cell rescue.

The American Intergroup trial randomized over 300 high-risk patients between standard or high-dose cisplatin with etoposide and bleomycin and achieved superior EFS in the high-dose group, but at the expense of significant renal toxicity and ototoxicity.[65]

CAN LONG-TERM COMPLICATIONS OF TREATMENT BE AVOIDED?

In the UK, renal toxicity and ototoxicity have been greatly reduced following the substitution of carboplatin for cisplatin, but whether JEB has the same efficacy as BEP has never been demonstrated in a controlled trial in children. Bleomycin lung has also been minimized by reducing the doses from three per course to one,[48] and a study of pulmonary function in survivors is planned. The German and Italian groups are substituting other agents for bleomycin, but both have introduced ifosfamide, a nephrotoxic drug.[68,74] A Brazilian group has achieved encouraging results with just cisplatin and etoposide.[75]

Secondary leukaemia may occur after chemotherapy but, as in adults, may in some cases have arisen from the same stem cell as did the germ cell tumour.[76] Among 1132 children treated in the German Malignant GCT trials, six developed acute myeloid leukaemia. There were no cases in children treated with only surgery or radiotherapy, but the cumulative risk at 10 years was 1 per cent for those who had chemotherapy and radiotherapy. Cytogenetic

abnormalities of the leukaemias suggested that four were therapy-related, associated with etoposide or alkylators.[77]

All groups are attempting to reduce the number of cycles of chemotherapy given, particularly in lower-risk groups, and ideally these modifications should be made within controlled trials.

For children with malignant intracranial tumours, attempts have been made to avoid irradiation, especially in younger children, to reduce damage to the cortex, spinal growth and pituitary function. Unfortunately, there was a high rate of incomplete response or relapse.[78] The SIOP CNS GCT 1996 is exploring chemotherapy with local instead of craniospinal radiotherapy.

KEY POINTS

- The majority of malignant GCTs produce AFP and/or β-hCG, which should be measured before treatment in all patients and also used to monitor response to treatment.
- While there are many similarities between GCTs in children and adults, the distribution of primary sites, histological subtypes and biological features differs according to age. Treatment protocols must take account of these differences and of other risk factors, such as AFP level.
- The prognosis for infants and children with mature and immature teratoma is excellent following surgical excision, which can be difficult but should avoid damage to neighbouring structures. Malignant yolk sac tumour recurrence occurs in around 10 per cent of cases of sacrococcygeal teratoma, so postoperative clinical and AFP monitoring to facilitate its early detection is recommended.
- Overall cure rates for children with extracranial malignant GCTs are now over 90 per cent, so current studies are exploring how to minimize surgical- and chemotherapy-induced late effects in survivors. Thus, a 'watch and wait' approach, with AFP monitoring, is now generally used after complete excision of (pT1) gonadal tumours, chemotherapy being reserved for recurrence. Also, in the UK, to reduce ototoxicity and renal toxicity, carboplatin is used instead of cisplatin, whereas modifications to cisplatin-based treatments are being made by other groups.
- Better 'salvage' therapy is being sought for children with refractory disease or relapse after standard platinum-based chemotherapy. Also, by multivariate analyses, attempts are being made to identify patients at very high risk of treatment

failure who might benefit from more intensive initial chemotherapy.
- Cure rates for intracranial pure germinomas are nearly 100 per cent and studies are in progress under the auspices of SIOP to determine whether patients treated with chemotherapy and localized irradiation will have fewer growth/endocrine and neurocognitive late effects than those given conventional craniospinal irradiation.
- The prognosis for 'secreting' intracranial GCTs has improved following cisplatin-based chemotherapy and radiotherapy but optimal therapy has still to be determined by clinical trials.

REFERENCES

♦1. Dehner LP. Gonadal and extragonadal germ cell neoplasms – teratomas in childhood. In: Finegold M, Benington JL, eds. *Pathology of Neoplasia in Children and Adolescents. Major Problems in Pathology*, vol. 18. Philadelphia: WB Saunders, 1986; 282–312.

♦2. Ablin A, Isaacs H. Germ cell tumors. In: Pizzo PA, Poplack DG, eds. *Principles and Practice of Pediatric Oncology*. Philadelphia: JB Lippincott, 1989; 713–32.

3. Mann JR, Stiller CA. Changing patterns of incidence and survival in children with germ cell tumours (GCTs). In: Jones WG, Harnden P, Appleyard I, eds. *Germ Cell Tumours III. Advances in the Biosciences*. Oxford: Pergamon Press, 1994; 59–64.

4. Parkin DM, Kramárova E, Draper GJ et al. *International Incidence of Childhood Cancer*. WHO IARC Scientific Publications No.144. Lyon: IARC, 1998; 428.

5. Li FP, Fraumeni JF. Testicular cancers in children: epidemiologic characteristics. *J Natl Cancer Inst* 1972; **48**: 1575–82.

6. Wakai S, Segawa H, Kitahara S et al. Teratoma in the pineal region in two brothers. *J Neurosurg* 1980; **53**: 239–43.

7. Fraumeni JF, Li FP, Dalager N. Teratomas in children: epidemiologic features. *J Natl Cancer Inst* 1973; **51**: 1425–30.

8. Johnston HE, Mann JR, Williams J et al. The Inter-Regional epidemiological study of childhood cancer (IRESCC): a case-control study in children with germ cell tumours. *Carcinogenesis* 1986; **7**: 717–22.

9. Taylor H, Barter RH, Jacobson CB. Neoplasms of dysgenetic gonads. *Am J Obstet Gynecol* 1966; **96**: 816–23.

10. Mann JR, Corkery JJ, Fisher HJW et al. The X-linked recessive form of XY gonadal dysgenesis with a high incidence of gonadal germ cell tumours: clinical and genetic studies. *J Med Genet* 1983; **20**: 264–70.

11. Krasna IH, Lee ML, Smilow P et al. Risk of malignancy in bilateral streak gonads: the role of the Y chromosome. *J Pediatr Surg* 1992; **27**: 1376–80.

12. Linder D, Kaiser-McCaw B, Hecht F. Pathogenetic origin of benign ovarian teratomas. *N Engl J Med* 1975; **292**: 63–6.

13. Quirke P, Dyson JED, Sutton J et al. Assessment of germ cell tumours of testis by flow cytometry and histopathology. In: Jones WG, Milford Ward A, Anderson CK, eds. *Germ Cell Tumours II. Advances in the Biosciences*, vol. 55. Oxford: Pergamon Press, 1985; 45–54.

14. Silver SA, Wiley JM, Perlman EJ. DNA-ploidy analysis of pediatric germ cell tumors. *Mod Pathol* 1994; **7**: 951–6.

15. Rodriguez E, Mathew S, Reuter VE et al. Cytogenetic analysis of prospectively ascertained male germ cell tumours. *Cancer Res* 1992; **52**: 2285–91.

16. Summersgill B, Goker H, Weber-Hall S et al. Molecular cytogenetic analysis of adult testicular germ cell tumours and identification of regions of consensus copy number change. *Br J Cancer* 1998; **77**: 305–13.

17. van Kessel AG, Suijkerbuijk RF, Sinke RJ et al. Molecular cytogenetics of human germ-cell tumors – i(12p) and related chromosomal anomalies. *Eur Urol* 1993; **23**: 23–9.

18. Suijkerbuijk RF, Sinke RJ, Meloni AM et al. Overrepresentation of chromosome 12p sequences and karyotype evolution in i(12p)-negative testicular germ cell tumours revealed by fluorescent *in situ* hybridisation. *Cancer Genet Cytogenet* 1993; **70**: 85–93.

19. Jenderny J, Koster E, Meyer A et al. Detection of chromosome-aberrations in paraffin sections of 7 gonadal yolk-sac tumors of childhood. *Hum Genet* 1995; **96**: 644–50.

20. Perlman EJ, Cushing B, Hawkins E, Griffin CA. Cytogenetic analysis of childhood endodermal sinus tumors: a Pediatric Oncology Group Study. *Pediatr Pathol* 1994; **14**: 695–708.

21. Stock C, Ambros IM, Lion T et al. Detection of numerical and structural chromosome abnormalities in pediatric germ cell tumors by means of interphase cytogenetics. *Genes Chromosomes Cancer* 1994; **11**: 40–50.

22. Looijenga L, Gillis A, van Putten W, Oosterhuis J. *In situ* numeric analysis of centromeric regions of chromosomes 1, 12 and 15 of seminomas, non-seminomatous germ cell tumours and carcinoma *in situ* of human testis. *Lab Invest* 1993; **68**: 211–19.

23. Soosay GN, Bobrow L, Happerfield L, Parkinson MCP. Morphology and immunohistochemistry of carcinoma *in situ* adjacent to testicular germ cell tumours in adults and children: implications for histogenesis. *Histopathology* 1991; **19**: 537–44.

24. Elwood JM, Elwood JH. *Epidemiology of Anencephalus and Spina Bifida*. Oxford: Oxford University Press, 1980; 255–67.

25. Tsuchida Y, Endo Y, Saito S et al. Evaluation of alpha-fetoprotein in early infancy. *J Pediatr Surg* 1978; **13**: 155–6.

26. Wu JT, Book L, Sudar K. Serum alphafetoprotein (AFP) levels in normal infants. *Pediatr Res* 1981; **15**: 50–2.

27. Blohm MEG, Verterling-Hörner D, Calaminus G, Göbel U. Alpha-1-fetoprotein (AFP) reference values in infants up to two years of age. *Klin Pädiatr* 1991; **203**: 246–50.

•28. Huddart SN, Mann JR, Gornall P et al. The UK Children's Cancer Study Group: testicular malignant germ cell tumours 1979–1988. *J Pediatr Surg* 1990; **25**: 406–10.

29. Mann JR, Lakin GE, Leonard JC et al. Clinical applications of serum carcinoembryonic antigen and alpha-fetoprotein levels in children with solid tumours. *Arch Dis Child* 1978; **53**: 366–74.

♦30. Rustin JS. Tumour markers in germ cell tumours. *Radiography* 1987; **53**: 229–32.

●31. Mann JR, Pearson D, Barrett A et al. Results of the United Kingdom Children's Cancer Study Group's malignant germ cell tumor studies. *Cancer* 1989; **63**: 1657–67.

32. Einhorn LH, Crawford ED, Shipley WU et al. Cancer of the testis. In: Devita VT, Hellman S, Rosenberg SA, eds *Cancer – Principles & Practice of Oncology*. Philadelphia: JB Lippincott, 1989; 1071–98.

♦33. Heifetz SA, Cushing B, Giller R et al. Immature teratomas in children: pathologic considerations. A report from the Combined Pediatric Oncology Group Children's Cancer Group. *Am J Surg Pathol* 1998; **22**: 1115–24.

34. Gonzalez-Crussi F. Extragonadal teratomas. *Atlas of Tumour Pathology*, second series, fascicle 18. Washington DC: Armed Forces Institute of Pathology, 1982; 48.

35. Thurlbeck WM, Scully RE. Solid teratoma of the ovary: a clinicopathological analysis of 9 cases. *Cancer* 1960; **13**: 804–11.

●36. Gobel U, Calaminus G, Blohm M et al. Extracranial non-testicular teratoma in childhood and adolescence: Introduction of a risk score for stratification of therapy. *Klin Pädiatr* 1997; **209**: 228–34.

●37. Marina NM, Cushing B, Giller R et al. Complete surgical excision is effective treatment for children with immature teratomas with or without malignant elements: a Pediatric Oncology Group/Children's Cancer Group Intergroup Study. *J Clin Oncol* 1999; **17**: 2137–43.

38. Kurman RJ, Norris HJ. Embryonal carcinoma of the ovary. A clinicopathologic entity distinct from endodermal sinus tumor resembling embryonal carcinoma of the adult testis. *Cancer* 1976; **38**: 2420–33.

39. Witzleben CL, Bruninga G. Infantile choriocarcinoma: a characteristic syndrome. *J Pediatr* 1968; **73**: 374–8.

40. Takeda A, Ishuzyka T, Goto T et al. Polyembryoma of ovary alpha-fetoprotein and HCG: Immunoperoxidase and electron microscopy study. *Cancer* 1982; **49**: 1878.

♦41. Scully RE. Gonadoblastoma. A review of 74 cases. *Cancer* 170; **25**: 1340–56.

♦●42. Mann JR. Germ cell tumours of childhood. In: Souhami RL, Tannock I, Hohenberger P, Horiot J-C, eds. *Oxford Textbook of Oncology*, 2nd edn. Oxford: Oxford University Press, 2002; 2638–55.

●43. Mann JR, Raafat F, Robinson K et al. Mature and immature extracranial teratomas in children: the UK Children's Cancer Study Group's experience. In: Jones WG, Appleyard I, Harnden P, Joffe JK, eds. *Germ Cell Tumours IV*. London: John Libbey, 1998; 237–46.

♦44. Altman RP, Randolph JG, Lilly JR et al. Sacrococcygeal teratoma. *J Pediatr Surg* 1974; **9**: 389–98.

45. Valdeserri RO, Yunis EJ. Sacrococcygeal teratomas: a review of 68 cases. *Cancer* 1981; **48**: 217–21.

46. Whalen T, Mahour G, Landing B, Wooleyt MM. Sacrococcygeal teratomas in infants and children. *Am J Surg* 1985; **150**: 373.

●47. Calaminus G, Schneider DT, Bokkerink JP et al. Prognostic value of tumor size, metastases, extension into bone, and increased tumor marker in children with malignant sacrococcygeal germ cell tumors: a prospective evaluation of 71 patients treated in the German cooperative protocols Maligne Keimzelltumoren (MAKEI) 83/86 and MAKEI 89. *J Clin Oncol* 2003; **21**: 781–6.

●48. Mann JR, Raafat F, Robinson K et al. The United Kingdom Children's Cancer Study Group's Second Germ Cell Tumor Study: carboplatin, etoposide and bleomycin are effective treatment for children with malignant extracranial germ cell tumors, with acceptable toxicity. *J Clin Oncol* 2000; **18**: 3809–18.

●49. Göbel U, Bamburg M, Budach V et al. Intracraniale Keimzelltumoren: analyse der Therapiestudie MAKEI 83/86 und Protokoländerungen für die Nachfolgestudie. *Klin Pädiatr* 1989; **201**: 261–8.

●50. Bouffet E, Baranzelli MC, Patte C et al. on behalf of the Société Française d'Oncology Pédiatrique. Combined treatment modality for intracranial germinomas: results of a multicentre SFOP experience. *Br J Cancer* 1999; **79**: 1199–204.

51. Allen JC. Controversies in the management of intracranial germ cell tumours. *Neurol Clin* 1991; **9**: 441–52.

♦●52. Calaminus G, Bamburg M, Baranzelli MC et al. Intracranial germ cell tumors: a comprehensive update of the European data. *Neuropediatrics* 1994; **25**: 26–32.

53. Brown NJ, Langley FA. Teratomas and other genital tumours. In: Marsden HB, Steward JK, eds. *Tumours in Children*. Berlin: Springer-Verlag, 1976; 383.

54. Bale PM, Painter DM, Cohen D. Teratomas in childhood. *Pathology* 1975; **7**: 209–18.

55. Young PG, Mount BF, Foote FW, Whitmore WF. Embryonal adenocarcinoma in the pubertal testis. *Cancer* 1970; **26**: 1065–75.

56. Ise T, Ohtsuki H, Matsumoto K, Sano R. Management of malignant testicular tumors in children. *Cancer* 1976; **37**: 1539–45.

57. Wollner N, Exelby PR, Woodruff JM et al. Malignant ovarian tumors in childhood: prognosis in relation to initial therapy. *Cancer* 1976; **37**: 1953–64.

58. Cangir A, Smith J, van Eys J. Improved prognosis in children with ovarian cancers following modified VAC (vincristine sulfate, dactinomycin and cyclophosphamide) chemotherapy. *Cancer* 1978; **42**: 1234–8.

59. Slayton RE, Hreshchyshyn MM, Silverberg SG et al. Treatment of malignant ovarian germ cell tumors. Response to vincristine, dactinomycin and cyclophosphamide (preliminary report). *Cancer* 1978; **42**: 390–8.

●60. Einhorn L, Donohue J. Cisdiamminedichloroplatinum, vinblastine and bleomycin combination chemotherapy in disseminated testicular cancer. *Ann Intern Med* 1977; **87**: 293–8.

61. Pinkerton CR, Pritchard J, Spitz L. High complete response rate in children with advanced germ cell tumors using cisplatin-containing combination chemotherapy. *J Clin Oncol* 1986; **4**: 194–9.

●62. Marina N, Fontanesi J, Kun L et al. Treatment of childhood germ cell tumors. *Cancer* 1992; **70**: 2568–75.

●63. Giller R, Cushing B, Lauer S et al. Comparison of high dose or standard dose cisplatin with etoposide and bleomycin (HDPEB vs PEB) in children with stage III and IV malignant germ cell tumors (MGCT) at gonadal primary sites: A Pediatric Intergroup trial (POG 9094/CCG8882). *Proc Am Soc Clin Oncol* 1998; **17**: 525a.

●64. Cushing B, Giller R, Lauer S et al. Comparison of high dose or standard dose cisplatin with etoposide and bleomycin

(HDPEB vs PEB in children with stage I–IV extragonadal malignant germ cell tumors (MGCT): A Pediatric Intergoup report (POG 9049/CCG8882). *Proc Am Soc Clin Oncol* 1998; **17**: 525a.

●65. Rescorla F, Billmire D, Stolar C *et al.* The effect of cisplatin dose and surgical resection in children with malignant germ cell tumors at the sacrococcygeal region: a Pediatric Intergroup Trial POG 9049/CCG8882). *J Pediatr Surg* 2001; **36**: 12–17.

●66. Baranzelli MC, Patte C. The French experience in paediatric malignant germ cell tumours. In: Jones WG, Appleyard I, Harnden P, Joffe JK, *eds. Germ Cell Tumours IV.* London: John Libbey, 1998; 219–26.

●67. Haas RJ, Schmidt P, Göbel U, Harms D. Testicular germ cell tumors, an update. *Klin Pädiatr* 1999; **211**: 300–4.

●68. Gobel U, Calaminus G, Engert J *et al.* On behalf of the GPOH MAKEI study group: malignant paediatric extracranial non-testicular germ cell tumours (GCTs), the German experience. In: Jones WG, Appleyard I, Harnden P, Joffe JK, eds. *Germ Cell Tumours IV.* London: John Libbey, 1998; 205–11.

69. Pinkerton CR, Broadbent V, Horwich A *et al.* JEB – a carboplatin based regimen for malignant germ cell tumours in children. *Br J Cancer* 1990; **62**: 257–62.

●70. Calaminus G, Andreussi L, Garré M-L *et al.* Secreting germ tumors of the central nervous system (CNS). First results of the cooperative German/Italian pilot study (CNSs GCT). *Klin Pädiatr* 1997; **209**: 222–7.

●71. Baranzelli MC, Kramar A, Bouffet E *et al.* Prognostic factors in children with localized malignant nonseminomatous germ cell tumors. *J Clin Oncol* 1999; **17**: 1212–18.

●72. Horwich A, Sleijfer DT, Fossa SD *et al.* Randomised trial of bleomycin, etoposide, and cisplatin compared with bleomycin, etoposide, and carboplatin in good-prognosis metastatic non-seminomatous germ cell cancer. A multi-institutional Medical Research Council/European Organization for Research and Treatment of Cancer Trial. *J Clin Oncol* 1997; **15**: 1844–52.

●73. Bokemeyer C, Kohrmann O, Tischler J *et al.* A randomised trial of cisplatin etoposide and bleomycin (PEB) versus carboplatin, etoposide and bleomycin (CEB) for patients with 'good risk' metastatic non-seminomatous germ cell tumors. *Ann Oncol* 1996; **7**: 1015–21.

●74. Lo Curto M, D'Angelo P, Arrighni A *et al.* Malignant germ cell tumours in childhood. The Italian experience. In: Jones WG, Appleyard I, Harnden P, Joffe JK, eds. *Germ Cell Tumours IV.* London: John Libbey, 1998; 227–31.

●75. Lopes LF, de Camargo B, Aguiar SS *et al.*, Cisplatin and etoposide regimen for germ cell tumor: preliminary results of the Brazilian germ cell study group – abstract of the joint meeting of the International Society of Paediatric Oncology and the American Society of Pediatric Hematology/Oncology. Montreal, Canada, September 1999. *Med Pediatr Oncol* 1999; **33**: 216.

76. Bosl GJ, Ilson DH, Rodriguez E *et al.* Isochromosome of chromosome 12: clinically useful marker for male germ cell tumors. *J Natl Cancer Inst* 1989; **81**: 1874–8.

◆77. Schneider DT, Behnisch W, Calaminus G *et al.* Acute myelogenous leukemia after treatment for malignant germ cell tumors in children. *J Clin Oncol* 1999; **17**: 3226–33.

●78. Balmaceda C, Heller G, Rosenblum M *et al.* for the First International Central Nervous System Gem Cell Tumor Study. Chemotherapy without irradiation – a novel approach for newly diagnosed CNS germ cell tumors: results of an international cooperative trial. *J Clin Oncol* 1996; **14**: 2908–15.

22

Liver tumours*

ELIZABETH A. SHAFFORD & JON PRITCHARD

Primary hepatic tumours in children are a heterogeneous group of neoplasms. Malignant tumours account for only 1.2–5 per cent of the totality of paediatric cancers, but occur more frequently than their benign counterparts (Box 22.1).[1,2] There are two main categories of malignant tumour, those of epithelial origin (hepatoblastoma and hepatocellular carcinoma) and the rarer mesenchymal tumours (sarcomas). Their relative frequency is approximately 9:1.[2]

Box 22.1 *Classification of liver tumours*

Malignant

Epithelial
- Hepatoblastoma
- Hepatocellular carcinoma

Mesenchymal
- Mixed mesenchymal
- Rhabdomyosarcoma
- Angiosarcoma
- Undifferentiated sarcoma

Benign

Epithelial
- Adenoma
- Focal nodular hyperplasia

Mesenchymal
- Haemangioma
- Haemangioendothelioma
- Hamartoma

HEPATOBLASTOMA AND HEPATOCELLULAR CARCINOMA

Aetiology

Hepatoblastoma is classified as an 'embryonal' tumour of the liver. There is now a considerable body of evidence to support the notion that embryonal tumours are the consequence of critical genetic changes in a single 'embryonic' cell, resulting in a derangement of normal mechanisms of cell proliferation and differentiation during organogenesis. The molecular pathogenesis of hepatoblastoma is poorly understood but some pointers come from the known associations between hepatoblastoma and Beckwith–Wiedemann syndrome and also familial adenomatous polyposis (FAP).

Most cases of hepatoblastoma are sporadic, but patients with Beckwith–Wiedemann syndrome have an increased risk of developing the embryonal tumours rhabdomyosarcoma, Wilms' tumour and hepatoblastoma. In 1985, Koufos et al.[3] suggested that this association might be due to loss of heterozygosity (LOH) from parts of chromosome 11p, thereby 'exposing' a mutated but otherwise silent (recessive) allele. Since then, there have been reports of LOH occurring in sporadic hepatoblastoma.[4] For instance, Albrecht et al.[5] found LOH from 11p in six of 18 hepatoblastomas. The common region of

*The authors acknowledge the contributions of Professor Lewis Spitz, Institute of Child Health, London, and Dr Jean Keeling, Royal Hospital for Sick Children, Edinburgh.

overlap was 11.15.5 and in all cases the maternal allele was absent. Other studies have identified LOH on chromosome 1, suggesting that this may also be a location for a putative tumour suppressor gene.[6,7]

The association between hepatoblastoma and FAP was first noted by Kingston et al.[8] in 1983. They reported five such cases occurring during a 50-year period, and calculated that FAP occurs around 100 times more frequently in parents of children with hepatoblastoma than in the general population. Children cured of hepatoblastoma who have a parent with FAP have a 50 per cent chance of developing this disease, so they must be screened regularly with colonoscopy, starting in their teens.[9] These patients often also have congenital hypertrophy of the retinal pigment epithelium, which can be used as a marker to identify carriers of the adenomatous polyposis coli (APC = FAP) gene, which has been located on chromosome 5.[10] Some APC gene mutations seem to be highly penetrant for hepatoblastoma, as well as for FAP.[10a] The APC tumour suppressor gene controls the degradation of beta-catenin, a protein involved in the Wnt signalling pathway. Koch et al.[11] examined 52 biopsies and three cell lines derived from sporadic hepatoblastoma for mutations in the APC and beta-catenin genes. In this study, 48 per cent of sporadic hepatoblastomas examined had beta-catenin mutations, suggesting that it has a role in the development of hepatoblastoma. No correlation was found with histological subtype or outcome. No APC mutations were identified in this study of hepatoblastomas from European patients, in contrast to a study of hepatoblastoma in Asian patients in which 69 per cent had alterations (LOH or somatic mutations) in the APC gene.[12]

Beta-catenin is found in the cytoplasmic membrane in normal liver but accumulates in the cytoplasm and nucleus of hepatoblastoma cells. Several studies have identified an association between predominantly nuclear staining and undifferentiated histology, and in one study multivariate analysis suggests that nuclear beta-catenin staining may be an important prognostic factor.[13–15]

Intriguingly, recent papers have suggested an association between low birth weight and the development of hepatoblastoma. Ikeda et al.[16] reviewed the birth weights of children in the Japanese children's cancer registry from 1985–1993 and found that hepatoblastoma accounted for 58 per cent of cancers occurring in children who were of very low birth weight (<1000 g). Data from the USA show an increase in the incidence of hepatoblastoma in children under the age of 5 years from 1973 to 1992, a period during which there was a marked improvement in the survival of infants of very low birth weight.[17] The Japanese group have confirmed their initial findings with a review of cancer registry data over a 26-year period[18] and have reported a case–control study in which they tried to identify possible risk factors for the development of hepatoblastoma in children with a very low birth

weight.[19] The duration of oxygen therapy was the only significant independent risk factor identified in multivariate analysis.

Hepatoblastomas almost always arise in an otherwise normal liver. Hepatocellular carcinoma, by contrast, is often associated with cirrhosis or another pre-existing parenchymal liver disorder.[20,21] For example, five of 32 children and adolescents with hepatocellular carcinoma studied by Lack et al.[22] had cirrhosis, two had an hepatic adenoma, and one had previously been treated with orthovoltage radiation for a Wilms' tumour. Twenty of 28 Taiwanese children with hepatocellular carcinoma had cirrhosis.[23] The association of hepatitis B infection and hepatocellular carcinoma in adults has been well documented, and there are increasing numbers of reports of this association in children.[24] Chen et al.,[23] for instance, demonstrated 100 per cent positivity for hepatitis B surface antigen (HBsAg) in 25 children with hepatocellular carcinoma in Taiwan. The HBsAg status of 15 of these patients' families was ascertained. Fourteen of 15 mothers were HBsAg-positive, indicating that vertical transmission from the mother is a very important source of hepatitis B infection in children. Administration of hepatitis B immune globulin at birth to infants of HBsAg-positive mothers, followed by hepatitis B vaccination, and vaccination of hepatitis B-negative children, in areas with a high incidence of hepatitis B infection, should reduce the incidence of the chronic HBsAg carrier state and thus the incidence of hepatocellular carcinoma in both children and adults. Since the introduction, in 1984, of a universal hepatitis B vaccination programme in Taiwan, there has been a significant decline in the incidence of hepatocellular carcinoma in children.[25] Southeast Asia is, of course, a high prevalence area for hepatitis B virus infection, but HBsAg in association with hepatocellular carcinoma in children has also been reported in Europe.[26,27]

Incidence

The incidence of hepatoblastoma is fairly constant throughout the world, with an annual incidence of 1–2 cases per million children.[28] In most countries, hepatocellular carcinoma is less common than hepatoblastoma, but there is considerable geographic variation, with rates ranging from 0.2 per million in England and Wales to 2.1 per million children in Hong Kong. In some populations (e.g. Hong Kong, Taiwan),[23,29] hepatocellular carcinoma occurs more frequently than hepatoblastoma. For unknown reasons, boys are more commonly affected by malignant epithelial liver tumours, especially hepatocellular carcinoma, than girls (male:female ratio approximately 2:1).[1,22,23,28,30] The vast majority of hepatoblastomas occur in children under the age of 5 years, with 50 per cent in children less than 18 months of age. Occasionally the tumour may be detected prenatally, by ultrasound, or at birth. Hepatocellular carcinoma, by contrast, is a tumour of older children, with a peak incidence between 10 and 14 years.[1,2,22,23,30,31]

Pathology

HEPATOBLASTOMA

The majority are unifocal and located in the right lobe of the liver. The macroscopic characteristics are variable (see Plate 21). Tumours may be encapsulated or unencapsulated, nodular or smooth, firm, soft or friable. Occasionally, they are pedunculated. The cut surface varies in colour from greyish-white to tan. Areas of haemorrhage, ossification and necrosis may be seen.[1]

Attempts have been made to divide hepatoblastoma into histopathological subtypes and to relate them to prognosis. In 1953, Willis[32] used the term 'hepatoblastoma' for all embryonal tumours containing hepatic epithelial parenchyma, subdividing them into three types: embryonic-pure epithelial; mixed-epithelial and mesenchymal; and rhabdomyoblastic mixed. In 1967, Ishak and Glunz[1] modified this classification, preferring two, rather than three, categories: epithelial, and 'mixed' epithelial and mesenchymal subtypes. In the pure epithelial tumours, which were usually nodular and had a cut surface of uniform appearance, they recognized two types of cells: fetal and embryonal.

Fetal-type cells resemble the cells of the fetal liver and are usually arranged in irregular plates, two cells thick. The cells vary in size but are smaller than normal hepatocytes and have acidophilic cytoplasm containing glycogen (Plate 22). Their nuclei are round or oval, and basophilic with few mitotic figures. Embryonal type cells are less well differentiated and arranged in sheets. The cells are small and darkly staining with scanty cytoplasm containing little or no glycogen. Nuclei are hyperchromatic and mitoses frequent (Plate 23).

The mixed tumours have a lobulated cut surface appearance, with bands of collagenous material separating the lobules. There are areas of fetal and embryonic type cells, as well as supporting reticulin fibres and blood vessels. Primitive mesenchyme, containing elongated spindle cells with scanty cytoplasm and areas of osteoid tissue, is another notable component of these tumours.

Kasai and Watanabe,[20] writing in 1970, suggested an alternative subclassification into fetal, embryonal and anaplastic varieties. Anaplastic tumours consist of small cells with scanty cytoplasm, with no glycogen, resembling neuroblasts. Mitoses are uncommon. They found that the morphologically poorly differentiated tumours, i.e. embryonal and anaplastic subtypes, had a worse prognosis than the better differentiated fetal tumours, a view supported by Lack et al.[30]

In a joint study by the Children's Cancer Study Group (CCSG), Southwest Oncology Group (SWOG), and Pediatric Oncology Group (POG),[33] tumours were classified according to Weinberg and Finegold,[34] as fetal, embryonal, macrotrabecular and small-cell undifferentiated (anaplastic). Because of the morphological similarity of small-cell undifferentiated tumours to other small round-cell tumours, particularly neuroblastoma, lymphoma and rhabdomyosarcoma, areas of epithelial (usually fetal) hepatoblastoma must be seen to confirm the diagnosis (Plate 24). In the macrotrabecular subtype, cells are arranged in trabeculae 10–20 or more cells thick (Plate 25). Cells may be larger than the surrounding normal liver cells, and resemble hepatocellular carcinoma, but fetal cells are always also present. There are overlaps between these classifications. A consensus on histopathological criteria for subclassification of hepatoblastoma (fetal, embryonal, macrotrabecular and small-cell undifferentiated) was reached at a workshop held in Bern in 1990,[35] but it is not universally used. Others prefer to add the additional categories of mixed epithelial and mesenchymal, with or without teratoid features.

Chemotherapy usually has a marked effect on the histology of hepatoblastoma. Necrosis, which may be present in primarily resected hepatoblastoma in small amounts, is generally more extensive in post-chemotherapy specimens, and in a few cases the tumour may be completely necrotic. Results from a small study by Saxena et al.[36] do not suggest preferential ablation of a particular morphological subtype. The most striking feature of that study was the extensive amount of osteoid noted – up to 40 per cent – in post-chemotherapy hepatoblastoma. The prognostic implication of this finding, if any, is as yet unclear.

HEPATOCELLULAR CARCINOMA

The majority of these tumours (70–80 per cent) are either multifocal or involve both lobes at the time of diagnosis.[2,22,23] Macroscopically, they are nodular and vary in consistency from soft to firm and in colour from yellow to green. Often there are areas of necrosis or haemorrhage. Microscopically, the tumours resemble hepatocellular carcinoma in adults, with a trabecular pattern up to 20 layers of cells thick. The cells are usually larger than those of the surrounding liver, but vary markedly in size. Giant cells are common and mitoses frequent (Plate 26).[1,20] Evidence of cirrhosis is seen in the non-tumorous liver in 10–70 per cent of cases depending on the geographic origin of the patients.[1,20,22,23]

The fibrolamellar variant of hepatocellular carcinoma, which is probably a distinct clinicopathological entity, invariably arises in a non-cirrhotic liver.[36a] The two distinctive features of this epithelial tumour are tumour cells with eosinophilic cytoplasm, and broad fibrous septa dividing the hepatocytes into thin columns of cells or large nodules. Mitotic figures are rare (Plate 27).[37]

'TRANSITIONAL LIVER CELL TUMOUR'

This new entity has recently been suggested for tumours that occur in older children and young adolescents, with a cell morphology intermediate between hepatoblastoma and hepatocellular carcinoma. Prokurat et al.[38] reported on eight such patients aged 5–18 years with a hepatocellular tumour, arising in a non-cirrhotic liver, with a poor outcome. Zimmerman and colleagues from the SIOPEL group share the same view, but further studies need to be done to confirm this finding.

Clinical presentation

The presenting symptoms of hepatoblastoma and hepatocellular carcinoma are similar. An abdominal mass and/or abdominal distension are the most common features. Anorexia and lethargy are also frequent. Jaundice and abdominal pain are unusual in patients with hepatoblastoma, but are more common (10–20 and 15–65 per cent, respectively) in patients with hepatocellular carcinoma, especially those with underlying liver disease. Rarely, presentation is with an 'acute abdomen' due to tumour rupture or intratumoral haemorrhage.[1,2,21–23,30,31,39] Precocious puberty is an unusual presentation of hepatoblastoma but has not been reported in hepatocellular carcinoma.[30,31,40] Virilization in such cases is due to gonadotrophin production by the tumour, which stimulates testosterone secretion by the testes. Testicular biopsy shows Leydig cell hyperplasia with no spermatogenesis. Generalized osteoporosis is present in about 20 per cent of patients with hepatoblastoma[30] and, when severe, may lead to multiple fractures. Presumably, the tumour cells secrete an 'osteoclast-activating factor'.

Hepatomegaly, with or without a distinct hepatic mass, is almost always present and pallor is common. There may be evidence of weight loss, dilated abdominal veins and jaundice. Features of the Beckwith–Wiedemann syndrome may be evident in patients with hepatoblastoma.[22,23,30,31,39]

Because of the aetiological implications, enquiry should seek to exclude a family history of FAP and a past history of hepatitis or other antecedent liver disease in the parents or the child.[21]

Laboratory investigations

Many patients are anaemic at diagnosis[22,30] and thrombocytosis is common, especially in hepatoblastoma.[22,30,31,41] The platelet count may be $>1000 \times 10^9$/L, probably due to production by the tumour of a circulating 'thrombopoietin'.[42] Liver function tests in hepatoblastoma are usually normal, but in hepatocellular carcinoma, serum bilirubin, aspartate aminotransferase (AST), alanine transaminase (ALT), and alkaline phosphatase levels may be elevated because of associated hepatitis or cirrhosis.[2,22,23,30] Alpha-fetoprotein (AFP) is produced by the normal fetal and neonatal liver and, although present in rapidly decreasing concentrations in the serum of babies up to 6–9 months old, only basal levels are present in the serum of older children and adults.[43] An elevated level of serum AFP is found in >90 per cent of cases of hepatoblastoma[31,44,45] and 60–90 per cent of hepatocellular carcinomas.[23] It is a very sensitive 'tumour marker' but not specific, as elevated levels are also found in patients with malignant germ cell tumours, especially those containing yolk sac elements and some immature teratomas. In patients with the fibrolamellar variant of hepatocellular carcinoma, serum AFP is normal but unsaturated vitamin B_{12} binding capacity (transcobalamin) is a useful tumour marker.[46] Increased excretion of cystathionine may be detected in the urine of children with hepatoblastoma, but it is not a specific tumour product and is not useful in diagnosis or follow-up.

Imaging

In a child with a suspected hepatic tumour, imaging should confirm the intrahepatic location, demonstrate the characteristics of the mass, identify metastases and give an indication of resectability (Figures 22.1 and 22.2).[47] In many cases, hepatomegaly is evident on plain abdominal X-ray, and in 10–20 per cent calcification is visible.[1,22,30,47] Calcification is usually coarse and dense, contrasting with the fine granular calcification seen in haemangioendothelioma. Abdominal ultrasound helps to define the site and extent of tumour. The inferior vena cava, portal vein and hepatic veins and arteries can also be identified. The majority of hepatocellular tumours are hyperechoic, whereas haemangioendotheliomas are usually hypoechoic, and mesenchymal hamartomas have large cystic areas.[48] Abdominal computed tomography (CT) scanning delineates the tumour, which is characteristically of low attenuation compared with the surrounding liver. Involvement of the hepatic veins, inferior vena cava or portal vein is best seen after contrast enhancement. Failure to recognize invasion (intraluminal tumour/thrombus) of hepatic veins or inferior vena cava may lead to pulmonary embolization at the time of operation with a possible fatal outcome.[49] Magnetic resonance imaging (MRI) gives definition of tumour and hepatic veins without intravenous contrast and permits assessment of the segmental extent of the tumour.[50] Some centres believe that angiography is essential for demonstrating the blood supply to the tumour and vascular anomalies, both of which may be important when assessing the resectability. Others, however, feel that

MRI or CT with intravenous enhancement is as useful, in this respect, as angiography. In around 10–15 per cent of patients, pulmonary metastases are visible on initial chest X-ray.[2,22,30] Lung CT scanning may reveal metastases not visible on chest X-ray.[31]

The osteoporosis seen in some patients with hepatoblastoma may be detected by plain X-rays.[30] When severe, fractures may be evident and a diagnosis of non-accidental injury or brittle bone disease may be suspected. Bone density returns to normal after successful treatment of the tumour.

Because of the rarity of bone and brain secondaries at diagnosis, scanning of these organs is not justified without a specific clinical indication. An exception to this may be patients with a congenital hepatoblastoma in whom systemic metastases, without lung involvement, may be more common.[51] Patients with a suspected primary liver malignancy should be investigated as indicated in Box 22.2.

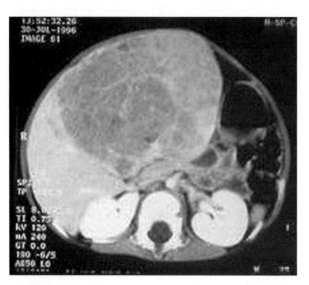

Figure 22.1 *Computed tomography (CT) scan of hepatoblastoma.*

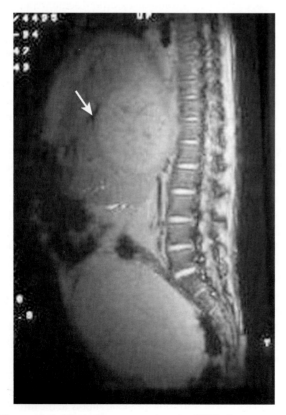

Figure 22.2 *Magnetic resonance imaging (MRI) of hepatoblastoma (arrow).*

Staging

Traditionally a post-surgical staging system has been used, with stage related to the amount of tumour removed at initial surgery as shown in Box 22.3.[33] The problem is that 'local' staging such as this is based on initial surgery and is dependent on the decision, (a) to attempt resection rather than give preoperative chemotherapy, and (b) the surgeon's expertise. These factors lessen the value of comparison of results from different studies.

Box 22.2 *Imaging investigation of a patient with a suspected malignant liver tumour*

Mandatory
- Abdominal X-ray
- Abdominal ultrasound
- Abdominal CT scan
- Chest X-ray
- Lung CT scan if chest X-ray is normal

Optional
- Angiography
- MRI scan
- Lung CT if chest X-ray shows metastases

Box 22.3 *Post surgical staging of hepatocellular tumours*

Stage I	Completely resected at initial surgery
Stage II	Resection with microscopic disease at the margin
Stage III	Unresectable or gross residual, but no metastases
Stage IV	Metastatic disease

A distinction may be made between stage IIIA (patients with a large unifocal unresectable tumour) and stage IIIB (patients with multifocal disease involving both lobes).

In the first liver tumour study of the International Society of Pediatric Oncology (SIOP), 'SIOPEL 1', a preoperative grouping system (PRETEXT – **pret**reatment **ext**ent of disease) was introduced.[52] PRETEXT describes the site and size of the tumour, invasion of vessels and distant spread, as judged by pretreatment imaging with ultrasound, CT scans and MRI. The liver is divided into four sectors. The left lobe consists of a lateral and medial sector, and the right lobe, an anterior and posterior sector. By establishing how many unaffected liver sector(s) there are, the tumour is classified in one of four groups (PRETEXT I–IV) (Figure 22.3):

In addition the letters V, P, E and M are used to indicate the extrahepatic extent of the tumour, as follows:

- V – involvement of the inferior vein cava and /or all three hepatic veins
- P – involvement of the main portal vein and /or both left and right portal veins
- E – extrahepatic intra-abdominal disease other than V or P
- M – distant metastases.

For example, II PM indicates a group II tumour with ingrowth into the portal vein and also distant metastases. Use of this system by other groups, alongside their own staging system, is becoming more common and facilitates comparison of results from different studies.[35]

Treatment

SURGERY

In a child with a liver mass and a markedly elevated serum AFP level for age, the diagnosis is almost certainly a hepatocellular tumour, but the distinction between hepatoblastoma and hepatocellular carcinoma and the exclusion of malignant germ cell tumour can only be made on histology.[53] However, tumour biopsy is not without risk, and a single core sample may not be representative of the tumour as a whole. If preoperative chemotherapy is to be given, most would favour a pretreatment biopsy either by percutaneous needle biopsy (Trucut or Menghini) or via a mini-laparotomy or laparoscopy so that several parts of the tumour may be sampled and the risk of bleeding reduced.[54] If no biopsy is done, there may never be histological confirmation of the diagnosis for one of two reasons. In a proportion of patients (1 in 10)[44] the tumour is completely necrotic after preoperative chemotherapy, and in others progression occurs, despite chemotherapy, and the tumour never becomes resectable. However, the limitations of biopsy must be recognized. On a small tissue sample, it may not be possible to differentiate between hepatoblastoma and hepatocellular carcinoma, nor to classify hepatoblastoma by histological subtype, as its histological appearance may vary from area to area. Fine-needle aspiration probably provides too little tissue to be of practical use.

Prior to surgery, detailed imaging of the tumour is necessary. The liver is divided into right and left lobes by the inferior vena cava and the gall bladder. The right lobe is subdivided into anterior and posterior sectors, and the left, by the falciform ligament, into medial and lateral sectors. The hepatic artery, a branch of the coeliac axis, usually divides into a right and a left branch, but variations occur in 25 per cent of the population, with the right hepatic artery arising from the superior mesenteric artery and the left from the gastric artery. The portal vein supplies all four lobes of the liver. Venous drainage is via the three hepatic veins to the inferior vena cava. The branches of the biliary tree usually follow those of the hepatic artery and the portal vein.

Complete tumour resection is of paramount importance for cure, but operative mortality, without prior

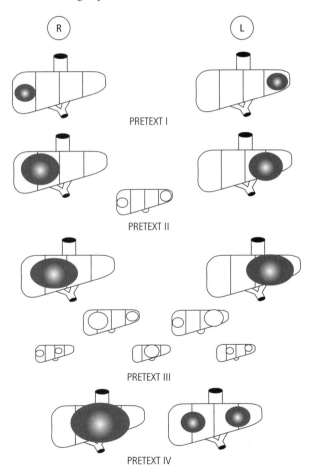

Figure 22.3 *SIOPEL **pret**reatment grouping system describing **ext**ent of disease (the PRETEXT system). PRETEXT I, one sector involved by tumour, three adjoining sectors free; PRETEXT II, two sectors involved by tumour, two adjoining sectors free; PRETEXT III, three sectors involved by tumour, one sector free, or two sectors involved by tumour, two non-adjoining sectors free; PRETEXT IV, all four sectors involved by tumour.*

chemotherapy, has been reported to be as high as 10–20 per cent.[1,2,22,30] In addition, fewer than 50 per cent of tumours are resectable at diagnosis[1,2,20,33,55] and survival of patients with unresectable tumours is rare.[56]

Blood loss is a major factor in the high operative mortality associated with hepatic resection, but improvements in anaesthetic and surgical techniques during recent years have substantially reduced the risk.[54,57,58] Isolation of the liver from the systemic circulation by vascular slings, hypothermia and hypotension can be used to reduce and control haemorrhage. The use of an ultrasonic dissector also reduces blood loss by permitting the surgeon to define and control the numerous vascular radicles in the raw surface of the liver at the line of resection. Resectability depends on the location and the vascular supply of the tumour, and in some instances this may only be determined at laparotomy. The usual types of resection are right lobectomy (anterior and posterior lobes) and left lobectomy (medial and lateral lobes). In children, because of the capacity of the remaining liver to regenerate, trisegmentectomy, e.g. an extended right hepatectomy, removing the left medial lobe as well as the right lobe, may be performed. Postoperatively patients need careful monitoring as they are at risk from hypoglycaemia, hypoproteinaemia, bleeding due to reduction in clotting factors, and infection. Damage to bile ducts during surgery may later cause stenosis and obstructive jaundice, or biliary fistula.[13,58]

Resection of pulmonary metastases is justified in patients who have shown a response to chemotherapy with complete resection of their primary tumour, but incomplete resolution of the secondaries. This kind of approach may be curative. Resection of pulmonary metastases should also be considered in patients who relapse in the lungs after complete excision of primary tumour when response to chemotherapy is incomplete.[54,59–61]

CHEMOTHERAPY

Most patients with hepatocellular tumours present with unresectable or metastatic disease. The possibility that chemotherapy could convert unresectable to resectable disease was first appreciated when, in 1970, Hermann and Lonsdale[62] reported a child with hepatoblastoma which became operable after treatment with vincristine, cyclophosphamide and radiotherapy. In 1975, Exelby et al.[2] reported three patients whose tumours responded to vincristine, actinomycin D and cyclophosphamide (VAC). At that time these were the drugs most commonly used in the treatment of hepatoblastoma. In 1982, Evans et al.[55] reported the response of hepatocellular tumours ('hepatomas') to a combination of vincristine, doxorubicin, cyclophosphamide and 5-fluorouracil. The response rate was 44 per cent in patients with measurable disease. Only one of 16 patients who had chemotherapy after complete resection relapsed compared with seven of 11 patients in an earlier study who were treated with surgery alone.

In the early 1980s, cisplatin and doxorubicin emerged as the most effective single agents in the treatment of hepatoblastoma.[63,64] This was a crucial advance and since then most studies have used these two drugs either as a two-agent regimen (cisplatin/doxorubicin = PLADO)[44,45,65] or in combination with other drugs. Ifosfamide, for example, was added as a third drug in the GPOH (German Society of Paediatric Oncology & Haematology) HB 89 study.[66] The combination of cisplatin and doxorubicin has been shown to be effective in converting unresectable to resectable disease, and in clearing lung metastases (Table 22.1).

There is a different emphasis amongst the three major groups running trials of treatment for hepatocellular tumours. The SIOPEL group treat all patients with four

Table 22.1 *Response of hepatoblastoma to preoperative chemotherapy*

Study	Chemotherapy	Number of patients	Partial response to chemotherapy	Resectable	Response of lung metastases
GOS/KCH[44]	Cisplatin/doxorubicin	14 (stage III, 9; stage IV, 5)	12/14	10/14	4/5 CR
GPOH HB 89[66]	Cisplatin/doxorubicin/ifosfamide	45 (stage III, 38; stage IV, 7)	44/45	39/45	Not known
POG 86 97[67]	Cisplatin/vincristine/5-fluorouracil	39 (stage III, 31; stage IV, 8)	36/39	25/39 +3 OLT	6/8
CCG 823F[45]	Cisplatin/doxorubicin	33 (stage II, 8; stage III 15; stage IV, 10)	25/33	Not known	Not known
SIOPEL 1[65]	Cisplatin/doxorubicin	138 (all patients given preoperative chemotherapy)	113/138	100/138 +6 OLT	24/31
HEPA 92[77]	Carboplatin/doxorubicin	19 (PRETEXT II, 3; PRETEXT III, 14; PRETEXT IV, 2)	15/20	14/20	No patients with metastases included

CR, complete response; OLT, orthotopic liver transplantation.

to six courses of preoperative chemotherapy.[65] They justify delayed surgery for the following reasons:

- Children are cured of hepatoblastoma/hepatocellular carcinoma only if complete resection can be achieved.
- Preoperative chemotherapy increases the resection rate.
- The operation becomes safer and easier after preoperative chemotherapy.
- There is no delay in treating micrometastases.

By contrast, both the GPOH and the American CCSG and POG have advocated primary resection of the tumour where feasible (although GPOH limit the resection to a standard lobectomy) followed by chemotherapy.[45,66,67]

Cisplatin and doxorubicin both have organ-threatening side-effects. Apart from the inevitable myelotoxicity, especially following doxorubicin, the toxicity of both drugs is cumulative and dose-related, so careful monitoring of cardiac function (measurement of left ventricular shortening fraction, or ejection fraction), renal function, (preferably, measurement of glomerular filtration rate by isotope clearance) and serial audiometry are necessary during therapy with these drugs. Cisplatin causes glomerular damage, which may be at least partly reversible, and irreversible high-frequency hearing loss. The median age at diagnosis for patients with hepatoblastoma is around 18 months, when children are developing language skills. Detection of high-frequency hearing loss in young children is difficult, so assessment by an expert audiologist is desirable. Brock et al.[68] proposed a grading system for ototoxicity in children treated with cisplatin, which facilitates comparison of the toxicity of different regimens. The definitive measurement of ototoxicity should be performed by pure tone audiometry after treatment, at around the age of 4 years, when the child is able to cooperate with the investigation. In adults there is evidence to suggest that continuous infusion of doxorubicin is less cardiotoxic than when it is administered as a bolus,[69] but a recent study by Lipschultz et al.[70] suggests that this does not hold true for children. Continuous infusion of cisplatin may be less ototoxic and nephrotoxic than bolus injection.[71]

Hepatocellular carcinoma is not as chemoresponsive as hepatoblastoma although clear-cut responses to PLADO chemotherapy have been documented. For example, eight out of 14 patients with hepatocellular carcinoma in the CCSG study had a partial response to PLADO,[45] although only two then achieved a complete resection. In the SIOPEL 1 study,[72] 49 per cent of patients with hepatocellular carcinoma showed some shrinkage of tumour and a fall in serum AFP level in response to PLADO. Thirty-six per cent of these patients had complete resection of primary tumour.

In summary, surgery and chemotherapy are both necessary in the treatment of most children with hepatoblastoma or hepatocellular carcinoma. Preoperative chemotherapy may convert unresectable to resectable disease and invariably makes the operation less hazardous. Postoperative chemotherapy after initial complete resection is effective against micrometastases and considerably reduces the risk of metastatic relapse.[55] Cisplatin and doxorubicin are the two most effective drugs.

RADIOTHERAPY

The role of radiotherapy, if any, in the treatment of hepatoblastoma and hepatocellular carcinoma has not yet been clearly defined.[73] The majority of patients who have radiotherapy also have chemotherapy, so it is difficult to attribute tumour shrinkage or cure to one or other modality.

Primary site

In a survey by Exelby et al.,[2] 27 out of 129 patients with hepatoblastoma were treated with radiotherapy to the primary site at some stage during their treatment programme. Three patients had complete resection of an initially unresectable tumour after treatment with radiotherapy and combination chemotherapy, but no patient with an inoperable tumour was cured by radiotherapy and chemotherapy alone. In the same survey, no patient with hepatocellular carcinoma treated with radiotherapy to the liver or whole abdomen survived. In a USA CCSG/SWOG study of combination chemotherapy in hepatoma,[55] seven out of 27 patients, four of whom had been treated with chemotherapy and radiotherapy, had a complete or good partial response. In three patients an initially unresectable tumour became resectable after chemotherapy and radiotherapy. In a report by Quinn et al.,[56] one patient, whose tumour remained unresectable after treatment with cisplatin and doxorubicin, was given 45 Gy to the tumour; afterwards, and without surgery, the serum AFP level fell to normal. Further chemotherapy was given and the child is alive and well over 6 years later. In the SIOPEL 1 study, patients who had 'miniscopic' (i.e. small volume macroscopic) residual disease after delayed surgery had two further courses of chemotherapy and the option of small field radiotherapy, but, in fact, only one patient received this treatment.

Metastases

Radiotherapy has also been used, in combination with chemotherapy, to treat pulmonary metastatic disease. In one series,[44] four out of five stage IV patients with lung metastases received whole-lung radiotherapy – three after complete radiological response to cisplatin and doxorubicin and complete resection of primary tumour, and one at the time of metastatic relapse. The dose was 12–15 Gy in eight to 10 fractions. Three are long-term survivors but the fourth died of metastatic disease.

Another patient was treated with doxorubicin, vincristine and whole-lung radiotherapy for pulmonary metastases which occurred 11 months after surgery, vincristine and cyclophosphamide treatment of a stage I tumour. She is a long-term survivor.[74]

Given the doubt about the value of adding lung radiotherapy with its attendant late morbidity to chemotherapy, especially when this includes doxorubicin, patients with lung metastases at diagnosis entered in the current SIOP, GPOH and American studies are not being given pulmonary radiation.

There are no randomized studies examining the value of radiotherapy in hepatoblastoma/hepatocellular carcinoma and no studies in which radiotherapy has been evaluated as a single agent. Most patients 'responding' to radiotherapy also received concomitant chemotherapy. Therefore, radiotherapy is probably not valuable in the management of lung secondaries or gross primary disease. Its role in postoperative residual disease was to be evaluated in SIOPEL 1, but in the event was hardly ever used. Therefore, radiation has little or no established role in the management these days, although, as with most other paediatric tumours, radiotherapy may be useful as part of palliative care.

Response

Patients given preoperative chemotherapy are assessed for response by clinical examination, imaging, with measurement of tumour dimensions, and serial serum AFP levels. To evaluate the response of a tumour to preoperative chemotherapy, and to compare the results of different studies, response must be clearly defined. Complete response (i.e. complete disappearance of all tumour) and no response (i.e. no measurable regression of disease) are clear-cut. The difficulty comes in defining partial response. Evans et al.[55] used two terms: 'good partial response' (objective regression of disease of >50 per cent, as measured by the sum of two diameters) and 'partial response' (objective regression of disease of <50 per cent).

In the SIOPEL 1 study, the terms used were 'complete response', 'partial response' (any tumour shrinkage), 'no response' and 'progressive disease' (unequivocal increase in one or more dimensions). For metastatic disease, a fifth category was added, 'minimal residual disease', which denoted complete clearing of posteroanterior and lateral chest X-ray with minimal residual change on lung CT scan.

In multifocal or metastatic disease, these criteria are applied to each tumour, and the patient's response is classified according to the 'worst responding' tumour. Allowance is made for the fact that, in the early stages of chemotherapy, real or apparent size increase may be due to intratumoral haemorrhage or oedema, and a temporary rise of serum AFP may reflect tumour lysis. To qualify as a partial response in the SIOPEL 1 study, the serum AFP level must have fallen from its initial elevated value, and for a complete response the serum AFP must fall to within the normal range. Patients with a good response to chemotherapy usually show a marked decrease in serum AFP level,[44,56,74] and a rising level is often the first indication of relapse.[31] Rarely, relapse may be AFP-negative. In fibrolamellar hepatocellular carcinoma, serum transcobalamin I level is a useful tumour marker and a rising level suggests disease recurrence.[75]

Patients in whom relapse is suspected should be re-investigated with chest and abdominal imaging, as at the time of their initial presentation, in order to determine the extent of recurrence. Relapse may be local (in the remaining liver) or metastatic. The commonest sites for metastases are the lungs. Rarely these tumours metastasize to brain or bone.[1,2,22,30,51]

Survival

The outlook for children with hepatocellular tumours in the past was poor, with overall survival (OS) between 9 and 35 per cent (Table 22.2), and in the series highlighted in the table no child with an initially unresectable tumour survived. Even in those patients with initial complete

Table 22.2 *Survival of children with hepatocellular tumours in studies up to and including 1982*

Study	Number of patients	Overall survival	Complete surgical resection	Survival after complete resection
Ishak and Glunz[1]	HB 35	28%	18	50%
	HCC 12	0	3	0
Kasai and Watanabe[20]	HB 57	21%	24	50%
	HCC 13	0	3	0
Exelby et al.[2]	HB 129	35%	78	58%
	HCC 98	12%	33	36%
Lack et al.[30]	HB 54	24%	32	40%
Lack et al.[22]	HCC 32	9%	7	42%

HB, hepatoblastoma; HCC, hepatocellular carcinoma.

Table 22.3 *Survival of children with hepatoblastoma in recent studies*

Study group	Number of patients	Treatment	Survival	Macroscopic surgical resection	Survival after surgical resection
CCG 823[45]	33 (stages II, III, and IV)	Primary surgery, cisplatin, doxorubicin	66.6% at 2 years	70%	83%
POG 8697[67]	60 (stages I UH, II, III and IV)	Primary surgery, cisplatin, vincristine, 5-fluorouracil	Stage I UH and stage II DFS 91% at 3 years, stage III 67% at 3 years, stage IV 12.5% at 3 years	76%	93%
GPOH HB 89[66]	72 (stages I, II, III and IV)	Primary surgery, ifosfamide, cisplatin, doxorubcin	Overall DFS 75% (stage I 100%, stage II 50%, stage III 71%, stage IV 29)	80%	81%
Intergroup 0098[83]	182 (stages I UH, II, III and IV)	Primary surgery cisplatin, vincristine, 5-fluorouracil vs. cisplatin, doxorubicin	EFS at 5 years – stage I UH 91%, stage II 100%, stage III 64%, stage IV 25%	Not known	83% for 41 stage III and IV patients
SIOPEL 1[65]	154 PRETEXT I, II, III and IV	Primary chemotherapy, cisplatin, doxorubicin, delayed surgery	Overall EFS at 5 years 66% (PRETEXT I 100%, PRETEXT II 83%, PRETEXT III 56%, PRETEXT IV 46%)	72%	81%
GPOH HB 94[86]	69 (stages I, II, III and IV)	Primary surgery, ifosfamide, cisplatin, doxorubicin	EFS (median follow-up 58 months) – stage I 89%, stage II 100%, stage III 68%, stage IV 21%	86%	DFS 95%

DFS, disease-free survival; EFS, event-free survival; UH, unfavourable histology.

tumour resection, survival for hepatoblastoma was only 40–60 per cent. Less than a third of patients with hepatocellular carcinoma had complete resection of tumour and survival was very poor (10–15 per cent at most). In all these studies, complete resection of tumour was a critical prognostic factor, but overall, only about 40 per cent of all patients had complete surgical resection.

Cisplatin and doxorubicin have had a major impact on survival by converting unresectable to resectable disease. Overall survival for hepatoblastoma in recent studies is over 60 per cent, and for patients having complete resection it is over 80 per cent (Table 22.3). Complete resection with clear margins is the 'gold standard', but there is a suggestion that microscopic residual disease does not necessarily imply a poor prognosis.[76] Although the combination of carboplatin/doxorubicin used in the HEPA 92 study produced response and resection rates equivalent to cisplatin/doxorubicin, the 5-year event-free survival (EFS) and OS of 55 and 60 per cent, respectively, were disappointing.[77] Of 14 children who had complete surgical resection after preoperative chemotherapy, four relapsed, three died and one was lost to follow-up.

Although the impact on prognosis for hepatocellular carcinoma has not been so great, there is a trend suggesting improvement both in OS and survival after complete resection (Table 22.4). The results of the various studies for hepatoblastoma and for hepatocellular carcinoma are similar, but these studies are not directly comparable as different treatment strategies (i.e. preoperative chemotherapy vs. primary surgery) and different grouping/staging systems are used (i.e. PRETEXT IV = tumour involving all four sectors of the liver; stage IV = metastatic tumour).

Prognostic factors

Weinberg and Finegold[34] reported an improved prognosis for patients with hepatoblastoma of pure fetal histology. A joint study by the CCSG, SWOG and POG[33] of 168 patients with hepatoblastoma demonstrated a better prognosis for those with tumours of pure fetal histology compared with other histological subtypes, although only in stage I disease. The proportion of patients with pure fetal histology was similar for stage I (28/55) and those with more advanced disease (60/113), indicating that the improved prognosis is not due to the fact that these patients have a lower tumour stage at diagnosis. Absence of mitotic figures was a good prognostic factor,

Table 22.4 *Survival of children with hepatocellular carcinoma in recent studies*

Study group	Number of patients	Treatment	Survival	Macroscopic surgical resection	Survival after resection
CCG 823[45]	14	Primary surgery, cisplatin, doxorubicin	21%	21%	33%
GPOH HB 89[96]	10	Primary surgery, ifosfamide, cisplatin, doxorubicin	33%	50%	60%
SIOPEL 1[72]	40	Primary chemotherapy, cisplatin, doxorubicin, delayed surgery	Overall survival 28% at 5 years, EFS 17% at 5 years	35%	57%
GPOH HB 94[97]	26	Primary surgery, ifo/CDDP/doxo, carbo/VP16, topo/doxo, taxol	Overall survival 34% at median follow-up of 20 months (stage I 2/3, stage II 2/2, stage III 3/9, stage IV 1/11)	42%	Not known
Intergroup[98]	46	Primary surgery CDDP, VCR 5FU, vs. CDDP + doxo	Overall EFS at 5 years 19% (stage I 7/8, stage III 2/25, stage IV 0/13)	Not known	Not known

5FU, 5-fluorouracil; carbo, carboplatin; CDDP, cisplatin; doxo, doxorubicin; EFS, event-free survival; ifo, ifosfamide; topo, topotecan; VCR, vincristine; VP16, etoposide.

whatever the tumour stage. Patients with advanced disease with chondroid or squamous epithelial metaplasia had a better prognosis than those whose tumours lacked this type of differentiation, whilst patients with a small-cell undifferentiated tumour, described by others as 'anaplastic', had a poorer prognosis.[20] These results are in contrast to the study by Conran et al.,[78] who classified hepatoblastoma according to their epithelial and mesenchymal components. To the four categories used by Weinberg and Finegold, they added two further subtypes: mixed epithelial and mesenchymal with and without teratoid features. Histological type was not found to be a significant prognostic factor, but stage of disease at presentation and complete resection of tumour were important. Recently Haas et al.[79] have suggested that small-cell undifferentiated histology may be unfavourable, even if only focal.[79] In 16 patients with such tumours among a group of 111 completely resected hepatoblastomas, there was a 63 per cent recurrence rate and five of the 10 patients who had a recurrence died from disease. In two patients, the small-cell histology comprised the bulk of the tumour, and in two it accounted for 25–60 per cent, but in the fifth patient there was only one small focus of small-cell undifferentiated histology. The authors recommend primary resection of all hepatocellular tumours, as such a small focus of undifferentiated histology will probably be missed on biopsy and might result in inappropriate treatment.

Other proposed prognostic variables include pTNM status, AFP level at diagnosis and post-treatment rate of fall. In a study from Germany of clinical data and histological specimens from 46 patients with hepatoblastoma,[80] pT status (according to the pTMN classification), involvement of both liver lobes, multifocality of tumour, vascular invasion and tumour residue after resection were found to be statistically significant factors. On multivariate analysis, however, only pT status and tumour residue maintained that significance.

A report from the CCG[81] suggests that serum AFP concentration at diagnosis of >10 000 mg/L and a rapid rate of fall of AFP in response to chemotherapy are favourable prognostic factors. They analysed serum AFP levels in 31 patients with unresectable or metastatic hepatoblastoma treated with chemotherapy after biopsy (20 patients), partial resection (two patients) or complete resection with microscopic residual disease (eight patients). They found that patients who had a striking early response (>2 log fall in serum AFP level) had a significantly better outcome than those who did not. There was also a trend for better survival of patients with a high serum AFP level at diagnosis, but these findings need to be confirmed in a larger group of patients.

The SIOPEL group has carried out an analysis of pretreatment prognostic factors in 154 hepatoblastoma patients treated in the SIOPEL 1 study.[82] The variables studied were age at diagnosis, serum AFP level, platelet count, histology, extent of intrahepatic tumour (PRETEXT), lung metastases, tumour multifocality, vascular invasion and hepatic hilar lymphadenopathy on imaging. PRETEXT and metastases at diagnosis were statistically significant for OS on univariate analysis, but only PRETEXT remained significant in multivariate analysis.

Lung metastases, PRETEXT, multifocal tumour and enlarged hilar lymph nodes on imaging were all statistically significant for EFS on univariate analysis, but only lung metastases and PRETEXT remained significant on multivariate analysis. There was also a statistically significant linear trend in the relationship between PRETEXT group and survival (PRETEXT I, 100 per cent; II, 83 per cent; III, 56 per cent; and IV, 46 per cent).

For patients with hepatocellular carcinoma treated on SIOPEL 1, both PRETEXT and lung metastases were identified as predictors of OS, but only metastases were identified as predictors of EFS.[72]

Recent and current trials

Concern over the potential cardiotoxicity of doxorubicin led to the design of the POG 8697 study,[67] in which cisplatin was used in combination with vincristine and 5-fluorouracil. Of 39 patients who presented with unresectable or metastatic disease, 92 per cent had a partial response to chemotherapy and in 64 per cent a complete resection was achieved. A randomized study (Intergroup 0098) of cisplatin/vincristine/fluorouracil vs. cisplatin/continuous-infusion doxorubicin followed.[83] All these patients had initial surgery and patients with a completely resected pure fetal hepatoblastoma with minimal mitotic activity were treated with just four courses of doxorubicin to a total dose of 240 mg/m^2. The remaining patients – the majority – were randomized. Outcome was not significantly different between the two arms, but the cisplatin/continuous-infusion doxorubicin regimen was more toxic, with more grade 3 and 4 toxicities reported and two toxic deaths, both from cardiomyopathy in patients each given doxorubicin to the high total dose of 640 mg/m^2.

These results have led the Americans to omit doxorubicin from their continuing studies of hepatoblastoma. Between 1993 and 1995, POG ran a study for unresectable and metastatic hepatoblastoma aimed at increasing efficacy and, at the same time, decreasing toxicity. Thirty-three patients were treated with one course of carboplatin alone followed by three courses of carboplatin/5-fluorouracil/vincristine. Patients whose tumours remained unresectable or who had stable disease or progression during this treatment were given two courses of high-dose cisplatin and etoposide. Fifty-five per cent of patients had a partial response to carboplatin alone, 24 of 30 assessable patients responded to carboplatin/5-fluorouracil/vincristine, and nine out of 12 patients had a response to high-dose cisplatin/etoposide. Complete tumour resection was achieved in 58 per cent and 5-year EFS was 48 ± 9 per cent.[84]

In a pilot study, Ortega et al.[85] investigated the efficacy of increasing the dose intensity of platinum compounds by alternating courses of carboplatin and cisplatin every 2 weeks. Thirteen newly diagnosed patients (two stage I, one stage II, seven stage III and three stage IV) were entered into the study, and after four courses of chemotherapy, 10 were evaluable for response. Two patients had a complete response and eight a partial response. Nine patients were alive, with no evidence of disease at a minimum follow-up of 21 months.[85] The US Children's Oncology Group (COG) is now running a randomized study of cisplatin/vincristine/5-fluorouracil vs. carboplatin/cisplatin for patients with unresectable hepatoblastoma. Patients with a completely resected pure fetal hepatoblastoma with a low mitotic rate are treated with surgery alone and observed carefully.

The German group (GPOH) has used carboplatin and etoposide in patients with advanced or recurrent hepatoblastoma. All these children had received prior treatment with ifosfamide/cisplatin/doxorubicin according to the HB 89 or HB 94 protocols.[66,86] Two patients with advanced disease only received carboplatin/etoposide after resection of the primary tumour and neither has relapsed. Five out of 12 patients treated after relapse showed a partial response; in one patient the lung metastases disappeared completely after two courses of carboplatin/etoposide. One patient had stable disease and five had progressive disease. Grade III/IV myelotoxicity was observed in seven patients. Seven patients eventually died of disease. The German group suggest that high doses of carboplatin and etoposide with stem cell rescue may be worthwhile investigating for the treatment of patients with recurrent hepatoblastoma.[87]

The SIOPEL group continues to recommend primary chemotherapy for all patients. In their second and third studies (SIOPEL 2 and 3), information on prognostic factors from SIOPEL 1 has been used to stratify patients as either 'standard risk' or 'high risk' of progression/relapse.[82] Standard-risk patients are those with tumour confined to the liver and involving no more than three sectors (PRETEXT I, II, III), and high-risk patients are those with PRETEXT IV tumours and/or with evidence of extrahepatic disease. SIOPEL 2 was a pilot study to test the efficacy of cisplatin alone for standard-risk patients, and to investigate the feasibility and toxicity of intensifying the PLADO regimen for high-risk patients. As in SIOPEL 1, all patients have delayed surgery, from 12 to 24 weeks after diagnosis. The rationale behind this plan was to eliminate the risk of cardiotoxicity for patients with a favourable outlook, using only the most active agent as monotherapy.[88] In the high-risk group, the intensity of treatment with platinum derivatives was increased, as in the pilot study of Ortega et al.,[85] by alternating the administration of cisplatin with carboplatin every 2 weeks. In the SIOPEL schedule, however, doxorubicin was also given with each course of carboplatin.

The results for the standard-risk study are extremely encouraging, with a response rate to cisplatin alone of

90 per cent, a complete macroscopic resection rate of 97 per cent, 3-year OS of 91 per cent and EFS of 89 per cent. The corresponding figures for the high-risk patients are 78, 67, 53 and 48 per cent, respectively.[89] Monotherapy with cisplatin followed by delayed surgery therefore seems to be effective treatment for most patients with 'standard risk' hepatoblastoma. Conclusive evidence for this should come from SIOPEL 3, the current randomized trial of the SIOPEL group comparing, again for 'standard risk' patients, cisplatin/surgery and cisplatin/doxorubicin/surgery (the SIOPEL 1 regimen). In SIOPEL 3, patients with a serum AFP level <100 µg/L are included in the 'high-risk' study regardless of PRETEXT category because results from SIOPEL 1 and 2 seem to indicate that these patients have a poor prognosis.[90]

The survival for hepatoblastoma patients has improved dramatically since the introduction of cisplatin and doxorubicin, but those who present with advanced disease, either an extensive primary tumour (PRETEXT IV) or lung metastases, still have only a moderate prognosis.[91] This may in part be due to the development of drug resistance,[92] so the search is now on for a more effective regimen for these patients. Xenograft models have already confirmed the activity of cisplatin, ifosfamide, doxorubicin, carboplatin and etoposide against hepatoblastoma.[93] In these experiments, the efficacy of chemotherapy was judged by analysis of decrease in serum AFP, decrease of proliferative activity in tumour cells, and histological regression of the tumour. Cisplatin and doxorubicin were the most effective agents, ifosfamide and carboplatin showed moderate activity, but etoposide as a single agent was ineffective. Paclitaxel, topotecan and irinotecan may also be useful agents in the treatment of hepatoblastoma.[94,95,95a] The COG and SIOPEL groups are planning a joint phase II study of irinotecan in relapsed and resistant hepatoblastoma.

At present, hepatocellular carcinomas are treated with the same protocols as hepatoblastoma, but survival for the majority of patients is poor (Table 22.4). In the SIOPEL 3 study, all patients with hepatocellular carcinoma are given the 'high-risk' chemotherapy, but primary surgery is advised, if feasible, as these tumours are not so chemosensitive as hepatoblastoma. Chemotherapy is justified because some patients have a definite response to PLADO and an unresectable tumour may become resectable. The problem is that many hepatocellular carcinomas are multifocal or metastatic, or both, so new treatment strategies are certainly needed for this tumour. Chemoembolization has been tried for both unresectable hepatoblastoma and hepatocellular carcinoma. In a feasibility study by Malogolowkin et al.,[99] nine patients (six with hepatoblastoma, and three with hepatocellular carcinoma) were treated with hepatic arterial chemoembolization. All nine patients responded to this treatment. Surgical resection was then achieved in five

patients, and three patients are alive with no evidence of disease. In another study by Arcement et al.,[100] 14 patients (seven with hepatoblastoma and seven with hepatocellular carcinoma) with unresectable tumours were treated with intra-arterial cisplatin and/or doxorubicin chemotherapy after failing systemic chemotherapy.[100] There was a response in some patients, but it was insufficient to enable complete resection of tumour by partial hepatectomy. Six patients then had an orthotopic liver transplant, three after a further decrease in AFP level, but only one patient had further tumour shrinkage. Another patient showed a response and is awaiting transplant. Four patients had progressive disease.

Immunotargeted chemotherapy is another new treatment under trial. Five children, three with hepatoblastoma and two with hepatocellular carcinoma, were treated with doxorubicin or cisplatin conjugated with anti-AFP antibody. Although two hepatoblastoma patients responded, there was no change in the volume of the hepatocellular carcinomas.[101]

In adults with hepatocellular carcinoma, a variety of treatments, including cryosurgery, thermotherapy, high-dose intra-arterial chemotherapy under hepatic venous isolation, and haemoperfusion, have been investigated, usually in a palliative setting.[102–104] Paclitaxel has also been used but with disappointing results.[105]

Although the survival for patients with hepatocellular carcinoma is poor, around 50 per cent of patients show a response to PLADO chemotherapy. The problem is that many tumours still remain unresectable. As yet, no other chemotherapeutic agent has been identified which produces a better response in hepatocellular carcinoma. Since increased expression of various angiogenesis factors is associated with hepatocellular carcinoma, and angiogenesis inhibitors have been shown to suppress growth and invasiveness of hepatocellular carcinomas, both in vitro and in vivo,[106] anti-angiogenesis agents are now under trial. A possible option is to combine cisplatin and/or doxorubicin with an anti-angiogenesis agent.

Orthotopic liver transplantation

The child with a unifocal or multifocal hepatocellular carcinoma or hepatoblastoma involving all four sectors of the liver (PRETEXT IV), or a tumour involving the hilum of the liver, presents a particular therapeutic challenge, as complete tumour resection may only be possible if liver transplantation is performed. These patients used to account for only a small percentage of liver transplants in children because the tumour recurrence rate was so high. In a study from Brussels in the mid-1980s, for instance, only two out of 52 patients were transplanted because of tumour.[107] However, recent studies have shown that orthotopic liver transplantation should be seriously considered for patients with hepatoblastoma who still have unresectable disease after response to chemotherapy. In the SIOPEL-1 study, 12 patients – five of whom had lung metastases at diagnosis – had liver transplantation after response to chemotherapy, including clearing of lung metastases. Six were transplanted after PLADO chemotherapy, three had additional chemotherapy, two were transplanted at relapse and one patient was transplanted because of left hepatic vein obstruction after right trisegmentectomy. Eight patients are alive with no evidence of disease at a median of 99 months from transplant. Two patients died from relapse, one of whom was transplanted for relapse. The two other patients died from tumour-unrelated causes.[108] In a series from the United States, six out of 12 children with hepatoblastoma treated by chemotherapy plus liver transplantation are alive 24–70 months after transplantation.[109] In this study, patients with unifocal, intrahepatic disease had a better prognosis than those with multifocal disease or extrahepatic spread. Because of the shortage of donor organs, patients should be selected for liver transplantation with extreme care, and the procedure carried out in a quaternary referral centre. Survival rates for children with hepatoblastoma treated with orthotopic liver transplantation have improved over recent years and are between 60 and 80 per cent, so there is now a strong feeling that patients who present with a tumour involving all four hepatic sectors should be referred to a transplant centre early in the course of their treatment if they show a response to chemotherapy.[110–112] Living related donors are being used in some centres. The advantage of this procedure is that the transplant can be timed precisely to fit in with the chemotherapy schedule.[113,114] Lung metastases that clear with chemotherapy are now not thought to be a contraindication to transplantation.[91,108]

The results for hepatocellular carcinoma are not so good but survival rates ranging from 44 to 63 per cent have been reported.[111,112] Patient selection is clearly crucial. Vascular invasion, distant metastases and lymph node involvement are adverse prognostic factors for recurrence.

MALIGNANT MESENCHYMAL TUMOURS

These tumours, which comprise 9–15 per cent of primary malignant childhood liver tumours,[2,115] include rhabdomyosarcoma, angiosarcoma,[116] fibrosarcoma and undifferentiated (embryonal) sarcoma. Rhabdomyosarcoma of the biliary tree – the only paediatric liver tumour commonly to present with jaundice – is discussed in Chapter 17. Undifferentiated sarcoma is the most common of the various types – absence of differentiated components, e.g. rhabdomyoblasts, precludes diagnosis by cell type. Undifferentiated sarcomas occur most often in children aged between 6 and 10 years. In the largest series,[113] the sex incidence was equal, but two smaller series[111,114] report a male predominance. The commonest presenting symptoms are an abdominal mass, abdominal pain and fever. Jaundice is unusual. Full blood count and liver function tests are usually normal, and serum AFP is never elevated. Imaging studies show a space-occupying lesion which may be solid or cystic, and hyper- or hypovascular. Tumours are well demarcated from the surrounding liver but are not encapsulated. The cut surface is gelatinous or glistening and yellowish-grey to tan in colour. Half the tumours have multiple cystic areas. Most of the tumour is made up of sarcomatous elements. The cells are stellate or spindle-shaped, with round, elongated or irregular-shaped nuclei, and may be closely packed or scattered loosely in an acid mucopolysaccharide material. Reticulin and collagen fibres may also be present. Multinucleate giant cells are seen and mitoses are frequent. Clusters of distorted 'normal' hepatocytes and bile duct-like structures may be found at the periphery of the tumour.[117]

The prognosis of these tumours used to be poor. In a retrospective study of 31 patients with undifferentiated sarcomas diagnosed between 1955 and 1975,[118] partial or complete resection was attempted in 23 patients, nine had chemotherapy, seven had chemotherapy and radiotherapy, and three had radiotherapy alone. Only six patients survived, with a median survival of 9 months (range 2–52 months). In an Italian study[115] of eight patients diagnosed between 1975 and 1981, and treated with surgery and chemotherapy, two had initial complete resection and a third had a complete resection after chemotherapy (doxorubicin, cyclophosphamide, vincristine and 5-fluorouracil) followed by radiotherapy to microscopic residual disease. Two of these patients survive at 14 and 60 months, but there were no survivors of unresectable disease. In a study by Horowitz et al.,[118] five patients with undifferentiated sarcoma and three with embryonal rhabdomyosarcoma, with no bile duct involvement, were treated with surgery and chemotherapy (vincristine, doxorubicin, actinomycin, cyclophosphamide ± DTIC). Six had measurable disease after surgery. Two had a complete response, two a partial response and one an 'objective response' to chemotherapy, and one had a partial response to combined chemotherapy and radiotherapy. Median survival was 19.5 months (range 6–73+ months). Two patients who had lung metastases at diagnosis had metastases to brain or bone at death.

Articles published in the 1990s suggest an improved survival for patients with undifferentiated sarcoma of the liver using a multimodal therapeutic regimen.[119,120] In the most recent study from the Italian and German groups, 17 patients were treated between 1979 and 1995, with conservative surgery at diagnosis, multiagent chemotherapy using combinations of vincristine, actinomycin D, cyclophosphamide, doxorubicin or ifosfamide, vincristine, actinomycin D and doxorubicin, and second-look surgery for residual disease.[121] Eight patients had complete tumour resection either at diagnosis or after preoperative chemotherapy and all survive. Six out of nine evaluable patients showed a response to preoperative chemotherapy. Twelve patients are alive with no evidence of disease 2.4–20 years from diagnosis. Treatment of these tumours with surgery and appropriate (sarcoma-type) multiagent chemotherapy may be curative. The role of radiotherapy has not yet been defined.

BENIGN TUMOURS

Benign tumours account for 33 per cent of primary liver tumours in children (Table 22.1).[2] The most common (40–60 per cent) are the vascular tumours haemangioma and haemangioendothelioma, although the distinction between the two is not always made in published reports.[2,122] Microscopically, haemangiomas are composed of dilated vascular spaces lined by one or more layers of endothelium, separated by connective tissue containing fibroblasts. Areas of thrombus, haemorrhage and calcification may be seen. Haemangioendotheliomas are composed of vascular channels lined by endothelial cells. Tumours may be single or multiple and the majority present within the first 6 months of life. Presenting symptoms are usually abdominal distension and/or congestive cardiac failure. Cutaneous haemangiomas may be present. Stippled calcification may be seen on plain abdominal X-ray. CT scanning or Doppler ultrasonography with a rapid scanning technique will demonstrate abnormal flow patterns. Abnormal vascular lesions retain contrast and appear brighter than the surrounding normal liver. Angiography confirms the highly vascular nature of the tumour.

Tumours commonly undergo spontaneous regression after the age of 12 months, but treatment may be necessary prior to this because of intractable cardiac failure and/or a Kasabach–Merritt syndrome. Ten out of 11 patients reported by Davenport et al. in a series from King's College Hospital, London, treated over a 20-year period, were symptomatic and the majority needed intensive medical treatment because of cardiac failure.[123] In this series, patients with bilobar disease were treated with ligation of the hepatic artery and those with localized haemangioendothelioma had the tumour resected. Other treatment options include corticosteroids, hepatic artery embolization, cytotoxic drugs, e.g. cyclophosphamide, or radiotherapy, but none of these approaches is reliable and it is often hard to be sure whether tumour regression is spontaneous or treatment-induced.[122,124,125]

Mesenchymal hamartoma is the second most common benign tumour (30 per cent) and usually occurs in children under 2 years old. These tumours have now been detected antenatally.[126] The commonest presenting symptom is abdominal distension, shown on imaging to be due to a solitary cystic avascular mass. Serum AFP level may be slightly elevated due to production by adjacent proliferating hepatocytes.[127] Tumours are well demarcated and composed of cysts of various sizes filled with clear fluid or mucoid material. Treatment is by resection or enucleation.[128]

Focal nodular hyperplasia and adenoma are both extremely rare and account for only 9 per cent of benign tumours.[2] They are either discovered incidentally or present with asymptomatic hepatomegaly. Focal nodular hyperplasia is a solitary lesion which, on angiography, is highly vascular, resembling haemangioma, in 10–15 per cent of cases. Microscopically the tumour has a nodular appearance, with aggregates of hepatocytes and stellate fibrous tissue. Resection of the lesion should be performed unless tumour anatomy suggests a particularly difficult technical procedure. In such cases, 'observation only' is a reasonable policy, since spontaneous regression may occur.[129–131] Adenoma may be associated with glycogen storage disease or androgen therapy. Tumours are usually multiple, may be vascular and are composed of cords of hepatocytes several cells thick. Differentiation from a well-differentiated hepatocellular carcinoma may be difficult, so resection of the tumour and careful follow-up are advised. There are no clear-cut reports of elevated serum AFP levels in adenoma patients but a rising AFP may indicate transformation of adenoma to hepatocellular carcinoma.

CONTROVERSY AND CHALLENGE

In the past 10 years or so, childhood liver cancer has achieved a high degree of exposure, disproportionate to its incidence. The reason seems to be the recent greatly improved prognosis for patients with hepatoblastoma – 'a quantum leap' brought about not by 'mega-chemotherapy' with stem cell rescue, monoclonal antibodies or gene therapy but by logical and simple readjustment of standard-dose chemotherapy! Nonetheless, a number of contentious issues and challenges remain and some of them will be summarized here.

AETIOLOGY AND PATHOGENESIS

The 'two-hit' hypothesis presumably applies as much to hepatoblastoma as to other 'embryonal' cancers. Over the past 10 years, molecular research has directly implicated the beta-catenin gene at chromosome 5q21/5q22 (the FAP/APC locus) in the pathogenesis of hepatoblastoma.[10–15] This finding corroborates the clinical insight of those researchers who, in 1983, identified an 800- to

900-fold increased incidence of hepatoblastoma in infants carrying this gene.[8,9] Molecular analysis of hepatoblastomas shows that this mutation is a 'necessary though insufficient' pathogenetic element of some hepatoblastomas. Other hepatoblastoma-associated mutations, in what is presumably a multistep oncogenic process, have yet to be identified.

The intriguing recent observations, from Japan and the USA, that very low birth weight (<1000 g) may predispose to hepatoblastoma have to be followed up and corroborated, since the number of subjects is so small.[16–19] If verified, a plausible explanation must be proposed. In particular, it is hard to understand why the association should be 'tissue-specific' – amongst childhood cancers, only hepatoblastoma has an increased incidence in these patients. Meanwhile, there need not be undue alarm, since, even if the association is eventually confirmed, it can only account for a small proportion (probably <5 per cent) of all hepatoblastomas.

In areas where hepatitis B is endemic, the incidence of paediatric hepatocellular carcinoma is unequivocally raised and it is not necessarily preceded by cirrhosis.[24,26] Presumably, an alteration in hepatocyte proliferation caused by the hepatitis B virus is all that is needed for the generation of the unrepaired 'molecular mistakes' (mutations) that initiate tumour development. Taiwanese researchers who have demonstrated a clear-cut reduction of childhood hepatocellular carcinoma – hopefully succeeded, in the future, by a reduction of adult hepatocellular carcinoma – following the introduction of hepatitis B immunization are 'unsung heroes' in the field of cancer prevention.[25] In 'non-endemic' areas of the world, other influences, possibly including other viruses, are presumably at work.

HEPATOBLASTOMA – HOW MANY SUBTYPES?

A number of histopathological classifications have been proposed but despite pleas, over at least the last 10 years, for a 'common language', none is as yet universally agreed.[35,132] 'Pure fetal' histology is regarded by the North American COG pathologists as a 'favourable' histology, and worldwide there is a growing feeling that the macrotrabecular (often difficult to distinguish from hepatocellular carcinoma) and 'small-cell' subtypes are 'unfavourable' and that more intensive than average chemotherapy is indicated.[33,34] Collaboration between the various international groups will be needed if useful information on histopathological subtypes is to be collected within a reasonable time-frame.

Infants with AFP-negative hepatoblastoma, which seems to metastasize readily, have a very poor prognosis at present, and possibly do not have hepatoblastoma at all.[90] Cytogenetic and molecular studies on these tumours are needed urgently so that they can be classified more appropriately.

THE TREATMENT APPROACH – HEPATOBLASTOMA

There is a good deal of agreement these days about the treatment of hepatoblastoma.

Surgery, with complete or near-complete excision (i.e. microscopic residual), and chemotherapy are necessary. Cisplatin and doxorubicin are the 'best' drugs. The role of other established drugs (carboplatin, etoposide, 5-fluorouracil, ifosfamide, the vinca alkaloids, cyclophosphamide and actinomycin D) is less well defined and many probably make little or no additional contribution. As yet, there is no reliable information on the taxoids or the topoisomerase II inhibitors. 'Alternative' approaches, such as intra-arterial or liposome-encapsulated chemotherapy, embolization and antibody-guided ('targeted') therapy, are experimental.

There is, however, a major difference of principle between collaborative groups concerning juxtaposition of treatments. The issue can be summarized thus: is 'up-front' (primary) or 'delayed' surgery better? The 'Up-fronters' – the German/Austrian group, the Japanese group and most North American centres – point out that delayed surgery means that the surgical stage of the tumour can never be established and may obscure 'unfavourable' histological features, as has similarly been claimed for Wilms' tumour. They also point out that needle biopsy cannot provide a representative tumour sample. However, the German/Austrian group has recently changed its approach and in the current study (HB 99) all stages of hepatoblastoma are treated with preoperative chemotherapy. The 'Delayers' – the multinational SIOPEL group – acknowledge the problems inherent in needle biopsy but point out that surgical staging is no longer strictly necessary when chemotherapy is so effective, and that 'unfavourable' subtypes of hepatoblastoma are rarer than in Wilms' (probably <5 per cent compared with 12–15 per cent) and that there is no uniform agreement, as yet, as to which hepatoblastoma variants are the 'bad actors'. They also point out several unequivocal advantages to preoperative chemotherapy: it makes the tumour much less vascular and more circumscribed, and thereby increases the likelihood of safe total resection.

The best way to sort out this issue would be a randomized controlled trial, but such a study is never likely to be carried out. Recruitment would be seriously affected by both the 'subjective' feelings of clinicians about individual cases, especially when randomization offers the surgical option that is less popular in their particular centre, and the real difficulty in persuading families to take part in a 'toss of a coin' trial offering two such disparate treatment options. These difficulties were certainly experienced in the third Wilms' trial of the UK Children's Cancer Study Group (UKW3; Mitchell CD et al., unpublished data), in which a similar question was posed.

THE TREATMENT APPROACH – HEPATOCELLULAR CARCINOMA

There is a general consensus in favour of 'up-front' (primary) surgery, probably because chemotherapy is not nearly so effective in hepatocellular carcinoma as in hepatoblastoma. No patient with hepatocellular carcinoma is cured without surgical removal of the primary tumour, and there is no consistent response to any specific chemotherapy regimen. Yet, in the SIOPEL studies at least, there are data showing that a sizeable fraction (around 50 per cent) show some degree of response to PLADO, with a serial fall of serum AFP and radiological tumour shrinkage, so there may be a clinical benefit in some patients.[72] This feeling is endorsed by the fact that, these days, with consistent use of chemotherapy – a cisplatin-based combination is favoured – the 5-year OS for hepatocellular carcinoma patients is around 20–30 per cent compared with ≤10 per cent in the whole pre-chemotherapy era.[72,97,98] The probable improvement is all the more surprising given that many hepatocellular carcinoma patients have multifocal primary tumours and many – not necessarily the same patients – have pulmonary and/or other metastases.

Are more 'experimental' approaches justified? That is certainly the case in patients not responding to standard treatment, preferably in a carefully thought-out multicentre phase 1 or 2 trial.

A practical approach to the hepatocellular carcinoma patient might therefore be as follows: careful scanning to detect any metastases in lungs or elsewhere; then patients without detectable secondary deposits and 'operable' tumours should be treated with primary surgery followed by six courses of PLADO or an equivalent regimen; and patients with metastases should receive treatment with PLADO, up to six courses providing there is a response, then surgery. In the case of treatment failure, either phase I/II therapy or palliative care might be appropriate. All these treatment plans should accord with any accessible multicentre trial.

BEST PRACTICE AND RESOURCE IMPLICATIONS

One definition of 'clinical governance' is 'the best treatment carried out in one or more suitably equipped and resourced centres by appropriately trained, experienced personnel'. Most European countries and many in other continents have a network of children's cancer centres that deliver effective and safe chemotherapy, usually linking up with others to participate in clinical trials to expand the 'evidence base'. The same arrangements are not necessarily optimal when specialized paediatric tumour surgery is the issue, including surgery for hepatoblastoma and hepatocellular carcinoma. For best results, childhood liver surgery should be focused in a few centres, each covering, perhaps, a total population of 10–15 million so that real expertise – in preoperative, anaesthetic and post-surgical care, as well as the surgery itself – is developed. In those cases in which imaging suggests difficulty with complete excision of the tumour, because of tumour involving all four liver sectors (PRETEXT IV), or proximity to great vessels, a transplant team should be forewarned and, preferably, to hand. The cost implications of this strategy – usually an overall saving, since the complication rate should be lower – should be attractive to managers.

KEY POINTS

- Malignant liver tumours in children are rare.
- Hepatoblastoma is more common than hepatocellular carcinoma, other than in hepatitis B virus endemic areas.
- Hepatoblastoma is a tumour of infants and young children, whereas hepatocellular carcinoma occurs in older children and adolescents.
- The prognosis for hepatoblastoma has improved dramatically over the past 20 years with the use of chemotherapy in addition to surgery.
- Cisplatin and doxorubicin are currently the 'best' drugs.
- Serum AFP level is a vital tumour marker for most hepatoblastomas and many hepatocellular carcinomas.
- Orthotopic liver transplantation should be seriously considered for hepatoblastoma patients who still have an unresectable primary tumour after a response to chemotherapy.
- Histopathological classification of subtypes of hepatoblastoma, which may have prognostic significance, is still a matter of debate.
- Primary liver sarcomas should be treated according to contemporary soft tissue sarcoma protocols.
- There are no standard treatment protocols for benign tumours.

REFERENCES

◆1. Ishak KG, Glunz PR. Hepatoblastoma and hepatocarcinoma in infancy and childhood. *Cancer* 1967; **20**: 396–422.

◆2. Exelby PR, Filler RM, Grosfeld JL. Liver tumours in children with particular reference to hepatoblastoma and hepatocellular carcinoma: American Academy of Pediatrics Surgical Section Survey-1974. *J Pediatr Surg* 1975; **10**: 329–37.

3. Koufos A, Hansen MF, Copeland NG *et al.* Loss of hetero-zygosity in three embryonal tumours suggests a common pathogenetic mechanism. *Nature* 1985; **316**: 330–4.

4. Bryne JA, Simms LA, Little MH *et al.* Three non-overlapping regions of chromosome arm 11p allele loss identified in infantile tumours of adrenal and liver. *Genes Chromosom Cancer* 1993; **8**: 104–11.

5. Albrecht S, von Schweinitz D, Waha A *et al.* Loss of maternal alleles on chromosome arm 11p in hepatoblastoma. *Cancer Res* 1994; **54**: 5041–4.

6. Kraus JA, Albrecht S, Wiestler OD *et al.* Loss of heterozygosity on chromosome 1 in human hepatoblastoma. *Int J Cancer* 1996; **67**: 467–71.

7. Parada LA, Limon J, Iliszko M *et al.* Cytogenetics of hepato-blastoma: further characterization of 1q rearrangements by fluorescence in situ hybridization. *Med Pediatr Oncol* 2000; **34**: 165–70.

♦8. Kingston JE, Herbert A, Draper GJ, Mann JR. Association between hepatoblastoma and polyposis coli. *Arch Dis Child* 1983; **58**: 959–62.

9. Garber JE, Li FP, Kingston JE *et al.* Hepatoblastoma and familial adenomatous polyposis. *J Natl Cancer Inst* 1988; **80**: 1626–8.

10. Bodmer WF, Bailey CJ, Bodmer J *et al.* Localisation of the gene for familial adenomatous polyposis on chromosome 5. *Nature* 1987; **328**: 614–16.

10a. Thomas D, Pritchard J, Davidson R *et al.* Familial hepatoblastoma and ADC gene mutations. *Eur J Cancer* 2003; **39**: 2200–4.

11. Koch A, Denkhaus D, Albrecht S *et al.* Childhood hepatoblastomas frequently carry a mutated degradation targeting box of the beta-catenin gene. *Cancer Res* 1999; **59**: 269–73.

12. Oda H, Imai Y, Nakatsuru Y *et al.* Somatic mutations of the APC gene in sporadic hepatoblastoma. *Cancer Res* 1996; **15**: 3320–3.

13. Takayasu H, Horie H, Hiyama E. Frequent deletions and mutations of the beta-catenin gene are associated with overexpression of cyclin D, and fibronectin and poorly differentiated histology in childhood hepatoblastoma. *Clin Cancer Res* 2001; **7**: 901–8.

14. Wei Y, Fabre M, Branchereau S *et al.* Activation of beta catenin in epithelial and mesenchymal hepatoblastoma. *Oncogene* 2000; **19**: 498–504.

15. Park WS, Oh RR, Park JY *et al.* Nuclear localization of beta catenin is an important prognostic factor in hepatoblastoma. *J Pathol* 2001; **193**: 483–90.

16. Ikeda H, Matsuyama S, Tanimura M. Association between hepatoblastoma and low birth weight: a trend or chance? *J Pediatr* 1997; **130**: 516–17.

17. Ross JA, Gurney JG. Hepatoblastoma incidence in the United States from 1973 to 1992. *Med Pediatr Oncol* 1998; **30**: 141–2.

18. Tanimura M, Matsui I, Abe J *et al.* Increased risk of hepatoblastoma among immature children with a lower birth weight. *Cancer Res* 1998; **58**: 3032–5.

19. Maruyama K, Ikeda H, Koizumi T *et al.* Case-control study of perinatal factors and hepatoblastoma in children with an extremely low birthweight. *Pediatr Int* 2000; **42**: 492–8.

20. Kasai M, Watanabe I. Histologic classification of liver cell carcinoma in infancy and childhood and its clinical evaluation. *Cancer* 1970; **24**: 551–63

21. Fraumeni JF, Miller RW, Hill JA. Primary carcinoma of the liver in childhood: an epidemiologic study. *J Natl Cancer Inst* 1968; **40**: 1087–99.

♦22. Lack EE, Neave C, Vawter GF. Hepatocellular carcinoma. Review of 32 cases in childhood and adolescence. *Cancer* 1983; **50**: 1500–15.

23. Chen WJ, Lee JC, Hung WT. Primary malignant tumour of liver in infants and children in Taiwan. *J Pediatr Surg* 1988; **23**: 457–61.

24. Hsu H-C, Wu M-U, Chang M-H *et al.* Childhood hepatocellular carcinoma develops exclusively in hepatitis B surface antigen carriers in three decades in Taiwan. *J Hepatol* 1987; **5**: 260–7.

♦25. Chang M-H, Chen C-J, Lai M-S *et al.* Universal hepatitis B vaccination in Taiwan and the incidence of hepatocellular carcinoma in children. *N Engl J Med* 1997; **336**: 1855–9.

26. Leuschner I, Harms D, Schmidt D. The association of hepatocellular carcinoma in childhood with hepatitis B infection. *Cancer* 1988; **62**: 2363–9.

27. Perilongo G, Pontisso P, Basso G. Can primary cancer of the liver in western countries be prevented? Pediatric point of view. *Med Pediatr Oncol* 1990; **18**: 57–60.

28. Parkin DM, Kramarova E, Draper GJ *et al.*, eds. *International Incidence of Childhood Cancer*, vol II. IARC Scientific Publications No.144. Lyon: IARC, 1998.

29. Stiller C. International variations in the incidence of childhood carcinoma. *Cancer Epidemiol Biomarkers Prev* 1994; **3**: 305–10.

●30. Lack EE, Neave C, Vawter GF. Hepatoblastoma – a clinical and pathologic study of 54 cases. *Am J Surg Pathol* 1982; **6**: 693–705.

31. Stringer MD, Hennayake S, Howard ER *et al.* Improved outcome for children with hepatoblastoma. *Br J Surg* 1995; **82**: 386–91.

32. Willis RA. *Pathology of Tumours*, 2nd edn. St Louis: CV Mosby, 1953.

33. Haas JE, Muczynski KA, Krailo M *et al.* Histopathology and prognosis in childhood hepatoblastoma and hepatocarcinoma. *Cancer* 1989; **64**: 1082–95.

34. Weinberg AG, Finegold MJ. Primary hepatic tumours in childhood. In: Milton Finegold, ed. *Pathology of Neoplasia in Children and Adolescents: Major Problems in Pathology.* Philadelphia: WB Saunders,1986; 333–72.

35. MacKinlay GA, Pritchard J. A common language for childhood liver tumours. *Pediatr Surg Int* 1992; **7**: 325–6.

♦36. Saxena R, Leake JL, Shafford EA *et al.* Chemotherapy effects on hepatoblastoma. A histological study. *Am J Surg Pathol* 1993; **17**: 1266–71.

36a. Katzenstein HM, Krailo MD, Malogolowkin MH *et al.* Fibrolamellar hepatocellular carcinoma in children and adolescents. *Cancer* 2003; **97**: 2006–12.

37. Craig JR, Peters RL, Edmonson HA, Omata M. Fibrolamellar carcinoma of the liver. *Cancer* 1980; **46**: 372–9.

38. Prokurat A, Kluge P, Kosciesza A *et al.* Transitional liver cell tumours in older children and adolescents: a novel group of aggressive heaptic tumours expressing beta-catenin. *Med Pediatr Oncol* 2002; **359**: 510–18.

39. Ni Y-H, Chang M-H, Hsu H-Y *et al.* Hepatocellular carcinoma in childhood. Clinical manifestations and prognosis. *Cancer* 1991; **68**: 1737–41.

40. Nakagawara A, Ikeda K, Tsureyoshi M *et al.* Hepatoblastoma producing both alpha feto-protein and human chorionic gonadotrophin. *Cancer* 1985; **56**: 1636–49.

41. Shafford EA, Pritchard J. Extreme thrombocytosis as a diagnostic clue to hepatoblastoma. *Arch Dis Child* 1993; **68**: 88–90.

42. Nickerson HJ, Silberman TL, McDonald TP. Hepatoblastoma thrombocytosis and increased thrombopoietin. *Cancer* 1980; **45**: 315–17.

43. Wu JT, Book L, Sudar K. Serum alpha fetoprotein (αFP) levels in normal infants. *Pediatr Res* 1981; **15**: 50–2.

44. Pritchard J, Shafford EA, Spitz L *et al.* Cis platinum, doxorubicin and surgery for advanced hepatoblastoma; a real chance for cure? ASCO abstracts. *J Clin Oncol* 1989; **8**: 298.

•45. Ortega JA, Krailo MD, Haas JE *et al.* Effective treatment of unresectable or metastatic hepatoblastoma with cisplatin and continuous infusion doxorubicin. A report from the Children's Cancer Study Group. *J Clin Oncol* 1991; **9**: 2167–76.

46. Paradinas FJ, Melia WM, Wilkinson ML *et al.* High serum vitamin B_{12} binding capacity as a marker of the fibrolamellar variant of hepatocellular carcinoma. *Br Med J* 1982; **285**: 840–2.

47. de Campo J, Phelan E. Imaging of liver tumours in childhood. *Pediatr Surg Int* 1988; **4**: 1–6.

48. Dachman AH, Pakter RL, Ros PR *et al.* Hepatoblastoma: radiologic-pathologic correlation in 50 cases. *Radiology* 1987; **164**: 15–19.

49. Dorman F, Sumner E, Spitz L. Fatal intraoperative tumour embolism in a child with hepatoblastoma. *Anaesthesiology* 1985; **63**: 692–3.

50. Finn JP, Hall-Craggs MA, Dicks-Mireaux C *et al.* Primary malignant liver tumors in childhood: assessment of resectability with high-field MR and comparison with CT. *Pediatr Radiol* 1990; **21**: 34–8.

51. Ammann RA, Plaschkes J, Leibundgut K. Congenital hepatoblastoma a distinct entity? *Med Pediatr Oncol* 1999; **32**: 466–8.

52. Vos A. Primary liver tumours in children. *Eur J Surg Oncol* 1995; **21**: 101–5.

53. Mann JR, Kasthuri N, Raafat F *et al.* Malignant hepatic tumours in children: incidence clinical features and aetiology. *Pediatr Perinat Epidemiol* 1990; **4**: 276–89.

54. Schnater JM, Aronson DC, Plaschkes J *et al.* Surgical view of the treatment of patients with hepatoblastoma. Results of the first prospective trial of the International Society of Pediatric Oncology Liver Tumour Study Group (SIOPEL-1). *Cancer* 2002; **94**: 1111–20.

•55. Evans AE, Land VJ, Newton WA *et al.* Combination chemotherapy (vincristine, adriamycin, cyclophosphamide and 5-fluorouracil) in the treatment of children with malignant hepatoma. *Cancer* 1982; **50**: 821–6.

56. Quinn JJ, Altman AJ, Robinson T *et al.* Adriamycin and cisplatin for hepatoblastoma. *Cancer* 1985; **56**: 1926–9.

57. Brown TCK, Davidson PD, Auldist AW. Anaesthetic considerations in liver tumour resection in children. *Pediatr Surg Int* 1988; **4**: 11–15.

58. Davidson PM, Auldist AW. Surgical anatomy and operative techniques for elective hepatic resection in children. *Pediatr Surg Int* 1988; **4**: 7–10.

59. Black CT, Luck SR, Musemeche CA *et al.* Aggressive excision of pulmonary metastases is warranted in the management of childhood hepatic tumours. *J Pediatr Surg* 1991; **26**: 1082–5.

60. Feusner JH, Kralio MD, Haas JE *et al.* Treatment of pulmonary metastases of initial stage I hepatoblastoma in childhood. *Cancer* 1993; **71**: 859–64.

61. Passmore SJ, Noblett HR, Wisheart JD, Mott MG. Prolonged survival following multiple thoracotomies for metastatic hepatoblastoma. *Med Pediatr Oncol* 1995; **24**: 58–60.

62. Hermann RE, Lonsdale D. Chemotherapy, radiotherapy, and hepatic lobectomy for hepatoblastoma in an infant: report of a survival. *Surgery* 1970; **68**: 383–8.

63. Weinblatt ME, Siegel SE, Siegel MM *et al.* Preoperative chemotherapy for unresectable primary hepatic malignancies in children. *Cancer* 1982; **50**: 1061–4.

64. Douglass EC, Green AA, Wrenn E *et al.* Effective cisplatin (DDP) based chemotherapy in the treatment of hepatoblastoma. *Med Pediatr Oncol* 1985; **13**: 187–90.

•65. Pritchard J, Brown J, Shafford E *et al.* Cisplatin, doxorubicin and delayed surgery for childhood hepatoblastoma: a successful approach – results of the first prospective study of the International Society of Pediatric Oncology. *J Clin Oncol* 2000; **18**: 3819–28.

•66. von Schweinitz D, Byrd DJ, Hecker H *et al.* Efficiency and toxicity of ifosfamide, cisplatin and doxorubicin in the treatment of childhood hepatoblastoma. *Eur J Cancer* 1997; **33**: 1243–9.

•67. Douglass EC, Reynolds M, Finegold M *et al.* Cisplatin, vincristine and fluorouracil therapy for hepatoblastoma: a Pediatric Oncology Group Study. *J Clin Oncol* 1993; **11**: 96–9.

68. Brock P, Pritchard J, Bellman S, Pinkerton CR. Ototoxicity of high-dose cisplatinum in children (letter). *Med Pediatr Oncol* 1988; **16**: 368–9.

69. Legha SS, Benjamin RS, Mackay B *et al.* Reduction of doxorubicin cardiotoxicity by prolonged continuous intravenous infusion. *Ann Intern Med* 1982; **96**: 133–9.

70. Lipshultz SE, Giantris AL, Lipsitz SR *et al.* Doxorubicin administration by continuous infusion is not cardioprotective: The Dana-Farber 91-01 acute lymphoblastic leukaemia protocol. *J Clin Oncol* 2002; **20**: 1677–82.

71. Vermorken JB, Kapteijn TS, Hart AA, Pinedo HM. Ototoxicity of cis-diamminedichloroplatinum (II): influence of dose, schedule and mode of administration. *Eur J Cancer Clin Oncol* 1983; **19**: 53–8.

•72. Czauderna P, MacKinlay G, Perilongo G *et al.* Hepatocellular carcinoma in children – results of the first prospective study of the International Society of Pediatric Oncology Group. *J Clin Oncol* 2002; **20**: 2798–804

73. Habrand JL, Nehme D, Kalifa C *et al.* Is there a place for radiation therapy in the management of hepatoblastoma and hepatocellular carcinomas in children? *Int J Radiat Oncol Biol Phys* 1992; **23**: 675–6.

74. Pritchard J, da Cunha A, Cornbleet MA, Carter CJ. Alpha feto protein monitoring of response to doxorubicin in hepatoblastoma. *J Pediatr Surg* 1982; **17**: 429–30.

75. Wheeler K, Pritchard J, Luck W, Rossiter M. Transcobalamin I as a 'marker' for fibrolamellar hepatoma. *Med Pediatr Oncol* 1986; **14**: 227–9.

76. Brugieres L, Plaschkes J, MacKinlay G *et al.* Hepatoblastoma – microscopic residual disease after delayed surgery; prognostic implications. Abstract O-33. *Med Pediatr Oncol* 2000; **35**: 177.

77. Dall'Igna P, Cecchetto G, Dominici C *et al.* Carboplatin and doxorubicin (CARDOX) for nonmetastatic hepatoblastoma: a

discouraging pilot study. *Med Pediatr Oncol* 2001; **36**: 332–4.

78. Conran RM, Hitchcock CL, Waclawiw MA *et al.* Hepatoblastoma: the prognostic significance of histologic type. *Pediatr Pathol* 1992; **12**: 167–83.

79. Haas JE, Feusner JH, Finegold MJ. Small cell undifferentiated histology in hepatoblastoma may be unfavourable. *Cancer* 2001; **92**: 3130–4.

•80. Von Schweinitz D, Wischmeyer P, Leuschner I *et al.* Clinico-pathological criteria with prognostic relevance in hepatoblastoma. *Eur J Cancer* 1994; **30**: 1052–8.

•81. Van Tornout JM, Buckley JD, Quinn J *et al.* Timing and magnitude of decline in alpha fetoprotein levels in treated children with unresectable or metastatic hepatoblastoma are predictors of outcome: a report from the Children's Cancer Group. *J Clin Oncol* 1997; **15**: 1190–7.

•82. Brown J, Perilongo G, Shafford E *et al.* Pretreatment prognostic factors for children with hepatoblastoma – results from the International Society of Pediatric Oncology (SIOP) study SIOPEL 1. *Eur J Cancer* 2000; **36**: 1418–25.

•83. Ortega JA, Douglass EC, Feusner JH *et al.* Randomised comparison of cisplatin/vincristine/fluorouracil and cisplatin/continuous infusion doxorubicin for the treatment of pediatric hepatoblastoma: a report from the Children's Cancer Group and the Pediatric Oncology Group. *J Clin Oncol* 2000; **18**: 2665–75.

84. Katzenstein HM, London WB, Douglass EC *et al.* Treatment of unresectable and metastatic hepatoblastoma: a Pediatric Oncology Group phase II study. *J Clin Oncol* 2002; **20**: 3438–44

85. Ortega JA, Rios P, Malogolowkin MH. Successful treatment of hepatoblastoma with an intensified platinum regimen. ASCO abstract 2091. *J Clin Oncol* 1998; **17**: 545a.

86. Fuchs J, Rydzynski J, von Schweinitz D *et al.* Pretreatment prognostic factors and treatment results in children with hepatoblastoma. A report from the German Cooperative Pediatric Liver Tumour Study HB 94. *Cancer* 2002; **95**: 172–82.

•87. Fuchs J, Bode U, von Schweinitz D *et al.* Analysis of treatment efficiency of carboplatin and etoposide in combination with radical surgery in advanced and recurrrent childhood hepatoblastoma: a report of the German Cooperative Pediatric Liver Tumor Study HB 89 and HB 94. *Klin Padiatr* 1999; **4**: 305–9.

88. Black CT, Cangir A, Choroszy M, Andrassy RJ. Marked response to preoperative high-dose cis-platinum in children with unresectable hepatoblastoma. *J Pediatr Surg* 1991; **26**: 1070–3.

•89. Perilongo G, Shafford E, Maibach R *et al.* Risk-adapted treatment for childhood hepatoblastoma. Final report of the second study of the International Society of Paediatric Oncology – SIOPEL 2. *Eur J Cancer* 2004; **40**: 411–21.

90. Brugieres L, Shafford E, Brock P *et al.* Hepatoblastoma presenting with low alpha foetoprotein value, an aggressive tumour. Abstract O-32. *Med Pediatr Oncol* 2000; **35**: 177.

•91. Perilongo G, Brown J, Shafford E *et al.* Hepatoblastoma presenting with lung metastases. Treatment results of the first cooperative prospective study of the International Society of Pediatric Oncology on childhood liver tumors. *Cancer* 2000; **89**: 1845–53.

92. von Schweinitz D, Hecker D, Harms D *et al.* Complete resection before development of drug resistance is essential for survival from advanced hepatoblastoma – a report from the German Cooperative pediatric Liver Tumor Study HB 89. *J Pediatr Surg* 1995; **30**: 845–52.

93. Fuchs J, Wenderoth M, von Schweinitz D *et al.* Comparative activity of cisplatin, ifosfamide, doxorubicin, carboplatin, and etoposide in heterotransplanted hepatoblastoma. *Cancer* 1998; **83**: 2400–7.

94. Fuchs J, Habild G, Leuschener I *et al.* Paclitaxel: an effective antineoplastic agent in the treatment of xenotransplanted hepatoblastoma. *Med Pediatr Oncol* 1999; **32**: 209–15.

95. Warmann SW, Fuchs J, Wilkens L *et al.* Successful therapy of subcutaneously growing human hepatoblastoma xenografts with topotecan. *Med Pediatr Oncol* 2000; **37**: 449–54.

95a. Palmer RD, Williams DM. Dramatic response of multiply relapsed hepatoblastoma to irinotecan (CPT 11). *Med Pediatr Oncol* 2003; **41**: 78–80.

96. von Schweinitz, Burger D, Bode *et al.* Results of the HB-89 study in treatment of malignant epithelial tumours in childhood and concept of a new HB-94 protocol. *Klin Padiatr* 1994; **206**: 282–8.

97. Fuchs J, Bode U, Rydzinsky J *et al.* Hepatocellular carcinoma in children: clinical review of the data of the German Cooperative Pediatric liver tumour Study HB-94. Abstract P-130. *Med Pediatr Oncol* 2000; **35**: 254.

98. Katzenstein HM, Krailo, Malogolowkin MH *et al.* Hepatocellular carcinoma in children and adolescents: results from the Pediatric Oncology Group and the Children's Cancer Group Intergroup study. *J Clin Oncol* 2002; **20**: 2789–97

99. Malogolowkin MH, Stanley P, Steele DA, Ortega JA. Feasibility and toxicity of chemoembolization for children with liver tumours. *J Clin Oncol* 2000; **18**: 1279–84.

100. Arcement CM, Towbin RB, Meza MP *et al.* Intrahepatic chemoembolization in unresectable pediatric liver malignancies. *Pediatr Radiol* 2000; **30**: 779–85.

101. Hata H, Takada N, Sasaki F *et al.* Immunotargeting chemotherapy for AFP-producing pediatric liver cancer using conjugates of anti-AFP antibody and anti-tumor agents. *J Pediatr Surg* 1992; **27**: 724–7.

102. Whang-Peng J, Chao Y. Clinical trials of HCC in Taiwan. *Hepatogastroenterology* 1998; **45**: 1937–43.

103. Adam R, Akpinar E, Johann M *et al.* Place of cryosurgery in the treatment of malignant liver tumours. *Ann Surg* 1997; **225**: 38–9.

104. Ravikumar TS, Pizzorno G, Bodden W *et al.* Percutaneous hepatic vein isolation and high-dose hepatic arterial infusion chemotherapy for unresectable liver tumours. *J Clin Oncol* 1994; **12**: 2723–36.

105. Chao Y, Chan WK, Birkhofer MJ *et al.* Phase II and pharmokinetic study of paclitaxel therapy for unresectable hepatocellular carcinoma patients. *Br J Cancer* 1998; **78**: 34–9.

106. Wang L, Tang ZY, Qin LX *et al.* High-dose and long-term therapy with interferon-alfa inhibits tumor growth and recurrence in nude mice bearing human hepatocellular carcinoma xenografts with high metastatic potential. *Hepatology* 2000; **32**: 43–8.

107. Otte JB, Yandza T, de Ville de Goyet J *et al.* Pediatric liver transplantation: report on 52 patients with a 2 year survival of 86%. *J Pediatr Surg* 1988; **23**: 250–3.

108. Otte JB, Pritchard J, Aronson DC *et al.* Liver transplantation for hepatoblastoma: results from the International Society of Pediatric Oncology (SIOP) study SIOPEL-1 and review of the world experience. *Pediatr Blood Cancer* 2004; **42**: 74–83.

109. Koneru B, Flye MW, Busuttil W *et al.* Liver transplantation for hepatoblastoma. The American Experience. *Ann Surg* 1991; **213**: 118–21.

110. Al-Qabandi W, Jenkinson HC, Buckels JA *et al.* Orthotopic liver transplantation for unresectable hepatoblastoma; a single center's experience. *J Pediatr Surg* 1999; **34**: 1261–4.

111. Reyes JD, Carr B, Dvorchik I *et al.* Liver transplantation and chemotherapy for hepatoblastoma and hepatocellular cancer in childhood and adolescence. *J Pediatr* 2000; **136**: 795–804.

112. Tagge EP, Tagge DU, Reyes J *et al.* Resection, including transplantation, for hepatoblastoma and hepatocellular carcinoma: impact on survival. *J Pediatr Surg* 1992; **27**: 292–7.

113. Chardot C, Saint Marie C, Gilles A *et al.* Living-related liver transplantation and vena cava reconstruction after total hepatectomy including the vena cava for hepatoblastoma. *Transplantation* 2002; **73**: 90–2.

♦114. Dower NA, Smith LJ. Liver transplantation for malignant liver tumours in children. *Med Pediatr Oncol* 2000; **34**: 136–40.

115. Perilongo G, Carli M, Sainati L *et al.* Undifferentiated (embryonal) sarcoma of the liver in childhood: results of a retrospective Italian study. *Tumori* 1987; **73**: 213–17.

116. Awan S, Davenport M, Portmann B, Howard ER. Angiosarcoma of the liver in children. *J Pediatr Surg* 1996; **31**: 1729–32.

117. Stocker JT, Ishak KG. Undifferentiated (embryonal) sarcoma of the liver: report of 31 cases. *Cancer* 1987; **42**: 336–48.

118. Horowitz ME, Etcubanas E, Webber BL *et al.* Hepatic undifferentiated (embryonal) sarcoma and rhabdomyosarcoma in children: results of therapy. *Cancer* 1987; **59**: 396–402.

119. Urban CE, Mache CJ, Schwinger W *et al.* Undifferentiated (embryonal) sarcoma of the liver in childhood. *Cancer* 1993; **72**: 2511–16.

120. Webber EM, Morrison KB, Pritchard SL, Sorensen PH. Undifferentiated embryonal sarcoma of the liver; results of clinical management in one centre. *J Pediatr Surg* 1999; **34**: 1641–4.

121. Bisogno G, Pilz T, Perilongo G *et al.* Undifferentiated sarcoma of the liver in childhood: a curable disease. *Cancer* 2002; **94**: 252–7.

122. Ehren H, Mahour GH, Isaacs H. Benign liver tumours in infancy and childhood: report of 48 cases. *Am J Surg* 1983; **145**: 325–9.

123. Davenport M, Hansen L, Heaton N, Howard ER. Hemangioendothelioma of the liver in infants. *J Pediatr Surg* 1995; **30**: 44–8.

124. Cornelius AS, Womer RB, Jakacki R. Multiple haemangioendotheliomas of the liver. *Med Pediatr Oncol* 1989; **17**: 501–4.

125. Prokurat A, Kluge P, Chrupek M *et al.* Haemangioma of the liver in children: proliferating vascular tumour or congenital vascular malformation? *Med Pediatr Oncol* 2002; **39**: 524–9.

126. Bessho T, Kubota K, Komori S *et al.* Prenatally detected hepatic hamartoma: another cause of non-immune hydrops. *Prenat Diagn* 1996; **16**: 337–41.

127. Ito H, Kishikawa T, Toda T *et al.* Hepatic mesenchymal hamartoma of an infant. *J Pediatr Surg* 1984; **19**(3): 315–17.

128. Murray JD, Ricketts RR. Mesenchymal hamartoma of the liver. *Am Surg* 1998; **64**: 1097–103.

129. Hutton KA, Spicer RD, Arthur RK, Batcup G. Focal nodular hyperplasia of the liver in childhood. *Eur J Pediatr Surg* 1993; **3**: 370–2.

130. Reymond D, Aebi C, Hirt A *et al.* Focal nodular hyperplasia of the liver in childhood. *Med Pediatr Oncol* 1993; **21**: 283–6.

131. Reymond D, Plaschkes J, Luthy AR *et al.* Focal nodular hyperplasia of the liver in children: review of follow-up and outcome. *J Pediatr Surg* 1995; **30**: 1590–3.

132. Rowland JM. Hepatoblastoma: assessment of criteria for histologic classification. *Med Pediatr Oncol* 2002; **39**: 478–83.

23

Langerhans cell histiocytosis

HELMUT GADNER & NICOLE GROIS

INTRODUCTION

Histiocytes originate from haemopoietic precursor cells in the bone marrow, circulate in the peripheral blood, and seed after maturation in almost every organ. They are of two types:

- mononuclear phagocytes, known as 'ordinary' histiocytes (blood monocytes and tissue macrophages, e.g. Kupffer cells in the liver)
- 'professional' antigen-presenting cells (dendritic cells and Langerhans cells in the skin).

Dendritic cells are intimately involved in the presentation of antigens to T lymphocytes, whereas the role of macrophages is phagocytosis and antigen processing. In 1987 the Writing Group of the Histiocyte Society proposed a new classification of histiocytosis syndromes with the aim of establishing specific criteria for definite diagnosis.[1,2] According to this recommendation, histiocytosis syndromes are grouped into three classes (Box 23.1):

- Class I diseases are of dendritic cell origin, with Langerhans cell histiocytosis as the most frequent form.
- Class II disorders, with ordinary histiocytes as lesional cells, include familial haemophagocytic lympho-histiocytosis, infection- or malignancy-associated

Box 23.1 *Classification of histiocytosis syndromes*

Class I (dendritic cell–related)
- Langerhans cell histiocytosis
- Secondary dendritic cell processes
- Juvenile xanthogranuloma
- Solitary dendritic histiocytoma

Class II (macrophage-related)
- Haemophagocytic lymphohistiocytosis
  - Primary:
    familiar
    sporadic
  - Secondary:
    infection-associated
    malignancy-associated
    others
- Sinus histiocytosis with massive lymphadenopathy (Rosai–Dorfman disease)
- Multicentric reticulohistiocytosis, often arthritis-associated

Class III (malignant disorders)
- Acute monocytic leukemia (FAB M5)
- Malignant histiocytosis
- True histiocytic lymphoma

---

haemophagocytic syndrome and sinus histiocytosis with massive lymphadenopathy.

- Class III comprises truly malignant histiocytic disorders characterized by the presence of histiocytes with malignant features, including acute monocytic leukaemia (FAB M5) and malignant histiocytosis, which is extremely rare, since large-cell anaplastic lymphoma has been recognized as a separate, non-histiocyte-related entity.

DESCRIPTION

Since the first description by Hand,[3] Langerhans cell histiocytosis (LCH) has remained a poorly understood disorder. The disease comprises a broad spectrum of clinical presentations, ranging from a spontaneously regressing solitary bone lesion to a widespread life-threatening disorder. In the past, several synonyms have been used to describe the disease, such as 'histiocytosis X', 'eosinophilic granuloma', 'Hand–Schueller–Christian disease' and 'Abt–Letterer–Siwe disease'.[4] Since 1985, 'Langerhans cell histiocytosis' has become the commonly accepted term,[1] which acknowledges the central role of the Langerhans cells in the various disease forms.[1,2]

INCIDENCE AND EPIDEMIOLOGY

Langerhans cell histiocytosis can present at any age, from birth to adulthood. Predominantly, young children between 1 and 3 years are affected. The incidence in different age groups is about 0.2–1.0/100 000 children per year (median 0.4/100 000), with males affected twice as frequently as females.[5,6] Although essentially sporadic, the disease has frequently been found associated with congenital anomalies,[7] and has been reported in twins and certain other family relations. However, there is little evidence for a strong genetic component.[8]

Only very few, and not consistent, data regarding associations between environmental exposure and LCH are available.[9] In adults there is evidence that cigarette smoking plays a key role in the development of pulmonary disease.[2,10]

AETIOLOGY AND PATHOGENESIS

Several studies in the 1970s and early 1980s described immunological abnormalities in patients with LCH, such as decreased lymphocyte function and dysplastic thymus changes,[11,12] but a consistent pattern has not been revealed. Currently LCH is regarded as a proliferative process characterized by an accumulation of dendritic cells with epidermal Langerhans cell (LC) phenotype in various tissues and organs. Although a clonal origin of the lesional LCs – in both single and multisystem disease – was found, the disease is widely regarded as a reactive process rather than a malignancy.[13]

Pathophysiologically, it has been postulated that an atypical immunological response to either an unidentified agent or a viral infection may cause a disequilibrium of cytokines, reflecting a deficient intercellular communication between T cells and LCs.[14] However, no specific agent has been consistently demonstrated.[15]

HISTOPATHOLOGY

Normal LCs reside primarily in the epidermis of the skin, in the orobuccal and vaginal epithelia, and in the bronchial mucosa. Within the skin they represent 1–2 per cent of all epidermal cells and play a critical role in cutaneous immunosurveillance. After antigen contact, the LCs migrate through the dermal lymphatics to regional lymph nodes, most probably to present antigen to paracortical T cells, and thereafter presumably become interdigitating dendritic cells[16] (Figure 23.1).

The aggregation of dendritic cells of Langerhans type in LCH with a variable admixture of other cells (eosinophils, neutrophils, lymphocytes, fibroblasts, multinucleated giant cells) forms granulomas with proliferative and locally destructive behaviour. These granulomas initially have a high cellular content, which decreases gradually, resulting in a xanthomatous and fibrotic pattern. The typical feature of a LC is a 'histiocytic' cell with abundant, homogeneous pink cytoplasma in the haematoxylin-eosin stained section, and a lobulated, 'coffee bean'-like nucleus. LCs express a number of phenotypic markers, which can be demonstrated by immunohistochemistry and electron microscopy.[16,17] Most important are class II MHC molecules and the CD1a complex. Furthermore, Birbeck granules, detectable in the cytoplasm by electron microscopy, are specific for LCs (Plate 28). Many of these markers may be implicated in the organ damage seen in LCH (e.g. fibrosis in the lungs and liver, gliosis in the brain).

To obtain a definitive diagnosis, immunohistochemical demonstration of CD1a epitopes on the cell surface and/or demonstration of Birbeck granules in the cytoplasm by electron microscopy is required, in addition to conventional light microscopy (Box 23.2).[1]

CLINICAL PRESENTATIONS AND DIFFERENTIAL DIAGNOSES

Symptoms and signs of LCH vary considerably depending on the localization and extent of the disease. Almost

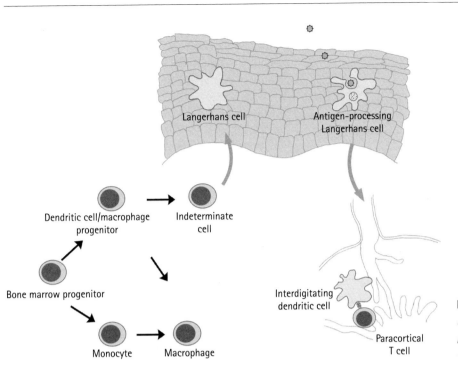

Dendritic cell/macrophage progenitor

Indeterminate cell

Bone marrow progenitor

Langerhans cell

Antigen-processing Langerhans cell

Monocyte

Macrophage

Interdigitating dendritic cell

Paracortical T cell

Figure 23.1 *Ontogeny of histiocytes (left) and migration pattern and maturation of Langerhans cells (right).*

Box 23.2 *Histopathological diagnosis of LCH*

> **Presumptive diagnosis**
> Conventional histology (light microscope)
>
> **Designated diagnosis**
> Conventional histology plus positive staining for two or more of the following:
> - ATPase
> - S100-protein
> - alpha-D-mannosidase
> - peanut agglutinin
>
> **Definitive diagnosis**
> Conventional histology plus:
> - CD1a staining or
> - Birbeck granules (electron microscope)

Box 23.3 *Stratification of LCH*

> **Single-system disease**
> - Single site
>   - single bone lesion
>   - isolated skin disease
>   - solitary lymph node involvement
> - Multiple site
>   - multiple bone lesions
>   - multiple lymph node involvement
>
> **Multisystem disease**
> Multiple organ involvement (with or without organ dysfunction)
> - 'Risk organs' – liver, lungs, haemopoietic system and spleen
> - 'Low-risk patients' – over 2 years old with no risk organ involvement
> - 'Risk patients' – of any age with involvement of at least one risk organ

every organ can be affected.[10,18] According to the number of organs and systems involved, 'single-system' and 'multisystem disease' are distinguished (Box 23.3).[19,20] Single-system involvement is found in more than half of the patients, mostly affecting bone or skin. Multisystem disease can involve bone, soft tissue, skin, liver, spleen, lungs, bone marrow, lymph nodes, thymus, thyroid glands or central nervous system (CNS) in various combinations and may be associated with very pronounced general symptoms (fever, pain, irritability, skin rash, weight loss, failure to thrive) and organ dysfunction.[21]

The involvement of haemopoietic system, spleen, liver and/or lungs has been shown to be associated with an increased risk of fatal outcome.[22,23] Therefore, these organs are referred to as 'risk organs', and depending on the involvement of risk organs, multisystem patients can be subdivided into 'low-risk' and 'risk' groups (see Boxes 23.3 and 23.4).

Box 23.4 *Definition of organ involvement 'risk' organs*

Haemopoietic involvement

(with or without bone marrow involvement*)

- Anaemia – haemoglobin <10 g/dL, infants <9 g/dL (exclusion of iron deficiency)
- Leucocytopenia – leucocytes <4.0 × 10⁹/L
- Thrombocytopenia – platelets <100 × 10⁹/L
- Spleen involvement
- Enlargement ≥2 cm below costal margin (proven by sonography)

Liver involvement

- Enlargement >3 cm below costal margin (proven by sonography) and/or liver dysfunction (hyperbilirubinaemia, hypoproteinaemia, hypoalbuminaemia, elevated γ-GT, alkaline phosphatase and transaminases, ascites, oedema) and/or histopathological diagnosis

Lung involvement

- Typical changes on high-resolution computed tomography (HR-CT) and/or histopathological diagnosis

---

γ-GT, gamma-glutamyl transferase.

*Bone marrow involvement is defined as demonstration of CD1a-positive cells on bone marrow smears. The clinical significance of CD1a positivity in the bone marrow remains to be proven. Hypocellularity, haemophagocytosis, myelodysplasia and/or myelofibrosis may be regarded as secondary phenomena. Haemophagocytosis may be prominent in severe progressive cases.

Bone and soft tissue involvement

In single and multiple site disease, the skeleton is involved in ~80 per cent of patients. Typically, bone lesions present on X-ray as well defined osteolytic areas, surrounded by a 'halo' of sclerosis and sometimes excessive periosteal reaction. Skeletal survey is superior to bone scan for the detection of bone lesions[24,25] (Figure 23.2). The disease most often affects the skull, long bones, pelvic and vertebral bones and ribs, and may lead to swelling, pain and functional impairment.[26–28] Jaw lesions may provoke premature eruption and loss of 'floating' teeth. Osteomyelitis and benign or malignant bone tumours must be ruled out. Computed tomography (CT) and magnetic resonance imaging (MRI) have become the procedures of choice for assessing vertebral or craniofacial lesions.[29]

Soft tissue swelling adjacent to a bone lesion caused by extension of the granuloma or by local oedema is a common finding and is usually not considered a separate organ involvement. Lesions in vertebrae may be associated

with significant intraspinal soft tissue extension, and must be differentiated from Ewing's sarcoma, neuroblastoma or lymphoma. Craniofacial bone lesions (mastoid or petrous bone including the paranasal, parameningeal or periorbital region) with intracranial extension are regarded as 'special sites', as they seem to be associated with an increased risk for diabetes insipidus.[30] Such lesions may resemble cholesteatoma, lymphoma, rhabdomyosarcoma, neuroblastoma or nasopharynx carcinoma.

Skin lesions

Skin rash, observed in one-third of children, can be the only manifestation in infants (~10 per cent) or can occur as part of multisystem disease. The cutaneous eruptions largely resemble seborrhoeic, atopic or infectious dermatitis. Areas of predilection are the trunk, abdomen and scalp, showing scattered pinkish-brown papules, often covered by a scale. When healing, depigmented areas or scars usually evolve. The granulomatous eruptions tend to become erosive and crusted, especially in the intertriginous regions (e.g. groin, perianal region, axilla, neck folds and retroauricular region), sometimes forming ulcers[31,32] (Plate 29). Skin rash with aural discharge may present as otitis externa. An underlying bone lesion with tissue extension into the ear canal and otorrhoea has to be ruled out.

A particular, purely cutaneous, manifestation in neonates, which tends to regress spontaneously within a few months, is 'congenital self-healing reticulohistiocytosis' (Hashimoto–Pritzker disease) with numerous firm skin nodules of brownish-red colour scattered over the trunk, head, palms and soles that may be similar to juvenile xanthogranuloma.[2,32,33]

Lymphohaemopoietic system

Lymph node involvement is observed in fewer than 10 per cent of children, either adjacent to bone or skin manifestations or in multisystem disease. In isolated cases, infectious or malignant lymphadenopathy has to be excluded. Cervical nodes, but also nodes in the mediastinum and abdomen, are most frequently affected, and may be markedly enlarged. Waldeyer's ring involvement, causing upper airway obstruction and compression of the superior vena cava, has been described.[34] Occasionally, morphological changes in the thymic tissue with or without organ enlargement are observed.[10,12]

LCs are not considered a normal component of the bone marrow; however, a few cells can be observed in single-system disease patients and in normal controls. In multisystem disease, diffuse infiltration and clustering of LCH cells in the bone marrow (together with haemophagocytic macrophages) may be present. Severe pancytopenia, frequently observed in infants, is usually associated with huge

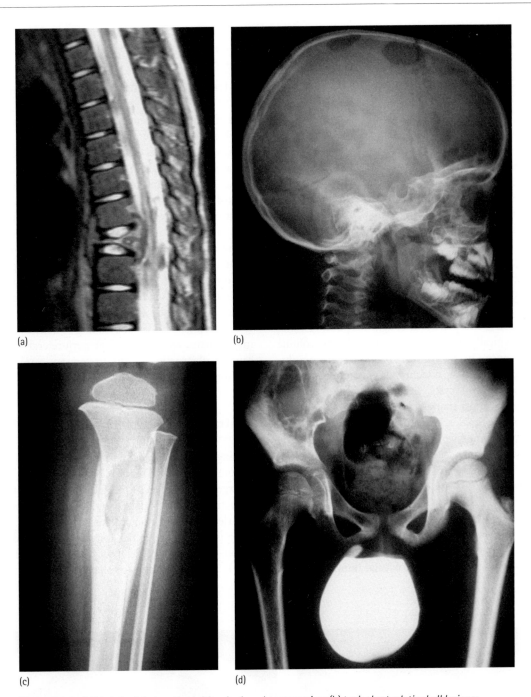

Figure 23.2 *(a) Vertebral destruction with spinal cord compression; (b) typical osteolytic skull lesions; (c) Langerhans cell histiocytosis lesion in the tibia with periosteal reaction; (d) huge osteolytic lesions in the right pelvis and femur.*

hepatosplenomegaly and is related to bone marrow dysfunction rather than infiltration.[35] In contrast, in cases with mild anaemia, iron deficiency and malabsorption related to occult gut disease have to be excluded.

Liver and spleen

Hepatomegaly due to infiltration with LCH cells, which are CD1a-positive but rarely contain Birbeck granules,

is common in multisystem disease, often associated with functional impairment. Ascites and oedema due to hypoalbuminaemia, which may be associated with coagulopathy [prolonged prothrombin time (PT)/partial thromboplastin time (PTT)] or hyperbilirubinaemia, are typical signs of liver dysfunction[21] (Box 23.4). The disease can progress from mild cholestasis to severe liver failure with fibrosis or even biliary cirrhosis.[36–38] The histological picture can resemble sclerosing cholangitis resulting from Kupffer cell hypertrophy and hyperplasia due to an activation of the cellular immune system by cytokine release.[16] The resulting fibrosis and cirrhosis may become self-perpetuating even when the active LCH regresses, and LCH cells may no longer be detectable.

Enlargement of the spleen is a typical sign of multi-system disease in very young children and may be an additional factor responsible for pancytopenia.

Lung disease

Lung involvement can occur at any age. In adolescents and young adults, lung disease may be an isolated manifestation strongly associated with smoking.[39–41] In children, pulmonary involvement usually occurs in multisystem disease. The natural history varies considerably, ranging from spontaneous resolution with disappearance of signs and symptoms to rapid progression.[42,43] The prominent clinical signs are tachypnoea with subcostal recession and persistent cough. Respiratory function tests typically show a decreased total lung volume and compliance. On chest X-ray, a bilateral reticulonodular interstitial shadowing is seen, and CT scanning demonstrates nodules and cystic lesions. Typically the lung involvement is most marked in the mid-zones, sparing the costophrenic angles. With advancing disease, all zones of the lung become involved, and cysts increase in number and size, forming 'honeycomb lungs' (Figure 23.3). Children with uncontrolled pulmonary LCH usually develop lung fibrosis with chronic functional incapacity. Rupture of bullae may result in multiple pneumothoraces with general symptoms such as fever and weight loss.[42] For confirmation of the diagnosis and to rule out other interstitial processes, e.g. infections, the finding of LCH cells on biopsy or in the bronchoalveolar fluid is required.

Only a significant increase of more than 5 per cent CD 1a-positive cells can be considered to be diagnostic.[44]

Gastrointestinal and genitourinary tract

Oral mucous membrane involvement (buccal mucosa, gingiva, palate) is common, with or without lesions in the jaw bones, and is diagnosed in more than 20 per cent of cases.[32,45] The localized or disseminated lesions present as whitish granulomatous plaques with a tendency towards ulceration and bleeding. Gastrointestinal involvement of the mucosa and submucosa, most often occurring in the small intestine but also in the colon, may be occult or lead to malabsorption with failure to thrive or chronic diarrhoea with protein-losing enteropathy. The diagnosis should be confirmed by endoscopic biopsy, including serosa and muscle coat, and by radiological evidence of stenotic areas.[46,47]

Anogenital LCH lesions leading to ulcers, genital tract involvement, and perirenal or periureteral infiltrations causing obstruction of the ureters are rarely found in children.[48]

Central nervous system

During the last decade, an increasing awareness of the various presentations of CNS disease in LCH has emerged.[49,50] CNS LCH may occur in all age groups, but the actual frequency and the pathogenesis are not known. A variety of intracranial lesions have been described, and there is a clear preference for structures outside of the blood–brain barrier. The most frequently involved structure is the hypothalamic–pituitary axis, leading to diabetes

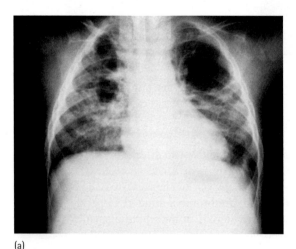

(a)

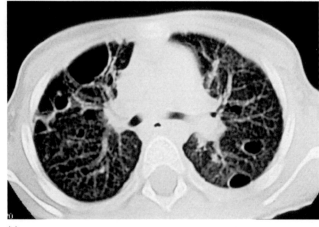

(b)

Figure 23.3 *(a) X-ray appearance of severe pulmonary disease with interstitial opacity and formation of bullae; (b) lung involvement on CT scan with multiple cysts.*

insipidus (DI) in about 10–20 per cent of the patients.[37,51–53] On MRI, typically, the lack of the normal signal in the posterior pituitary ('bright spot') and a thickening of the pituitary stalk are seen, which can progress to mass lesions involving the pituitary gland and hypothalamus and resembling granulomatous infections, germ cell or other tumours (Figure 23.4a).[54,55] Up to 50 per cent of DI patients develop further deficiencies of the anterior pituitary hormones.[56–59] Infiltrative lesions may also be found in the meninges, the pineal gland and the choroid plexus, and as single or multiple foci in the brain parenchyma or even in the spinal cord.[50,60–63] Clinical symptoms depend on the size and location of these lesions, and comprise headaches, seizures, visual abnormalities or other focal symptoms, and a variety of benign or malignant tumours are in the range of differential diagnoses. Apart from active LCH lesions, neurodegenerative lesions in the cerebellum, brainstem or basal ganglia are detected on MRI, often many years after the initial diagnosis of LCH (Figure 23.4b). These lesions may resemble degenerative brain diseases. Some patients are without symptoms over several years, while others develop progressive neurological dysfunction with gait disturbance, tremor, dysarthria, dysmetria, motor spasticity, palsy, and intellectual and behavioural deficits[50,58,64]

PERMANENT CONSEQUENCES AND LATE EFFECTS

Permanent consequences are irreversible long-term disabilities linked to sites of active LCH. The frequency is related to the disease extent, and correlates with a prolonged disease activity, reactivations and recurrences.[36,65] In more than half of patients with permanent consequences, these are already present at diagnosis of LCH. They are usually minimal in single-system disease, but are reported in 30–50 per cent in multisystem disease.[65,66] A great variety of permanent consequences have been observed, including small stature, growth hormone deficiency, hypothyroidism, DI, partial deafness, cerebellar ataxia, loss of dentition, orthopaedic problems, pulmonary fibrosis and biliary cirrhosis with portal hypertension.[37,53] Endocrine dysfunction or neurological disease may become apparent years or even decades after the initial diagnosis of LCH.[50]

Various malignancies have been reported in 5 per cent of long-term survivors of LCH.[67,68] In a retrospective analysis, a high association of malignancy and LCH, even without any treatment and not infrequently preceding the diagnosis of LCH, was recognized.[68] Recently, there has been concern regarding an association of secondary acute myeloblastic leukemia (sAML) with etoposide. However,

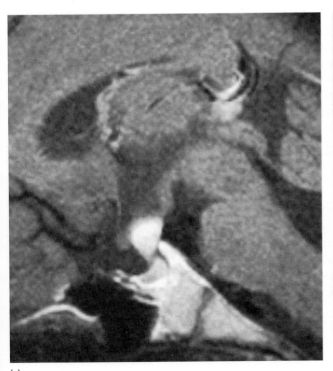

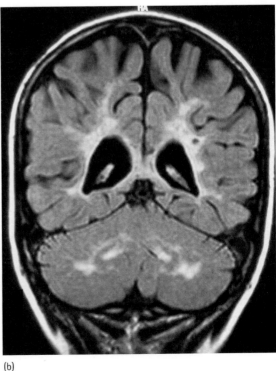

(a)

(b)

Figure 23.4 *Sagittal and coronal T1-weighed images after gadolinium-DTPA: (a) thickened infundibulum and a partial empty sella; (b) diffuse atrophy and bilateral patchy areas of strong enhancement in the periventricular and cerebellar white matter.*

it has been shown that sAMLs occurred only when etoposide was used in high cumulative doses with a short interval or in combination with other cytotoxic drugs[19,69,70]

DIAGNOSTIC MANAGEMENT

The diagnosis of LCH can only be established by a lesional biopsy. The definitive diagnosis of LCH according to the criteria of the Writing Group of the Histiocyte Society requires the demonstration of CD1a antigen or Birbeck granules[1] (Box 23.2).

Due to the highly variable clinical presentation, it is crucial to use uniform guidelines for clinical evaluation and assessment of disease extent at diagnosis and during the follow-up period. Mandatory baseline investigations based on an exact history and a thorough clinical examination should be performed uniformly in every newly diagnosed patient, and in selected cases diagnostic procedures are required upon specific indication (Boxes 23.5 and 23.6).[71]

CURRENT MANAGEMENT

Evaluation of response to therapy

The biological behaviour of LCH differs from malignant processes. Terms such as remission and relapse do not adequately describe the frequently fluctuating disease activity in LCH. For the purpose of cooperative clinical trials, in 1990 the LCH Study Group adopted a simple system for uniform assessment of disease activity and response to a given therapy.[71] Response was defined as a measurable regression or resolution of symptoms and signs at defined time points after start of therapy and during follow-up (Box 23.7).[22,23,65] It may take several months to document a clear disease regression on X-ray, especially in bone disease, even though the disease process itself has been inactive for a while.

Single–system disease

The clinical course of LCH in patients with single-system disease is generally benign with a high chance of spontaneous remission and favourable outcome over a period of months to years.[26,72] There is neither a general consensus nor an ongoing clinical trial for treatment of patients with single-system LCH.

Isolated skin disease

Congenital LCH confined to skin tends to regress spontaneously within a few months in most cases. However, progression to multisystem involvement with fatal out-

Box 23.5 *Baseline diagnostic evaluations*

Clinical evaluation

Complete history
Fever, pain, irritability, failure to thrive, loss of appetite, diarrhoea, polydipsia, polyuria, recurrent otitis, skin rashes, activity level, behavioural changes, neurological changes

Complete physical examination
Measurement of temperature, height, weight, head circumference, pubertal status, skin and scalp rashes, purpura, bleeding, jaundice, pallor, aural discharge, orbital abnormalities, gum and palatal lesions, dentition, soft tissue swelling, lymphadenopathies, dyspnoea, tachypnoea, intercostal retractions, liver and spleen size, ascites, oedema, neurological examination (including papilloedema, cranial nerve abnormalities, cerebellar dysfunction)

Laboratory and radiographic evaluation

Mandatory minimum baseline evaluations for all patients
- Haemoglobin and/or haematocrit, ferritin, iron, transferrin
- White blood count and differential, platelet count
- Erythrocyte sedimentation rate (ESR), renal function test, liver enzymes and function tests (SGOT, SGPT, γ-GT, alkaline phosphatase, bilirubin, total protein, albumin), coagulation studies (PT, PTT, fibrinogen)
- Chest radiograph, posteroanterior and lateral
- Skeletal radiograph survey/skeletal scan (radionuclide bone scan is not as sensitive as the skeletal radiograph survey in most patients)
- Urine osmolality (measurement after overnight water deprivation)

Mandatory for multisystem 'risk' patients
Bone marrow aspiration and trephine with CD1a staining, HLA-typing

γ-GT, gamma-glutamyl transferase; PT, prothrombin time; PTT, thromboplastin time; SGOT, serum glutamic oxaloacetic transaminase; SGPT, serum glutamate pyruvate transaminase.

come may occur, and therefore close observation during a longer follow-up period is mandatory.[33] Surgical excision is the treatment of choice for skin nodules. Erythematous lesions usually respond to topical steroids; in severe persisting or progressing skin involvement topical 20 per cent solution of nitrogen mustard or psoralen and ultraviolet A irradiation photochemotherapy may be useful, but can be recommended only for short-term therapy due to

Box 23.6 *Evaluations required upon specific indication*

- Abnormal chest radiograph, tachypnoea, intercostal retractions
  - high-resolution CT,
  - pulmonary function test (if age appropriate)
- Patients with abnormal pulmonary high-resolution CT – to yield a diagnosis in case of isolated lung involvement or to exclude infection
  - lung biopsy
  - branchoalveolar lavage (when diagnostic, obviates lung biopsy)
- Unexplained chronic diarrhoea or failure to thrive, evidence of malabsorption
  - endoscopic biopsy
  - small bowel series
- Liver dysfunction – to differentiate active LCH of the liver from sclerosing cholangitis
  - sonography
  - liver biopsy
- Visual or neurological abnormalities
  - MRI of brain with i.v. gadolinium-DTPA
  - neurological evaluation, psychological tests
- Polyuria, polydipsia, short stature, growth failure, hypothalamic syndromes, galactorrhoea, precocious or delayed puberty
  - endocrine evaluation, including water deprivation test, dynamic tests of the anterior pituitary
  - MRI of brain with i.v. gadolinium-DTPA
- Gingival involvement, loose teeth
  - panoramic dental radiography and CT of mandible and maxilla, oral surgery consultation
- Aural discharge, deafness
  - otolaryngology consultation and audiogram,
  - MRI of brain with i.v. gadolinium-DTPA

Box 23.7 *Disease state and response as defined by the LCH Study Group*

Definition of disease state

Non-active disease
No evidence of disease

Active disease
Better
Intermediate
  Mixed ± complications
  Stable ± complications
Worse

Definition of response criteria
Better
  Complete resolution
  Continuous regression of the disease
Intermediate
  Mixed ± complications
  Unchanged ± complications
Worse
  Progression of disease

multisystem patients. As in adults, in adolescents, refraining from smoking is mandatory, and mild systemic therapy with steroids with or without vinblastine can be effective.[39–41] In progressing disease cyclosporin A or bisphosphonates anecdotally have shown positive effect.[42,75,76]

CNS disease

Tumorous active LCH lesions in the CNS usually respond to conventional LCH chemotherapy. The choice of therapy depends on the individual case and possible pretreatment. A beneficial effect of combined chemotherapy (prednisone, vinblastine, etoposide and 2-chlorodeoxyadenosine) has been reported.[50,60] Radiotherapy and systemic therapy are usually not able to restore pituitary function, and hormone replacement therapy is required.[77,78] For neurodegenerative CNS disease, no specific therapy can be recommended to date.

Unifocal bone disease

In cases with single bone lesions, often simple curettage or just the biopsy will result in ultimate healing.[20,79] Besides conservative surgery, intralesional instillation of steroids (75–150 mg crystalline methylprednisolone) has been shown to be an effective and safe treatment modality.[80] Indications for systemic treatment (e.g. prednisone, vinblastine) include risky locations with imminent spontaneous fracture, spinal cord compression and huge non-resectable tumour mass.[18,26,28,65,79]

possible carcinogenicity.[73,74] In severe resistant disease, mild systemic steroid therapy with or without vinca alkaloids is needed.[26]

Lymph node involvement

For isolated lymph node involvement, excisional biopsy may be sufficient. Systemic steroid therapy with or without vinblastine is preferred if multiple or bulky lymph nodes are present.[19,20,26]

Lung disease

In young children, isolated lung involvement should be treated with chemotherapy according to protocols for

The use of radiation therapy for localized bone or soft tissue disease has continuously been restricted in the last decades, due to the risk of late sequelae and secondary malignancy. Emergency low-dose radiation (6–12 Gy) should be reserved for critical circumstances (e.g. optic nerve or spinal cord).[81–83]

Special site involvement

Surgical removal of lesions in the craniofacial region (skull base, temporal or zygomatic bones, mastoids, sphenoidal and ethmoidal bones, orbits, anterior and middle cranial fossae) or spinal column would be a risky and incomplete procedure due to prominent intracranial or intraspinal soft tissue components. In such cases of 'special site involvement' impending impairment of critical organ function may require urgent treatment with low-dose radiation therapy (6–10 Gy).[81–83] According to the LCH-III study protocol, systemic chemotherapy with prednisone and vinblastine is recommended even for isolated lesions.

Multifocal bone disease

Over recent decades, there has been an ongoing discussion about the appropriate treatment for patients with multifocal bone disease. It is known that osseous lesions tend to regress spontaneously ('wait and see' strategy) or respond to minimal treatment. However, there is also a tendency to recur, though reactivation usually remains restricted to the skeleton.[18,65,72,84] The frequency of reactivation in single-system bone disease is 4–30 per cent, much lower than in multisystem LCH (50–80 per cent).[72,85] Various systemic regimens have been used in polyostotic disease, including steroids (40 mg/m^2/day), vinblastine (6 mg/m^2/week) and etoposide. Combining these drugs, the reactivation frequency was only 18 per cent in the DAL-HX 83 study.[26] Recently, indomethacin (2 mg/m^2/day), bisphosphonates and also a combination of 6-mercaptopurine and methotrexate have shown beneficial effect.[76,86,87] So far, no data on standardized clinical studies are available, and therefore the Histiocyte Society has adopted the concept of systemic chemotherapy for the ongoing LCH-III protocol.[30]

Multisystem disease

A wide range of therapies, including antibiotics, anti-inflammatory agents, radiation therapy, and a number of single- and multiagent cytotoxic regimens (steroids, alkylating agents, antimetabolites, anthracyclines, vinca alkaloids, cytosine arabinoside, epiphyllotoxins), have been applied in multisystem disease with variable success.[19,20,84,88–90] During the last 20 years it has been shown in several therapeutic trials that prompt initiation of systemic combination therapy yields better results with respect to prevention of recurrences and permanent consequences when compared with conservative approaches delivering chemotherapy to only severe progressive cases.[65,72,85,91]

INTERNATIONAL TRIALS

In 1991, the Histiocyte Society initiated the first international cooperative trial for the treatment of multisystem disease. In this prospective randomized trial, two treatment arms compared monotherapy with etoposide (VP-16) with vinblastine given for 6 months. There was no significant difference between the two treatment arms with respect to initial response, the probability of reactivation or mortality. The overall survival rate was 78 per cent, but was 91 per cent for patients who responded well to initial treatment after 6 weeks, whereas it was only 34 per cent for non-responders. This finding clearly indicated the prognostic impact of response to initial therapy.[22]

The LCH-I study was retrospectively compared with the DAL-HX 83/90 studies in which initial chemotherapy (vinblastine, VP-16, prednisone) followed by 1 year of continuation therapy (prednisone, vinblastine, VP-16, 6-mercaptopurine and methotrexate for patients with organ dysfunction) was given.[23,65] The results showed a clear superiority of combination therapy given for 1 year over monotherapy for 6 months with respect to initial response and rate of reactivation (Figures 23.5 and 23.6). Interestingly, the mortality rate of about 20 per cent did not differ between the two studies. All fatalities were under 2 years old and were multisystem patients with involvement of liver, spleen, lungs or haemopoietic system, which were called 'risk organs'.

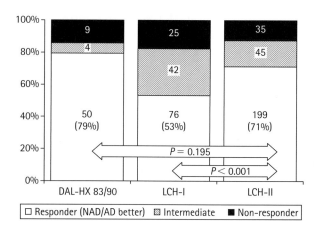

Figure 23.5 *Comparison of response at week 6 between DAL-HX 83/90 studies and LCH-I and LCH-II studies. AD, active disease; NAD, non-active disease.*

Therefore, in the consecutive LCH-II study, patients were stratified into a 'risk group' with 'risk organ' involvement and age under 2 years, and a 'low-risk group' without such organs involved and age over 2 years.[20] LCH-II aimed to match the good results of the DAL-HX studies and intended to clarify the value of the addition of VP-16 to prednisone and vinblastine in a randomized way. Continuation treatment was given for 24 weeks. The comparison between the two- and three-drug arms did not show any significant difference with respect to response, survival, reactivation rate or toxicity. The results in the 'low-risk group' were encouraging, as there were 89 per cent responders to the initial treatment and no fatalities. The response in the 'risk group' was 65 per cent and better than in LCH-I (53 per cent), but less than in DAL-HX (76 per cent). Evaluation of the correlation of response and survival revealed that, independent of age, 22 per cent of 'risk patients' did not show a response after 6 weeks of initial therapy, and a further 35 per cent did not show improvement within the next 6 weeks. After 12 weeks of treatment, about 50 per cent of 'risk patients' still had active or progressive disease. These patients had a 75 per cent probability of mortality and seem to need intensified therapy.[30]

After achieving a non-active disease state, the probability of experiencing a disease reactivation was 62 per cent in LCH-II, which was much worse than in the DAL-HX study with 27 per cent (Figure 23.6). The main difference between the two studies was a duration of continuation therapy of 6 months in LCH-II and 12 months in DAL-HX, indicating a preventive effect of prolonged therapy.

Based on the experience of these three trials, the concept for the ongoing LCH-III study was developed.[22,23,65] The goal of this study is to deliver risk-adapted therapy to three groups: multisystem 'risk' and 'low-risk' patients and single-system patients with multifocal bone or 'special site' involvement. The aims are to decrease the mortality and the morbidity, i.e. rate of reactivation and permanent consequences, by intensifying the initial therapy and introducing methotrexate as a new agent for 'risk' patients, and by prolongation of continuation therapy. This ongoing international study LCH-III was opened in April 2001, and the study protocol is available at the study reference centre (Figure 23.7).

SALVAGE AND EXPERIMENTAL THERAPIES

Only preliminary data exist as to the efficacy of alternative treatment approaches in resistant multisystem disease.[18–20,92] A few studies suggest that cyclosporin A may be a potent immunomodulator, especially in young children with advanced disease. Persistent response, however, was rarely seen in patients with risk organ involvement, and often was obtained only by adding other drugs such as steroids or vinblastine.[42,93,94] Early reports on thymic hormone or extract therapy, resulting in clinical response with improvement or correction of immunological abnormalities, could not been confirmed by further experience.[12,89] Alpha-interferon (IFN-alpha), used in the past with inconsistent success, is only sporadically reported in recent publications.[95] Monoclonal antibody therapy against CD1a antigen on LCs seems to be a promising new approach of interest for future studies.[96]

Only few and inconsistent data are available regarding bone marrow transplantation in resistant multisystem disease. Transplantation mortality in severely affected children is high. In 1991, the Salvage Therapy Group of the Histiocyte Society proposed two experimental treatment approaches (LCH-I-S protocol)[30] for the poorest

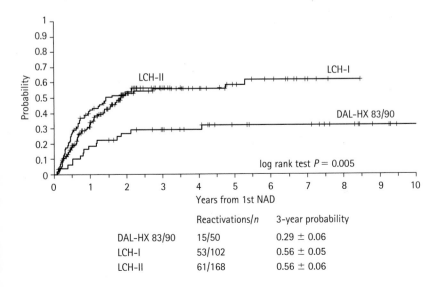

Figure 23.6 *Comparison of the probability of recurrence after having achieved complete resolution and disappearance of symptoms and signs (NAD). n = number of included patients.*

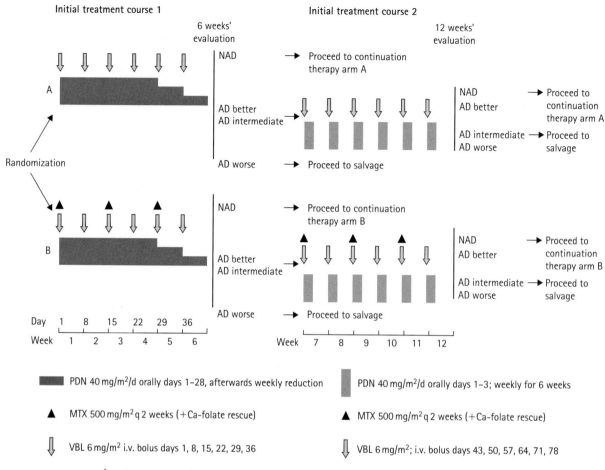

Figure 23.7 *Treatment plan and stratification of risk groups in the LCH–II study. AD, active disease; MTX, methotrexate; NAD, non-active disease; PDN, prednisone; VBL, vinblastine.*

prognostic group of patients (risk organ involvement, non-response by weeks 6 and 12, early recurrence or progression under conventional chemotherapy):

- high-dose immunosuppressive therapy with steroids, cyclosporin A and antithymocyte globulin to interrupt the abnormal cellular immune response
- stem cell transplantation to replace the abnormal clonal LCH cells.

Unfortunately, this study had to be closed due to lack of patients.[92]

According to preliminary reports, 2-chlorodeoxyadenosine (2-CdA) or 2′-deoxycoformycin promise to be successful in refractory LCH.[60,97–99] The ongoing LCH-S 98 study of the Histiocyte Society offers 2-CdA (5 mg/m²/day given at 3- to 4-weekly intervals for two, four or six courses) to non-responding multisystem patients or patients with recurrent disease.

Further studies will clarify if an early switch to new salvage therapy approaches, including stem cell transplantation with reduced intensity conditioning, can improve

therapy response and survival by avoiding treatment-related mortality.

KEY POINTS

- LCH is considered a clonal proliferation of Langerhans cells as a reactive rather than a malignant process.
- Definite diagnosis is based on histopathology, including detection of CD1a surface antigen and/or Birbeck granules in the lesional cells.
- The incidence of LCH is low and predominates in children aged 1–3 years.
- Clinical presentation of LCH varies considerably, and almost every organ can be involved.
- Single-system disease (bone, skin or lymph node, lung, CNS) and multisystem disease (more than two organs involved) can be distinguished.

- Patients with single-system disease have an excellent prognosis.
- Involvement of 'risk organs', i.e. liver, spleen, haemopoietic system and lungs, correlates with poor outcome.
- 'Low-risk' multisystem patients have an excellent survival probability, whereas 'risk' patients who do not respond adequately to initial therapy have a high risk of dying.
- Rapid response to initial therapy within 12 weeks has been shown to be an independent prognostic factor in multisystem disease.
- A prednisone/vinblastine combination is accepted as the standard approach for multisystem disease; the optimal combination and duration of chemotherapy is under investigation.
- The role of intensified immunosuppressive therapy or stem cell transplantation in resistant disease as salvage approach has not been clarified yet.

REFERENCES

♦1. Writing Group of the Histiocyte Society. Histiocytosis syndromes in children. *Lancet* 1987; **1**: 208–9.

♦2. Favara BE, Feller AC, Pauli M *et al.* A contemporary classification of histiocytic disorders. The WHO Committee on Histiocytic/Reticulum Cell Proliferations. Reclassification Working Group of the Histiocytic Society. *Med Pediatr Oncol* 1997; **29**: 157–66.

3. Hand A. Polyuria and tuberculosis. *Arch Pediatr* 1893; **10**: 673–5.

●4. Lichtenstein L. Histiocytosis X, integration of eosinophilic granuloma of bone, 'Letterer–Siwe Disease' and 'Schüller–Christian Disease' as related manifestations of a single nosologic entity. *AMA Arch Pathol* 1953; **56**: 84–102.

●5. Carstensen H, Ornvold K. The epidemiology of Langerhans cell histiocytosis in children in Denmark, 1975–1989. *Med Pediatr Oncol* 1993; **21**: 387–8.

6. Kaatsch P, Spix C, Michaelis J. *Annual Report 2000. 700. 2002.* University of Mainz: German Childhood Cancer Registry, JMBEI.

7. Sheils C, Dover GJ. Frequency of congenital anomalies in patients with histiocytosis X. *Am J Hematol* 1989; **31**: 91–5.

8. Arico M, Haupt R, Russotto VS *et al.* Langerhans cell histiocytosis in two generations: a new family and review of the literature. *Med Pediatr Oncol* 2001; **36**: 314–16.

●9. Bhatia S, Nesbit ME Jr, Egeler RM *et al.* Epidemiologic study of Langerhans cell histiocytosis in children. *J Pediatr* 1997; **130**: 774–84.

♦10. Broadbent V, Egeler RM, Nesbit ME. Langerhans cell histiocytosis – clinical and epidemiological aspects. *Br J Cancer* 1994; **70**(Suppl XXIII): 11–16.

●11. Nesbit ME Jr, O'Leary M, Dehner LP, Ramsay NK. The immune system and the histiocytosis syndromes. *Am J Pediatr Hematol Oncol* 1981; **3**: 141–9.

12. Osband ME, Lipton JM, Lavin P *et al.* Histiocytosis X: demonstration of abnormal immunity, T-cell histamine H2-receptor deficiency and successful treatment with thymic extract. *N Engl J Med* 1981; **304**: 146–53.

●13. Willman C, Busque L, Griffith B *et al.* Langerhans cell histiocytosis (histiocytosis X) – a clonal proliferative disease. *N Engl J Med* 1994; **331**: 154–60.

14. Kannourakis G, Abbas A. The role of cytokines in the pathogenesis of Langerhans cell histiocytosis. *Br J Cancer* 1994; **70**(Suppl. XXIII): 37–40.

15. McClain K, Weiss RA. Viruses and Langerhans cell histiocytosis: is there a link? *Br J Cancer* 1994; **70**(Suppl XXIII): 34–6.

♦16. Schmitz L, Favara BE. Nosology and pathology of Langerhans cell histiocytosis. *Hematol Oncol Clin North Am* 1998; **12**: 221–46.

♦17. Chu T, Jaffe R. The normal Langerhans cell and the LCH cell. *Br J Cancer* 1994; **70**(Suppl XXIII): 4–10.

♦18. Egeler RM, D'Angio GJ. Langerhans cell histiocytosis. *J Pediatr* 1995; **127**: 1–11.

♦19. Ladisch S, Gadner H. Treatment of Langerhans cell histiocytosis – evolution and current approaches. *Br J Cancer* 1994; **70**(Suppl XXIII): 41–6.

♦20. Broadbent V, Gadner H. Current therapy for Langerhans cell histiocytosis. *Hematol Oncol Clin North Am* 1998; **12**: 327–38.

●21. Lahey E. Histiocytosis X: an analysis of prognostic factors. *J Pediatr* 1975; **87**: 184–9.

●22. Gadner H, Grois N, Arico M *et al.* A randomized trial of treatment for multisystem Langerhans' cell histiocytosis. *J Pediatr* 2001; **138**: 728–34.

●23. Minkov M, Grois N, Heitger A. Response to initial treatment: an important prognostic predictor in multisystem Langerhans cell histiocytosis. *Med Pediatr Oncol* 2002; **39**: 581–5.

♦24. Meyer JS, De Camargo B. The role of radiology in the diagnosis and follow-up of Langerhans cell histiocytosis. *Hematol Oncol Clin North Am* 1998; **12**: 307–26.

25. Parker BR, Pinckney L, Etcubanas E. Relative efficacy of radiographic and radionuclide bone surveys in the detection of the skeletal lesions of histiocytosis X. *Radiology* 1980; **134**: 377–80.

●26. Titgemeyer C, Grois N, Minkov M *et al.* Pattern and course of single-system disease in Langerhans cell histiocytosis. *Med Pediatr Oncol* 2001; **37**: 1–7.

●27. Kilpatrick SE, Wenger DE, Gilchrist GS *et al.* Langerhans' cell histiocytosis (histiocytosis X) of bone. A clinicopathologic analysis of 263 pediatric and adult cases. *Cancer* 1995; **76**: 2471–84.

♦28. Slater JM, Swarm OJ. Eosinophilic granuloma of bone. *Med Pediatr Oncol* 1980; **8**: 151–64.

●29. Moore JB, Kulkarni R, Crutcher DC, Bhimani S. MRI in multifocal eosinophilic granuloma: staging disease and monitoring response to therapy. *Am J Pediatr Hematol Oncol* 1989; **11**: 174–7.

30. Writing Group of the Histiocyte Society. Treatment protocol of the third international study for Langerhans cell histiocytosis. Vienna: LCH Study Reference Centre, St Anna's Children's Hospital, 2001.

♦31. Munn S, Chu AC. Langerhans cell histiocytosis of the skin. *Hematol Oncol Clin North Am* 1998; **12**: 269–86.

♦32. Gadner H, Grois N. The histiocytosis syndromes. In: Fitzpatrick TB, Eisen AZ, Wolff K *et al.*, eds. *Dermatology in General Medicine*. New York: McGraw-Hill, 1993; 2003–17.

33. Hashimoto K, Pritzker MS. Electron microscopic study of reticulohistiocytoma. An unusual case of congenital, self-healing reticulohistiocytosis. *Arch Dermatol* 1973; **107**: 263–70.

34. Mogul M, Hartman G, Donaldson S *et al.* Langerhans' cell histiocytosis presenting with the superior vena cava syndrome: a case report. *Med Pediatr Oncol* 1993; **21**: 456–9.

●35. McClain K, Ramsey NKC, Robison L *et al.* Bone marrow involvement in histiocytosis X. *Med Pediatr Oncol* 1983; **11**: 167–71.

●36. Braier J, Chantada G, Rosso D *et al.* Langerhans cell histiocytosis: retrospective evaluation of 123 patients at a single institution. *Pediatr Hematol Oncol* 1999; **16**: 377–85.

●37. The French Langerhans cell Histiocytosis Group. A multicentric retrospective survey of Langerhans' cell histiocytosis: 348 cases observed between 1983 and 1993. *Arch Dis Child* 1996; **75**: 17–24.

●38. Heyn RM, Hamoudi A, Newton WA. Pretreatment liver biopsy in 20 children with Histiocytosis X: a clinicopathologic correlation. *Med Pediatr Oncol* 1990; **18**: 110–18.

39. Tazi A, Soler P, Hance AJ. Adult pulmonary Langerhans' cell histiocytosis. *Thorax* 2002; **55**: 405–16.

40. McClain KL, Gonzalez JM, Jonkers R *et al.* Need for a cooperative study: Pulmonary Langerhans cell histiocytosis and its management in adults. *Med Pediatr Oncol* 2002; **39**: 35–9.

♦41. Vassallo R, Ryu JH, Colby TV *et al.* Pulmonary Langerhans'-cell histiocytosis. *N Engl J Med* 2000; **342**: 1969–78.

42. Zeller B, Storm-Mathisen I, Smevik B, Lie SO. Multisystem Langerhans-cell histiocytosis with life-threatening pulmonary involvement – good response to cyclosporine A. *Med Pediatr Oncol* 2000; **35**: 438–42.

43. Bernstrand C, Cederlund K, Sandstedt B *et al.* Pulmonary abnormalities at long-term follow-up of patients with Langerhans cell histiocytosis. *Med Pediatr Oncol* 2001; **36**: 459–68.

44. Auerswald U, Barth J, Magnussen H. Value of CD-1-positive cells in bronchoalveolar lavage fluid for the diagnosis of pulmonary histiocytosis X. *Lung* 1991; **169**: 305–9.

●45. Filocoma D, Needleman HL, Arceci R *et al.* Pediatric histiocytosis; characterization, prognosis, and oral involvement. *Am J Pediatr Hematol Oncol* 1993; **15**: 226–30.

46. Egeler RM, Schipper MEI, Heymans HSA. Gastrointestinal involvement in Langerhans' cell histiocytosis (Histiocytosis X): a clinical report of three cases. *Eur J Pediatr* 1990; **149**: 325–9.

47. Gilmore BS, Cohen M. Barium enema findings in a case of Langerhans cell histiocytosis involving the colon. *Pediatr Radiol* 1993; **23**: 589–90.

♦48. Axiotis CA, Merino MJ, Duray PH. Langerhans cell histiocytosis of the female genital tract. *Cancer* 1991; **67**: 1650–60.

49. Barthez MA, Araujo E, Donadieu J. Langerhans cell histiocytosis and the central nervous system in childhood: evolution and prognostic factors. Results of a collaborative study. *J Child Neurol* 2000; **15**: 150–6.

♦50. Grois N, Favara BE, Mostbeck G, Prayer D. Central nervous system disease in Langerhans cell histiocytosis. *Hematol Oncol Clin North Am* 1998; **12**: 287–305.

51. Grois N, Flucher-Wolfram B, Heitger A *et al.* Diabetes insipidus in Langerhans cell histiocytosis: results from the DAL-HX 83 study. *Med Pediatr Oncol* 1995; **24**: 248–56.

●52. Dunger DB, Broadbent V, Yeoman E *et al.* The frequency and natural history of diabetes insipidus in children with Langerhans cell histiocytosis. *N Engl J Med* 1989; **321**: 1157–62.

●53. Willis B, Ablin A, Weinberg V *et al.* Disease course and late sequelae of Langerhans cell histiocytosis: 25-year experience at the University of California, San Francisco. *J Clin Oncol* 1996; **14**: 2073–82.

54. Tien RD, Newton TH, McDermott MW *et al.* Thickened pituitary stalk on MR images in patients with diabetes insipidus and Langerhans cell histiocytosis. *Am J Neuroradiol* 1990; **11**: 703–8.

55. Kucharczyk J, Kucharczyk W, Berry I *et al.* Histochemical characterization and functional significance of the hyperintense signal on MR images of the posterior pituitary. *Am J Radiol* 1989; **152**: 153–7.

●56. Broadbent V, Dunger DB, Yeomans E, Brian K. Anterior pituitary function and computed tomography/magnetic resonance imaging in patients with Langerhans cell histiocytosis and diabetes insipidus. *Med Pediatr Oncol* 1993; **21**: 31–5.

57. Dean HJ, Bishop A, Winter JSD. Growth hormone deficieny in patients with Histiocytosis X. *J Pediatr* 1986; **109**: 615–18.

58. Braunstein GD, Kohler PO. Endocrine manifestations of histiocytosis. *Am J Pediatr Hematol Oncol* 1981; **3**: 67–75.

59. Nanduri VR, Bareille P, Pritchard J, Stanhope R. Growth and endocrine disorders in multisystem Langerhans' cell histiocytosis. *Clin Endocrinol (Oxf)* 2000; **53**: 509–15.

60. Watts J, Files B. Langerhans cell histiocytosis: central nervous system involvement treated successfully with 2-chlorodeoxyadenosine. *Pediatr Hematol Oncol* 2001; **18**: 199–204.

61. Whelan HT, Clinton ME, Fogo A, Smith H. Histiocytosis-X isolated to the cervical spinal cord. *Am J Pediatr Hematol Oncol* 1987; **9**: 228–32.

62. Gizewski ER, Forsting M. Histiocytosis mimicking a pineal gland tumour. *Neuroradiology* 2001; **43**: 644–6.

63. Kepes JJ. Histiocytosis X. In: Vinken PJ, Bruyn GW, eds. *Handbook of Clinical Neurology, Neurological Manifestations of Systemic Diseases*. Amsterdam: North Holland, 1989.

●64. Whitsett St, Kneppers K, Coopes MJ, Egeler RM. Neuropsychologic deficits in children with Langerhans cell histiocytosis. *Med Pediatr Oncol* 1999; **33**: 486–92.

●65. Gadner H, Heitger A, Grois N *et al.* Treatment strategy for disseminated Langerhans cell histiocytosis. *Med Pediatr Oncol* 1994; **23**: 72–80.

♦66. Komp DM, Mahdi AE, Starling KA *et al.* Quality of survival in histiocytosis X: a Southwest Oncology Group Study. *Med Pediatr Oncol* 1980; **8**: 35–40.

●67. Greenberger JS, Crocker AC, Vawter G *et al.* Results of treatment of 127 patients with systemic histiocytosis (Letterer–Siwe Syndrome, Schuller–Christian Syndrome and multifocal eosinophilic granuloma). *Medicine* 1981; **60**: 311–38.

♦68. Egeler RM, Neglia JP, Arico M *et al.* The relation of Langerhans cell histiocytosis to acute leukemia, lymphomas, and other solid tumors. The LCH-Malignancy Study Group of the Histiocyte Society. *Hematol Oncol Clin North Am* 1998; **12**: 369–78.

●69. Haupt R, Fears TR, Heise A *et al.* Risk of secondary leukemia after treatment with etoposide (VP-16) for Langerhans' cell histiocytosis in Italian and Austrian–German populations. *Int J Cancer* 1997; **71**: 9–13.

70. Smith MA, Rubinstein L, Ungerleider RS. Therapy-related acute myeloid leukemia following treatment with epipodophyllotoxins: estimating the risks. *Med Pediatr Oncol* 1994; **23**: 86–98.

♦71. Writing Group of the Histiocyte Society. Histiocytosis syndromes in children: II. Approach to the clinical and laboratory evaluation of children with Langerhans cell histiocytosis. *Med Pediatr Oncol* 1989; **17**: 492–5.

●72. McLelland J, Broadbent V, Yeomans E *et al.* Langerhans cell histiocytosis: the case for conservative treatment. *Arch Dis Child* 1990; **65**: 301–3.

●73. Sheehan MP, Atherton DJ, Broadbent V, Pritchard J. Topical nitrogen mustard: an effective treatment for cutaneous Langerhans cell histiocytosis. *J Pediatr* 1991; 119: 317–21.

74. Neumann G, Kolde G, Bonsmann G. Histiocytosis X in an elderly patient. Ultrastructure and immunochemistry after PUVA photochemotherapy. *Br J Dermatol* 1988; **119**: 385–91.

75. Brown RE. Bisphosphonates as antialveolar macrophage therapy in pulmonary Langerhans cell histiocytosis? *Med Pediatr Oncol* 2001; **36**: 641–3.

76. Farran RP, Zaretski E, Egeler RM. Treatment of Langerhans cell histiocytosis with pamidronate. *J Pediatr Hematol Oncol* 2001; **23**: 54–6.

77. Broadbent V, Pritchard J. Diabetes insipidus associated with Langerhans cell histiocytosis: is it reversible? *Med Pediatr Oncol* 1997; **28**: 289–93.

♦78. Howell SJ, Wilton P, Shalet SM. Growth hormone replacement in patients with Langerhan's cell histiocytosis. *Arch Dis Child* 1998; **78**: 469–73.

●79. Berry DH, Gresik M, Maybee D, Marcus R. Histiocytosis X in bone only. *Med Pediatr Oncol* 1990; **18**: 292–4.

♦80. Egeler RM, Thompson RC, Voute PA, Nesbit ME. Intralesional infiltration of corticosteroids in localized Langerhans cell histiocytosis. *J Pediatr Orthop* 1992; **12**: 811–14.

81. Selch MT, Parker RG. Radiation therapy in the management of Langerhans cell histiocytosis. *Med Pediatr Oncol* 1990; **18**: 97–102.

●82. Greenberger JS, Cassady JR, Jaffe N *et al.* Radiation therapy in patients with histiocytosis: management of diabetes insipidus and bone lesions. *Int J Radiat Oncol Biol Phys* 1979; **5**: 1749–55.

83. Gramatovici R, D'Angio GJ. Radiation therapy in soft-tissue lesions in histiocytosis X (Langerhans' cell histiocytosis). *Med Pediatr Oncol* 1988; **16**: 259–62.

●84. Feldges A. Childhood histiocytosis X: clinical aspects and therapeutic approaches. *Haematol Blood Transfus* 1981; **27**: 225–8.

●85. Berry DH, Gresik MV, Humphrey B *et al.* Natural history of histiocytosis X: a Pediatric Oncology Group Study. *Med Pediatr Oncol* 1986; **14**: 1–5.

86. Munn SE, Olliver L, Broadbent V, Pritchard J. Use of indomethacin in Langerhans cell histiocytosis. *Med Pediatr Oncol* 1999; **32**: 247–9.

87. Womer RB, Anunciato KR, Chehrenama M. Oral methotrexate and alternate-day prednisone for low-risk Langerhans cell histiocytosis. *Med Pediatr Oncol* 1995; **25**: 70–3.

●88. Egeler RM, Kraker JD, Voute PA. Cytosine-arabinoside, vincristine, and prednisolone in the treatment of children with disseminated Langerhans cell histiocytosis with organ dysfunction: experience at a single institution. *Med Pediatr Oncol* 1993; **21**: 265–70.

89. Ceci A, deTerlizzi M, Colella R *et al.* Etoposide in recurrent childhood Langerhans' cell histiocytosis: an Italian Cooperative Study. *Cancer* 1988; **62**: 2528–31.

●90. Broadbent V, Pritchard J, Yeomans E. Etoposide (VP16) in the treatment of multisystem Langerhans cell histiocytosis (Histiocytosis X). *Med Pediatr Oncol* 1989; **17**: 97–100.

●91. Ceci A, Terlizzi MD, Colella R *et al.* Langerhans cell histiocytosis in childhood: results from the Italian Cooperative AIEOP-CNR-HX'83 Study. *Med Pediatr Oncol* 1993; **21**: 259–64.

●92. Minkov M, Grois N, Braier J *et al.* Immunosuppressive treatment for chemotherapy-resistant multisystem Langerhans cell histiocytosis. *Med Pediatr Oncol* 2003; **40**(4): 253–6.

●93. Mahmoud HH, Wang WC, Murphy SB. Cyclosporine therapy for advanced Langerhans cell histiocytosis. *Blood* 1991; **77**: 721–5.

♦94. Minkov M, Grois N, Broadbent V *et al.* Cyclosporine A therapy for multisystem Langerhans cell histiocytosis. *Med Pediatr Oncol* 1999; **33**: 482–5.

95. Culic S, Jakobson A, Culic V *et al.* Etoposide as the basic and interferon-alpha as the maintenance therapy for Langerhans cell histiocytosis: a RTC. *Pediatr Hematol Oncol* 2001; **18**: 291–4.

96. Kelly KM, Pritchard J. Monoclonal antibody therapy in Langerhans cell histiocytosis – feasible and reasonable? *Br J Cancer* 1994; **70**(Suppl XXIII): 54–5.

●97. Stine KC, Saylors RL, Williams LL, Becton DL. 2-Chloro-deoxyadenosine (2-CDA) for the treatment of refractory or recurrent Langerhans cell histiocytosis (LCH) in pediatric patients. *Med Pediatr Oncol* 1997; **29**(4): 288–92.

♦98. Weitzman S, Wayne AS, Arceci R *et al.* Nucleoside analogues in the therapy of Langerhans cell histiocytosis: a survey of members of the histiocyte society and review of the literature. *Med Pediatr Oncol* 1999; **33**: 476–81.

99. McCowage GB, Frush DP, Kurtzberg J. Successful treatment of two children with Langerhans' cell histiocytosis with 2'-deoxycoformycin. *J Pediatr Hematol Oncol* 1996; **18**: 154–8.

24

Rare tumours

R. G. GRUNDY & PIERS N. PLOWMAN

INTRODUCTION

The previous chapters in this book have reviewed the management of the commonest childhood cancers. There remains a heterogeneous group of tumours, which, whilst rarely encountered, often present significant management challenges. These tumours are discussed here and, where possible, treatment recommendations are made.

Paediatric oncologists will occasionally encounter examples of common adult cancers such as malignant melanoma and gastrointestinal tract cancers. Reviews of these conditions have not been included here as the management is identical to that in adults. We have therefore chosen to concentrate on tumours that are, perhaps, no more common than those just cited, but whose management contains an element of controversy in the paediatric versus the adult patient population. The overriding plea in this chapter is that we should move to international trials in order to better understand and better treat these rare but important tumours of childhood.

NASOPHARYNGEAL CARCINOMA

Nasopharyngeal carcinoma (NPC) is the commonest epithelial cancer of childhood, accounting for approximately 30 per cent of the nasopharyngeal malignancies that occur in this age group.

The nasopharynx has a rich vascular and lymphatic supply and drainage system. It is defined anatomically by the posterior choanae anteriorly, by the clivus superiorly and the first two cervical vertebra posteriorly. The declivity of the sphenoid defines the superior margin, while the lower boundary is defined by the soft palate. It is these characteristics that define the route of tumour spread, the clinical symptoms and the treatment.

Epidemiology

Nasopharyngeal carcinoma exhibits a wide disparity in gender, age, racial and geographic incidence. For example, males are twice as likely as females to develop NPC.[1,2] NPC is endemic in the southern parts of China, other parts of south-east Asia and the Mediterranean littoral. Aetiological factors of endemic NPC include environmental risk factors, genetic susceptibility and the Epstein–Barr virus (EBV).[3] Migration seems to reduce the incidence of NPC, being lower in US-born Chinese than in native-born Chinese. Furthermore, there are distinct geographic variations in the incidence of NPC, suggesting that environmental differences are important. Prior exposure to EBV is clearly implicated in the aetiology of poorly differentiated NPC in children and adults. The aetiological link between NPC and EBV was first based on serological evidence with elevated levels of IgG and IgA antibodies against the EBV early antigen complex. Large population screening trials have validated the use of EBV serology for NPC, particularly in high-risk groups in southern China.[4,5] The antibody levels seem to provide an indicator of initial tumour burden, with high levels corresponding with advanced disease, while declining levels of IgG to viral capsid antigen (VCA) correspond with the response to treatment remaining high or increasing in non-responders.[4,5] Rising antibody titres can predict clinical relapse by 1–6 months.[4,5] It has now been shown that EBV DNA is present in the NPC tumour cells and that NPC is clonal and arises from a single EBV-infected cell.[6] Furthermore, EBV has been detected in premalignant nasopharyngeal lesions, including carcinoma *in situ*,[7] suggesting that EBV infection is an early event in NPC. From the current data the most tenable hypothesis involves the action of EBV, a genetically determined susceptibility and environmental factors that vary from population to population. EBV is ubiquitous, and whilst this virus clearly plays a role in nasopharyngeal oncogenesis, it is not the sole causative agent.

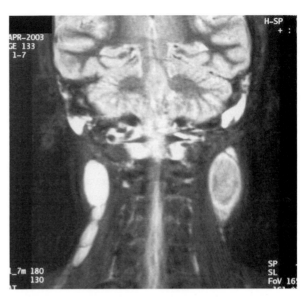

Figure 24.1 *Bilateral nodal involvement in nasopharyngeal carcinoma on magnetic resonance imaging.*

Histopathology

The majority of NPCs in childhood are of the subgroup undifferentiated (type 3). Undifferentiated NPCs are associated with the greater likelihood of advanced disease at presentation, despite having a lower stage primary disease.[8]

Clinical features

The characteristic presentation in the paediatric age group is with advanced locoregional disease. Symptoms are often relatively short and may initially be non-specific and attributed to upper respiratory tract infections. The most common presentation is cervical lymphadenopathy, which may be tender and bilateral (Figure 24.1). Unilateral or bilateral otitis media may result from tumour obstructing the eustachian tubes, which open into the lateral walls of the nasopharynx. Rarely, upward extension of the tumour towards the middle cranial fossa may result in the involvement of cranial nerves III–V, while lymphadenopathy or invasion of the base of the skull may affect the lower cranial nerves. Nasal obstruction or epistaxis occurs in approximately one-third of cases. Headache is a more common finding in young patients and is thought to reflect the higher stage disease seen at this age.[9] Delays in diagnosis are frequent and a high index of suspicion for this tumour in children with cervical lymphadenopathy, nasal symptoms or headache is essential so that examination of the nasopharynx is not unduly delayed.

Although around 80 per cent of NPCs in children have spread to local cervical lymph nodes by the time of diagnosis, some primaries are so small that the nasopharynx appears normal and only a blind biopsy reveals primary tumour. Overt distant metastases, present in less than 10 per cent of children at diagnosis, are most commonly to bone followed by liver and lung.[9–11] In childhood, the presence of cervical lymphadenopathy at diagnosis does not adversely affect the prognosis.[11] Poor prognosis factors include skull base involvement, cranial nerve involvement and extensive primary tumours.[11–13]

An unusual paraneoplastic syndrome may occur with widespread disease or metastatic relapse. This includes a marked osteoarthropathy with joint swelling and pain and clubbing of the fingers. This syndrome may also be seen in lymphoepithelioma of the thymus.

Staging

No single staging system has been widely accepted for NPC.[14–16] The staging system of the American Joint Committee on Cancer (AJCC) accommodates oropharyngeal malignancies of all ages and does not take into account the distinct characteristics of nasopharyngeal cancer in young people. Thus, in the fourth edition of the AJCC staging, more than 70 per cent of young patients are stage III or IV, mainly due to the high incidence of lymph node metastasis at diagnosis. Nor does it take into account the lack of association between T and N stage or the relatively good prognosis in children despite presenting with more 'advanced disease'.[17–19] Difficulty in examining the nasopharynx means that it is often difficult to assess whether the tumour involves one or more sites, an important factor in AJCC staging. Cranial nerve involvement in children carries a worse prognosis than base of skull involvement,[20] a factor not accounted for in the

AJCC classification. An alternative staging system proposed by Ho, specifically designed for NPC, accounts for some of these deficiencies.[14] The fifth edition of AJCC is an improvement on the previous versions.[21] However, a generally accepted staging system that allows accurate assessment of prognosis and planning of appropriate treatment for children with nasopharyngeal carcinoma is still required.

The size of the primary appears to be the most important prognostic factor in young patients.[17,18] Most studies in childhood have analysed the data according to the T stage, and thus results can be compared. Children less than 15 years and females tend to have a better prognosis, albeit not statistically significant.[18,22]

Evaluation

Clinical evaluation should define the extent of the cervical lymphadenopathy and involvement of cranial nerves. Indirect nasopharyngoscopy should be performed to assess the size and extent of the primary tumour. Surgical biopsy is recommended for histological evaluation and for assessment of EBV DNA. In view of the pattern of presentation and metastatic spread to mediastinum and lung, and later bone, staging investigations should include a magnetic resonance (MR) scan of the head, (concentrating on the base of the skull) and neck and chest X-ray or CT (computed tomography) of the chest, and for advanced disease a radionucleotide bone scan and abdominal ultrasound. Cerebrospinal fluid examination is indicated in those presenting with cranial nerve palsies. EBV serology, including IgG and IgA to VCA, should be assayed; the 'monospot' test is not adequate.

Treatment

The major obstacle to the cure of young patients with NPC is distant metastasis. As in adults, the mainstay of treatment hitherto has been high-dose radiotherapy to the nasopharynx and involved cervical nodes, plus moderate-dose radiation to uninvolved nodes. One randomized study has shown that chemotherapy, using cisplatinum and 5-fluorouracil (5-FU) and radiotherapy, is superior to radiotherapy alone in patients with advanced disease.[23] In addition, several prospective but non-randomized studies have shown a benefit for adjuvant chemotherapy in children.[10,19,24–29] Using a similar chemotherapy protocol to Al-Sarraf et al.,[23] the German co-operative group have also reported extremely good results.[27] Gasparini et al.,[24] using three cycles of cyclophosphamide, doxorubicin and vincristine prior to radiotherapy, reported a 75 per cent 3-year relapse-free survival (RFS) for patients with T3 and T4 tumours, compared with 8 per cent in the historical control group. The use of pre-irradiation chemotherapy led to a 50 per cent reduction in the size of the primary, and identified a group of non-responders who relapsed early despite further therapy. More recently, Kim et al.[26] reported a RFS of 85 per cent, median follow-up 4 years, using cyclophosphamide, doxorubicin, vincristine and 5-FU.

Radiotherapy is the critical component of curative treatment for NPC. The treatment volume should include the nasopharynx, posterior nasal cavity and any MR imaged spread, as well as prophylactic radiation to both sides of the neck – usually requiring generous coverage of the skull base. Current recommended prescriptions require at least 45 Gy to the clinical target volume, which should include a 1 cm margin around the MRI-detected primary site and regional lymph nodes where involved in the cervical region. Although the total radiation dose to the tumour appears to be an important prognostic factor regarding outcome in adults, the significance of dose is less clear in the paediatric population. Lombardi et al.[11] noted that the incidence of relapse is not directly related to dose of radiotherapy given, and doses as low as 35 Gy may achieve cure.[18] Studies relying on radiotherapy alone favour high doses, i.e. >60 Gy.[22] The optimal radiation dose for sustained local control is thus unclear. Some studies have shown that the volume of tissue irradiated may be important since the majority of patients with locoregional relapse have recurrent disease of, or at the margin of, the treatment portal;[18,19] this has not been universally found especially in studies using adjuvant chemotherapy.[24,26,28] Pre-radiation chemotherapy has shown that a reduction in the volume of tissue irradiated is possible, and clearly this would be of benefit in terms of reducing late morbidity. Those children whose disease responds poorly to pre-irradiation chemotherapy[17] may represent a subgroup with more aggressive disease, and should perhaps be singled out for more intensive therapy. Radiotherapy alone may be sufficient for patients with stage I or II disease, as in adults, with some controversy as to the continuing need for 'current standard practice' prophylactic lower neck irradiation.[29] A retrospective analysis using Ho's classification and stage grouping showed a 100 per cent disease-free survival (DFS) in groups A and B using total neck irradiation – this is the benchmark against which new approaches will be assessed.

Interferon has been used successfully in a child who relapsed with widespread metastasis after treatment with radiotherapy and chemotherapy. In addition to resolution of disease, the titre of EBV antibodies also normalized.[30] The use of this antiviral agent has not been tested in a prospective randomized manner.

The optimal chemoradiotherapy regimen for children with NPC is unclear and attempts to produce an international protocol are now overdue. The acceptance of synchronous chemoradiation in adult head and neck cancer treatment protocols cannot be immediately applied to paediatric practice. There is a well defined late morbidity from concurrent use of sensitizing drugs with radiation therapy that has led to many severe late effects.

TREATMENT TOXICITY

Acute toxicity depends upon the nature of the combination of chemotherapy and radiotherapy used. Acute encephalopathy has been reported in 20 per cent of adults when doses of radiotherapy exceed 60 Gy without attention to meticulous technique.[31] Long-term toxicity is primarily due to high doses of radiotherapy, and includes soft tissue, bone and endocrine change.[19,24,26] Neck atrophy and fibrosis commonly occur and may be severe. Chronic oral problems include xerostomia and trismus.[19,24,26] Intensive dental care may reduce these problems. Reduced final height, especially in those treated prepubertally, when the pituitary was included in the radiation field provides indirect evidence of pituitary dysfunction.[19] Hypothyroidism is relatively rare but should be regularly assessed. Second malignant neoplasms in the radiation field may be a risk[32] but have not occurred in most series.[19,24,26,33] Documentation is required rather than any change in practice at present.

Future directions

There are many questions outstanding with regard to epidemiology, staging and treatment of NPC. The involvement of EBV in oncogenesis merits further study, as does the role of biological response modifiers, such as interferon, and that of adoptive immunotherapy. A staging system appropriate to NPC in young patients is essential. Prospective international collaborative randomized trials to define optimal chemotherapy, the timing of chemotherapy and radiotherapy, the role of hyperfractionated radiotherapy and the possibility of reduction in radiation dose depending on tumour response need to be organized.

SALIVARY GLAND TUMOURS

Of all salivary gland tumours, 2–4 per cent occur in patients under 16 years of age.[34,35] Fortunately, the majority of these are not true neoplasms, and those that are neoplastic are usually benign.

There were 430 paediatric cases in the series of salivary swellings analysed by the American Armed Forces Institute of Pathology (AFIP).[35] Of these cases (from which mumps was virtually excluded), 262 were non-neoplastic and, among those, mucoceles comprised the majority (185 cases). However, there were 168 true neoplasms of the salivary glands. The majority (124 cases) occurred in the parotid gland, and 124 of those were benign (45 pleomorphic adenomas and 40 vascular tumours).

Pleomorphic adenoma in children, as in adults, occurs predominantly in the parotid gland. It is more common in females, the sex ratio being 2:1 in one series.[36] Teenagers are more commonly affected than younger children. Presentation is with a slowly enlarging smooth mass.

The treatment of choice is parotidectomy with preservation of the facial nerve. Tumours lateral to the facial nerve or in the tail of the parotid gland are managed by a lateral (superficial) parotidectomy, while deep-seated tumours are managed by total parotidectomy with preservation of the nerve. Local excision alone or with radiotherapy can be regarded as inferior management schemes.

In the Ann Arbor experience, 18 previously untreated patients underwent conservation parotidectomy with preservation of the facial nerve. All patients remained free of disease at the time of reporting. However, these authors also reported 12 children referred to them with recurrent tumour following surgery at other institutions, and only one of those patients had received surgery as major as superficial parotidectomy.[36] The authors point out that not only does local excision carry a risk of a high local recurrence rate, but that with further surgery it is less easy to preserve the facial nerve. Moreover, there is a risk of true malignancy (carcinoma ex-pleomorphic adenoma): two of the 12 children referred with local recurrence developed distant metastases.

Of salivary gland tumours, the group of vascular tumours comprises: juvenile cellular haemangioendothelioma (in infants), haemangioma and lymphangioma. The parotid is the most common site of occurrence, and females are affected more often than males. These lesions give rise to smooth, soft, slowly enlarging (to a plateau size) masses that fluctuate (Figure 24.2). Surgical excision of large masses, or radiotherapy in exceptional circumstances (see below), is the treatment of choice.

Of 168 paediatric true salivary neoplasms assimilated by the AFIP, 54 were malignant epithelial tumours and the remaining 19 cases were a heterogeneous collection of primary and secondary sarcomas (rhabdomyosarcoma, fibrosarcoma, anaplastic tumours). In a recently reported series of 19 children with malignant salivary tumours, there were six primary carcinomas and nine rhabdomyosarcomas.[37]

From the Memorial Hospital series, it seems unlikely that undiagnosed neoplasms in the submandibular gland are more likely to be malignant than those in the parotid. The rare neoplasms in the sublingual gland were all malignant.[34]

Mucoepidermoid carcinoma, the most common salivary carcinoma, accounted for 20 out of 35 malignant epithelial cancers in the AFIP series (14 out of 20 cases in the parotid). The majority of patients presented only

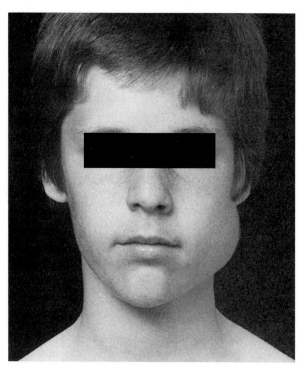

Figure 24.2 *Haemangioma of the parotid gland (courtesy of Professor L. Spitz).*

because of swelling, and pain or facial nerve paresis was rare. A histological grading system (grades I–III) was found to be prognostically useful, and patients with facial nerve dysfunction or positive cervical nodes were more likely to have low-grade (I) histology. However, although these tumours were often felt to be clinically mobile and discrete, histologically they had no true capsule. In this large study that embraced all age groups, prognosis was clearly better in younger patients.[38]

Treatment recommendations for childhood mucoepidermoid carcinoma are the same as in adult practice. The recommended surgical strategy is complete removal of the neoplasm with minimum morbidity to normal tissue. The type of operation depends on the extent of the lesion. A subtotal parotidectomy with sparing of the facial nerve is optimal if it complies with this strategy, but for more extensive growths, total parotidectomy with nerve sacrifice and postoperative radiotherapy may be necessary. In general, the results of surgery for paediatric salivary gland carcinoma are good and the majority of children are cured.[39] Limited surgery, when histology shows disease at or close to the margins, and postoperative radiotherapy probably represent an inferior treatment strategy to radical surgery, as outlined above. However, postoperative radiotherapy does decrease the local relapse rate in higher-risk patients.[40]

Mucoepidermoid carcinoma of submandibular and sublingual glands is treated by radical gland resection.

Block dissection of cervical lymph nodes is indicated either at presentation or at relapse when these nodes are clinically involved. Overall, with optimal management, the expected survival rate for children with salivary mucoepidermoid carcinoma should exceed 90 per cent.

Three very rare malignant epithelial salivary tumours, in decreasing incidence and worsening prognosis, are actinic cell carcinoma, adenoid cystic carcinoma and adenocarcinoma. The clinical presentation and principles of therapy are exactly as for mucoepidermoid carcinoma.

True neoplasms of the minor salivary glands are extremely rare in childhood, but they comprise the same tumours with similar relative incidence as those discussed above.[41] Treatment principles are also similar.

AMELOBLASTOMA

The ameloblastoma is a rare tumour of the enamel organ stem cells. It usually presents as a cystic mass, much more commonly in the mandible (85 per cent of cases) than in the maxilla. On section, there may be both cystic and solid components. Surgical resection is the treatment of choice, but incomplete excision frequently leads to local recurrence. Wide surgical clearance is therefore the optimal treatment, with radiotherapy reserved only for failure to achieve microscopically clear margins. Metastatic spread is extremely rare.

THYROID CANCER

Although children with differentiated thyroid carcinomas often present with extensive disease, it is rarely fatal. This paradox has created uncertainty regarding the optimal surgical and adjuvant therapies for differentiated thyroid carcinomas in childhood.

Epidemiology

The incidence of childhood thyroid cancer is 0.5/million per year, equal to five new cases in England and Wales per year. Only 5–10 per cent of all thyroid cancers occur in childhood. Peak incidence is in adolescents (main age around 15 years).[42,43] Tumours occur more frequently in girls of all races and of all ages.[43]

Histopathology

Most children with thyroid carcinoma have well differentiated papillary tumours (80–90 per cent). The proportion of follicular cancers (5–15 per cent) is much lower than in adults, these two making up the group of tumours referred to as differentiated thyroid cancer (DTC). Medullary carcinomas of the thyroid (MTCs) comprise 5–10 per cent. Anaplastic carcinoma is extremely rare. Most radiation-induced tumours are papillary.

Aetiology

Ionizing radiation is strongly implicated in the oncogenesis of DTC. Evidence for this emanates from clinical reports describing excess risk of DTC in those who had previously received therapeutic irradiation.[44,45] The impact of environmental irradiation has been intensively studied since atmospheric testing of nuclear weapons after the Second World War and more recently after the radiation leak at Chernobyl.[46] Incidence rates after the accident were raised by up to 10-fold[47] and are thought to be related to exposure to radioactive iodine. Younger children, some of whom were irradiated *in utero*, were more vulnerable than adolescents.[48] The tumours have been reported as being more aggressive in their clinical behaviour.

Ret proto-oncogene mutations with oncogenic rearrangements of the ret tyrosine kinase receptor have been characterized in patients with both differentiated papillary thyroid cancer and MTC.[49,50] Specific somatic rearrangements (ret/PTC1, ret/PTC2 and ret/PTC3) have been identified. All are formed by the fusion of the truncated tyrosine kinase domain of ret to the aminoterminus of different gene fragments. Their frequency varies according to geographic area, the highest being in Italy (33–35 per cent) and lowest in Saudi Arabia (2.5 per cent) and Japan (0–9 per cent). ret/PTC1 mutation was most common in sporadic cases, whilst ret/PTC3 was most common in those in radiation-induced cases in both adults and children.[51]

Clinical findings

Enlargements of a cervical lymph node or a painless thyroid nodule are the commonest presenting complaints and occur in up to 60 per cent of cases. A solitary nodule in a child's thyroid gland is always a matter of concern and between 15 and 20 per cent of such nodules are malignant. Metastatic disease occurs in less than 10 per cent of patients at diagnosis. The lungs are the commonest extranodal sites for secondary disease, which are more frequent with follicular than with papillary tumours.

Investigations

Fine-needle aspiration biopsy is used in children, although it is controversial as to whether it is as sensitive or specific as in adult practice. This is related to difficulties in discriminating cytologically between follicular

adenoma and carcinoma.[52,53] Clearly the interpretation of such samples is a matter of great expertise.

Conventional imaging with X-rays, CT/MRI scans and bone scans will also demonstrate local spread to the mediastinum, lung and distant metastases. Distant metastases can be demonstrated by radioiodine uptake studies after radical thyroidectomy and ablation of the thyroid remnant by radioiodine.

Surgery

The evidence favours a radical surgical approach in childhood.[54,55] Radical neck dissection, with its attendant risks, is generally avoided in children with differentiated tumours.[56]

Total thyroidectomy is also recommended for MTC in view of the high incidence of multifocal tumours. It is recommended that in individuals affected by multiple endocrine neoplasia (MEN) type 2A, prophylactic thyroidectomy should be carried out before the age of 5 years; and in those with MEN type 2B it should be considered in the first year of life.[57]

Treatment and prognosis

Apart from the rare anaplastic tumours, most thyroid cancers have a 'slow' natural history, particularly in children. The corollary to the indolent course of this disease is that there may be very late recurrences, 20–30 years from diagnosis. A sensible and prolonged follow-up strategy is essential.

Children with microcarcinomas less than 1.5 cm in the greatest diameter have a low risk of recurrence (<5 per cent), which is almost always locoregional. Lobectomy is treatment of choice for unifocal disease of this size and total thyroidectomy for patients with multifocal disease. This may be the group of small, intrathyroidal papillary and microangioinvasive/non-angioinvasive follicular thyroid cancers (FTCs), for which a less than radical surgical policy (and no radioiodine ablation) is appropriate. The treatment of children with larger intrathyroidal disease remains somewhat controversial; however, until evidence accrues to the contrary, radical surgery plus adjunctive therapy is recommended.

There is little published evidence in childhood and adolescent DTC that radioiodine ablation is indicated, although this is often the recommended treatment. The largest reported group of children, adolescents and young adults with DTC includes 170 patients (137 papillary and 33 follicular) and has shown that the risk of recurrence was more common in multifocal or large tumours and in those with palpable cervical lymphadenopathy or metastases at diagnosis. By multivariate analysis, multifocal tumours showed the greatest risk of recurrence.[54] However, none of these risk factors pertains to children <16 years.[54] These findings would suggest that it is difficult to extrapolate from adults to children, although the sample size in the childhood series tends to be small by comparison. These same authors found that the recurrence rate was similar for children, adolescents and young adults whether they were treated with thyroid hormone suppression alone or with thyroid hormone suppression plus radioactive iodine.[54]

Massimino et al.[58] also suggest that surgery and thyroid-stimulating hormone (TSH) suppression by thyroid hormone was adequate treatment for DTC in childhood albeit from a considerably smaller study. Similar findings were reported by Newman et al.,[59] who found that ^{131}I therapy was not a determinant of progression-free survival (PFS).

Furthermore, a report from Landou et al.[60] from the Royal Marsden Hospital suggested that thyroxine therapy, resulting in TSH suppression, was the only intervention shown to reduce the recurrence rate. Radioiodine used as part of the initial management for ablation of residual thyroid tissue in this series was associated with a lower recurrence rate; however, this did not reach statistical significance ($P = 0.13$). Moreover, the follow-up in patients who received radioiodine is only 7 years compared with 30 years for the rest of the group. As the median time to recurrence was 7 years, it is possible that recurrence in the iodine-treated group will increase and reduce any difference between these treatment modalities. It may also be that in time a benefit is seen.

There is some evidence that FTC is less aggressive than papillary thyroid cancer (PTC) in children.[54,61–63] Children with FTC are less likely to have either total or distant metastases at diagnosis than those with PTC. Indeed, the majority (66 per cent) have disease localized to the tumour at diagnosis. In one of these series with long follow-up, no children with FTC died of disease.[54] The risk of relapse was greater in those with multifocal disease among the adolescents and young adults but this did not hold true for those <16 years. However, the patients with recurrence of FTC tended to be younger than those in whom recurrence did not occur. The risk of recurrence was not associated with gender, palpable cervical lymphadenopathy at diagnosis, the interval between initial symptoms and diagnosis, metastatic disease at diagnosis or tumour size.[54] Earlier reports also showed a lower rate of recurrence for FTC vs. PTC.[61–63]

The major concern over the use of ^{131}I is the risk of late effects especially to children. In terms of toxicity and late effects the available data suggest that fertility is not impaired.[64] The paper by Landou et al.[60] suggested that with ^{131}I delivering 3 GBq the dose to each testis is 9.2 cGy, a level that should not cause azoospermia. The dose of ^{131}I is clearly of importance; from Mazzaferri's paper[64a] it would seem that when using ^{131}I to ablate remnant thyroid tissue after thyroidectomy, low doses (29–50 mCi) were as effective as higher doses (51–200 mCi), the lower doses having the additional benefit of reduced side-effects. There appears to be a relatively low risk of second tumour.[65,66] Clearly, in a tumour with a very high overall survival rate, we have to be sure that the lifetime risk of secondary cancer is low.

Local and distant metastatic disease is more common in PTC than in FTC.[67] For such patients, the evidence is in favour of radical thyroidectomy (one clear indication for early radical surgery to primary tumour despite the establishment of metastatic disease) and repeated ^{131}I therapy applications (for as long as there is uptake on post-therapy body scanning and reduction in thyroglobulin measurements or other assessments) and long-term TSH suppression; regular monitoring of serum thyroglobulin and iodine scanning is mandatory.

Serum thyroglobulin levels should be unrecordable in the athyroid patient (i.e. after radical surgery and radio-iodine ablation). Any increase in the thyroglobulin is therefore due to recurrence.[68] The use of radioiodine scanning (^{123}I or ^{131}I) is also facilitated by radioablation of remnant thyroid tissue, as, in general, metastatic disease is less avid in terms of iodine avidity than normal thyroid tissue.

Future directions

The role of DNA aneuploidy as an indicator of malignant potential in thyroid cancer of childhood requires further evaluation. The precise influence of the ret/PTC mutation type may provide biological markers of tumour behaviour as well as act as an indicator of aetiology.

The use of serum thyroglobulin as a tumour marker in localized PTCs/FTCs is well established in adult practice and may permit disease monitoring without the use of radioisotopes. Such an approach could reserve these established investigations and treatments for those at greatest risk of life-threatening disease progression.

BREAST TUMOURS IN CHILDHOOD AND ADOLESCENCE

Breast tumours are far more likely to be benign than malignant throughout childhood and into adolescence. However, because carcinoma of the breast is the most common neoplasm in adult women, any breast lump raises understandable fears for both the child and the parents. A clear understanding of normal and abnormal breast development is essential in order to avoid needless diagnostic evaluation and the potential physical and psychological damage done by unnecessary surgery. It is essential that a biopsy is taken before radical surgery is undertaken.

Due to the rarity of breast carcinoma in childhood, breast masses need not be immediately excised unless rapidly growing or fixed. Biopsy undertaken by a specialist breast surgeon, with careful pathological review by a paediatric pathologist, can help to decide appropriate therapy. There is usually very little breast tissue in young patients, and thus excessively wide excision may lead to disfigurement and potentially considerable psychological trauma, particularly in females. Conservation of the breast bud is crucial in prepubertal children. Accurate pathological diagnosis and an understanding of the behaviour of the various tumours of the breast in childhood are essential so that excessive surgery and adjuvant therapy are avoided. Careful pathological study of all breast cancers in children, including receptor assays, are indicated in order to further our understanding of these neoplasms.

In cases where the pathology of the breast mass is identical to adult cases, the treatment recommendations are as for adults.

Fibroadenoma is the commonest breast mass occurring before and during puberty and usually presents as a freely mobile, asymptomatic lump, most commonly in the upper outer quadrant of the breast.[69] Although clearly related to hormonal activity, the cause of these tumours is unknown. Bilateral tumours of fibroadenomatosis may occur but are uncommon.[69] Observation of any breast mass in this age group through a menstrual period is recommended; benign lesions are more likely to show an increase in size and tenderness at menstruation.

Intraductal papillomas usually present with a bloody or sero-sanguineous discharge from the nipple; local excision of the involved ductal system is curative.

Clearly, in dealing with these essentially benign conditions, emotional and cosmetic considerations are paramount. The culture of breast self-examination from adolescence should be encouraged.

Breast malignancy may be primary, metastatic or arise as a second malignant neoplasm (SMN). Over a 25-year period at a single institution 18 patients were seen with malignancy of the breast; two had primary disease, 13 had metastatic involvement and three were SMNs.[70] It is axiomatic that this ratio needs to be considered in the investigation of children and adolescents with a suspected breast cancer. Primary malignancies include breast carcinomas, rhabdomyosarcomas and non-Hodgkin's lymphoma.[70] Breast cancer as a SMN usually follows irradiation, e.g. as given for low-stage Hodgkin's disease.[71]

Several large series have reported that fewer than 0.1 per cent of all primary carcinomas of the breast occur in children under 15 years of age.[69] Interestingly, approximately 15 per cent of children with this cancer are male, compared with only 1 per cent of adults with this condition.[69] It is now recognized that the majority of primary cancers of the breast in childhood and adolescence are clinically and histologically distinct from those seen in older patients. Histologically, the so-called, juvenile secreting carcinoma (JSC) grossly resembles the infiltrating type of carcinoma seen in adults, but the similarity is less marked at the histological level where a sheet-like arrangement of proliferating cells is characteristic. Furthermore, the cytoplasm stains less intensely with eosin, often appearing clear and homogeneous. Eosinophilic periodic acid-Schiff (PAS) positivity is seen within the cytoplasm of the tumour cells and within the rudimentary ductal spaces formed by the tumour.[72]

Juvenile secreting carcinoma is a slow-growing, locally recurring tumour and a long-standing asymptomatic breast lump in the subareolar region is the usual presenting symptom.[69,72,73] Nipple discharge and lymphadenopathy rarely, if ever, occur. Prognosis is clearly related to age and histopathological type. To date, no patient with JSC under 12 years at diagnosis has died, whereas, seven of 16 patients presenting in the adolescent period have died from disease.[69,72,74]

Cystosarcoma phyllodes is a related but rapidly growing tumour and is usually, but not exclusively, benign. Approximately 5 per cent of phyllodes tumours occur in adolescence. Phyllodes tumour has not been reported in males. Large tumours do not seem to bear a higher risk of recurrence.[75] Macroscopically these tumours contain firm fibrous areas alternating with soft fleshy or cystic areas. Histopathologically, they show greater cellularity, particularly of the fibrous tissue stroma, than fibroadenomas. Atypical cellular appearance, increased mitotic activity, haemorrhage, necrosis and infiltrative margins help to distinguish the malignant phyllodes tumour.[76] A study of 40 cases of phyllodes tumour in adolescents has shown that 84 per cent of cases are benign, 3 per cent borderline and 13 per cent malignant.[77] However, histology does not always accurately predict future behaviour and so-called 'benign' tumours may relapse.[76–78] Wide local excision is the primary treatment of choice.[69,76,79] Axillary clearing is usually unnecessary as the possibility of lymphadenopathy is remote.[76,79] More radical surgery should be reserved for malignant phyllodes tumours or multi-recurrent disease.[79] Metastasis predominantly to the lungs followed by the bones may occur.[79] In the rare instances of progressive disease, responses to chemotherapy, cyclophosphamide, and radiotherapy have been reported.[80] As phyllodes tumours can recur, regardless of their histology, long-term follow-up is necessary.[76,78]

THORACIC TUMOURS

Primary tumours of the lung are uncommon in childhood, most cases being bronchial adenomas of which fewer than 100 have been reported.[81–85] Bronchial adenomas are a heterogeneous group encompassing four distinct tumours only one of which is truly benign.[81,84,86–91] As these tumours involve major bronchi, presentation is usually that of bronchial obstruction with repeated or non-resolving pulmonary infections and chronic cough; haemoptysis may occur and wheezing may be heard on auscultation. Delays in diagnosis are common.

Bronchial carcinoid

Although these represent 80–85 per cent of bronchial adenomas, only 36 proven cases have been reported in children.[81,84,87,88,91] These tumours arise from the multipotential neural crest cells known as Kutschinsky cells. It is postulated that oat cell carcinomas arise from the same cells, and thus electron microscopy often helps to make the diagnosis. This histology largely predicts the behaviour, with atypical carcinoids having a greater metastatic potential (66 per cent of cases) compared with the more benign typical carcinoid that metastasizes in only 5 per cent of cases.[92] Carcinoid syndrome rarely occurs with pulmonary tumours. The treatment is surgical resection. The overall survival in children is 90 per cent.[86]

Cylindroma

These are the most malignant thoracic tumours and account for 12–25 per cent of all adenomas. They are derived from mucus-secreting cells of the bronchial mucosa and histologically resemble tumours of salivary glands.[86] The treatment is surgical.

Mucoepidermoid

The least common and least malignant, fewer than 20 cases have been reported in children.[81,88,89,91,93,94] One of these was associated with a lymph node metastasis; however, this tumour, diagnosed at 4 years of age, was, in retrospect, present on chest X-rays taken at 3 months and 2.5 years of age. It is a slow-growing, locally invasive disease with a more favourable outcome in children.[81,88,89,91,93,94] Once again, the treatment is surgical.

Mucous gland adenoma

This is the only truly benign lesion and also the rarest.[86,89,90] Therapy is surgical.

Primary carcinoma of the lung

Fewer than 50 cases of primary carcinoma of the lung have now been reported, the youngest being 5 months at diagnosis. No firm aetiological factors have been identified, and only two patients ever smoked.[83,86,89] Undifferentiated carcinoma is the commonest histological type followed by adenocarcinoma, unclassified and squamous cell carcinoma. This latter tumour comprises 12 per cent of all cases compared with 35 per cent in adults.[83,86,89,95]

Although many children have symptoms related to their primary disease there may be metastatic symptoms of weight loss, bone pain and anaemia. In Japan a series of bronchogenic carcinomas were discovered by mass screening for tuberculosis.[83] Despite the chest X-ray appearances, the malignant nature of the underlying condition was not always immediately recognized.[83] Trials of chemotherapy have not been undertaken in this very small group, and standard treatment is radical surgery.[95]

Pleuropulmonary blastoma (PPB)

Pleuropulmonary blastoma (PPB) is a distinct clinicopathological entity that only occurs in children.[96,97] PPBs are now considered to be true embryonic neoplasms that arise from the thoracopulmonary mesenchyme.[96] PPB is an aggressive disease with a poor prognosis.

PPBs may be predominately cystic or exclusively solid. At the microscopic level, a mixed picture is usually seen with condensed blastematous islands of high mitotic activity and areas of undifferentiated loose mesenchymal spindle cells. The stroma in the blastema often blends into spindle cell sarcoma areas. In other cases, the stoma may be sharply demarcated from the blastematous islands and resemble the stroma surrounding the blastema of a Wilms' tumour.[96] Histopathologically, PPBs may recapitulate fetal lung tissue.[98] PPBs are subclassified as purely cystic (type I), cystic and solid (type II) and purely solid (type III). Rhabdomyoblastic differentiation is observed in most type I PPBs, whilst cartilaginous differentiation is seen in the majority of type II and type III PPBs. Areas of anaplasia occur in almost 70 per cent of type II and type III PPBs. Because of the histological variability of the solid component of a PPB, the differential diagnosis may be wide and, depending on the degree of mesenchymal differentiation, may be misdiagnosed. Immunopositivity to desmin and S-200 confirm myogenic origin.[96]

The occurrence of PPB marks a familial predisposition to neoplastic and dysplastic disease.[99] In approximately 25 per cent of cases of PPB, there is a family history of childhood neoplasms or congenital dysplastic conditions of the lung, kidney and thyroid gland.[99] Two instances of familial PPB are also documented. Associated conditions include those in two children with PPB and cystic adenomatoid malformation of the lung, one of whom also had intralobar nephroblastomatosis, a developmental abnormality associated with Wilms' tumour.[100] To date, no constitutional DNA abnormalities are reported, and limited molecular analyses of TP53 and WT1 have likewise revealed no abnormalities.[99] Partial and complete trisomy of chromosomes 2 and 8 are reported, with trisomy 2 being associated with embryonal rhabdomyosarcoma.[99,101–103] Further molecular analysis of familial and sporadic PPB is likely to be fruitful and aid our understanding of this malignancy.

The most common clinical symptom is respiratory difficulty such as cough or breathlessness; fever may or may not be present, and children are usually treated with antibiotics for a suspected chest infection but fail to respond.[96,103–107] Chest or abdominal pain may be present, as may more non-specific symptoms such as anorexia and malaise. Congenital pulmonary cystic disease may predispose to PPB in children.[106–108] Chest X-rays may reveal the presence of pulmonary cysts. This raises the possibility that PPB may arise in a pre-existing developmental abnormality (c.f. nephroblastomatosis and Wilms' tumour). PPB has also been reported to masquerade as an empyema.

Type I PPB is the least complex tumour and presents at an earlier age than type II or type III PPB. The prognosis would appear to be better for type I PPB, with an 83 per cent 5-year survival; however, the small number of cases reported makes this suggestion hard to confirm. The 5-year survival for type II and type III PPB is 42 per cent.[96] Mediastinal or pleural involvement is associated with a worse outcome, and the size of the primary tumour is also an important risk factor with tumours >5 cm having a worse outcome.[96,109] PPB metastasizes preferentially to the CNS and to the skeletal system. Type I PPB is the least common of the three tumour types and typically occurs in young children and, rarely, in the neonatal period.[96,108]

Treatment guidelines are difficult to establish, with only around 50 cases reported in the literature. Most patients undergo initial surgical resection, which is often incomplete due to tumour involvement of adjacent tissues.[96] This suggests a potentially valuable role for pre-operative chemotherapy, particularly as PPBs are chemosensitive tumours.[96,103,105–107,110] As this tumour arises from mesenchyme, it responds to agents used to treat malignant mesenchymal tumours (MMTs). Gadolinium scanning is useful in the detection of recurrence or metastatic disease.[111]

THYMIC TUMOURS

A number of primary malignancies can involve the thymus, including Hodgkin's, non-Hodgkin's lymphoma, germ cell tumour, thymoma, thymolipoma and carcinoid in relative order of frequency. It is now recognized that paraneoplastic phenomena such as myasthenia gravis, red cell aplasia and hypogammaglobulinaemia occur in children as well as adults with thymomas or thymolipomas.[112,113]

Thymolipomas

This is a slow-growing benign tumour that represents less than 10 per cent of all thymic neoplasms. Thymolipomas can achieve a massive size prior to discovery, and insidious breathlessness and long-standing symptoms of asthma have been reported.[114]

This lobular, fleshy tumour is composed of mature fatty and thymic tissue, but the histogenesis is uncertain. Due to the high fat content, thymolipomas have a characteristic appearance on CT and MRI. As the treatment of choice is surgical, a generous biopsy to confirm the diagnosis should precede surgical resection.

Thymoma

The distinction between benign and malignant thymomas depends upon clinical behaviour and pathology. Some thymomas behave in a malignant fashion despite a benign histological appearance. The distinction between benign and malignant thymomas depends on the demonstration of local invasion or metastases. Thymomas are usually slow-growing tumours, with up to 40 per cent being found serendipitously on chest X-ray. Symptoms may be respiratory in nature due to the slowly growing compressive mediastinal mass. To date, fewer than 30 cases of this highly aggressive tumour have been reported. Clinical presentation of malignant thymoma is attributable to a rapidly expanding mediastinal mass and to local invasion. The occurrence of periosteal new bone formation and clubbing has also been reported in thymomas, a paraneoplastic phenomenon reminiscent of children with NPC which may reflect the fact that both the thymus and nasopharynx arise from the primitive foregut.

AETIOLOGY

The demonstration of EBV in lymphoepithelial-like carcinoma arising in the thymus suggests a role for EBV in the aetiology of this condition as well as in NPC.[115,116]

PATHOLOGY

Malignant thymomas in children are defined as tumours that derive exclusively from epithelial cells. Lymphocytes are usually abundant and may cause some difficulty in distinguishing thymomas from lymphomas, but are not part of the neoplastic process. Due to the variety of thymomas in children the histopathological subclassification has not been established. Two distinct groups of thymic tumours are recognized (Box 24.1).[117]

Box 24.1 *Pathological classification of malignant thymomas*

> I Low-grade well differentiated tumours
> II High-grade tumours (thymic carcinoma)
> – squamous cell carcinoma
> – lymphoepithelial-like carcinoma
> – clear cell carcinoma
> – sarcomatoid
> – undifferentiated

High-grade tumours are characterized by a diffuse growth pattern with sheets of tumour cells containing large vesicular nuclei and prominent nucleoli surrounded by a dense lymphoid infiltrate; neuroendocrine differentiation may be seen. Differentiated/paraneoplastic changes with pronounced cellular pleomorphism, bizarre nuclei and atypical mitosis may also be seen.

SURGICOPATHOLOGICAL STAGING OF THYMOMA

 I Intact capsule
 II Pericapsular growth into adjacent mediastinal fat or tissue, including adjacent pleura or pericardium
 III Invasion into surrounding structures
 IV Extrathoracic metastases

TREATMENT

As these tumours are uncommon in children, it is necessary to extrapolate from the adult experience in order to provide treatment guidelines. A number of studies in adults have now shown that combination chemotherapy is an effective treatment for invasive thymoma.[116,118–120] Patients with stage I disease are curable by resection alone. Patients with stage II disease should be treated with postoperative radiotherapy. Those patients with advanced disease stages III or IV require a multidisciplinary approach that includes preoperative chemotherapy, surgical resection, postoperative radiotherapy and consolidation chemotherapy. The most impressive results reported in the literature to date are those from Shin *et al.*[120] Responses to similar therapy in advanced thymomas in children have been reported.[116]

MESOTHELIOMA

Introduction and epidemiology

Mesothelioma arises from the surface mesothelial layer that covers the pleura and peritoneal cavities, but may also arise from other serosal surfaces such as the tunica vaginalis and the pericardium.[121–124] Mesotheliomas are exceedingly rare primary malignancies in children. Indeed, no case of malignant mesothelioma was diagnosed from 3645 tumours in the population-based Manchester Children's Tumour Registry.[125] In adults, the incidence is 2.2 per million with only 2–5 per cent of all cases occurring in the first two decades,[125,126] whilst the incidence of malignant pleural tumours in those younger than 15 years is 0.13/million per year.[127] It should be noted, however, that any figures for the incidence of mesothelioma are unreliable, particularly as there is no internationally recognized code for mesothelioma and since these tumours present a diagnostic dilemma to the pathologist, with as many as 45 per cent of all cases being misdiagnosed.[128]

In adults there is the strong link to prior exposure to asbestos, particularly crocidolite, as first noted by Pliny. The latent period between exposure and cancer is estimated to be 12–20 years.[129] Accordingly, there is a strong male predominance in adults, with three times as many males as females developing mesothelioma, whereas only a slight male predominance (ratio of 1.7:1) has been reported in childhood pleural mesothelioma.[128] In the largest study so far reported in children, only four out of 80 were found to have identifiable risk factors, two of whom had prior asbestos exposure.[128] Asbestos-induced childhood mesothelioma is a theoretical possibility and asbestos bodies have been reported in the lungs of young children.[130] However, there is no clear evidence for prior exposure to asbestos in children who develop pleural mesothelioma, nor in over 20 per cent of men and 90 per cent of women, suggesting other aetiological factors are important.[131] The absence of geographical clustering in a study from the USA is a feature against environmental influence.[132] A cluster of cases of childhood mesothelioma in the West Midlands regions has been reported but still requires explanation.[133] Exposure to SV40-contaminated polio virus vaccine has, however, been implicated in the aetiology of a number of cancers including mesothelioma, but a recent study with 30-year follow-up failed to show an increased rate in this tumour in children so exposed.[134]

A number of patients have now been reported who have developed pleural mesothelioma as a SMN. These patients all received radiation therapy as part of their initial treatment.[135–138] Out of a total of 30 patients reported in the literature, 18 were treated in childhood. Of note, nine of these children had Hodgkin's disease and five had Wilms' tumour.

Biology

Cytogenetic analysis of pleural malignant mesothelioma has revealed complex clonal abnormalities.[139] Most tumours displayed multiple numeral and structural alterations. The most frequent changes were loss of chromosomal material from 1p and 9p and the shortest region of overlap was 1p21–p22 and 9p21–p22.[139] Most tumours had loss of multiple chromosomal regions, including 3p, 6q, 14, 16, 18 and 22, suggesting a multistep pathogenic process. The *WT1* tumour suppressor gene is expressed in the mesothelial lining during embryological development.[140] Mutations in *WT1* have been detected in some sporadic mesotheliomas,[141] but the role of this gene in the progression to malignancy is unclear. Those children with a mesothelioma as a SMN did not have any clinical features of a germ line mutation in the *WT1* gene.

Pathology

Difficulties in making the pathological diagnosis of mesothelioma are well recognized in both adults and children.[128,129] In children, as many as 45 per cent of all cases may be misdiagnosed.[125] In children, most cases have a predominant tubular papillary pattern with solid areas, whilst some tumours show foci of single cells. The immunohistochemical profile shows reactivity for antibodies to cytokeratin, epithelial membrane antigen and vimentin. These may be helpful in the differential diagnosis.[125] As tissue diagnosis is difficult, the diagnosis of malignant mesothelioma is best made by a panel of pathologists.

Clinical presentation

Approximately 75–85 per cent of all mesotheliomas arise from the pleura, 15–20 per cent from the peritoneal cavity and a small percentage from either the pericardium or the tunica vaginalis.

Tumours arising from the pleural cavity usually present with gradually increasing diffuse chest pain. Shortness of breath and cough arise following the development of a pleural effusion, and hoarseness and haemoptysis may also occur.

Peritoneal mesotheliomas (PMs) usually present with vague symptomatology of abdominal pain, distension, weight loss and ascites. Approximately 65 per cent of PMs occur in girls. PMs have variable clinical behaviour, with multicystic PMs appearing to carry a more favourable outcome.[142–144] These tumours present either as multiple, translucent, fluid-filled cysts or, less commonly, as a free-floating mass. They are well differentiated with scattered or cuboid mesothelial lined cysts. Immunohistochemical staining with Cam 5.2 confirms mesothelial origin.[143] These tumours may recur locally but do not progress to malignancy.[142–144] By contrast the prognosis for patients with malignant PM is poor, eight out of 12 patients in one review dying as a consequence of local disease progression.[144] Chemotherapy using

doxorubicin and cisplatin was effective with one child.[142] Congenital peritoneal mesothelioma has been described.[145]

CT and MRI are essential in order to determine the extent of the disease.

Staging

The UICC-TNM staging should be adopted.[146]

Treatment

Mesothelioma is a difficult tumour to treat and cure. Surgery alone, even when radical, is rarely curative. Malignant mesothelioma tends to be a locally aggressive tumour recurring at the surgical site after resection. The role of radiotherapy is uncertain in this often diffuse disease and difficulties are encountered in administering a therapeutic dose without concomitant damage to normal tissues. Treatment failure is usually locoregional in adults, but distant metastases occur if systemic therapy is not used. However, there are no adequate published trials of chemotherapy on which to base treatment guidelines; patient numbers are usually small and follow-up short. The most active drugs are doxorubicin, cisplatin, cyclophosphamide and mitomycin-C. A complete response to ifosfamide has been reported in a phase 1 study by Pratt *et al.*[147] and a complete response to vincristine, doxorubicin and cyclophosphamide has been reported in one child.[126] It is therefore recommended that any patient with a malignant pleural or peritoneal mesothelioma be treated on the EICESS protocol with VAIA (vincristine, doxorubicin, ifosfamide, actinomycin D).

Intrapleural or intraperitoneal cisplatin has also been used to good effect in cases of recurrent malignant pleural or peritoneal effusions or peritoneal disease, as has bleomycin.[146] Brachytherapy and instillation of radioactive gold or phosphorus into the pleural and peritoneal cavities are experimental at present with no long-term results available for consideration.

The treatment of peritoneal mesothelioma depends on the clinical behaviour of the disease and its histological appearance. Treatment choices need to be individualized. Those with cystic mesothelioma may not require treatment other than surgical debulking, which may be necessary on more than one occasion. Chemotherapy and radiotherapy have been used to treat malignant peritoneal mesothelioma. There is, however, no clear role for radiotherapy in this condition. Chemotherapy has been administered either systemically or directly into the peritoneal cavity. Intraperitoneal chemotherapy using cisplatinum appears to be effective, but side-effects may be considerable with the formation of extensive abdominal adhesions.[142] In view of the considerable side-effects that may ensue from intraperitoneal administration, systemic therapy is advised.

Recommendations

If pleural or peritoneal mesothelioma is suspected, or even considered, it is essential to obtain as much tumour tissue as is possible. Histological diagnosis is difficult and best made by a panel of histopathologists. Surgical resection should be as extensive as possible. It is therefore recommended that any patient with a malignant pleural or peritoneal mesothelioma is treated on the Ewing's protocols with VAIA or equivalent. The combination of chemotherapy and radiotherapy appears to be more affective than radiotherapy or chemotherapy alone.[146] Therefore, combined therapy should be considered in these patients. The use of intrapleural/intraperitoneal cisplatin should be considered in patients with pleural or peritoneal mesothelioma.

ABDOMINAL TUMOURS

Adrenocortical tumours

Adrenocortical tumours (ACTs) comprise 0.2 per cent of childhood malignancies with an international incidence of 0.5/million and occurs far more commonly in girls than in boys (ratio 1.5:1).[148] A bimodal age distribution curve with a peak incidence at 3.5 and 57 years of age is seen. Most ACTs in children and adolescents are hormone-secreting and the clinical presentation reflects the pattern of adrenocortical hormones secreted by that tumour. Signs and symptoms of virilization are present in over 90 per cent of cases (Table 24.1). Hirsutism, acne and deepening of the voice may be apparent in both sexes. The development of acne in a child under 6 years

Table 24.1 *Clinical manifestations of adrenocortical tumours (ACTs) in children*[149,150,246]

Manifestation	Percentage affected
Premature/secondary sexual hair	90
Cliteromegaly	92
Phallomegaly	81
Hirsutism	62.5
Palpable abdominal mass	61
Hypertension	54
Acne	47
Plethora	42
Deep voice	42
Moon face	35
Seizure (hypertensive)	17
Headache	12

should make the exclusion of ACT a priority. Girls may also present with clitoromegaly and facial hair, while boys present with penile enlargement and virilization. Cushing's syndrome occurs in a third of cases, with moon facies, centripetal fat distribution and plethora being the most common signs. Hypertension is often present and children may present in hypertensive crisis. Generally, ACTs are inefficient in producing cortisol, and the secretion of androgens and intermediates such as 11-deoxycortisol and 11-deoxycorticosterone can dominate their activity. About half of ACTs will be large enough to palpate at diagnosis. In a recent retrospective study of 54 children with an ACT referred to a regional centre, 60 per cent had endocrine symptoms and virilization, and 40 per cent had an abdominal mass.[149] Careful examination of this cohort revealed endocrine signs and symptoms in 81 per cent.[149] There is often a considerable delay between presentation with endocrine dysfunction and diagnosis.[149–151] In one large series only 11 per cent of the patients were diagnosed within 6 months of their initial presentation.

AETIOLOGY AND BIOLOGY

The adrenal cortex arises from the mesenchyme. At term, the 'fetal' cortex represents about 80 per cent of the adrenal gland. Within a few days there is rapid involution by apoptosis with little cortex remaining by 6 months of age.

In the original description of a familial cancer syndrome, Li *et al.*[152] documented four out of 151 affected family members with ACT, all of whom were under 14 at diagnosis. The diagnosis of sarcoma in one individual, the proband, under 45 years of age, a first-degree relative with cancer before 45 and another first- or second-degree relative in the lineage with any cancer diagnosed during the interval, or a sarcoma at any age now constitutes the classic Li–Fraumeni syndrome (LFS) family. Although a rare component of this syndrome, ACT occurs 100 times more frequently than would be expected. Germ line mutations of the *TP53* gene have been identified in most but not all of the families with classic LFS.[153,154] Molecular analysis has shown that 50 per cent of children with ACT carried germ line *TP53*, suggesting that presentation with ACT in childhood may be the first manifestation of this familial cancer syndrome within a family.[155]

There is also an increased incidence of ACT in patients with isolated hemihypertrophy and the Beckwith–Wiedemann syndrome.[149–156] A number of children with congenital adrenal hyperplasia (CAH) who have subsequently developed ACT have also been reported.[157] Mutations in the *CYP21* gene are responsible for most cases of CAH.[158] Molecular analysis of CYP21 in 27 cases of sporadic ACT revealed no mutations, excluding this gene in the aetiology of ACT and of mild undiagnosed

CAH as a predisposing factor.[159] The gene for MEN type 1 has been localized to 11q13; although deletions in this chromosomal region are frequently found in ACT, no mutations in the *MEN1* gene have been detected. Loss of heterozygosity studies have also implicated region 2p16, particularly in malignant tumours. Whether this region contains a tumour suppressor gene important in adrenocortical carcinoma remains to be evaluated.

The incidence of ACT in Brazil is 1.5/million, more than three times the international rate for reasons that are currently unclear.[148,150] A retrospective study noted that seven fathers and four mothers of the 14 children with ACT in the Manchester Children's tumour registry were exposed to potentially toxic substances during the pregnancy.[160] This finding raises the possibility that environmental as well as genetic factors are important in the aetiology of some ACTs. Clearly case–control studies are now indicated in order to determine which environmental factors are important.

DIAGNOSIS

Any child who presents with signs and symptoms of adrenal dysfunction, however mild, such as virilization, Cushing's syndrome or precocious puberty, should alert the paediatrician to the possible diagnosis of ACT. Abdominal ultrasound is a simple and useful screening test and is recommended in such cases. More sophisticated scanning such as CT or MRI will be required presurgery. The suspected diagnosis of ACT can be confirmed by checking serum and urine for elevated levels of androgens and/or cortisol and their precursors. Less than 10 per cent of adrenocortical tumours are non-secreting.[149] It is important to measure free cortisol, 17-hydroxycorticosteroids (17-OHCS) and androgens in a 24-hour urinary collection as well as plasma cortisol, dehydroepiandrosterone sulphate (DHEA-S), testosterone, androstenedione, deoxycorticosterone and 17-hydroxyprogesterone. ACTH levels will be low due to pituitary suppression in ACT. It is important to determine each tumour's characteristic endocrine profile for monitoring of response to treatment and detection of relapse. Virilizing adrenal tumours commonly secrete 11β-hydroxyandrostenedione,[161] for which there is no readily available blood assay. Characteristic steroid profiles have been found for ACT[161] and the urine profile analysis excludes CAH as a cause of virilization. Dexamethasone will not suppress the output of abnormal steroids in the case of ACT. This test is important because some tumours secrete 17-hydroxyprogesterone, mimicking CAH. Steroid metabolites present in the urine at the time of diagnosis provide a useful test of surgical success and they should normalize postoperatively. The urinary steroid profile can act as a useful tumour marker.

HISTOPATHOLOGY AND PROGNOSTIC FACTORS

The histopathological distinction between adrenal adenomas and carcinomas is difficult. A modification of the Weiss criteria based on mitotic index, atypical mitoses, confluent necrosis and nuclear grade is reported by some to predict clinical outcome.[162] It is, however, widely accepted that tumour size is the best available predictor of biological behaviour; tumours greater than 100 g/200 cm^3 are associated with a worse prognosis.[150] Other adverse prognostic factors include older age at presentation, increased urinary steroid levels and delay in diagnosis.[150] Capsular and vascular invasion has been associated with a high frequency of recurrence.[149]

INVESTIGATIONS

- blood serum levels – DHEA-S, androstenedione, testosterone, cortisol (and ACTH if cortisol is raised with loss of diurnal rhythm), 17-OH progesterone, aldosterone, oestradiol
- 24-hour urine steroid profile
- follow-up – 24-hour urine collections for steroid metabolites; should normalize following adrenalectomy.

IMAGING

Abdominal ultrasound, CT and MRI scans are all useful modalities with some evidence that MRI is preferable if available. As 20 per cent of ACTs have metastasized at diagnosis, usually to lung or bone, early diagnosis offers the best hope for curing this disease. Intrahepatic metastases are frequently observed followed by spread to lung and bone.

STAGING

I   Total excision of tumour, tumour volume <200 cm^3; absence of metastases and normal hormone levels after surgery

II Microscopic residual tumour, tumour volume >200 cm^3, persistently elevated adrenocortical hormone levels after surgery

III Gross residual or inoperable tumour

IV Distant metastases.

In a recent series, 78 per cent had local disease (stage I and II), 9 per cent had stage III disease and 13 per cent had stage IV disease.[149]

TREATMENT

Joint patient management between a paediatric surgeon, an oncologist and an endocrinologist is recommended. Complete, radical surgical resection is the treatment of choice and may be curative, especially in small tumours. Patients achieving complete resection survive significantly longer than those with residual disease.[163] In one recent series, survival rate reached 70 per cent if resection was complete, but was a dismal 7 per cent if complete resection was not achieved.[149] Surgical resection of isolated recurrence and metastatic disease is also indicated where possible.

Surgical guidelines

Most paediatric oncology surgeons are familiar with the approach to the adrenal glands because of their experience with neuroblastoma. However, unlike neuroblastoma, adrenal tumours are more often a discrete entity, less likely to encase adjacent vessels and invade the vascular wall. For this reason, the preoperative cross-sectional images may draw the surgeon to the inaccurate conclusion that the tumour will be easily resected. This is not necessarily true, mainly because of the multiple routes of venous drainage from the tumour. This is particularly true for right-sided lesions which drain directly into the inferior vena cava; the uppermost of the three main venous channels may be hard to control because of the proximity of the vessel to the undersurface of the liver, particularly with a large tumour. Equally, the lowest venous channel on the left drains directly into the renal vein and, if torn inadvertently, may result in damage to the left renal vein (LRV) and compromise of the left kidney.

Surgical resection should be preceded by full laparotomy, including the contralateral adrenal. Biopsy of the apparently normal side is controversial, but may reveal an unexpected adenoma. Resection of the affected side should include any obvious lymph nodes whether apparently involved or not.

The entire operative specimen, which should not be sectioned in the operating theatre, should be transferred fresh directly to the pathology department. Use of formalin solution will render the specimen useless for biological studies.

Immediate postoperative care will require corticosteroid supplementation and close observation of both mineralocorticoid and glucocorticoid effects. Later surveillance of the adrenal bed by physical examination and ultrasound, with cross-sectional imaging as required, is essential. This approach can be supplemented by endocrine surveillance, measuring any marker adrenal hormones that were elevated during initial presentation.

Postoperative guidelines

Complete resection Follow-up should involve regular clinical examination and estimations of urinary steroid profiles.

Incomplete resection In patients with incomplete resection or metastatic spread, treatment options include chemotherapy and/or mitotane. Due to the rarity of this condition, no randomized or controlled studies have been performed. It is not even completely clear whether chemotherapy or mitotane should be the initial treatment of choice, although an international registry of adrenocortical tumours coordinated at St Jude Hospital recommends the use of mitotane (www.stjude.org/ipactr).

Mitotane, the ortho-para derivative of an insecticide, dichlorodiphenyl-dichloroethane (DDD), was serendipitously noted to cause adrenal necrosis, leading to its use in ACT.[164] The efficacy of radiotherapy has not been established. Mitotane is usually effective in controlling the endocrine symptoms and may cause tumour regression but is not an antineoplastic agent and a recent large retrospective study in adults concluded that mitotane did not have a significant effect on survival.[165] There is, however, some evidence that mitotane is more effective in children than adults,[166–168] particularly if the neoplasm is hormonally active.[169] There is no clear evidence base for a treatment dose; most series give mitotane within the range 5–10 g/m^2 per day, but dose levels will depend on symptoms.[149,170,171] A role for low-dose mitotane 0.5–1 g/m^2 per day has been suggested due to unacceptable side-effects, but the evidence for this is weak.[172] Mitotane should be started at 2 g/m^2 per day, aiming to reach 10 g/m^2 per day or until therapeutic levels are achieved. Mitotane absorption is enhanced when given with fats, e.g. in a chocolate milkshake. Unpleasant side-effects, including gastrointestinal, neurological and dermal, are common and very careful monitoring is essential. Recent studies have shown that mitotane exhibits a clear dose–response curve, being most effective when the serum level is >14 mg/L.[173] Side-effects can be minimized by keeping the serum mitotane level below 20 mg/L.[173] It is possible that the equivocal results achieved with mitotane reflect the administration of subtherapeutic levels of this drug, particularly as it has a narrow therapeutic window.[163,174]

It is also important to recognize that higher than normal doses of mineralocorticoid and glucocorticoid therapy are required due to an increased serum steroid-binding capacity during mitotane therapy.[175] Recommended replacement therapy is as follows:

- hydrocortisone: 10–15 mg/m^2/day as two or three divided doses
- fludrocortisone: 100–150 μg/m^2/day as a single daily dose.

Functional recovery of the zona glomerulosa and zona fasiculata has been reported following mitotane therapy.[166] Thyroid function may also be impaired, and therefore free T$_4$ should be checked whilst children are on mitotane therapy.

Effective chemotherapeutic agents include cisplatinum, etoposide, doxorubicin, 5-FU and cyclophosphamide.[149,174,176–181] The combination of cisplatin/etoposide and mitotane, whilst tolerable, may confer a survival advantage over chemotherapy according to one adult study; however, no randomised trials have been performed.[176]

Due to the rarity of ACT in children, it is unlikely that a randomized question can be asked even with international collaboration.

Treatment recommendation

Cisplatinum, etoposide and cyclophosphamide all appear to have activity against ACT. It is therefore recommended that patients are treated on the OPEC/OJEC regimen used in the UK for stage 4 neuroblastoma. The notion of giving mitotane concurrently with chemotherapy is attractive, especially as there seems to be no additional adverse effects and the prognosis is so poor.

Radiotherapy has been used, but the use of this modality in the presence of a high risk of genetic predisposition to cancer due to germ line *TP53* mutations is not generally advised; indeed, secondary tumours have been reported within the radiation field.[182]

CONCLUSIONS

There is still much to be learnt concerning the biology of ACT, in particular the relationship between genetic predisposition and environmental factors. The optimum treatment is still unclear and enrolment of patients in the International Paediatric Adrenocortical Tumour registry is recommended if we are to make further progress in the management of this tumour (www.stjude.org/ipactr).

Renal cell carcinoma

Also known as Grawitz tumour or hypernephroma, this tumour is occasionally reported in children, particularly older children and adolescents. Renal cell carcinomas (RCCs) arise from the proximal tubular cells and are, therefore, ultimately derived from metanephric blastema.[183] The incidence of this tumour is estimated at between 0.3 and 3 per cent of all renal tumours in children. By contrast to adults, there is little evidence for gender preference. Clinical presentation is usually with an abdominal mass and often with haematuria. Tumours are usually of advanced stage at diagnosis. The mean age at presentation is 10 years compared with 4 years of age in Wilms' tumour.[184] Metastasis is to liver, lungs, bone and abdominal lymph nodes. A recent report of childhood RCC noted that five out of 16 patients (31 per cent) presented with various paraneoplastic phenomena, a far higher figure than that found in adults.[185,186] RCC is associated with von Hippel–Lindau syndrome (hereditary angiomatosis of the retina and cerebellum). The *VHL* gene is a tumour suppressor gene and is located on the short arm of chromosome 3.[187] Familial RCC is associated with a constitutional translocation involving chromosome

3p, t(3;8) (p14;q24). Abnormalities of the short arm of chromosome 3 have also been reported in 66 per cent of sporadic RCCS of clear cell histology, suggesting that loss of genes on 3p are a necessary step in tumour development.[188] Translocations involving the X chromosome, t(Xp11.2), have been reported in male children with RCC and in isolated cases in adults. The significance of this finding is not yet clear.[185] An association with tuberous sclerosis has been reported.[186]

HISTOPATHOLOGY

Based on morphological, histochemical and ultrastructural analysis, five histological types of RCC are now recognized in adults. The most prevalent subtype is the clear cell carcinoma (75–80 per cent), followed by chromophobic (papillary) (12–15 per cent), chromophobic (4–6 per cent), oncocytic (2–4 per cent) and collecting duct carcinoma (1 per cent). There is no clear evidence for a different histological profile in children compared with adults.[189]

CLINICOPATHOLOGICAL STAGING (MODIFIED ROBSON STAGING)

  I Confined to renal parenchyma
  II Extension onto peripheral fat
IIIA Involvement of renal vein, inferior vena cava
IIIB Involvement of regional lymph nodes
 IV Metastatic disease.

PROGNOSIS AND TREATMENT

There is some evidence that the prognosis for childhood RCC is more favourable than for adults, with an overall 5-year survival of 60 per cent in children compared with 40 per cent in adults.[190] Radical nephrectomy is the treatment of choice and, since prognosis is stage-related, may be sufficient in well-encapsulated tumours. The role of regional lymphadenectomy is unclear.[191] Chemotherapy and radiotherapy have been used in patients with stage II and III tumours. However, due to small patient numbers and mixing of therapies, the relative merits of radiotherapy and chemotherapy are unclear.[189,191,192] Surgery alone was curative in a recent series of patients with stage II and III tumours.[193] Those presenting with stage 4 disease fare as badly with no proven curative regimen. The occasional dramatic response to immunotherapy and rare cure suggest this novel treatment is worth trying in patients with metastatic disease.[194]

PANCREATIC TUMOURS

In addition to the tumour types commonly seen in adults but rarely seen in children, two important histologically distinct pancreatic tumours are recognized in childhood and adolescence: pancreaticoblastoma and Frantz's tumour.

Pancreaticoblastoma

The term pancreaticoblastoma was first suggested in the 1970s by Horie *et al.* and has now largely replaced the confusing term, infantile pancreatic carcinoma.[195,196] Pancreaticoblastoma is the most common malignant pancreatic tumour of early life. The main age of presentation is 4.5 years and it is rare in children over 10 years at diagnosis. There appears to be a predominance of Asian children in the reported literature, but no case studies have been done. Children present with non-specific symptoms of pain, nausea, vomiting and an abdominal mass. Obstructive jaundice is only seen in around one-third of children, compared with two-thirds of adults presenting with pancreatic neoplasms. Endocrine symptoms have been noted, including Cushing's syndrome and inappropriate ACTH secretion.[197] Elevation of serum levels of alpha-fetoprotein have been noted in under half of the cases so far reported.[198,199] A number of patients with Beckwith–Wiedemann syndrome have also presented with pancreaticoblastomas, suggesting a link between these two rarely occurring conditions.[200–202] The incidence of this tumour is difficult to assess.

Pancreaticoblastomas are large tumours that are often well circumscribed. They are characterized histologically by relatively dense cellularity, a nesting growth pattern, acinar differentiation and the characteristic finding of squamoid corpuscles (cords or nodules of squamoid cells with elongated nuclei arranged in a parallel fasciculating pattern). Immunohistochemical staining for acinar differentiation is characteristically found in these tumours. Immunohistochemical staining for alpha-fetoprotein may be seen even in patients in whom the serum levels of this hormone are not elevated. The histological differential diagnosis rests between adenocarcinoma, mixed acinar–endocrine carcinoma and Frantz's tumour. There is a close embryological relationship between the development of the liver and of the pancreas; both trace a common ancestry in the foregut. There is thus a close kinship between the primary blastomas of the liver and pancreas, leading to similar choice of therapy for both these conditions.

Pancreaticoblastoma is clearly a malignant neoplasm with frequent local invasion occurrence and metastases. A recent review has shown that 35 per cent of patients present with metastases, most commonly to liver, regional lymph nodes or lungs.[199] In this same review, 19 out of 45 (42 per cent) evaluable patients died from the tumour. However, many of these children received what would now be considered inadequate therapy and it is now clear that pancreaticoblastoma is a potentially curable malignancy.[203–206] Chemotherapy protocols developed for hepatoblastomas have been used with some success in pancreaticoblastoma.[204–206] Furthermore, preoperative chemotherapy for an advanced unresectable pancreaticoblastoma, allowing subsequent complete resection of the tumour, has also been reported.[203] To date, surgical resection has been the recommended treatment. However, the surgery required has often been extensive, resulting in short-term and long-term morbidity. It is therefore suggested that unless patients have tumours that are easily resectable at diagnosis, preoperative chemotherapy is given according to the SIOPEL III protocol, using continuous doses of cisplatinum and doxorubicin (PLADO). At delayed surgery, tumours should then be resectable with minimal morbidity. If complete excision is obtained, with metastases with falling alpha-fetoprotein levels (if elevated), the option of continuing treatment with cisplatinum alone should be considered as in the SIOPEL III protocol. Those patients with metastases at diagnosis or residual disease at delayed surgery should receive treatment according to the high-risk tumour arm of SIOPEL III. Second-look surgery is advised in patients in whom there is still radiological or tumour marker evidence of residual disease following treatment on the above strategy. Radiotherapy may be of benefit in tumour control of minimal residual disease of the tumour bed.[207]

Frantz's tumour

Papillary and cystic tumours of the pancreas, also known as Frantz's tumours, predominately affect young women, with approximately one-third occurring in children under 16 years of age.[208–218] Despite its histological appearance, this tumour has a low malignant potential and usually behaves in a benign fashion. In the rare cases presenting with metastatic disease, prognosis remains good with surgery alone.[208–218] However, the outcome in older patients, especially those aged over 40 years, is not as good.[211,214] Clinical presentation is usually with progressive abdominal pain often of several months' duration. Clinical examination may reveal an epigastric mass.

Frantz's tumour, a somewhat misunderstood pancreatic neoplasm, has attracted several synonymous titles (Box 24.2).[218] Frantz's tumour is not a new entity but more likely one that has been misclassified in the past; it may even explain the relatively good prognosis of series of pancreatic carcinomas in children compared with adults. The almost exclusive female predominance of Frantz's tumour suggests that hormonal factors are likely to be important in this tumour.

Imaging studies usually indicate a well-defined large mass with varying degrees of cystic change; calcification may be seen.

Box 24.2 *Synonyms of Frantz's tumour*

- Papillary tumour, benign or malignant[247]
- Papillary epithelial neoplasm[248]
- Papillary-cystic neoplasm
- Solid and papillary epithelial neoplasm
- Solid and cystic acinar cell tumour
- Papillary and solid neoplasm[249]
- Papillary-cystic carcinomas

Macroscopically, there is often focal or extensive haemorrhage and necrotic change, the cut surface showing areas of cystic and solid patterns. The tumour is often encapsulated. Microscopically, two distinct types of cellular arrangements – solid and papillary – are evident. In the papillary areas, the tumour cells characteristically form papillary structures around a central fibrovascular stalk. PAS-positive granules are seen. The areas of cystic degeneration stain with alcian blue, and the solid areas may have a pseudorosette pattern, similar to that seen in acinar cell tumours. Immunohistochemical studies for endocrine cells are negative. Cholesterol crystals and giant cells are frequently observed around the areas of cystic degeneration. Mitoses are rare. Ultrastructural analysis supports an acinar origin for this tumour by the demonstration of zymogen granules.[215] Overall, metastases are rare. Capsular invasion has been reported. Although Frantz's tumour has been reported in boys, there is some question over the histological diagnosis in at least one of these cases.[215]

TREATMENT

The clinical behaviour of this tumour is that of a low-grade malignancy that is locally invasive and rarely metastatic. The prognosis is better in children than in adults. The literature attests to the fact that Frantz's tumour is a potentially curable surgical lesion[212,214–218] and extensive surgical operations, including a pancreaticoduodenectomy, are indicated, as is metastectomy, whenever possible. Although this tumour is reported to respond to both chemotherapy and radiotherapy,[219,220] such treatment should be restricted to those patients who have inoperable residual or progressive disease. Oestrogen and progesterone receptor status should be sought as this might provide a therapeutic option.

Carcinomas of the pancreas

As in adults, ductal adenocarcinoma is the more common exocrine tumour of the pancreas followed by acinar cell carcinoma. However, due to a continued refinement in histological diagnosis, there are very few true cases of exocrine carcinoma.[221] The prognosis for these tumours seems similar to that of adults, i.e. an almost uniformly fatal outcome, although there is some evidence that acinar tumours have a better prognosis in children than in adults.[222] Treatment of choice is by surgical resection.

Endocrine tumours of the pancreas

Exocrine tumours are the least common pancreatic tumour in childhood.[223–225] Clinical presentation depends upon the islet cell of origin of the tumour (Table 24.2). A plasma insulin:glucose ratio greater than 1 with a normal C-peptide level is diagnostic of an insulinoma. Tumour localization may, however, prove difficult. Surgical resection is usually curative, as over 90 per cent of these tumours are benign.

Gastrinomas, by contrast, are predominantly malignant, albeit slow-growing. Diagnosis can be made by demonstrating elevated serum levels of gastrin. Treatment involves a combination of medical and surgical measures; if the lesion is solitary, surgical resection is advisable, whereas medical treatment is indicated in the face of multiple adenomatosis or metastatic disease. Powerful proton pump inhibitors are effective but compliance with this lifelong treatment may be difficult in children.

Most VIP (vasoactive intestinal polypeptide)-producing tumours in children are of neurogenic origin, either neuroblastomas or ganglioneuroblastomas rather than primary liver tumours. A number of these endocrine tumours can occur as part of familial MEN syndromes.

Clear cell sarcoma or malignant melanoma of soft parts

Clear cell sarcoma (CCS) is a rare soft tissue malignancy that most commonly occurs on the extremities of young adults.[226–231] It commonly presents as a painless mass or swelling. The period of time from the onset of symptoms to diagnosis is highly variable and attests to the relatively indolent nature of this tumour. The long latent period between symptoms and final presentation belies the relatively high incidence of local recurrence and distant metastases.[226–231]

HISTOPATHOLOGY

This tumour is characterized by variably sized nests of uniform plump spindle cells; clear to pale cytoplasm and clear nuclei with prominent nucleoli are consistent findings.[226,227,230] The clusters are separated by delicate fibrous septae; however, considerable variation occurs in this histological pattern. The tumour often appears to be intimately associated with tendons and the aponeuroses.[226,227,230] Melanin production has been reported in a number of these tumours and gives rise to the alternative

Table 24.2 *Islet cell tumours*

Cell type	Hormone secreted	Tumour	Clinical presentation
A	Glucagon	Glucagonoma	Primarily occur in adults
B	Insulin	Insulinoma	Hypoglycaemia
G	Gastrin	Gastrinoma	Peptic ulceration, Zollinger–Ellison syndrome
D	Somatostatin	Somatostatinoma	Primarily occur in adults
D_1	Vasoactive intestinal polypeptide	Vipoma	Diarrhoea

name for this tumour. Biologically this tumour is closer to sarcoma than melanoma in nature and is characterized by a t(12:22)(q13:q12) translocation which interrupts the Ewing's sarcoma gene on chromosome 22.[227]

Approximately 20 per cent of CCS tumours occur on the extremities.[229,231] The duration of symptoms is an unreliable indicator of outcome. Tumours less than 5 cm diameter are associated with good prognosis. Initial tumour involvement of regional lymph nodes is an extremely poor prognostic factor. Treatment options are essentially surgical[229–231] and radical local resection is indicated.[228–231] There is no clear evidence for chemosensitivity in patients with residual disease after surgery but treatment on the SIOP malignant mesenchymal tumour protocol is advised (MMT 95).

Once the diagnosis of CCS is made, the patient is at risk of recurrent disease for a considerable number of years. Many reports attest to a considerably poorer outcome at 20 years than at 5 years.

In conclusion, CCS is a slow-growing but highly malignant tumour. There is frequently a long latent period between symptoms and diagnosis as well as between diagnosis and death.

FIBROMATOSIS

The fibromatoses are a heterogeneous collection of clinical conditions with similar histopathological appearances that may be difficult to distinguish from fibrosarcoma.[232] Aggressive fibromatosis (desmoid tumour) is a fibroblastic condition behaving like a locally invasive tumour, but rarely metastasizing, and it may occur in any musculoaponeurotic structure – head and neck, trunk and limb tumours are all encountered. The condition tends to affect younger age groups. For example, of 25 patients presenting to the Massachusetts General Hospital (MGH), 76 per cent were under 40 years of age.[233]

Radical surgical excision is curative, but if these dense growths tie in vital structures, this may not be possible. In 1977, Stein[234] reported that aggressive fibromatoses responded to vincristine, actinomycin and cyclophosphamide (VAC) chemotherapy, and responses are seen in paediatric patients to vincristine and actinomycin alone (see Chapter 17) and weekly vinblastine/methotrexate.[234]

The observation that desmoids occurred in caesarian section scars led to the discovery of sex steroid receptors in these tumours, and subsequently to case reports of regression with tamoxifen therapy. More recently, endocrine inactive derivatives of tamoxifen have caused major regressions in patients with aggressive fibromatoses.[235]

Radiotherapy is also an effective form of therapy. In the MGH experience, eight out of 10 patients treated primarily by radiotherapy achieved complete remission without an attempt at resection (five cases), or achieved stabilization (three cases) of their disease after some regression. Regression post-radiotherapy was slow.[233] Kiel and Suit[233] recommend radiotherapy where wide field resection is not possible.

COMPLICATED ANGIOMAS

Several types of angiomas are seen in infancy and childhood. The 'neonatal stain' on the head and neck fades spontaneously, while the 'salmon patch' remains unchanged. The 'port wine' stain is a sharply defined area of intense intradermal erythema that persists throughout life.

The 'strawberry' (capillary) haemangioma presents at birth or soon afterwards, most commonly in the head and neck region. Initially, this lesion may grow rapidly, and the fast response to low doses of radiotherapy led to widespread application of this method in the past. However, after the age of 9 months, most lesions involute spontaneously, and it is only lesions that threaten severe complications, such as amblyopia, that justify active therapy.

Cavernous haemangiomas are subcutaneous lesions with less easily distinguishable margins on the skin. They are present at birth or appear in the first 6 months of life, and may occur anywhere in the body (vertebrae, liver, pericardium, orbit, subglottis, etc.). Cavernous haemangiomas may also be complicated by thrombocytopenia and consumption coagulopathy due to sequestration within the lesion (Kasabach–Merritt syndrome).

'Alarming haemangioma' is a term introduced by Enjolras et al.[236] to designate haemangiomas that impair vital structures with life-endangering complications. High-dose corticosteroids are the primary means of treatment in this situation. The rate of response to the systemic or intralesional administration is 30–60 per cent.[237–239]

However, the mortality rate can be as high as 50 per cent among alarming haemangioma patients, despite steroids.[240–241] Recently, the value of alpha-interferon in this situation has been appreciated. Ezekowitz *et al.*[242] reported that 18 out of 20 patients with alarming haemangiomas responded to alpha-interferon ($3 \times 10^6 \, \text{U/m}^2$ s.c. daily). Alpha-interferon has undoubtedly become an important therapeutic modality that is appropriate for serious haemangiomas. Low-dose radiotherapy is the third method of treatment for alarming haemangiomas, and should not be withheld if steroids and alpha-interferon have failed; dramatic responses can occur.

The natural history of other cavernous haemangiomas is similar to that of strawberry naevi, with a growth phase, a plateau phase and a subsequent involution phase. No treatment may be necessary.

Treatment of complicated haemangiomas depends on the site, size and complicating factors. For instance, steroid therapy may raise the platelet count in Kasabach–Merritt syndrome (Figure 24.3), although it does not significantly alter the size of the underlying haemangioma. Surgical excision of a cavernous haemangioma may offer cure but can be hazardous. Embolization may also be effective but carries risks; one child presented to us

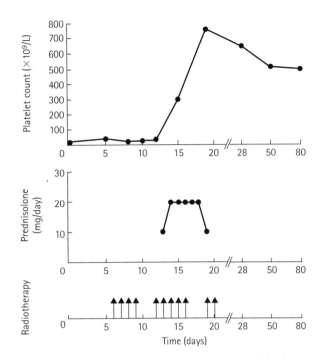

Figure 24.3 *Cavernous haemangioma with Kasbach–Merritt syndrome; response of platelet count to steroid and radiotherapy.*

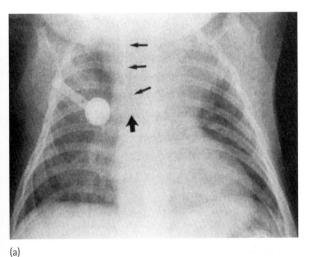

(a)

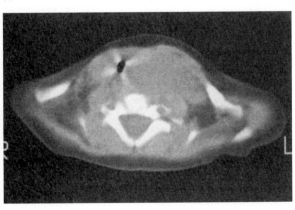

(b)

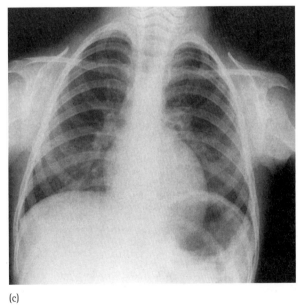

(c)

Figure 24.4 *Massive cavernous haemangioma of the thoracic inlet with tracheal compression. (a) Plain chest radiography and (b) transaxial CT scanning at this level. Following low-dose radiotherapy, an excellent response occurred rapidly. (c) Chest X-ray 3 years later.*

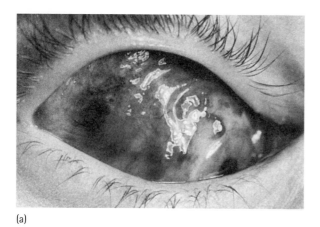
(a)

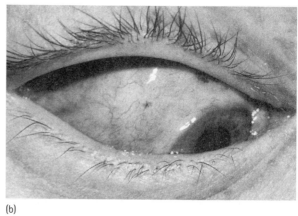
(b)

Figure 24.5 *(a) Conjunctival angioma. (b) After strontium plaque beta radiotherapy.*

recently with infarction and gangrene of the arm following unsuccessful embolization attempts for an upper thoracic giant cavernous haemangioma.

Low-dose radiotherapy remains an important therapeutic weapon against haemangiomas presenting with complications. If steroid therapy and alpha-interferon have failed to control an inoperable lesion, radiotherapy can be highly effective (Figures 24.4 and 24.5).[243,244] Focal stereotactic radiotherapy now has an established place in the management of inoperable cerebral arteriovenous malformations, and is perhaps particularly useful in childhood cases.[245]

KEY POINTS

- Nasopharyngeal carcinoma: localised ($\pm$ regional nodes) disease is usually curable with careful radiotherapy. Concomitant cisplatinum chemotherapy (as in adult practice) may further increase the cure rate.
- Salivary gland tumours of childhood are reviewed; in particular, the role of expert surgery is stressed.
- Thyroid cancer: there is controversy as to whether all patients with differentiated thyroid cancer require total thyroidectomy and radioiodine ablation, as well as fully TSH suppressive thyroid hormone replacement and careful follow-up.
- The rare occurrences of 'adult' type cancers of lung, breast, kidney, adrenal and pancreas are reviewed and differences from adult practice highlighted. Tumours arising in these sites are more typical of the paediatric age group (e.g. pancreaticoblastoma and pulmonary blastoma).
- Benign conditions such as angiomas and fibromatosis are reviewed.

REFERENCES

1. Fernandez, Sangara A, Samana A, Riverar A. Nasopharyngeal carcinoma in children. *Cancer* 1996; **37**: 2787–91.
2. Baker SD, McClatchey KD. Carcinoma in the nasopharynx in childhood. *Otolaryngology* 1981; **89**: 555–9.
3. Henderson BE, Louie E, SooHoo Jing J *et al*. Risk factors associated with nasopharyngeal carcinoma. *N Engl J Med* 1976; **295**: 1101–6.
4. Henle W, Ho HC, Burtin P *et al*. Antibodies to Epstein–Barr virus in nasopharyngeal carcinoma, other head and neck cancers and control groups. *J Natl Cancer Inst* 1970; **44**: 551–5.
5. de-Valnaire F, Sancho-Garnier H, de-The H *et al*. Prognostic value of EBV markers in the clinical management of nasopharyngeal carcinoma (NPC): a multicentre follow-up study. *Int J Cancer* 1988; **42**: 176–81.
6. Traub NR, Flynn K. The structure of the termini of the Epstein–Barr virus as a marker of clonal cellular proliferation. *Cell* 1986; **47**: 883–9.
7. Pathmanathan R, Prasad U, Sadler R *et al*. Clonal proliferations of cells infected with Epstein–Barr virus in pre-invasive lesions related to nasopharyngeal carcinoma. *N Engl J Med* 1995; **333**: 693–8.
8. Shanmugaratman K, Cobin L. *Histological Typing of Upper Respiratory Tract Tumours*. Geneva: WHO, 1978.
9. Sham JST, Poon YF, Wei WI, Choy D. Nasopharyngeal carcinoma in young patients. *Cancer* 1990; **65**: 2606–10.
10. Lobo-Sanahuja F, Garcia I, Carranza A, Camacho A. Treatment and outcome of undifferentiated carcinoma of the nasopharynx in childhood: a 13 year experience. *Med Pediatr Oncol* 1986; **14**: 6–11.
11. Lombardi F, Gasparinin M, Giannic C *et al*. Nasopharyngeal carcinoma in childhood. *Med Pediatr Oncol* 1982; **10**: 243–50.
12. Jerab B, Huvous AG, Steinherzp P, Unal A. Nasopharyngeal carcinoma in children: review of 16 cases. *Int J Radiat Oncol Biol Phys* 1979; **6**: 487–91.
13. Baker SR, Wolf RA. Prognostic factors of nasopharyngeal malignancy. *Cancer* 1982; **49**: 163–9.
14. Ho HJC, ed. *Stage Classification of Nasopharyngeal Carcinoma: A Review*. Lyon: IARC, 1978.

15. Flemming ID, Cooper JS, Henson DE *et al. AJCC Cancer Staging Manual*, 5th edn. Philadelphia: Lippincott-Raven, 1997.

16. Bears OH, Henson DE, Hutter RVP *et al. Manual for Staging for Cancer*, 4th edn. Philadelphia: JB Lippincott, 1992.

17. Berry MP, Smith CR, Brown TC *et al.* Nasopharyngeal carcinoma in the young. *Int J Radiat Oncol Biol Phys* 1980; **6**: 415–21.

18. Jenkin RDT, Anderson JR, Jereb B *et al.* Nasopharyngeal carcinoma – a retrospective review of patients less than thirty years of age: a report from the Children's cancer study group. *Cancer* 1981; **47**: 360–6.

19. Pao WJ, Hustu HO, Douglass EC *et al.* Pediatric nasopharyngeal carcinoma: long term follow up of 29 patients. *Int J Radiat Oncol Biol Phys* 1989; **17**: 299–305.

20. Jereb B, Huvous AG, Steinherzp P, Unal A. Nasopharyngeal carcinoma in children: review of 16 cases. *Int J Radiat Oncol Biol Phys* 1979; **6**: 487–91.

21. Cooper JS, Cohen R, Stevens RE. A comparison of staging systems for nasopharyngeal carcinoma. *Cancer* 1997; **83**: 213–19.

22. Huang TB. Cancer of the nasopharynx in childhood. *Cancer* 1990; **47**: 360–6.

23. Al-Sarraf M, LeBlanc M, Giri PGS *et al.* Chemoradiotherapy versus radiotherapy in patients with advanced nasopharyngeal cancer: phase III randomised intergroup study 0099. *J Clin Onc* 1998; **16**: 1310–17.

24. Gasparini M, Lombardi F, Rottoli L *et al.* Combined radiotherapy and chemotherapy in stage T3 and T4 nasopharyngeal carcinoma in children. *J Clin Oncol* 1988; **6**: 491–4.

25. Ghim TT, Briones M, Mason P *et al.* Effective adjuvant chemotharapy for advanced nasopharyngeal carcinoma in children: a final update of a long-term prospective study in a single institution. *J Pediatr Hematol Oncol* 1998; **20**: 131–5.

26. Kim TH, McLaren J, Alvarado CS *et al.* Adjuvant chemotherapy for advanced nasopharyngeal carcinoma in childhood. *Cancer* 1989; **63**: 1922–6.

27. Mertens R, Granzen B, Lassay L *et al.* Nasopharyngeal carcinoma in childhood and adolescence. *Cancer* 1997; **80**: 951–9.

28. Roper HP, Carter AE, Marsden HB *et al.* Nasopharyngeal carcinoma in children. *Pediatr Hematol Oncol* 1986; **3**: 143–52.

29. Strojan P, Benedick MD, Kragelj B, Jereb B. Combined radiation and chemotherapy for advanced undifferentiated nasopharyngeal carcinoma in chlidren. *Med Pediatr Oncol* 1997; **28**: 366–9.

30. Treuner J, Nierhamer D, Dannecker G *et al.* Successful treatment of nasopharyngeal carcinoma with interferon. *Lancet* 1980; **i**: 817–18.

31. Quin D, Yuhua H, Jiehuaa Y *et al.* Analysis of 1379 patients with nasopharyngeal carcinoma treated by radiation. *Cancer* 1988; **61**: 1117–24.

32. Ayan I, Altun M. Nasopharyngeal carcinoma in children: retrospective review of 50 patients. *Int J Radiat Oncol Biol Phys* 1996; **35**: 485–92.

33. Ingersoll L, Woo SY, Donaldson S *et al.* Nasopharyngeal carcinoma in the young: a combined M D Anderson and Stanford experience. *Int J Radiat Oncol Biol Phys* 1989; **19**: 881–7.

34. Castro ED, Huvos AG, Strong EW, Foote FW. Tumours of the major salivary glands in children. *Cancer* 1972; **29**: 312–17.

35. Krolls SO, Trodahl JN, Boyers RC. Salivary gland lesions in children. *Cancer* 1972; **30**: 459–69.

36. Malone B, Baker SR. Benign pleomorphic adenomas in children. *Ann Otol Rhinol Laryngol* 1984; **93**: 210–14.

37. Rogers DA, Lobe TE, Rao BN *et al.* Breast malignancy in children. *J Pediatr Surg* 1994; **29**: 48–51.

38. Spiro RH, Huvos AC, Strong EW. Cancer of the parotid gland. A clinicopathological study of 288 primary cases. *Am J Surg* 1975; **130**: 452–9.

39. Taylor RE, Cattamaneni HR, Spooner D. Salivary gland carcinomas in children: a review of 15 cases. *Med Pediatr Oncol* 1993; **21**: 429–32.

40. Iriaperato JP, Weichselbaum RR, Ervin TJ. The role of post-operative radiation therapy in the treatment of malignant tumours of the parotid gland. *J Surg Oncol* 1984; **27**: 163–7.

41. Buduick SD. Minor salivary gland tumours in children 1. *Dent Child* 1984; **49**: 44–7.

42. Harach HR, Williams ED. Childhood thyroid cancer in England and Wales. *Br J Cancer* 1995; **72**: 777–83.

43. Stiller CA. International variations in the incidence of childhood carcinomas. *Cancer Epidemiol Biomarkers Prev* 1984; **3**: 305–10.

44. Tucker MA *et al.* Therapeutic radiation at a young age is linked to secondary thyroid cancer. *Cancer Res* 1991; **51**: 2885–8.

45. Black P, Straaten A, Gutjahr P. Secondary thyroid cancer after treatment for childhood cancer. *Med Pediatr Oncol* 1998; **31**: 91–5.

46. Baverstock K, Egloff B, Pinchera A *et al.* Thyroid cancer after Chernobyl. *Nature* 1992; **359**: 21–2.

47. Jacob P, Goulko G, Heidenreich WF *et al.* Thyroid cancer risk to children calculated. *Nature* 1998; **392**: 31–2.

48. Sobolev B, Heidenreich WF, Kairo I *et al.* Thyroid cancer incidence in the Ukraine after the Chernobyl accident: comparison with spontaneous incidences. *Radiat Environ Biophys* 1997; **36**: 195–9.

49. Mulligan LM, Kwok JBJ, Healey CS *et al.* Germ-line mutations of the RET proto-oncogene in multiple endocrine neoplasia type 2A. *Nature* 1993; **363**: 458–60.

50. Donis-Keller H, Dou S, Chi D *et al.* Mutations in the RET proto-oncogene are associated with MEN 2A and FMTC. *Hum Mol Genet* 1993; **2**: 851–6.

51. Motomura T, Nikiforov YE, Namba H *et al.* ret Rearrangements in Japanese pediatric and adult papillary thyroid cancers. *Thyroid* 1998; **8**: 485–9.

52. Raab SS, Silverman JF, Elsheikh TM. Pediatric thyroid nodules: disease demographics and clinical management as determined by fine needle aspiration biopsy. *Pediatrics* 1995; **95**: 46–9.

53. Degnan BM, McClellan DR, Francis GL. An analysis of fine needle aspiration biopsy of the thyroid in children and adolescents. *J Pediatr Surg* 1996; **31**: 903–7.

54. Dinauer CW, Tuttle R, Robie D *et al.* Clinical features associated with metastasis and recurrence of differentiated thyroid cancer in children, adolescents and young adults. *Clin Endocrinol* 1998; **49**: 619–28.

55. Hallwirth U, Flores J, Kaserer K *et al.* Differentiated thyroid cancer in children and adolescents: the importance of

adequate surgery and review of literature. *Eur J Pediatr Surg* 1997; **9**: 359–63.

56. Robie DK, Dinauer CW, Tuttle RM *et al.* The impact of initial surgical management on outcome in young patients with differentiated thyroid cancer. *J Pediatr Surg* 1998; **33**: 1134–40.

57. Pacini F, Martino E, Romei C *et al.* Treatment of pre-clinical medullary thyroid carcinoma in MEN 2A gene carrier. *Lancet* 1994; **344**: 1084–5.

58. Massimino M, Gasparini M, Ballerini E *et al.* Primary thyroid carcinoma in children: a retrospective study of 20 patients. *Med Pediatr Oncol* 1995; **24**: 13–17.

59. Newman K, Black T, Heller G *et al.* Differentiated thyroid cancer: determinance of disease progression in patients less than 21 years of age at diagnosis. *Ann Surg* 1998; **227**: 533–41.

60. Landou D, Vini L, Hern R, Harmer C. Thyroid cancer in children: the Royal Marsden Hospital experience. *Eur J Cancer* 2000; **36**: 214–20.

61. Farahati J, Bucsky P, Parlowsky T *et al.* Characteristics of differentiated thyroid carcinoma in children and adolescents with respect to age, gender and histology. *Cancer* 1997; **80**: 2156–62.

62. LaQuaglia M, Corbally M, Heller G *et al.* Recurrence and morbidity in differentiated thyroid cancer in children. *Surgery* 1988; **104**: 1149–56.

63. Schlumberger M, Vathaire FD, Travagli J *et al.* Differentiated thyroid cancer in childhood: long term follow up of 72 patients. *J Clin Endocrinol Metab* 1987; **65**: 1088–94.

64. Al-Saadi A, McCready V, Harmer C. Fertility after iodine ^{131}I therapy for thyroid cancer. *Br J Cancer* 1998; **78**(Suppl 2): 16.

64a. Mazzaferri EL, Young RL, Oertel JE *et al.* Papillary thyroid carcinoma: the impact of therapy in 576 patients. *Medicine (Baltimore)* 1977; **56**: 171–96.

65. Dottorini M, Vigniti A, Mazzucchelli L *et al.* Differentiated thyroid carcinoma in children and adolescents: a 37 year study in 85 patients. *J Nucl Med* 1997; **38**: 669–75.

66. Vatharie F, Schlumberger M, Delisle M *et al.* Leukaemias and cancers following iodine 131 administration for thyroid cancer. *Br J Cancer* 1997; **75**: 734–9.

67. Zimmerman D, Hay I, Gough I *et al.* Papillary thyroid carcinoma in children and adults: long term follow up of 1039 patients conservatively treated at one institution during three decades. *Surgery* 1988; **104**: 1157–66.

68. Kirk J, Mort C, Grant D *et al.* The usefulness of serum thyroglobulin in the follow-up of differentiated thyroid carcinoma in children. *Med Pediatr Oncol* 1992; **20**: 201–8.

69. Seashore JH. Breast enlargements in infants and children. *Pediatr Ann* 1975; **4**: 7–46.

70. Rogers DA, Lobe TE, Rao BN *et al.* Breast malignancy in children. *J Pediatr Surg* 1994; **29**: 48–51.

71. Bhatia S, Robinson LL, Oberlin O *et al.* Breast cancer and other second neoplasms after childhood Hodgkins disease. *N Engl J Med* 1996; **334**: 745–51.

72. McDivitt RW, Stewart FW. Breast carcinoma in children. *J Am Med Assoc* 1966; **195**: 144–6.

73. Masse SR, Roiux A, Beauchesne C. Juvenile carcinoma of the breast. *Hum Pathol* 1981; **12**: 1044–6.

74. Serour F, Gilad A, Kopolovic J, Krispin M. Secretory breast cancer in childhood and adolescence: report of a case and review of the literature. *Med Pediatr Oncol* 1992; **20**: 341–4.

75. Norris HY, Taylor H. Relationship of histological features to behavior in cystosarcoma phyllodes: analysis of ninety-four cases. *Cancer* 1967; **41**: 1974–83.

76. Salvadori B, Cusumano F, Bo RD *et al.* Surgical treatment of phyllodes tumour of the breast. *Cancer* 1989; **63**: 2532–6.

77. Briggs RM, Walters M, Rosenthal D. Cystosarcoma phyllodes in adolescent female patients. *Am J Surg* 1983; **146**: 712–14.

78. Pietruska M, Barnes L. Cystosarcoma phyllodes: a clinico-pathologic analysis of 42 cases. *Cancer* 1974; **41**: 1974–83.

79. Leveque J, Meunier B, Wattier E *et al.* Malignant cystosarcomas phyllodes of the breast in adolescent females. *Eur J Obstet Gynaecol* 1994; **54**: 197–203.

80. Hoover HC, Trestioranu A, Ketcham AS. Metastatic cystosarcoma phyllodes in an adolescent girl. *Ann Surg* 1975; **181**: 279–81.

81. McDougall JC, Unni K, Gorenstein A, O'Connell EJ. Carcinoid and mucoepidermoid carcinoma of the bronchus in children. *Ann Otol* 1980; **89**: 425–7.

82. Pettinato G, Manivel JC, Wick MR, Dehner LP. Classical and cellular (atypical) mesoblastic nephroma: a clinicopathologic, ultrasound, immunohistochemical and flowcytometric study. *Hum Pathol* 1989; **6**: 682–90.

83. Niitu Y, Kubota H, Hasegewa S *et al.* Lung cancer in adolescence. *Am J Dis Child* 1974; **127**: 108–11.

84. Rael J, Misra RP. Carcinoid tumorlet of the bronchus in a child. *South Med J,* 1990; **83**: 1104–5.

85. Salle AJL, Andrassy RJ, Stanford W. Bronchogenic squamous cell carcinoma in childhood: a case report. *J Pediatr Surg* 1977; **12**: 519–21.

86. Hartman GE, Shochat SJ. Primary pulmonary neoplasms of childhood. A review. *Ann Thoracic Surg* 1982; **36**: 108–17.

87. Andrassy RJ, Feltman RW, Stanford W. Bronchial carcinoid tumours in children. *J Pediatr Surg* 1977; **12**: 513–16.

88. Archer RL, Grogg SE, Sanders SP. Mucoepidermoid bronchial adenoma in a 6 year old girl: a case report and review of the literature. *J Thorac Cardiovasc Surg* 1987; **94**: 452–4.

89. Cohen MC, Kaschula ROC. Primary pulmonary tumours in childhood: a review of 31 years experience and the literature. *Pediatr Pulmonol* 1992; **140**: 222–32.

90. Emory WB, Mitchell WT, Hatch HB. Mucous gland adenoma of the bronchus. *Am Rev Respir Dis* 1973; **108**: 1407–10.

91. Lack EE, Harris GBC, Eraklis AJ, Vawter GF. Primary bronchial tumours in childhood. *Cancer* 1983; **51**: 492–7.

92. Okike N, Bernatz PE, Woolner LB. Carcinoid tumours of the lung. *Ann Thorac Surg* 1976; **22**: 269–77.

93. Liberman A, Bar-Ziv J, Zirkin HJ. Low grade mucoepidermoid tumour of the bronchus in childhood: a therapeutic dilemma. *Eur J Pediatr* 1986; **145**: 130–2.

94. Seo S, Warren J, Mirkin D *et al.* Mucoepidermoid carcinoma of the bronchus in a 4 year old child. *Cancer* 1984; **53**: 1600–4.

95. Keita O, Lagrange J-L, Michiels J-F *et al.* Primary bronchogenic squamous cell carcinoma in children: report of a case and review of the literature. *Med Pediatr Oncol* 1995; **24**: 50–2.

96. Priest JR, McDermott MB, Bhatia S *et al.* Pleuropulmonary blastoma. *Cancer* 1997; **80**: 147–61.

97. Manivel JC, Priest JR, Watterson J *et al.* Pleuropulmonary blastoma: the so-called pulmonary blastoma of childhood. *Cancer* 1988; **62**: 1516–26.

98. Yousem SA, Hochholzer L, Randhawa P, Manivel JC. Pulmonary blastoma. An immunohistochemical analysis with comparison with fetal lung in its pseudoglandular stage. *Am J Clin Pathol* 1990; **93**: 167–75.

99. Priest JR, Watterson J, Strong L *et al.* Pleuropulmonary blastoma: a marker for familial disease. *J Pediatr* 1996; **128**: 220–4.

100. Beckwith JB. Precursor lesions of Wilms' tumor: clinical and biological implications. *Med Pediatr Oncol* 1993; **21**: 158–68.

101. Wang-Wuu S, Soukup S, Ballard E *et al.* Chromosomal analysis of sixteen human rhabdomyosarcomas. *Cancer Res* 1988; **48**: 983–7.

102. Novak R, Dasu S, Agamanolis D *et al.* Trisomy 8 is a characteristic finding in pleuropulmonary blastoma. *Pediatr Pathol Lab Med* 1997; **17**: 99–103.

103. Kelsey AM, McNally K, Birch J *et al.* Case of extrapulmonary, pleuro-pulmonary blastoma in a child: pathological and cytogenetic findings. *Med Pediatr Oncol* 1997; **29**: 61–4.

104. Yang P, Hasegawa T, Hirose T *et al.* Pleuropulmonary blastoma: fluorescence in situ hybridisation. *Am J Surg Pathol* 1997; **21**: 854–9.

105. Schmaltz C, Sauter S, Opitz O *et al.* Pleuro-pulmonary blastoma: a case report and review of the literature. *Med Pediatr Oncol* 1995; **25**: 479–84.

106. Tagge EP, Mulvihill D, Chandler JC *et al.* Childhood pleuropulmonary blastoma: caution against non-operative management of congenital lung cysts. *J Pediatr Surg* 1996; **31**: 187–90.

107. Manivel JC, Priest JR, Watterson J *et al.* Pleuropulmonary blastoma: the so-called pulmonary blastoma of childhood. *Cancer* 1988; **62**: 1516–26.

108. Cappuccino H, Helotis T, Krumerman M. Pulmonary blastoma as a unique case of fatal respiratory distress in a newborn. *J Pediatr Surg* 1995; **30**: 886–8.

109. Kummet TD, Doll DC. Chemotherapy of pulmonary blastoma: a case report and review of the literature. *Med Pediatr Oncol* 1982; **10**: 27–33.

110. Lobo-Sanahuja F, Santamaria S, Barrantes JC. Case report: pulmonary blastoma in children – response to chemotherapy. *Med Pediatr Oncol* 1996; **26**: 196–200.

111. Howman-Giles R, Dalla-Pozza L, Uren R. Ga-67 scintigraphy in pleuropulmonary blastoma in children. *Clin Nucl Med* 1993; **18**: 120–2.

112. Souadjian JV, Enriquez P, Silverstein MN, Pepin J-M. The spectrum of diseases associated with thymoma. *Arch Intern Med* 1974; **134**: 374–9.

113. Furman WL, Buckley PJ, Green AA *et al.* Thymoma and myaesthenia gravis in a 4-year old child. *Cancer* 1985; **56**: 2703–6.

114. Gregory AK, Connery CP, Resta-Flarer F *et al.* A case of massive thymolipoma. *J Pediatr Surg* 1997; **32**: 1780–2.

115. Dimery IS, Blick M, Pearson G *et al.* Association of the Epstein–Barr virus with lymphoepithelioma of the thymus. *Cancer* 1988; **61**: 2475–80.

116. Niehues T, Harms D, Jurgens H, Gobel U. Treatment of pediatric malignant thymoma: long term remission in a 14 year old boy with EBV associated thymic carcinoma by aggressive combined modality treatment. *Med Pediatr Oncol* 1996; **26**: 419–24.

117. Levine GD, Rosai J. Thymic hyperplasia and neoplasia: a review of current concepts. *Hum Pathol* 1978; **9**: 495–515.

118. Fornasiero A, Daniele O, Ghiotta C *et al.* Chemotherapy of invasive thymoma. *J Clin Oncol* 1990; **8**: 1419–23.

119. Gripp S, Hilgers K, Wurn R, Schmidt G. Thymoma: prognostic factors and treatment outcome. *Cancer* 1998; **83**: 1495–503.

120. Shin DM, Walsh GL, Komaki R *et al.* A multidisciplinary approach to therapy for unresectable malignant thymoma. *Ann Intern Med* 1998; **129**: 100–4.

121. Khan M, Puri P, Devaney D. Mesothelioma of the tunica vaginalis testis in a child. *J Urol* 1997; **158**: 198–9.

122. Jones M, Young R, Scully R. Malignant mesothelioma of the tunical vaginalis: a clinicopathologic analysis of 11 cases with a review of the literature. *Am J Surg Pathol* 1995; **19**: 815–25.

123. Henkes D, Stein N. Mesothelioma of the testicle in a child. *J Urol* 1986; **135**: 794.

124. Eker R, Cantez T, Dogan O *et al.* Pericardial mesothelioma. A pediatric case report. *Turk J Pediatr* 1989; **31**: 305–9.

125. Kelsey A. Mesothelioma of childhood. *Pediatr Hematol Oncol* 1994; **11**: 461–2.

126. Brenner J, Sordillo P, Magill G. Malignant mesothelioma in children: report on 7 cases and review of the literature. *Med Pediatr Oncol* 1981; **9**: 367–73.

127. Young J, Gloeckler Ries L, Silverberg E *et al.* Cancer incidence, survival and mortality for children younger than age 15 years. *Cancer* 1986; **58**: 598–602.

128. Fraire A, Cooper S, Greenberg D *et al.* Mesothelioma of childhood. *Cancer* 1988; **62**: 838–47.

129. Cooper S, Fraire A, Buffler P *et al.* Epidemiologic aspects of childhood mesothelioma. *Pathol Immunopathol Res* 1989; **8**: 276–86.

130. Haque AK, Hernandez JC, Dillard EA. Asbestos bodies found in infant lungs. *Arch Pathol Lab Med* 1985; **109**: 212.

131. Peterson JT, Greenberg SD, Buffler PA. Non-asbestos related malignant mesothelioma. *Cancer* 1984; **54**: 951–60.

132. Grundy G, Miller R. Malignant mesothelioma in childhood. *Cancer* 1972; **30**: 1216–18.

133. Powell J, Stevens M, Stiller C. Clustering of childhood peritoneal mesothelioma in the Midlands. *Lancet* 1995; **345**: 66–7.

134. Srickler H, Rosenberg P, Devesa S *et al.* Contamination of polio virus vaccines with Simian virus 40 (1955–1963) and subsequent cancer rate. *J Am Med Assoc* 1998; **279**: 292–5.

135. Antman K, Ruxer R, Aisner J, Vawter G. Mesothelioma following Wilms' tumour in childhood. *Cancer* 1984; **54**: 367–9.

136. Anderson K, Hurley W, Hurley B, Ohrt D. Malignant pleural mesothelioma following radiotherapy in a 16 year old boy. *Cancer* 1985; **56**: 273–6.

137. Cavazza A, Travis L, Travis W *et al.* Post-irradiation malignant mesothelioma. *Cancer* 1996; **77**: 1379–85.

138. Hoffmann J, Mintzer D, Warhol M. Malignant mesothelioma following radiation therapy. *Am J Med* 1994; **97**: 379–82.

139. Taguchi T, Jhanwar S, Siegfries J *et al.* Recurrent deletions of specific chromosomal sites in 1p, 3p, 6q & 9p in human mesothelioma. *Cancer Res* 1993; **53**: 4349–55.

140. Pritchard-Jones K, Fleming S, Davidson D *et al.* The candidate Wilms' tumour gene is involved in genitourinary development. *Nature* 1990; **346**: 194–7.

141. Park S, Scalling M, Bernard A *et al.* The Wilms' tumour gene is expressed in murine mesoderm-derived tissues and mutated in a human mesothelioma. *Nat Genet* 1993; **4**: 415–20.

142. Niggli F, Gray T, Raafat F, Stevens M. Spectrum of peritoneal mesothelioma in childhood: clinical and histopathological features. *Pediatr Hematol Oncol* 1994; **11**: 399–408.

143. McCullagh M, Keen C, Dykes E. Cystic mesothelioma of peritoneum: a rare cause of ascites in children. *J Pediatr Surg* 1994; **29**: 1205–7.

144. Geary W, Mills S, Frierson H, Pope T. Malignant peritoneal mesothelioma in childhood with long term survival. *Am J Clin Pathol* 1991; **95**: 493–8.

145. Silberstein M, Lewis J, Blair J *et al.* Congenital peritoneal mesothelioma. *J Pediatr Surg* 1983; **18**: 243–5.

146. Antman K, Schiff P, Pass H, eds. *Benign and Malignant Mesothelioma*, 5th edn. Philadelphia: Lippincott-Raven, 1997.

147. Pratt CB, Meyer WH, Douglass EC *et al.* A phase I study of ifosphamide with mesna given daily for 3 consecutive days to children with malignant solid tumours. *Cancer* 1993; **71**: 3661–5.

148. Stiller CA. International variations in the incidence of childhood carcinomas. *Cancer Epidemiol Biomarkers Prev* 1984; **3**: 305–10.

149. Teinturier C, Pauchard MS, Brugieres L *et al.* Clinical and prognostic aspects of adrenocortical neoplasms in childhood. *Med Pediatr Oncol* 1999; **32**: 106–11.

150. Ribeiro RC, Sandrini R, Schell MJ *et al.* Adrenocortical carcinoma in children: a study of 40 cases. *J Clin Oncol* 1990; **8**: 67–74.

151. Michalkiewcz EL, Sandrini R, Bugg MF *et al.* Clinical characteristics of small functioning adrenocortical tumours in children. *Med Pediatr Oncol* 1997; **28**: 175–8.

152. Li FP, Fraumeni JF, Mulvihill JJ *et al.* A cancer family syndrome in twenty-four kindreds. *Cancer Res* 1988; **48**: 5358–62.

153. Malkin D, Li FP, Strong LC *et al.* Germ line p53 mutations in a familial syndrome of breast cancer, sarcomas, and other neoplasms. *Science* 1990; **250**: 1233–8.

154. Birch JM, Hartley AL, Blair V. Cancer in the families of children with soft tissue sarcoma. *Cancer* 1990; **66**: 2239–48.

155. Wagner J, Portwine C, Rabin K *et al.* High frequency of germline mutations in childhood adrenocortical cancer. *J Natl Cancer Inst* 1994; **86**: 1707–10.

156. Wiedemann HR. Tumours and hemihypertrophy associated with Wiedemann–Beckwith syndrome. *Eur J Pediatr* 1983; **141**: 129.

157. Hanwi GJ, Serbin RA, Kruger FA. Does adrenocortical hyperplasia result in adrenocortical carcinoma? *N Engl J Med* 1957; **257**: 1153–7.

158. Wedell A, Luthman H. Steroid 21-hydroxylase deficiency two additional mutations and a rapid screening of disease causing mutations. *Hum Mol Genet* 1993; **2**: 499–504.

159. Kjellman M, Holst M, Backdahl M *et al.* No overrepresentation of congenital adrenal hyperplasia in patients with adrenocortical tumours. *Clin Endocrinol* 1999; **50**: 3443–46.

160. Hartley AL, Birch JM, Marsden HB *et al.* Adrenal cortical tumours: epidemiological and familial aspects. *Arch Dis Child* 1987; **62**: 683–9.

161. Abraham SC, Wu TT, Klimstra DS *et al.* Distinctive molecular genetic alterations in sporadic and familial adenomatous polyposis-associated pancreatoblastomas – frequent alterations in the APC/beta-catenin pathway and chromosome 11p. *Am J Pathol* 2001; **159**: 1619–27.

162. Bugg MF, Ribeiro RC, Roberson PK *et al.* Correlation of pathologic features with clinical outcome in pediatric adrenocortical neoplasia. *Am J Clin Pathol* 1994; **101**: 625–9.

163. Haak HR, Hermans J, van de Velde CJH *et al.* Optimal treatment of adrenocortical carcinoma with mitotane: results in a consecutive series of 96 patients. *Br J Cancer* 1994; **69**: 947–51.

164. Wood AA, Woodward G. Severe adrenal cortical atrophy (cytotoxic) and hepatic damage produced in dogs by feeding 2,2-bis(parachlorophenyl) = 1,1 dichloroethane (DDD or TDE). *Arch Pathol* 1949; **48**: 387–94.

165. van Slooten H, Moolenaar AJ, van Seters AP, Smeenk D. The treatment of adrenocortical carcinoma with o,p'-DDD: the prognostic implications of serum monitoring. *Eur J Clin Oncol* 1984; **20**: 47–53.

166. Greig F, Oberfield SE, Levine LS *et al.* Recovery of adrenal function after treatment of adrenocortical carcinoma with o,p'-DDD. *Clin Endocrinol* 1984; **20**: 389–99.

167. Korth-Schutz S, Levine LS, Roth JA *et al.* Virilizing adrenal tumor in a child suppressed with dexamethasone for 3 years. Effect of o,p'-DDD on serum and urinary androgens. *J Clin Endocrinol Metab* 1977; **44**: 433–9.

168. Helson L, Wollner N, Murphy L, Schwartz MK. Metastatic adrenal cortical carcinoma: biochemical changes accompanying clinical regression. *Clin Chem* 1971; **17**: 1191–3.

169. Hogan TF, Gilchrist KW, Westring DW, Citrin DL. A clinical and pathological study of adrenocortical carcinoma. *Cancer* 1980; **45**: 2880–3.

170. Bonacci R, Gigliotti A, Baudin E *et al.* Cytotoxic therapy with etoposide and cisplatin in advanced adrenocortical carcinoma. *Br J Cancer* 1998; **78**: 546–9.

171. Lubitz JA, Freeman L, Okun R. Mitotane use in inoperable adrenal cortical carcinoma. *J Am Med Assoc* 1973; **223**: 1109–12.

172. Dickstein G, Shechner C, Arad E, Best L-A. Is there a role for low doses of mitotane as adjuvant therapy in adrenocortical carcinoma? *J Clin Endocrinol Metab* 1998; **83**: 3100–3.

173. Moolenaar AJ, van Slooten H, van Seters AP, Smeenk D. Blood levels of o,p'-DDD following administration in various vehicles after a single dose and in long treatment. *Cancer Chemother Pharmacol* 1981; **7**: 51–4.

174. van Slooten H, van Oosterom AT. CAP (cyclophosphamide, doxorubicin and cisplatin) regimen in adrenal cortical carcinoma. *Cancer Treat Rep* 1983; **67**: 377–9.

175. van Seters AP, Moolenaar AJ. Mitotane increases the blood level of hormone-binding proteins. *Acta Endocrinol* 1991; **124**: 526–33.

176. Bonnacci R, Gigliotti A, Wion-Barbot H *et al.* Cytotoxic therapy with etoposide and cisplatin in advanced adrenocortical carcinoma. *Br J Cancer* 1998; **78**: 546–9.

177. Ayass M, Gross S, Harper J. High-dose carboplatinum and VP-16 in the treatment of metastatic adrenal carcinoma. *Am J Pediatr Hematol Oncol* 1991; **13**: 470–2.

178. Crock PA, Clark ACL. Combination chemotherapy for adrenal carcinoma: response in a 5½ year old male. *Med Pediatr Oncol* 1989; **17**: 62–5.

179. Johnson DH, Greco FA. Treatment of metastatic adrenal cortical carcinoma with cisplatin and etoposide. *Cancer* 1986; **58**: 2198–202.

180. Schlumberger M, Brugieres L, Gicquel C *et al.* 5-Fluorouracil, doxorubicin and cisplatin for the treatment of adrenal cortical carcinoma. *Cancer* 1991; **67**: 2997–3000.

181. Haq MM, Legha SS, Samaan NA *et al.* Cytotoxic chemotherapy in adrenal cortical carcinoma. *Cancer Treat Rep* 1980; **64**: 909–13.

182. Squire RA, Bianchi A, Jakate SM. Radiation induced sarcoma of the breast in a female adolescent. *Cancer* 1988; **60**: 2444–7.

183. Holtoefer H, Miettinen A, Paasivuo R *et al.* Cellular origin and differentiation of renal carcinomas. A fluorescence microscopic study with kidney specific antibodies, anti-intermediate filament antibodies and lectins. *Lab Invest* 1983; **49**: 317–62.

184. Breslow N, Olshan A, Beckwith J, Green D. Epidemiology of Wilms' tumour. *Med Pediatr Oncol* 1993; **21**: 172–82.

185. Carcao MD, Taylor GP, Greenberg ML *et al.* Renal-cell carcinoma in children: a different disorder from its adult counterpart? *Med Pediatr Oncol* 1998; **31**: 153–8.

186. Motzer RJ, Bander NH, Nanus DM. Renal-cell carcinoma. *N Engl J Med* 1996; **335**: 865–75.

187. Crossey PA, Foster K, Richards FM *et al.* Molecular genetic investigations of the mechanism of tumourigenesis in von Hippel-Lindau disease: analysis of allele loss in VHL tumours. *Hum Genet* 1994; **93**: 53–8.

188. Yoshida MA, Ohyashiki K, Ochi H *et al.* Cytogenetic studies of tumour tissue from patients with non-familial renal cell carcinoma. *Cancer Res* 1986; **46**: 2139–47.

189. Lack EE, Cassady JR, Sallan SE. Renal cell carcinoma in children and adolescence: a clinical and pathological study of 17 cases. *J Urol* 1985; **133**: 822–8.

190. Erkschlager T, Kodet R. Renal cell carcinoma in children. *Med Pediatr Oncol* 1994; **23**: 36–9.

191. Raney RB, Palmer N, Sutow WW *et al.* Renal cell carcinoma in children. *Med Pediatr Oncol* 1983; **11**: 91–8.

192. Booth CM. Renal parenchymal carcinoma in children. *Br J Surg* 1986; **73**: 313–7.

193. Freedman AL, Vates TS, Stewart T *et al.* Renal cell carcinoma in children: the Detroit experience. *J Urol* 1996; **155**: 1708–10.

194. Bukowski RM. Natural history and therapy of metastatic renal cell carcinoma. *Cancer* 1997; **80**: 1198–220.

195. Frable WJ, Still WJS, Kay S. Carcinoma of the pancreas, infantile type. *Cancer* 1971; **27**: 667–73.

196. Horie A, Yano Y, Kotoo Y, Miwa A. Morphogenesis of pancreatoblastoma, infantile carcinoma of the pancreas. *Cancer* 1977; **39**: 247–54.

197. Passmore SJ, Berry PJ, Oakhill A. Recurrent pancreatoblastoma with inappropriate adrenocorticotrophic hormone secretion. *Arch Dis Child* 1988; **63**: 1494–6.

198. Iseki M, Suzuki T, Koizumi Y *et al.* Alpha-fetoprotein-producing pancreatoblastoma: a case report. *Cancer* 1986; **57**: 1833–5.

199. Klimstra DS. Pancreatoblastoma: a clinicopathologic review of the literature. *Am J Surg Pathol* 1995; **19**: 1371–89.

200. Potts SR, Brown S, O'Hara MD: Pancreatoblastoma in a neonate associated with Beckwith–Wiedemann syndrome. *Z Kinderchir* 1986; **41**: 56–7.

201. Koh T, Cooper J, Newman C *et al.* Pancreatoblastoma in a neonate with Wiedemann–Beckwith Syndrome. *Eur J Pediatr* 1986; **145**: 435–8.

202. Drut R, Jones MC. Congenital pancreatoblastoma in Beckwith–Wiedemann syndrome: an emerging association. *Pediatr Pathol* 1988; **8**: 331–9.

203. Inomata Y, Nishizawa T, Takasan H *et al.* Pancreatoblastoma resected by delayed primary operation after effective chemotherapy. *J Pediatr Surg* 1992; **12**: 1570–2.

204. Eden OB, Shaw MP. Chemotherapy for pancreaticoblastoma. *Med Pediatr Oncol* 1992; **20**: 357–8.

205. Morgan ER, Perryman JH, Reynolds M *et al.* Pancreatic blastomatous tumour in a child responding to therapy used for hepatoblastoma: case report and review of the literature. *Med Pediatr Oncol* 1996; **26**: 284–92.

206. Vannier J-P, Flamant F, Hemet J *et al.* Pancreatoblastoma: response to chemotherapy. *Med Pediatr Oncol* 1991; **19**: 187–91.

207. Griffin BR, Wisbeck WM, Schaller RT, Benjamin DR. Radiotherapy for recurrent infantile pancreatic carcinoma (Pancreatoblastoma). *Cancer* 1987; **60**: 1734–6.

208. Boor PJ, Swanson MR. Papillary cystic neoplasm of the pancreas. *Am J Surg Pathol* 1979; **3**: 69–75.

209. Compagno J, Oertel JE, Kremzer M. Solid and papillary epithelial neoplasms of the pancreas, probably of small duct origin: a clinicopathologic study of 52 cases. *Lab Invest* 1979; **40**: 248–9.

210. Dales RL, Garcia JC, Davis RS. Papillary-cystic carcinoma of the pancreas. *J Surg Oncol* 1983; **22**: 115–17.

211. Horisawa M, Niinomi N, Sato T *et al.* Frantz's tumour (solid and cystic tumour of the pancreas) with liver metastasis: successful treatment and long term follow up. *J Pediatr Surg* 1995; **30**: 724–6.

212. Jeng L-BB, Chen M-F, Tang R-P. Solid and papillary neoplasm of the pancreas. *Arch Surg* 1993; **128**: 433–6.

213. Kloppel GK, Morohoshi T, John HD *et al.* Solid and acinar cell tumour of the pancreas: a tumour in young women with favourable prognosis. *Virchows Archiv A* 1981; **392**: 171–83.

214. Matsunou H, Konishi F. Papillary cystic neoplasm of the pancreas. *Cancer* 1990; **65**: 283–91.

215. Rafaat F, PArkes SE, McLachlan K *et al.* Papillary and solid epithelial neoplasm(PSEN) of the pancreas: an often misdiagnosed benign tumour of young women. *Ann Diagn Paediatr Pathol* 1997; **1**: 271–8.

216. Rustin RB, Broughan TA, Hermann RE *et al.* Papillary cystic epithelial neoplasms of the pancreas. *Arch Surg* 1986; **121**: 1073–6.

217. Sanfey H, Mandelsohn G, Cameron JL. Solid and papillary neoplasm of the pancreas: a potentially curable surgical lesion. *Ann Surg* 1982; **197**: 272–5.

218. Todani T, Shimada K, Watanabe Y *et al.* Frantz's tumour: a papillary and cystic tumour of the pancreas in girls. *J Pediatr Surg* 1988; **23**: 116–21.

219. Fried P, Cooper J, Balthazar E *et al.* A role for radiotherapy in the treatment of solid and papillary epithelial neoplasms of the pancreas. *Cancer* 1985; **56**: 2783–5.

220. Strauss JF, Hirsch VJ, Rubey CN, Pollock M. Resection of a solid and papillary epithelial neoplasm of the pancreas following treatment with cis-platinum and 5-fluorouracil: a case report. *Med Pediatr Oncol* 1993; **21**: 365–7.

221. Klimstra DS, Heffess CA, Oertel JE, Rosai J. Acinar cell carcinoma of the pancreas. *Am J Surg Pathol* 1992; **16**: 815–37.

222. Mah P-T, Loo DC, Tock EPC. Pancreatic acinar cell carcinoma in childhood. *Am J Dis Child* 1974; **128**: 101–4.

223. Lewis MA, Lilleyman JS, Variend S. Benign metastatic islet cell tumour of the pancreas. *Med Pediatr Oncol* 1985; **13**: 97–100.

224. Ichijima K, Akaishi K, Toyoda M *et al.* Carcinoma of the pancreas with endocrine component in childhood. *Am J Clin Pathol* 1983; **83**: 95–100.

225. Cubilla AL, Hajdu SI. Islet cell carcinoma of the pancreas. *Arch Pathol* 1975; **99**: 204–7.

226. Chung EB, Enzinger FM. Malignant melanoma of soft parts. *Am J Surg Pathol* 1983; **7**: 405–13.

227. d'Amore ESG, Ninfo V. Clear cell tumours of somatic soft tissues. *Semin Diag Pathol* 1997; **14**: 270–80.

228. Eckardt JJ, Pritchard DJ, Soule EH. Clear cell sarcoma. *Cancer* 1983; **52**: 1482–8.

229. Lucas DR, Nascimento AG, Sim FH. Clear cell sarcoma of soft tissues. *Am J Surg Pathol* 1992; **16**: 1197–204.

230. Pavlides NA, Fisher C, Wiltshaw E. Clear-cell sarcoma of tendons and aponeuroses: a clinicopathologic study. *Cancer* 1984; **54**: 1412–17.

231. Sara AS, Evamns HL, Benjamin RS. Malignant melanoma of soft parts (clear cell sarcoma). *Cancer* 1990; **65**: 367–74.

232. Stout AP, Lattes R. Tumours of the soft tissues. In: *Atlas of Tumor Pathology*, second series, Fascicle I. Washington, DC: Armed Forces Institute of Pathology, 1967; 17–30.

233. Kiel KD, Suit HD. Radiation therapy in the treatment of aggressive fibromatosis (desmoid tumour). *Cancer* 1984; **54**: 2051–5.

234. Stein R. Chemotherapeutic response in fibromatosis of the neck. *J Paediatr* 1977; **90**: 482–3.

235. Brooks MD, Ebbs SR, Colletta AA, Baum MD. Desmoid tumours treated by triphenylethylenes. *Eur J Cancer* 1992; **28a**: 1014–18.

236. Enjolras O, Riche MC, Merland JJ, Escaude JP. Management of alarming hemangiomas of infancy: a review of 25 cases. *Pediatrics* 1990; **85**: 491–8.

237. Bartoshesky LE, Bull M, Feingold M. Corticosteroid treatment of cutaneous hemangiomas: how effective? A report of 24 children. *Clin Pediatr (Phila)* 1978; **17**: 625–8.

238. Kushner BJ. The treatment of periorbital infantile haemangioma with intralesional corticosteroid. *Plast Reconstr Surg* 1985; **76**: 517–26.

239. Sloan GM, Reinisch JF, Nichter S *et al.* Intralesional corticosteroid therapy for infantile haemangiomas. *Plast Reconstr Surg* 1989; **83**: 459–67.

240. Berman B, Lim HW-P. Concurrent cutaneous and hepatic haemangiomata in infancy: report of a case and review of the literature. *J Dermatol Surg Oncol* 1978; **4**: 869–73.

241. El-Dessouky M, Azny AF, Raine PAM, Young D. Kasbach–Merritt syndrome. *J Pediatr Surg* 1988; **23**: 109–11.

242. Ezekowitz RA, Mulliken JB, Folkman J. Interferon alpha-2a therapy for life threatening hemangiomas of infancy. *N Engl J Med* 1992; **326**: 1456–63.

243. Plowman PN, Harnett AN. Radiotherapy in benign orbital disease 1: Complicated ocular angiomas. *Br J Ophthalmol* 1986; **72**: 286–8.

244. Dutton SC, Plowman PN. Paediatric haemangiomas: the role of radiotherapy. *Br J Radiol* 1991; **64**: 261–9.

245. Sebag-Monteflore DS, Biggs D, Dean E *et al.* Inoperable pediatric cerebral angiomas successfully treated by stereotactic radiotherapy. *Proc Am Soc Clin Oncol* 1994; **13**: abstract 1445.

246. Sabbaga CC, Avilla SG, Schultz C *et al.* Adrenocortical carcinoma in children. *J Pediatr Surg* 1993; **28**: 841–3.

247. Frantz VK. Tumours of the pancreas. In: *Atlas of Tumour Pathology*. Washington, DC: Armed Forces Institute of Pathology, 1959.

248. Hamoudi AB, Misugi K, Grosfeld JL, Reiner CB. Papillary epithelial neoplasm of pancreas in a child. *Cancer* 1970; **26**: 1126–33.

249. Schlosnagle DC, Campbell WG. The papillary and solid neoplasm of the pancreas: a report of two cases with electron microscopy, one containing neurosecretory granules. *Cancer* 1981; **47**: 2603–10.

Advances in therapy: megatherapy

25

Allogeneic stem cell transplantation

PAUL VEYS & KANCHAN RAO

The concept that haemopoietic stem cells could rescue irreversibly damaged bone marrow was first proposed in the 1950s when it was shown that mice could recover from lethal irradiation if the haemopoietic areas in their spleens were shielded by lead foil.[1] It was initially believed that recovery was prompted by humoral factors produced from shielded cells; however, subsequent experiments, which established that haemopoiesis could also be restored by transfused bone marrow cells,[2] suggested that it was repopulation of the irradiated marrow spaces by protected stem cells that mediated recovery. Consequently, investigators realized the potential of marrow transplantation to rescue patients from the myeloablative effects of chemoradiotherapy and the use of both autologous and allogeneic bone marrow transplantation (BMT) was vigorously pursued.

Allogeneic BMT was initially plagued by the immunological problems of graft rejection and graft-versus-host disease (GvHD), and only 1 in 10 of the early allogeneic BMTs achieved a clinical improvement.[3] Much of the early pioneering work was performed by Thomas et al.[4] using dogs to develop effective total body irradiation schedules and introducing methotrexate to prevent GvHD. The characterization of the HLA system opened a new era in BMT, with transplants being carried out between matched sibling donor (MSD)/recipient pairs. Throughout the 1970s and 1980s there was a rapid expansion in the number of allogeneic BMT procedures performed, facilitated by the introduction of cyclosporin A prophylaxis against GvHD.[5] Only about 30 per cent of children

requiring BMT have HLA-MSDs, and the 1990s saw an increase in the use of alternative donors, particularly the use of volunteer unrelated donors (UDs). In recent years, there has been an increasing use of umbilical cord blood cells[6,7] and megadoses of purified peripheral blood stem cells[8] as an alternative source of stem cells to bone marrow, and both techniques have facilitated stem cell transplantation (SCT) from HLA-mismatched donors. The development of reduced-intensity, non-myeloablative conditioning has permitted SCT in children with organ dysfunction coexisting at the time of transplantation.[9]

There have been parallel advances in supportive care, including new generations of broad-spectrum antibiotics, ganciclovir for treatment of cytomegalovirus (CMV) infection, a wide availability of recombinant growth factors, new antifungal agents, including imidazoles and liposomal amphotericin, and the availability of high-efficiency particulate air filtration (HEPA). The application of these new therapies has been facilitated by rapid and sensitive diagnosis of infection by DNA amplification techniques using the polymerase chain reaction (PCR). Together, these technological advances have led to a slow but sustained improvement in the outcome of SCT over recent decades.

CURE OF LEUKAEMIA BY SCT

The original concept of cure by SCT was through dose intensification, allowing rescue from myeloablative doses of chemotherapy and radiotherapy by infusion of autologous or allogeneic bone marrow cells. Cure of leukaemia by this mechanism depends on the number and chemosensitivity of leukaemic cells present at the time of transplantation, and the original concept is strongly supported by the lower relapse rates achieved by carrying out SCT when patients are in 'remission' rather than 'relapse' from their underlying disease. Hence, most indications for SCT in childhood acute leukaemia now carry the prerequisite that the child has achieved remission prior to SCT.

There are also several lines of evidence to suggest that alloreactive donor cells can exert an important anti-leukaemic action.[10] One mechanism of this graft-versus-leukaemia (GvL) effect is mediated by cytotoxic T cells recognizing major and/or minor histocompatibility antigen differences on recipient cells; hence it may also involve cells responsible for GvHD, although other GvL mechanisms may be more leukaemia-specific.[11] Consequently, GvL reactions are more pronounced in the presence of GvHD and/or with increasing donor/recipient HLA disparity, e.g. in transplants from UDs.[12] GvL also appears to be disease-specific, with the most powerful GvL effect being observed in chronic myeloid leukaemia (CML), and the smallest effect in acute lymphoblastic leukaemia (ALL), presumably owing to coexpression or not of target antigens.[13]

PROBLEMS IN ASSESSING RESPONSE TO SCT

Much debate continues over which children should receive SCT. This problem arises because of the paucity of prospective randomized trials. This occurs frequently because the patient groups have not been large enough to enable randomized studies, and because randomization, often at the end stage of the child's disease, is complicated by both patient/family and physician preferences. Much of the available data are, therefore, subject to the bias of patient selection, in particular selection of patients who have achieved and maintained a complete remission until the time of SCT and who, therefore, might fall into a better prognostic group. This can be somewhat offset by censoring patients from 'intent to transplant' or by comparing the outcome of those 'with and without donors' from the outset.

Further problems arise because favourable results of a treatment are more likely to be reported than unfavourable results, giving the impression of greater success from SCT than may be warranted. Conversely, any comparison of the outcome of SCT with chemotherapy requires a prolonged follow-up, because of late leukaemia relapses following chemotherapy.

TYPES OF STEM CELL DONOR

Over the last decade, the number of donors available for transplant procedures has increased enormously. The expanded number comes from the worldwide pool of UDs, which is now approaching six million. If a MSD is not available (70 per cent of children), then a matched (10/10 HLA antigens including A, B, C, DRβ1, DQβ1 × 2) or single locus mismatched UD can now be found for greater than 90 per cent of Caucasian children within the UK. The survival after UD SCT in children is 40–50 per cent, significantly better than that in adults, and comparable to that after MSD SCT.[14–17] With the increasing number of UDs, any one search may reveal several fully matched donors; it then becomes important to consider other factors, such as age, CMV status and sex of the donor. Wherever possible, the donor should be young, the CMV status of the donor and recipient should be matched to minimize the risk of post-transplant viral reactivation and disease, and male donors are preferable to avoid sensitization by pregnancy. If no closely matched donor is available then encouraging survival has also been reported from small studies using haplotype mismatched family donors (usually parents) following preparation with highly immunosuppressive regimens and megadoses of purified peripheral blood stem cells (PBSCs).[18–20] Alternatively, mismatched SCT for children may be facilitated by the use of umbilical cord blood (UCB) cell transplantation, and growing UCB banks around the world now store over 100 000 UCB donations. Nearly 2000 UCB transplants had been carried out by the year 2000 from sibling and unrelated donors in children with both genetic and malignant diseases. Engraftment of UCB is generally slower than conventional BMT, but rates of GvHD are reduced, permitting a greater degree of HLA mismatch (4/6 HLA antigens – A, B, DRβ1), and overall survival is equivalent to that of BMT.[21]

While the use of purified PBSCs and naïve UCB cells facilitates the use of mismatched donors, there is ensuing debate about the best source of stem cells for matched related and unrelated donors. The higher cell yield with PBSCs is offset by the greater incidence of chronic GvHD. There is concern over the administration of granulocyte colony-stimulating factor (G-CSF) to childhood donors, and hence, for paediatric donors bone marrow is recommended as the preferred source of stem cells, while adult related and unrelated donors may make an informed choice. Some prefer to receive G-CSF and undergo leukapheresis to avoid a bone marrow harvest under general anaesthesia. Guidelines as to the appropriate choice of donor have been drawn up by the United Kingdom Children's Cancer Study Group Bone Marrow Transplant Group (UKCCSG BMT Group), and are listed in Box 25.1.

Box 25.1 *United Kingdom Children's Cancer Study Group Bone Marrow Transplant Group (UKCCSG BMT) donor selection guidelines*

HLA hierarchy[a]

1. Matched sibling donor = phenotypic matched family donor = fully matched related cord blood[b]
2. 10/10 molecular matched unrelated donor = 6/6 matched unrelated cord blood[b]
3. One allelic mismatched unrelated donor = 5/6 matched family donor, ≤2/6 mismatched unrelated cord blood[b]
4. Two allelic mismatched unrelated donor = ≥2 mismatched family donor

Stem cell source

1. MSD[c] – BM > PBSC
2. MUD[c] – BM = PBSC
3. MMUD/MMFD – PBSC > BM

Cytomegalovirus status

Patient   Donor
Positive   Positive > negative
Negative Negative > positive

Age

Young > old

Gender

Patient   Donor
Male   Male > female
Female   Male > female

ABO

Aim for a match in heavily pre-transfused patients.

BM, bone marrow; MMFD, mismatched family donor; MMUD, mismatched unrelated donor; MSD, matched sibling donor; MUD, matched unrelated donor; PBSC, peripheral blood stem cell.
[a]Options 3 and 4 should only be considered in poor-risk patients for whom alternative treatment is unavailable or has failed.
[b]With nucleated cell dose >3.7 × 10^7/kg recipient weight.
[c]Adult sibling and unrelated donors should be allowed a choice after non-directive counselling by a physician independent of the transplant programme.
>, preferred to ; =, equivalent to.

INDICATIONS FOR SCT

The indications for SCT in paediatric malignancies have been under close scrutiny for the last decade.[22] The disease-free survival (DFS) following front-line chemotherapy protocols has improved, and SCT appears to be no longer advantageous in many first remission paediatric leukaemias. Although transplant-related mortality may now be as low as 10 per cent in many paediatric transplant centres,[23] late effects – including infertility, growth retardation, neuropsychometric learning difficulties and second tumours – remain a considerable problem.[24] A clear benefit in DFS from SCT should therefore exist before the procedure is undertaken. Specific indications for allogeneic SCT are given in Table 25.1.

ALL

HIGH-RISK ALL IN FIRST COMPLETE REMISSION (CR)

Children with ALL at high risk of relapse may be considered for SCT in first remission. This remains a controversial area which has recently been reviewed in some detail.[25] A recent large American study examined the outcome of higher-risk ALL based on age, leucocyte count and immunophenotype, excluding patients with Philadelphia chromosome positive (Ph+) ALL and t(4,11) translocations. Non-T-ALL patients who received MSD SCT had a significantly better leukaemia-free survival (LFS) (58 vs. 39 per cent) but no difference in overall survival (OS) (61 vs. 55 per cent) compared with patients receiving only chemotherapy. The group with T-ALL showed no significant difference in LFS between chemotherapy (53 per cent) and SCT (63 per cent) and no difference in OS.[26] A similar decrease in relapse and increase in treatment-related death in the transplant group (including both MSDs and UDs) was also shown in a recent update of the MRC UKALL X and XI studies with no overall benefit for SCT.[27] Consequently, there is no evidence at present that SCT is superior to conventional treatment in the broad group of children with higher-risk ALL. There may, however, be a case for evaluation of SCT from both sibling and unrelated donors in clearly defined subsets of the highest-risk patients, including failure to achieve remission at 28 days,[28] Ph+ ALL,[29–31] near-haploid ALL, and infants with t(4,11)[32] who show a poor response to steroids. Collectively this highest-risk group comprises 8–9 per cent of children with ALL, in whom the event-free survival (EFS) is under 40 per cent. It is recommended that a transplant be performed early in Ph+ ALL at approximately 6–8 months from diagnosis.

ALL IN SECOND CR

The prognosis of children who suffer a relapse of ALL depends on the site of the relapse and the duration of the first remission.[33] Thus, while the 5-year EFS of children treated according to the MRC UKALL R1 protocol was 46 per cent, it was only 7 per cent for those suffering a bone marrow relapse on therapy. This is in marked contrast to the 77 per cent EFS in those relapsing without bone marrow involvement. The place of SCT remains uncertain in relapsed ALL. Results from the MRC[33] and

Table 25.1 *Proposed indications for transplant procedures in children (developed through the UKCCSG BMT group and modified from Cornish et al.[150])*

Disease	Disease status	Allogeneic matched related[a]	Allogeneic unrelated[b]	Haploidentical related	Autologous blood or marrow
AML	CR1	R[e]	CRP	NR	NR
	CR2	R	CRP	CRP[c]	R[d]
	Relapse/refractory	D	D	CRP[h]	NR
ALL	High-risk CR1	R[f]	R[f]	NR	NR
	CR2[g]	R[g]	R[g]	CRP[g]	CRP
	CR3	R	R	R	NR
	Relapse/refractory	NR	NR	NR	NR
CML	Chronic phase	R	R	CRP[i]	CRP
	Advanced phase	R	R	CRP[i]	CRP
	Blast crisis	D	NR	CRP[i]	NR
T-NHL	As ALL				
Hodgkin's disease	CR1	NR	NR	NR	NR
	CR2	CRP	D	NR	CRP
	CR3	D	D	NR	D
	Refractory	NR	NR	NR	D
Myelodysplasia	JMML, RA[j], RARS, CMML,	R	R	CRP	NR
	RAEB/T, sAML[k]	R	CRP	CRP	NR

CRP, to be undertaken in approved clinical research protocols; D, developmental or pilot studies can be approved in specialist units; NR, not generally recommended; R, in routine use for selected patients.

ALL, acute lymphoblastic leukaemia; AML, acute myeloid leukaemia; CMML, chronic myelomonocytic leukaemia; CML, chronic myeloid leukaemia; CR1–3, first/second/third complete remission; JMML, juvenile myelomonocytic leukaemia; T-NHL, T-cell non-Hodgkin's lymphoma; RA, refractory anaemia; RAEB/T, refractory anaemia with excess blasts in transformation; RARS, refractory anaemia with ringed sideroblasts; sAML, secondary AML.

[a]Also includes 5/6 matched related donors in certain cases.
[b]Includes 9/10, 10/10 from HLA A, B, C, DRB1, DQB1.
[c]If relapse <1 year from diagnosis.
[d]If relapse >1 year from diagnosis.
[e]Only poor-risk patients (see Box 25.2).
[f]Philadelphia-positive t(9,22), near haploid, >25% blasts in BM at day 28.
[g]For high-risk patients by BFM classification (see Table 25.2), any standard- or intermediate-risk patient with MRD >10^4 at week 5 of re-induction will be offered BMT if a closely matched related/unrelated donor is available; otherwise the patient will receive chemotherapy.
[h]Worth considering if a KIR mismatched donor is available due to graft-versus-leukaemia effect of natural killer cells.
[i]If no haematological response to imatinib of IFN, or haematological relapse on imatinib.
[j]If cytogenetics are abnormal or blood product-dependent.
[k]RAEB/T, sAML eligible for AML trials, except Down's syndrome where BMT is not necessary.

BFM groups[34] suggest that the groups that benefit the most are those with early bone marrow relapse and those with T-cell disease. Most centres in Europe are about to adopt a simplified BFM risk stratification, shown in Table 25.2.

All high-risk patients will be offered a SCT procedure. The previous recommended UK approach was to proceed to either a MSD or UD; in the absence of a donor, the recommendation was to continue with chemotherapy. However, haploidentical transplants are now being successfully performed,[18,19] and since transplantation appears to have a survival advantage over those who receive chemotherapy in the high-risk group,[35] those without closely matched related or unrelated donors will undergo haploidentical PBSC transplant (PBSCT). Just prior to SCT, minimal residual disease (MRD) positivity >10^3 is associated

with a very high subsequent relapse rate,[36] and such patients should be selected to receive other experimental approaches which may or may not involve transplantation.

It is unclear as to the best strategy for the intermediate-risk group. It is probable that transplantation will not benefit those with isolated extramedullary relapse,[37] but it is equally possible that it may improve survival in those with medullary disease. Ideally a randomization of chemotherapy versus SCT would be appropriate for this group, but previous attempts at this have failed due to patient and physician preferences. At the present time in the UK, intermediate-risk and standard-risk children will be treated with chemotherapy/radiotherapy, except for those who are MRD-positive >10^4 at week 5, who will be offered SCT.

Table 25.2 *Simplified BFM therapeutic risk stratification for relapsed acute lymphoblastic leukaemia (ALL) of childhood*

	Non-T ALL			Pre-T ALL		
	Extramedullary	Combined	Marrow	Extramedullary	Combined	Marrow
Very early diagnosis <18 months	I	H	H	I	H	H

Early
  diagnosis >18 months,
  off treatment <6 months
	I	I	H	I	H	H

Late off treatment >6 months	S	I	I	S	H	H

S, standard risk; I, intermediate risk; H, high risk.

If a further relapse occurs after salvage chemotherapy and patients achieve a third CR, as long as there is not significant organ dysfunction at that stage, SCT should be considered in all patients.

AML

AML IN FIRST CR

Since most younger patients with AML enter a CR, the major therapeutic issue is to prevent relapse. Univariate and multivariate analyses of MRC AML 10[38] indicated that two parameters were of very highly significant prognostic importance in relation to relapse: cytogenetic group and percentage of blasts in the bone marrow after the first chemotherapy course (see Box 25.2). Prior to AML 10, it was assumed that all children would benefit from an allogeneic SCT if a MSD was available. This was supported by a recent multicentre study by the Children's Cancer Group (CCG) that compared SCT with chemotherapy. This showed a moderate survival advantage for patients eligible for transplantation versus those without a sibling donor, significant at 3 years (53 vs. 41 per cent), 5 years (50 vs. 36 per cent) and at 8 years (47 vs. 34 per cent).[39] The results from AML 10 disputed the concept that all children with AML were candidates for SCT and emphasised the constant requirement to reappraise the need for SCT in the face of improving chemotherapy. It was clear from AML 10 that more intensive chemotherapy had improved DFS to 56 per cent at 7 years, with substantially lower relapse rates than both its predecessor, AML 9, and the CCG study. Using a comparison of donor versus non-donor, AML 10 demonstrated that there was no overall survival benefit for first CR SCT in adults over 35 years of age or in children. This has been confirmed in AML 12, and in AML 15 a transplant will only be offered to patients under 15 years of age in the poor-risk category. However, even in this group SCT did not produce a survival advantage in either MRC 10 or MRC 12, but both MSD and matched unrelated donor (MUD) SCT are being pursued as SCT has the greatest antileukaemic effect, and attempts will be made to

Box 25.2 *Risk categories for acute myeloid leukaemia (AML)*

Good risk
Any patient with favourable genetic abnormalities, e.g. t(8;21), inv(16), t(15;17) including those molecularly detected, irrespective of marrow status after course 1 or the presence of other genetic abnormalities

Standard risk
Any patient not in good-risk or poor-risk groups, e.g. neither favourable nor adverse genetic abnormalities and not more than 15 per cent blasts in the bone marrow after course 1

Poor risk
Any patient with more than 15 per cent blasts in the bone marrow after course 1 or with adverse genetic abnormalities, e.g. −5, −7, del(5q), abn(3q), complex, and without favourable genetic abnormalities

reduce the toxicity associated with SCT. Conventional allografts will be brought forward to course 3, so reducing the amount of prior chemotherapy. This is particularly relevant as a recent International Bone Marrow Transplant Registry (IBMTR) analysis has shown that the result of a transplant was not improved by prior consolidation chemotherapy.[40] In adults but not in children at this stage, the concept of 'mini-allografting' (non-myeloablative, low-morbidity pretransplant regimen, usually fludarabine based[40a]) will be examined in MRC AML15. The use of peripheral blood rather than bone marrow has been suggested to be more effective,[41,42] although in the sibling setting this would involve administration of G-CSF to childhood donors and is unlikely to be pursued in the paediatric setting.

AML IN SECOND CR

The prognosis following relapse of AML is again dependent on the time to relapse. If relapse occurs within 1 year from diagnosis, the outlook is extremely poor (second remission rate 36 per cent, 3-year survival 11 per cent). Children relapsing after longer periods may be salvaged with further intensive chemotherapy with or without SCT if they achieve a remission (second remission rate 75 per cent, 3-year survival 49 per cent). For children who have not undergone SCT and do not have a sibling donor, reinduction (avoiding cardiotoxic agents), e.g. with FLAG (fludarabine, cytarabine, G-CSF), followed by autologous SCT (if late relapse) or UD or haploidentical SCT (if early relapse) in second CR is a worthwhile approach.[43] The role of Mylotarg (anti-CD33)[44] to achieve remission prior to SCT is being tested in refractory AML. The overall strategy for the treatment of relapsed AML is summarised in Table 25.3.

Myelodysplastic and myeloproliferative syndromes

MYELODYSPLASTIC SYNDROME

Myelodysplastic syndromes (MDS) in children/adolescents have eluded a generally agreed system of classification or diagnosis. In 1999/2000 some consensus was achieved and a recent proposal for the classification of paediatric myelodysplastic diseases distinguishes three main categories (see Box 25.3).[45] Juvenile myelomonocytic leukaemia (JMML) accounts for most patients in category I, but this remains a rare disorder, accounting for about 2 per cent of all childhood malignancies.[46,47] Diagnostic guidelines for JMML are given in Box 25.4.[48]

The initial course of JMML is varied, with approximately one-third of patients developing a rapidly progressive course leading to early death, while others remain stable without any treatment.[49] Although survival for 12 years after diagnosis without treatment has been described, the 10-year DFS is only 6 per cent and median survival time is approximately 10 months.[50,51] Treatment of JMML with chemotherapy has been unsuccessful, with

Box 25.3 *Diagnostic categories of myelodysplastic diseases*

I Myelodysplastic/myeloproliferative disease
1. Juvenile myelomonocytic leukaemia (JMML)
2. Chronic myelomonocytic leukaemia (CMML) (secondary only)
3. *BCR-ABL*-negative chronic myeloid leukaemia (Ph– CML)

II Down's syndrome (DS) disease
4. Transient abnormal myelopoiesis (TAM)
5. Myeloid leukaemia of DS

III Myelodysplastic syndrome (MDS)
6. Refractory cytopenia (RC) (PB blasts <2 per cent and BM blasts <5 per cent)
7. Refractory anaemia with excess blasts (RAEB) (PB blasts 2–19 per cent, or BM blasts 5–19 per cent)
8. RAEB in transformation (RAEB-T) (PB or BM blasts 20–29 per cent)

Box 25.4 *Criteria for the diagnosis of juvenile myelomonocytic leukaemia*

Mandatory
- Absence of the Philadelphia chromosome
- Blood monocytes $>1 \times 10^9$/L
- Bone marrow blasts <20 per cent

+two or more of:
- Raised Hb F for age
- White cell count $>10 \times 10^9$/L
- Peripheral immature myeloid cells
- Hypersensitivity of myeloid precursors to granulocyte monocyte colony-stimulating factor (GM-CSF)
- Bone marrow clonal abnormalities (e.g. -7).

In addition there may be:
- Hepatosplenomegaly (almost invariable)
- Skin rash (usually a facial butterfly rash)
- Lymphadenopathy
- Fever
- Pallor

Table 25.3 *Management of relapsed acute myeloid leukaemia (AML) in second complete remission*

Previous treatment	Management
No SCT	MSD SCT
	If not available consider UD/Haplo SCT if relapse <1 year from diagnosis
	Auto SCT if relapse >1 year from diagnosis (with CR1 marrow)
Autologous SCT	Consider UD/Haplo SCT if relapse >6 months since autologous SCT
MSD SCT	Donor T-cell infusion or second 'mini' SCT
	Second MSD SCT (myeloblative) if >12 months since first SCT

CR, complete remission; Haplo, haploidentical (parental) donor; MSD, matched sibling (or family) donor (including 5/6 HLA matches in certain cases); SCT, stem cell transplantation; UD, unrelated donor.

no sustained response to even high-dose chemotherapy protocols.[52,53] SCT has offered a chance of cure, but relapse rates and transplant-related mortality remain higher than with other haematological malignancies.[51,54–56] However, unlike most other paediatric leukaemias, JMML may be susceptible to the GvL effect, with lower relapse rates with reduced GvHD prophylaxis,[51] acute GvHD[54,55] and chronic GvHD.[57] There are a few reports of post-SCT relapse of JMML responding to withdrawal of immunosuppression,[55,57,58] but there has been only one successful report of the use of donor lymphocyte infusions (DLIs) in this setting, presumably due to rapid pace of disease.[56] Therefore the current approach to treatment of JMML is to use debulking chemotherapy with or without splenectomy for rapidly progressive disease followed by SCT, and to consider SCT up front for indolent disease.

Myeloid leukaemia of Down's syndrome responds well to AML-type chemotherapy, and these patients do not require SCT in first remission. The few patients who relapse should proceed to SCT in second CR, but Down's syndrome patients tolerate SCT poorly, with increased rates of transplant-related morbidity and mortality.[59]

There is controversy as to the best approach to paediatric MDS (category III). One approach is to treat these patients as for AML, proceeding to transplant only in those patients who relapse or make a poor response to initial chemotherapy.[60] This approach led to an OS of 51 per cent at 5 years, although those patients with refractory anaemia with excess blasts (RAEB) and those with monosomy 7 had a particularly poor prognosis in this patient study. Other groups proceed to SCT in all children with or without prior intensive chemotherapy.[61] Either approach may be reasonable, although it may be more advisable to consider early transplant in the presence of monosomy 7.

Patients with MDS occurring secondary to a constitutional (Fanconi) or acquired aplastic anaemia or secondary to chemotherapy require transplantation as the only curative option. Recent promising results were reported in a small group of children with secondary MDS.[62]

In all JMML/MDS patients undergoing SCT, an attempt should be made to exploit a GvL effect where possible, by early withdrawal of immunosuppression or introduction of DLI.

CML

Classical Ph+ CML is rare in childhood. Despite the recent remarkable successes reported with STI571 (imatninib),[63] the treatment of choice for both chronic-phase and accelerated-phase CML is a sibling allograft. This should be performed as soon as possible in accelerated phase and not more than 12 months from diagnosis of chronic phase. If there are no MSDs available then a full MUD should be sought and, if found, then SCT performed as above. If no matched donors are found on the registry then STI should be commenced ±interferon or ±Ara-C while the search is continued. If cytogenetic remission is achieved then the patient can be continued on STI. If only partial remission is achieved, transplantation with a mismatched volunteer donor, or indeed a haploidentical parental donor, should be considered.[64] If cytogenetic remission is achieved with STI, it remains uncertain how long remission will be sustained, although long-term cure is thought to be unlikely. Data from the UK BMT Registry show that survival rates after MSD SCT and MUD SCT are 66 and 60 per cent, respectively, but there are very few survivors after mismatched unrelated SCT.

PREPARATIVE REGIMENS AND THEIR TOXICITIES

The aim of the preparative regimen pre-transplant is to eradicate residual malignant cells and to provide sufficient immunosuppression to facilitate engraftment of donor stem cells. There is a fine line, however, between achieving these goals and increasing early mortality from over-intensification.[65] In children over the age of 2 years, the combination of cyclophosphamide with total body irradiation (Cy/TBI)[66] remains the most commonly used conditioning therapy for haematological malignancy. Later variations have concentrated on hyperfractionation of the TBI dose[67] with the aim of achieving equivalent disease eradication and immunosuppression with less toxicity, particularly less interstitial pneumonitis and fewer long-term sequelae. Leukaemic relapse still remains a problem, however, and other investigators have explored the substitution of different chemotherapeutic agents for cyclophosphamide (Table 25.4). High-dose cytarabine in combination with TBI[68] and melphalan (Melph)/TBI[69] have equivalent antileukaemic efficacy but are associated with considerable toxicity. Etoposide (VP-16)/TBI[70] has shown considerable promise in refractory leukaemias, and may be the most suitable alternative to Cy/TBI. More recently, fludarabine (Flu) has been added to Cy/TBI to permit the engraftment of profoundly T-cell-depleted haploidentical stem cell grafts.[18]

The use of radiation in children under the age of 2 years may result in severe neurological sequelae, and for this reason chemotherapy-only protocols are usually employed. Busulphan and cyclophosphamide (Bu/Cy),[71] first introduced for the treatment of AML, is now also the

Table 25.4 *Transplant preparative schedules and their toxicities*

Disease	Donor	Age (years)	Protocol	Agents	Doses	Toxicity
ALL >2 years CML (ap) CML (cp), AML	MSD, MUD MSD MUD	>2 >2 >2	Cy/TBI[a]	Cyclophosphamide	60 mg/kg × 2	Haemorrhagic cystitis, inappropriate ADH, cardiac failure
				TBI	1200/6[b] 1440/8[b]	Parotitis, erythema, mucositis, somnolence
ALL >2 years	MSD, MUD	>2	VP-16/TBI	VP-16	60 mg/kg	Mucositis, veno-occlusive disease, haemorrhagic cystitis
				TBI	1200/6[b] 1320/11[b]	As above
ALL AML MDS	MMUD Haplo	>2 >2	Flu/Cy/TBI[a]	Fludarabine Cyclophosphamide TBI	120 mg/m² 60 mg/kg × 2 1440/8[b]	Occasional neurotoxicity As above As above
ALL <2 years CML (cp) AML	MSD, MUD MSD MSD		Bu/Cy	Busulphan	16–20 mg/kg	Veno-occlusive disease, seizures, pulmonary fibrosis, skin changes
				Cyclophosphamide	50 mg/kg × 4	As above
AML, ALL JMML/MDS	Haplo	<2	Flu/Bu/Cy	Fludarabine Busulphan Cyclophosphamide	120 mg/m² 14 mg/kg 50 mg/kg × 4	As above As above As above
AML (cardiac dysfunction)	MSD	<2	Bu/Melph	Busulphan Melphalan	16–20 mg/kg 140 mg/kg	As above Mucositis, renal impairment
JMML/MDS AML	MFD/UD		Bu/Cy/Melph	Busulphan Cyclophosphamide Melphalan	16 mg/kg 120 mg/kg 140 mg/kg	As above As above As above
Poor organ function, second SCT	MFD/UD		Flu/Melph	Fludarabine Melphalan	150 mg/m² 140 mg/m²	As above As above

[a] Order reversed to TBI/Cy in some centres
[b] Fractions
ap, accelerated phase; cp, chronic phase.
ALL, acute lymphoblastic leukaemia; AML, acute myeloid leukaemia; CML, chronic myeloid leukaemia; Haplo, haploidentical; JMML, juvenile myelomonocytic leukaemia; MDS, myelodysplastic syndrome; MMUD, mismatched unrelated donor; MSD, matched sibling donor; MUD, matched unrelated donor; SCT, stem cell transplant.
Protocols – Bu, busulphan; Cy, cyclophosphamide; Flu, fludarabine; Melph, melphalan; TBI, total body irrigation; VP-16, etoposide.

most widely used pre-SCT chemotherapy in other paediatric malignancies as well as in non-malignant diseases. Busulphan exhibits different kinetics in children from those in adults, and a wider volume of distribution and more rapid drug excretion results in relatively lower plasma levels of busulphan in children.[72] This may also predispose to graft rejection and, theoretically, disease relapse. Many paediatric centres consequently increase the dose of busulphan from 16 to 20 mg/kg, and even 24 mg/kg in children under the age of 3 years. Not surprisingly, this also tends to increase the incidence of side-effects, particularly hepatic veno-occlusive disease (VOD). There is also considerable interpatient variation in the busulphan levels achieved at

equivalent doses, and in critical patients, or where high doses are given, monitoring busulphan levels may be helpful (Figure 25.1). The addition of fludarabine or melphalan is occasionally used to intensify Bu/Cy; Flu/Bu/Cy has been used in young children <2 years with haemophagocytic lymphohistiocytosis (HLH) and leukaemia undergoing haploidentical SCT. Bu/Cy/Melph is now widely used in children with JMML and other paediatric myelodysplasias.[51] Radiotherapy is no longer recommended for conditioning in JMML[56] Melphalan can also be used in combination with busulphan (Bu/Melph) in order to reduce the additional cardiotoxicity of cyclophosphamide when significant cardiac dysfunction

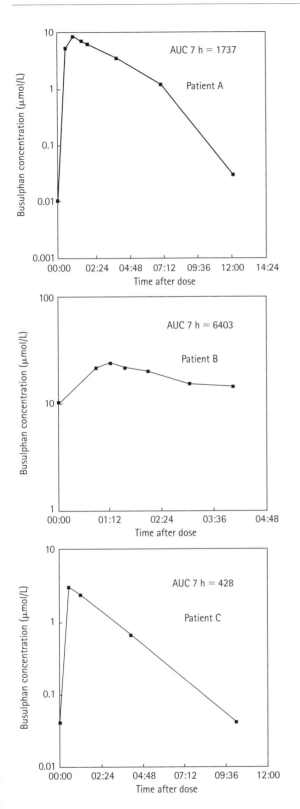

Figure 25.1 *Busulphan levels in three children receiving 16 mg/kg total dose in preparation for stem cell transplantation. Samples taken around first dose of 2 mg/kg. Exposure to the drug has been calculated from the area under the curve (AUC). Patient A engrafted successfully, patient B died of fulminating VOD, and patient C rejected the graft.*

exists pre-SCT. This latter combination is also becoming popular for autologous PBPCT in solid tumours such as neuroblastoma. The combination of fludarabine and melphalan is being examined as a reduced-intensity conditioning (RIC) regimen to facilitate SCT in children with genetic diseases with significant co-morbidities at the time of transplant.[9] A similar approach could be taken for children with malignant disease unable to tolerate conventional ablative preparation as long as a GvL process might be expected. RIC may be particularly useful to reduce toxicity in any child undergoing a second SCT procedure within a year of the first SCT. Typically, with the use of unrelated or haploidentical donors, serotherapy in the form of Campath 1H or antithymocyte globulin (ATG) is given with the chemoradiotherapy schedule to enhance removal of recipient T cells, so reducing rejection while also exerting a degree of *in vivo* T-cell depletion to reduce GvHD.

The choice of TBI versus non-TBI protocols in older children is not resolved. The incidence of certain early toxicities, such as idiopathic interstitial pneumonitis, may be lower with non-TBI-containing preparations, although other complications such as VOD are more common with Bu/Cy regimens. Initial indications that longer-term complications, including growth, endocrine, and neuropsychometric problems, would be fewer with Bu/Cy are not apparent as yet. While chemotherapeutic regimens may be equivalent to TBI-containing protocols in terms of disease eradication, in certain instances, e.g. ALL, the use of TBI remains preferable.[73] For myeloid diseases such as AML and JMML/MDS, non-TBI regimens are now favoured.[51] Recommended conditioning for a MSD SCT for chronic phase CML is Bu/Cy, and for a sibling transplant in accelerated phase Cy/TBI. Children undergoing UD transplantation should receive Cy/TBI and Campath 1H pre-infusion, and patients in blast crisis should receive appropriate chemotherapy to achieve chronic phase and then proceed to transplant as above. TBI is more immunosuppressive and appears to facilitate better engraftment of heavily T-cell-depleted mismatched SCTs (see Table 25.4).

STEM CELL HARVESTING AND ENGRAFTMENT

Stem cell harvest

In the autologous setting, it is usual practice to transplant at least 1×10^8 nucleated cells per kg of the recipient's weight to ensure engraftment, and $2–5 \times 10^8$/kg nucleated cells in matched sibling and unrelated donor transplants, respectively. Around $3–4 \times 10^7$/kg nucleated cells are required to secure engraftment in UCB transplantation

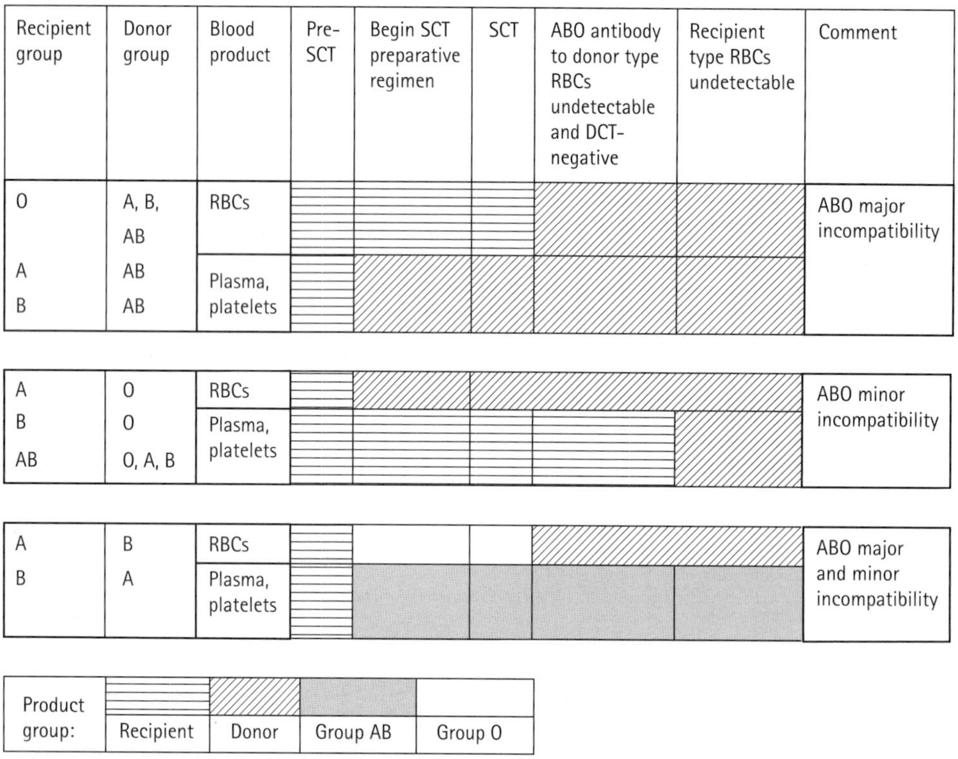

Recipient group	Donor group	Blood product	Pre-SCT	Begin SCT preparative regimen	SCT	ABO antibody to donor type RBCs undetectable and DCT-negative	Recipient type RBCs undetectable	Comment
O	A, B, AB	RBCs						ABO major incompatibility
A	AB	Plasma, platelets						
B	AB							
A	O	RBCs						ABO minor incompatibility
B	O	Plasma, platelets						
AB	O, A, B							
A	B	RBCs						ABO major and minor incompatibility
B	A	Plasma, platelets						

Product group:	Recipient	Donor	Group AB	Group O

Figure 25.2 *Blood product support throughout transplant. DCT, direct Coombs test; RBCs, red blood cells; SCT, stem cell transplant.*

(i.e. × 1 log less than bone marrow). Transplantation of sufficient numbers of primitive self-replicating progenitor cells, characterized by the phenotype CD34+, HLA DR–, lineage-, is crucial to successful long-term marrow reconstitution; these constitute only about 5 per cent of all CD34+ cells. Clinical experience has shown that engraftment can readily be achieved with $1–2 \times 10^6$ CD34+ cells/kg recipient weight, implying that $10^4–10^5$ primitive 'stem' cells/kg are required. In the heavily T-cell-depleted haploidentical setting, $\geq 10 \times 10^6$ CD34 cells/kg secure rapid engraftment.

Concern is frequently expressed about harvesting small donors for larger recipients, but in fact, because of the increased cellularity of paediatric marrow, harvesting 20–25 per cent of the blood volume of a 6-month-old child with small 3–5 mL harvests can usually provide sufficient nucleated cells for an adult recipient. Adequate blood replacement for the donor is essential in such harvests, and this can be provided by pre-harvest deposit or irradiated, genotyped, leucocyte-depleted, CMV-negative allogeneic blood.

Marrow reinfusion and blood product support

Transplantation across ABO barriers requires careful consideration. If there is major incompatibility between recipient and donor (e.g. group O recipient of group A red cells), then removal of red cells from the donor marrow will suffice and plasmapheresis of the recipient is not generally required in the paediatric setting. Minor ABO incompatibility (e.g. group A recipient of group O red cells) requires removal of plasma from the donation. Following infusion of the marrow, transfusion of appropriate group red cells, platelets and fresh frozen plasma is determined by the multiple considerations of the blood groups and red cell antibodies in both recipient and donor, which will change with progress through the transplant procedure (a summary of current recommendations is shown in Figure 25.2). Cellular blood products, i.e. red cells and platelets, should be of the correct CMV status and irradiated with 2500 cGy. Red cells should be transfused if the haemoglobin falls below 8 g/dL, or at higher levels if the child is symptomatic. The specific volume to be given should be calculated in millilitres from the desired rise in haemoglobin × the patient's weight (kg) × 4. Prophylactic platelets should be administered if the count falls below 10×10^9/L; if there are petechiae, bruising, bleeding or fever, a higher cut-off of 30×10^9/L should be used. The dosage of platelets required is 10 mL/kg. For children with documented refractoriness to random platelets (poor 1-hour and 24-hour increments, i.e. failure to rise above 50 and trough level <10), HLA-matched platelets may be required. In anticipation of this event, children undergoing autologous transplantation should have their HLA-A, B status determined before the transplant procedure.

Table 25.5 *Factors determining engraftment*

	Best	Moderate	Worst
Histocompatibility	Twin	Sib/MFD/MUD	MMUD/Haplo
Recipient	No transfusion	<40 units	>40 units
	TBI	Bu/Cy	Cy alone
	Immunodeficient	Leukaemia, haemoglobinopathy	Bone marrow failure
	High CD34 count	$1–2 \times 10^6$ CD34	$<10^6$ CD34
	PBSC	BM	Cord blood
		Undepleted marrow	T-depleted marrow

BM, bone marrow; Bu, busulphan; Cy, cyclophosphamide; Haplo, haploidentical; MFD, matched family donor ; MMUD, mismatched unrelated donor; MUD, matched unrelated donor; PBSC, peripheral blood stem cell; TBI, total body irradiation.

Colony-stimulating factors

The use of G-CSF or granulocyte monocyte colony-stimulating factor (GM-CSF) accelerates neutrophil recovery following autologous progenitor cell transplantation. Their benefit following allogeneic SCT is less conclusive, probably due to the myelosuppressive effects of cyclosporin and methotrexate employed for GvHD prophylaxis. However, many centres utilize G-CSF from 6 to 8 days post-stem cell infusion until neutrophil engraftment is secured. There does appear to be a more definite role for G-CSF in patients experiencing delayed or inadequate neutrophil engraftment following transplantation.[74] Recent studies showed delayed immune reconstitution following G-CSF, and therefore the role of G-CSF in haploidentical transplants needed to be reviewed.[75]

Graft rejection

Graft rejection after SCT may be manifested as either lack of initial engraftment suggested by a neutrophil count <0.5 continuing beyond day 28, often with the re-emergence of host T cells, or the development of pancytopenia and marrow aplasia after initial engraftment (reviewed by Wolff[76]). With HLA-genotypically identical SCT, the risk of graft rejection is less than 1 per cent, with a 2 per cent risk of secondary graft failure. With unrelated or non-HLA-identical related donors, the risk of rejection rises to 3–20 per cent, and in these situations it may be wise to save cryopreserved autologous marrow as a back-up. Other factors that increase the risk of rejection include less immunosuppressive regimens pre- (e.g. no TBI) and post-transplant (e.g. no cyclosporin), and T-cell depletion of the marrow. Reduced immunosuppression allows the survival of larger numbers of host lymphocytes, while the presence of T cells in the donor marrow helps to eliminate or inactivate these residual host cells. Graft failure occurs in approximately 10 per cent of patients when T cells are removed to prevent GvHD in HLA-identical recipients.[77] Factors determining the likelihood of successful engraftment are listed in Table 25.5.

COMPLICATIONS AFTER SCT

Complications occurring within the first 100 days of transplantation are referred to as 'early' complications. Collectively they contribute to substantial morbidity and an early mortality rate ranging from 5 per cent in autologous transplantation up to 20 per cent in complex allogeneic procedures.[23] Complications fall into three main categories: regimen-related toxicity, infectious complications and GvHD.

Regimen-related toxicity

Most children suffer significant nausea and vomiting, which can usually be controlled by antiemetic combinations (e.g. $5-HT_3$ antagonist and dexamethasone). Mucositis is also predictable and particularly problematic following TBI, melphalan and VP-16. Mucosal damage may also be exacerbated by the use of methotrexate for GvHD prophylaxis, although this can be offset to some extent by the use of folinic acid 12–24 hours after each dose of methotrexate.[78] Management of mucositis involves adequate pain relief, preferably with patient-controlled analgesia (PCA), the early institution of parenteral nutrition and appropriate treatment of superadded infection, especially with herpes simplex virus or *Candida*.

VENO-OCCLUSIVE DISEASE

Hepatic veno-occlusive disease (VOD) occurs in 5–20 per cent of paediatric transplants and is a consequence of endothelial injury leading to terminal venular occlusion and hepatocyte necrosis. The clinical features are diagnostic in 90 per cent of cases and include jaundice, unexplained weight gain, painful hepatomegaly and ascites;[79] there may be associated renal failure and refractory thrombocytopenia. Additional information may be gained non-invasively by Doppler ultrasound, which may reveal altered hepatic artery indices or, in more severe cases, reversal of hepatoportal blood flow, but the findings are inconsistent, and clinical features are more important. Liver biopsy can provide confirmation in atypical cases, but percutaneous biopsy is hazardous and transvenous biopsy is advisable if expertise is locally available.

Predisposing factors for VOD include higher doses of busulphan in the preparative regimen (>16 mg/kg), pre-transplant biochemical hepatitis and allogeneic transplantation. If sufficient risk factors are present, prophylactic ursodeoxycholic acid[80] or defibrotide[81] may be warranted. Recent studies[82] suggest that prophylaxis with low-dose heparin (1000 units/kg/day) does not appear to be reduce VOD, and although prostaglandin E_1 may reduce the incidence of VOD, it has unacceptable toxicity.[83] Treatment is usually supportive, with reduced sodium intake, fluid restriction, frusemide $\pm$ low-dose dopamine and an aldosterone antagonist, e.g. spironolactone, accompanied by salt-poor albumin infusions to maintain intravascular volume. Occasionally, careful paracentesis is required to improve patient comfort and maintain adequate respiratory function. Resolution has been achieved in severe cases with the fibrinolytic agent tissue plasminogen activator (tPA),[84] but such therapy can induce catastrophic bleeding. Defibrotide may be more efficacious and is associated with few side-effects. Antithrombin III has been shown to be useful in occasional patients, but there are no data from randomized prospective studies.[85] The prognosis of VOD is very variable, ranging from complete recovery to fulminant hepatic failure and death. Peak bilirubin concentrations >215 μmol/L and ALT levels >394 U/L are associated with a 60 per cent mortality, whereas peak bilirubin concentrations <105 μmol/L and ALT <286 U/L usually indicate less aggressive disease.[86] Early-onset VOD has a worse prognosis.

HAEMORRHAGIC CYSTITIS

Haemorrhagic cystitis that occurs during or shortly after the preparative therapy is a recognized complication of high-dose cyclophosphamide, and is caused by urothelial damage from contact with acrolein, a metabolite of the parent drug. The haematuria may vary from microscopic to life-threatening haemorrhage. Treatment is unsatisfactory and preventive measures are paramount. Bladder irrigation and/or massive hyperhydration are not practical solutions in children, and a combination of moderate hyperhydration ($\times 2$ maintenance) with mesna infusion (which forms an inactive complex with acrolein) may be preferable. Diuretics may be required to maintain a high urinary flow, and frequent voiding should be encouraged. Other drugs, including busulphan and etoposide, may be implicated in haemorrhagic cystitis, and in late-onset haematuria a viral aetiology, e.g. CMV, adenovirus or BK virus, or even GvHD may be instrumental. Onset of haemorrhagic cystitis during cyclophosphamide infusion should be treated by further increasing fluids and mesna,

including irrigation if resolution does not occur. At a later stage, treatment options in order of priority include:

- continuing hydration
- bladder irrigation (through suprapubic catheter if required)
- intravesical alum infusion[87]
- intravesical prostaglandins[88]
- formalin[89] (which results in a small fibrotic bladder) and cystectomy as last resorts.

More recently, oestrogen has been used with some success.[90]

PULMONARY OEDEMA

Pulmonary oedema is not uncommon in the early stages after SCT, due to the large amount of fluid required to deliver the appropriate drugs and nutrition; it is exacerbated in the presence of hypoalbuminaemia. The presence of basal crepitations, in keeping with other features of fluid overload, is suggestive; appropriate treatment includes frusemide $\pm$ albumin infusions.

IDIOPATHIC PNEUMONIA SYNDROME

Idiopathic pneumonia syndrome (IPS) is used to define acute lung injury post-SCT for which no infectious agent can be found. It typically occurs around 50 days and before 100 days post-SCT (see Figure 25.3). Chest X-ray and computed tomography (CT) typically show diffuse airspace and/or interstitial infiltrates. The aetiology is thought to be multifactorial, including chemoradiotherapeutic insults and GvHD. Because the lung is typically not a target organ in acute GvHD, another inciting factor is believed to be important for the development of lung injury. Some studies suggest that this factor may be a latent viral infection, e.g. CMV or HHV6.[91,92] Potential risk factors for IPS are higher dose and dose rate of TBI, older age, HLA disparity and GvHD. There is no specific treatment, although steroids may be useful in some cases. Overall mortality of patients with this syndrome is high (50–70 per cent), with most dying from progressive/recurrent respiratory failure or from infection. The presence of hepatic failure and the need for ventilatory support are associated with poor outcome.

DIFFUSE ALVEOLAR HAEMORRHAGE

Diffuse alveolar haemorrhage (DAH) refers to the diffuse alveolar damage with alveolar erythrocytes in the context of thrombocytopenia. DAH occurs mostly during the first weeks after SCT, often at the time of granulocyte recovery, and is uncommon after 2 months. Clinical presentation includes a sudden onset of dyspnoea, cough, fever and hypoxia with or without a drop in the haemoglobin level in blood. Haemoptysis is rare. X-rays show

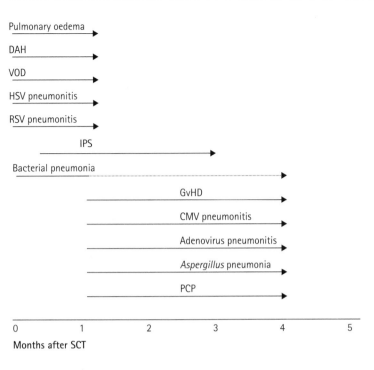

Figure 25.3 *Approximate time of onset of respiratory disorders in the first 4 months after stem cell transplant (SCT). CMV, cytomegalovirus; DAH, diffuse alveolar haemorrhage; GvHD, graft-versus-host disease; HSV, herpes simplex virus; IPS, idiopathic pneumonia syndrome; PCP, pneumocystis carinii pneumonia; RSV, respiratory syncytial virus; VOD, veno-occlusive disease. Dotted arrow, risk of bacterial pneumonia continues due to impaired synthesis of immunoglobulins.*

a normal heart with basilar patchy alveolar opacifications. Bronchoalveolar lavage (BAL) demonstrates a blood alveolar fluid without evidence of airway bleeding, with haemosiderin-loaded macrophages on microscopic examination. DAH has been shown to be associated with older patient age, malignancy, severe oral mucositis, renal insufficiency, TBI and grade II or more acute GvHD. Supportive treatment attempts to correct thrombocytopenia, while the use of steroids remains a controversial issue. Mortality ranges from 15 to 80 per cent. One must keep in mind that DAH may also be an accompanying syndrome during the course of pneumonia of other origin, including IPS and infection.

THROMBOTIC MICROANGIOPATHY/HAEMOLYTIC URAEMIC SYNDROME

Thrombotic microangiopathy (TMA) is biologically defined by the association of microangiopathic haemolytic anaemia,[93] which is characterized by the presence of ≥1.2 per cent fragmented red cells and elevated lactate dehydrogenase (LDH) and thrombocytopenia. Renal insufficiency is the rule. Patients may suffer from various degrees of hypertension, neurological disturbances and oedema.

The incidence is around 5–15 per cent in retrospective adult studies, and possibly lower in the paediatric setting. TMA may occur as early as 4 days post-SCT and as late as 30 months, but mostly within 2 months. Although risk factors for TMA for any individual patient are not well defined, TBI, cyclosporin A and GvHD play an important role in its pathogenesis, probably through diffuse endothelial damage. TMA ranges in severity from a self-limiting to a fatal disorder. Treatment involves discontinuation of cyclosporin A, supportive care with transfusions and anti-hypertensive drugs. There may be a role for apheresis in the treatment of severe disease. Overall, TMA-associated mortality has been reported to be around 30 per cent (0–87 per cent). Survivors may suffer from progressive renal impairment.

Infections following transplantation

Children undergoing SCT are particularly prone to infectious complications due to the combined myelosuppression of aggressive chemoradiotherapy and the immunosuppressive effects of pre-transplant therapy, and, in the allogeneic setting, subsequent GvHD, its prophylaxis and treatment. The spectrum of infections is determined by the pattern of haematological and immunological recovery following SCT, and can be divided into those occurring in the neutropenic period, those occurring following engraftment and throughout the first 100 days, and late infections.

NEUTROPENIC PERIOD

Infections during the neutropenic period (day 0 to days 12–21) are largely bacterial and fungal, and are described in Chapter 30. Viral infections may cause morbidity during the neutropenic period. These may be mild, including oropharyngeal mucositis due to reactivation of herpes simplex virus, rotavirus gastroenteritis, and upper respiratory tract infection due to respiratory syncytial virus (RSV), although RSV can lead to a fulminant pneumonitis (see below). The exception is adenovirus, which may cause severe infection, usually in the post-engraftment period, manifesting with bloody diarrhoea, pneumonitis, hepatitis and marrow suppression. Methods used as prophylaxis against infection during this period vary greatly between transplant units; benefit is probably afforded by strict handwashing by all visitors and staff, the use of chlorhexidine mouthwashes, the use of imidazole antifungal agents,[94] and HEPA (to reduce *Aspergillus* infection). However, the role of laminar air flow cubicles, strict reverse barrier nursing, sterile diets and oral gut decontamination, and surveillance cultures remains largely unproven.[95]

Respiratory Syncytial Virus

Respiratory syncytial virus (RSV) is a common cause of respiratory tract infections in infants and children. Although RSV may be confined to upper respiratory tracts in SCT, it not infrequently leads to a devastating primary viral pneumonia. The true incidence of RSV pneumonia in SCT is unknown, although figures as high as 11 per cent have been suggested.[96] RSV pneumonia is most common in the very early period after transplantation during the pre-engraftment period (see Figure 25.3). In most cases, pneumonia occurs in the spring and winter months and is usually preceded by the symptoms and signs of rhinitis. Chest X-ray initially shows diffuse infiltrates, and progression to diffuse air space disease is common. Despite antiviral therapy, RSV pneumonia is associated with a high mortality rate of around 50 per cent.[97] A diagnosis of RSV is usually made by detection of RSV antigens within infected cells from a nasopharyngeal aspirate (NPA) or from BAL fluid using fluorescent monoclonal antibodies. In view of the high mortality rate, therapy should be started as soon as RSV is isolated from the upper respiratory tract during the transplant course. Appropriate therapy consists of nebulized ± intravenous ribavirin and RSV-specific hyperimmune globulin/intravenous immunoglobulin.[98,99] Better still, if RSV can be detected prior to SCT in an NPA, it is prudent to defer the procedure if at all possible. RSV is highly contagious and may spread rapidly throughout the transplant unit. Aggressive policies for prevention of nosocomial infection is paramount and may reduce the incidence of RSV disease during outbreaks in transplant centres.

Candida

Although *Candida* is a common pathogen in the immediate post-transplant period, and invasive infection (either fungaemia or visceral organ involvement) occurs in 11–16 per cent of patients, candidal pneumonia is rare, occurring in only 1 per cent of patients.[100] Candidal pneumonia may result from haematogenous dissemination or from aspiration from the oral pharynx. Most SCT patients would routinely receive fungal prophylaxis with itraconazole/fluconazole and therapy for breakthrough candidaemia is usually with AmBisome 3–5 mg/kg ± flucytosine in refractory patients.

POST-ENGRAFTMENT PERIOD

During the period after engraftment (usually days 30–100), cell-mediated and humoral immunity continue to be depressed. The total number of lymphocytes usually normalizes after 2 months, but T-cell subsets, and T-cell function, may take considerably longer. Normal immunoglobulin levels are frequently not achieved until 1 year after transplantation. The presence of ongoing GvHD delays these processes further.

Cytomegalovirus

Infection with CMV used to account for approximately 40 per cent of all pneumonias occurring after SCT.[101] A large series reported incidence rates ranging from 10–20 per cent in allogeneic SCT and 1–4 per cent in recipients of autologous transplants.[102] Acquisition of CMV may be via primary infection from donor cells or blood products in a previously seronegative patient, reactivation of endogenous virus, or reinfection with a different strain of CMV in a previously seropositive patient. With the introduction of CMV-negative and/or filtered blood products, the most likely source in practice is reactivation of endogenous virus, from either a seropositive recipient or a donor. A combination of reduced prevalence of CMV in children and their childhood donors and better recent prophylaxis for CMV during the at-risk period has reduced the incidence of CMV pneumonitis in the paediatric SCT setting. Most cases of CMV pneumonia occur after marrow engraftment during the first 100 days of transplantation, and almost all within 180 days[103] (see Figure 25.3). With the more recent successful prophylaxis of CMV during the early post-SCT period, there has been a resurgence of late CMV infection occurring beyond the first 100 days.[104] CMV pneumonia is very uncommon prior to marrow engraftment. In the setting of a seropositive child or donor, additional risk factors for occurrence of CMV reactivation/disease include higher pre-transplant total doses of TBI and chemotherapy, presence and severity of acute GvHD and the use of intensive T-cell depletion strategies.[105]

Clinical manifestations of CMV pneumonia are not specific and include non-productive cough, fever, progressive dyspnoea and hypoxaemia. Chest X-ray typically shows diffuse interstitial alveolar infiltrates, and numerous small nodules may be evident on CT.[106]

CMV pneumonia is usually diagnosed by detection of virus in BAL fluid. Monoclonal antibodies can rapidly detect the presence of CMV antigen within infected cells, and typical CMV inclusions may be evident on histological examination. Recently DNA amplification methods using PCR has been shown to be a very sensitive method for detecting CMV.[107] CMV may be isolated from the lower respiratory tract of both immunocompetent and immunocompromised children in the absence of pneumonia, and hence detection of virus in respiratory samples does not necessarily establish a diagnosis of CMV pneumonia. Nevertheless, CMV must always be considered a pathogen in patients undergoing SCT, and CMV in pneumonia should be diagnosed in any patient with suspicious clinical findings.

The best therapeutic regimen consists of combination therapy with intravenous ganciclovir and immune globulin (either CMV-specific or pooled). However, although this approach has been shown to decrease mortality significantly, response rates may be as low as 35 per cent and mortality rates in patients requiring mechanical ventilation continue to approach 100 per cent.[108] Consequently, approaches designed to prevent CMV pneumonia are essential in the management of patients undergoing SCT. In seronegative patients, the best approach is to transplant stem cells and transfuse blood products from seronegative donors.[109] Leucodepleted products may be used in an emergency if no CMV-negative blood products are available. In seropositive patients and seronegative patients who received a transplant from a seropositive donor, prophylactic administration of immunoglobulin and high-dose acyclovir therapy[110] comprises the most widely used regimen in paediatrics at the present time. In patients at risk of CMV infection, the viral load is monitored weekly with PCR methods and a rising titre is treated promptly with ganciclovir.[111] If therapy with ganciclovir is not successful in reducing the viral load, or indeed causes excess myelosuppression, it may be substituted for foscarnet; a combination of 50 per cent of both drugs is currently being assessed.

Further studies are also underway to assess the efficacy of CMV-specific cytotoxic T cells which have been generated *in vivo* using donor T cells. At the present time it seems most appropriate to use such technology in patients in whom CMV loads are rising despite therapy with ganciclovir or foscarnet.

Adenoviruses

Members of this virus group are common causes of respiratory and gastrointestinal illnesses in children. Reactivation of latent virus or primary infection has now been widely described after SCT, during both the neutropenic and post-engraftment periods. Serotypes belonging to subgroups B and C are most commonly isolated. Incidental detection in the stool of an asymptomatic patient is becoming increasingly common with institution of specific screening. In some patients undergoing SCT, gastrointestinal infection may lead to severe diarrhoea, which must be rapidly differentiated from gastrointestinal GvHD as steroid therapy may exacerbate adenoviral infection. Some of these children will go on to develop

disseminated adenoviral infection, which may be suspected by the detection of adenovirus in the peripheral blood using PCR techniques. Within a variable period extending from days to several weeks, some of these children will develop rapidly fatal forms of hepatitis often accompanied by pneumonitis.[112] Progression from asymptomatic excretion to fulminant fatal infection is exacerbated by profound T-cell depletion of the graft and ongoing immunosuppressive therapy, particularly with high doses of steroids. This is therefore most frequently seen in the setting of mismatched SCT, particularly haplotype mismatched transplants.

There are currently two antiviral drugs that show some promise in the setting of adenoviral infection, namely ribavirin and cidofovir. However, both of these drugs are only virustatic and neither therapy is effective in fulminant disease, but may be useful in the early stages of disseminated infection when PCR for adenovirus first becomes positive in the peripheral blood. Reduction of immunosuppression is crucial and may be sufficient to eliminate the virus if lymphocytes increase to $>0.3 \times 10^9$/L. However, following profound T-cell depletion of the graft, some form of T-cell add-back may be required to eliminate disseminated virus.

Aspergillus

Aspergillus spores are ubiquitous and, because of their small size, are commonly inhaled and reach the alveoli. Most SCT units in the UK are HEPA-filtered and are generally free of spores, but patients may be harbouring *Aspergillus* spores on entry to the unit. Under normal circumstances, spores are eradicated by alveolar macrophages, and if fungal hyphae are formed, neutrophils enter the lungs and destroy them. Major risk factors for invasive pulmonary aspergillosis (IPA) therefore include steroid therapy, which impairs alveolar macrophage function, and prolonged neutropenia, both of which are frequent occurrences in patients undergoing SCT. In the absence of neutrophils, *Aspergillus* hyphae proliferate and invade the pulmonary parenchyma, invading local blood vessels and resulting in thrombosis and haemorrhagic infarction of lung tissue, and distant spread of the disease.[113] In previous studies, the incidence of aspergillosis was estimated at around 4 per cent of patients undergoing SCT, and the most common causes were *Aspergillus fumigatus* and *Aspergillus flavus*.[114] Infection usually becomes evident in the post-engraftment period and is almost always associated with prolonged neutropenia and the use of steroids to treat GvHD.

Clinical symptoms may be non-specific but the presence of pleuritic chest pain, haemoptysis and/or pleural rub should raise suspicion. There may be evidence of disseminated infection, including meningitis, sinusitis or a space-occupying cerebral lesion. Chest X-ray typically shows solitary or multiple pulmonary nodules or mass-like infiltrates (mycotic lung sequestrum), and cavitation, which is frequently present in the adult population, may also be seen in the paediatric population, although less frequently. CT often reveals frank disease not evident on chest X-ray and may demonstrate the presence of a rim of ground glass attenuation surrounding a parenchymal nodule (halo sign).

The definitive diagnosis of IPA can only be made when histological specimens show characteristic hyphae involving lung tissue. *Aspergillus* is present in less than half of sputum cultures, although culture and staining of BAL fluid may offer a significantly higher yield. Consequently, appropriate therapy should begin with the presence of a strong clinical suspicion of IPA, as all cultures, including percutaneous needle biopsy, may be negative for *Aspergillus*. The use of *Aspergillus* PCR and galactomannan assays in predicting the presence of early *Aspergillus* infection is presently under investigation.

In terms of treatment for IPA, the best current approach includes high-dose liposomal amphotericin (e.g. AmBisome 5–10 mg/kg/day), usually given in conjunction with voriconazole/caspofungin. In the presence of localized lesions and for worsening haemoptysis, surgical resection with lobectomy or even pneumonectomy has been attempted. However, once established, the prognosis for IPA remains dismal. Consequently, prevention rather than therapy of IPA must be the goal. Within paediatric practice in the UK, there is a consensus approach which includes the use of oral itraconazole solution 5 mg/kg/day from 2 weeks prior to SCT until neutrophil recovery is well established. During the SCT procedure, the presence of a fever unresponsive to 96 hours of broad-spectrum antibiotics should be treated empirically with AmBisome 1–3 mg/kg. CT may be used at this point to determine escalation or de-escalation of antifungal therapy. If *Aspergillus* PCR proves to be a reliable marker, this may allow the earlier institution of higher doses of liposomal amphotericin in patients with early infection.

Other Fungi

Trichosporon fusarium and *Zygomycetes* organisms are occasionally seen in patients undergoing SCT. As with other fungal infections, major risk factors include prolonged neutropenia and steroid therapy.

LATE INFECTIONS

In the absence of continuing GvHD, late infections occurring beyond day 100 are usually caused by encapsulated organisms, including *Streptococcus pneumoniae* and *Haemophilus influenzae*. IgG2 is the predominant antibody that is directed against encapsulated organisms, and it may be deficient for up to 2 years after transplant. This has led to the widespread practice of commencing penicillin prophylaxis from the time of stopping trimethoprim-sulfamethoxazole (TMP-SMX) up until 2 years from transplant or even for life. Up to 50 per cent of transplant patients will develop varicella zoster virus infections in the

first year following transplant. Most infections are mild and respond to treatment with acyclovir. Continuing prophylaxis with acyclovir beyond the period indicated for CMV prophylaxis (up to 3–6 months) is therefore not warranted.

Both regimen-related toxicity and infections post-SCT contribute to a significant number of respiratory complications, which can occur in up to 50 per cent of patients and account for over 40 per cent of all deaths;[115,116] those patients who require admission to intensive care and needing intubation and mechanical ventilation have a particularly poor prognosis,[115,117,118] with less than 10 per cent becoming long-term survivors.

The range of potential differential diagnoses is given in Figure 25.3, while Figure 25.4 summarizes the key points for clinical management of respiratory problems post-SCT.[119]

Graft–versus–host disease

AETIOLOGY

The initiation of GvHD is through the recognition by donor T lymphocytes of major HLA class I or II antigen mismatches in the host, or of minor histocompatibility antigen differences in the case of MSDs. In addition to donor recipient mismatching, immune imbalance during recovery of immunity may also play a role in GvHD, as illustrated by an imbalance in T-cell subset recovery following administration of cyclosporin A.[71] The afferent pathway of GvHD is amplified by interleukin-2 (IL-2) production by T-helper lymphocytes acting on effector cells, which may be T4, T8 and/or natural killer (NK) lymphocyte subsets. The contribution of cytotoxic lymphocytes, macrophages and cytokines (e.g. tumour necrosis factor, TNF) in mediating damage during the efferent phase of GvHD remains unknown. Target cells for GvHD include proliferating cells of the skin, gut and liver ducts, as well as bone marrow and the lymphoid system. Proliferating cells susceptible to GvHD may also express HLA DR antigens, which may be upregulated by viral and bacterial infections. This may explain the close relationship between adenoviral and CMV infection on the one hand, and exacerbation of GvHD on the other.[120]

RISK FACTORS AND PROPHYLAXIS

While there remains a considerable degree of unpredictability in the occurrence of GvHD, there are many recognized risk factors, including:

- HLA disparity between donor and recipient
- minor MHC antigen differences, e.g. Y chromosome in male recipients of parous female marrow[121]
- intensity of the pre-transplant treatment[121]
- increasing donor and recipient age
- viral infection after transplant.[122]

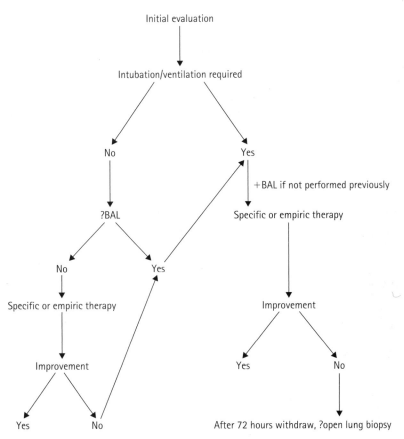

Initial evaluation

Intubation/ventilation required

No — Yes

+BAL if not performed previously

?BAL — Specific or empiric therapy

No — Yes

Specific or empiric therapy — Improvement

Improvement

Yes — No

Yes — No

After 72 hours withdraw, ?open lung biopsy

Figure 25.4 *Key points for clinical management of respiratory disease following stem cell transplant (SCT). BAL, bronchoalveolar lavage.*

Among recipients of UCB transplants, there was no acute GvHD (aGvHD) of severity greater than grade I in recipients who were HLA-matched or -mismatched for one or two antigens.[123] Depending on all these factors, the risk of GvHD can vary from 15 to 70 per cent.[124] There are some guidelines to the appropriate selection of prophylaxis against GvHD: identical twin transplants require no GvHD prophylaxis; CYA and short-course methotrexate is adequate in standard-risk MSD transplants in children under 16 years of age;[125] while *in vivo* T-cell depletion with Campath 1H or ATG is usually required with UD transplants. For haplotype mismatched (parental) transplants, profound 4–5 log T-cell depletion is required; this is now readily achieved by CD34 selection techniques (e.g. CliniMACS), which usually ensure that no more than 1×10^5 CD3-positive cells/kg are returned with the graft. In the absence of chronic GvHD (cGvHD), prophylactic immunosuppression can be discontinued at about 3–6 months after SCT without complications, indicating either that the originally infused T cells, which recognize host alloantigens, have a limited life span, or that regulatory mechanisms develop to prevent the T cells from causing immune damage. T cells that develop in the host thymus after SCT do not cause GvHD because of induction of anergy and negative selection mediated by host thymic epithelial cells. A GvL effect may, to some extent, parallel GvHD, and complete abolition of GvHD may therefore not be desirable.[126,127]

ACUTE GRAFT-VERSUS-HOST DISEASE

Acute graft-versus-host disease classically occurs in the first 100 days following transplant and varies in degree of seriousness from a mild self-limiting condition requiring no treatment to a severe and fatal disorder. The three organs commonly involved in aGvHD are skin, gut and liver. The first manifestation is of a rash involving the extensor surface of the limbs, face (including ears), neck, palms and soles. The more severe rashes become confluent, spreading to most of the body surface, and subsequent epidermolysis with the formation of bullae may occur. If gut GvHD occurs, it usually follows skin GvHD and manifests with diarrhoea accompanied by anorexia, nausea, vomiting and abdominal cramps. Liver GvHD usually develops last, often 5–6 weeks after transplantation, as a continuation of, or following on from, resolution of skin and gut GvHD; occasionally liver GvHD may occur as an isolated manifestation. It is accompanied by a mixed hepatitic/obstructive pattern of liver biochemistry with rising bilirubin, alkaline phosphatase, aspartate aminotransferase and alanine aminotransferase.

The diagnosis of aGvHD is largely clinical, but can be confirmed by the finding of a single cell necrosis on skin, gut (jejunal or rectal) or liver biopsy. The differential diagnosis includes drug effects or viral infection, and biopsy may be equally valuable in ruling out important differentials including VOD and CMV colitis. Individual organ system grading and calculation of an overall GvHD grade are shown in Table 25.6. Patients with GvHD limited to grade I or II severity have a 6-month transplant-related mortality, comparable with patients with no GvHD. Patients with grade III GvHD, however, have a 50 per cent risk of mortality at 6 months, whereas grade IV GvHD is usually fatal.[77]

Systemic treatment is required for skin GvHD if the patient is constitutionally unwell with fever, or there is rapid progression of skin lesions. Treatment should also be given if there is a suspicion of hepatic or gastrointestinal GvHD. The mainstay of treatment is steroids, usually 2–4 mg/kg/day of prednisolone, increasing to 30 mg/kg/day of methylprednisolone in severe or refractory cases. Doses are generally halved at 2- to 3-day intervals depending on the response. The treatment of steroid refractory GvHD is unsatisfactory, but further, albeit temporary, responses have been achieved in severe disease with ATG and various monoclonal antibodies, including Campath 1H, anti-IL-2 receptor,[128] anti-CD5,[129] anti-CD2 and anti-TNF (infliximab). With less aggressive disease, FK506 can be substituted for cyclosporin A, or indeed mycophenolate mofetil (MMF) added to either drug.

CHRONIC GRAFT-VERSUS-HOST DISEASE

Chronic graft-versus-host disease is defined as GvHD occurring beyond day 100, although features characteristic of cGvHD may occur much earlier and overlap aGvHD. Chronic GvHD may follow on from acute GvHD, or it may arise after a quiescent phase.[130] HLA disparity, increasing age and prior aGvHD involvement are the major risk factors for its development. Sometimes, possibly associated with discontinuation of cyclosporin or prior T-cell depletion, cGvHD may appear without a preceding acute phase.

Among recipients of HLA-identical marrow receiving conventional cyclosporin/methotrexate GvHD prophylaxis, the probability for the development of cGvHD is 13 per cent in children under 10 years old, and 28 per cent in adolescents aged 10–19 years.[131] The clinical features of cGvHD, which are summarized in Box 25.5, are much broader than aGvHD, and involve other organ systems, including the lungs and musculoskeletal system. There are similarities with autoimmune diseases such as scleroderma and primary biliary cirrhosis, including the presence of autoantibodies. The major histological feature of cGvHD is an increase in collagen deposition, with the development of sclerosis and dermal atrophy. The most effective treatment that minimizes drug-related

---

Box 25.5 *Clinical features of chronic graft-versus-host disease*

- *Skin* – hypo/hyperpigmentation, patchy sclerosis, scaling, erythroderma, alopecia, nail dystrophy and nail loss
- *GI tract* – weight loss, malabsorption, mucosal ulceration, lichenoid lesions
- *Exocrine glands* – ocular and oral sicca, anhydria
- *Lungs* – recurrent chest infections, restrictive-obstructive bronchiolitis
- *Bone marrow* – hypoplasia, autoimmune cytopenia
- *Liver* – intrahepatic cholestasis, cirrhosis, liver failure
- *Immune system* – immunodeficiency with recurrent infections with encapsulated organisms, fungi and viruses

---

Table 25.6 *Grading of graft-versus-host disease*

	Individual system		
Skin rash (% BSA)	GI tract (diarrhoea, mL/kg/day)	Liver (bilirubin, μmol/L)	Grade
<25	8–15	12–20	1
25–50	16–25	20–50	2
>50	>25	>50	3
Desquamation	Pain/ileus	Raised AST/ALT	4

	Overall grading		
Skin	GI tract	Liver	Grade
1–2	–	–	I
1–3	1	1	II
2–3	2–3	2–3	III
2–4	2–4	2–4	IV

ALT, alanine aminotransaminase; AST, aspartate aminotransferase; BSA, body surface area.

side-effects is daily treatment with alternating prednisolone and cyclosporin.[132] The addition of thalidomide sometimes achieves a further response in patients refractory to this therapy,[133] and other options include FK506, MMF,[134] extracorporeal photopheresis,[135] PUVA,[136] and anti-TNF.[137] They also need immunoglobulin replacement and prophylactic antibiotics because of the associated immunodeficiency. The likelihood of treatment response depends upon whether single or multiorgan systems are affected and on the platelet count, thrombocytopenia $<50 \times 10^9$/L carrying a worse prognosis.[138]

TREATMENT OF RELAPSE FOLLOWING TRANSPLANTATION

Relapse after an uncomplicated SCT presents a difficult problem and is the most common cause of SCT failure now that transplant-related mortality is decreasing. Parents frequently wish to pursue further attempts at cure. The toxicity of a second SCT using conventional conditioning is considerable, and LFS is very poor, <10 per cent if the relapse is within 6 months of the first SCT. LFS may be better for later relapses, and conventional second SCT should not be considered unless relapse occurs at least 1 year after initial SCT. The use of RIC SCT may permit a second procedure at minimal separation from the first. If a second SCT is undertaken, attempts should be made to increase GvL activity[139] by using a T-replete graft and/or reducing GvHD prophylaxis. In relapse of CML, infusion of donor T lymphocytes may achieve a further remission without further preparative treatment,[140] although induction of severe GvHD and marrow aplasia may be problematic. This is best avoided by detection of relapse at a molecular level by monitoring post-SCT for an increasing BCR-ABL ratio, and, if progressive, treating with incremental infusions of DLI, starting at 10^6 CD3-positive cells/kg in the sibling setting, and 10^5 CD3-positive cells/kg in the UD setting. One log incremental infusions of DLI can be given at 12-weekly intervals in the absence of GvHD if no response has occurred. In rapidly progressive disease, STI may be used as a holding measure. The benefits of DLI following relapse of acute leukaemia after SCT, particularly when the initial graft is T-cell replete, remain unknown. Such approaches may be more successful in AML, although there are anecdotal successes reported with Ph+ ALL and infant ALL. An alternative to DLI in this setting is a second RIC SCT procedure.[141] DLI in acute leukaemia is only effective in the MRD setting, and therefore prior chemotherapy to induce a further remission may be essential. DLI is of doubtful benefit in the treatment of extramedullary relapse following SCT.

FUTURE PROSPECTS

Preparative regimens

In the last few years, studies in adult patients with malignancies undergoing SCT have demonstrated that RIC is feasible and is associated with a significantly reduced transplant-related mortality. The role of RIC in children with malignancies is not yet clear and there have only been a few reports with limited follow-up. Conventional SCT procedures are more easily tolerated in children and the GvL response which eradicates disease after RIC procedures is less prominent in paediatric malignancies. At present RIC can only be considered for children who are not eligible for conventional conditioning regimens, although as our strategies for augmenting GvL responses improve, we may see a bigger role for RIC in paediatric malignancies.

A promising future approach is the use of monoclonal antibodies (MAbs) directed against haemopoietic cells in ablative and partially ablative marrow conditioning regimens to provide a safe and effective means of achieving donor cell engraftment. Investigators have evaluated the use of anti-CD45, anti-CD33 (Mylotarg) and anti-CD66 MAbs either naked or conjugated to toxins or radioisotopes in pre-transplant conditioning regimens for malignant and non-malignant diseases.[142] These MAbs may permit intensification of the antileukaemic effects of ablative preparative regimens without increasing toxicity, or alternatively produce a sufficiently high level of host immunosuppression in the non-ablative/reduced intensity transplant setting to permit mixed chimerism.

Toxicity/infection

As mentioned earlier, VOD occurs in 5–20 per cent of paediatric transplants. Due to the differences in the kinetics of busulphan in children, it is often difficult to get the balance right between risking rejection due to low busulphan levels and VOD due to high levels.[142] Intravenous busulphan has recently been introduced to reduce interpatient variability[143] and treosulphan may be associated with less toxic side-effects.[144]

A problem area for CMV infection post-SCT in children has recently been defined where most cases of lethal CMV disease occurred in CMV seropositive recipients of CMV seronegative grafts.[145] Seropositive donors should be sought for such patients (see Box 25.1).

Treatment and prevention of relapse

The exquisite specificity of cytotoxic T lymphocytes (CTLs) has made the goal of isolating cells with anti-tumour activity an attractive option. The potential clinical efficacy of CTLs has been demonstrated in pilot studies directed against viral targets such as CMV and Epstein–Barr virus.[146] Whether these types of results can be extended to patients with malignancies where these clearly defined antigens are lacking remains to be determined. A number of groups have successfully identified and expanded CTLs against leukaemia cells. In some instances, these CD8+ and CD4+ CTL clones recognized the minor histocompatibility antigens HA-1 and HA-2 present on leukaemic cells[147] and relatively restricted to haemopoietic tissues of the recipient. Such approaches are likely to enhance GvL without GvHD.

In the haploidentical setting, donor NK cells which engraft rapidly after purified CD34 peripheral blood progenitor cell infusion have been shown to exert a GvL effect in the absence of GvHD by targeting 'KIR' mismatches on recipient haemopoietic cells and AML blasts.[148] Because of their specificity for haemopoietic tissues, NK cells may in future be utilized as part of the conditioning regimen prior to SCT.[149]

KEY POINTS

- There is a lack of randomized studies comparing BMT with chemotherapy protocols.
- The GvL effect in CML and JMML is greater than in AML, which is greater than in ALL.
- There is a small and controversial role of SCT for first CR ALL.
- In relapsed ALL, the benefit of SCT is mostly seen in those with early relapse and those with T-cell disease.
- The role of SCT in first CR AML is doubtful.
- SCT is the optimal approach for AML in second CR.
- JMML requires SCT + GvL effect to achieve cure.
- Despite availability of STI571 (imatinib), MSD or MUD SCT remains the treatment of choice for CML in childhood.
- TBI is avoided in children <2 years of age. The choice between TBI and non-TBI conditioning in older children is not resolved.
- Complications of SCT fall into three main categories:
  - regimen-related toxicity
  - infectious complications
  - GvHD.
- The spectrum of infections is determined by the pattern of haematological and immunological recovery.
- Regimen-related toxicity and infections post-SCT contribute to a significant number of respiratory complications.

> - Relapsed leukaemia after SCT is the most common cause of SCT failure now that transplant-related mortality is decreasing.

REFERENCES

1. Jacobsen LO, Simmons EL, Marks EK et al. The role of the spleen in radiation injury. J Lab Clin Med 1950; **35**: 746–51.
2. Lorenz E, Congdon CC, Uphoff D. Modification of acute irradiation injury in mice and guinea pigs by bone marrow injections. Radiology 1952; **58**: 863–77.
♦3. Pegg DE. Allogeneic bone marrow transplantation in man. In: Pegg DE, ed. Bone Marrow Transplantation. London: Lloyd-Luke Books, 1966; 77–101.
4. Thomas ED, Lochte HL, Lu WC et al. Intravenous infusion of bone marrow in patients receiving radiation and chemotherapy. N Engl J Med 1957; **257**: 491.
5. Powles RL, Clink HM, Spence D et al. Cyclosporin A to prevent GvHD in man after allogeneic bone marrow transplantation. Lancet 1980; **1**: 327–9.
●6. Gluckman E, Rocha V, Boyer-Chammard A et al. Outcome of cord blood transplantation from related and unrelated donors. N Engl J Med 1997; **337**: 373–81.
●7. Kurtzberg J, Laughlin M, Graham M et al. Placental blood as a source of haemopoietic stem cells for transplantation into unrelated recipients. N Engl J Med 1996; **335**: 157–66.
●8. Aversa F, Tabilio A, Terenzi A et al. Successful engraftment of T cell depleted haploidentical 'three-loci' incompatible transplants in leukaemia patients by addition of recombinant human granulocyte colony-stimulating factor-mobilised peripheral blood progenitor cells to bone marrow inoculum. Blood 1994; **84**: 3948–55.
9. Amrolia P, Gaspar B, Hassan A et al. Non-myeloablative stem cell transplantation for congenital immunodeficiencies. Blood 2000; **96**: 1239–46.
♦10. Antin JH. Graft versus leukaemia: no longer an epiphenomenon. Blood 1993; **82**(8): 2273–7.
11. Sullivan KM, Weiden PL, Storb R et al. Influence of acute and chronic graft versus host disease after relapse and survival after bone marrow transplantation from HLA matched siblings as treatment of acute and chronic leukaemia. Blood 1989; **73**: 1720–8.
12. Gajewski JL, Champlin RE. Enhanced graft versus leukaemia effect in patients receiving matched unrelated donor bone marrow transplants. In: Champlin RE, Gale RP, eds. New Strategies in Bone Marrow Transplantation. New York: Wiley-Liss, 1991; 281–4.
♦13. Horowitz MM, Gale RP, Sondel PM et al. Graft versus leukaemia reactions after bone marrow transplantation. Blood 1990; **75**: 555–62.
●14. Casper J, Camitta B, Truitt R et al. Unrelated bone marrow donor transplants for children with leukaemia or myelodysplasia. Blood 1995; **85**(9): 2354–63.
●15. Oakhill A, Pamphilon D, Potter MN et al. Unrelated donor bone marrow transplantation for children with relapsed

acute lymphoblastic leukaemia in second complete remission. *Br J Haematol* 1996; **94**(3): 574–8.

●16. Davies SM, Shu XO, Wagner JE *et al.* Unrelated donor bone marrow transplantation for acute leukaemia in children. *Blood* 1995; **86**(10): 383a.

●17. Balduzzi A, Gooley T, Anasetti C *et al.* Unrelated donor marrow transplantation in children. *Blood* 1995; **86**(8): 3247–56.

18. Ortin M, Raj R, Kinning E *et al.* Partially matched related donor peripheral blood progenitor cell transplantation in paediatric patients adding fludarabine and anti-lymphocyte gamma-globulin. *Bone Marrow Transplant* 2002; **30**(6): 359–66.

19. Handgretinger R, Klingerbiel T, Lang P *et al.* Megadose transplantation of purified peripheral blood CD34(+) progenitor cells from HLA-mismatched parental donors in children. *Bone Marrow Transplant* 2001; **27**(8): 777–83.

●20. Veys PA, Meral A, Hassan A *et al.* Haploidentical related transplants and unrelated donor transplants with T cell addback. *Bone Marrow Transplant* 1998; **21**(Suppl. 2): S42–4.

♦21. Laughlin MJ. Mini-review: umbilical cord blood for allogeneic transplantation in children and adults. *Bone Marrow Transplantation* 2001; **27**: 1–6.

♦22. Pinkel D. Bone marrow transplantation in children. *J Pediatr* 1993; **122**: 331–41.

23. Psiachou E, Hann IM, Morgan G *et al.* Early deaths in children undergoing marrow ablative therapy and bone marrow transplantation. *Bone Marrow Transplant* 1994; **14**: 975–80.

♦24. Leiper AD. Non-endocrine late complications of bone marrow transplantation in childhood: part 1. *Br J Haematol* 2002; **118**: 3–22.

♦25. Chessells JM. The role of bone marrow transplantation in first remission of paediatric ALL. *Front Biosci* 2001; **6**: G38–42.

26. Warwick AB, Zhang M-J, Camitta BM *et al.* Chemotherapy versus HLA-identical sibling bone marrow transplantation for high risk childhood acute lymphoblastic leukaemia in first remission (abstract). *Blood* 1999; **94**(Suppl. 1): 350a.

●27. Wheeler K, Richards S, Bailey C *et al.* Comparison of bone marrow transplantation with chemotherapy for high risk childhood acute lymphoblastic leukaemia in first remission: from Medical Research Council UKALL X and XI. *Blood* 2000; **96**(7): 2412–18.

28. Biggs JC, Horowitz MM, Gale PR *et al.* Bone marrow transplants may cure patients with acute lymphoblastic leukaemia never achieving remission with chemotherapy. *Blood* 1992; **80**: 1090–3.

●29. Arico M, Valsecchi MG, Camitta BM *et al.* Outcome of treatment in children with Philadelphia chromosome-positive acute lymphoblastic leukaemia. *N Engl J Med* 2000; **342**: 998–1006.

30. Sierra J, Radich J, Hansen JA *et al.* Marrow transplants from unrelated donors for treatment of Philadelphia-positive acute lymphoblastic leukaemia. *Blood* 1997; **90**: 1410–14.

31. Marks DI, Bird JM, Cornish JM *et al.* Unrelated donor bone marrow transplantation for children and adolescents with Philadelphia-positive acute lymphoblastic leukaemia. *J Clin Oncol* 1998; **16**: 931–6.

32. Dordelmann M, Harbott J, Reiter A *et al.* Prednisolone response is the strongest predictor of treatment outcome in infant acute lymphoblastic leukaemia, regardless of presenting age. *Blood* 1999; **94**: 1209–17.

●33. Lawson SE, Harrison G, Richards S *et al.* The UK experience in treating relapsed childhood acute lymphoblastic leukaemia: a report on the Medical Research Council UKALL R1 study. *Br J Haematol* 2000; **108**(3): 531–43.

♦34. Uderzo C, Conter V, Dini G *et al.* Treatment of childhood acute lymphoblastic leukaemia after the first relapse: curative strategies. *Haematologica* 2001; **86**(1): 1–7.

●35. Harrison G, Richards S, Lawson S *et al.* Comparison of allogeneic transplant versus chemotherapy for relapsed childhood acute lymphoblastic leukaemia in the MRC UKALL R1 trial. MRC Childhood Leukaemia Working Party. *Ann Oncol* 2000; **11**(8): 999–1006.

36. Knechtli CJ, Goulden NJ, Hancock JP *et al.* Minimal residual disease status before allogeneic bone marrow transplantation is an important determinant of successful outcome for children and adolescents with acute lymphoblastic leukaemia. *Blood* 1998; **92**(11): 4072–9.

37. Dini G, Cornish JM, Gadner H *et al.* Bone marrow transplant indications for childhood leukaemias: achieving a consensus. The EBMT Paediatric Diseases Working Party. *Bone Marrow Transplant* 1996; **18** (Suppl. 2): 4–7.

●38. Wheatley K, Burnett AK, Goldstone AH *et al.* A simple, robust, validated and highly predictive index for the determination of risk-directed therapy in acute myeloid leukaemia derived from the MRC AML 10 trial. United Kingdom Medical Research Council's Adult and Childhood Leukaemia Working Parties. *Br J Haematol* 1999; **107**(1): 69–79.

●39. Nesbit ME Jr, Buckley JD, Feig SA *et al.* Chemotherapy for induction of remission of childhood acute myeloid leukaemia followed by marrow transplantation or multiagent chemotherapy: a report from the Children's Cancer Group. *J Clin Oncol* 1994; **12**(1): 127–35.

40. Tallman MS, Rowlings PA, Milone G *et al.* Effect of post-remission chemotherapy before human leukocyte antigen-identical sibling transplantation for acute myeloid leukaemia in first complete remission. *Blood* 2000; **96**(4): 1254–8.

40a. Schwartz JE, Yeager AM. Reduced-intensity allogeneic hematopoietic cell transplantation: graft versus tumor effects with decreased toxicity. *Pediatr Transplant* 2003; **7**: 168–78.

●41. Cassileth PA, Harrington DP, Appelbaum F *et al.* Chemotherapy compared with autologous or allogeneic bone marrow transplantation in the management of acute myeloid leukaemia in first remission. *N Engl J Med* 1998; **23**: 1649–56.

42. Suciu S. The value of BMT in ALL patients in first remission: a statistician's view point. *Ann Haematol* 1991; **62**: 41–4.

●43. Webb DKH, Wheatley K, Harrison G *et al.* Outcome for children with relapsed acute myeloid leukaemia following initial therapy in the Medical Research Council (MRC) AML 10 trial. *Leukaemia* 1999; **13**: 25–31.

44. Sievers EL, Larson RA, Stadtmauer EA *et al.* Efficacy and safety of Gemtuzumab Ozogamicin in patients with CD33-positive acute myeloid leukaemia in first relapse. *J Clin Oncol* 2001; **19**: 3244–54.

45. Hasle H, Niemeyer C, Chessells J *et al.* Proposal for the diagnosis and classification of myelodysplastic diseases in children. *Leukaemia* 2003; **17**: 277–82.

46. Passmore SJ, Hann IH, Stiller CA *et al.* Paediatric myelodysplasia: a study of 68 children and a new prognostic scoring system. *Blood* 1995; **85**: 1742–50.

47. Hasle H, Kerndrup G, Jacobsen BB. Childhood myelodysplastic syndrome in Denmark: incidence and predisposing conditions. *Leukaemia* 1995; **9**: 1569–72.

48. Niemeyer CM, Fenu S, Hasle H *et al.* Differentiating juvenile myelomonocytic leukaemia from infectious disease. *Blood* 1998; **91**: 365–7.

49. Arico M, Biondi A, Pui CH. Juvenile myelomonocytic leukaemia. *Blood* 1997; **90**: 479–88.

50. Niemeyer CM, Arico M, Basso G *et al.* Chronic myelomonocytic leukaemia in childhood: a retrospective analysis of 110 cases. *Blood* 1997; **89**: 3534–43.

●51. Locatelli F, Niemeyer CM, Angelucci E *et al.* Allogeneic bone marrow transplantation for chronic myelomonocytic leukaemia in childhood: a report from the European working group on myelodysplastic syndrome in children. *J Clin Oncol* 1997; **15**: 566–73.

52. Festa RS, Shende A, Lanzkowsky P. Juvenile chronic myelomonocytic leukaemia: experience with intensive combination chemotherapy. *Med Pediatr Oncol* 1990; **18**: 311–16.

53. Chan HSL, Estrov Z, Weitzmann SS *et al.* The value of intensive combination chemotherapy for juvenile chronic myelogenous leukaemia. *J Clin Oncol* 1987; **5**: 1960–7.

54. Sanders JE, Buckner CD, Stewart P *et al.* Successful treatment of juvenile chronic granulocytic leukemia with bone marrow transplantation. *Pediatrics* 1979; **63**: 44–6.

55. MacMillan ML, Davies SM, Orchard PJ *et al.* Haemopoietic cell transplantation in children with juvenile myelomonocytic leukaemia. *Br J Haematol* 1998; **103**: 552–8.

♦56. Matthes-Martin S, Mann G, Peters C *et al.* Allogeneic bone marrow transplantation for juvenile myelomonocytic leukaemia: a single centre experience and review of the literature. *Bone Marrow Transplant* 2000; **26**: 377–82.

57. Veys P, Saunders JE, Calderwood S *et al.* The role of graft-versus-leukaemia in bone marrow transplantation for juvenile chronic myeloid leukaemia. *Blood* 1994; **84**(Suppl. 1): 201a.

●58. Orchard PJ, Miller JS, McGlennan R *et al.* Graft versus leukaemia is sufficient to induce remission in juvenile myelomonocytic leukaemia. *Bone Marrow Transplant* 1998; **22**: 201–3.

♦59. Rubin CM, Mick R, Johnson FL. Bone marrow transplantation for the treatment of haematological disorders in Down's syndrome: toxicity and outcome. *Bone Marrow Transplant* 1996; **18**: 533–40.

●60. Webb DK, Passmore SJ, Hann IM *et al.* Results of treatment for children with refractory anaemia with excess blasts (RAEB) and RAEB in transformation (RAEBt) in Great Britain. *Br J Haematol* 2002; **117**(1): 33–9.

●61. Niemeyer U, Duffner C, Bender-Gotze C *et al.* AML-type intensive chemotherapy prior to stem cell transplantation (SCT) does not improve survival in children and adolescents with primary myelodysplasia syndromes (MDS) for the European Working Group of MDS in Childhood (EWOG-MDS) (Abstract). *Blood* 2000; **96**: 5212.

62. Niemeyer CM, Kontny U, Strahm B *et al.* Stem cell transplantation (SCT) for children with secondary MDS: report from a multicentre study of the European Working Group of MDS in childhood (EWOG-MDS). *Bone Marrow Transplant* 2002; **29** (Suppl. 2): S89

63. Mughal TI, Goldman JM. Chronic myeloid leukaemia. STI571 magnifies the therapeutic dilemma. *Eur J Cancer* 2001; **37**(5): 561–8.

64. Roberts I. CML in children. *Bone Marrow Transplant* 2002: **30**(suppl. 1): S9–10.

65. Kanfer E. Bone marrow transplant conditioning schedules. In: Treleaven J, Barrett J, eds. *Bone Marrow Transplantation in Practice.* Edinburgh: Churchill Livingstone, 1992; 247–55.

●66. Thomas ED, Buckner CD, Banaji M *et al.* One hundred patients with acute lymphoblastic leukaemia treated by chemotherapy, total body irradiation and allogeneic bone marrow transplantation. *Blood* 1977: **49**: 511–23.

67. Brochstein JA, Kernan NA, Groshen S *et al.* Allogeneic bone marrow transplantation after hyperfractionated total body irradiation and cyclophosphamide in children with acute leukaemia. *N Engl J Med* 1987; **317**: 1624–8.

68. Coccia PF, Strandjord SE, Warkentin PI *et al.* High dose cytosine arabinoside and fractionated total body irradiation: an improved preparative regimen for bone marrow transplantation of children with acute lymphoblastic leukaemia in remission. *Blood* 1988; **71**: 888–93.

●69. Helenglass G, Powles RL, McElwain TJ *et al.* Melphalan and total body irradiation (TBI) versus cyclophosphamide and TBI as conditioning for allogeneic matched sibling bone marrow transplants for acute myeloblastic leukaemia in first remission. *Bone Marrow Transplant* 1988; **3**: 21–31.

70. Blume KG, Forman SJ, O'Donnell MR *et al.* Total body irradiation and high dose etoposide: a new preparatory regimen for bone marrow transplantation in patients with advanced haematological malignancies. *Blood* 1987; **69**: 1015–20.

♦71. Santos GW, Hess AD, Vogelsgang GB. Graft versus host reactions and disease. *Immunol Rev* 1983; **88**: 169–92.

72. Grochow LB, Jones RJ, Brundrett RB *et al.* Pharmacokinetics of busulphan: correlation with veno-occlusive disease in patients undergoing bone marrow transplantation. *Cancer Chemother Pharmacol* 1989; **25**: 55–61.

♦73. Davies SM, Ramsay NK, Klein JP *et al.* Comparison of preparative regimen in transplants for children with acute lymphoblastic leukaemia. *J Clin Oncol* 2000; **18**(2): 340–7.

♦74. American Society of Clinical Oncology. Recommendations for the use of haematopoietic colony-stimulating factors: evidence-based, clinical practice guidelines. *J Clin Oncol* 1994; **12**(11): 2471–508.

75. Volpi I, Perruccio K, Tosti A *et al.* Postgrafting administration of granulocyte colony-stimulating factor impairs functional immune recovery in recipients of human leukocyte antigen haplotype-mismatched haemopoietic transplants. *Blood* 2001; **97**(8): 2514–21.

♦76. Wolff SN. Mini review: second haematopoietic stem cell transplantation for the treatment of graft failure, graft rejection or relapse after allogeneic transplantation. *Bone Marrow Transplant* 2002; **29**: 545–52.

♦77. Martin P. Overview of marrow transplantation immunology. In: Forman SJ, Blume KG, Thomas ED, eds. *Bone Marrow Transplantation.* Oxford: Blackwell Scientific Publications, 1994; 16–21.

78. Neville TJ, Tirgan MH, Deeg HJ et al. Influence of post-methotrexate folinic acid rescue on regimen-related toxicity and GvHD after allogeneic bone marrow transplant. *Bone Marrow Transplant* 1992; **9**: 349–54.

79. McDonald GB, Sharma P. Matthews DE et al. Venoocclusive disease of the liver after bone marrow transplantation: diagnosis, incidence and predisposing factors. *Hepatology* 1984; **4**: 116–22.

●80. Essell JH, Schroeder MT, Harman GS et al. Ursodiol prophylaxis against hepatic complications of allogeneic bone marrow transplantation. A randomised, double-blind, placebo-controlled trial. *Ann Intern Med* 1998; **128**: 975–81.

●81. Chopra R, Eaton JD, Grassi A et al. Defibrotide for the treatment of hepatic veno-occlusive disease: result of the European compassionate use study. *Br J Haematol* 2000; **111**: 1122–9.

●82. Rosenthal J, Sender L, Secola R et al. Phase II trial of heparin prophylaxis for veno-occlusive disease of the liver in children undergoing bone marrow transplantation. *Bone Marrow Transplant* 1996; **18**: 185–91.

●83. Gluckman E, Jolivet I, Scrobohaci ML et al. Use of prostaglandin E1 for prevention of liver veno-occlusive disease in leukaemic patients treated by allogeneic bone marrow transplantation. *Br J Haematol* 1990; **74**: 277–81.

84. Baglin TP, Harper P, Marcus RE. Venoocclusive disease of the liver complicating ABMT successfully treated with recombinant tissue plasminogen activator (rt-PA). *Bone Marrow Transplant* 1990; **5**, 439–41.

●85. Morris JD, Harris RE, Hashmi R et al. Antithrombin III for the treatment of chemotherapy-induced organ dysfunction following bone marrow transplantation. *Bone Marrow Transplant* 1997; **20**: 871–8.

♦86. Baglin TP. Veno-occlusive disease of the liver complicating bone marrow transplantation. *Bone Marrow Transplant* 1994; **13**(1): 1–4.

87. Kennedy L, Snell ME, Witherow RO. Use of alum to control intractable vesical haemorrhage. *Br J Urol* 1984; **56**: 673–5.

88. Mohiuddin J, Prentice HG, Schey S et al. Treatment of cyclophosphamide induced cystitis with prostaglandin E2. *Ann Intern Med.* 1984: **101**(1): 142.

89. Shrom SH, Donaldson MH, Duckett JW et al. Formalin treatment for intractable haemorrhagic cystitis. *Cancer* 1976: **38**: 1785–9.

90. Kawakami M, Ueda S, Maeda T et al. Vidarabine therapy for virus-associated cystitis after allogeneic bone marrow transplantation. *Bone Marrow Transplant* 1997; **20**: 485–90.

91. Clark JG, Hansen JA, Hertz MI, et al. Idiopathic pneumonia syndrome after bone marrow transplantation. *Am Rev Respir Dis* 1993; **147**(6 Pt 1): 1601–6.

92. Muller CA, Hebart H, Roos A et al. Correlation of interstitial pneumonia with human cytomegalovirus-induced lung infection and graft vs. host disease after bone marrow transplantation. *Med Microbiol Immunol* 1995 **184**(3); 115–21.

93. Pettitt AR, Clark RE. Thrombotic microangiopathy following bone marrow transplantation. *Bone Marrow Transplant* 1994; **14**: 495–504.

●94. Ninane J and the Multicentre Study Group. A multicentre study of fluconazole versus oral polyenes in the prevention of fungal infection in children with haematological or oncological malignancies. *Eur J Clin Microbiol Infect Dis* 1994: **13**(4): 330–7.

♦95. Barnes R. Infections following bone marrow transplantation. In: Treleaven J, Barrett J, eds. *Bone Marrow Transplantation in Practice.* Edinburgh: Churchill Livingstone, 1994: 281–8.

96. Hertz MI, Englung JA, Snover D et al. Respiratory syncytial virus-induced acute lung injury in adult patients with bone marrow transplant: a clinical approach and review of the literature. *Medicine* 1989; **68**: 269–81.

97. Englund JA, Sullivan CJ, Jordan MC et al. Respiratory syncytial virus infection in immunocompromised patients. *Ann Intern Med* 1988; **109**: 203–8.

98. DeVincenzo JP, Hirsch RL, Fuentes RJ et al. Respiratory syncytial virus immune globulin treatment of lower respiratory tract infection in paediatric patients undergoing bone marrow transplantation – a compassionate use experience. *Bone Marrow Transplant* 2000; **25**(2): 161–5.

99. Ghosh S, Champlin RE, Englund J et al. Respiratory syncytial virus upper respiratory tract illnesses in adult blood and marrow transplant recipients: combination therapy with aerosoled ribavirin and intravenous immunoglobulin. *Bone Marrow Transplant* 2000; **25**: 751–5.

100. Goodrich JM, Reed EC, Mori M et al. Clinical features and analysis of risk factors for invasive candidal infection after marrow transplantation. *J Infect Dis* 1991; **164**: 731–40.

101. Wingard JR, Mellits ED, Sostrin MB et al. Interstitial pneumonitis after allogeneic bone marrow transplantation. *Medicine* 1988; **67**: 175–86.

102. Ljungman P, Biron P, Bosi A et al. Cytomegalovirus interstitial pneumonia in autologous bone marrow transplant recipients. *Bone Marrow Transplant* 1994; **13**: 209–12.

103. Weiner RS, Bortin MM, Gale RP et al. Interstitial pneumonitis after bone marrow transplantation. *Ann Intern Med* 1986; **104**: 168–75.

104. Li CR, Greemberg PD, Gilbert MJ et al. Recovery of HLA-restricted Cytomegalovirus-specific T cell responses after allogeneic bone marrow transplant: correlation with CMV disease and effect of ganciclovir prophylaxis. *Blood* 1994; **83**: 1971–9.

105. Meyers JD, Flournoy N, Thomas ED. Risk factors for cytomegalovirus infection after human marrow transplantation. *J Infect Dis* 1986; **153**: 478–88.

106. Janzen DL, Padley SPG, Adler BD et al. Acute pulmonary complications in immunocompromised non-AIDS patients: comparison of diagnostic accuracy of CT and chest radiography. *Clin Radiol* 1993; **47**: 159–65.

107. Cathgomas G, Morris P, Pekle K et al. Rapid diagnosis of cytomegalovirus pulmonary pneumonia in marrow transplant recipients by bronchoalveolar lavage using the polymerase chain reaction, virus culture, and the direct immunostaining of alveolar cells. *Blood* 1993; **81**: 1909–14.

108. Enright H, Haake R, Weisdorf D et al. Cytomegalovirus pneumonia after bone marrow transplantation. *Transplantation* 1993; **55**: 1339–46.

109. Rowe JM, Ciobanu N, Ascensao J et al. Recommended guidelines for the management of autologous and allogeneic bone marrow transplantation. *Ann Intern Med* 1994; **120**: 143–58.

●110. Prentice HG, Gluckman E, Powles RL et al. Long term survival in allogeneic bone marrow transplant recipients following Aciclovir prophylaxis for CMV infection. Bone Marrow Transplant 1997; 19: 129–133.

●111. Goodrich JM, Mori M, Gleaves CA. Early treatment with ganciclovir to prevent cytomegalovirus disease after allogeneic bone marrow transplantation. N Engl J Med 1991; 325: 1601–7.

112. Blanke C, Clark C, Broun R et al. Evolving pathogens in allogeneic bone marrow transplantation: increased fatal adenovirus infections. Am J Med 1995; 99: 326–8.

♦113. Kreit JW. Respiratory complications. In: Ball ED, Lister JL, Law PL, eds. Haemopoietic Stem Cell Therapy. Philadelphia: Churchill Livingstone, 2000: 563–77.

114. McWhinney PHM, Kibbler CC, Hamon MD et al. Progress in the diagnosis and management of aspergillosis in bone marrow transplantation: 13 years experience. Clin Infect Dis 1993; 17: 397–404.

115. Cordonnier C, Bernaudin J, Bierling P et al. Pulmonary complications occurring after allogeneic bone marrow transplantation. Cancer 1986; 58: 1047–54.

116. Quabeck K. The lung as a critical organ in marrow transplantation. Bone Marrow Transplant 1994; 14(Suppl. 4): S19–28.

117. Afessa B, Tefferi A, Hoagland HC et al. Outcome of recipients of bone marrow transplants who require intensive care unit support. Mayo Clin Proc 1992; 67(2): 117–22.

118. Paz HL, Crilley P, Weinar M et al. Outcome of patients requiring medical ICU admission following bone marrow transplantation. Chest 1993; 104(2): 527–31.

♦119. Veys P, Owens C. Respiratory infections following haemopoietic stem cell transplantation in children. Br Med Bull 2002; 61: 151–74.

♦120. Meyers JD, Flournay N, Thomas ED. Risk factors for cytomegalovirus infection after human marrow transplantation. J Infect Dis 1986; 153(3): 478–88.

♦121. Gale RP, Bortin MM, van Bekkum D et al. Risk factors for acute graft versus host disease. Br J Haematol 1987; 67: 397–406.

122. Lonqvist B, Ringden O, Wahren B et al. Cytomegalovirus infection associated with and preceding chronic graft versus host disease. Transplantation 1984; 38: 465–8.

♦123. Apperley JF. Umbilical cord blood progenitor cell transplantation. Bone Marrow Transplant 1994; 14: 187–96.

♦124. Weisdorf D, Hakke R, Blazar B et al. Risk factors for acute graft versus host disease in histocompatible donor bone marrow transplantation. Transplantation 1991; 5: 1197–203.

♦125. Poynton C. T cell depletion in bone marrow transplantation. In: Pegg DE, ed. Bone Marrow Transplantation in Practice. Edinburgh: Churchill Livingstone, 1992; 227–37.

126. Sullivan KM, Weiden PL, Storb R et al. Influence of acute graft versus host disease after relapse and survival after bone marrow transplantation from HLA identical siblings as treatment of acute and chronic leukaemia. Blood 1989; 73: 1720–8.

127. Veys P, Sanders F, Calderwood S et al. The role of graft versus leukaemia in bone marrow transplantation for juvenile chronic myeloid leukaemia. Blood 1994; 84(Suppl.): 337A.

128. Hervé P, Wijdens J, Bergerat JP et al. Treatment of acute graft versus host disease with monoclonal antibody to the IL-2 receptor. Lancet 1988; 2: 1072–3.

129. Fay, JW, Burkeholder S, Stone M. Treatment of allogeneic bone marrow with anti T cell antibody prior to transplantation. Bone Marrow Transplant 1987; 2(Suppl. 2): 127.

♦130. Atkinson KA. Chronic graft versus host disease – review. Bone Marrow Transplant 1990; 5: 69–82.

131. Sullivan KM, Agura E, Anasetti C et al. Chronic graft versus host disease and other late complications of bone marrow transplantation. Semin Hematol 1991; 28: 250–9.

●132. Sullivan KM, Witherspoon RP, Storb R et al. Alternating day cyclosporin and prednisolone for treatment of high risk chronic graft versus host disease. Blood 1988; 72: 555–61.

133. McCarthy DM, Kanfer EJ, Barrett AJ. Thalidomide for the therapy of graft versus host disease following allogeneic bone marrow transplantation. Biomed Pharmacother 1989; 43: 693–7.

134. Gross TG, Egeler RM, Smith FO. Pediatric hematopoietic stem cell transplantation. Hematol Oncol Clin North Am 2001; 15(5): 795–808.

135. Greinix HT, Volc-Platzer B, Watkins P et al. Successful use of extracorporeal photopheresis (ECP) in the treatment of chronic graft versus host disease. Blood 1998; 92: 3098–104.

136. Vogelsang GB, Wolff D, Altomonte V et al. Treatment of chronic graft versus host disease with PUVA. Bone Marrow Transplant 1996; 17: 1061–7.

137. Couriel DR, Hicks K, Ippoliti C et al. Infliximab for the treatment of graft versus host disease in allogeneic transplant recipients: an update. Abstract 1724. Blood 2001; 96: 400a.

138. Sullivan KM, Witherspoon RP, Storb R et al. Prednisolone and azathioprine compared with prednisolone and placebo for treatment of chronic graft versus host disease: prognostic influence of prolonged thrombocytopenia after allogeneic bone marrow transplantation. Blood 1988; 72: 546–54.

139. Gale RP, Champlin RE. How does bone marrow transplantation cure leukaemia? Lancet 1984; 2: 28–30.

●140. Kolb HJ, Mittermüller J, Clemm C et al. Donor leukocyte transfusions for treatment of recurrent chronic myelogenous leukaemia in marrow transplant patients. Blood 1990; 76: 2462–5.

141. Pawson R, Potter MN, Theocharous P et al. Treatment of relapse after allogeneic bone marrow transplantation with reduced intensity conditioning (FLAG ± IDA) and second allogeneic stem cell transplant. Br J Haematol 2001; 115(3): 622–9.

142. Pagel JM, Matthews DC, Appelbaum FR et al. The use of radioimmunoconjugates in stem cell transplantation: mini review. Bone Marrow Transplant 2002; 29: 807–16.

143. Schuler US, Renner UD, Kroschinsky F et al. Intravenous busulphan for conditioning before autologous or allogeneic human blood stem cell transplantation. Br J Haematol 2001; 114(4): 944–50.

144. Casper J, Wilhelm S, Steiner B et al. Treosulphan and fludarabine conditioning for allogeneic blood stem cell

transplantation. *Bone Marrow Transplant* 2000; **25**(Suppl. 1): S129.

145. Matthes-Martin S, Lion T, Aberle SW *et al.* Pre-emptive treatment of CMV DNAemia in paediatric stem cell transplantation: the impact of recipient and donor CMV serostatus on the incidence of CMV disease and CMV-related mortality. *Bone Marrow Transplant* 2003; **31**: 803–8.

146. Rooney CM, Smith CA, Ng CYC *et al.* Use of gene modified virus-specific T lymphocytes to control Epstein Barr virus-related lymphoproliferation. *Lancet* 1995; **345**(8941): 9–13.

147. Faber LM, Van Der Hoeven J, Goulmy E *et al.* Recognition of clonogenic leukaemic cells, remission bone marrow and HLA-identical bone marrow by CD8 + or CD4 + minor histocompatibility antigen-specific cytotoxic T lymphocytes. *J Clin Invest* 1995; **96**(2): 877–83.

148. Ruggeri L, Capanni M, Casucci M *et al.* Role of natural killer cell alloreactivity in HLA-mismatched haemopoietic stem cell transplantation. *Blood* 1999; **94**(1): 333–9.

149. Ruggeri L, Capanni M, Urbani E *et al.* Effectiveness of donor natural killer cell alloreactivity in mismatched haemopoietic transplants. *Science* 2002; **295**(5562): 2097–100.

150. Cornish J, Goulden N, Potter M. Unrelated donor bone-marrow transplantation. In: Barrett J, Treleaven JG, eds. *The Clinical Practice of Stem Cell Transplantation.* St Louis: Mosby Year Book, 1998, 363–91.

26

Megatherapy with stem cell rescue in solid tumours

RUTH LADENSTEIN, OLIVIER HARTMANN, EWA KOSCIELNAK & THIERRY PHILIP

INTRODUCTION

In contrast to adult malignancies, most paediatric solid tumours show high response rates to, and may be cured by, conventional chemotherapy. One way to increase dose level and intensity is to use megatherapy (MGT) followed by haemopoietic stem cell reinfusion (SCR) for poor prognosis or relapsed childhood solid tumours. In the future, the use of growth factors (GFs) and new purging techniques may decrease morbidity and relapse, respectively. Several extensive or critical reviews[1–5] reflect the persistent effort to establish more successful drug combinations in terms of response and survival. Within the past 24 years, more than 5000 paediatric transplantations have been reported to the European Bone Marrow Transplant Solid Tumour Registry (EBMT-STR).

DOSE–EFFECT RELATIONSHIP

The Goldie–Coldman theories[6–8] support multimodality treatment, including, in sequence, chemotherapy, radiotherapy and delayed surgery to excise any residual chemoresistant tumour mass. High-dose chemotherapy should preferably be applied in a situation of minimal residual disease (MRD).[9–11]

Dose escalation of single agents or drug combinations may be a key factor in the attempt to convert response into cure. The Ridgeway sarcoma model in dogs suggested that the dose–response curve was steep and that modest modifications of dose intensity and/or dose rate of many cytostatic drugs could convert response into cure.[12] However, in clinical practice the doses are limited by a variety of organ toxicities.[13] Among children receiving MGT, 11 per cent suffer early death (before day 100); one-third of these deaths are due to disease progression and two-thirds to toxicity. However, this early toxic death rate has been consistently reduced and is now about half that previously reported, as a result of experience and better patient selection. The monitoring of drug pharmacokinetics is one way to decrease toxicity and optimize drug efficacy.[14]

HIGH-DOSE THERAPY WITH HAEMOPOIETIC PROGENITOR RESCUE

Reinfusion of *in vitro* gene-marked marrow has proven that autologous reinfusion contributes to long-term haemopoietic recovery after myeloablative therapy.[15] SCR rescue thus permits the administration of active agents at doses limited only by extramedullary toxicity. It may be used to shorten the period of aplasia after non-ablative high-dose chemotherapy or as a rescue after myeloablative chemotherapy, often with total body irradiation (TBI). Doses may be increased three- to 10-fold above levels normally used in cancer treatment.[16] Toxicities particularly involve tissues with a rapid cellular proliferation rate, such as oral and intestinal mucosa.

The essential problem of overcoming mechanisms of drug resistance is complex and multifactorial.[17–23] Alkylating agents may overcome resistance when applied in high dose.[24] High-dose cisplatin can overcome membrane transport constraints and saturate other mechanisms, such as detoxification and DNA repair.[25] In vivo, the majority of phase II studies show impressive response rates in progressive disease resistant to conventional doses.[26,27] However, in contrast to leukaemia or lymphoma, most patients with solid tumours achieve only incomplete remissions. Repeated MGT has been used to overcome this apparent resistance of solid tumours. However, with data now available (EBMT 2002 analysis; see below), this approach is hard to justify taking forward to randomized studies.

Alternative ways of increasing tumour cell kill include the use of post-megatherapy immunotherapy or chemotherapy. Allogeneic bone marrow transplantation (BMT) may induce a graft-versus-tumour (GvT) effect in Hodgkin's and non-Hodgkin's lymphomas. An 18 per cent relapse rate has been described for allogeneic BMT compared with 45 per cent for autologous BMT in lymphoma.[28] However, this GvT effect may not apply if tumour cells do not express the major HLA class II antigens. Furthermore, in young children there is a lower incidence of GvT effect after allogeneic BMT.[29] The GvT effect may be mimicked pharmacologically, e.g. by cyclosporin A.

Although no graft-versus-leukaemia effect is expected, reinfusion of autologous bone marrow (BM), autologous peripheral blood stem cell (PBSC) or umbilical cord progenitors[30] has become the method of choice in solid tumours because of its practicality and the fact that only 25 per cent of patients have HLA and DR matched donors. The choice between BM and/or PBSC rescue is still a matter for debate. Either cells may be safely collected, even in young children aged under 1 year.[31] The contamination by malignant cells may be less in PBSCs.[32] Several critical problems remain unsolved:

- What is the best induction regimen to achieve good-quality remission and adequate progenitors where marrow has initially been involved?
- What is the ideal time for harvesting?
- What is the real significance of MRD in the sample collected?

PURGING

A possible limitation of stem cell rescue is the potential contamination of the transplanted BM or PBSCs by malignant cells. Considerable efforts have therefore been made to detect[33,34] and remove tumour (negative purging) or select progenitor cells (positive purging) before reinfusion.

Non-specific purging techniques such as Percoll or bovine serum albumin gradients and counterflow centrifugation have been reported. Sheep red blood rosetting and soya bean lectin separation have been used for T-cell and neuroblastoma depletion.[35] Chemotherapeutic agents destroy malignant cells with at least a partial preservation of normal haemopoietic progenitors;[36] active derivatives of cyclophosphamide are now extensively used in leukaemia and neuroblastoma.[37,38] Some non-chemotherapeutic agents are of potential interest, e.g. merocyanine 540, a DNA dye with lytic activity after photoactivation,[39,40] or 6-hydroxydopamine.[41] Desferrioxamine may be used against neuroblastoma contamination.[42] Malignant cells may be removed by immunomagnetic depletion[43–46] or be absorbed in a column via monoclonal antibodies (MoAbs) attached to a solid phase through avidin-biotin linkages.[47,48] Another possibility is complement lysis. MoAbs (IgM or IgG$_{2a}$ isotypes) lyse targeted cells in the presence of rabbit or human complement.[49] Finally, MoAbs can also be conjugated to various plant toxins (ricin). Immunological purging by addition of interleukin-2 (IL-2) in long-term cultures (1–2 weeks) is efficient and generates anti-tumour cytotoxic effects.[50] Purging with antisense oligomers is feasible providing that malignant cells have a specific target such as oncogene or translocation.

Positive selection purging has been described more recently. The CD34 antigen is expressed by 1–4 per cent of human marrow cells, including virtually all haemopoietic progenitors, but has not been detected in most solid tumours. Positive selection of CD34+ cells may thus be used to provide marrow cells that are capable of engraftment but depleted of tumour cells.[51,52] The positive purging obtained by CD34 purification can be further increased by the association with immunotoxins.[53] In the chronic myeloid leukaemia model, short-term culture allows the preferential growth of normal progenitors. Ex vivo long-term cultures may be performed in bioreactors: more than 3 billion cells containing 12×10^6 CFU-GM may be reproducibly generated from the equivalent of a 10–15 mL BM aspirate.[54] Ex vivo-expanded CD34+ PBPCs could allow the long-term reconstitution of haemopoiesis.[51] Retroviral transfer of genes such as the multidrug resistant gene (MDR) is possible, which could protect marrow stem cells and allow post-consolidation chemotherapy using MDR-related drugs.

A minimal count of 0.5×10^8 mononuclear cells/kg is necessary after autologous BMT.[55] For PBSC collection, if the preharvest number of circulating CD34+ cells is more than 10^5/mL, a single standardized leukapheresis is sufficient to obtain the minimum of 5×10^4 CFU-GM/kg that usually provides safe engraftment in children.[56] The haematological toxicity observed with delays of engraftment in the double graft programme of the LMCE2[57] suggests that both previous damage to the BM microenvironment by heavy and prolonged pre-treatment and toxic stem cell damage by purging procedures share responsibility.

The efficacy of purging procedures has been demonstrated *in vitro* for adult acute leukaemia,[37] Burkitt lymphoma[44,58] and neuroblastoma cells.[59,60] The need for purging procedures in practice remains a controversial issue, as the clonogenic potential of reinfused tumour cells is difficult to demonstrate. Clinical observations demonstrate that relapses emerge from residual tumour sites rather than from reinfused malignant cells in the BM. However, the rare pulmonary relapses after autologous BMT for neuroblastoma suggest that malignant cells in reinfused marrow may have been trapped by the lungs.[61,62] A retrospective comparison between two groups of patients who received similar induction and high-dose therapy regimens with either purged or unpurged marrow[63] failed to show any significant difference in the outcome. The most convincing evidence that contaminated marrow may participate in relapse comes from the detection of the *Neo R* transfected gene in tumour cells at relapse when autologous BM had been transfected with this gene prior to reinfusion.[64] A clear demonstration by a clinical randomized study is still lacking. However, an ongoing Children's Oncology Group (COG) trial is currently investigating this particular question.

THE ROLE OF HAEMOPOIETIC GROWTH FACTORS

The normal steady-state haemopoiesis is locally regulated by the specific microenvironment in the bone marrow. The stromal cells secrete and can bind exogenous GFs, thus supplying them to stem cells and committed precursors.[65] After BMT, several alterations have been reported. Stromal cells have a reduced capacity to produce granulocyte colony-stimulating factor (G-CSF) and probably other GFs.[66,67] There is a coordinated pattern of interleukin cytokine release with fluctuations of interleukin (IL)-3 related to stem cell recruitment, whereas the increase in IL-6, G-CSF and IL-8 may underlie neutrophil recovery.[68] In contrast, there is no correlation with circulating Steel factor, a multilineage haemopoietic stimulating factor.[69] The insufficient production and response of T cells to IL-2 is well documented. Overactive mononuclear cells expressing Leu 7 and CD8 may explain some cases of delayed engraftment after autologous BMT.[70]

Timed administration of GFs could help obtain a better stem cell harvest from BM or PBSCs for autograft.

Recombinant human granulocyte colony-stimulating factor (rhG-CSF) administered in children prior to marrow harvesting may increase myeloid cellularity.[71] Even in patients with extensive prior radiotherapy and chemotherapy that preclude bone marrow harvest, the use of rhGM-CSF improves the collection of PBSCs after chemotherapy.[72] The use of these factors, either during the rapid upswing of white blood cells following conventional chemotherapy or as a steady-state procedure, results in the enriched collection of PBSCs. However, their use after PBSC reinfusion is associated with only modest clinical benefit in neutrophil recovery.[73–76]

Myeloid recovery is accelerated after autologous BMT in patients receiving either G-CSF or GM-CSF (granulocyte/monocyte colony-stimulating factor). The theoretical risks of depleting the stem cell pool[77] and stimulating neoplastic residual cells[78] have not been confirmed. GM-CSF stimulates myelopoiesis at the level of bone marrow CFU-GM, while G-CSF causes earlier neutrophil recovery peripherally.[79] In adults, G-CSF post-autologous BMT enhances the engraftment of neutrophils and platelets significantly more than GM-CSF.[80] For paediatric solid tumours, addition of GM-CSF or G-CSF after MGT may not speed up engraftment, but G-CSF significantly reduces the rate of documented bacteraemias.[81] Since GM-CSF and IL-6 may act through different mechanisms post-transplant, their sequential administration may be worthwhile.[82] Erythropoietin treatment post-allogeneic BMT in adults significantly accelerates erythroid recovery, although conflicting results have been published in children receiving purged autologous marrow. The administration of G-CSF after autologous BMT is as effective when initiated at day +1 as it is at day +6.[83] Growth factors also have a potential role in dose escalation without marrow rescue.

TOTAL BODY IRRADIATION

Until 1990 there was a general consensus that patients with leukaemia/lymphoma who were treated with TBI did better.[84] Busulphan-containing regimens are now considered as equivalent,[2,85,86] although TBI may have a role in advanced disease.[87]

Neuroblastoma shows *in vitro* radiosensitivity to the low radiation dose of 2 Gy.[88,89] Thus TBI seemed to be an appropriate component of MGT regimens for some solid tumours. The advantages of fractionated TBI remain controversial, although pulmonary toxicity is reduced. The relative cytotoxic effect in tumours with shouldered response curves remains to be clarified.[90] Characterization of the genetic control of radiation damage repair may have far-reaching implications for therapy and radiation-related carcinogenesis. If TBI regimens are to be offered to patients in first complete remission as a consolidation treatment, late effects such as growth disturbances, sterility, hormone imbalances and potential second malignancies must be considered.

Alternative ways of delivering radiation directly to malignant cells include ^{131}I-labelled antibodies (CD45 antibody) and ^{131}I-mIBG (^{131}I meta-iodobenzylguanidine). However, limitations in availability and associated radioprotection measures limit the role of the latter in a multicentre setting.

PRINCIPAL CONCLUSIONS FROM THE EBMT

Up to the present date, the EBMT registry in paediatric solid tumours remains an important information resource. It reflects the experience gathered in 33 countries on 5200 patients aged below 18 years at stem cell transplantation (SCT) as reported from 243 centres. European prospective randomized trials investigating the value of MGT/SCR in solid tumours are the ultimate goal in some but not all indications, due to the rarity of some malignancies. In view of evolving treatment strategies within international and national treatment studies, the characterization of high-risk patients has to be constantly reviewed and the eligibility for MGT/SCR approaches regularly revised and questioned.

Neuroblastoma is still the only tumour in which MGT has been explored in a randomized fashion.[91] In other indications, evidence-based data are still scarce and the EBMT registry still serves as a reference source (see Table 26.1).

The main conclusions that can be drawn from the EBMT Paediatric Solid Tumour Registry data are as follows:

- Response status prior to MGT/SCT has a crucial influence on final outcome. First-line patients with good responding disease in complete, very good partial or partial remission (CR/VGPR/PR) as well as patients with sensitive relapse (SR) are usually good indications in most high-risk solid tumour patients,

while stable disease (SD) and minor response (MR, <50 per cent) are at least questionable indications. Any patients with no response (NR) or tumour progression as well as resistant relapse (RR) have a very short life expectancy even after MGT/SCT and thus should not undergo this procedure.

- First-line patients fare significantly better than relapse patients. If criteria clearly define the high-risk patient at diagnosis or during the early treatment phase (i.e. poor histological response), MGT/SCR should be part of the first-line treatment strategy and not be reserved until the occurrence of relapse. For many tumour types, the potential benefit of MGT/SCTR over conventional approaches awaits demonstration in randomized studies.
- Age has to be considered since it may have a significant influence (i.e. in neuroblastoma patients under 2 years of age or in soft tissue sarcoma in those over 10 years).
- There is no detectable advantage of repetitive MGT approaches over a single MGT course.
- No advantage for the use of TBI can be shown. TBI should thus be avoided in children with solid tumours in view of late effects.
- Busulphan/melphalan was highlighted as the most successful MGT combination in the EBMT Solid Tumour Registry data, resulting in significantly better survival rates in neuroblastoma and Ewing's tumours. This regimen is currently under investigation in randomized European trials.

NEUROBLASTOMA

For many years, the management of neuroblastoma relied on simple clinical staging. Advances in nuclear medicine and the extension of bone marrow investigations have thrown the classic staging systems somewhat into disarray and encouraged the development of the new International Neuroblastoma Staging System (INSS) staging system.[92,93]

Children with metastatic disease over the age of 1 year represent the largest neuroblastoma subgroup. Their prognosis remains poor in most cases and the ability to predict the clinical course and the outcome of the individual patient is modest, so there is little indication at the moment for a reduction in treatment intensity whatever the biological pattern. Age and response to induction are major prognostic factors in stage 4. For stage 4 patients under 1 year at diagnosis, cure rates may exceed 70 per cent with conventional therapy if the tumour is not *MYCN* non-amplified. In non-metastatic disease, MGT should be considered if the tumour shows *MYCN* amplification, irrespective of age, since in the presence of this biological marker, prognosis is as bad as in stage 4 disease.

Table 26.1 *Overall survival (OS) rates of paediatric high-risk solid tumours in Europe according to the European Bone Marrow Transplant Group registry data in 2002*

Tumour type	Patient numbers	5-year OS
Neuroblastoma	2285	0.34 ± 0.01
Ewing's tumour	924	0.37 ± 0.02
Osteosarcoma	137	0.22 ± 0.05
Soft tissue sarcoma	647	0.28 ± 0.02
Brain tumour	528	0.27 ± 0.02
Germ cell tumour	197	0.39 ± 0.04
Wilms' tumour	197	0.52 ± 0.04
Retinoblastoma	66	0.60 ± 0.06
Miscellaneous	53	0.35 ± 0.08

OS, overall survival.

Long-term survival of children with stage 4 disease over the age of 1 year used to be rare (<5 per cent of the cases).[94–99] The great improvement in supportive care that occurred in the early 1980s led to the widespread use of dose-intensive regimens.[100–106] Treatment intensification usually included an intensified induction regimen followed by the resection of the primary tumour and a final cycle of MGT combined with SCT.[107–114] The addition of platinum derivatives and epipodophyllotoxins to the conventional drugs used in induction has contributed to more than 70 per cent complete or partial remission rates prior to MGT. Prolongation of conventional chemotherapy, dose increases and schedule modifications have not produced additional major advances.[115]

Early results from the UK and the USA[116–119] were confirmed by several reports from France, Italy, Germany, Japan and other national groups.[120–126] The expectation that the refinement of these strategies would progressively improve patient outcome was frustrated by a number of trials that failed to increase the 5-year event-free survival (EFS) above 30 per cent.[127–135] In addition, even 5-year survivors showed only an 80 per cent chance of continued remission.[136–138] Following MGT, 20 per cent of relapses occur in the primary site alone, and 45 per cent in distant sites only, highlighting the role of local treatment.[139–141] A few reports on smaller patient series claiming superior results appeared most likely to be related to limited statistical power due to small numbers and, possibly, patient selection.[142]

Few clinical factors seem to have prognostic significance in children treated with modern high-dose protocols. It has been suggested that lack of skeletal involvement at diagnosis may increase 6-year progression-free survival (PFS) post-autologous BMT (50 vs. 5 per cent).[132] The most consistent factor is the disappearance of all detectable metastatic disease.[138,143–144]

The lack of uniform criteria to document the regression of skeletal and bone marrow disease (the most common sites of metastatic disease) has made it difficult to compare results[145–149] and the clearance of bone marrow deposits has no significant value in the EBMT database. The most discriminatory feature is the disappearance of skeletal metastases on mIBG scintigraphy at the end of induction: nearly 40 per cent of patients are in such a situation and their 5-year overall survival is 40 per cent, compared with 15 per cent otherwise.[94,133] The latter criteria may currently be the most appropriate one to separate two prognostic groups.

Biological studies[150–154] as well as some serological factors, i.e. lactate dehydrogenase, ferritin and neuron-specific enolase,[92,155–157] which are of great prognostic value for localized disease, are of less value for high-risk patients. However, this may be related to the inconsistent evaluation of data sets of these factors in most studies. A non-randomized study by the US Children's Cancer Group

(CCG) suggested that autologous BMT is more effective for patients with genomic amplification of *MYCN*.[158–162]

A very large number of MGT regimens have been employed since this therapeutic modality was introduced in the early 1980s. The large variety, and consequently the limited number of patients treated with each individual regimen, has hindered the ability to reach firm conclusions as to their respective anti-tumour effect and toxicity.

In patients with stage 3 or 4 neuroblastoma who achieved at least partial remission after a standardized cisplatin-containing induction regimen, a prospective randomized study of high-dose melphalan demonstrated a significant advantage at 2 years for the melphalan group, in terms of both median survival and length of the progression-free interval.[163] Most conditioning regimens proposed since then have combined melphalan with drugs and/or radiation therapy: VM-26 (teniposide), BCNU and melphalan; BCNU, cisplatin, VP-16 (etoposide) and melphalan and thiothepa; cisplatin, etoposide, adriamyacin and melphalan plus TBI; vincristine, melphalan, VP-16 and carboplatin (OMEC); melphalan plus TBI; VM-26, doxorubicin, cisplatin, melphalan and TBI; vincristine, melphalan and TBI; high-dose carboplatin and etoposide; and VAMP TBI, PEM TBI and carboplatin, etoposide, melphalan (CEM) TBI. The use of a triple alkylator regimen seems worthwhile, since despite its toxicity, the EFS of bad responders is similar to that of good responders. A double MGT procedure has been proposed in view of the frequency of early relapse following BMT. Among selected patients who are in partial remission after induction therapy and who received a double graft without TBI, there were no survivors at 2 years. This differs from the LMCE2 pilot study in which a double graft and TBI were used, which had survivors for up to 5 years. No clear advantage of a double graft was seen when compared with two additional courses prior to final MGT.[130]

TBI is still included in pre-transplant regimens to a total dose of 14 Gy. This is predicted to achieve a cell kill that is likely to eradicate micrometastases smaller than 1 mm in diameter. Tumours measuring more than 1 cm are likely to be detectable by imaging and may be treated by local radiation therapy. For tumours of intermediate size, mIBG, with its optimum cure size in millimetres, used in addition to TBI and local radiotherapy, may increase the chance of eradicating small tumour deposits. The use of mIBG in place of TBI has been proposed in pilot studies.[163] Preliminary results of the association of melphalan with TBI and mIBG demonstrate the feasibility of such a regimen.[164] The acute haematological toxicity is similar for all these regimens. The EBMT analysis does not show any significant difference in the overall toxic death rate between different regimens, but TBI may produce more long-term complications.

There is no significant difference in the PFS of patients who received an allograft rather than an autograft in either the EBMT[119] data or the International Bone Marrow Transplant Registry data. Any potential anti-tumour effect was probably lost through the increased toxicity observed, resulting in no progression-free or survival advantage in the allogeneic group. Attempts to treat MRD after MGT with IL-2 have so far not been convincing and were associated with major toxicities.[165,166] In contrast, the efficacy of differentiating agents, in particular of retinoic acid, has recently been demonstrated by a randomized CCG study.[91]

Although widely used, the role of megatherapy as a first-line treatment for all neuroblastomas in children older than 1 year at diagnosis remains, after 20 years, a matter of debate. Preliminary results from a non-randomized study of the German Neuroblastoma Study Group showed no significant advantage for autologous BMT over maintenance therapy.[156] Results from a non-randomized CCG study suggest an advantage for BMT only for patients older than 2 years at diagnosis with *MYCN* amplified tumours and at least partial remission after induction therapy.[134] The important randomized CCG trial investigated the advantage of TBI-containing high-dose chemotherapy followed by autologous SCT with purged bone marrow compared with continued therapy. Evaluating 379 patients randomly assigned to standard continuation therapy or autologous SCT, Matthay *et al.*[91] confirmed the superiority of autologous SCT over continuous consolidation chemotherapy (EFS at 3 years: 34 vs. 22 per cent; $P = 0.034$). These data provided, for the first time, evidence on the positive effect of autologous SCT in children over 1 year with high-risk neuroblastoma, confirming previously published results obtained in a retrospective comparison of two consecutive CCG studies (EFS at 4 years: 40 per cent in the autologous SCT group vs. 19 per cent in the chemotherapy group) and ENSG 1.

The EBMT analysis on MGT in relapsed disease suggests that responding patients who relapse more than 12 months from diagnosis and had not received previous MGT benefit from salvage MGT.[137] Relapse patients who do not fulfil these criteria gain no advantage from this intensive procedure.

EBMT DATA

A total of 2285 neuroblastoma patients with a median age of 3.9 (0.4–18) years at MGT are registered in the EBMT database. EBMT data represent a selected patient cohort reflecting the outcome only in patients reaching the decision point to undergo the MGT procedure. The latter is quite variable in terms of indication, pretreatment response status and type of MGT. Nonetheless, the data may be used as an instrument to design forthcoming prospective studies to investigate certain questions in depth.[161] The EBMT data analysis on behalf of the Paediatric Working Party (PWP) confirms for

Table 26.2 *Paediatric Working Party – European Bone Marrow Transplant Group 2002 analysis for neuroblastoma*

Factors	Patient numbers	5-year OS	P
MGT during primary treatment	1882	0.38 ± 0.01	<0.001
MGT after relapse	222	0.28 ± 0.03	
CR1	809	0.40 ± 0.02	<0.001
PR, VGPR	964	0.36 ± 0.02	
PD	40	0.32 ± 0.09	
SD	47	0.32 ± 0.09	
CR2	97	0.48 ± 0.06	<0.001
Relapse untreated	19	0	
SR	81	0.18 ± 0.05	
RR	23	0.07 ± 0.06	
<1 year	12	0.78 ± 0.14	<0.001
1–2 years	265	0.58 ± 0.03	
≥2 years	2008	0.33 ± 0.13	
Single MGT	1984	0.37 ± 0.01	0.071
Repetitive MGT	301	0.31 ± 0.03	
Single MGT			
TBI−	830	0.37 ± 0.02	0.002
TBI+	351	0.32 ± 0.03	
MGT during primary treatments			
Busulphan/melphalan without CYC/TTP	205	0.53 ± 0.05	<0.001
Busulphan/melphalan with CYC/TTP	98	0.35 ± 0.05	
Melphalan alone	157	0.35 ± 0.04	
Melphalan+	194	0.32 ± 0.04	
TBI	297	0.33 ± 0.03	
Others	39	0.46 ± 0.08	

CR, complete remission (CR1 = first, CR2 = second); CYC, cyclophosphamide; MGT, megatherapy; OS, overall survival; PD, progressive disease; PR, partial remission; RR, resistant relapse; SD, stable disease; SR, sensitive relapse; TBI, total body irradiation; TTP, thiotepa; VGPR, very good partial remission.

neuroblastoma the necessity of responding disease prior to the MGT procedure, the influence of age and the lack of impact of repetitive MGT approaches or TBI-containing regimens. The most interesting result from the registry is that, with growing statistical power, the busulphan/melphalan approach leads to a significantly improved survival rate in comparison with any other combination (Table 26.2).

Most investigators currently agree on the following:

- Peripheral blood progenitor cells are preferable to bone marrow progenitors, particularly because of the rapid recovery of the peripheral blood count they induce, which lowers the procedure-related morbidity.[162–160]
- Children should be spared TBI, given its severe toxicity on organ development and risk of secondary cancer.[138]

Box 26.1 *The definition of high-risk neuroblastoma patients and eligibility for megatherapy (MGT) in 2002*

First-line high-risk patients

Neuroblastoma patients over the age of 1 year are eligible for MGT as part of first-line treatment if they are stage 4 at diagnosis or stages 2–4 when diagnosed at any age with *MYCN* amplified tumour

At relapse

Any metastatic relapse in patients over the age of 1 year and any patient with *MYCN* amplified tumour, not having received previous MGT

- Data from a number of sources support the use of myeloablative therapy.[62,75] The most encouraging of these is the CCG 3891 protocol (although limited to the 3-year EFS).[91]

The definition of high-risk patients and eligibility for MGT in 2002 are given in Box 26.1.

EUROPEAN PROSPECTIVE RANDOMIZED TRIAL: THE HR-NBL-1/ESIOP STUDY

Currently the European Neuroblastoma SIOP Study Group is investigating (i) two MGT regimens and (ii) the role of additional immunotherapy. After a rapid dose induction schedule (rapid COJEC), based on the results of the randomized study ENSG5, and surgery, two MGT regimens are randomized. CEM (carboplatin, etoposide, melphalan) is considered as the US standard MGT regimen and is currently used in the US in the ongoing COG study for high-risk neuroblastoma. Its background is the observation that the CEM-LI regimen as published by Villablanca *et al.*, based on 77 patients in first response, resulted in a 3-year EFS of 65 per cent, whereas the CEM-TBI regimen (as used in the CCG trial), including 43 patients, had a 3-year EFS rate of only 40 per cent.

The busulphan/melphalan (BUMEL) approach is regarded as the 'European' regimen. The single centre multivariate analysis on prognostic factors as published by Hartmann *et al.* was performed on data sets of 218 metastatic neuroblastoma patients over 1 year of age[143] with skeletal disease in 79 per cent of cases and bone marrow involvement in 93 per cent. *MYCN* oncogene amplification was found in 27 per cent of the patients studied. The probability of EFS at 5 years post-diagnosis was 29 per cent in this series. Three major favourable prognostic factors were significant and independent: age under 2 years at diagnosis ($P < 0.01$), absence of bone marrow metastases at diagnosis ($P < 0.04$) and the MGT regimen containing the BUMEL combination ($P = 0.001$).

The quality of response to conventional primary chemotherapy was close to significance ($P = 0.053$).

The hypothesis in the HR-NBL-1/ESIOP study is that, based on the Institut Gustave Roussy and EBMT data, BUMEL may provide an improvement in the 3-year EFS after rapid COJEC induction. MGT toxicity-related risks are, in particular, gut and pulmonary toxicity for the CEM regimen, while in the BUMEL regimen anticipated risks are particularly related to veno-occlusive disease (VOD),[167–170] pulmonary toxicity (although this is very unusual without the use of alkylating agents prior to the BUMEL regimen), cutaneous acute toxicities and the additional disadvantage of infertility, in particular ovarian failure in females.

Those eligible are first-line patients in CR/VGPR/PR with both a morphologically cleared BM and a skeletal mIBG response of more than 50 per cent and not more than a maximum of three residual mIBG-positive spots. MGT is followed by local radiation treatment and differentiation treatment. The rationale for using 13-cis-retinoic acid as adjuvant treatment is based on numerous reports that it is effective in inducing neuroblastoma differentiation and apoptosis *in vitro*. The result of the CCG trial revealed a clear increase in the survival rate 3 years after randomization among the 130 patients assigned to receive 13-cis-retinoic acid, in contrast to the 129 patients receiving no further therapy (46 ± 6 vs. 29 ± 5 per cent, $P = 0.027$).[134]

The second randomization will investigate additional immunotherapy in randomizing the application of the chimeric monoclonal antibody ch 4.18, which recognizes the ganglioside GD_2 expressed by virtually all neuroblastoma cells.[80] This antibody induces killing of tumour cells *in vitro* by both antibody-dependent cellular cytotoxicity and complement-dependent cellular cytotoxicity.[171]

SARCOMAS

Soft tissue sarcomas

Soft tissue sarcomas (STSs) are highly malignant tumours that constitute 5–6 per cent of all malignant childhood neoplasms. Of these, rhabdomyosarcoma (RMS) is the most common in children and has a characteristic two-peak age incidence, at 2–5 and 15–19 years. In STSs, diagnosis and therapy are complicated by their large inherent heterogeneity. Major progress in the accuracy of diagnosis and classification has been made by the identification of specific, recurring genetic alterations: t(2;13)(q35;q14) and t(1;13)(p36;q14) in alveolar RMS; t(X;18)(p11;q11) for synovial sarcoma (SS); and t(11;22)(q24;q12) or t(21;22)(q22;q12) for Ewing's family of tumours. As a result of large multicentre STS studies, such as the North American Intergroup Rhabdomyosarcoma Study, the German Paediatric Soft Tissue Sarcoma Study Group (CWS), the Gruppo Cooperativo Italiano study and the Société Internationale d'Oncologie Pédiatrique (SIOP) Malignant Mesenchymal Tumours study,[172] more effective treatment strategies have been identified and an improvement in prognosis has been achieved in the last 30 years.[173] STSs have an EFS of between 50 and 80 per cent: RMS, 70 per cent; extraosseous Ewing's sarcoma (EOE) and peripheral primitive neuroectodermal tumour (pPNET), ~50 per cent; and SS, 70–80 per cent.[174]

About one-fifth of patients with newly diagnosed RMS-like STSs have metastatic disease. The 5-year survival rate among these patients is low (20–30 per cent). Even with recent regimens that include platinum compounds, etoposide and ifosfamide, the long-term survival decreases to 20 per cent in patients with metastases or unfavourable alveolar histology. A recent study from the Intergroup Rhabdomyosarcoma Study Group based on 128 patients investigated two novel drug pairs in a phase II window therapy of 12 weeks [vincristine and melphalan (VM) vs. ifosfamide and etoposide (IE)], followed by vincristine, dactinomycin and cyclophosphamide (VAC) chemotherapy, surgery and irradiation, with continuation of either VM or IE in patients with initial response. Failure-free survival (FFS) and overall survival (OS) at 3 years were significantly better with the IE-containing regimen (FFS: 33 vs. 19 per cent; $P = 0.043$; OS: 55 vs. 27 per cent; $P = 0.012$). IE is included in current treatment strategies for metastatic RMS.[175]

In relapsed or resistant patients, high-dose melphalan achieved good response rates in phase II studies. However, only short durations of response were experienced, and there were only a few long-term survivors. Thus there is a need for salvage programmes in patients with resistant disease prior to MGT. One of these is the use of escalated doses of topotecan and cyclophosphamide to enhance anti-tumour effect (cyclophosphamide $4200 \, mg/m^2$ by 48-hour infusion, and topotecan $6 \, mg/m^2$ by 72-hour infusion). The recommended dosages of topotecan and cyclophosphamide in combination for prior-treated patients (3.75 and $1250 \, mg/m^2$ in children, and 5 and $600 \, mg/m^2$ in adults, respectively) are well below those of each agent when used singly. Partial or minor responses were noted in neuroblastoma, desmoplastic small round-cell tumour, Ewing's sarcoma, RMS and osteosarcoma.

The VETOPEC regimen [comprising vincristine, $0.05 \, mg/kg$, on days 1 and 14; etoposide, $2.5 \, mg/kg$ on days 1, 2 and 3; and fractionated, dose-escalated cyclophosphamide on days 1, 2 and 3 – the initial cyclophosphamide dose was $90 \, mg/kg$ ($2.7 \, g/m^2$) per cycle escalated to a maximum (over six cycles) of $165 \, mg/kg$ ($5.0 \, g/m^2$ per cycle)], with its intense scheduling, produced a high response rate and appreciable survival in patients with a variety of recurrent, progressive or advanced solid tumours of childhood. The combined and partial response rates were 66 per cent (25 of 38 patients) and 91 per cent (10 of 11 patients), respectively.

There are still many phase II studies on MGT reported in this subset of patients, all indicating that response rates to MGT approaches are observed but translate to prolonged survival only in a very few patients.

High-dose chemotherapy regimens use either melphalan alone within a dose range of $180–220 \, mg/m^2$, sometimes preceded by a priming cycle of low-dose cyclophosphamide, or etoposide intensified with carboplatin.[176–179]

The European Collaborative MMT4-91 trial was conducted as a prospective non-randomized study to evaluate the potential benefit of high-dose melphalan as consolidation of first complete remission in children with stage IV RMS. Fifty-two patients in complete remission after six courses of chemotherapy received 'megatherapy': 42 received melphalan alone, and 10 received melphalan in combination with etoposide, carboplatin/etoposide or thiotepa/busulphan and etoposide. The outcome of this group of patients was compared with that observed in 44 patients who were also in complete remission after six courses of identical chemotherapy (plus surgery or radiotherapy) but who went on to receive a total of up to 12 courses of conventional chemotherapy (four cycles). The groups were comparable regarding clinical characteristics and presentation of disease, chemotherapy received before complete remission, and response to chemotherapy. The 3-year EFS and OS rates were 29.7 and 40 per cent, respectively, for those receiving high-dose melphalan or other multiagent high-dose regimens, and 19.2 and 27.7 per cent, respectively, for those receiving standard chemotherapy. The difference was not statistically significant ($P = 0.3$ and $P = 0.2$ for EFS and OS, respectively). There was, however, a significant prolongation in the time from the last day of high-dose chemotherapy or the end of chemotherapy cycle 4 to the time of relapse in those receiving MGT. The addition of a high-dose alkylating agent to consolidation therapy may have prolonged PFS in this poor-risk patient group, but it did not significantly improve the ultimate outcome in this series.[180]

Nineteen high-risk patients (RMS, undifferentiated sarcomas, Ewing's sarcoma) in complete or partial remission received consolidation with high-dose melphalan and etoposide followed by autologous BMT. The 2-year OS was 56 per cent [95 per cent confidence interval (CI), 36–76 per cent] and the PFS was 53 per cent for the whole group (95% CI = 33–73 per cent). Consolidation of response by myeloablative chemotherapy was well tolerated.[181]

A phase II study of high-dose thiotepa ($900\,mg/m^2$) and SCR in 18 patients previously treated with conventional therapy for metastatic or refractory malignant mesenchymal tumours gave a response rate of 33 per cent. This encouraged the combination of thiotepa with further drugs known to be effective at high dose.[182,183]

In patients with extensive, unresectable RMS at diagnosis who could not receive radiation to all areas of disease based on concerns of marrow reserve, but who were in CR prior to MGT, a combination of thiotepa $900\,mg/m^2$, cyclophosphamide $4500\,mg/m^2$ and carboplatin $1200\,mg/m^2$ followed by SCR was investigated. Only one of the four patients was alive without evidence of disease 53 months post-PBSCR; the others died of progressive disease.[184,185]

A Japanese study increased the dose intensity to nearly the maximum for each drug, using a double regimen with a single graft, i.e. two cycles of administration of a combination of thiotepa ($300–600\,mg/m^2$) plus melphalan ($70–150\,mg/m^2$) with a 1-week interval (and busulphan in addition in brain tumour patients). Advanced or chemotherapy-resistant solid tumour patients were included (seven RMS, four hepatoblastoma, three neuroblastoma and four other). According to the results of the dose-escalating study, the maximum tolerable doses of TEPA and melphalan for children aged 2 years or older were 1000 and $280\,mg/m^2$, respectively. This approach seemed to reduce adverse effects compared with previously reported regimens with these drugs. Among 13 patients who received MGT during CR, 10 were alive with no evidence of disease (15–59 months, median, 35 months), and in 13 evaluable patients without CR, six were alive without regrowth of the disease (14–59 months, median 39 months). With regard to the effect on outcome, the results of this study seem to be encouraging.[186]

The data on busulphan/melphalan in STS are very limited and no conclusion may be drawn today on the efficacy of this regimen. This is a particularly interesting question since this combination appears superior when used in Ewing's tumours and neuroblastoma according to the EBMT data.[187]

Based on the high response rate described in the recent phase II trial by the US Pediatric Oncology Group (POG), MGT with the ifosfamide/carboplatin/etoposide (ICE) regimen was designed.[188] Despite a high morbidity, the association of carboplatin with cyclophosphamide and etoposide obtained a 70 per cent response rate in 28 paediatric sarcomas.[189]

Other groups have chosen TBI-containing regimens in combination with melphalan or the high-dose VACA (vincristine, Adriamycin, cyclophosphamide, actinomycin D), strategy reported by Miser.[190–193] The VACA/TBI regimen produced a response rate of 93 per cent and a survival rate of 45 per cent, but it was observed at a rather short median follow-up of 1 year.

In the German Cooperative Soft Tissue Sarcoma Studies CWS-81, CWS-86, CWS-91 and CWS-96, patients with primary metastatic tumours represent about 20 per cent of registered patients with RMS-like STS (RMS, Ewing's sarcoma family of tumours and undifferentiated sarcoma). The 5-year survival rate among these patients is low (20–30 per cent) despite the use of intensive chemotherapy with or without haemopoietic stem cell rescue (HSCR). In the ongoing study CWS-96, the CEVAIE regimen (carboplatin, vincristine, ifosfamide, VP-16, epirubicin) was followed by two therapy options: double MGT (MGT1, cyclophosphamide/thiotepa; and MGT2, melphalan/VP-16) with HSCR or oral maintenance therapy with VP-16/idarubicin and trophosphamide. A preliminary analysis did not show any advantage for MGT. The median time to relapse in patients with clinical remission after double MGT was 5.7 (3–9) months. In comparison, the median time to relapse in patients on oral maintenance was 7 months. The major cause of treatment failure was malignancy, recurring in one of the previously known tumour sites. Thus the good response, as measured by reduction of tumour mass, was not translated into improved survival. The prognostic factors in 201 patients with primary metastatic tumours treated according to CWS-81, CWS-86, CWS-91 and CWS-96 were age (>10 years, $P < 0.003$) and bone/bone marrow metastases ($P < 0.014$). Patients with stage IV, >10 years with bone and/ or bone marrow (B/BM) metastases had a survival rate at 5 years of 6 ± 4 per cent. In contrast, the outcome of metastatic patients <10 years of age without B/BM metastases was much better, with a cure rate of 41 ± 7 per cent. Histology, single vs. multiorgan metastases and consolidation with MGT were not related to prognosis.

Thirty-six patients (22 alveolar RMS, 13 embryonal RMS and one undifferentiated sarcoma) underwent MGT for primary metastatic disease (27 patients) or a relapse of a primary localized tumour (nine patients). Patients were given MGT $\pm$ TBI and SCR in first or second CR or VGPR. MGT consisted of melphalan ($120–180\,mg/m^2$), VP-16 ($40–60\,mg/kg$), carboplatin ($3 \times 400–500\,mg/m^2$) in 26 patients, 10 of whom received additional fractionated TBI. Ten patients had modifications of the above regimen. Nine patients are alive and free of disease with a median observation time of 57 (32–108) months. The median time from MGT to relapse was 4 (1–17) months. The tumour recurred in the majority of patients at previously known sites; in three cases new metastatic sites were observed. Patients with primary localized tumours who had been treated with high-dose chemotherapy because of relapse did slightly better [four out of nine alive with no evidence of disease (NED)] than patients with primary metastatic disease (five out of 27 alive with NED).[194]

A recent review summarized the published data on the use of MGT/SCR in the treatment of 389 recurrent or metastatic RMS patients; 177 patients had stage 4 disease and were treated during first complete remission (CR1). The remaining patients were treated during CR1/first partial remission (PR1) (110 patients), CR2/PR2 (53 patients), CR2 (12 patients), CR3 (one patient) or treated with disease (36 patients). Patients treated during CR1 or CR1/PR1 had EFS rates ranging from 24 to 29 per cent at 3–6 years from diagnosis and OS rates ranging from 20 to 40 per cent at 2–6 years after diagnosis according to data provided as Kaplan–Meier estimates. Patients treated during CR2, CR3 or with evidence of disease had a worse outcome with an estimated 3-year OS of 12 per cent ($n = 51$). Based on these data, there does not appear to be a significant advantage to undergoing MGT with SCR for patients with relapsed or refractory high-risk RMS. Thus, there is a need for incorporating new treatment strategies for patients with high-risk RMS.[195]

Studies in STS have been reviewed recently by different authors and should be translated into cooperative trials.[196–198] Further pilot studies are currently underway but there is a need for a randomized international study based on clear definitions of poor prognosis patients and evaluating the place of TBI and/or immunotherapy.[199]

EBMT DATA

The EBMT analysis now includes almost 600 patients in the age group up to 18 years (Table 26.3) and suggests that the following factors predict a better outcome:

- treatment in first remission
- complete response status prior to the MGT procedure
- age <10 years.

No improved survival is seen either with the use of repetitive regimens or with TBI. So far no superior MGT regimen may be identified in the data sets.

The EBMT–CWS experience

A multivariate analysis of the 269 patients with metastatic RMS registered in the EBMT data base or in the German/Austrian/Swiss Paediatric Stem Cell Transplantation Registry and treated with MGT revealed similar prognostic factors: age ($\geq$10 years, $P < 0.0001$) and B/BM involvement ($P < 0.019$) as the most important predictors for fatal outcome. The 3-year EFS for 78 patients with B/BM metastases of RMS or EOE/pPNET registered in CWS-81–91 and/or the EBMT registry was 9 per cent. The survival rate in patients with MGT it was 16 per cent, and in patients without MGT it was 6 per cent ($P < 0.01$).

Table 26.3 *Paediatric Working Party – European Bone Marrow Transplant Group 2002 data on soft tissue sarcomas*

Factors	Patient numbers	5-year OS	P
MGT during primary treatment	379	0.35 ± 0.03	0.018
MGT after relapse	201	0.25 ± 0.04	
Primary treatment			
Local disease	56	0.46 ± 0.07	0.049
Metastatic disease	149	0.37 ± 0.04	
Response			
CR1	251	0.42 ± 0.04	<0.001
PR	92	0.23 ± 0.05	
SD, PD	31	0.12 ± 0.07	
CR2	115	0.29 ± 0.06	<0.001
RR	33	0.16 ± 0.07	
SR	48	0.23 ± 0.07	
<3 years	81	0.37 ± 0.06	<0.001
3–10 years	274	0.41 ± 0.03	
≥10 years	288	0.19 ± 0.03	
Single MGT	543	0.31 ± 0.02	
Repetitive MGT	104	0.29 ± 0.07	
Single MGT			
TBI−	258	0.37 ± 0.04	0.024
TBI+	30	0.16 ± 0.07	

CR, complete remission (CR1 = first, CR2 = second); MGT, megatherapy; OS, overall survival; PD, progressive disease; PR, partial remission; RR, resistant relapse; SD, stable disease; SR, sensitive relapse; TBI, total body irradiation.

A similar poor prognosis was seen in patients with alveolar RMS and all patients with RMS-like tumours who developed metastatic or combined relapse. In the CWS studies, the 5-year EFS rates were only 6–8 per cent. Thus, it became evident that neither the conventional dose escalation nor the intensification of chemotherapy with a dose level which requires SCR altered the prognosis of patients with primary metastatic STS, especially the high-risk group with B/BM metastases (see Box 26.2) or patients with metastatic relapse.

FUTURE DIRECTIONS

Identification of novel strategies which could eradicate chemotherapy-resistant tumour cells is needed. Several therapeutic approaches are currently investigating whether residual tumour cells can be eradicated by autologous or allogeneic cellular immunotherapy and/or by prolonged low-dose chemotherapy. Many types of STS are characterized by specific chromosomal translocations which may be considered as targets for immunotherapeutic approaches. Allogeneic transplantation avoids the risk of reinfusion of malignant cells, and may

Box 26.2 *High-risk features in soft tissue sarcoma*

At diagnosis
- Primary refractory disease
- Metastatic disease
- Age ≥10 years at diagnosis
- Bone/bone marrow metastases

At relapse
- Any metastatic if no previous megatherapy
- Histologies at high risk: alveolar rhabdomyosarcoma (RMS)/RMS-like tumours

Box 26.3 *High-risk features in osteosarcoma*

- Histology poor or non-response in the primary tumour at the time of definitive surgery
- Inoperable, central tumours (large volume)
- Primary metastatic patients (in particular those without complete surgical resection and with multiple metastases)
- Relapse patients other than isolated, late lung metastases

act in addition to the cytoreduction from MGT through a potential GvT effect (although evidence for this is still scarce and limited to small numbers of single case report observations).

Recently, peripheral allogeneic, not fully HLA-compatible stem cells mobilized with cytokines and highly purified have been established as a very promising source of haemopoietic progenitors. This type of haemopoietic rescue has several advantages over conventional sources for many reasons:

- the high numbers of progenitors available
- facilitation of engraftment across the MHC barrier by 10- to 60-fold doses of CD34+ cells
- avoidance of GvHD (without immunosuppressive therapy) but maintaining possible GvT effects
- rapid and functionally competent reconstitution of the T, B and NK compartment in paediatric recipients
- novel GvT effector mechanism, unique to HLA haplotype-mismatched SCR
- possibility of adoptive transfer of donor effector cells.

As consolidation therapy, several experimental therapeutic options are of interest:

- high-dose busulphan-containing therapy with autologous SCR and vaccination with autologous dendritic cells
- oral maintenance therapy
- alloimmunotherapy with reduced intensity conditioning and HLA-matched related donor (common EBMT, PWP and STWP study)
- chemo-alloimmunotherapy (busulphan-containing dose-intensive regimen) and HLA-matched or 1–3 loci mismatched familial donor.

Chimeric genes can be used as genetic markers in highly sensitive polymerase chain reaction (PCR)-based assays for detecting minimal metastatic disease (MMD) and MRD. This type of monitoring should be used for all patients with translocation-positive sarcomas to evaluate whether the molecular remission status could be useful in evaluating adjuvant therapies.

Osteosarcoma

The patients at high risk based on the results of prospective cooperative trials are well defined and alternative rescue strategies for these patients are under investigation (see Box 26.3).[200]

A total of 1702 consecutive newly diagnosed patients with high-grade osteosarcoma of the trunk or limbs registered into the neoadjuvant studies of the Cooperative Osteosarcoma Study Group before July 1998 were entered into an analysis of demographic, tumour-related and treatment-related variables, response and survival. Actuarial 10-year OS and EFS rates were 59.8 and 48.9 per cent, respectively. Among the variables assessable at diagnosis, patient age (actuarial 10-year survival ≥40, 41.6 per cent; <40, 60.2 per cent; $P = 0.012$), tumour site (axial, 29.2 per cent; limb, 61.7 per cent; $P < 0.0001$) and primary metastases (yes, 26.7 per cent; no, 64.4 per cent; $P < 0.0001$), and, for extremity osteosarcomas, size (≥one-third, 52.5 per cent; <one-third, 66.7 per cent; $P < 0.0001$) and location within the limb (proximal, 49.3 per cent; other, 63.9 per cent; $P < 0.0001$), had significant influence on outcome. Two additional important prognostic factors were treatment-related: response to chemotherapy (poor, 47.2 per cent; good, 73.4 per cent; $P < 0.0001$) and the extent of surgery (incomplete, 14.6 per cent; macroscopically complete, 64.8 per cent; $P < 0.0001$). All factors except age maintained their significance in multivariate testing, with surgical remission and histological response emerging as the key prognostic factors. Thus tumour site and size, primary metastases, response to chemotherapy and surgical remission are of independent prognostic value in osteosarcoma.[201,202]

Recently Kager *et al.*[203] reported prognostic factors in 186 patients with high-grade osteosarcoma with clinically detectable metastases at presentation and treated on neoadjuvant Cooperative Osteosarcoma Study Group protocols.[203] Complete surgical remission was achieved in 96 patients, who reached a 5-year OS rate of 49 ± 5 per cent, while 90 patients in whom no surgical remission was achieved had an OS rate of only 4 ± 2 per cent. The site of the primary tumour (axial: $n = 20$, OS $= 5 \pm 5$ per cent vs. extremity: $n = 166$, OS $= 30 \pm 4$, $P < 0.001$) and the number of metastases (solitary: $n = 30$, OS $= 72 \pm 8$ per cent; two to five: $n = 65$, OS $= 21 \pm 5$ per cent, greater than five: $n = 89$, OS $= 18 \pm 4$ per cent, $P < 0.001$) correlated with survival. Patients whose metastases involved only one organ system had a better outcome than those with more disseminated disease (OS: 32 ± 4 per cent vs. 9 ± 5 per cent, $P < 0.001$). Patients with metastases confined to the lung had an OS of 35 ± 4 per cent (59 ± 7 per cent if unilateral involvement, and 22 ± 5 per cent if bilateral involvement, $P < 0.001$). In a multivariate Cox regression model, macroscopically incomplete surgical resection [relative hazard rate (RH) = 5.6] and multiple metastases (2–5 vs. 1: RH = 1.9, >5 vs. 1: RH = 2.3) were significantly associated with inferior outcome.

EBMT DATA

The experience with MGT in osteosarcoma is limited but growing (EBMT 2002 analysis), although disappointing. In the EBMT experience, over 100 patients in the age group up to 18 years have been submitted to a MGT procedure (Table 26.4).

Patients with osteosarcoma refractory to standard multiagent chemotherapy, including platinum compounds, doxorubicin and high-dose methotrexate, are in need of new therapeutic strategies. Combinations of carboplatin, etoposide ± ifosfamide (CE, ICE) and high-dose cyclophosphamide, etoposide (HD-CYC/VP-16) have been explored and produced response rates of up to 28 per cent.[204] However, this does not translate into cure and different strategies need further exploration. Even in responding high-risk patients treated in first or second remission, the length of remission is short and relapse occurs early after MGT.[205]

The Italian sarcoma group recently published data of a prospective study exploring the feasibility and activity of two courses of high-dose chemotherapy in patients in metastatic relapse, i.e. multiple metastases or solitary metastasis at intervals of less than 30 months. High-dose chemotherapy consisted of carboplatin and etoposide followed by stem cell rescue. The relapse or progressive disease rate was 84.4 per cent, the 3-year OS rate was 20 per cent and the 3-year disease-free survival (DFS) rate was only 12 per cent.[206]

NOVEL STRATEGIES

First reports on high-dose samarium treatment in combination with SCR suggest this as a promising option which may potentially be combined with radiosensitizing drugs.

Samarium-153 ethylene diamine tetramethylene phosphonate (^{153}Sm-EDTMP), a bone-seeking radiopharmaceutical, provides therapeutic irradiation to osteoblastic bone metastases. Because the dose-limiting toxicity of ^{153}Sm-EDTMP is thrombocytopenia, a dose-escalation trial using peripheral blood progenitor cells (PBPCs) or marrow support was conducted in patients with osteosarcoma. Patients with locally recurrent or metastatic osteosarcoma or skeletal metastases avid on bone scan were treated with 1, 3, 4.5, 6, 12, 19 or 30 mCi/kg of ^{153}Sm-EDTMP. Thirty patients were treated with ^{153}Sm-EDTMP. Transient symptoms of hypocalcaemia were seen at 30 mCi/kg. Estimates of radioisotope bound to bone surfaces and marrow radiation dose were linear with injected amount of ^{153}Sm-EDTMP. After PBPC or marrow infusion on day 14 after ^{153}Sm-EDTMP, recovery of haemopoiesis was problematic in two patients at the 30 mCi/kg dose infused with less than 2×10^6 CD34+/kg on day 14, but not in other patients. Reduction or elimination of opiates for pain was seen in all patients. Patients had no adverse changes in appetite or performance status. ^{153}Sm-EDTMP with PBPC support can provide bone-specific therapeutic irradiation (estimates of 39–241 Gy). Haematological toxicity at 30 mCi ^{153}Sm-EDTMP/kg requires PBPC grafts with more than 2×10^6 CD34+/kg to overcome myeloablative effects of skeletal irradiation. Non-haematological side-effects are minimal.[207]

The COSS study group use high activity of ^{153}Sm-EDTMP (150 MBq/kg body weight) and autologous PBSC support in patients with unresectable osteosarcomas or skeletal metastases. The combination with external radiation and polychemotherapy seems to be promising. Although osteosarcoma is believed to be relatively radio-resistant, the total focal dose achieved may delay local progression or even achieve permanent local tumour control in patients with a surgically inaccessible primary or relapsing tumours.[208–211]

Ewing's sarcoma

Since the 1970s, aggressive cytotoxic treatment regimens have increased survival rates to 55–65 per cent in localized disease, and up to 35 per cent in primary metastatic

Table 26.4 *European Bone Marrow Transplant Group 2002 data on osteosarcoma*

Factors	Patient numbers	5-year OS	P
Megatherapy (MGT) during primary treatment	50	0.24 ± 0.09	NS
MGT after relapse	72	0.17 ± 0.07	
Single MGT	94	0.19 ± 0.06	NS
Repetitive MGT	43	0.17 ± 0.09	

OS, overall survival.

disease. Staging procedures as presently applied identify 20–25 per cent of cases as metastatic at diagnosis.

The following drugs and/or combinations of drugs proved to be effective and are in current use: VAC (vincristine, actinomycin D, cyclophosphamide), VACA (VAC plus doxorubicin alternating with actinomycin D), the Intergroup Ewing's Sarcoma Study (IESS) II schedule (alternating the combination of ifosfamide plus etoposide and VACA), VAIA and EVAIA (ifosfamide replacing cyclophosphamide in VACA, either without or with additional etoposide).[212–216]

RISK FEATURES ACCORDING TO PROSPECTIVE NATIONAL TRIALS

Recent publications suggest that the type of chromosomal rearrangement has an independent prognostic impact. Other known prognostic factors in localized disease include tumour volume, tumour site (pelvic/non-pelvic, axial/extremity, bone/soft tissue), histological response to chemotherapy, and factors related to feasibility and choice of local treatment options.[217–221] In the UK ET-2 trial, increasing the dose of ifosfamide from 6 to 9 g/m^2 per course as compared with ET-1, and application of doxorubicin in all initial four courses ('IVAD3': ifosfamide 3 g/m^2/day × 3, vincristine 2 mg/m^2 × 1 dose, doxorubicin 20 mg/m^2/day × 3 days) substantially improved EFS for localized disease from 0.44 in ET-1 to 0.62.[222]

Ten to 20 per cent DFS has been reported in patients with initial metastatic disease who received conventional therapy.[223–225] The prognosis for patients with newly diagnosed metastatic Ewing's sarcoma depends on the site. Patients with lung and multifocal primary bone metastases have a 35 and 0 per cent EFS, respectively, at 5 years.[128] Prognostic factors include site(s) of metastatic disease and responsiveness to chemotherapy. The prognosis of patients with bone or bone marrow metastases (B/BM) remains poor (11 per cent at 3 years) despite the addition of new agents in induction.[129] In the US CCG 7881 study, patients with B/BM metastases at diagnosis had a 3-year DFS of less than 15 per cent compared with 22 per cent for any metastatic site (CCG 7951 treatment manual, 1996). Kushner et al. reported that patients with pulmonary metastases fared better than patients with BM involvement.[215] These findings are comparable to experiences from previous CESS and EICESS studies.[226–230]

The EFS is 31 per cent at 5 years for late relapses (more that 2 years post-diagnosis) compared with 5 per cent for those relapsing earlier. Despite a 54 per cent response rate to phase II trials with ifosfamide and etoposide, only 10 per cent of relapse patients survive.

Conventional treatment regimens induce remission, but cannot prevent relapse in patients with initial metastases. Clinically undetectable MRD leads to relapse at a median time of 1–2 years after completion of therapy. In order to consolidate remission by reduction of MRD/MMD, regimens of high-dose (myeloablative) intensification with stem cell rescue have been piloted.

High-dose melphalan as a single agent resulted in a very high response rate of more than 75 per cent, but with mainly partial responses of short duration.[231] Some patients benefit from such consolidation therapy, as evidenced by reports of up to 35 per cent 3-year survivors with primary B/BM-metastases.[226] Several myeloablative regimens including melphalan, may be effective.[232–245]

Pilot studies in patients with high-risk Ewing's sarcoma suggested that TBI may be of benefit. A regimen based on TBI combined with vincristine, doxorubicin and cyclophosphamide obtained a 26 per cent survival at 8 years for 31 metastatic patients, and 44 per cent for 34 high-risk non-metastatic patients.[227] For patients with multifocal primary or early relapse, the probability of relapse-free survival 7 years after the last event is 40 per cent (compared with 0 per cent in a comparable control group) after a MGT regimen that obtained fractionated TBI with melphalan and etoposide.[226]

Promising data are available with the use of high-dose busulphan combined with melphalan or other agents.[234,239–241] Preliminary results using triple alkylating therapy (melphalan, busulphan, thiotepa) followed by TBI, administered after recovery of the triple alkylating megatherapy, are encouraging.[229]

The German CESS/EICESS reported on 131 Ewing's tumour patients who underwent MGT, 79 with primary metastases and 52 with relapsed tumours. MGT was mainly based on melphalan and/or etoposide (92 per cent). The subgroup of patients with initial lung and bone metastases seemed to benefit from MGT with an EFS 5 years after diagnosis of 34 per cent compared with 5 per cent ($P = 0.0001$). The outcome of patients with an early Ewing's tumour relapse (<2 years) was also improved by MGT (EFS 4 years after relapse: 17 vs. 2 per cent, $P = 0.0001$). The total group of metastatic Ewing's tumour patients showed no obvious benefit from high-dose chemotherapy, based on melphalan and/or etoposide. However, patients with metastases to multiple organ systems and early relapse seemed to benefit from high-dose chemotherapy.[242]

Therapy of metastatic Ewing's sarcomas was recently reviewed by Pinkerton et al.,[243] who compared the results of 12 papers on conventional dose chemotherapy and seven papers on autologous SCT. Although tolerable for high-risk patients, megatherapy regimens followed by autologous SCT have failed to show a clear benefit (EFS between 14 per cent at 6 years, and 21 per cent at 5 years in metastatic disease) over more recent chemotherapy regimens, including increased doses of alkylating agents and anthracyclines (relapse-free survival 20–30 per cent).

Furthermore, a CCG study could not demonstrate any benefit of autologous SCT in CR/VGPR high-risk patients, with only 24 per cent DFS at 2 years.[244] This is in contrast to the EBMT registry updated data (Table 26.5).

In order to evaluate a possible therapeutic benefit after allogeneic SCT in patients with advanced Ewing's tumours, outcomes after autologous and allogeneic SCT were compared in patients treated with the myeloablative hyper-ME protocol (hyperfractionated TBI, melphalan, etoposide ± carboplatin); 10/36 patients were treated with allogeneic haemopoietic stem cells. According to the type of graft, EFS was 0.25 ± 0.08 after autologous SCT and 0.20 ± 0.13 after allogeneic SCT. Incidence of toxic death was more than twice as high after allogeneic SCT (40 per cent) than after autologous (19 per cent) SCT.[245]

Additional benefit has been claimed for immuno-therapy post-transplant, either through the graft-versus-host effect of allogeneic transplant, or by IL-2/LAK therapy.

Table 26.5 *Paediatric Working Party – European Bone Marrow Transplant Group 2002 data on Ewing's tumours*

Factors	Patient numbers	5-year OS	*P*
MGT during primary treatment	589	0.47 ± 0.03	<0.001
MGT after relapse	262	0.29 ± 0.03	
Primary treatment			
Metastatic disease	195	0.38 ± 0.04	0.002
Local disease	63	0.63 ± 0.08	
Response			
CR1, VGPR	374	0.53 ± 0.03	<0.001
PR	179	0.39 ± 0.04	
SD, PD	32	0.19 ± 0.07	
CR2	133	0.40 ± 0.05	<0.001
Relapse untreated	14	0	
RR	33	0.13 ± 0.07	
SR	76	0.21 ± 0.06	
Single MGT	799	0.41 ± 0.02	0.036
Repetitive MGT	125	0.25 ± 0.06	
TBI−	378	0.44 ± 0.03	0.038
TBI+	89	0.35 ± 0.05	
Primary treatments			
Busulphan	200	0.60 ± 0.04	<0.001
Melphalan	31	0.29 ± 0.10	
TBI	52	0.34 ± 0.07	
Other	16	0.35 ± 0.17	

CR, complete remission (CR1 = first, CR2 = second); MGT, megatherapy; PR, partial remission; OS, overall survival; PD, progressive disease; RR, resistant relapse; SD, stable disease; SR, sensitive relapse; TBI, total body irradiation; VGPR, very good partial remission.

Considering the reported results of conventional chemotherapy, the place of high-dose chemotherapy and autologous BMT is still unclear.[155,246] There is an evident need for randomized studies comparing aggressive conventional protocols with MGT to define the best approach for these patients.

EBMT DATA

In 1995, 65 high-risk Ewing's tumour patients registered on the EBMT data base and achieving a first or second CR (CR1 or CR2) were analysed. Thirty-two patients with metastatic disease at diagnosis (22 had B/BM metastases) and consolidated in CR1 reached an EFS of 21 per cent at 5 years. Thirty-one patients in CR2 achieved an actuarial EFS of 32 per cent at 5 years. Favourable outcome was limited to relapsed patients with localized disease at initial diagnosis. Distant relapse had a more favourable prognosis than local failure. At that time it appeared that MGT may contribute to improved EFS rates in high-risk patients in comparison with historical experience.[235]

By 2002 the data had grown to more than 800 patients below the age of 18 and the EBMT registry data now hold important messages (Table 26.5). In the EBMT data set, busulphan as part of various MGT regimens appears to improve results in high-risk patients. Its role is even more pronounced when used during primary treatment. The Euro Ewing 99 study is currently investigating prospectively the role of busulphan/melphalan in high-risk patients eligible for a MGT approach (see Box 26.4). Overall the survival data appear improved in comparison with earlier analysis, which is probably related to the wider use of busulphan in MGT approaches throughout Europe. No advantage, either for TBI or for repetitive MGT courses, is suggested by this data set.

Box 26.4 *Definition of high-risk Ewing's tumour patients and eligibility for megatherapy (MGT)*

First-line high-risk patients
- Patients with poor histological response after induction (≥ 10 per cent viability in resected tumour) (R2 Euro Ewing 99)
- Patients with a tumour volume ≥ 200 ml (R2 Euro Ewing 99)
- Patients with primary lung metastases only (R2 Euro Ewing 99)
- Patients with primary metastatic disease other than lungs only (R3 in Euro Ewing 99)

At relapse
- Any metastatic if no previous MGT

ONGOING EUROPEAN PROSPECTIVE TRIAL

Cooperative groups participating in the Euro-Ewing 99 protocol are the UKCCSG (United Kingdom Children's Cancer Study Group), GPOH (Gesellschaft für Pädiatrische Onkologie und Hämatologie), SFOP (Société Française d'Oncologie Pédiatrique), EORTC-STBSG (European Organisation for Research and Treatment of Cancer – Soft Tissue and Bone Sarcoma Group), and SIAK (Schweizerisches Institut für Angewandte Krebsforschung). The high-dose therapy and stem cell rescue part of this study is carried out in cooperation with the EBMT.

Based on the experience of ET-1, ET-2, EW88, EW93, CESS81, CESS86, EICESS92 and other European studies, patients are stratified according to the following prognostic indicators:

- presence or absence of metastatic disease (CESS/ EICESS EFS rates: no metastases 0.41, lung metastases 0.31, other metastases 0.18, $P = 0.0001$)
- site of metastases – pulmonary/pleural only metastases or other sites of metastatic involvement (bone, bone marrow)
- feasibility of local therapy options and histological response to chemotherapy (in locoregional disease)
- initial tumour volume (in locoregional disease) of <200 mL or >200 mL in patients not eligible for surgery as primary modality of local control.

The relevance of the histological response of the primary tumour to initial chemotherapy in both localized and systemic disease stresses the value of high-intensity induction treatment in Ewing's tumour patients.

Patients with more than 10 per cent viable tumour cells at surgery following neoadjuvant chemotherapy (not radiochemotherapy) in the previous CESS/EICESS studies had a less favourable outcome, with an EFS of 0.47 after 10 years. Patients with good histological response (<10 per cent viable tumour cells) after chemotherapy alone had a prognosis of about 0.70 after 10 years. In a combined analysis, accumulating data on surgically treated patients from the CESS/EICESS and the SFOP EW studies (Euro-Ewing 99 protocol, analysis dated August 1998), the impact of histological response was more prominent than the impact of tumour volume. The 5-year EFS rates according to tumour volume and response showed the following correlations: patients with good response, i.e. less than 10 per cent of viable tumour cells, had a comparable outcome after 5 years independent of their tumour size, while patients with poor histology response had a worse outlook with EFS rates of 45–50 per cent according to tumour volume. Histological response was thus demonstrated to have significant influence on outcome ($P < 0.0001$).

Selected high-risk patients will be randomly assigned to either consolidation therapy or MGT with busulphan/melphalan (so-called R2 randomization). Those eligible for this R2 randomization are patients with resected localized tumours of any initial tumour volume but poor histological response to induction (≥10 per cent viability), unresectable localized tumours and all patients with pulmonary/pleural metastases at diagnosis. Patients with metastases at other sites are excluded.

WILMS' TUMOUR

Major multi-institutional studies [International Society of Paediatric Oncology (SIOP), National Wilms' Tumor Studies in the US (NWTS) and the Medical Research Council in the United Kingdom (MRC)] have adapted the intensity of multimodal treatment to the characteristics of initial disease. These efforts have raised the expectation for cure up to approximately 85 per cent of children with Wilms' tumours (WT). Hence, very few patients now experience failure, defined as local relapse, secondary metastases or refractory disease. However, even with the combination of surgery, radiotherapy and salvage multiagent chemotherapy, two-thirds of patients with these treatment failures remain incurable. In the SIOP studies 1, 2 and 5, among 293 patients with initial or subsequent metastatic disease, only 38 per cent of survivors were disease-free.[247]

Also in the NWTS 2 and 3 studies, which focused on 367 cases of stage I–IV recurrent WT, the 3-year post-relapse survival rate was only 30 ± 3 per cent.[248] Tumour histology, length of initial remission, initial therapy with two vs. three drugs, and site of relapse were each independently predictive of post-relapse survival. Subgroups with 3-year post-relapse survival rates of greater than 40 per cent included patients who had tumours of favourable histology (FH) that recurred (i) only in the lungs; (ii) in the abdomen when radiotherapy was not initially given; or (iii) that were originally stage I; (iv) that were originally treated with only two drugs; or (v) that recurred 12 months or more after diagnosis. These results were achieved with the use of standard treatments, i.e. surgery, radiotherapy and chemotherapy using dactinomycin, vincristine and doxorubicin.

Fairly similar results were observed in the first UKCCSG WT study in 17 surviving patients among 71 patients with a recurrent WT (24 per cent).[249]

High-dose melphalan produced a high rate of complete remission in relapsed patients.[179] The efficacy of thiotepa or a cisplatin-etoposide plus whole-lung irradiation or local radiotherapy regimen has also been reported.[250]

SFOP used adverse prognostic factors to select patients with very poor-risk recurrent WT. In a group of 29 paediatric high-risk recurrent (HRR) WT patients with chemotherapy-responsive disease, as well as in two additional patients with stage IV anaplastic WT consolidated in first complete response, a three-drug MGT was prospectively explored. MEC consisted of melphalan 180 mg/m^2 for 1 day, etoposide 200 mg/m^2/day for 5 days, and carboplatin at a daily targeted area under the concentration–time curve (AUC) of 4 mg/min/mL for 5 days. Autologous stem cells were reinfused 48 hours after melphalan.[251]

Twelve out of 28 assessable patients with HRR WT are still in continuous complete response at a median of 48.5 months (range, 36 to 96 months) after consolidation. DFS and OS at 3 years, as estimated by the Kaplan–Meier method, were 50 ± 17 and 60 ± 18 per cent, respectively. The MEC regimen led to a high morbidity, i.e. grade III and IV toxicities including haematological side-effects, haemorrhage, mucositis, diarrhoea, renal disorders and pneumonitis. Patient outcome is statistically better when high-dose chemotherapy is performed as early as the second complete response or partial response.

The above experience was confirmed by the German group applying the same study strategy, reporting an EFS of 51 ± 17 per cent in a cohort of defined high-risk WT patients.[252]

EBMT DATA

The first EBMT publication on WTs in 1994 referred to 25 children registered.[253] Eight out of the 17 who were grafted in complete remission remained alive and event-free 3 years post-BMT. The relapses occurred early, at a median of 6 months. The risk of pulmonary and renal toxicities was high in those patients who have been submitted to nephrectomy.

Since the last EBMT publication on WTs (2002), the EBMT cohort has increased to 184 patients under the age of 18; 57 patients have received MGT during primary treatment and 127 patients after relapse (Table 26.6).

FUTURE DIRECTIONS

Adverse prognostic factors define patients with a probability of cure of 30 per cent at best and are based on the overall experience with WT failures of the SIOP, NWTS and MRC groups over the last 20 years. The high-risk population comprises patients with unfavourable histology, those with metastatic disease and patients resistant to or relapsing after first-line treatment (Box 26.5). In the latter subgroup, poor prognostic risk factors include unfavourable histology and one of the following criteria: extrapulmonary relapse or abdominal relapse after radiation; stage IV; more than a two drug regimen; relapse

Table 26.6 *Paediatric Working Party – European Bone Marrow Transplant Group 2002 data on Wilms' tumours*

Factors	Patient numbers	5-year OS	P
MGT during primary treatment	57	0.53 ± 0.07	NS
MGT after relapse	127	0.58 ± 0.05	
Response			
CR1, VGPR	36	0.73 ± 0.08	<0.001
PR, SD	19	0.20 ± 0.11	
CR2	86	0.66 ± 0.06	
SR	25	0.38 ± 0.11	
RR, relapse untreated	15	0.37 ± 0.14	

CR, complete remission (CR1 = first, CR2 = second); MGT, megatherapy; OS, overall survival; PR, partial remission; RR, resistant relapse; SD, stable disease; SR, sensitive relapse; VGPR, very good partial remission.

Box 26.5 *High-risk features identified in Wilms' tumours*

- Metastatic disease and patients resistant to or relapsing after first-line treatment
- Unfavourable histology relapse (anaplasia, clear-cell sarcoma, rhabdoid)
- Early relapse ≤12 months
- Two or more relapses
- Thoracic or abdominal site of recurrence
- Bone or brain metastases
- Lymph nodes including relapse
- Post-irradiation, in-field relapse

within 1 year. These patients appear eligible for consolidation with MGT if response is achieved with intense two- to three-drug second-line regimens.

Recurrent WT forms a heterogeneous group because initial therapies vary widely. Given the complexity of the problem, there is a great need for a consensus with respect to a standard approach to management.[254]

The current proposal of the NWT and SFOP is a randomized study evaluating prolonged consolidation chemotherapy vs. MGT/SCR in children with recurrent tumours. Induction chemotherapy should include four ICE chemotherapy cycles, a stem cell harvest followed by surgery on the primary and/or metastatic sites. Responding patients (CR/PR) will be randomized either to receive three more ICE cycles or to undergo CEM as MGT followed by SCR. MGT dose intensity is to be modified when glomerular filtration rate is ≤100 ml/min/ 1.73m^2 or if body weight ≤12 kg. CEM consists of melphalan, etoposide (4-day continuous infusion) and carboplatin (4-day continuous infusion adapted according to the modified Calvert formula).

BRAIN TUMOURS

The outcome for children with malignant brain tumours has improved modestly in recent years. Notable is the improved 5-year DFS for those children with 'standard-risk' medulloblastoma and other primitive neuroectodermal tumours (PNET) without neuraxis dissemination at presentation. For many other children with newly diagnosed malignant brain tumours, especially in the absence of radical surgical resection, the outcome remains poor despite irradiation and conventional chemotherapy.[3] DFS for medulloblastoma and ependymoma ranges from 40 to 70 per cent. The prognosis for children with high-grade astrocytomas, including anaplastic astrocytoma and glioblastoma multiforme, is, however, hardly better than for their adult counterparts.[136] Up to 30 per cent of children with supratentorial gliomas will remain disease-free at 3 years, whereas 2-year survival is unusual for children with intrinsic diffuse brainstem gliomas. Thus, more than half of the children and adolescents with malignant brain tumours will relapse following initial therapy. Irrespective of the therapeutic modalities, the prognosis of patients with recurrent or metastatic brain tumours is still poor. These patients experience a dismal outlook with the conventional strategies of treatment. High-dose radiation therapy given to the whole neuraxis leads to major failures in growth and development failures. An additional objective of MGT in children is to delay, or even avoid, radiation therapy.

Poor prognosis of certain types of central nervous system (CNS) tumours and unacceptable long-term sequelae of radiotherapy, especially in young children, led to the development of new treatment strategies in paediatric brain tumours. In this respect, there has been much recent interest in the use of MGT. Alkylating agents appear to be the most appropriate class of drugs to be used in a high-dose setting, since they are among the most active drugs against CNS tumours and are characterized by a steep log-linear response relationship. The protocols tested in children have assessed combinations that include nitrosoureas, etoposide, thiotepa, carboplatin, busulphan, cyclophosphamide and melphalan in two- or three-drug schedules.[255-263]

Thiotepa and its major metabolite, TEPA, reach cerebrospinal fluid (CSF) concentrations that are approximately equivalent to the plasma concentrations. They show *in vitro* cytocidal activity with a steep dose–response curve against medulloblastoma and glioma CNS tumour cell lines.[259-261]

Busulphan crosses the blood–brain barrier with a cerebrospinal fluid (CSF): plasma ratio of 1.39 when given at a dose of 600 mg/m² and has displayed anti-tumour activity against medulloblastoma xenografts in athymic nude mice.

Table 26.7 *Paediatric Working Party – European Bone Marrow Transplant Group 2002 data on brain tumours*

Factors	Patient numbers	5-year OS	P
MGT during primary treatment	272	0.33 ± 0.04	NS
MGT after relapse	203	0.27 ± 0.04	
CR1	95	0.59 ± 0.07	<0.001
PR	109	0.31 ± 0.05	
SD, PD	67	0.16 ± 0.06	
CR2	77	0.37 ± 0.07	<0.001
RR	60	0.19 ± 0.06	
SR	63	0.24 ± 0.06	
<2 years	50	0.61 ± 0.08	<0.001
2–5 years	126	0.31 ± 0.05	
≥5 years	351	0.24 ± 0.03	

CR, complete remission (CR1 = first, CR2 = second); MGT, megatherapy; NS, not significant; OS, overall survival; PD, progressive disease; PR, partial remission; RR, resistant relapse; SD, stable disease; SR, sensitive relapse.

Tolerance, pharmacokinetics and pharmacodynamics of high-dose single-agent melphalan administered over two consecutive courses (C1 and C2) in children were recently investigated in those with a cerebral PNET. The melphalan AUC ranged from 177 to 475 μg min/mL (no difference between C1 and C2). Partial remission was observed in 11/14 patients with measurable cerebral PNET. Tandem high-dose melphalan is feasible and safe in children and has achieved a high response rate.[263]

Results of several of these studies have been reviewed, demonstrating durable DFS for a proportion of patients with recurrent malignant gliomas and medulloblastoma/PNETs, as well as encouraging preliminary data in newly diagnosed patients.[260,262,264–267]

EBMT DATA ON BRAIN TUMOURS

The EBMT data have been constantly growing, reaching almost 600 transplant procedures by 2002 (Table 26.7), and reflect the fairly high frequency of the use of MGT in brain tumours in the age group up to 18 years. More detailed analysis on the subtype of tumours and distinct risk factors is currently not possible on the basis of the EBMT data set. Complete response in high-risk patients and young age are the important favourable indications from these data. The eligibility for MGT in brain tumours in 2002 is shown in Box 26.6.

Malignant gliomas

The majority of schedules have included thiotepa. The association of thiotepa with busulphan, etoposide or cyclophosphamide gives a 30 per cent response rate. The addition of a third agent (BCNU or carboplatin) does

Box 26.6 *Eligibility for megatherapy in brain tumours in 2002*

Good indications
- Medulloblastoma (in CR2)
- PNETs (in CR2)
  - metastasis at diagnosis
  - additional high-risk features: incomplete resection, age (<3 years)

No indication
- Ependymoma
- Brainstem glioma

Much work is still required to define the optimal high-dose chemotherapy for each tumour type. The full impact of high-dose chemotherapy in terms not only of survival but also of quality of life of children with CNS tumours must be determined by prospective collaborative national and international studies. It is noteworthy that most groups work with similar MGT regimens, i.e. BU-TTP (± repetitive L-PAM) (SFOP, Spain), VP-16/TTP/±CBDCA (US/CCG, Germany, Spain) and a tandem approach VP-16/CBDCA-TTP/L-PAM (Italy).

not increase the response rate, but is associated with 20–30 per cent toxic deaths. The association of BCNU, thiotepa and etoposide[268] in children with glioblastomas or incompletely resected anaplastic astrocytomas, excluding brainstem lesions, produces a 50 per cent EFS, although the median follow-up is only 8 months. The toxicity of this regimen is high, particularly in patients with relapsed disease.[269] Thus MGT compares favourably with conventional chemotherapy, but the median OS and PFS durations do not demonstrate an improvement in newly diagnosed patients.[270,271] For patients with recurrent tumours, the objective response rate was similar.[272,273]

Brainstem gliomas

These have been excluded from MGT studies until recently because of the patients' poor clinical condition. SFOP has proposed the use of thiotepa and busulphan in an unselected population of children with diffuse brainstem gliomas. This MGT administered 2–3 months after focal radiotherapy in 24/35 eligible patients with brainstem glioma failed to improve their median survival time (10 months, range, 3 to 26 months). This aggressive treatment modality did not appear to be any better than that reported with conventional radiotherapy.[274,275]

Medulloblastoma

This is a chemosensitive disease, and conventional polychemotherapy [mechlorethamine, vincristine,

procarbazine, prednisone (MOPP), 'eight in one' regimen, or etoposide-carboplatin] gives response rates up to 60 per cent. Several drug combinations have been assessed with MGT. They give similar response rates (60–80 per cent) in newly diagnosed or relapsing patients. Initial encouraging evaluations of this technique in patients with recurrent disease have prompted testing of its feasibility in infants and young children.[276]

Long-term survival is unusual among relapse patients, and progression generally occurs early after MGT. This suggests that cure in medulloblastoma requires radiation therapy. However, some cases of long-term survival in newly diagnosed infants treated with MGT have been reported, using limited field radiotherapy alone to the posterior fossa. MGT might avoid the need for craniospinal radiation therapy and thus reduce subsequent neurocognitive or growth deficits. Further studies will be required to confirm these preliminary data. More recently, the use of high-dose carboplatin, thiotepa and etoposide with autologous SCR was reported in 23 patients with recurrent medulloblastoma, aged 2–44 years (median, 13 years). Seven out of 23 patients (30 per cent) are event-free survivors at a median of 54 months post-autologous SCR (range, 24 to 78 months). This strategy may provide long-term survival for some patients with recurrent medulloblastoma.[277]

The SFOP group has paid specific attention to the development of MGT in this indication. In children aged <3 years with local relapse of a medulloblastoma after surgery and conventional chemotherapy alone, the 5-year EFS after treatment with busulphan-thiotepa followed by autologous SCT and irradiation limited to the posterior fossa was 80 per cent. This high salvage rate was the basis on which to increase the age limit for a chemotherapy alone strategy at diagnosis to 5 years. The prognosis of young patients with metastatic medulloblastoma treated according to this strategy remained poor. Thus, for this group of patients, a more aggressive therapeutic schedule was developed. After surgery, patients were planned to receive two courses of etoposide (500 mg/m^2) and carboplatin (800 mg/m^2), and then two courses of melphalan (100 mg/m^2) and busulphan (480 mg/m^2) and thiotepa (720 mg/m^2). These three courses were followed by autologous SCT and irradiation of the posterior fossa alone. Eighteen patients entered this programme, and tumour response was evaluable in 13/16 who received the whole treatment (four CR and nine PR). Four patients are alive with a 5-year median follow-up. However, a very high visceral toxicity was observed after the last course, with three toxic deaths, six patients with pulmonary haemorrhage and nine with hepatic veno-occlusive disease. Despite the very high response rate and possible improvement in survival, this approach appeared too toxic. A strategy with less dose intensity of alkylating agents is in progress for young patients with metastatic medulloblastoma and PNETs.[278]

Ependymoma

Chemotherapy has been used extensively in the management of children with intracranial ependymoma, although there is little evidence that it is effective. The response rate to single agents is 11 per cent, with less than 5 per cent complete responses, cisplatin being the most active agent in phase II studies. With conventional chemotherapy, response rates do not exceed 20 per cent, and chemotherapy plays no part in standard protocols, except in very young children, in which case its primary objective is to delay radiation therapy. Only a small number of reports have described MGT in this tumour. It does not demonstrate any benefit for patients with recurrent tumours, and for newly diagnosed patients the only long-term survivors were treated in an adjuvant setting after a complete resection of their primary. Similar results have been obtained using conventional therapy. For children with residual tumours, MGT does not achieve responses that are sufficient for radiation therapy to be avoided.[279]

Sixteen patients with refractory or relapsed ependymoma were treated in the SFOP group with busulphan/thiotepa. Eight of them had previously received irradiation at the tumour site, while the eight others, <3 years at diagnosis, were treated with postoperative conventional chemotherapy. At the time of MGT, nine patients were in first relapse, five in second relapse and two in third relapse or more; all had measurable disease. Fifteen patients were evaluable for response. No radiological response >50 per cent was observed. Stable disease and progressive disease were documented in 10 and five cases, respectively. The duration of response to this treatment, which lasted for a median time of 7 months (range, 5 to 8 months), was only evaluable in five patients who did not receive further treatment after autologous BMT. There were three disease-free survivors at 15, 25 and 27 months, all of whom were treated with second complete surgical resection and local radiotherapy (55 Gy). Thus, unlike medulloblastomas, ependymomas do not appear to be sensitive to this combination therapy. As with the CCG protocol using a combination of etoposide, thiotepa ± carboplatin, no tumour response or prolonged survival was attributable to high-dose chemotherapy.[280]

Intensive chemotherapy with thiotepa, etoposide ± carboplatin and autologous BMT was not an effective strategy in heavily pretreated children with recurrent ependymoma.[281] New therapeutic approaches are warranted in this situation.

RETINOBLASTOMA

Retinoblastoma usually has a good prognosis in western countries. Survival is achieved in 90 per cent of patients by surgery and/or radiotherapy. Conventional chemotherapy is reserved for cases with locally extensive disease or disseminated disease. In some circumstances, retinoblastoma is a high-risk disease, e.g. where there is involvement of the cut end or subarachnoidal space of the optic nerve after enucleation.[282] Optic nerve invasion of retinoblastoma beyond the lamina cribrosa is associated with a greater metastatic risk. Large exophytic retinoblastoma with secondary glaucoma is at highest risk for optic nerve invasion. In addition, retrolaminar optic nerve involvement, with free resection line, and massive choroidal invasion significantly increase the risk for orbital and/or metastatic disease.[283]

Orbital involvement is a rare occurrence in retinoblastoma but still carries a bad prognosis, with a survival of 34 per cent (±8 per cent). The disease-free interval was longer when patients had no CNS disease ($P < 0.05$); 95 per cent of recurrences occurred within 1 year after diagnosis of orbital involvement. Intensive chemotherapy using cyclophosphamide, platinum compounds, epipodophyllotoxins, doxorubicin and vincristine was effective in orbital involvement of retinoblastoma, even with associated extra-CNS metastases, but still carries a bad prognosis. In addition, long-term follow-up is necessary to evaluate the risk of a second tumour.[284]

Cyclophosphamide has been shown to be very active as a single drug in extraocular retinoblastoma. A more recent study of the activity of a combination of etoposide and carboplatin in extraocular retinoblastoma showed a very high response rate. The response rates achieved with conventional chemotherapy[285–288] are the basis for using MGT in high-risk retinoblastoma, and some anecdotal reports have been published.[289,290]

The SFOP group investigated the role of MGT/SCR as consolidation treatment in high-risk retinoblastoma (extraocular disease at diagnosis or relapse or invasion of the cut end of the optic nerve; see Box 26.7). The CARBOPEC regimen (carboplatin, etoposide and cyclophosphamide) was used in 25 patients. Nineteen patients received this drug combination for chemosensitive extraocular relapse, while the other six patients with histological high-risk factors were given this treatment as consolidation after enucleation and conventional chemotherapy. The 3-year DFS was 67 per cent. In seven of the nine relapsing patients, the first site of relapse was the CNS. All patients with CNS disease died except one. The CARBOPEC regimen seems to be a promising therapeutic strategy in patients with high-risk retinoblastoma, especially those with bone and/or bone marrow involvement. However, this treatment did not improve the outcome of patients with CNS disease.[291]

EBMT DATA

Megatherapy in retinoblastoma patients was reported to the EBMT as part of primary treatment in 33 patients

Box 26.7 *High-risk features of retinoblastoma*

- Involvement of the cut end or subarachnoidal space of the optic nerve after enucleation
- Orbital involvement
- Distant metastatic disease
- Central nervous system disease

(40 per cent with locoregional disease and 60 per cent with metastatic disease) and in 32 patients after relapse. MGT approaches achieved a 5-year probability of survival of 0.76 ± 0.08 during primary treatment and 0.55 ± 0.10 after relapse.

The advocated MGT approach by the SFOP is CARBOPEC-MGT (carboplatin/etoposide/cyclophosphamide). However, since the outcome of CNS-positive patients was not improved, the addition of thiotepa or busulphan is proposed but needs a prospective collaborative study for sufficient recruitment.

GERM CELL TUMOURS

In germ cell tumours (GCTs), there is continuing controversy over the relative merits of dose dense therapy (increased frequency over a given time) vs. vertical intensification (increased dose per fraction).[292–296]

The prognosis of metastatic non-seminomatous GCTs has considerably improved since the introduction of multidrug chemotherapy involving cisplatin and either etoposide or vinblastine followed by surgery. The prognosis is still poor for patients in whom residual malignant GCT persists in spite of conventional cisplatin-based induction chemotherapy, especially in patients who initially present with large or very large volume disease and/or preoperatively elevated tumour markers. More effective treatment modalities have to be developed for these patients.[297]

Equally, relapse patients who fail to achieve a second complete remission on conventional regimens have a dismal prognosis and need more aggressive treatment. Several agents – carboplatin, ifosfamide, cyclophosphamide and etoposide – are known to have a steep dose–response curve in this tumour, achieving remissions in pretreated patients who are refractory to conventional doses. In patients with malignant GCTs progressing after platinum-based induction chemotherapy with or without surgery, the following factors most importantly predicted a poor prognosis:

- progression-free interval <2 years
- initial poor prognosis category (MRC criteria)
- $<$CR to induction chemotherapy
- inadequate initial chemotherapy.

Three prognostic factors remained in the multivariate analysis: progression-free interval, response to induction treatment and the level of serum human chorionic gonadotrophin (hCG) and alpha-fetoprotein (AFP) at relapse. Results of high-dose salvage chemotherapy must be interpreted against the background of these prognostic factors.[298]

A total of 150 adult patients with relapsed and/or refractory GCT were treated with conventional-dose salvage chemotherapy followed by one cycle of high-dose chemotherapy with carboplatin 1500–2000 mg/m^2, etoposide 1200–2400 mg/m^2 and ifosfamide 0–10 g/m^2. The projected EFS and OS are 29 per cent (CI 22–37 per cent) and 39 per cent (CI 31–47 per cent), respectively. The relevance of prognostic variables for long-term survival after high-dose chemotherapy were prospectively confirmed. Treatment intensification with high-dose chemotherapy resulted in a significant proportion of the long-term survivors lending support to trials to evaluate high-dose chemotherapy prospectively.[299–302]

A randomized phase III trial comparing standard chemotherapy with additional MGT as first-line treatment in adults with poor-risk GCTs failed to show advantage for the latter subgroup in terms of complete remission and survival rate.[303] In contrast, patients with poor-prognosis, non-seminomatous GCTs who received induction with BEP (bleomycin, etoposide, cisplatin) followed by one cycle of high-dose CEC (carboplatin, etoposide, cyclophosphamide) had an OS at 4 years of 66 per cent with a durable complete response rate of 50 per cent. These results support the case for first-line high-dose chemotherapy. The excellent toxicity profile of BEP/CEC and the 2-year OS of 78 per cent were encouraging and support further the ongoing randomized US Intergroup Study evaluating this regimen.

For relapse patients and patients in first partial remission, an international cooperative group has recently compared a standard salvage regimen with or without MGT as consolidation treatment. No significant benefit was found for MGT.[304] In patients relapsing following MGT, the outcome was poor, with many of them relapsing in the CNS and at other new sites of disease. Further responses were seen to chemotherapy or radiotherapy but these were not sustained. The failure to improve results when high-dose chemotherapy was used as second-line rather than third-line chemotherapy consolidation was disappointing and adds further uncertainty to the role of this approach as far as timing and the ideal regimen are concerned.[305,306]

EBMT DATA ON GCTs

For PWP-EBMT 2002 data on GCTs in patients aged <18 years, (see Table 26.8).

Table 26.8 *Paediatric Working Party – European Bone Marrow Transplant Group 2002 data on GCT < 18 years*

Factor	Patient numbers	5–year OS
MGT during primary treatment	88	0.52 ± 0.06
MGT after relapse	86	0.39 ± 0.07

MGT, megatherapy; OS, overall survival.

CNS Germ cell tumours

In ongoing protocols, the frequency of relapses in malignant CNS GCTs after platin-based treatment regimens is about 15 per cent for germinoma and 30 per cent for secreting CNS GCTs. Recurrent malignant intracranial CNS GCTs, especially those of non-germinomatous histology, carry a poor prognosis. According to published series, nearly all patients with recurrence of a non-germinomatous CNS GCT died. Therefore, the attempt of recent protocols is to evaluate treatment strategies for recurrent malignant CNS GCTs to achieve better overall outcome.[307–309]

Within the SFOP protocols of the 1990s, 73 patients with germinoma were treated. In SIOP CNS GCT 96, 150 patients with germinoma were registered. Patients were treated with platinum compounds (CDDP or carboplatin), etoposide and ifosfamide, and with focal or craniospinal irradiation as indicated (local or metastatic).

Seventeen of 223 patients developed recurrent disease. All were treated with standard dose chemotherapy again [etoposide, ifosfamide, cisplatin (VIP) or etoposide, carboplatin], and all responded very well. One had residual tumour which turned out to be mature teratoma.

For secreting tumours in the SFOP studies, 10 patients with relapse received additional chemotherapy (etoposide, cisplatin or VIP). Biological remission was obtained in seven. In SIOP CNS GCT 96, 25 relapses occurred. Relapses were mainly local (14), spinal (four) and combined (six local and spinal), while one had an abdominal relapse. Additional platin-based chemotherapy again led to a complete or nearly complete biological response in most cases.

PATIENTS WITH MGT/SCR

Eight patients with germinoma in the SFOP series received MGT with two cycles of VP-16/thiotepa (VP-16, 3×500 mg/m^2; thiotepa, 3×300 mg/m^2). Four achieved a long-term remission, four relapsed again, of whom one died, two were salvaged by high-dose methotrexate and radiotherapy, and one is under third-line treatment. Three others had high-dose treatment with carboplatin/etoposide/thiotepa or etoposide/thiotepa. Two out of three

are alive, and the other five out of eight had irradiation after conventional treatment: three survived and two died of disease.

Seven out of 10 relapsed patients with secreting tumours in the SFOP series received high-dose chemotherapy after recurrence and second-line treatment. Three are alive after etoposide/thiotepa. In SIOP CNS GCT96, nine out of 25 received high-dose chemotherapy; two are in remission, and two have short follow-up.

The optimal treatment of intracranial GCTs is controversial. The late sequelae of craniospinal radiotherapy and the high response rate to chemotherapy have led to new treatment strategies. Chemoradiotherapy has the potential for a gradual reduction in treatment intensity but high cure rates must be maintained. MGT in recurrent CNS GCTs is a possible treatment option when biological remission is achieved prior to high-dose chemotherapy. In the new SIOP protocol, MGT/SCR will be used within the first line in patients with insufficient response to primary chemotherapy.

KEY POINTS

- MGT/SCR is widely used in paediatric malignancies. It is now well established as a major component in the treatment of children with metastatic neuroblastoma over the age of 1 year at diagnosis.
- Its place for other tumours such as Ewing's tumours and rhabdomyosarcoma needs to be better established and is currently under investigation.
- MGT may replace craniospinal irradiation in the treatment of medulloblastoma in young children and represents an important strategy for retrieval therapy in relapsed Wilms' tumour and retinoblastoma.
- More cooperative studies are needed in order to clarify the population of patients who may benefit from this approach and to determine the optimal chemotherapy regimen for each disease.
- The concept of high-dose therapy is still based on the Goldie–Coldman hypothesis. In the field of paediatric oncology, two conclusions are clear:
  - The concept of consolidation at the time of MRD is still appropriate. However, high relapse rates show that we are not yet able to overcome resistance in most cases. The purging question is not the major one at this time.
  - The concept of combining non-cross-resistant agents in a single regimen may have been

counterproductive in the field of high-dose therapy. In multidrug regimens, the dose for each effective drug is often reduced, and multiple drug regimens have frequently proven no better than using one drug at maximum dose. Future directions will involve either multiple graft programmes with a regimen that uses each effective drug at maximum dosage, or single-agent high-dose regimens with or without autologous BMT. The concept of maximum tolerated dose of each single agent should be emphasized in new strategies.

REFERENCES

1. Armitage JO, Gale RP. Bone marrow autotransplantation. *Am J Med* 1989; **86**: 203–6.
2. Hartmann O. New strategies for the application of high-dose chemotherapy with haematopoietic support in paediatric solid tumours. *Ann Oncol* 1995; **6**(Suppl 4): 13–16.
3. Atra A, Pinkerton R. Autologous stem cell transplantation in solid tumours of childhood. *Ann Med* 1996; **28**: 159–64.
4. Michon J, Schleiermacher G. Autologous haematopoietic stem cell transplantation for paediatric solid tumours. *Baillieres Best Pract Res Clin Haematol* 1999; **12**: 247–59.
5. Ladenstein R, Hartmann O, Pinkerton CR. The role of megatherapy with autologous bone marrow rescue in solid tumours of childhood. *Ann Oncol* 1993; **4**(Suppl. 1): 45–58.
6. Goldie JH, Coldman AJ. A mathematic model for relating the drug sensitivity of tumors to their spontaneous mutation rate. *Cancer Treat Rep* 1979; **63**: 1727–33.
7. Goldie JH, Coldman AJ. Quantitative model for multiple levels of drug resistance in clinical tumors. *Cancer Treat Rep* 1983; **67**: 923–31.
8. Goldie JH, Coldman AJ. Genetic instability in the development of drug resistance. *Semin Oncol* 1985; **12**: 222–30.
9. Norton L, Simon R. Tumor size, sensitivity to therapy, and design of treatment schedules. *Cancer Treat Rep* 1977; **61**: 1307–17.
10. Norton L. Implications of kinetic heterogeneity in clinical oncology. *Semin Oncol* 1985; **12**: 231–49.
11. Skipper HE, Schabel FMJ, Wilcor WS *et al.* Experimental evaluation of potential anticancer agents. On the criteria and kinetics associated with 'curability' of experimental leukemia. *Cancer Chemother Rep* 1964; **35**: 1–111.
12. Gehan EA. Dose-response relationship in clinical oncology. *Cancer* 1984; **54**: 1204–7.
13. Garaventa A, Porta F, Rondelli R *et al.* Early deaths in children after BMT. Bone Marrow Transplantation Group of the Italian Association for Pediatric Hematology and Oncology (AIEOP) and Gruppo Italiano Trapianto di Midollo Osseo (GITMO). *Bone Marrow Transplant* 1992; **10**: 419–23.
14. Vassal G. Pharmacologically-guided dose adjustment of busulfan in high-dose chemotherapy regimens: rationale and pitfalls (review). *Anticancer Res* 1994; **14**: 2363–70.
15. Brenner MK, Rill DR, Holladay MS *et al.* Gene marking to determine whether autologous marrow infusion restores long-term haemopoiesis in cancer patients. *Lancet* 1993; **342**: 1134–7.
16. De Vita V. Dose response is alive and well. *J Clin Oncol* 1986; **4**: 1157.
17. Chabner BA, Fojo A. Multidrug resistance: P-glycoprotein and its allies – the elusive foes. *J Natl Cancer Inst* 1989; **81**: 910–13.
18. Philip T, Bouffet E, Biron P *et al.* [Dose factors/time factors in chemotherapy]. *Bull Cancer* 1989; **76**: 979–94.
19. Philip T. Overview of current treatment of neuroblastoma. *Am J Pediatr Hematol Oncol* 1992; **14**: 97–102.
20. Philip T, Lasset C, Ladenstein R *et al.* European bone marrow registry in solid tumors: 10 years of experience. *Bone Marrow Transplant* 1995; **15**(Suppl 2).
21. Rothenberg M, Ling V. Multidrug resistance: molecular biology and clinical relevance. *J Natl Cancer Inst* 1989; **81**: 907–10.
22. Waxman S. The importance of the induction of gene expression and differentiation by cytotoxic chemotherapy. *Cancer Invest* 1988; **6**: 747–53.
23. Lum BL, Kaubisch S, Yahanda AM *et al.* Alteration of etoposide pharmacokinetics and pharmacodynamics by cyclosporine in a phase I trial to modulate multidrug resistance. *J Clin Oncol* 1992; **10**: 1635–42.
24. Frei E, III, Teicher BA, Holden SA *et al.* Preclinical studies and clinical correlation of the effect of alkylating dose. *Cancer Res* 1988; **48**: 6417–23.
25. Canon JL, Humblet Y, Symann M. Resistance to cisplatin: how to deal with the problem? *Eur J Cancer* 1990; **26**: 1–3.
26. Roberts I. Bone marrow transplantation in children: current results and controversies. Meeting, Hilton Head Island, SC, March 1994. *Bone Marrow Transplant* 1994; **14**: 197–9.
27. Shpall EJ, Jones RB, Bearman S. High-dose therapy with autologous bone marrow transplantation for the treatment of solid tumors. *Curr Opin Oncol* 1994; **6**: 135–8.
28. Jones RJ. The existence of a clinical graft-versus-lymphoma effect. The Johns Hopkins Oncology Center. *Exp Hematol* 1990; **18**.
29. Ladenstein R, Lasset C, Hartmann O *et al.* Comparison of auto versus allografting as consolidation of primary treatments in advanced neuroblastoma over one year of age at diagnosis: report from the European Group for Bone Marrow Transplantation. *Bone Marrow Transplant* 1994; **14**: 37–46.
30. Vanlemmens P, Plouvier E, Amsallem D *et al.* Transplantation of umbilical cord blood in neuroblastoma. *Nouv Rev Fr Hematol* 1992; **34**: 243–6.
31. Demeocq F, Kanold J, Chassagne J *et al.* Successful blood stem cell collection and transplant in children weighing less than 25 kg. *Bone Marrow Transplant* 1994; **13**: 43–50.
32. Miyajima Y, Kato K, Numata S *et al.* Detection of neuroblastoma cells in bone marrow and peripheral blood at diagnosis by the reverse transcriptase-polymerase chain reaction for tyrosine hydroxylase mRNA. *Cancer* 1995; **75**: 2757–61.
33. Chan WC, Wu GQ, Greiner TC *et al.* Detection of tumor contamination of peripheral stem cells in patients with lymphoma using cell culture and polymerase chain reaction technology. *J Hematother* 1994; **3**: 175–84.

34. Combaret V, Favrot MC, Kremens B et al. Immunological detection of neuroblastoma cells in bone marrow harvested for autologous transplantation. Br J Cancer 1989; **59**: 844-7.

35. Berthold F, Schumacher R, Schneider A et al. Removal of neuroblastoma cells from bone marrow by a direct monoclonal antibody rosetting technique. Bone Marrow Transplant 1989; **4**: 273-8.

36. Korbling M, Hess AD, Tutshka PJ et al. 4-Hydroperoxycyclo-phosphamide: a model for eliminating residual human tumour cells and T-lymphocytes from the bone marrow graft. Br J Haematol 1987; **52**: 89-90.

37. Gorin NC, Douay L, Laporte JP et al. Autologous bone marrow transplantation using marrow incubated with Asta Z 7557 in adult acute leukemia. Blood 1986; **67**: 1367-76.

38. Hartmann O, Kalifa C, Beaujean F et al. Treatment of advanced neuroblastoma with two consecutive high-dose chemotherapy regimens and ABMT. In: Evans AE, D'Angio O, Seeger RC, eds. Advances in Neuroblastoma Research. New York: Alan Liss, 1985; 565-8.

39. Mulroney CM, Gluck S, Ho AD. The use of photodynamic therapy in bone marrow purging. Semin Oncol 1994; **21**: 24-7.

40. Sieber F, Spivak JL, Sutcliffe AM. Selective killing of leukemic cells by merocyanine 540-mediated photosensitization. Proc Natl Acad Sci USA 1984; **81**: 7584-7.

41. Reynolds CP, Reynolds DA, Frenkel EP et al. Selective toxicity of 6-hydroxydopamine and ascorbate for human neuroblastoma in vitro: a model for clearing marrow prior to autologous transplant. Cancer Res 1982; **42**: 1331-6.

42. Skala JP, Rogers PC, Chan KW et al. Deferoxamine as a purging agent for autologous bone marrow grafts in neuroblastoma. Prog Clin Biol Res 1992; **377**: 71-8.

43. Combaret V, Favrot MC, Chauvin F et al. Immunomagnetic depletion of malignant cells from autologous bone marrow graft: from experimental models to clinical trials. J Immunogenet 1989; **16**: 125-36.

44. Favrot M, Philip I, Combaret V et al. Experimental evaluation of an immunomagnetic bone marrow purging procedure using the Burkitt lymphoma model. Bone Marrow Transplant 1987; **2**: 59-66.

45. Kemshead JT. Monoclonal antibodies to the small round cell tumours of childhood: an international workshop. In: Evans AE, D'Angio O, Seeger RC, eds. Advances in Neuroblastoma Research 2. New York: Alan Liss, 1988; 535-46.

46. Poynton CH, Dicke KA, Culbert S et al. Immunomagnetic removal of CALLA positive cells from human bone marrow. Lancet 1983; **1**: 524.

47. Berenson RJ, Bensinger WI, Kalamasz D et al. Elimination of Daudi lymphoblasts from human bone marrow using avidin-biotin immunoadsorption. Blood 1986; **67**: 509-15.

48. Favrot MC, Philip T. Bone marrow purging. In: Magrath I, ed. New Directions in Cancer Treatment. Berlin: UICC, 1989; 343-57.

49. Favrot MC, Philip I, Philip T et al. Bone marrow purging procedure in Burkitt lymphoma with monoclonal antibodies and complement: quantification by a liquid cell culture monitoring system. Br J Haematol 1986; **64**: 161-8.

50. Verma UN, Bagg A, Brown E et al. Interleukin-2 activation of human bone marrow in long-term cultures: an effective strategy for purging and generation of anti-tumor cytotoxic effectors. Bone Marrow Transplant 1994; **13**: 115-23.

51. Henschler R, Brugger W, Luft T et al. Maintenance of transplantation potential in ex vivo expanded CD34(+)-selected human peripheral blood progenitor cells. Blood 1994; **84**: 2898-903.

52. Holyoake TL, Alcorn MJ. CD34+ positive haemopoietic cells: biology and clinical applications. Blood Rev 1994; **8**: 113-24.

53. Lemoli RM, Tazzari PL, Fortuna A et al. Positive selection of hematopoietic CD34+ stem cells provides 'indirect purging' of. Bone Marrow Transplant 1994; **13**: 465-71.

54. Koller MR, Emerson SG, Palsson BO. Large-scale expansion of human stem and progenitor cells from bone marrow mononuclear cells in continuous perfusion cultures. Blood 1993; **82**: 378-84.

55. Bouffet E, Philip I, Chauvin F et al. Analysis of parameters influencing recovery from aplasia following autologous bone marrow transplantation (ABMT). (XXII SIOP meeting, Rome). Med Pediatr Oncol 1990; **18**: 386.

56. Leibundgut K, von Rohr A, Brulhart K et al. The number of circulating CD34+ blood cells predicts the colony-forming capacity of leukapheresis products in children. Bone Marrow Transplant 1995; **15**: 25-31.

57. Philip T, Ladenstein R, Zucker JM et al. Double megatherapy and autologous bone marrow transplantation for advanced neuroblastoma: the LMCE2 study. Br J Cancer 1993; **67**: 119-27.

58. Philip I, Favrot MC, Philip T. Use of a liquid cell culture assay to quantify the elimination of Burkitt lymphoma cells from the bone marrow. J Immunol Methods 1987; **97**: 11-17.

59. Beck D, Maritaz O, Gross N et al. Immunocytochemical detection of neuroblastoma cells infiltrating clinical bone marrow samples. Eur J Pediatr 1988; **147**: 609-12.

60. Combaret V, Viehl P, Bouffet E et al. Immunological detection of minimal residual disease in the bone marrow of neuroblastoma patients: interest and limit for therapeutic strategies. Med Pediatr Oncol 1990; **18**: 369.

61. Glorieux P, Bouffet E, Philip I et al. Metastatic interstitial pneumonitis after autologous bone marrow transplantation. A consequence of reinjection of malignant cells? Cancer 1986; **58**: 2136-9.

62. Graeve JL, de Alarcon PA, Sato Y et al. Miliary pulmonary neuroblastoma. A risk of autologous bone marrow transplantation? Cancer 1988; **62**: 2125-7.

63. Garaventa A, Ladenstein R, Chauvin F et al. High-dose chemotherapy with autologous bone marrow rescue in advanced stage IV neuroblastoma. Eur J Cancer 1993; **29A**: 487-91.

64. Brenner MK, Rill DR, Moen RC et al. Gene marking and autologous bone marrow transplantation. Ann NY Acad Sci 1994; **716**: 204-14.

65. Athanasou NA, Quinn J, Brenner MK et al. Origin of marrow stromal cells and haemopoietic chimaerism following bone marrow transplantation determined by in situ hybridisation. Br J Cancer 1990; **61**: 385-9.

66. Cayeux S, Meuer S, Pezzutto A et al. T-cell ontogeny after autologous bone marrow transplantation: failure to synthesize interleukin-2 (IL-2) and lack of CD2- and CD3-mediated proliferation by both CD4− and CD8+ cells even in the presence of exogeneous IL-2. Blood 1989; **74**: 2270-7.

67. Migliaccio AR, Migliaccio G, Johnson G *et al*. Comparative analysis of hematopoietic growth factors released by stromal cells from normal donors or transplanted patients. *Blood* 1990; **75**: 305–12.

68. Testa U, Martucci R, Rutella S *et al*. Autologous stem cell transplantation: release of early and late acting growth factors relates with hematopoietic ablation and recovery. *Blood* 1994; **84**: 3532–9.

69. Cairo MS, Gillan ER, Weinthal J *et al*. Decreased endogenous circulating steel factor (SLF) levels following allogeneic and autologous BMT: lack of an inverse correlation with post-BMT myeloid engraftment. *Bone Marrow Transplant* 1993; **11**: 155–61.

70. Favrot M, Philip T, Combaret V *et al*. Effect of in vivo therapy with a CD8 monoclonal antibody on delayed engraftment after autologous bone marrow transplantation. *Bone Marrow Transplant* 1990; **5**: 33–8.

71. Lopez JL, Gonzalez-Requejo A, Lopez-Botet M *et al*. Treatment with rhG-CSF pre and post-autologous bone marrow transplantation in children. *Bone Marrow Transplant* 1992; **12**(4): 422.

72. Haas R, Hohaus S, Egerer G *et al*. Recombinant human granulocyte-macrophage colony-stimulating factor (rhGM-CSF) subsequent to chemotherapy improves collection of blood stem cells for autografting in patients not eligible for bone marrow harvest. *Bone Marrow Transplant* 1992; **9**: 459–65.

73. Brice P, Divine M, Marolleau JP *et al*. Comparison of autografting using mobilized peripheral blood stem cells with and without granulocyte colony-stimulating factor in malignant lymphomas. *Bone Marrow Transplant* 1994; **14**: 51–5.

74. Quinones RR. Hematopoietic engraftment and graft failure after bone marrow transplantation. *Am J Pediatr Hematol Oncol* 1993; **15**: 3–17.

75. Spitzer G, Adkins DR, Spencer V *et al*. Randomized study of growth factors post-peripheral-blood stem-cell transplant: neutrophil recovery is improved with modest clinical benefit. *J Clin Oncol* 1994; **12**: 661–70.

76. Suzue T, Takaue Y, Watanabe A *et al*. Effects of rhG-CSF (filgrastim) on the recovery of hematopoiesis after high-dose chemotherapy and autologous peripheral blood stem cell transplantation in children: a report from the Children's Cancer and Leukemia Study Group of Japan. *Exp Hematol* 1994; **22**: 1197–202.

77. Ho AD, Haas R, Wulf G *et al*. Activation of lymphocytes induced by recombinant human granulocyte-macrophage colony-stimulating factor in patients with malignant lymphoma. *Blood* 1990; **75**: 203–12.

78. Dexter TM, White H. Growth factors. Growth without inflation. *Nature* 1990; **344**: 380–1.

79. Laughlin MJ, Kirkpatrick G, Sabiston N *et al*. Hematopoietic recovery following high-dose combined alkylating-agent chemotherapy and autologous bone marrow support in patients in phase-I clinical trials of colony-stimulating factors: G-CSF, GM-CSF, IL-1, IL- 2, M-CSF. *Ann Hematol* 1993; **67**: 267–76.

80. Bolwell BJ, Goormastic M, Yanssens T *et al*. Comparison of G-CSF with GM-CSF for mobilizing peripheral blood progenitor cells and for enhancing marrow recovery after autologous bone marrow transplant. *Bone Marrow Transplant* 1994; **14**: 913–18.

81. Baethman M, Peters C, Laws HJ *et al*. Comparison of G-CSF versus GM-CSG after myeloablative radiochemotherapy and hematopoietic stem cell rescue in children with solid tumours. *Bone Marrow Transplant* 1994; **14**.

82. Albin N, Douay L, Fouillard L *et al*. In vivo effects of GM-CSF and IL-3 on hematopoietic cell recovery in bone marrow and blood after autologous transplantation with mafosfamide-purged marrow in lymphoid malignancies. *Bone Marrow Transplant* 1994; **14**: 253–9.

83. Vey N, Molnar S, Faucher C *et al*. Delayed administration of granulocyte colony-stimulating factor after autologous bone marrow transplantation: effect on granulocyte recovery. *Bone Marrow Transplant* 1994; **14**: 779–82.

84. Cabanillas F, Jagannath S, Philip T. Management of recurrent or refractory disease. In: Magrath I, ed. *The Non Hodgkin Lymphomas*. London: Edward Arnold, 1990; 359–72.

85. Armitage JO, Bierman PJ. Is there an optimum conditioning regimen for patients with lymphoma undergoing autologous bone marrow transplantations? In: Dicke KA, Spitzer G, Jagannath S *et al*., eds. *ABMT. Proceedings of the Fourth International Symposium*. Houston: 1989; 299–303.

86. Hartmann O, Benhamou E, Beaujean F *et al*. High-dose busulfan and cyclophosphamide with autologous bone marrow transplantation support in advanced malignancies in children: a phase II study. *J Clin Oncol* 1986; **4**: 1804–10.

87. Dusenbery KE, Daniels KA, McClure JS *et al*. Randomized comparison of cyclophosphamide-total body irradiation versus busulfan-cyclophosphamide conditioning in autologous bone marrow transplantation for acute myeloid leukemia. *Int J Radiat Oncol Biol Phys* 1995; **31**: 119–28.

88. Deacon JM, Wilson PA, Peckham MJ. The radiobiology of human neuroblastoma. *Radiother Oncol* 1985; **3**: 201–9.

89. Weichselbaum RR, Schmit A, Little JB. Cellular repair factors influencing radiocurability of human malignant tumours. *Br J Cancer* 1982; **45**: 10–16.

90. Kinsella TJ, Glaubiger D, Diesseroth A *et al*. Intensive combined modality therapy including low-dose TBI in high-risk Ewing's sarcoma patients. *Int J Radiat Oncol Biol Phys* 1983; **9**: 1955–60.

91. Matthay KK, Villablanca JG, Seeger RC *et al*. Treatment of high-risk neuroblastoma with intensive chemotherapy, radiotherapy, autologous bone marrow transplantation, and 13-cis-retinoic acid. Children's Cancer Group. *N Engl J Med* 1999; **341**: 1165–73.

92. Evans AE, D'Angio GJ, Propert K *et al*. Prognostic factor in neuroblastoma. *Cancer* 1987; **59**: 1853–9.

93. Brodeur GM, Pritchard J, Berthold F *et al*. Revisions of the international criteria for neuroblastoma diagnosis, staging, and response to treatment. *J Clin Oncol* 1993; **11**: 1466–77.

94. Berthold F, Burdach S, Kremens B *et al*. The role of chemotherapy in the treatment of children with neuroblastoma stage IV: the GPO (German Pediatric Oncology Society) experience. *Klin Padiatr* 1990; **202**: 262–9.

95. Finklestein JZ, Hittle RE, Hammond GD. Evaluation of a high dose cyclophosphamide regimen in childhood tumors. *Cancer* 1969; **23**: 1239–42.

96. Finklestein JZ, Klemperer MR, Evans A *et al*. Multiagent chemotherapy for children with metastatic neuroblastoma: a report from Children's Cancer Study Group. *Med Pediatr Oncol* 1979; **6**: 179–88.

97. Pinkerton CR, Lewis IJ, Pearson AD *et al*. Carboplatin or cisplatin? [letter; comment]. *Lancet* 1989; **2**: 161.

98. Rosen EM, Cassady JR, Frantz CN *et al*. Neuroblastoma: the Joint Center for Radiation Therapy/Dana-Farber Cancer Institute/Children's Hospital experience. *J Clin Oncol* 1984; **2**: 719–32.

99. Shafford EA, Rogers DW, Pritchard J. Advanced neuroblastoma: improved response rate using a multiagent regimen (OPEC) including sequential cisplatin and VM-26. *J Clin Oncol* 1984; **2**: 742–7.

100. Bernard JL, Philip T, Zucker JM *et al*. Sequential cisplatin/ VM-26 and vincristine/cyclophosphamide/doxorubicin in metastatic neuroblastoma: an effective alternating non-cross-resistant regimen? *J Clin Oncol* 1987; **5**: 1952–9.

101. Coze C, Hartmann O, Michon J *et al*. NB87 induction protocol for stage 4 neuroblastoma in children over 1 year of age: a report from the French Society of Pediatric Oncology. *J Clin Oncol* 1997; **15**: 3433–40.

102. Kushner BH, Helson L. Coordinated use of sequentially escalated cyclophosphamide and cell-cycle-specific chemotherapy (N4SE protocol) for advanced neuroblastoma: experience with 100 patients. *J Clin Oncol* 1987; **5**: 1746–51.

103. Pearson ADJ, Craft AW. Ultra high dose induction regime for disseminated neuroblastoma – 'Napoleon'. *Med Pediatr Oncol* 1988; **16**: 414.

104. Pinkerton CR, Zucker JM, Hartmann O *et al*. Short duration, high dose, alternating chemotherapy in metastatic neuro-blastoma. (ENSG 3C induction regimen). The European Neuroblastoma Study Group. *Br J Cancer* 1990; **62**: 319–23.

105. Dini G, Lanino E, Garaventa A *et al*. Myeloablative therapy and unpurged autologous bone marrow transplantation for poor-prognosis neuroblastoma: report of 34 cases. *J Clin Oncol* 1991; **9**: 962–9.

106. Matthay KK, Atkinson JB, Stram DO *et al*. Patterns of relapse after autologous purged bone marrow transplantation for neuroblastoma: a Children's Cancer Group pilot study. *J Clin Oncol* 1993; **11**: 2226–33.

107. August CS, Serota FT, Koch PA *et al*. Treatment of advanced neuroblastoma with supralethal chemotherapy, radiation, and allogeneic or autologous marrow reconstitution. *J Clin Oncol* 1984; **2**: 609–16.

108. Berthold F, Bender-Gotze C, Dopfer R *et al*. [Myeloablative chemo- and radiotherapy with autologous and allogenic bone marrow reconstitution in children with metastatic neuroblastoma]. *Klin Padiatr* 1988; **200**: 221–5.

109. Corbett R, Pinkerton R, Pritchard J *et al*. Pilot study of high-dose vincristine, etoposide, carboplatin and melphalan with autologous bone marrow rescue in advanced neuroblastoma. *Eur J Cancer* 1992; **28A**: 1324–8.

110. Hartmann O, Benhamou E, Beaujean F *et al*. Repeated high-dose chemotherapy followed by purged autologous bone marrow transplantation as consolidation therapy in metastatic neuroblastoma. *J Clin Oncol* 1987; **5**: 1205–11.

111. McElwain TJ, Hedley DW, Gordon MY *et al*. High dose melphalan and non-cryopreserved autologous bone marrow treatment of malignant melanoma and neuroblastoma. *Exp Hematol* 1979; **7**(Suppl 5): 360–71.

112. Philip T, Bernard JL, Zucker JM *et al*. High-dose chemoradiotherapy with bone marrow transplantation as consolidation treatment in neuroblastoma: an unselected group of stage IV patients over 1 year of age. *J Clin Oncol* 1987; **5**: 266–71.

113. Pritchard J, McElwain TJ, Graham-Pole J. High-dose melphalan with autologous marrow for treatment of advanced neuroblastoma. *Br J Cancer* 1982; **45**: 86–94.

114. Kushner BH, O'Reilly RJ, Mandell LR *et al*. Myeloablative combination chemotherapy without total body irradiation for neuroblastoma. *J Clin Oncol* 1991; **9**: 274–9.

115. Pinkerton CR. Where next with therapy in advanced neuroblastoma? *Br J Cancer* 1990; **61**: 351–3.

116. Evans AE, August CS, Kamani N *et al*. Bone marrow transplantation for high risk neuroblastoma at the Children's Hospital of Philadelphia: an update. *Med Pediatr Oncol* 1994; **23**: 323–7.

117. Kletzel M, Becton DL, Berry DH. Single institution experience with high-dose cyclophosphamide, continuous infusion vincristine, escalating doses of VP-16-213, and total body irradiation with unpurged bone marrow rescue in children with neuroblastoma. *Med Pediatr Oncol* 1992; **20**: 64–7.

118. Pole JG, Casper J, Elfenbein G *et al*. High-dose chemoradiotherapy supported by marrow infusions for advanced neuroblastoma: a Pediatric Oncology Group study [published erratum appears in *J Clin Oncol* 1991; **9**(6): 1094]. *J Clin Oncol* 1991; **9**: 152–8.

119. Pritchard J, Germond S, Jones D *et al*. Is high dose melphalan of value in treatment of advanced neuroblastoma? Preliminary results of a randomization trial by the European neuroblastoma study group. *Proc ASCO* 1986; **5**: 205–8.

120. Garaventa A, Rondelli R, Lanino E *et al*. Myeloablative therapy and bone marrow rescue in advanced neuroblastoma. Report from the Italian Bone Marrow Transplant Registry. Italian Association of Pediatric Hematology-Oncology, BMT Group. *Bone Marrow Transplant* 1996; **18**: 125–30.

121. Hartmann O, Kalifa C, Benhamou E *et al*. Treatment of advanced neuroblastoma with high-dose melphalan and autologous bone marrow transplantation. *Cancer Chemother Pharmacol* 1986; **16**: 165–9.

122. Kremens B, Klingebiel T, Herrmann F *et al*. High-dose consolidation with local radiation and bone marrow rescue in patients with advanced neuroblastoma. *Med Pediatr Oncol* 1994; **23**: 470–5.

123. McCowage GB, Vowels MR, Shaw PJ *et al*. Autologous bone marrow transplantation for advanced neuroblastoma using teniposide, doxorubicin, melphalan, cisplatin, and total-body irradiation. *J Clin Oncol* 1995; **13**: 2789–95.

124. Mugishima H, Harada K, Suzuki T *et al*. Comprehensive treatment of advanced neuroblastoma involving auto-logous bone marrow transplant. *Acta Paediatr Jpn* 1995; **37**: 493–9.

125. Philip T, Zucker JM, Bernard JL *et al*. Improved survival at 2 and 5 years in the LMCE1 unselected group of 72 children with stage IV neuroblastoma older than 1 year of age at

diagnosis: is cure possible in a small subgroup? *J Clin Oncol* 1991; **9**: 1037–44.

126. Zucker JM, Philip T, Bernard JL *et al*. Single or double consolidation treatment according to remission status after initial therapy in metastatic neuroblastoma: first results of LMCE 3 study in 40 patients. *Prog Clin Biol Res* 1991; **366**: 543–51.

127. Boogaerts M, Cavalli F, Cortes-Funes H *et al*. Granulocyte growth factors: achieving a consensus. *Ann Oncol* 1995; **6**: 237–44.

128. Burdach SE, Muschenich M, Josephs W *et al*. Granulocyte-macrophage-colony stimulating factor for prevention of neutropenia and infections in children and adolescents with solid tumors. Results of a prospective randomized study. *Cancer* 1995; **76**: 510–16.

129. Kamani N, August CS, Bunin N *et al*. A study of thiotepa, etoposide and fractionated total body irradiation as a preparative regimen prior to bone marrow transplantation for poor prognosis patients with neuroblastoma. *Bone Marrow Transplant* 1996; **17**: 911–16.

130. Kushner BH, Heller G, Kramer K *et al*. Granulocyte-colony stimulating factor and multiple cycles of strongly myelosuppressive alkylator-based combination chemotherapy in children with neuroblastoma. *Cancer* 2000; **89**: 2122–30.

131. Matthay KK, O'Leary MC, Ramsay NK *et al*. Role of myeloablative therapy in improved outcome for high risk neuroblastoma: review of recent Children's Cancer Group results. *Eur J Cancer* 1995; **31A**: 572–5.

132. Michon JM, Hartmann O, Bouffet E *et al*. An open-label, multicentre, randomised phase 2 study of recombinant human granulocyte colony-stimulating factor (filgrastim) as an adjunct to combination chemotherapy in paediatric patients with metastatic neuroblastoma. *Eur J Cancer* 1998; **34**: 1063–9.

133. Newell DR, Pearson AD, Balmanno K *et al*. Carboplatin pharmacokinetics in children: the development of a pediatric dosing formula. The United Kingdom Children's Cancer Study Group. *J Clin Oncol* 1993; **11**: 2314–23.

134. Stram DO, Matthay KK, O'Leary M *et al*. Consolidation chemoradiotherapy and autologous bone marrow transplantation versus continued chemotherapy for metastatic neuroblastoma: a report of two concurrent Children's Cancer Group studies. *J Clin Oncol* 1996; **14**: 2417–26.

135. Santana VM, Schell MJ, Williams R *et al*. Escalating sequential high-dose carboplatin and etoposide with autologous marrow support in children with relapsed solid tumors. *Bone Marrow Transplant* 1992; **10**: 457–62.

136. Cervera A, Kingston JE, Malpas JS. Late recurrence of neuroblastoma: a report of five cases and review of the literature. *Pediatr Hematol Oncol* 1990; **7**: 311–22.

137. Ladenstein R, Lasset C, Hartmann O *et al*. Impact of megatherapy on survival after relapse from stage 4 neuroblastoma in patients over 1 year of age at diagnosis: a report from the European Group for Bone Marrow Transplantation. *J Clin Oncol* 1993; **11**: 2330–41.

138. Ladenstein R, Philip T, Lasset C *et al*. Multivariate analysis of risk factors in stage 4 neuroblastoma patients over the age of one year treated with megatherapy and stem-cell transplantation: a report from the European Bone Marrow Transplantation Solid Tumor Registry. *J Clin Oncol* 1998; **16**: 953–65.

139. Madero L, Muonz A, Diaz DH *et al*. G-CSF after autologous bone marrow transplantation for malignant diseases in children. Spanish Working Party for Bone Marrow Transplantation in Children. *Bone Marrow Transplant* 1995; **15**: 349–51.

140. Schaison G, Eden OB, Henze G *et al*. Recommendations on the use of colony-stimulating factors in children: conclusions of a European panel. *Eur J Pediatr* 1998; **157**: 955–66.

141. Ikeda H, August CS, Goldwein JW *et al*. Sites of relapse in patients with neuroblastoma following bone marrow transplantation in relation to preparatory 'debulking' treatments. *J Pediatr Surg* 1992; **27**: 1438–41.

142. Ladenstein R, Lasset C, Philip T. Treatment duration before bone marrow transplantation in stage IV neuroblastoma. European Bone Marrow Transplant Group Solid Tumour Registry [letter]. *Lancet* 1992; **340**: 916–17.

143. Hartmann O, Valteau CD, Vassal G *et al*. Prognostic factors in metastatic neuroblastoma in patients over 1 year of age treated with high-dose chemotherapy and stem cell transplantation: a multivariate analysis in 218 patients treated in a single institution. *Bone Marrow Transplant* 1999; **23**: 789–95.

144. Ladenstein R, Favrot M, Lasset C *et al*. Indication and limits of megatherapy and bone marrow transplantation in high-risk neuroblastoma: a single centre analysis of prognostic factors. *Eur J Cancer* 1993; **29A**: 947–56.

145. Carlsen NL, Christensen IJ, Schroeder H *et al*. Prognostic value of different staging systems in neuroblastomas and completeness of tumour excision. *Arch Dis Child* 1986; **61**: 832–42.

146. Faulkner LB, Garaventa A, Paoli A *et al*. In vivo cytoreduction studies and cell sorting–enhanced tumor-cell detection in high-risk neuroblastoma patients: implications for leukapheresis strategies. *J Clin Oncol* 2000; **18**: 3829–36.

147. Mehes G, Luegmayr A, Ambros IM *et al*. Combined automatic immunological and molecular cytogenetic analysis allows exact identification and quantification of tumor cells in the bone marrow. *Clin Cancer Res* 2001; **7**: 1969–75.

148. Moss TJ, Cairo M, Santana VM *et al*. Clonogenicity of circulating neuroblastoma cells: implications regarding peripheral blood stem cell transplantation. *Blood* 1994; **83**: 3085–9.

149. Moss T. Sensitive detection of metastatic tumor cells in bone marrow. *Prog Clin Biol Res* 1994; **389**: 567–77.

150. Ambros IM, Zellner A, Roald B *et al*. Role of ploidy, chromosome 1p, and Schwann cells in the maturation of neuroblastoma. *N Engl J Med* 1996; **334**: 1505–11.

151. Ambros PF, Ambros IM, Ladenstein R *et al*. Neuroblastoma: impact of biological characteristics on treatment strategies. *Onkologie* 1995; **18**: 548–55.

152. Ambros PF, Ambros IM, Strehl S *et al*. Regression and progression in neuroblastoma. Does genetics predict tumour behaviour? *Eur J Cancer* 1995; **31A**: 510–15.

153. Berthold F, Sahin K, Hero B et al. The current contribution of molecular factors to risk estimation in neuroblastoma patients. Eur J Cancer 1997; 33: 2092–7.

154. Brodeur GM, Azar C, Brother M et al. Neuroblastoma. Effect of genetic factors on prognosis and treatment. Cancer 1992; 70: 1685–94.

155. Hartmann O, Oberlin O, Beaujean F et al. Place de la chimiothérapie à hautes doses suivie d'autogreffe médullaire dans le traitement des sarcomes d'Ewing métastatiques de l'enfant. Bull Cancer 1990; 77: 181–7.

156. Berthold F, Trechow R, Utsch S et al. Prognostic factors in metastatic neuroblastoma. A multivariate analysis of 182 cases. Am J Pediatr Hematol Oncol 1992; 14: 207–15.

157. Shuster JJ, McWilliams NB, Castleberry R et al. Serum lactate dehydrogenase in childhood neuroblastoma. A Pediatric Oncology Group recursive partitioning study. Am J Clin Oncol 1992; 15: 295–303.

158. Gordon SJ, Pearson AD, Reid MM et al. Toxicity of single-day high-dose vincristine, melphalan, etoposide and carboplatin consolidation with autologous bone marrow rescue in advanced neuroblastoma. Eur J Cancer 1992; 28A: 1319–23.

159. Benedetti PP, Pierelli L, Scambia G et al. High-dose carboplatin, etoposide and melphalan (CEM) with peripheral blood progenitor cell support as late intensification for high-risk cancer: non-haematological, haematological toxicities and role of growth factor administration. Br J Cancer 1997; 75: 1205–12.

160. Graham-Pole JG, Casper J, Elfenbein G et al. High-dose chemoradiotherapy supported by marrow infusions for advanced neuroblastoma: a Pediatric Oncology Group study. J Clin Oncol 1991; 9: 152–8.

161. Philip T, Ladenstein R, Lasset C et al. 1070 myeloablative megatherapy procedures followed by stem cell rescue for neuroblastoma: 17 years of European experience and conclusions. European Group for Blood and Marrow Transplant Registry Solid Tumour Working Party. Eur J Cancer 1997; 33: 2130–5.

162. Hartmann O, Le Corroller AG, Blaise D et al. Peripheral blood stem cell and bone marrow transplantation for solid tumors and lymphomas: hematologic recovery and costs. A randomized, controlled trial. Ann Intern Med 1997; 126: 600–7.

163. Saarinen UM, Hovi L, Juvonen E et al. Granulocyte-colony-stimulating factor after allogeneic and autologous bone marrow transplantation in children. Med Pediatr Oncol 1996; 26: 380–6.

164. Klumpp TR, Mangan KF, Goldberg SL et al. Granulocyte colony-stimulating factor accelerates neutrophil engraftment following peripheral-blood stem-cell transplantation: a prospective, randomized trial. J Clin Oncol 1995; 13: 1323–7.

165. Tarella C, Castellino C, Locatelli F et al. G-CSF administration following peripheral blood progenitor cell (PBPC) autograft in lymphoid malignancies: evidence for clinical benefits and reduction of treatment costs. Bone Marrow Transplant 1998; 21: 401–7.

166. Bensinger WI, Longin K, Appelbaum F et al. Peripheral blood stem cells (PBSCs) collected after recombinant granulocyte colony stimulating factor (rhG-CSF): an analysis of factors correlating with the tempo of engraftment after transplantation. Br J Haematol 1994; 87: 825–31.

167. Attal M, Huguet F, Rubie H et al. Prevention of hepatic veno-occlusive disease after bone marrow transplantation by continuous infusion of low-dose heparin: a prospective, randomized trial. Blood 1992; 79: 2834–40.

168. Essell JH, Schroeder MT, Harman GS et al. Ursodiol prophylaxis against hepatic complications of allogeneic bone marrow transplantation. A randomized, double-blind, placebo-controlled trial. Ann Intern Med 1998; 128: 975–81.

169. McDonald GB, Sharma P, Matthews DE et al. Venocclusive disease of the liver after bone marrow transplantation: diagnosis, incidence, and predisposing factors. Hepatology 1984; 4: 116–22.

170. Brugieres L, Hartmann O, Benhamou E et al. [Hepatic complications after high-dose chemotherapy and bone marrow autograft in solid tumors in children]. Presse Med 1988; 17: 1305–8.

171. Barker E, Mueller BM, Handgretinger R et al. Effect of a chimeric anti-ganglioside GD2 antibody on cell-mediated lysis of human neuroblastoma cells. Cancer Res 1991; 51: 144–9.

172. Flamant F, Rodary C, Rey A et al. Treatment of non-metastatic rhabdomyosarcomas in childhood and adolescence. Results of the second study of the International Society of Paediatric Oncology: MMT84. Eur J Cancer 1998; 34: 1050–62.

173. Donaldson SS, Meza J, Breneman JC et al. Results from the IRS-IV randomized trial of hyperfractionated radiotherapy in children with rhabdomyosarcoma – a report from the IRSG. Int J Radiat Oncol Biol Phys 2001; 51: 718–28.

174. Koscielniak E, Morgan M, Treuner J. Soft tissue sarcoma in children: prognosis and management. Paediatr Drugs 2002; 4: 21–8.

175. Breitfeld PP, Lyden E, Raney RB et al. Ifosfamide and etoposide are superior to vincristine and melphalan for pediatric metastatic rhabdomyosarcoma when administered with irradiation and combination chemotherapy: a report from the Intergroup Rhabdomyosarcoma Study Group. J Pediatr Hematol Oncol 2001; 23: 225–33.

176. Pinkerton CR, Philip T, Hartmann O et al. High-dose chemo-radiotherapy with autologous bone marrow rescue in pediatric soft tissue sarcomas. In: Dicke KA, Spitzer G, Jagannath S et al., eds. ABMT. Proceedings of the Fourth International Symposium. Houston: 1989; 617–20.

177. Pinkerton CR. Megatherapy for soft tissue sarcomas. EBMT experience. Bone Marrow Transplant 1991; 7(Suppl 3): 120–2.

178. Pinkerton CR, Groot-Loonen J, Barrett A et al. Rapid VAC high dose melphalan regimen, a novel chemotherapy approach in childhood soft tissue sarcomas. Br J Cancer 1991; 64: 381–5.

179. Pinkerton R, Philip T, Bouffet E et al. Autologous bone marrow transplantation in paediatric solid tumours. Clin Haematol 1986; 15: 187–203.

180. Carli M, Colombatti R, Oberlin O et al. High–dose melphalan with autologous stem-cell rescue in metastatic rhabdomyosarcoma. J Clin Oncol 1999; 17: 2796–803.

181. Boulad F, Kernan NA, LaQuaglia MP et al. High–dose induction chemoradiotherapy followed by autologous bone

marrow transplantation as consolidation therapy in rhabdomyosarcoma, extraosseous Ewing's sarcoma, and undifferentiated sarcoma. *J Clin Oncol* 1998; **16**: 1697–706.

182. Lafay-Cousin L, Hartmann, Plouvier P *et al.* High-dose thiotepa and hematopoietic stem cell transplantation in pediatric malignant mesenchymal tumors: a phase II study. *Bone Marrow Transplant* 2000; **26**: 627–32.

183. Lucidarme N, Valteau-Couanet D, Oberlin O *et al.* Phase II study of high-dose thiotepa and hematopoietic stem cell transplantation in children with solid tumors. *Bone Marrow Transplant* 1998; **22**: 535–40.

184. Saarinen UM, Hovi L, Makipernaa A, Riikonen. High-dose thiotepa with autologous bone marrow rescue in pediatric solid tumors. *Bone Marrow Transplant* 1991; **8**: 369–76.

185. Walterhouse DO, Hoover ML, Marymont MA *et al.* High-dose chemotherapy followed by peripheral blood stem cell rescue for metastatic rhabdomyosarcoma: the experience at Chicago Children's Memorial Hospital. *Med Pediatr Oncol* 1999; **32**: 88–92.

186. Hara J, Osugi Y, Ohta H *et al.* Double-conditioning regimens consisting of thiotepa, melphalan and busulfan with stem cell rescue for the treatment of pediatric solid tumors. *Bone Marrow Transplant* 1998; **22**: 7–12.

187. Diaz MA, Vicent MG, Madero L. High-dose busulfan/melphalan as conditioning for autologous PBPC transplantation in pediatric patients with solid tumors. *Bone Marrow Transplant* 1999; **24**: 1157–9.

188. Kung FH, Desai SJ, Dickerman JD *et al.* Ifosfamide/carboplatin/etoposide (ICE) for recurrent malignant solid tumors of childhood: a Pediatric Oncology Group Phase I/II study. *J Pediatr Hematol Oncol* 1995; **17**: 265–9.

189. Wiley JM, Cohen K, Gold S *et al.* High dose chemotherapy and bone marrow/peripheral blood stem cell rescue. Experience in pediatric sarcomas. In: Dicke KA, Keating A, eds. *Autologous Marrow and Blood Transplantation* 1994; 439–49.

190. Horowitz ME, Kinsella TJ, Wexler LH *et al.* Total-body irradiation and autologous bone marrow transplant in the treatment of high-risk Ewing's sarcoma and rhabdomyosarcoma. *J Clin Oncol* 1993; **11**: 1911–18.

191. Miser JS, Kinsella TJ, Triche TJ *et al.* Treatment of peripheral neuroepithelioma in children and young adults. *J Clin Oncol* 1987; **5**: 1752–8.

192. Philip T, Pinkerton R. Very high dose therapy in lymphomas and solid tumors. In: Magrath I, ed. *New Directions in Cancer Treatment.* Berlin: Springer-Verlag, 1989; 119–42.

193. Yaniv I, Bouffet E, Irle C *et al.* Autologous bone marrow transplantation in pediatric solid tumors. *Pediatr Hematol Oncol* 1990; **7**: 35–46.

194. Koscielniak E, Klingebiel TH, Peters C *et al.* Do patients with metastatic and recurrent rhabdomyosarcoma benefit from high-dose therapy with hematopoietic rescue? Report of the German/Austrian Pediatric Bone Marrow Transplantation Group. *Bone Marrow Transplant* 1997; **19**: 227–31.

195. Weigel BJ, Breitfeld PP, Hawkins D *et al.* Role of high-dose chemotherapy with hematopoietic stem cell rescue in the treatment of metastatic or recurrent rhabdomyosarcoma. *J Pediatr Hematol Oncol* 2001; **23**: 272–6.

196. Atra A, Pinkerton R. High-dose chemotherapy in soft tissue sarcoma in children. *Crit Rev Oncol Hematol.* 2002; **41**: 191–6.

197. Dallorso S, Manzitti C, Morreale G *et al.* High dose therapy and autologous hematopoietic stem cell transplantation in poor risk solid tumors of childhood. *Haematologica* 2000; **85**: 66–70.

198. Mackall CL, Helman LJ. High-dose chemotherapy for rhabdomyosarcoma: where do we go from here. *J Pediatr Hematol Oncol* 2001; **23**: 266–7.

199. Bonig H, Laws HJ, Wundes A *et al.* In vivo cytokine responses to interleukin-2 immunotherapy after autologous stem cell transplantation in children with solid tumors. *Bone Marrow Transplant* 2000; **26**: 91–6.

200. Mesia R, Sola C, Lopez PA *et al.* [High-dose chemotherapy and autologous bone marrow transplantation in high-grade metastatic sarcomas]. *Rev Clin Esp* 1994; **194**: 960–5.

201. Bielack SS, Kempf-Bielack B, Delling G *et al.* Prognostic factors in high-grade osteosarcoma of the extremities or trunk: an analysis of 1,702 patients treated on neoadjuvant cooperative osteosarcoma study group protocols. *J Clin Oncol* 2002; **20**: 776–90.

202. Winkler K, Bielack SS, Delling G *et al.* Treatment of osteosarcoma: experience of the Cooperative Osteosarcoma Study Group (COSS). *Cancer Treat Res* 1993; **62**: 269–77.

203. Kager L, Zoubek A, Potschger U *et al.* Evaluating prognostic factors for outcomes in 186 patients presenting with high-grade metastatic osteosarcoma treated on neoadjuvant COSS protocols. *Proc ASCO* 2002; **21**: 392a.

204. Rodriguez-Galindo C, Daw NC, Kaste SC *et al.* Treatment of refractory osteosarcoma with fractionated cyclophosphamide and etoposide. *J Pediatr Hematol Oncol* 2002; **24**: 250–5.

205. Colombat P, Biron P, Coze C *et al.* Failure of high-dose alkylating agents in osteosarcoma. Solid Tumors Working Party. *Bone Marrow Transplant* 1994; **14**: 665–6.

206. Fagioli F, Aglietta M, Tienghi A *et al.* High-dose chemotherapy in the treatment of relapsed osteosarcoma: an Italian sarcoma group study. *J Clin Oncol* 2002; **20**: 2150–6.

207. Anderson PM, Wiseman GA, Dispenzieri A *et al.* High-dose samarium-153 ethylene diamine tetramethylene phosphonate: low toxicity of skeletal irradiation in patients with osteosarcoma and bone metastases. *J Clin Oncol* 2002; **20**: 189–96.

208. Bruland OS, Skretting A, Solheim OP *et al.* Targeted radiotherapy of osteosarcoma using 153 Sm-EDTMP. A new promising approach. *Acta Oncol* 1996; **35**: 381–4.

209. Franzius C, Bielack S, Sciuk J *et al.* High-activity samarium-153-EDTMP therapy in unresectable osteosarcoma. *Nuklearmedizin* 1999; **38**: 337–40.

210. Franzius C, Bielack S, Flege S *et al.* High-activity samarium-153-EDTMP therapy followed by autologous peripheral blood stem cell support in unresectable osteosarcoma. *Nuklearmedizin* 2001; **40**: 215–20.

211. Franzius C, Schuck A, Bielack SS. High-dose samarium-153 ethylene diamine tetramethylene phosphonate: low toxicity of skeletal irradiation in patients with osteosarcoma and bone metastases. *J Clin Oncol* 2002; **20**: 1953–4.

212. Craft AW, Cotterill SJ, Bullimore JA *et al.* Long-term results from the first UKCCSG Ewing's Tumour Study (ET-1). United

Kingdom Children's Cancer Study Group (UKCCSG) and the Medical Research Council Bone Sarcoma Working Party. *Eur J Cancer* 1997; **33**: 1061–9.

213. Evans R, Nesbit M, Askin F *et al.* Local recurrence, rate and sites of metastases, and time to relapse as a function of treatment regimen, size of primary and surgical history in 62 patients presenting with non-metastatic Ewing's sarcoma of the pelvic bones. *Int J Radiat Oncol Biol Phys* 1985; **11**: 129–36.

214. Jurgens H, Exner U, Gadner H *et al.* Multidisciplinary treatment of primary Ewing's sarcoma of bone. A 6-year experience of a European Cooperative Trial. *Cancer* 1988; **61**: 23–32.

215. Kushner BH, Meyers PA, Gerald WL *et al.* Very-high-dose short-term chemotherapy for poor-risk peripheral primitive neuroectodermal tumors, including Ewing's sarcoma, in children and young adults. *J Clin Oncol* 1995; **13**: 2796–804.

216. Miser JS, Kinsella TJ, Triche TJ *et al.* Preliminary results of treatment of Ewing's sarcoma of bone in children and young adults: six months of intensive combined modality therapy without maintenance. *J Clin Oncol* 1988; **6**: 484–90.

217. Hayes FA, Thompson EI, Meyer WH *et al.* Therapy for localized Ewing's sarcoma of bone. *J Clin Oncol* 1989; **7**: 208–13.

218. Oberlin O, Patte C, Demeocq F *et al.* The response to initial chemotherapy as a prognostic factor in localized Ewing's sarcoma. *Eur J Cancer Clin Oncol* 1985; **21**: 463–7.

219. Sandoval C, Meyer WH, Parham DM *et al.* Outcome in 43 children presenting with metastatic Ewing sarcoma: the St Jude Children's Research Hospital experience, 1962 to 1992. *Med Pediatr Oncol* 1996; **26**: 180–5.

220. Sauer R, Jurgens H, Burgers JM *et al.* Prognostic factors in the treatment of Ewing's sarcoma. The Ewing's Sarcoma Study Group of the German Society of Paediatric Oncology CESS 81. *Radiother Oncol* 1987; **10**: 101–10.

221. Terrier P, Llombart-Bosch A, Contesso G. Small round blue cell tumors in bone: prognostic factors correlated to Ewing's sarcoma and neuroectodermal tumors. *Semin Diagn Pathol* 1996; **13**: 250–7.

222. Craft A, Cotterill S, Malcolm A *et al.* Ifosfamide-containing chemotherapy in Ewing's sarcoma: The Second United Kingdom Children's Cancer Study Group and the Medical Research Council Ewing's Tumor Study. *J Clin Oncol* 1998; **16**: 3628–33.

223. Cangir A, Vietti TJ, Gehan EA *et al.* Ewing's sarcoma metastatic at diagnosis. Results and comparisons of two intergroup Ewing's sarcoma studies. *Cancer* 1990; **66**: 887–93.

224. Marcus RB Jr, Graham-Pole JR, Springfield DS *et al.* High-risk Ewing's sarcoma: end-intensification using autologous bone marrow transplantation. *Int J Radiat Oncol Biol Phys* 1988; **15**: 53–9.

225. Pinkerton CR. Intensive chemotherapy with stem cell support – experience in pediatric solid tumours. *Bull Cancer* 1995; **82**(Suppl 1): 61–5s.

226. Burdach S, Jurgens H, Pape Hea. Myeloablative radiochemotherapy and stem cell rescue in poor prognosis Ewing sarcoma. A 1994 update of the German-Austrian cooperative study. *Bone Marrow Transplant* 1994; **14**(Suppl 1).

227. Miser JS, Sanders J. High dose chemotherapy and systemic adjuvant irradiation in Ewing's sarcoma. *Bone Marrow Transplant* 1994; **14**(Suppl 1).

228. Paulussen M, Braun-Munzinger G, Burdach S *et al.* [Results of treatment of primary exclusively pulmonary metastatic Ewing sarcoma. A retrospective analysis of 41 patients]. *Klin Padiatr* 1993; **205**: 210–16.

229. Paulussen M, Ahrens S, Burdach S *et al.* Primary metastatic (stage IV) Ewing tumor: survival analysis of 171 patients from the EICESS studies. European Intergroup Cooperative Ewing Sarcoma Studies. *Ann Oncol* 1998; **9**: 275–81.

230. Wessalowski R, Jurgens H, Bodenstein H *et al.* [Results of treatment of primary metastatic Ewing sarcoma. A retrospective analysis of 48 patients]. *Klin Padiatr* 1988; **200**: 253–60.

231. Cornbleet MA, Corringham RE, Prentice HG *et al.* Treatment of Ewing's sarcoma with high-dose melphalan and autologous bone marrow transplantation. *Cancer Treat Rep* 1981; **65**: 241–4.

232. Graham-Pole J, Lazarus HM, Herzig RH *et al.* High-dose melphalan therapy for the treatment of children with refractory neuroblastoma and Ewing's sarcoma. *Am J Pediatr Hematol Oncol* 1984; **6**: 17–26.

233. Burdach S, Jurgens H, Peters C *et al.* Myeloablative radiochemotherapy and hematopoietic stem-cell rescue in poor-prognosis Ewing's sarcoma. *J Clin Oncol* 1993; **11**: 1482–8.

234. Hartmann O, Oberlin O, Beaujean F *et al.* [Role of high-dose chemotherapy followed by bone marrow autograft in the treatment of metastatic Ewing's sarcoma in children]. *Bull Cancer* 1990; **77**: 181–7.

235. Ladenstein R, Lasset C, Pinkerton R *et al.* Impact of megatherapy in children with high-risk Ewing's tumours in complete remission: a report from the EBMT Solid Tumour Registry. *Bone Marrow Transplant* 1995; **15**: 697–705.

236. Young MM, Kinsella TJ, Miser JS *et al.* Treatment of sarcomas of the chest wall using intensive combined modality therapy. *Int J Radiat Oncol Biol Phys* 1989; **16**: 49–57.

237. McCann SR, Reynolds M, Meldrum R *et al.* High dose melphalan with autologous bone marrow transplantation in the treatment of metastatic Ewing's sarcoma. *Ir J Med Sci* 1983; **152**: 160–4.

238. Samuels BL, Bitran JD. High-dose intravenous melphalan: a review. *J Clin Oncol* 1995; **13**: 1786–99.

239. Atra A, Whelan JS, Calvagna V *et al.* High-dose busulphan/melphalan with autologous stem cell rescue in Ewing's sarcoma. *Bone Marrow Transplant* 1997; **20**: 843–6.

240. Ladenstein R, Gadner H, Hartmann O *et al.* [The European experience with megadose therapy and autologous bone marrow transplantation in solid tumors with poor prognosis Ewing sarcoma, germ cell tumors and brain tumors]. *Wien Med Wochenschr* 1995; **145**: 55–7.

241. Vassal G, Challine D, Koscielny S *et al.* Chronopharmacology of high-dose busulfan in children. *Cancer Res* 1993; **53**: 1534–7.

242. Frohlich B, Ahrens S, Burdach S *et al.* [High-dosage chemotherapy in primary metastasized and relapsed Ewing's sarcoma. (EI)CESS]. *Klin Padiatr* 1999; **211**: 284–90.

243. Pinkerton CR, Bataillard A, Guillo S et al. Treatment strategies for metastatic Ewing's sarcoma. Eur J Cancer 2001; 37: 1338–44.

244. Meyers PA, Krailo MD, Ladanyi M et al. High-dose melphalan, etoposide, total-body irradiation, and autologous stem-cell reconstitution as consolidation therapy for high-risk Ewing's sarcoma does not improve prognosis. J Clin Oncol 2001; 19: 2812–20.

245. Burdach S, van Kaick B, Laws HJ et al. Allogeneic and autologous stem-cell transplantation in advanced Ewing tumors. An update after long-term follow-up from two centers of the European Intergroup study EICESS. Stem-Cell Transplant Programs at Dusseldorf University Medical Center, Germany and St. Anna Kinderspital, Vienna, Austria. Ann Oncol 2000; 11: 1451–62.

246. Hayes FA, Thompson EI, Parvey L et al. Metastatic Ewing's sarcoma: remission induction and survival. J Clin Oncol 1987; 5: 1199–204

247. Jereb B, Issac R, Tournade MF et al. Survival of patients with metastases from Wilms' tumour (SIOP1, SIOP2 and SIOP5). Eur J Paediatr Hematol Oncol 1985; 2: 71–6.

248. Grundy P, Breslow N, Green DM et al. Prognostic factors for children with recurrent Wilms' tumor: results from the Second and Third National Wilms' Tumor Study. J Clin Oncol 1989; 7: 638–47.

249. Pritchard J, Imeson J, Barnes J et al. Results of the United Kingdom Children's Cancer Study Group first Wilms' Tumor Study. J Clin Oncol 1995; 13: 124–33.

250. Saarinen UM, Hovi L, Makipernaa A et al. High-dose thiotepa with autologous bone marrow rescue in pediatric solid tumors. Bone Marrow Transplant 1991; 8: 369–76.

251. Pein F, Michon J, Valteau-Couanet D et al. High-dose melphalan, etoposide, and carboplatin followed by autologous stem-cell rescue in pediatric high-risk recurrent Wilms' tumor: a French Society of Pediatric Oncology study. J Clin Oncol 1998; 16: 3295–301.

252. Kremens B, Gruhn B, Hasan C et al. High-dose chemotherapy in children with nephroblastoma. Bone Marrow Transplant 2002; 29(Suppl 2): S44.

253. Garaventa A, Hartmann O, Bernard JL et al. Autologous bone marrow transplantation for pediatric Wilms' tumor: the experience of the European Bone Marrow Transplantation Solid Tumor Registry. Med Pediatr Oncol 1994; 22: 11–14.

254. Miser JS, Tournade MF. The management of relapsed Wilms' tumor. Hematol Oncol Clin North Am 1995; 9: 1287–302.

255. Biron P, Bouffet E. High-dose chemotherapy and hematopoietic cell support in brain tumours. In: Dicke KA, Keating A, eds. Autologous Marrow and Blood Transplantation. Proceedings of the VII International Symposium. 1995; 451–2.

256. Abrey LE, Rosenblum MK, Papadopoulos E et al. High dose chemotherapy with autologous stem cell rescue in adults with malignant primary brain tumors. J Neurooncol 1999; 44: 147–53.

257. Finlay JL, August CS, Packer R et al. High dose chemotherapy with autologous bone marrow rescue in children with recurrent brain tumors. In: Dicke KA, Spitzer G, Jagannath S et al., eds. ABMT. Proceedings of the Fourth International Symposium. Houston: , 1989; 449–55.

258. Busca A, Miniero R, Besenzon L et al. Etoposide-containing regimens with autologous bone marrow transplantation in children with malignant brain tumors. Childs Nerv Syst 1997; 13: 572–7.

259. Fleischhack G, Popping K, Hasan C et al. [High dose chemotherapy with thiotepa, carboplatin, VP16 and autologous stem cell transplantation in treatment of malignant brain tumors with poor prognosis. Results of a mono-center pilot study]. Klin Padiatr 1998; 210: 248–55.

260. Graham ML, Herndon JE, Casey JR et al. High-dose chemotherapy with autologous stem-cell rescue in patients with recurrent and high-risk pediatric brain tumors. J Clin Oncol 1997; 15: 1814–23.

261. Heideman RL, Packer RJ, Reaman GH et al. A phase II evaluation of thiotepa in pediatric central nervous system malignancies. Cancer 1993; 72: 271–5.

262. Mahoney DH, Jr., Strother D, Camitta B et al. High-dose melphalan and cyclophosphamide with autologous bone marrow rescue for recurrent/progressive malignant brain tumors in children: a pilot pediatric oncology group study. J Clin Oncol 1996; 14: 382–8.

263. Morikawa N, Mori T, Kawashima H et al. Pharmacokinetics of etoposide in plasma and cerebrospinal fluid in the space left by tumor removal. Ann Pharmacother 1999; 33: 115–16.

264. Vassal G, Tranchand B, Valteau-Couanet D et al. Pharmacodynamics of tandem high-dose melphalan with peripheral blood stem cell transplantation in children with neuroblastoma and medulloblastoma. Bone Marrow Transplant 2001; 27: 471–7.

265. Finlay JL. The role of high-dose chemotherapy and stem cell rescue in the treatment of malignant brain tumors. Bone Marrow Transplant 1996; 18(Suppl 3): S1–5.

266. Finlay JL. The role of high-dose chemotherapy and stem cell rescue in the treatment of malignant brain tumors: a reappraisal. Pediatr Transplant 1999; 3(Suppl 1): 87–95.

267. Kuttesch JF Jr Advances and controversies in the management of childhood brain tumors. Curr Opin Oncol 1997; 9: 235–40.

268. Dunkel IJ, Finlay JL. High dose chemotherapy with autologous bone marrow rescue for high-grade astrocytomas. Bone Marrow Transplant 1994; 14(Suppl 1).

269. Papadakis V, Malkin M, Thompson SJ et al. Autologous bone marrow transplantation following thiotepa, etoposide and BCNU in patients with malignant brain tumors. Med Pediatr Oncol 1994; 23: 185.

270. Heideman RL, Douglass EC, Krance RA et al. High-dose chemotherapy and autologous bone marrow rescue followed by interstitial and external-beam radiotherapy in newly diagnosed pediatric malignant gliomas. J Clin Oncol 1993; 11: 1458–65.

271. Kedar A, Maria BL, Graham-Pole J et al. High-dose chemotherapy with marrow reinfusion and hyperfractionated irradiation for children with high-risk brain tumors. Med Pediatr Oncol 1994; 23: 428–36.

272. Bouffet E, Mottolese C, Jouvet A et al. Etoposide and thiotepa followed by ABMT (autologous bone marrow transplantation) in children and young adults with high-grade gliomas. Eur J Cancer 1997; 33: 91–5.

273. Bouffet E, Foreman N. Chemotherapy for intracranial ependymomas. *Childs Nerv Syst* 1999; **15**: 563–70.

274. Kalifa C, Hartmann O, Vassal G *et al.* High-dose busulfan and thiotepa following radiation therapy in childhood malignant brain stem glioma. *VI International Symposium on Pediatric Neuro-Oncology*, 1994.

275. Bouffet E, Raquin M, Doz F *et al.* Radiotherapy followed by high dose busulfan and thiotepa: a prospective assessment of high dose chemotherapy in children with diffuse pontine gliomas. *Cancer* 2000; **88**: 685–92.

276. Dunkel IJ, Finlay JL. High dose chemotherapy with autologous stem cell rescue for patients with medulloblastoma. *J Neurooncol* 1996; **29**: 69–74.

277. Dunkel IJ, Boyett JM, Yates A *et al.* High-dose carboplatin, thiotepa, and etoposide with autologous stem-cell rescue for patients with recurrent medulloblastoma. Children's Cancer Group. *J Clin Oncol* 1998; **16**: 222–8.

278. Kalifa C, Valteau D, Pizer B *et al.* High-dose chemotherapy in childhood brain tumours. *Childs Nerv Syst* 1999; **15**: 498–505.

279. Mason R, Goldman S, Grovas A *et al.* Intensive chemotherapy and autologous bone marrow reconstitution for children with new or recurrent ependymoma. *Proc ASCO* 1995; **14**: 145.

280. Grill J, Kalifa C, Doz F *et al.* A high-dose busulfan-thiotepa combination followed by autologous bone marrow transplantation in childhood recurrent ependymoma. A phase-II study. *Pediatr Neurosurg* 1996; **25**: 7–12.

281. Mason WP, Goldman S, Yates AJ *et al.* Survival following intensive chemotherapy with bone marrow reconstitution for children with recurrent intracranial ependymoma – a report of the Children's Cancer Group. *J Neurooncol* 1998; **37**: 135–43.

282. Shields CL, Shields JA, Baez K *et al.* Optic nerve invasion of retinoblastoma. Metastatic potential and clinical risk factors. *Cancer* 1994; **73**: 692–8.

283. Schvartzman E, Chantada G, Fandino A *et al.* Results of a stage-based protocol for the treatment of retinoblastoma. *J Clin Oncol* 1996; **14**: 1532–6.

284. Doz F, Khelfaoui F, Mosseri V *et al.* The role of chemotherapy in orbital involvement of retinoblastoma. The experience of a single institution with 33 patients. *Cancer* 1994; **74**: 722–32.

285. Doz F, Neuenschwander S, Plantaz D *et al.* Etoposide and carboplatin in extraocular retinoblastoma: a study by the Société Française d'Oncologie Pédiatrique. *J Clin Oncol* 1995; **13**: 902–9.

286. Pratt CB, Crom DB, Howarth C. The use of chemotherapy for extraocular retinoblastoma. *Med Pediatr Oncol* 1985; **13**: 330–3.

287. White L. The role of chemotherapy in the treatment of retinoblastoma. *Retina* 1983; **3**: 194–9.

288. Zucker JM, Lemercier N, Schlienger P *et al.* Chemotherapeutic conservative management in 23 patients with locally extended bilateral retinoblastoma. *Eur J Cancer Clin Oncol* 1982; **10**: 1046–53.

289. Ekert H, Ellis WM, Waters KD *et al.* Autologous bone marrow rescue in the treatment of advanced tumors of childhood. *Cancer* 1982; **49**: 603–9.

290. Saleh RA, Gross S, Cassano W *et al.* Metastatic retinoblastoma successfully treated with immunomagnetic purged autologous bone marrow transplantation. *Cancer* 1988; **62**: 2301–3.

291. Namouni F, Doz F, Tanguy ML *et al.* High-dose chemotherapy with carboplatin, etoposide and cyclophosphamide followed by a haematopoietic stem cell rescue in patients with high-risk retinoblastoma: a SFOP and SFGM study. *Eur J Cancer* 1997; **33**: 2368–75.

292. Shamash J, Oliver RT, Ong J *et al.* Sixty percent salvage rate for germ-cell tumours using sequential m-BOP, surgery and ifosfamide-based chemotherapy. *Ann Oncol* 1999; **10**: 685–92.

293. Ledermann JA, Holden L, Newlands ES *et al.* The long-term outcome of patients who relapse after chemotherapy for non-seminomatous germ cell tumours. *Br J Urol* 1994; **74**: 225–30.

294. Barnett MJ, Coppin CM, Murray N *et al.* High-dose chemotherapy and autologous bone marrow transplantation for patients with poor prognosis nonseminomatous germ cell tumours. *Br J Cancer* 1993; **68**: 594–8.

295. Kattan J, Mahjoubi M, Droz JP *et al.* High failure rate of carboplatin-etoposide combination in good risk non-seminomatous germ cell tumours. *Eur J Cancer* 1993; **29A**: 1504–9.

296. Droz JP, Pico JL, Ghosn M *et al.* Long-term survivors after salvage high dose chemotherapy with bone marrow rescue in refractory germ cell cancer. *Eur J Cancer* 1991; **27**: 831–5.

297. Hollender A, Stenwig EA, Ous S *et al.* Survival of patients with viable malignant non-seminomatous germ cell tumour persistent after cisplatin-based induction chemotherapy. *Eur Urol* 1997; **31**: 141–7.

298. Fossa SD, Stenning SP, Gerl A *et al.* Prognostic factors in patients progressing after cisplatin-based chemotherapy for malignant non-seminomatous germ cell tumours. *Br J Cancer* 1999; **80**: 1392–9.

299. Broun ER, Belinson JL, Berek JS *et al.* Salvage therapy for recurrent and refractory ovarian cancer with high-dose chemotherapy and autologous bone marrow support: a Gynecologic Oncology Group pilot study. *Gynecol Oncol* 1994; **54**: 142–6.

300. Lotz JP, Andre T, Donsimoni R *et al.* High dose chemotherapy with ifosfamide, carboplatin, and etoposide combined with autologous bone marrow transplantation for the treatment of poor-prognosis germ cell tumors and metastatic trophoblastic disease in adults. *Cancer* 1995; **75**: 874–85.

301. Droz JP, Pico JL, Biron P *et al.* French experience with high dose chemotherapy and hematopoietic stem-cell support in germ cell tumors. *Bone Marrow Transplant* 1994; **14**(Suppl): S39.

302. Rick O, Beyer J, Kingreen D *et al.* High-dose chemotherapy in germ cell tumours: a large single centre experience. *Eur J Cancer* 1998; **34**: 1883–8.

303. Decatris MP, Wilkinson PM, Welch RS *et al.* High-dose chemotherapy and autologous haematopoietic support in poor risk non-seminomatous germ-cell tumours: an effective first-line therapy with minimal toxicity. *Ann Oncol* 2000; **11**: 427–34.

304. Rosti G, Pico J-L, Wandt H *et al.* High-dose chemotherapy (HDC) in the salvage treatment of patients failing first-line platinum chemotherapy for advanced germ cell tumors (GCT): first results of a prospective randomised

trial of the European Group for Blood and Marrow Transplantation (EBMT): IT-94 study. *Proc ASCO* 2002; 21.

305. Shamash J, O'Doherty CA, Oliver RT *et al*. Should high-dose chemotherapy be used to consolidate second or third line treatment in relapsing germ cell tumours? *Acta Oncol* 2000; **39**: 857–63.

306. Lampe H, Dearnaley DP, Price A *et al*. High-dose carboplatin and etoposide for salvage chemotherapy of germ cell tumours. *Eur J Cancer* 1995; **31A**: 717–23.

307. Nishizaki T, Kajiwara K, Adachi N *et al*. Detection of craniospinal dissemination of intracranial germ cell tumours based on serum and cerebrospinal fluid levels of tumour markers. *J Clin Neurosci* 2001; **8**: 27–30.

308. Plowman PN, Kingston JE, Sebag-Montefiore D *et al*. Clinical efficacy of perceived 'CNS friendly' chemoradiotherapy for primary intracranial germ cell tumours. *Clin Oncol (R Coll Radiol)* 1997; **9**: 48–53.

309. Nicholson JC, Punt J, Hale J *et al*. Neurosurgical management of paediatric germ cell tumours of the central nervous system – a multi-disciplinary team approach for the new millennium. *Br J Neurosurg* 2002; **16**: 93–5.

PART **3B**

Advances in therapy: targeted therapy

Novel approaches to therapy

LINDA S. LASHFORD

Much of the improved survival from common childhood malignancies has been achieved by the judicious use of a relatively small number of anti-cancer drugs. The majority of these are anti-proliferative in action and a substantial number exert their action through direct DNA damage. Consequently, almost all children with cancer will experience significant collateral toxicity during therapy, and a proportion will experience delayed end-organ damage and secondary malignancy. The challenges for the future are twofold: to increase survival from tumours where classical agents have had limited therapeutic impact (e.g. metastatic neuroblastoma and sarcomas, central nervous tissue tumours) and to reduce the early and late morbidity of treatment. Strategies such as the use of high-dose and dose-intensive chemotherapy have been widely explored with some tangible benefits; however, further study is unlikely to radically change outcome and will certainly not improve a child's experience of treatment. Changing the pharmacological properties of old agents to achieve a better biodistribution may improve the therapeutic index but is also unlikely to achieve more than an incremental benefit in overall survival.

OPPORTUNITIES

During the last few decades there have been a number of important developments providing opportunities to evolve a new therapeutic landscape. The first of these is the growth in our understanding of the molecular events and biological consequences that underpin tumour development. The opportunity to exploit an understanding of the molecular drivers of the cancer phenotype is best exemplified by the development of the tyrosine kinase inhibitor imatinib. This compound was rationally designed to target the dominant molecular abnormality underpinning chronic myeloid leukaemia (CML).[1]

Chronic myeloid leukaemia is characterized by a reciprocal translocation of chromosomes 9 and 22 to produce the diagnostic Philadelphia chromosome. The translocation results in the genesis of the Bcr-Abl fusion protein, which is a constitutively active tyrosine kinase. The presence of the Bcr-Abl fusion protein is both necessary and sufficient to cause CML and the drug imatinib was rationally designed to exploit this observation by interfering with the active site and modulating its tyrosine kinase activity. The early experience of the drug has been encouraging and has resulted in fast-tracking of its regulatory approval. In a study which enrolled 532 patients with chronic-phase CML and who had failed previous therapy with alpha-interferon, 60 per cent achieved a major cytogenetic response and 95 per cent a complete haematological response.[2]

The developmental pathway of Glivec raises a number of interesting points that bear closer examination. These include the rationale for adopting a new paradigm for therapeutic intervention, i.e. the development of a therapeutic programme that emphasizes a hypothesis-driven, mechanistic drug development programme versus the more intuitive approach of chemical screening for a biological effect, perhaps starting with crude mixtures of natural products and subsequent fractionation, identification and purification of compounds with relevant activity. These two processes are not mutually exclusive, but one of the major criticisms levelled against the latter, more serendipitous process, is the time taken to achieve a therapeutic product. In general it takes approximately

15 years to move a compound from initial discovery through to marketing approval. Thus the development of paclitaxel from identification of activity in a crude extract through to regulatory approval took almost 30 years, and inhibitors of the *ras* oncogene are just entering clinical evaluation approximately 20 years after the description of *ras*'s pivotal role in oncogenesis.

So where will the new targets come from? To date, approximately 30 tumour suppressor genes and 100 dominant oncogenes have been reported.[3] These probably reflect a fraction of the identifiable molecular abnormalities that drive the cancer phenotype. More subtle and lower penetrance molecular abnormalities will take time to identify, but may prove to provide new and important functional information on tumour genesis. Technological developments and organizational change, such as the widespread availability of DNA microarrays and cooperative efforts to organize centralized and widely accessible tumour tissue collections, are essential to achieve a mechanistic understanding of the cancer phenotype.

The UK-based Cancer Genome Project is currently undertaking a systematic, genome-wide sequencing project which should yield many new targets for therapeutic intervention. The important business of collecting and storing high-quality biological material in childhood cancer is being undertaken in parallel, and a joint initiative between the United Kingdom Children's Cancer Study Group (UKCCSG) and Cancer Research UK, a major cancer charity, is systematically banking tumour specimens in paediatric tumours. Similar initiatives are underway in the USA, where there is also a central repository for childhood tumour specimens. These initiatives should help speed the process of identifying novel targets in paediatric tumours and hopefully will lead to a situation in which selection of targets around which it might prove useful to build a drug discovery programme will be the major challenge.

The characteristics that help to identify a potential target for launching a therapeutic evaluation programme can be summarized as follows:

- experimental evidence that the molecular abnormality plays a role in tumour development
- frequent expression in the tumour of interest
- demonstration that the molecular abnormality has a relevant, functional consequence
- target interference results in reversal of the malignant phenotype
- modulating the target is pharmacologically feasible
- appropriate assays are available to demonstrate target interference
- the necessary resources are identified to select and modify a lead molecule for therapeutic development.

These principles are widely applicable, whether the therapeutic development pathway might result in a small molecular weight inhibitor or a biological modulator such as a monoclonal antibody.

MODULATING NOVEL TARGETS

Whilst the Cancer Genome Project may throw up some unique molecular targets in childhood cancer, it is those genes and pathways that are commonly dysregulated in a variety of cancers that will be the most commercially viable and thus represent the immediate and clinically realistic targets for drug discovery. Many opportunities can already be identified where new agents are under development. These include agents that interfere with the receptor tyrosine kinase proliferation pathway [e.g. dysregulated in neuroblastoma (Trk-A), medulloblastoma (HER2) and Ewing's tumours (PDGF1-c)], *ras* farnesylation (gliomas), the cyclin-dependent kinase (CDK; retinoblastoma-mediated control of cellular proliferation), and telomerase, for which there is evidence that its overexpression relates to adverse outcome in neuroblastoma. Broader classes of agents that may be of value essentially contain groupings of compounds directed against both well characterized molecular targets and some less well elucidated mechanisms of action, including anti-angiogeneic agents, inducers of apoptosis and anti-metastatic agents. One way of looking at the opportunities for experimental approaches is illustrated in Figure 27.1, where the ovals represent broad classes of biological effector functions within which are multiple,

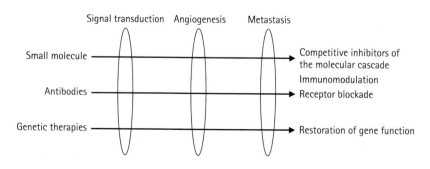

Figure 27.1 *Therapeutic approaches and opportunities.*

interdependent molecular cascades. Some of these will be novel therapeutic targets. Not all of the targets within any biological domain are known, and even where a putative target is identified, its exact role in the biological cascade may be imperfectly understood. Modulating these targets may be undertaken through a number of pharmacological approaches, represented here by small molecules, antibodies and genetic therapies. These are only examples of specific approaches and others, such as cell-based therapies and vaccines, are also important. Examples of the most important features of each therapeutic class are given on the right side of the figure.

Small molecules

As exemplified by imatinib, the first wave of compounds entering the therapeutic arena are primarily small-molecular-weight compounds developed against a molecular event which leads to a gain in function. Many of the resultant protein targets are enzymes, such as telomerase. This reflects the relative technical ease of developing small-molecular-weight inhibitors against a well characterized active site, compared with the more challenging problem of disrupting large protein:protein or protein:oligonucleotide domains by small molecules. The recent acceleration in the development of small-molecular-weight inhibitors has benefited from advances in combinatorial chemistry and production of large compound libraries, the development of high-throughput screening techniques for identification of a lead compound with biological activity from these libraries, and the subsequent molecular modelling and chemical modification to optimize the potency and pharmacological characteristics of the lead compound.[4]

The process is illustrated by the development of a range of inhibitors against the transforming oncogene *ras*. Mutated *ras* has been well validated as a potential therapeutic target. Mutations are common across many important tumour types and have been shown to transform normal cells *in vitro*, as well as driving tumour formation in transgenic animals. Conversely, inhibition of function leads to reversal of the malignant phenotype, cytostasis or apoptosis.

The critical post-translational modification of *ras* that produces its biological activity is prenylation. Prenylation, primarily through farnesylation, occurs at the carboxy terminal tetrapeptide or 'CaaX' box and permits membrane localization of the biologically active protein.[5] High-throughput screening, lead identification and subsequent optimization of compounds have resulted in a range of molecules which compete for CaaX binding of the enzyme responsible for farnesylation, farnesyl transferase, and based on these structures a new class of agents, the farnesyl transferase inhibitors, has entered early-phase clinical trials in adults. These compounds are just entering the evaluation stage in the paediatric arena. A summary of the toxicity profile of three compounds in adults is given in Table 27.1.

Some important features of these new compounds are as follows:

- the dominance of oral, protracted schedules, which should be welcomed for ease of administration and the potential for home use; this may mean some modification of their formulation for widespread paediatric use
- a trend towards a different toxicity profile for many classical chemotherapy agents (in this case, neuro-toxicity and fatigue)
- the incorporation of pharmacodynamic as well as pharmacokinetic end-points in clinical trials. Studies of both R115777 and L-778,123 have incorporated end-points investigating the proposed mechanism of action, although this is done largely through observations of the farnesylation state of surrogate proteins in surrogate tissues such as peripheral blood lymphocytes.

Table 27.1 *A summary of the toxicity profile of three compounds, R115777, SCH66336 and L-778,123*

Study	Inhibitor	Route	Schedule	Maximal tolerated dose	Dose–limiting toxicities
Zujewski *et al.*[6]	R115777	Oral	b.d. × 5 days	500 mg b.d.	Neuropathy
Karp *et al.*[7]	R115777	Oral	b.d. × 21 days	500 mg b.d.	Central neurotoxicity
Punt *et al.*[8]	R115777	Oral	b.d. × 28 days	300 mg b.d.	Myelosuppression
Ferry *et al.*[9]	SCH66336	Oral	b.d. continuous	200 mg b.d.	Vomiting Myelosuppression Neurotoxicity Fatigue Gastrointestinal
Britten *et al.*[10]	L-778,123	i.v.	Continuous × 7	560 mg/m²	Thrombocytopenia Fatigue Cardiac

Antibodies

The second class of experimental agents to show significant development during the last 5–10 years are the monoclonal antibodies. The issues surrounding development of these agents have been extensively reviewed in previous editions of this title. Many of the problems associated with developing antibodies as a therapeutic class were related to the species origin (primarily murine) and consequent immunogenicity, poor tumour penetration and unfavourable pharmacokinetics. Despite these issues, the original goals of the pioneers in this field have remained relatively constant: to develop highly specific compounds against tumour-associated antigens and to utilize these as immunoeffectors or to amplify therapeutic response through their development as vectors for other agents, such as radionuclides or toxins.

Over the last 15 years, technical capability has increased and it is now much easier to humanize antibodies and, by utilizing phage display techniques, to select for higher affinity reagents. Issues surrounding adequate and uniform tumour penetration remain a problem, but a more realistic understanding of limitations and opportunities, such as a potential role in the eradication of minimal residual disease and in treating tumours of the reticuloendothelial system, has helped develop a therapeutic niche. Since 1995, five antibodies have been licensed for clinical use in cancer and at least 16 have reached late-phase clinical trial.[11] These are shown in Table 27.2 and include the anti-GD2 antibody, 3F8, which has been developed primarily for a paediatric indication. The products continue to reflect the aspirations of the field, containing a mixture of effector functions, including the use of radionuclides with varying properties (^{131}I and ^{90}Yt), the modulation of surface receptors (e.g. against HER2) and exploring an immunomodulatory strategy (anti-idiotypic monoclonal antibody utilized as a vaccine).

The development of trastuzumab (Herceptin) is generally accepted as the proof of principle for the field. This is a humanized monoclonal antibody directed against the oncogenic tyrosine kinase, the HER2 receptor. This receptor is overexpressed in 20–30 per cent of breast cancer patients. Two pivotal trials have been undertaken:[12] a study of the antibody as monotherapy in 222 women, all with HER2-positive, metastatic breast cancer; and a study of combined antibody/chemotherapy vs. chemotherapy alone in 489 patients previously untreated for the disease. Results of the randomized study of combined modality treatment were particularly encouraging, demonstrating both a significantly higher objective response rate and prolonged median survival. Outcome correlated with HER2 status and the therapy was generally well tolerated. These impressive results resulted in the fast-tracking of trastuzumab for Food and Drug Administration approval, taking 4.5 months from submission to the granting of a licence for clinical use.

Antibodies against other receptor tyrosine kinases are in development, most notably against the epidermal growth factor receptor. As for trastuzumab, a number of these antibodies show synergy with classical chemotherapy or radiotherapy in xenograft systems.

Table 27.2 illustrates the interest in the commercial and adult sector of utilizing antibody therapy in the management of haematological malignancies, and also provides examples of the range of development strategies for advancing this class of agents. The addition of a second active moiety as the principle effector strategy adds a layer

Table 27.2 *Antibodies that have reached late-phase clinical trial since 1995 (adapted from Carter[11])*

Antibody	Antigen	Origin and isotype	Tumour target	Effector strategy
Tositumomab	CD20	Mu IgG$_{2a}$	NHL	^{131}I
Epratuzumab	CD22	Hu IgG	NHL	Antibody alone
Rituximab	CD20	Ch IgG$_1$	NHL	Adjuvant with chemotherapy
Zevalin	CD20	Mu IgG$_1$	NHL	^{90}Yt
Zarnyl	CD33	Hu IgG$_1$	AML	Adjuvant with chemotherapy
Gemtuzumab	CD33	Hu IgG$_4$	AML	Toxin
Alemtuzumab	CD52	Hu IgG$_1$	B-cell CLL	Antibody alone
Trastuzumab	Her2	Hu IgG$_1$	Breast cancer	Adjuvant with chemotherapy
MDX-210	Her2x CD64	Mu (Fab)$_2$	Ovarian	Antibody alone
Pentumomab	Polymorphic epithelial mucin	Mu IgG$_1$	Ovarian	^{90}Yt
Edrecolomab	Epithelial cell adhesion molecule	Mu IgG$_{2a}$	Colorectal	Adjuvant with chemotherapy
Cetuximab	Epidermal growth factor	Ch IgG	Colorectal, head and neck	Adjuvant with chemotherapy
CeaVac	Anti-idiotypic CEA mimetic	Mu IgG	Colorectal, NSCLC	Vaccine
Bevacizumab	VEGF	Hu IgG$_1$	NSCLC	Adjuvant with chemotherapy
BEC2	Anti-idiotype GD3 mimetic	Mu IgG	SCLC, melanoma	Vaccine
3F8	GD2	Mu IgG$_3$	Neuroblastoma	Antibody/^{131}I antibody

AML, acute myeloid leukaemia; CLL, chronic lymphocytic leukemia; NHL, non-Hodgkin's lymphoma; NSCLC, non-small-cell lung cancer; SCLC, small-cell lung cancer.

of complexity to treatment development. Thus, for radioimmunotherapeutic approaches, as exemplified by tositumomab and Zevalin, efficacy is dependent on three interdependent variables: (1) antibody characteristics such as specificity, affinity, avidity, species origin, (2) the effector strategy (in the case of radioimmunotherapy, isotope characteristics including isotopic half-life, nature of the particle emission, particle range and (3) energy transfer – see Table 27.3). Tumour host factors that influence effect include heterogeneity, level and distribution of antigen expression within the tumour, presence of circulating tumour shed antigen, tumour size and vascularity.

No single radiolabel is necessarily optimal for tumour eradication, as differing path lengths offer different opportunities to match range of particle emission to tumour size. However, the most widely used radionuclides remain the beta emitters ^{131}I and ^{90}Yt, reflecting their ease of production and handling as well as the fact that they both produce a relatively stable chemical conjugate *in vivo*.^{131}I has a relatively short path length over which to deposit its energy (~ 2 mm), which makes it more suitable for targeting relatively small tumour deposits, whilst ^{90}Yt has higher energy, is a pure beta emitter and has a longer path length (~ 12 mm), making it more suitable for larger tumours. Compared with ^{90}Yt, ^{131}I-labelled compounds are less stable *in vivo*, and the production of penetrating gamma emissions during the decay process results in a greater environmental hazard than ^{90}Yt. Depending on starting dose, this necessitates containment and shielding of patients in specialized facilities for a number of days after treatment. This presents difficulties for many paediatric centres, as specialized facilities are usually located in distant radiotherapy centres which may not have a permanent paediatric nursing establishment.

Both tositumomab (^{131}I) and Zevalin (^{90}Yt) are targeted against the CD20 antigen, which is expressed on malignant and normal B lymphocytes, and a number of studies have shown impressive response rates to these agents in chemoresistant follicular low-grade lymphoma and also in transformed non-Hodgkin's lymphoma (NHL). Depending on the study objective, responses range between 65 and 97 per cent for tositumomab, and 74 and 80 per cent for Zevalin. A substantial number of these responses are both significant and durable. A recent review[13] of these two approaches to lymphoma therapy suggested the following tentative conclusions:

- Responses can be achieved at relatively low radiation doses.
- Patients with lower volume disease fare better than those with advanced lymphoma.
- Combination strategies with unlabelled antibodies or chemotherapy or in high dose with stem cell support may be particularly effective.

However, as unlabelled antibody is also effective as a single agent (although less so than the radiolabelled product), there is still a debate as to the relative value of using the radiolabelled conjugate with its additional toxicity.

There is one phase I paediatric study currently open in the UK, testing the value of an antibody–toxin conjugate (BU12-Saporin) in relapsed haematological malignancy. The study is still in the early phase of recruitment but should provide some interesting data on the stability, kinetics, safety and feasibility of an alternative effector strategy in a paediatric population. However, it is the anti-GD2 strategy in neuroblastoma that is furthest developed as a clinical entity in paediatric practice. GD2 is a ganglioside that is widely expressed in normal neural tissue and at high level in neuroblastoma. The murine antibody 3F8 was developed first as an imaging agent and then subsequently as a vector for ^{131}I to target radiotherapy. 3F8 is also able to activate complement and mediate cellular cytotoxicity and has been developed as an immunotherapeutic strategy in its own right. More recently, a second reagent, the chimeric human/murine anti-GD2 monoclonal ch 14.18, has undergone phase I evaluation.[14]

Early experience with both anti-GD2 strategies indicate that the principle side-effects reflect cross-reactivity with normal neural tissue, producing neuropathic pain in addition to the well recognized side-effects which tend to accompany immunomodulatory strategies, such as

Table 27.3 *Characteristics of radionuclides currently under evaluation for radioimmunotherapy*

Isotope	Effective half-life (hours)	Therapeutic emission	Maximum energy (keV)	Maximum particle range (mm)
Iodine-131	193	Beta	610	2.0
Yttrium-90	64	Beta	2280	12.0
Lutetium-177	161	Beta	496	1.5
Copper-67	62	Beta	577	1.8
Rhenium-186	91	Beta	1080	5.0
Rhenium-188	17	Beta	2120	11.0
Bismuth-212	1	Alpha	8780	0.09
Bismuth-213	0.77	Alpha	>6000	<0.1
Astatine-211	7.2	Alpha	7450	0.08

capillary leak syndrome, fever, fatigue, urticaria and hypotension. On a 5-day schedule of 3F8 and at a dose of $10\,mg/m^2$, 16 out of 16 patients experienced grade 4 pain and 13 out of 16 grade 4 hypotension.[15] A similar spectrum of side-effects was experienced in a second study when 3F8 was combined with granulocyte/macrophage colony-stimulating factor (GM-CSF) at the same dose but in a more protracted schedule.[16] In the later study, acute effects were found to be manageable and it was possible to administer treatment as part of an outpatient regimen. Both studies suggest some activity against low-volume disease but no efficacy against larger tumour deposits. Thus 3/13 patients cleared bone marrow disease with 3F8 alone and 12/15 patients in combination with GM-CSF. Two important national and international phase III studies are now open to assess the value of anti-GD2 therapy in neuroblastoma. The developmental process to get this far has taken over 20 years.

'Gene medicine'

A third class of agents that have taken a long time to evolve into clinical development are the nucleic acid-based approaches to therapy. For a long time these compounds have been flagged as potentially exciting for therapeutic development, offering the potential to restore the activity of tumour suppressor genes and to directly modulate transcription and translation. Within this broad therapeutic class are the non-catalytic antisense deoxyribonucleotides, ribozymes, transcription factor decoys and DNA-based 'gene therapies'.[17] Many of the problems associated with bringing these compounds forward into clinical trial have had to do with obtaining stable products *in vivo* and efficient and effective cellular targeting.

For example, the antisense oligonucleotides modulate translation through complementary base pairing at specific mRNA sites. The first generation of compounds were highly susceptible to degradation by exonucleases and subsequent chemical modification of the phosphate backbone by substitution of the non-bridging oxygen for sulphur has significantly increased resistance to exonuclease degradation.

A summary of the first generation of single-agent antisense clinical trials in cancer is given in Table 27.4. These studies have demonstrated the relative safety of oligonucleotide strategies, although serious dose-dependent complement activation was observed with ISIS 5132, producing a range of potentially serious side-effects, including a haemolytic anaemia. Complement activation appeared to be schedule-dependent and was not seen in two other studies of alternative dosing schemes. Importantly, two of the studies have indicated that oligonucleotide strategies are capable of target modulation and individual studies have produced evidence of target depletion of both Raf-1 and bcl-2.

Alternative nucleic acid strategies such as ribozymes and transcription factor decoys are less well advanced. Ribozymes are catalytic RNAs which have the capacity to bind complementary sequences and cleave and ligate target RNA through the catalytic domain. Thus, a ribozyme may be designed to cleave a target upstream of a mutated sequence and then ligate a wild-type version of the sequence into the upstream cleavage product. Consequently, these are a potentially exciting class of agents as they have the potential to act as 'molecular scissors' and snip out abnormal sequences that result from mutations in DNA. Whilst ribozymes may be theoretically engineered to cleave any DNA sequence, there are a number of issues that need to be solved to produce a therapeutic

Table 27.4 *Summary of single-agent phase I studies of antisense therapy*

Oligonucleotide	Target	Study design	Schedule	Output
ISIS 5132[18]	Raf-1	Phase I	2-hour infusion three times per week	Dosed to 6 mg/kg No MTD Raf-1 depletion at doses > 2.5 mg/kg
ISIS 5132[19]	Raf-1	Phase I	Continuous infusion × 21 days	No DLT at 4.0 mg/kg/day
ISIS 5132[20]	Raf-1	Phase I	Weekly 24-hour infusion	Dose-dependent complement activation
GEM-231[21]	Alpha subunit protein kinase A	Phase I	2-hour infusion twice per week	Reversible transaminitis at 360 mg/m²
G3139[22]	Bcl-2	Phase I	Subcutaneous infusion over 14 days	MTD 147.2 mg/m²/day Thrombocytopenia, hypotension, fever, asthenia Downregulation of bcl-2 in 7/16 patients
ISIS 2503[23]	H-ras	Phase I	Continuous infusion × 14 days	Dosed to 10 mg/kg/day No DLT

DLT, dose-limiting toxicity; MTD, maximal tolerated dose.

product. These include an incomplete understanding of cellular RNA structure, optimization of the binding characteristics of any particular ribozyme, such as the length of the antisense arms that flank the catalytic domain, and stability *in vivo*.

There are two principle approaches for producing a useful therapeutic product. The first is to adopt the approach of the 'gene therapists' and clone the ribozyme mini-gene into a viral or non-viral vector. These approaches make use of non-integrating vectors such as disabled adenoviruses or condensation strategies with cationic polymers and thus share with other DNA-based gene replacement strategies problems of satisfactory nucleic acid delivery to multiple tumour sites.

The initial therapeutic gains of 'gene therapy' approaches have largely been achieved through *ex vivo* manipulation of target tissue, such as bone marrow and subsequent re-engraftment, e.g. gene replacement for adenosine deaminase deficiency, or where a relatively modest level of gene expression at a single site can result in secretion of an important circulating protein and restore function, e.g. the clotting disorders. Thus, whilst it is relatively easy to demonstrate clinical utility in a narrow range of inherited disorders and the pre-clinical utility of these approaches for cancer, either in cell lines or through direct intratumoral instillation of vector, it is difficult to obtain widespread and efficient tumour delivery through systemic administration of the naked vector. These are all problems that troubled the early development of antibodies, and given the size of the research effort in attempting to develop effective vectors for gene delivery, it should be possible to chart some major progress in this area within the next decade.

The alternative approach to ribozyme development is to follow the lead of the antisense field and to chemically modify nucleotides to enhance resistance to ribonucleases. At present, generic modifications, such as uniformly modifying a single amino group throughout the ribozyme, appear to compromise cleavage activity. Site-specific modifications appear to be more successful and have generated the first potential product for clinical development, an anti-angiogenic ribozyme targeted to the Flt-1 VEGF receptor mRNA.[24]

Thus, it is possible to discern the beginning of a multilayered approach to modulating tumour biology, from restoration of tumour suppressor gene activity, through modulation of gene expression as well as classical (small molecule) and innovative inhibitors of cellular proteins. These approaches are not necessarily mutually exclusive – a good example is reactivation of the *p53* tumour suppressor gene.[25] Mutated *p53* is well recognized as a common contributor to the molecular signature of the cancer phenotype and is also the primary abnormality underlying the genetic predisposition to cancer that occurs in the Li–Fraumeni syndrome. Functional *p53* is essential to mediate normal cellular stress responses to DNA damage, hypoxia and nucleotide deprivation, and acts either to check cell cycle and permit repair or to activate an apoptotic cellular response. Loss of wild-type *p53* activity results in accumulation of genetic damage and promotes tumour development.

Perhaps the most intuitive approach for restoration of function is to attempt gene replacement through a variety of targeting strategies, including viral gene delivery and composite synthetic vectors. Correction of an underlying genetic disorder, as in Li–Fraumeni syndrome, has different therapeutic goals than attempting to manipulate the *p53* status of a given tumour. Thus, the objective for Li–Fraumeni is 100 per cent somatic reconstitution of a normal genotype, which is probably only achievable through germ line manipulation. Tumour-specific gene delivery should be a more realistic goal, but awaits further refinement of targeting strategies. As this field develops, parallel strategies for gene reactivation are being pursued and may be relevant to the treatment of both Li–Fraumeni syndrome and *p53* loss as a part of tumour evolution. These include the development of antibodies, peptides and small-molecular-weight compounds which can result in regain of wild-type activity. For example, the monoclonal antibody Pab421 can restore specific DNA binding to a variety of mutant p53 proteins. More potent still are peptides derived from the C-terminal domain. The problem of translocating peptides to the nucleus is being addressed through fusion of the peptide with nuclear localizing proteins such as the *Drosophila* Antennapedia protein. Recently, utilizing the techniques outlined in the earlier section on 'Small molecules', a novel compound was identified from screening a chemical library for restoration of *p53* function (PRIMA-1).[26] The compound is able to mediate restoration of *p53* function both *in vitro* and in mice-bearing tumour xenografts, and would appear to be a useful lead molecule around which to launch a drug development programme.

Similar examples can be cited right across the therapeutic landscape, with complementary approaches available, for example, against receptor tyrosine kinase[27] pathways, modulating telomerase expression[28] and angiogenesis.

SPECIFIC ISSUES FOR CLINICAL DEVELOPMENT IN CHILDREN

Access to new agents

Historically there have been problems persuading industry of the need to undertake a dedicated paediatric development programme for new drugs. A combination of small market size and the ethical issues surrounding early-phase studies in childhood has limited the number of compounds being brought forward for clinical evaluation. The dosing and schedules of the majority of classical cytotoxic agents in paediatric use have been extrapolated from adult studies and modified through experience. The pressures to change are twofold. Firstly, regulatory authorities have recognized the need for adequate safety data in childhood and have put in place incentives for industry to integrate a paediatric development programme into their pre-registration research and development. A programme is now established in the USA and this has had a marked influence on the number of compounds being brought forward for clinical trial. The EU is currently considering the framework that should be in place in Europe and this should help drive forward paediatric drug testing in the member states.

The second issue is the influence of market size. In the past, products were frequently dropped from the development process unless they demonstrated efficacy in a relatively common adult tumour. Action has been taken to protect the patent position of companies who develop drugs for small markets, so-called 'orphan indications'. The additional marketing time before competition from generic drugs kicks in has proven useful and a number of 'orphan products', such as Neupogen, have been profitable. With the development of more rational therapeutics, perhaps based on molecular stratification at the outset, there may be an overall effect of reducing expected profitable market size, and thus the paediatric sector may become a more attractive prospect to the pharmaceutical industry for clinical development.

Influence of new compounds on study design

The classical process for developing a novel agent is through a dose-ranging study in which the dose-limiting toxicity is established. This is the dose level at which a statistically significant number of life-threatening events are seen following exposure to the drug. A lower dose level (the maximum tolerated dose, MTD) is selected for further studies which seek to establish the efficacy of the compound. Whilst it will be necessary to continue with a dose-escalation strategy for many of the new compounds, studies are more likely to incorporate a measure of the biological effect of the compound, such as target depletion or activation. Thus the concept of a biologically effective dose is likely to assume prominence in many studies and, with time, may replace the notion of a toxicity-related end-point. It is particularly important to ensure that the chosen biological end-point is directly related to the putative mechanism of action. The potential impact on current paediatric resources for new drug development will be profound, and will include the need to develop academic and industrial partnerships to collect, store and screen tissue samples, establish well validated

assays of biological effect, and consider the implications of these end-points on cohort size and on data management and analysis.

Will a classical phase II evaluation of efficacy be required? Following the first dose-ranging study, the usual approach is to design a second study in which tumour shrinkage is taken as evidence of cytotoxicity and a specific drug effect. The sample size is predetermined by the desired probability of accepting or rejecting a response rate which is indicative of desirable activity. Many of the newer compounds are expected to be primarily cytostatic rather than cytotoxic; others, such as telomerase inhibitors, may require multiple rounds of cellular replication to achieve any effect and responses may have a delayed time course, whilst some drugs may only be active in combination with another rationally designed inhibitor. These issues are likely to require much more flexibility in study design, which may range from rapid transition following establishing a biologically effective dose, through a combination strategy and straight into a phase III evaluation. Alternatively, the combination of disease stabilization and a surrogate marker of biological effect may go forward as an adequate demonstration of efficacy.

Implications for patients

At one level, patients should profit both from any initial biological screen which would maximize their chances of benefiting from an experimental therapy and from exposure to new classes of compounds rather than analogues of previously tried treatments. A rather different spectrum of side-effects may be welcome, particularly if the patient is being dosed below MTD but at a biologically effective level. Alternatively, side-effects such as severe fatigue may be more difficult to recognize in the paediatric population.

One of the inescapable conclusions is that there will be an increased need and pressure for studies with mechanistic end-points, either by direct tissue sampling or through functional imaging. The first approach would argue for an increase in the number of invasive procedures in a child in a terminal phase and is likely either to prove unethical in certain situations or to reduce the willingness of patients to participate in certain study designs. Compromises include the use of accessible surrogate tissues to provide evidence of target modulation (which might include peripheral blood lymphocytes and buccal scrapings), the study of novel compounds much earlier in the disease, scheduling a novel compound immediately before routine and necessary surgery, and development of non-invasive functional imaging techniques for evidence of biological effects. Drawbacks of using surrogate end-points include the question of their reliability in reflecting accurately what is happening in the tumour and the difficulty of taking into account the levels of target in both tumour and surrogate tissue, as well as any differential exposure to drugs, e.g. as may occur in the CNS compared with other tissues following intravenous administration.

Trans-national and international alliances for drug development

To date, there are two main trans-national alliances for paediatric drug development, the Children's Oncology Group, phase I alliance, and EuroNAG, a grouping of centres straddling the UK, France, Germany and the Netherlands. These research groupings have common tasks:

- to prevent duplication of effort through regular exchange of information
- to build a sophisticated laboratory infrastructure which is responsive to establishing new pharmacokinetic and pharmacodynamic end-points
- to work towards an iterative development process that is able rationally to select both new single agents and novel synergistic combinations, and integrating this process into phase III studies.

Both alliances have grown out of earlier coordinated activity, but have been reconstituted to reflect new needs. Each grouping consists of a moderate number of centres that contain the necessary skills and infrastructure for safe drug evaluation and are an important resource to families and physicians seeking access to novel therapeutics.

KEY POINTS

- The challenge of improving cancer cure rates whilst reducing late morbidity in a growing child remains a priority.
- The move is away from traditional chemotherapy drugs towards new agents aimed at molecular genetic targets.
- The potential for immunotherapy (and particularly targeting with monoclonal antibodies) is beginning to be exploited.
- The potential for gene therapy remains limited owing to target access shortfalls.

REFERENCES

1. Gambacorti C. ST1571 (Glivec): a new paradigm for the development of innovative therapeutics in onco-hematology. *Tumori* 2001; **87**: 510–12.

2. Kantarjian H, Sawyers C, Hochhaus A *et al*. Hematological and cytogenetic responses to imatinib mesylate in chronic myelogenous leukemia. *N Engl J Med* 2002; **346**: 645–52.

3. Futreal PA, Ksprzyk A, Birney E *et al*. Cancer and genomics. *Nature* 2001; **40a**: 850–5.

4. Aherne W, Garret M, McDonald T, Workman P. Mechanism-based high-throughput screening for novel anticancer drug discovery. In: Baguley BC, Kerr DJ, eds. *Anticancer Drug Development*. San Diego: Academic Press, 2002; 249–67.

5. Prendergast GC, Oliff A. Farnesyl transferase inhibitors: antineoplastic properties, mechanisms of action and clinical prospects. *Cancer Biol* 2000; **10**: 443–52.

6. Zujewski J, Horak ID, Bol CJ *et al*. Phase I and pharmacokinetic study of farnesyl protein transferase inhibitor R115777 in advanced cancer. *J Clin Oncol* 2000; **18**: 927–41.

7. Karp JE, Lancet LE, Kaufman SH *et al*. Clinical and biologic activity of the farnesyl transferase inhibitor R115777 in adults with refractory and relapsed acute leukaemias: a phase I clinical-laboratory correlative trial. *Blood* 2001; **97**: 3361–9.

8. Punt CJ, van Maanen L, Bol CJ *et al*. Phase I and pharmacokinetic study of the orally administered farnesyl transferase inhibitor R115777 in patients with advanced solid tumours. *Anticancer Drugs* 2001; **12**: 193–7.

9. Ferry ALM, Awada A, Cutter DL *et al*. Phase I and pharmacokinetic study of the oral farnesyl transferase inhibitor SCH66336 given twice daily to patients with advanced solid tumours. *J Clin Oncol* 2001; **19**: 1167–75.

10. Britten CD, Rowinsky EK, Soignets *et al*. A phase I study and pharmacological study of farnesyl protein transferase inhibitor L-778, 123 in patients with solid malignancies. *Clin Cancer Res* 2001; **7**: 3894–903.

11. Carter P. Improving the efficacy of antibody based cancer therapies. *Nat Rev Cancer* 2001; **1**: 118–29.

12. Smith IE. Efficacy and safety of Herceptin in women with metastatic breast cancer, results from pivotal clinical studies. *Anticancer Drugs* 2001; **12**(Suppl. 4): S3–10.

13. Goldenberg DM. Targeted therapy of cancer with radio labelled antibodies. *J Nucl Med* 2002; **43**: 693–713.

14. Ozkayn MF, Sandel PM, Krailo MD *et al*. Phase I study of chimeric human/murine anti-ganglioside GO_2 monoclonal antibody (ch14–18). *J Clin Oncol* 2000; **18**: 4077–85.

15. Cheung NK, Kushner BH, Yeh SDJ, Larson SM. 3F8 monoclonal antibody treatment of patients with stage 4 neuroblastoma: a phase II study. *Int J Oncol* 1998; **12**: 1299–306.

16. Kushner BH, Kramer K, Cheung NK. Phase II trial of the anti GD2 monoclonal antibody 3F8 and granulocyte–macrophage colony stimulating factor for neuroblastoma. *J Clin Oncol* 2001; **19**: 4189–94.

17. Santiago FS, Khachigian LM. Nucleic based strategies as potential therapeutic tools: mechanistic considerations and implications to restenosis. *J Mol Med* 2001; **79**: 695–706.

18. Stevenson JP, Yao KS, Gallagher M *et al*. Phase I clinical/pharmacokinetic and pharmacodynamic trial of c-raf-I antisense oligonucleotide ISIS 5132. *J Clin Oncol* 1999; **17**: 2227–36.

19. Cunningham CC, Holmlund JT, Schiller JH *et al*. A phase I trial of c-Raf kinase antisense oligonucleotide ISIS 5132

administered as a continuous infusion in patients with advanced cancer. *Clin Cancer Res* 2000; **6**: 1626–31.

20. Rudin CM, Holmlund J, Fleming GF *et al*. Phase I trial of ISIS 5132 an antisense oligonucleotide inhibitor of c-raf-I, administered by 24 hour weekly infusion to patients with advanced cancer. *Clin Cancer Res* 2001; **7**: 1214–20.

21. Chen HX, Marshall JL, Ness E *et al*. A safety and pharmacokinetic study of a mixed backbone oligonucleotide (GEM 231) targeting the type I protein kinase by two hour infusions in patients with refractory solid tumours. *Clin Cancer Res* 2000; **6**: 1259–66.

22. Waters JS, Webb A, Cunningham D *et al*. Phase I clinical and pharmacokinetic study of bcl-2 antisense oligonucleotide therapy in patients with non Hodgkins lymphoma. *J Clin Oncol* 2000; **18**: 1812–23.

23. Cunningham CC, Holmlund JT, Geary RS *et al*. A phase I trial of H-ras antisense oligonucleotide ISIS 2503 administered as a continuous infusion in patients with advanced carcinoma. *Cancer* 2001; **92**: 1265–71.

24. Sandberg JA, Parker VP, Blanchard KJ *et al*. Pharmacokinetics and tolerability of an antiangiogenic ribozyme (angiozyme) in healthy volunteers. *J Clin Pharmacol* 2000; **40**: 1462–9.

25. Selivanova C, Kawasaki T, Ryabchenko L, Wiman KG. Reactivation of mutant p53: a new strategy for cancer. *Cancer Biol* 1988; **8**: 369–78.

26. Bykov VJN, Issaeva N, Shilov A *et al*. Restoration of the tumour suppressor function to mutant p53 by a low molecular weight compound. *Nat Med* 2002; **8**: 282–8.

27. Shawver LK, Slamon D, Ullrich A. Smart drugs: tyrosine kinase inhibitors in cancer therapy. *Cancer Cell* 2002; **1**: 117–23.

28. Hedler MN, Wisman GBA, van der Zee AGJ. Telomerase and telomere from basic biology to cancer treatment. *Cancer Invest* 2002; **20**: 82–101.

28

Recent advances in cancer chemotherapy

GARETH J. VEAL & DAVID NEWELL

INTRODUCTION

Although the management of paediatric cancer is often heralded as one the success stories of cancer treatment, in truth there is no childhood malignancy for which therapy can be deemed completely satisfactory. Thus, cure rates of 100 per cent are never achieved and, even when patients are cured, therapy is often associated with significant acute and late effects. There is, therefore, an unequivocal need for improved therapies for childhood cancers.

Therapies for cancer can be classified into five broad categories:

- surgery
- radiotherapy
- chemotherapy
- immunotherapy
- gene therapy.

The central problem with cancer in both adults and children is that, at diagnosis, the majority of patients already have disseminated disease, even though it may not be detectable using standard procedures. As a consequence, local or regional therapies such as surgery, radiotherapy or intratumoral gene therapy cannot, by definition, be curative. Immunotherapy and gene therapy are discussed in Chapter 27 and, whilst holding considerable promise, neither approach has an established role in the treatment of either adult or paediatric cancer. In contrast,

chemotherapy has a major role in the management of the disease, with curative activity in a number of solid and haematological childhood cancers.

As reviewed in Chapter 8, cancer chemotherapy was introduced in the 1940s and the first 50 years of treating cancer with drugs has taught us that, although some types of cancer can be cured by chemotherapy, and hence there is nothing inherently incurable about the disease, cure is the exception rather than the rule. Cancer chemotherapy, as with any drug, is only as good as the target against which it is directed – and therein lies the problem with cytotoxic agents. Cytotoxic anticancer agents work by preventing cell division: by depriving the cells of the nucleotides required for DNA replication, damaging the DNA template or preventing chromosome segregation during mitosis. Thus, predictably, cytotoxic drugs are toxic to replicating normal tissues (notably the bone marrow, gastrointestinal tract epithelium and hair follicles) as well as tumour cells. The challenge is to develop cancer treatments which, in contrast to cytotoxic drugs, are selective for tumour cells.

The development of selective cancer chemotherapies requires the identification of pathways and processes, and the genes and proteins underlying these, that are to a greater or lesser extent specific for the tumour cell. Ideally, these processes should be those that maintain the malignant phenotype such that intervention is not only specific for the cancer cell or tumour, but damaging to its growth and survival. Recognition that the development of selective therapy for cancer is intimately linked to the molecular and cellular pathology of the disease has given birth to the era of 'targeted therapy', which foresees a future scenario in which each patient's tumour is analysed at a molecular level, for gene mutations, amplifications, rearrangements, deletions and polymorphisms, and gene expression at the mRNA and protein levels, following which selective treatment appropriate to each patient is prescribed. Looking somewhat further into the future, such analyses as applied to somatic cells in healthy individuals might identify cancer predisposition with sufficient accuracy to allow intervention with targeted chemopreventive agents. Since the last edition of this textbook, the above vision has moved considerably closer. There are now two well established registered examples of targeted therapies for established tumours (i.e. imatinib for Bcr/Abl- and c-Kit-positive malignancies, and trastuzumab for HER-2-positive breast cancers), and these and the many other agents in clinical development are reviewed in detail below. Furthermore, the study of chemoprevention in high-risk patient populations is being systematically evaluated.

Although these recent results are extremely encouraging, the new wave of cancer treatments has yet to have a major impact in paediatric oncology, and there are structural as well as clinical/scientific reasons for this. Firstly, the molecular and cellular processes underlying paediatric malignancies, and hence the targets for intervention, are often different from those found in the common adult cancers. Hence, from a commercial perspective, the development of drugs to exploit targets in paediatric cancers is an unattractive proposition. Secondly, with the relatively good response and cure rates obtained with conventional therapies in many childhood cancers, paediatric oncologists are understandably reluctant to relinquish well tried and tested protocols. As a result, even when a new drug is available, it is often only offered to patients who have multiply relapsed, and hence very chemo-insensitive, disease.

There is considerable optimism that the future of cancer chemotherapy will be the use of more active, less toxic drugs selected on the basis of the molecular and cellular pathology of each individual patient's tumour. Nevertheless, conventional cytotoxic drugs will remain the mainstay of paediatric cancer treatment for the foreseeable future and hence, in addition to developing targeted agents, attempts to use conventional drugs more effectively must continue to be explored. In this chapter, progress towards the improved use of established agents and the development of novel targeted drugs will be reviewed. In the majority of cases, for the reasons alluded to above, examples will be drawn from studies in adult patient populations; however, there is no reason to believe that similar approaches will not ultimately be equally effective in children.

APPROACHES TO OPTIMIZING THE USE OF ESTABLISHED CYTOTOXIC TREATMENTS

Over the last decade essentially only one new class of cytotoxic drugs has been identified, the topoisomerase I inhibitors, of which irinotecan (pictured below) is the lead molecule. Irinotecan has established activity in the management of recurrent and primary colorectal cancer, and adjuvant studies are ongoing as are trials in other tumour types.[1] Modifications to existing cytotoxic drugs such as capecitabine (pictured), an oral flouropyrimidine prodrug that avoids gastrointestinal catabolism and exploits tumour-related thymidine phosphorylase expression,[2] and temozolomide (pictured), an oral methylating agent that does not require metabolic activation,[3] are examples of incremental advances that improve patient convenience without compromising activity. However, the consensus is that the development of further cytotoxic drugs is very unlikely to have any additional major impact on cancer treatment. Instead, approaches to optimizing the activity of existing cytotoxic drugs are being explored, and these include the evaluation of new combinations of cytotoxic drugs, high-dose therapy, pharmacologically guided treatment and the use of resistance-modifying agents.

Irinotecan

Capecitabine

Temozolomide

Recently developed combinations, with improved activity or reduced toxicity in the treatment of paediatric malignancies, are reviewed in the appropriate disease-specific chapters (Chapters 11–24), as are high-dose therapy and megatherapy (Chapter 26). Here, it is sufficient to note that, in adults, high-dose therapy for breast cancer was not the breakthrough that was hoped for in the early 1990s.[4] Data from a number of large studies are still maturing and these may yet show that high-dose adjuvant chemotherapy does confer a modest survival benefit in breast cancer. However, what is already clear is that any benefit will only have been achieved in the face of considerable toxicity, and hence any future trials must target high-dose treatments to those patients who are likely to benefit.

The use of pharmacologically guided cytotoxic drug therapy to optimize the use of conventional agents has been covered in Chapter 8. In pharmacologically guided dosing, each patient is given the drugs and drug doses that are most likely to produce therapeutic benefit whilst at the same time avoiding unacceptable toxicity. An expanding aspect of pharmacologically guided dosing is the use of pharmacogenetic data where patients with genetic polymorphisms that predispose, for example, to impaired systemic drug clearance can have pre-emptive dose reductions.[5–7] Integration of host and tumour pharmacogenetic information with the use of appropriate targeted therapies (e.g. those discussed below) represents the 'Holy Grail' of cancer chemotherapy, and recent developments are consistent with this being an achievable goal.

Resistance modifiers to optimize the activity of existing agents

The presence of inherent resistance, i.e. failure to respond to initial treatment with anti-cancer drugs, or the development of acquired resistance, i.e. relapse after initially successful treatment, is a common phenomenon in cancer therapy. A large number of cellular resistance mechanisms have been defined (see Chapter 8), including impaired drug uptake, enhanced drug efflux, intracellular detoxification, amplification or mutation of the drug target, enhanced repair of drug-induced damage and resistance to drug-induced apoptosis. Many of these mechanisms have been defined in detail in pre-clinical model systems, notably tumour cell lines; however, only rarely have clinical studies been performed in which a direct relationship between tumour response or patient survival and the presence or absence of a defined resistance mechanism has been established.

Notwithstanding a potential lack of target validation, a number of drug resistance modifiers or reversing agents have reached the stage of clinical evaluation.[8] Amongst these, inhibitors of the p-glycoprotein multidrug resistance protein (MDR-1) drug efflux pump are the most numerous. The MDR-1 transporter is a member of the ATP-binding cassette family of membrane pumps which now extends to the multidrug resistance-associated transporters and lung resistance-related protein. MDR-1 has a broad substrate specificity, which includes anthracyclines, epipodophyllotoxins, vinca alkaloids and taxanes, and plays an endogenous secretory role in the apical efflux of compounds of epithelia, e.g. the lining of the gastrointestinal tract, and in maintaining important biological barriers such as the blood–brain barrier. Building on the initial observations that the immunosuppressive agent cyclosporin A and the calcium channel blocker verapamil were inhibitors of MDR-1-mediated cytotoxic drug efflux, a number of 'second generation' MDR-1 modulators have entered clinical trials. PSC833, a non-immunosuppressive derivative of cyclosporin A, and the amido-keto-pipecolinate VX710 are amongst the more widely studied compounds and phase II trials in patients with paclitaxel-resistant breast (VX710) or ovarian (PSC833) cancer have been reported.[9,10] In addition, randomized phase III clinical trials are ongoing and these will provide definitive evidence of the value of MDR-1 modulation. However, on the basis of trials reported to date, it does not appear that co-administration of the MDR-1 modulator has any profound effect on drug resistance. Non-invasive imaging of MDR-1 activity and its modulation have been shown by using ^{99}Tc-sestamibi,[11] and the pharmacokinetic interaction between many cytotoxic drugs and MDR-1 modulators, i.e. reduced cytotoxic drug clearance as a result of impaired MDR-1-mediated elimination, confirms that pharmacologically active levels of MDR-1 modulators can be achieved in patients at tolerated doses. Given that active levels of modulators can be achieved in patients, yet these appear to be associated with only limited therapeutic benefit, the validity of MDR-1 as a target is called into question.

A second class of resistance modulators that are currently under intense investigation are inhibitors of DNA damage repair. DNA repair mechanisms are being defined in increasing detail and, importantly, certain inherited cancer predisposition syndromes are associated with DNA repair defects, e.g. familial breast and ovarian cancer due to BRCA1 and 2 mutations, patients with ATM-related malignancies and individuals with hereditary non-polyposis colon cancer. In addition, many sporadic tumours have been shown to have DNA repair defects. In DNA repair-defective tumours, redundancy in repair pathways may be lost, and such individuals should be particularly sensitive to treatment with a DNA-damaging agent in combination with a DNA repair inhibitor that removes the remaining pathway on which the tumour is presumably dependent for survival. Inhibitors of the repair protein methylguanine methyltransferase have reached phase II clinical trials,[12] as have approaches to reactivate the expression of mismatch repair proteins,[13] and many other repair inhibitors are in pre-clinical development. These approaches may, for the first time, allow the rational and selective use of DNA-damaging drugs and radiation.

THE DEVELOPMENT OF TARGETED ANTI-CANCER DRUGS

Generic approaches used in the development of targeted therapies

Contemporary approaches to the development of a new drug follow the path outlined in Figure 28.1. The initial stage in the process is target discovery and this involves showing that the target is present in human tumours, using genomic and/or proteomic analyses as appropriate for the target, and demonstrating that the presence of the target is related to the clinical behaviour of the tumour. For example, using the clinically validated example of the HER-2 growth factor receptor in breast cancer, immunohistochemical and fluorescent *in situ* hybridization (FISH) experiments have shown that HER-2 is expressed on the tumour cell surface and that gene amplification, and hence high levels of expression, is associated with a poor prognosis.[14,15] Similarly, in neuroblastoma, *MYCN* amplification is a good example of a well-characterized poor prognostic factor (see Chapter 19).

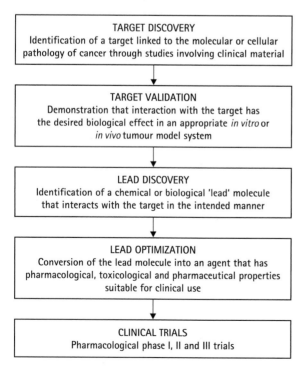

Once a potential target is identified, the next stage is to validate the target, and this is frequently the most difficult stage in the drug development process. Target validation involves demonstrating a clear, and preferably mechanistic, link between the presence of the target, its function and the biology of the tumour. Such a demonstration usually involves showing that adding or activating the target enhances the 'cancer' phenotype, whereas inhibition or removal of the target results in loss of the phenotype. The exact phenotype will depend on the target, but could include cellular proliferation, immortality, invasion, angiogenesis or metastasis. The addition or removal of the target can be achieved by genetic means in either cellular or whole animal models (e.g. transgenic or knock-out animals), or may involve transient modulation with antisense constructs, siRNA or antibodies. Again, using HER-2 as an example, it was shown that HER-2 transfection of breast cancer cells that had normal levels of the gene, with additional copies, resulted in increased proliferation *in vitro* and tumorigenicity *in vivo*. Conversely, antibodies to HER-2 produced tumour cell growth inhibition both *in vitro* and *in vivo*, and the ultimate clinical therapeutic, trastuzumab, is a derivative of the murine antibody used in the pre-clinical target validation studies.[16]

Once a validated target has been identified, the next stage is to identify and develop an agent that interacts with the target to produce the required effect on tumour biology. Although antibodies possess exquisite specificity, they have limited potential as drugs because their size (~150 000 kDa in the case of an intact immunoglobulin molecule) limits penetration into solid tumour deposits, and poor cellular uptake precludes interaction with intracellular targets. For these reasons, the development of a small molecule drug is required for the exploitation of the majority of novel targets, and two generic approaches are usually employed: structure-based drug design and high-throughput screening. Structure-based drug design requires information on the structural biology of the target, which is usually provided by either X-ray protein crystallography or macromolecular nuclear magnetic resonance spectroscopy. Guided by structural information of the target, often with a prototype ligand bound which may be a natural substrate, it is possible to optimize potential inhibitors rapidly. Structure-based drug design was first successfully applied to the development of antimetabolite thymidylate synthase inhibitors[17] and is now widely used as exemplified by the development of kinase inhibitors (see p. 587). An alternative approach is the screening of many thousands of small (molecular weight <1000 kDa) 'drug-like' molecules against the target using a robotic assay for target function (e.g. enzyme activity, receptor-ligand binding, protein conformation) in the hope of finding a lead molecule for subsequent optimization. A combination of high-throughput screening followed by optimization using structure-based design

Figure 28.1 *Stages in the development of anti-cancer therapies.*

is now often used, and the development of the Bcr/Abl tyrosine kinase inhibitor imatinib is an example of the success of this approach (see p. 592).

Once an inhibitor of a validated target has been identified, it is usual to demonstrate that the agent can interact with the intended target, and produce the required biological effect, in an *in vivo* model at tolerated doses. Historically, evidence of activity in a number of *in vivo* tumour models was sought, but with targeted therapies this is not necessary. Instead, activity in, for example, two models with the drug target and lack of activity in one model without the target are probably sufficient. More importantly, the *in vivo* models should be used to develop and validate the pharmacokinetic and pharmacodynamic assays that will be used in early clinical trials with the new agent. In the past, the major objectives of early clinical trials were to identify the maximum tolerated dose (MTD) and dose-limiting toxicities, describe the pharmacokinetics of the drug and seek evidence of activity. With targeted therapies, the objectives are to demonstrate that tumour drug concentrations and levels of drug–target interaction associated with activity in pre-clinical models can be achieved and maintained in patients at tolerated doses. Describing side-effects and clinical response is a secondary objective. To facilitate the required pharmacokinetic and pharmacodynamic studies, it is necessary to have robust and well validated methods, and the primary function of *in vivo* pre-clinical studies is the development of these assays.

The remainder of this chapter will focus on the development of drugs designed to exploit the molecular and cellular pathology of cancer. In a landmark paper, Hanahan and Weinberg[18] summarized the six characteristics of cancer that constitute the malignant phenotype, and these are summarized in Figure 28.2. Each of these processes is potentially amenable to therapeutic intervention, and the following sections describe progress to date in each case. With the exception of therapies designed to overcome the immortality of tumour cells, compounds have reached clinical trials in every other area. The most successful so far have been agents designed to inhibit oncogene function, and in general it is easier to devise therapies where the tumour has a gain of function (e.g. oncogene activation, stimulation of angiogenesis) than a loss of function (e.g. deletion of tumour suppressor genes). A second general feature of targeted drug development to date is that the most tractable targets have been those that have enzymatic activity, with kinase inhibitors being particularly successful.

Inhibitors of activated oncogenes

Proto-oncogenes encode proteins involved in the transduction of mitogenic and survival signals, and are converted to oncogenes by mutation, amplification, translocation or other mechanisms of overexpression, events which serve to activate signalling inappropriately. Oncogene products can be classified into the following categories (and well-defined examples of oncogenes are given):

- growth factors, e.g. platelet-derived growth factor overexpression in glioma
- growth factor receptors, e.g. *HER-2* amplification in breast cancer
- intracellular signal transduction molecules, e.g. *Ras* mutation in multiple tumour types
- transcription factors, e.g. c-*MYC* in Burkitt's lymphoma
- secondary effectors, e.g. cyclin D1 overexpression in multiple tumour types.

In some cases, oncogenes play a dual role in promoting both replication and survival pathways, as exemplified by mutant *Ras*, which stimulates proliferation by activating the mitogen-activated protein (MAP) kinase pathway whilst at the same time inhibiting apoptosis by activating phosphatidylinositol 3-kinase (PI3-K).

GROWTH FACTOR AND GROWTH FACTOR RECEPTOR ANTAGONISTS

The binding of polypeptide growth factors to the extracellular domain of cognate transmembrane receptors leads to the activation of the intracellular tyrosine kinase activity of the receptor, which in turn signals to adapter and intracellular signal transduction molecules. Over 50 membrane receptor tyrosine kinases are known and oncogenic activation of at least half of these has been described in a wide range of tumour types.[19] Although theoretically

MOLECULAR PATHOLOGY	CELLULAR PATHOLOGY
Loss of tumour suppressor gene function	Local tissue invasion and tumour cell migration
Evasion of apoptosis and tolerance of genome damage	Activation of matrix degrading enzymes
	Induction of sustained angiogenesis
Activation of oncogenes	Vascular endothelial cell mitogenesis and invasion
Self-sufficiency in growth signals	
	Metastasis
Activation of immortality genes	Haematological and lymphatic dissemination
Limitless replicative potential	and distant invasion and metastatic angiogenesis

Figure 28.2 *The molecular and cellular pathology of cancer. Adapted from Hanahan and Weinberg (2000).*[18]

possible, the development of low-molecular-weight drugs that prevent the extracellular binding of a growth factor to its receptor has proved challenging, and the vast majority of therapies have targeted the intracellular tyrosine kinase domain. Two notable exceptions are antibodies to the extracellular domain of growth factor receptors and suramin, a polyanion that binds to a range of growth factors. Suramin has modest activity in the treatment of hormone refractory prostate cancer in combination with hydrocortisone,[20] and monoclonal antibodies to growth factor receptors, trastuzumab in particular, are seen as key 'proof of principle' agents that demonstrate that a knowledge of the molecular pathology of cancer can be exploited for therapeutic benefit.

With the exception of anti-endocrine therapies for the treatment of hormone-dependent tumours, where anti-oestrogenic and anti-androgenic agents are successfully used for the treatment of breast and prostate cancer, respectively, trastuzumab has the distinction of being the first targeted therapy to be widely registered for the treatment of a solid tumour. The *HER-2* transmembrane growth factor receptor gene (also known as c-*erbB-2* or *neu*) is a member of the epidermal growth factor receptor (EGFr) family, which is amplified in 20–30 per cent of human breast cancers and is a poor prognostic indicator.[21] Trastuzumab was developed as the humanized form of a mouse monoclonal antibody that had been shown to prevent HER-2-mediated cell and tumour growth in pre-clinical models. The exact mechanism of action of trastuzumab remains controversial and, in addition to direct inhibition of growth factor binding and hence receptor dimerization and tyrosine kinase activation, antibody-dependent cell-mediated cytotoxicity and receptor loss due to internalizaton have also been proposed.[22] Regardless of its mechanism of action, trastuzumab produces single agent response rates of 20–30 per cent in patients whose tumours are classified as being HER-2 overexpressing, on the basis of immunohistochemical analyses, and in some patients complete regressions have been observed.[23] In combination with cytotoxic chemotherapy (an anthracycline plus cyclophosphamide or paclitaxel alone in anthracycline-pretreated patients) for the first-line treatment (excluding adjuvant therapy) of HER-2-overexpressing metastatic breast cancer patients, trastuzumab improved both response rates and time to disease progression in comparison to cytotoxic chemotherapy alone.[24]

On the basis of these data, trastuzumab has been registered for the treatment of HER-2-overexpressing breast cancer in a number of countries, and clinical experience with the drug has highlighted two critical features in the development of targeted therapies. The first lesson is that targeted therapies only work in the appropriate patient population; trastuzumab is ineffective against breast cancer that does not overexpress HER-2. The second lesson is that, despite being a targeted drug and hence, in theory, more tumour-selective, trastuzumab is not without side-effects, most notably cardiotoxicity in patients previously or concurrently treated with anthracyclines. The exact mechanism of this toxic interaction is not known, although cardiac myocytes do express HER-2 at low levels.[25] More generally, the experience with trastuzumab counsels caution when cytotoxic drugs and targeted agents are combined.

The second member of the EGFr family to be targeted is the EGFr itself, also known as erbB-1. Both antibodies to extracellular domain of EGFr and small-molecule EGFr tyrosine kinase inhibitors have been developed. The antibodies include IMC-C225, MDX-447, h-R3 and ABX-EGF, of which IMC-C225 is the most advanced, with phase III clinical trials ongoing (see Table 28.1).[22,26] In pre-clinical models, combinations of IMC-225 with conventional therapy have shown synergy, and in a clinical trial in colorectal cancer of the topoisomerase I inhibitor irinotecan in combination with IMC-C225, in patients with documented progression on irinotecan alone, an impressive overall response rate of 22.5 per cent was observed.[27] Importantly, unlike trastuzumab, there was no relationship between the level of EGFr and response in the latter study, and the key question of the relationship between EGFr expression and response to EGFr-targeted therapies has not been resolved. Nevertheless, clinical pharmacodynamic studies with the small-molecule EGFr tyrosine kinase inhibitors, e.g. ZD1839 (pictured), have shown that tyrosine kinase inhibition can be achieved in patients.[28] Again in contrast to HER-2, EGFr expression is not driven by gene amplification and high levels of EGFr expression could either reflect dependency of the tumour cell on the receptor for division/survival, and hence predict sensitivity to EGFr-targeted drugs, or alternatively predispose the cancer cell to resistance to these agents. Results from ongoing translational research studies will hopefully resolve this issue.

ZD1839

A number of small-molecule EGFr tyrosine kinase inhibitors have entered clinical trials (Table 28.1), of which ZD1839 and OSI-774 (pictured) are the most advanced. The inhibitors differ in their specificity for the members of the EGFr family, and in their mechanism of enzyme inhibition (Table 28.1). Anticipating that receptor tyrosine

Table 28.1 *EGF receptor-targeted therapies undergoing clinical evaluation. Adapted from Baselga[22] and de Bono and Rowinsky[26]*

Compound	Class	Receptor target and mechanism of action	Stage of clinical development
Small molecule			
ZD1839	Quinazoline	EGFr – reversible ATP competitive	Phase II–III/registered
OSI-774	Quinazoline	EGFr – reversible ATP competitive	Phase II–III
PKI 116	Pyrrolopyrimidine	EGFr – reversible ATP competitive	Phase I
GW2016	Quinazoline	EGFr and ErbB2 – reversible ATP competitive	Phase I
CI-1033	Quinazoline	Pan-ErbB family – irreversible ATP site	Phase I
EKB-569	3-Cyanoquinoline	Pan-ErbB family – irreversible ATP site	Phase I
Monoclonal antibodies			
IMC-C225	Chimeric	EGFr	Phase III
MDX-447	Bispecific	EGFr and CD64	Phase II
h-R3	Humanized	EGFr	Phase II
ABX-EGF	Human	EGFr	Phase I

EGFr, epidermal growth factor receptor.

kinase inhibitors will require chronic administration, oral formulations are being developed, with daily dosing representing the most common schedule. Side-effects are manageable, with rash and diarrhoea being common toxicities, the former presumably as a result of EGFr inhibition in the skin. Phase II clinical trials with ZD1839 and OSI-774 have been completed, and both drugs have activity against solid malignancies.[22,26] Two phase III studies of ZD1839 with carboplatin/paclitaxel or gemcitabine/cisplatin in non-small-cell lung cancer (NSCLC) have completed accrual, with more than 1000 previously untreated patients entered into each study;[29] however, there was no survival benefit in the ZD1839 arms. Similarly, phase III combination studies with OSI-774 are ongoing in NSCLC and pancreatic cancer. Mechanistically, the reasons for positive interactions between erbB-targeted therapies and cytotoxic agents are not fully defined but could include both prevention of MAP kinase signalling or impairment of survival signalling through the PI-3 kinase pathway and inhibition of the repair of drug-induced damage.[30] Regardless, an understanding of the underlying mechanisms will ultimately be important for the optimum use of these drugs.

OSI774

The second growth factor receptor to be successfully targeted with a small-molecule inhibitor is the c-Kit receptor. The c-Kit receptor is expressed in a wide range of human malignancies; however, it is an activating K642E mutation in the first of the two tyrosine kinase domains that has been implicated as the key carcinogenic event in 50–70 per cent of gastrointestinal stromal tumours (GISTs).[31] The natural ligand for the c-Kit receptor is Steel factor, which induces c-Kit homodimerization and ligand-dependent tyrosine kinase activation. In contrast, the K652E mutant form of c-Kit has ligand-independent tyrosine kinase activity. During the development of the Bcr-Abl tyrosine kinase inhibitor imatinib (see p. 592) it was recognized that the compound also inhibited c-Kit and the platelet-derived growth factor (PDGF) receptor kinase activities. Following demonstration of the excellent tolerability and outstanding activity of imatinib in chronic myeloid leukaemia (CML), imatinib was therefore rapidly evaluated in patients with GIST. In two separate phase I trials, a high level of activity was observed with imatinib in GIST, with 59 and 36 per cent of patients having partial responses and many others showing clinical benefit.[31] Phase III trials in GIST have therefore been performed, although the level of activity is such that imatinib has already been registered for the treatment of GIST in some countries.

In addition to c-Kit and the EGF/c-erbB receptor family, inhibitors of a number of other transmembrane growth factor receptor antagonists have been developed, in many cases as antiangiogenic therapies. Thus a number of compounds have been developed which target the vascular endothelial growth factor receptors (VEGFr; KDR and flt-1, e.g. SU5416, SU6668, ZD4190, ZD6474 and PTK 787) and some of these agents also target the PDGF and fibroblast growth factor (FGF) receptors. PDGF receptors (PDGFr) have a well established role in the autocrine loop for mitogenic signalling in glioma, in which overexpression of PDGF by the tumour cells directly signals to PDGFr on the tumour cell surface. SU101 (pictured), also know as leflunomide and originally developed as an antimetabolite inhibitor of the pyrimidine biosynthetic enzyme dihydroorotate dehydrogenase, was the first inhibitor of the VEGFr and FGFr kinases to enter clinical trials. A phase I study demonstrated that SU101 is well tolerated, but extensive conversion to an active metabolite (SU0020) was observed, a metabolite that also has antipyrimidine effects.[32] A partial response was observed in a patient with anaplastic astrocytoma; however, it has been reported that phase III trials in glioblastoma have been abandoned.[33] In general, the pharmacology of SU101 complicates the interpretation of clinical results with the compound, and more selective agents have been developed.

SU101

An alternative approach to modulating growth factor receptor-mediated signalling is the use of drugs that activate inhibitory receptors. One such receptor, the somatostatin receptor, has been extensively studied and some encouraging clinical data have been reported. Somatostatin (SST) is a 14-amino acid peptide that has a broad range of exocrine, endocrine, autocrine and paracrine effects. In general, SST-14 and its 28-amino acid precursor, SST-28, are inhibitory peptides which reduce the release of certain hormones, notably growth hormone, as well as gastric acid and pancreatic enzymes.[34] SST acts by binding to a family of cell surface receptors (SSTr), activation of which reduces adenyl cyclase activity, and hence cellular cyclic AMP levels. In addition, SSTr 2, the receptor subtype most frequently found on neoplastic cells, upregulates phosphoprotein phosphatase activity and is linked to membrane ion channels.[34] Phosphoprotein phosphatases can antagonize the effects of receptor tyrosine kinase activation (see above), and hence there is a good rationale for the growth inhibitory activity of SSTr agonists. In addition to direct effects on SSTr-expressing tumour cells, SSTr agonists have been shown to have activity in SSTr-negative tumour models and hence an indirect effect is implicated. Specifically, SST can reduce insulin-like growth factor (IGF) survival and mitogenic signalling by a number of mechanisms, including inhibition of pituitary growth hormone secretion. In pre-clinical models, SST analogues have growth inhibitory activity and at least three compounds have undergone widespread clinical evaluation, namely, octreotide, lantreotide and vapreotide (RC-160). A wealth of clinical experience with neuroendocrine tumours (e.g. carcinoid and pancreatic islet cell tumours) has shown that SST agonists have both direct clinical anti-tumour activity as well as palliating symptoms associated with inappropriate neuropeptide secretion.[35] Conversely, single-agent phase II trials in patients with common solid and certain haematological malignancies have failed to show significant activity, particularly in an advanced disease setting. More limited phase III randomized trials, which report a survival benefit in gastric and hepatocellular carcinoma for patients treated with SST analogues, require repeating with larger patient numbers. Hence, at this time, the role of SST agonists in cancer therapy, beyond the management of neuroendocrine tumours, is not clear.

In conclusion, proof of principle studies with EGFr family and c-Kit antagonists have shown that disrupting membrane growth factor receptor signalling can lead to clinically significant anti-tumour activity. To date, inhibitors of only a small fraction of the receptors implicated in cancer are available and these vary in their selectivity for receptor subtypes. As a consequence, the development of receptor antagonists remains a very active area of drug development with considerable promise.

INHIBITORS OF INTRACELLULAR MITOGENIC SIGNAL TRANSDUCTION PATHWAYS

Following growth factor receptor activation, mitogenic signals are transmitted to the nucleus by intracellular signal transduction pathways. As reviewed by Adjei,[36] the Ras family of GTP-binding proteins are key players in mitogenic signal transduction and are mutated and activated in a high proportion of certain human malignancies (e.g. 90 per cent in pancreatic cancer, 33 per cent in NSCLC and 44 per cent in colorectal cancer). The three major Ras proteins, H-Ras, K-Ras and N-Ras, translocate to the intracellular surface of the plasma membrane following post-translational prenylation, i.e. farnesylation (H-, K- and N-Ras) or geranylgeranylation (K- and N-Ras only). Biochemically, Ras is a guanine nucleotide binding protein, which is activated in the GTP-bound form and inactive in the GDP-bound form. Through interactions with adaptor proteins, activated growth factor receptors cause dissociation of GDP, binding of GTP, Ras activation and hence signal transduction to downstream targets such as Raf-1, Rac, Rho, PI-3 kinase and MEKK1 (see pp. 591–2). Signalling by Ras is terminated by the inherent GTPase activity of the protein, an activity which is stimulated by cytosolic GTPase-activating proteins or GAPs. In mutant Ras, both intrinsic and GAP-stimulated GTPase activities are reduced, and as a consequence Ras is constitutively activated.

Therapeutic approaches to treating mutant Ras-expressing tumours primarily involve prevention of Ras prenylation, and hence membrane localization, or inhibition of targets downstream from Ras. To date, molecules designed to promote or restore the GTPase activity of mutant Ras have not been described. Inhibitors of Ras prenylation include both farnesyl and geranylger-anyl transferase inhibitors (FTIs and GGTIs, respectively), and with both classes of inhibitor, a key factor is the lack of selectivity of the agents for mutant Ras. A large number of proteins undergo post-translational modification by prenylation, including both wild-type and mutant Ras, and hence it is not surprising that in pre-clinical models both mutant and wild-type Ras-expressing cell lines are sensitive to FTIs. The intracellular targets of FTIs remain to be defined, although in at least some cell lines, the pro-metaphase cell cycle arrest produced by FTIs is consistent with inhibition of the farnesylation of the centromere-associated proteins CENP-E and CENP-F.[37]

Three classes of FTIs can be defined:[36,37]

- CAAX competitive inhibitors (e.g. R115777, SCH66336; pictured) – where the inhibitor competes with the Ras substrate by mimicking the cysteine/aliphatic amino acid/aliphatic amino acid/X (where X is methionine, leucine, serine or glutamine) tetra-peptide which directs the farnesyl or geranylgeranyl group to the X position
- farnesyl pyrophosphate competitive inhibitors
- bisubstrate analogues (BMS214662; pictured) – which mimic the farnesyl pyrophosphate–peptide transition state.

Certain of these compounds have entered clinical trials, of which R115777 (pictured) is amongst the more advanced, whereas GGTIs have yet to undergo clinical evaluation. In a phase II trial of oral R115777 (300 mg twice daily), in patients with metastatic breast cancer, a 12 per cent partial response rate and 35 per cent stable disease rate were observed in 27 evaluable patients.[36] Similarly, single-agent R115777 activity has been seen in patients with refractory leukaemia.[38] The dose-limiting side-effects of FTIs include manageable diarrhoea, myelo-suppression and fatigue, although the clinical development of one compound, L778,123 (pictured), has been discontinued because of cardiotoxicity.[39] Combination studies are ongoing with a range of conventional drugs, and SCH66336 (pictured) combined with paclitaxel has shown interesting activity in patients with taxane-resistant disease.[36]

R115777

L778,123

SCH66336

BMS214662

Excellent clinical pharmacodynamic studies have shown that FTIs, at clinically tolerated doses, can inhibit farnesyl transferase, as shown by inhibition of HDJ2 or lamin A prenylation. However, these events are surrogate markers of FTI activity and at present the FTIs cannot claim to be targeted drugs in the strict sense of the definition. Consistent with the general philosophy of targeted drug development, the full clinical utility of FTIs is unlikely to be realized without a firmer understanding of their mechanism of action; however, it is already clear that these drugs do not selectively target mutant Ras.

Components of the MAP kinase signal transduction pathway downstream of Ras have also been targeted and both Raf-1 and MEK (MAP/ERK kinase) inhibitors are in clinical trials.[40] The first of these targets, Raf-1, is mutated in a range of tumour types as well as being activated in tumours with increased mitogenic signalling via growth factor receptors. As reviewed by Herrera and Sebolt-Leopold,[41] Raf-1 is, like Ras, involved in both mitogenic and anti-apoptotic signalling, and surprisingly the latter effect may be independent of the kinase activity of the enzyme. The Raf-1 kinase inhibitor Bay 43-9006 (pictured) is currently in clinical trials,[42] as is the anti-Raf-1 antisense ISIS 5132 (see p. 599). It is too early to comment on the clinical potential of these drugs; however, toxicities to date have been manageable. MEK is one of the downstream targets of Raf-1 which has the advantage of only signalling to the MAP kinases ERK1 (extracellular signal-regulated kinase) and ERK2, and as such MEK has been described as a master gatekeeper.[41] CI-1040 (previously known as PD184352; pictured) is a non-ATP competitive orally active MEK inhibitor, which produces tumour growth inhibition in a number of pre-clinical models at doses that cause a reduction in activated MAP kinase levels in tumour material, and clinical trials with CI-1040 are ongoing.

BAY 43-9006

CI-1040 (previously PD184352)

In addition to intracellular MAP kinase pathways linked directly to growth factor receptor signalling, additional cytoplasmic kinases are also well established as oncogenes and hence targets for therapeutic intervention. Amongst these, *Bcr-Abl*, *c-Src* and protein kinase C have been the subject of intense study, and *Bcr-Abl* has provided unequivocal proof of principle that small-molecule drugs targeted at the molecular lesions that underlie the pathology of cancer can have clinically significant activity.

As reviewed by Mauro *et al.*[43] the *Bcr-Abl* oncogene is formed during the reciprocal translocation between the long arms of chromosomes 9 and 22, the resultant shortened chromosome 22 being known as the Philadelphia chromosome. The Philadelphia chromosome is detected in 90 per cent of patients with CML, and 20 per cent of adults and 5 per cent of children with acute lymphoblastic leukaemia (ALL). The 9:22 translocation results in the constitutive activation of the kinase domain of the Abl protein, and the downstream effects of kinase activation include stimulation of the proliferation via the Ras pathway, inhibition apoptosis via PI-3 kinase and altered cellular adhesion via phosphorylation of Crk1. During the late 1980s and 1990s, Drs Lydon, Matter and colleagues at Novartis initiated the development of Bcr-Abl inhibitors, and the lead compound STI571 (imatinib mesylate or

Glivec; pictured) entered clinical trial in 1998. In preclinical *in vitro* and *in vivo* models of CML, imatinib displayed potent activity, and this activity was rapidly confirmed in clinical studies. The drug was given daily as a single oral dose and, once doses were escalated to 300 mg/day and above, 53/54 patients with interferon-α refractory CML in chronic phase achieved a complete haematological remission, and cytogenetic responses were seen in 17/31 patients. Toxicities were in general mild (grade 1 periorbital oedema, muscle cramps, skin rashes and diarrhoea) with grade 2 or 3 myelosuppression in 16/54 patients treated with ≥300 mg imatinib daily. The outstanding activity and tolerability of imatinib are unprecedented in cancer chemotherapy. Furthermore, the clear mechanistic understanding of the reasons for the activity of the drug hold out real hope for the future management of cancer, as lesions equivalent to *Bcr-Abl* become identified in an ever-increasing number of solid and haematological malignancies.

Imatinib (STI571)

Building on the results of the phase I trial in CML, phase II studies have confirmed that the drug has activity in chronic-phase, accelerated-phase and even myeloid blast crisis CML, and phase III combination studies are ongoing. Perhaps predictably, with a potent and specific enzyme inhibitor analogous in many ways to conventional antimetabolite cytotoxic drugs, clinical resistance to imatinib has already been observed due to both amplification and mutation of the *Bcr-Abl* gene. The use of imatinib in combination with other drugs may limit the development of resistance, and analogues which retain activity against the mutant forms of the Bcr-Abl protein may ultimately be more useful drugs. The development of imatinib has been so rapid that evidence of a survival benefit in the setting of a large randomized trial is only now becoming available; however, 18-month follow-up data on patients treated in the phase II trial of imatinib in interferon-α refractory CML in chronic phase show that remission is maintained in 84 per cent of cases who have a major response, with an overall progression-free survival (PFS) rate of 89 per cent.

In addition to Bcr-Abl, other cytoplasmic kinases that are being explored as targets include c-Src and protein kinase C (PKC). c-Src is a tyrosine kinase that is the cellular homologue of the well characterized viral oncogene v-*Src*.[44] In common with other signal transduction kinases, c-*Src* is involved in a large number of pathways, including proliferation (e.g. via PDGFr, Ras, MAPK and erbB), migration (e.g. via integrin) and survival (e.g. via nuclear factor kB) signalling. Inhibitors of the kinase activity of c-Src have been developed as potential anti-cancer and anti-osteoporosis drugs, although clinical data have not yet been reported. The protein kinase C family of enzymes are, like c-Src, potentially involved in a range of events related to the molecular pathology of cancer, including growth factor signalling, cell cycle control and nuclear oncogene activation.[45] PKC412 (pictured) is an N-benzoyl derivative of staurosporine, a naturally occurring and well characterized kinase inhibitor, which has recently completed phase I clinical trials in adults.[46] PKC412 is, like staurosporine, a relatively promiscuous kinase inhibitor with activity against at least six of the PKC isoforms as well as a number of tyrosine kinases, including VEGFr tyrosine kinase. PKC412 has single-agent activity in a number of pre-clinical tumour models, and enhances the activity of established agents. In patients, nausea, vomiting, fatigue and diarrhoea were the most common toxicities of PKC412, and were dose-limiting at daily oral doses of 225 and 300 mg in the phase I trial. A partial response was observed in a patient with cholangiocarcinoma, and parallel pharmacodynamic studies using peripheral blood cells provided evidence of PKC inhibition at tolerated doses.

PKC412

However, avid binding to plasma α_1-acid glycoprotein was a notable property of PKC412, which may complicate the clinical utility of the agent, particularly in relation to dose optimization in individual patients.

NUCLEAR ONCOGENES

As described in Chapter 2, many of the genes whose role in childhood cancer has been most clearly defined at the molecular genetic level are those in which amplification (e.g. *MYCN* in neuroblastoma), overexpression

(e.g. c-*Myc* in Burkitt lymphoma), translocation to form fusion proteins (e.g. *PML-RARA* in acute myeloid leukaemia and *EWS/FLI-1* in Ewing's sarcoma) or inactivating deletions (e.g. *WT1* in Wilms' tumours) involve transcription factors. Transcription factors interact with DNA as part of multi-protein complexes, and hence disrupting or promoting their activity requires an ability to bind to either specific DNA sequences or large protein/protein interaction surfaces. Designing such binding properties into small-molecule drugs is extremely challenging and has yet to be systematically realized. Building on experience with small-molecule DNA interactive cytotoxic agents, progress has been made in the development of drugs that target specific DNA sequences as well DNA–protein complexes.[47] Such agents may ultimately be very important in the treatment of paediatric tumours, although drugs with the required specificity and biological activity are still some way from clinical trials.

PROTEASOME INHIBITION

Recently, a novel approach to the control of proliferation has reached the stage of clinical evaluation, namely, the inhibition of proteasome activity.[48] A number of cell cycle regulatory and cell cycle-related proteins (e.g. certain cyclins, CDK inhibitors, cdc25 phosphatase, p53), nuclear oncogenes (e.g. c-*Fos*/c-*Jun*, c-*Myc* and *MYCN*) and enzymes (e.g. topoisomerases I and IIα) are degraded by the 26s proteasome. Inhibition of proteasome activity by the dipeptidyl boronic acids such as PS-341 (pictured) causes cell growth inhibition and apoptosis. For reasons that are not well understood, apoptosis induced by proteasome inhibition shows tumour cell selectivity, and proteasome inhibitors are active in a number of pre-clinical tumour models. PS-341 has entered clinical trials and phase I studies have shown that once or twice weekly PS-341 is well tolerated provided proteasome inhibition does not exceed 80 per cent, which is achieved by doses in the range 1–1.5 mg/m^2. Side-effects include low-grade fever, fatigue, diarrhoea and, in patients previously treated with neurotoxins, reversible peripheral neuropathy. Importantly, evidence of activity has been seen in a number of tumour types, with 50 per cent of myeloma patients with relapsed or refractory disease showing evidence of a response, and a large clinical programme of single-agent and combination studies is ongoing.[48]

PS-341

Therapies to restore or replace tumour suppressor gene function

The molecular pathology of cancer involves three key events: the activation of oncogenes and immortality genes, and the loss of function of tumour suppressor genes, the latter due to mutation, deletion or epigenetic gene silencing. Therapeutically, a disease process that involves loss of function is a more challenging target in comparison to events that involve gain of function, where enzyme inhibitors or receptor antagonists can be made. In the case of tumour suppressor gene loss of function, three major approaches to restoring activity have been explored:

- the reactivation of tumour suppressor genes that have been epigenetically silenced
- the 'reshaping' of mutant proteins such that normal function is restored
- the inhibition of downstream targets whose activity is deregulated in the absence of normal tumour suppressor gene function.

TUMOUR SUPPRESSOR GENE REACTIVATION BY EPIGENETIC MODULATORS

The regulation of gene expression is extremely complex and involves multiple levels of control and large numbers of gene products that often function in multiprotein complexes. Two important covalent modifications are the 5-methylation of cytosine residues in cytosine-guanine (CpG) doublets in the promoter regions of certain genes, and the acetylation of histones in chromatin.[13,49] Therapeutic agents that inhibit both of these epigenetic modifications are currently in clinical trials.

The 5-methylation of cytosine in CpG-containing promoter regions of genes leads to gene silencing, and important tumour suppressor genes that are regulated by methylation include *p16* and *p15*, inhibitors of cyclin-dependent kinases (CDK), and the retinoblastoma gene, the protein that maintains the E2F transcription factors in an inactive form (see Figure 28.3). The enzyme family members responsible for 5-methylation of cytosine are the DNA methyltransferases (DNMTs), and these can be irreversibly inhibited by the nucleoside 5-azadeoxy-cytidine (pictured) once it is incorporated into DNA. In addition, an antisense molecule that targets DNMT1 is undergoing clinical evaluation (see below). Clinical trials with 5-azadeoxycytidine and DNMT1 antisense have yet to demonstrate marked single-agent activity in common tumours, and the use of the agents in combination with cytotoxic drugs, in order to restore tumour suppressor gene function in the face of DNA damage, may be the more fruitful.

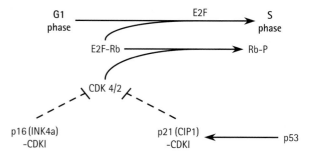

Figure 28.3 *Control of G1→S phase cell cycle progression by the p53-Rb tumour suppressor gene pathway. E2F, E2F transcription factors; Rb, retinoblastoma protein; P, phosphorylation; CDK4/2, cyclin-dependent kinases 4 and 2; p16 and p21, endogenous peptide CDK inhibitors (CDKI). Solid arrows indicate activation and broken lines inhibition.*

5-Azadeoxycytidine

The acetylation of histones is a second major transcriptional control mechanism.[50] Following acetylation, the electrostatic interaction between positively charged histones and negatively charged DNA is greatly reduced, and as a consequence the chromatin relaxes and the DNA becomes more accessible to transcription complexes. As a result, a wide range of genes are activated, including the gene for p21, a further endogenous peptide CDK inhibitor (see Figure 28.3), one that is normally regulated by p53. Acting in opposition to histone acetylation is histone deacetylation, and histone deacetylases (HDACs) have also been targeted in an attempt to prevent the epigenetic silencing of tumour suppressor genes. HDAC inhibitors have entered clinical trials and pre-clinical data, particularly when HDAC inhibitors are used in combination with cytotoxic drugs, are impressive; whether or not this promise will be borne out in patients remains to be seen.

THE RESHAPING OF MUTANT TUMOUR SUPPRESSOR PROTEINS

The *p53* tumour suppressor gene is often cited as the gene most frequently disrupted in human cancer. As indicated in Figure 28.3, *p53* indirectly controls transition from the G1 to the S phase of the cell cycle by regulating, amongst many other genes, levels of the *p21* peptide CDK inhibitor. In normal cells, DNA damage causes G1/S cell cycle arrest via *p53* activation and *p21* induction, whilst in *p53*-deficient cells, arrest is not seen. In addition, *p53* plays a key role in apoptotic signalling, and lack of *p53* function can be associated with reduced cytotoxic drug-induced cell killing, although the effect is highly cell line/tumour-dependent. In tumours which express mutant, non-functional *p53*, a possible therapeutic approach is the use of molecules that can induce a conformational shift in the mutant protein, such that a functional conformation is adopted. Studies with the PAb421 monoclonal antibody have shown that *p53* can be activated by external non-covalent ligands, and this observation has stimulated the screening of chemical collections for small molecules capable of reactivating mutant forms of *p53*.[51] These screens have apparently yielded 'hits' and the resultant molecules have been shown to inhibit tumour cell growth *in vitro* and *in vivo*; however, clinical trials with these agents have yet to be reported.[52,53]

Other approaches to restoring the function of *p53* include preventing premature MDM2-mediated degradation[51] and the promotion of active *p53* tetramerization through the inhibition of molecular chaperone function, e.g. heat-shock protein 90 inhibition by the ansamycin 17-allylaminogeldanamycin.[54]

INHIBITION OF DOWNSTREAM TARGETS OF TUMOUR SUPPRESSOR GENES

As illustrated in Figure 28.3, the CDKs are key targets for endogenous peptide CDK inhibitors such as *p16* and *p21*, and hence CDKs are being intensively studied as potential drug targets for the treatment of tumours where endogenous *p53*/*p21* or *p16* is non-functional. The cyclin partners of CDKs are frequently overexpressed in human cancers, and CDK mutations have been described. As kinases, CDKs are excellent targets for drug development, and a large number of inhibitors have been developed. Clinical trials with at least three CDK inhibitors, flavopiridol (pictured), UCN-01 (pictured) and R-roscovitine (pictured), are underway and the first mentioned agent has completed phase II single-agent trials, although no significant activity was detected in a range of solid adult malignancies.[55,56] In general, these first-generation CDK inhibitors lack the level of kinase specificity that is likely to be required to exploit CDKs as targets; nevertheless, they are important probe molecules that will facilitate the development of more selective compounds.

UCN-01

R-roscovitine

Flavopiridol

Tumour cell immortality and telomerase inhibitors

As indicated in Figure 28.2, cellular immortality is a key hallmark of cancer and there is significant current interest in telomerase because of the role this enzyme plays in the immortalization of tumour cells. Telomerase is a ribonucleoprotein DNA polymerase required for the replication of the ends of eukaryotic chromosomes that are characterized by tandem nucleotide repeats which, in humans, have the sequence TTAGGG. Telomeres composed of these tandem repeats may be up to 15 000 bases in length, and, in a normal cell population, successive divisions are associated with a progressive shortening of the length of the telomere as telomeric repeats are lost. This observation has led to the proposal that telomere length is the 'biological clock' that ultimately limits the number of divisions that any one cell can undergo. When telomeres become sufficiently short, cells enter an irreversible growth arrest called cellular senescence. In most cases, senescence occurs before cells can accumulate enough mutations to become transformed, and thus the growth arrest induced by short telomeres may be a potent tumour suppressor mechanism. A pivotal observation is that most normal cells, either taken directly from patients or following short-term culture, lack telomerase activity, whereas tumour cell lines and primary tumour material have detectable telomerase activity in the majority of cases. Indeed, telomerase activity has been detected in 85 per cent of all cancers studied.[57] Therefore, whereas normal cells undergo a limited number of rounds of replication and telomere shortening before senescence, tumour cells have a potentially unlimited capacity to divide and can thus be immortalized.

Studies of normal tissue have shown that telomerase activity is only detectable in the testis, ovary and, probably, tissue stem cells. This would be consistent with the need to ensure that germ cells have full-length telomeres for progeny to inherit and stem cells for tissue renewal. The current hypothesis is, therefore, that tumour cells must reactivate telomerase in order to sustain indefinite cell proliferation, whereas normal tissues do not require this enzyme activity.[58] Of relevance to paediatric oncology is the observation that low telomerase activity was found in stage 4S neuroblastoma tumours that spontaneously regressed, and in good prognosis stage 3 and 4 neuroblastoma tumours, whereas patients whose tumours had high levels of the enzyme had an unfavourable outcome. Overall, only two out of 63 patients with low or undetectable levels of telomerase activity died of their disease compared with 12 out of 16 who had high levels.[59] This preliminary finding in neuroblastoma has been supported by several publications suggesting that telomerase activity may act as a useful prognostic factor for neuroblastoma progression. Similar studies in Wilms' tumour have indicated significant levels of telomerase activity in tumour samples and a correlation between high levels of telomerase reverse transcriptase messenger RNA and tumour recurrence in patients with favourable histology Wilms' tumour.[60] Telomerase activation has also been investigated in haematological malignancies with considerable increases in enzyme activity observed during progression of myeloid leukaemias.[61] This latter study also suggested a tendency for higher telomerase activity to be observed in relapsed cases. A study in children with acute myeloid leukaemia (AML) or ALL showed high telomerase activity in mononuclear cells from all leukaemia patients, at levels comparable to those in biopsy specimens from paediatric solid tumour patients. Furthermore, telomerase was consistently and highly upregulated in bone marrow and peripheral blood specimens in leukaemia at diagnosis, but decreased after induction chemotherapy and correlated with patient remission.[62]

These findings have led to the concept of telomerase as a highly selective, albeit challenging, target for the development of new anti-tumour agents.[63] Inhibition of telomerase would be expected to exhibit a lag period, as cell growth will not be arrested until cells have undergone sufficient cell divisions to give critical telomere shortening. Treatment may have to be given continuously for many weeks or months and, even then, telomerase inhibition alone may well not be sufficient for the treatment of large tumour masses.[64] Despite these limitations, however, telomerase inhibitors may prove to be an effective adjuvant treatment in combination with other anti-cancer drugs, and may offer a unique approach to the treatment of minimal residual disease (MRD).

Several approaches to telomerase inhibition have been reported, including peptide nucleic acids and oligonucleotides targeted to the telomerase RNA template, nucleoside reverse transcriptase inhibitors and compounds that target telomeric DNA such as cationic porphyrins or anthraquinones.[65–67] Recently, a novel structural class of non-peptide, non-nucleoside inhibitors of human telomerase have been shown to be highly potent and selective *in vitro* and to result in a marked reduction of the tumorigenic potential of drug-treated tumour cells when used in a mouse xenograft model.[68] Similarly encouraging preclinical results have been published by several groups and candidate telomerase inhibitors are now being selected for clinical trials. The success of this approach to anticancer treatment will require good tolerability of continuous treatment, a low toxicity profile and a practical route of administration.

Retinoids in cancer

The past decade has seen the emergence of a class of compounds known as retinoids for use in the treatment of a number of different paediatric malignancies. Retinoids are naturally occurring and synthetic analogues related to retinol, or vitamin A, that exert biological effects related to control of cell proliferation, differentiation and fetal development.[69] Retinoids are believed to exert most of their effects by binding to specific nuclear receptors, the retinoic acid receptors (RAR-α, β and γ) and the retinoid X receptors (RXR-α, β and γ), thereby modulating gene expression.[70] Specific cellular retinoid-binding proteins, cellular retinol-binding protein (CRBP) and cellular retinoic acid-binding protein (CRABP), have also been identified and are involved in regulating the availability of the retinoids for nuclear receptor binding.[71] The clinical use of retinoids has been investigated predominantly in studies involving patients with premalignant lesions and patients with a high risk of developing a second primary cancer. Trials with all-*trans*-retinoic acid (ATRA; pictured) have been carried out in a number of different cancers, including squamous cell carcinoma, high-risk myelodysplastic syndromes and multiple myeloma. 13-*cis*-retinoic acid (13-*cis*RA; pictured) has been shown to be clinically beneficial in the treatment of early-stage head and neck squamous cell carcinoma and phase II trials have also been carried out in metastatic renal cell carcinoma and for high-risk myelodysplastic syndromes. A phase I study with 9-*cis*RA has also recently been completed in paediatric patients with refractory cancer.[72] However, the most dramatic clinical benefits from the use of retinoids in paediatric oncology have been observed with ATRA in children with acute promyelocytic leukaemia (APL) and with 13-*cis*RA in the treatment of high-risk neuroblastoma.

All-trans-retinoic acid

13-cis-retinoic acid

APPLICATION OF ATRA IN THE TREATMENT OF APL

The possible clinical use of ATRA for the treatment of APL was based on *in vitro* studies showing terminal differentiation of human promyelocytic cells in response to this retinoid. The clinical activity of ATRA in patients with APL was first shown in a study of 24 patients with APL who were either non-responsive or resistant to chemotherapy, or were previously untreated. All patients studied, including both children and adults, attained complete remission following treatment with ATRA at doses of 45–100 mg/m²/day.[73] Similar results have since been published from several phase II trials with ATRA, all confirming that this retinoid effectively induces complete remission in the majority of patients studied. However, these trials have also shown that the period of complete remission with ATRA is usually short and relapse is commonly seen unless ATRA treatment is consolidated with post-remission intensive chemotherapy. Studies investigating possible resistance mechanisms to ATRA have indicated that continuous daily treatment is associated with a marked decrease in plasma drug concentrations at the time of relapse, as compared with systemic concentrations when ATRA therapy is initiated.[74] In an attempt to overcome this problem, a number of techniques have been investigated to modulate the induction of ATRA clearance, including the use of liposomal drug formulations, inhibitors of cytochrome P450 induction and intermittent dosing strategies.

APPLICATION OF 13-*cis*RA IN THE TREATMENT OF NEUROBLASTOMA

The clinical benefits of 13-*cis*RA for the treatment of high-risk neuroblastoma were not established until the publication of data from the US Children's Cancer Group (CCG) study by Matthay *et al*. in 1999.[75] The 13-*cis*RA dosing regimen used in this clinical study, a dose of 160 mg/m²/day administered orally in two divided doses

for 14 consecutive days in a 28-day treatment course (six courses in total), was based on results from a phase I trial of 13-*cis*RA in neuroblastoma patients. This dose of 13-*cis*RA was shown to result in plasma levels known to be effective against neuroblastoma cells *in vitro*. The CCG randomized study demonstrated a significant improvement in the 3-year event-free survival (EFS), from 29 to 47 per cent, for patients receiving 13-*cis*RA after myeloablative chemotherapy as opposed to those assigned to no further treatment. Previous studies in similar patient populations, but with lower doses of 13-*cis*RA given continuously, had shown 13-*cis*RA to have no clinical benefit for the treatment of advanced neuroblastoma. These findings raise the possibility that high-dose intermittent retinoid schedules may be effective in other diseases where low-dose continuous administration has shown no benefit.

NOVEL RETINOIDS AND FUTURE USES

In addition to the use of naturally occurring retinoids, a number of novel retinoids have been synthesized. Currently the most promising of these would appear to be fenretinide (pictured) which has been shown to be more effective than either 13-*cis*RA or ATRA in inhibiting growth and inducing apoptosis in many different tumour cell types.[76] This synthetic retinoid has also been shown to be effective in neuroblastoma cell lines resistant to 13-*cis*RA and to act synergistically with cytotoxic drugs such as carboplatin, cisplatin and etoposide *in vitro*.[77] Fenretinide is currently being investigated in several clinical trials as a therapeutic and chemopreventive agent.

Preliminary data from these early clinical studies suggest that the retinoids will be useful clinical tools in both chemoprevention and advanced disease, or as adjuvant therapy in combination with other chemotherapeutic agents. Ongoing and future studies will determine the optimal retinoic acid isomers to use for individual tumour types, and the most effective way to combine retinoids with established cytotoxic agents.

Fenretinide

ANTISENSE TECHNOLOGY TO TARGET THE MOLECULAR PATHOLOGY OF CANCER

The promise of antisense technology for cancer treatment lies in its potential selectivity for target oncogenes.

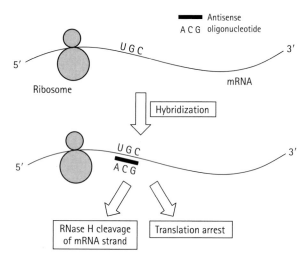

Figure 28.4 *Proposed mechanisms of action of antisense oligonucleotides.*

An antisense oligodeoxynucleotide has a sequence that is opposite to that of the normal mRNA transcript for a given gene, such that a duplex forms between the mRNA and the antisense DNA oligonucleotide.[78,79] Once the antisense oligonucleotide has bound to the target mRNA sequence, there are a number of potential mechanisms of action. Firstly, the direct binding of the antisense oligonucleotide to the mRNA, by Watson–Crick hybridization, may lead to the steric inhibition of translation by ribosomes. Alternatively, or additionally, protein production may be inhibited by the action of RNase H, an ubiquitous ribonuclease that degrades the RNA strand of the formed RNA–DNA duplex (see Figure 28.4). Other possible mechanisms of action include inhibition of mRNA splicing or transport to the cell cytoplasm.[80,81] Depletion of target gene mRNA levels leads to a cessation of translation and, if the gene is required for cell growth or survival, cytostasis and/or cell death will be produced. This approach allows the expression of a single member of a gene family to be specifically inhibited and should lead to less non-specific toxicity than observed with more conventional cytotoxic anti-cancer drugs. An example of this specificity was demonstrated in a study in neuroepithelioma cells, where antisense inhibition of single copy *MYCN* expression resulted in decreased cell growth without any reduction of C-Myc protein levels.[82]

The development of antisense drugs in general has been complicated by a variety of methodological limitations, many of which have still not been adequately resolved. Initial stability problems with phosphodiester oligonucleotides were overcome with the synthesis of phosphorothioate oligonucleotides, in which a non-bridging oxygen in the oligonucleotide is replaced by a sulphur atom. Such modifications, however, whilst increasing oligonucleotide resistance to nucleases, result in a decreased hydrophobicity and hence problems with cellular uptake.

Liposomal delivery systems are frequently used to maximize intracellular accumulation of antisense oligonucleotides *in vitro* but have not been widely studied *in vivo*. Additional obstacles can be encountered once the oligonucleotide is inside the cell, with entrapment in endosomes and lysosomes being a frequent problem, and access to the target sequence of the intricately folded nuclear RNA also potentially limiting the efficacy of these drugs. However, despite these difficulties, progress has been made in the treatment of many different diseases and an antisense drug has now been licensed for use in the treatment of cytomegalovirus-induced retinitis in AIDS patients.

The application of antisense to cancer

With respect to their potential use in cancer treatment, antisense oligonucleotides have been designed to target many different oncogenes, and in a number of cases development has progressed to clinical trials (summarized below). These include phase I and phase II trials with antisense monotherapy in patients with a variety of different malignancies, as well as studies investigating the use of antisense oligonucleotides in combination with conventional chemotherapeutic agents.

bcl-2 ANTISENSE (G3139)

The *bcl-2* gene is overexpressed in the majority of low-grade non-Hodgkin's lymphoma (NHL) patients and 50 per cent of high-grade NHL cases, commonly due to a translocation between chromosomes 14 and 18. The cellular resistance to apoptosis caused by *bcl-2* overexpression leads to drug resistance and a poor clinical prognosis,[83] thus making *bcl-2* an attractive target for antisense strategies. The phosphorothioate antisense oligonucleotide G3139, targeted to the first six codons of the *bcl-2* mRNA open reading frame, has demonstrated effectiveness in a variety of tumour models *in vitro* and *in vivo*, and a phase I clinical trial has been completed in patients with NHL.[84] This phase I study involved 21 patients with *bcl-2*-positive relapsed NHL receiving a 14-day subcutaneous infusion of G3139. A MTD of 6 mg/kg/day was determined with dose-limiting toxicities of leucopenia and thrombocytopenia. This dose is well within the therapeutic range observed in animal model studies with G3139. A complete clinical remission was achieved in one patient, two had partial responses and eight had stabilization of disease. In addition, levels of *bcl-2* expression were reduced in peripheral blood lymphocytes and lymph nodes of patients following treatment with G3139. Based on the results of this clinical study, a phase II trial is currently in progress using G3139 in combination with standard chemotherapy regimens for patients with relapsed, chemotherapy-resistant NHL. A phase I–II trial of G3139 in advanced malignant melanoma, a disease in which chemoresistance has been linked to expression of *bcl-2*, has also recently been completed. Significant decreases in bcl-2 protein levels in melanoma samples were observed concomitantly with increased tumour cell apoptosis and clinical responses in six out of 14 patients studied.[85] This anti-tumour effect was improved further when the antisense oligonucleotide was co-administered with dacarbazine and the combination regimen was well tolerated.

PROTEIN KINASE C-α ANTISENSE (ISIS 3521)

Protein kinase C-α (PKC-α) is a member of a family of serine/threonine kinases involved in the initiation of cellular responses such as cellular proliferation and differentiation (see p. 593). Changes in PKC expression have been linked to the growth and progression of some human tumours, and inhibitors of PKC have demonstrated anti-tumour activity both *in vitro* and *in vivo*.[45] Specific inhibition of PKC-α has been shown to inhibit the growth of medulloblastoma cells[86] and this PKC isozyme is thought to be involved in mediating the effects of the *Ras* oncogene.[87] ISIS 3521, a 20-base antisense oligonucleotide specifically targeting PKC-α, demonstrated anti-tumour activity in a number of different *in vitro* cell types and pre-clinical models and has now completed phase I clinical studies.[88,89] Modest side-effects of thrombocytopenia and fatigue were seen in these phase I studies and a dose of 2 mg/kg/day given as a continuous i.v. infusion over a period of 21 days was recommended for phase II studies. Evidence of anti-tumour activity was also observed in patients with NHL and ovarian cancer.

H–ras ANTISENSE (ISIS 2503)

Deregulation or mutation of the *Ras* oncogene is thought to occur more frequently than in any other oncogene in human cancer (see above). The antisense oligonucleotide ISIS 2503, which binds to the translation initiation region of human H-ras mRNA, has demonstrated a selective reduction in expression of H-ras mRNA and protein in cell culture. A phase I study of this oligonucleotide, using similar dosing regimens to those used in the phase I trial of ISIS 3521, showed the drug to be well tolerated at doses up to 10 mg/kg/day by 14-day continuous intravenous infusion, with several patients having stabilization of disease.[90] A phase I study of ISIS 2503 in combination with gemcitabine has also been completed and phase II studies are in progress.

c–Raf KINASE ANTISENSE (ISIS 5132)

c-*Raf* kinase, a serine/threonine kinase that regulates the mitogen-activated protein kinase pathway that transmits signals from *Ras* and is thought to be involved in the regulation of apoptosis and proliferation, represents another attractive target for antisense technology (see above). Prolonged disease stabilization was observed in two patients in a phase I trial with ISIS 5132, with doses up to 6 mg/kg given as a 2-hour infusion, and this was associated with a reduction in c-Raf kinase mRNA levels in peripheral blood mononuclear cells.[91] Phase II trials are ongoing but initial results have shown little indication of single-agent efficacy in patients with recurrent ovarian cancer or lung cancer.

c-Myb ANTISENSE IN LEUKAEMIA

The proto-oncogene c-*Myb* is a widely studied transcription factor important in the proliferation and differentiation of haemopoietic cells. c-*Myb* regulates a number of genes required for cell maintenance and the progression of the cell through DNA replication and cell division. A key gene controlled by c-*Myb* is the stem cell factor c-*Kit*, which plays an important role in the development of haemopoietic cells as well as GISTs (see p. 589). Antisense oligonucleotides targeted to c-*Myb* have been shown to be inhibitory to human bone marrow mononuclear cells and leukaemic cells *in vitro* and in animal models.[92] This approach is based on the assumption that leukaemic cells are more dependent on Myb protein than normal, non-transformed haemopoietic cells. Two different clinical approaches have been initiated with c-*Myb* antisense oligonucleotides in CML patients. A clinical trial is currently ongoing to look at *ex vivo* antisense treatment of marrow mononuclear cells following removal from patients. It is hoped that this approach will lead to the elimination of CML cells prior to autologous bone marrow transplantation. In addition, a clinical study is being carried out to investigate the effects of a c-*Myb* antisense oligonucleotide administered at a dose of 2 mg/kg/day for 7 days as a continuous infusion to CML patients.

HUMAN DNA METHYLTRANSFERASE I ANTISENSE (MG98)

Human DNA methyltransferase I, an enzyme involved in the epigenetic inactivation of tumour suppressor genes (see p. 594), has also been selected as a target for the development of antisense oligonucleotides. A second-generation phosphorothioate antisense oligonucleotide, MG98, was shown to delay tumour cell growth and cause regression in xenograft models, and has recently completed phase I clinical studies. An MTD of 480 mg/m^2 was determined following a twice-weekly 2-hour infusion, for 3 weeks out of four, and a dose of 360 mg/m^2 has been taken forward to phase II studies using this dosing schedule.[93] DNA methyltransferase levels measured in PBLs isolated before and after dosing on the phase I study showed sustained suppression of message in a limited number of patients.

Future prospects for antisense therapy in cancer treatment

In summary, significant advances have recently been made in the development of antisense technology for the treatment of cancer and the results of phase II clinical trials are awaited with interest. Promising results from clinical studies with *bcl-2* antisense drugs, showing downregulation of target protein at the site of the tumour in addition to a clinical benefit in patients with advanced melanoma, encourage an optimistic view for the future of antisense technology. The development of second-generation antisense oligonucleotides, to improve the physicochemical and biochemical properties of these drugs, and the careful selection of potential new targets are likely to be important factors in determining the future success of this approach to cancer treatment.

TARGETING THE CELLULAR PATHOLOGY OF CANCER – ANGIOGENESIS AND METASTASIS

Despite the significant advances made in the diagnosis and treatment of cancer in children, there remains a significant reduction in the chance of recovery once a solid tumour enters the metastatic phase. For this reason, the prevention of tumour metastasis is an attractive approach to cancer management. For metastatic spread, two interrelated processes are required to take place: tumour cells must first gain access to the surrounding vasculature and, once tumour cells have reached the distant site, they must be able to invade the normal tissue and establish a new tumour mass. Two processes are involved in both of these events: the degradation of normal tissue during both the escape of tumour cells from the primary tumour and their invasion of distant sites, and the formation of new blood vessels.[94]

Angiogenesis or neovascularization refers to the proliferation of new capillaries and can occur under normal conditions, e.g. when damage occurs to a tissue in the body or during menstruation. However, the general turnover of endothelial cells in adult tissues is very slow as compared with endothelial cell proliferation during tumour angiogenesis. Under abnormal conditions, angiogenesis can be 'switched on' by tumour cells, a key factor in creating a permissive environment for tumour growth. Indeed, this process is likely to be essential for the formation of large malignant growths capable of metastasis to other parts of the body from an initial small mass of transformed cells. For example, it has been estimated that a tumour is unable to grow beyond approximately 1 mm^3 in the absence of neovascularization.[95] Clearly, therefore, an understanding of the mechanism of angiogenesis, and the development of ways of interfering with this process, may provide an effective and novel approach to anti-tumour chemotherapy.

The initiation of angiogenesis in tumour cells is brought about by an alteration of the balance of angiogenesis regulation, both downregulation of endogenous angiogenesis inhibitors and overexpression of positive angiogenic factors.[96] Despite the fact that different types of cancer can, in many regards, be treated as distinctive diseases, the endothelial cells of the tumour, being derived from host tissue, are relatively uniform. An increasing number of angiogenic growth factors have been identified as being involved in the initiation of angiogenesis in a number of different tumour types.[97] These include members of the vascular endothelial growth factor (VEGF) gene family, basic-fibroblast-like growth factor (bFGF) and interleukin-8 (IL-8) (a more extensive list of these factors is given in Box 28.1), and it is likely that numerous factors are involved in the regulation of the angiogenic process in a particular tumour type. With direct relevance to paediatric oncology, studies have recently been carried out to determine which angiogenic factors contribute to neuroblastoma angiogenesis. Induction of angiogenesis in a variety of experimental neuroblastoma models has been

Box 28.1 *Selected angiogenic growth factors and angiogenesis inhibitors found in the body*

Endogenous angiogenic growth factors
- Angiogenin
- Angiopoietin (Ang-1)
- Follistatin
- Granulocyte colony-stimulating factor (G-CSF)
- Hepatocyte growth factor (HGF)
- Interleukin-8 (IL-8)
- Leptin
- Placental growth factor
- Platelet-derived growth factor (PDGF)
- Transforming growth factor-α (TGF-α)
- Tumour necrosis factor-α (TNF-α)
- Vascular endothelial growth factor (VEGF)

Endogenous angiogensis inhibitors
- Angiostatin
- Endostatin
- Heparinases
- Human chorionic gonadotrophin
- Interferon-α/β/γ
- Interleukin-12 (IL-12)
- Metalloproteinase inhibitors (TIMPs)
- Plasminogen activator inhibitor
- Retinoids
- Tumistatin
- Vasculostatin
- Vasostatin

shown to involve VEGF, bFGF, transforming growth factor-α (TGF-α), platelet-derived growth factor (PDGF) and the angiopoietins, Ang-1 and Ang-2. In addition, a recent study designed to determine the angiogenic profile of neuroblastoma has indicated that several different angiogenic factors are expressed in neuroblastoma primary tumours. The expression levels of the majority of these factors were correlated with each other, suggesting cooperation in the regulation of angiogenesis, and significantly higher expression levels of several angiogenic factors were found in advanced-stage tumours.[98] Serum VEGF has been shown to be elevated in children with several solid tumour types, including Ewing's sarcoma, primitive neuroectodermal tumours, malignant lymphoma and medulloblastoma. Elevated levels of VEGF declined to levels present in healthy children following successful treatment, suggesting that VEGF may contribute to the progression of paediatric solid malignancies, and that serum levels of this angiogenic growth factor may be used to monitor therapeutic response.[99]

Rationale for the inhibition of angiogenesis as an anti–cancer therapy

The idea that tumour cell growth may be inhibited by treatment with antiangiogenic drugs was originally put forward by Folkman around 30 years ago. However, it is only recently that significant advances have been made in this area, leading to the progression of an increasing number of agents designed to inhibit angiogenesis into clinical trials. There are several reasons why antiangiogenic therapy may offer advantages over more conventional approaches to the treatment of cancer. Firstly, the target endothelial cells should provide a uniform and easily accessible target for drug treatment with similar characteristics in a range of different types of solid tumour. Secondly, there is a great diversity of molecular targets which may provide opportunities for combination antiangiogenic therapy as well as the potential for designing treatment with limited host toxicity. In addition, and arguably the biggest advantage of the antiangiogenic approach to cancer treatment, it may avoid acquired drug resistance due to the fact that the genetically unstable, and hence resistance-prone, cancer cells themselves are not being directly targeted.[100]

Two basic approaches have been used in the design of drugs to target tumour blood vessels. Firstly, agents can be devised to inhibit the formation of new blood vessels, thus leading to a slowing or cessation of tumour growth. Whilst this approach can lead to difficulties in assessing efficacy in phase I and II clinical studies, it is important to note that these drugs are likely to be used in a combination therapy setting, possibly with more conventional cytotoxics. Alternatively, agents can be designed with a more direct mechanism of action, i.e. to cause the degradation of existing tumour blood vessels. This latter approach allows efficacy to be assessed in a more conventional way by measuring quantitative tumour responses. However, whilst measuring tumour response may provide a more satisfactory way of determining which agents to take forward clinically, it will not necessarily be advantageous in selecting those that will have clinical benefit in terms of prolongation of patient survival.

Of those agents that are designed to exert their antiangiogenic effect by inhibition of the formation of new blood vessels, which represent the vast majority of drugs studied to date, the following different classes of compounds have been investigated:

- endogenous angiogenesis inhibitors, i.e. agents that physiologically inhibit the switch to angiogenesis, e.g. angiostatin, endostatin, IL-12
- inhibitors of endothelial cell growth, e.g. TNP-470, thalidomide, interferon-α
- VEGFr tyrosine kinase inhibitors, i.e. agents designed to block the activity of VEGFr autocrine pathways, resulting in a decreased production of angiogenic factors, e.g. SU5416
- inhibition of angiogenic peptides by inactivation of endothelial cell growth factors, e.g. suramin, antibodies to VEGF/bFGF
- metalloproteinase inhibitors – agents which target proteinases involved in the degradation and remodelling of the extracellular matrix, the overexpression of which are associated with tumour growth and metastasis, e.g. batimastat, marimastat, COL-3.

Antiangiogenic drugs in clinical trials

There are currently over 50 agents being tested as antiangiogenic drugs in phase I, phase II and phase III clinical trials for the treatment of various different types of cancer.[100] Selected examples are discussed below with regard to their development and clinical evaluation.

ENDOGENOUS ANGIOGENESIS INHIBITORS (ANGIOSTATIN/ENDOSTATIN)

In vitro and *in vivo* angiogenesis models have been used to identify a large number of endogenous inhibitors targeting the tumour vasculature (see Box 28.1). Inhibitors such as angiostatin and endostatin appear to exhibit specific effects on the proliferation and migration of endothelial cells of newly formed blood vessels, whilst other endogenous angiogenesis inhibitors display a broader spectrum of activity in numerous biological systems.[101,102] The vast majority of endogenous angiogenesis inhibitors suppress the growth of a variety of tumours and metastases in animal models, although relatively few have yet progressed to clinical trials. There are many reasons why the clinical use of these agents may prove to be problematic. For example, doses required to inhibit tumour growth in animal studies may be too high for use in patients, and repeat injections and prolonged treatment with antiangiogenic peptides and proteins may also compromise their clinical use. However, despite the fact that the endogenous angiogenesis inhibitors are in their clinical infancy, some clinical effectiveness has been shown with interferon-2α for the treatment of haemangiomas in children.[103] The future use of these agents may be in combination with chemotherapy, immunotherapy or radiotherapy, and combining agents with different mechanisms of action has produced enhanced efficacy in animal xenograft studies. Potential benefits of such an approach include a decreased likelihood of the development of acquired drug resistance and a lack of overlapping toxicity profiles. Alternatively, the use of gene therapy with endogenous angiogenesis inhibitors may allow some of the problems described above to be overcome,[104] and this approach with both angiostatin and endostatin has again proved to be effective in animal studies.

TNP-470

TNP-470 (pictured) is a synthetic analogue of the antibiotic fumagillin, which was first shown to be a potent inhibitor of angiogenesis *in vitro* approximately 10 years ago.[105] TNP-470 exerts it antiangiogenic effects by preventing endothelial cells from moving into the G1 phase of the cell cycle and also suppresses the activation of CDK1 and CDK2. Animal studies have shown inhibition of both primary tumour growth and the development of metastasis in several different experimental models.[106] For example, results from neuroblastoma xenograft studies have shown a significant inhibition of tumour growth rate and inhibition of tumorigenicity when administered shortly after xenograft inoculation, and when administered following cyclophosphamide. These data suggest that this approach may provide a useful adjuvant therapy for the treatment of high-risk neuroblastoma, particularly in the setting of MRD,[107] although the specific cellular pathways involved in neuroblastoma tumour growth inhibition by TNP-470 are at present unclear.

TNP-470

TNP-470 was the first of this class of drugs to go into clinical trials based on its efficacy as an inhibitor of angiogenesis and its lack of major side-effects in preclinical studies. A phase I study in patients with advanced squamous cell cancer of the cervix determined an MTD of $60 \, mg/m^2$ given as a 1-hour intravenous infusion every other day for 28 days, followed by a 14-day rest period.[108] A comparable MTD of $177 \, mg/m^2/week$ was determined in a phase I study of TNP-470, administered as a 4-hour weekly infusion, in patients with various different types of advanced solid tumour.[109] Pharmacokinetic studies indicated a very short plasma half-life for this drug, with low levels in the systemic circulation 60 minutes after the end of infusion. Plasma concentrations were significantly in excess of those required for *in vitro* inhibition of endothelial cell proliferation and were comparable to those required for the inhibition of tumour-induced neovascularization in animal studies. Neurotoxicity was observed to be the dose-limiting toxicity in both of these phase I studies, but was completely reversible when treatment was discontinued. No myelosuppression was reported and a clinical response or stabilization of disease was seen in a small number of patients. TNP-470 is currently in phase II and III studies for the treatment of a number of different types of malignancy and a phase I study is currently ongoing in children with recurrent or refractory paediatric solid tumours, lymphomas and acute leukaemias.

SU5416

Several tyrosine kinase receptors have been identified as having important roles to play in the formation of new tumour blood vessels, and thus representing potential targets for chemotherapy. SU5416 (pictured) is a potent inhibitor of the kinase activities of both VEGFr and PDGFr, resulting in inhibition of endothelial cell proliferation *in vitro* and anti-tumour efficacy in human xenograft and animal tumour models.[110] The first phase I clinical trial with SU5416, involving 69 patients with advanced disease, showed the drug to be well tolerated with dose limiting toxicity being observed at a dose of $190 \, mg/m^2/day$ when given intravenously twice weekly.[111] This dose of SU5416 results in the attainment of systemic drug concentrations equivalent to those required to effectively inhibit tumour growth in animal models. Partial responses were observed in 3 patients enrolled onto this study and several patients remained on study for more than 6 months. This has led to the opening of phase II and III clinical trials at a dose of $145 \, mg/m^2$, both as a single agent and in combination with established cytotoxic therapy, for the treatment of various haematological malignancies and solid tumours.

SU5416

ANTIBODIES TO VEGF/bFGF

The use of monoclonal antibodies targeted to specific angiogenic factors represents another distinct approach to the inhibition of angiogenesis. Monoclonal antibodies specific for VEGF have been developed and shown to be active in various animal xenograft models, including human rhabdomyosarcoma cell lines transplanted into nude mice.[112] Also of relevance to paediatric oncology are results from an experimental model of Wilms' tumour, showing a significant reduction in primary tumour growth and the development of metastases following treatment with an anti-VEGF antibody.[113] However, whilst clinical trials are ongoing with humanized monoclonal antibody to VEGF, and other angiogenic factors, targeting a single angiogenic peptide in this manner may not be sufficient to induce tumour remission, due to the fact that several of these factors are likely to be involved in tumour progression and metastasis. Therefore, determining which angiogenic factors are expressed in individual tumours may well be required for this approach to be successful.

The use of anti-VEGF monoclonal antibodies in combination with cytotoxic chemotherapy may be a more productive way forward for these agents, with promising data having been published from animal tumour models. For example, the recombinant humanized anti-VEGF monoclonal antibody bevacizumab, in combination with doxorubicin, has been shown to result in significantly increased efficacy relative to either agent alone, in some cases inducing complete regression of tumours derived from MCF-7 breast carcinoma cells in nude mice. Phase I studies with this agent have been carried out with doses up to 3 m/kg weekly for 8 weeks, in combination with various different chemotherapy regimens, with good tolerability observed.[114]

METALLOPROTEINASE INHIBITORS

Metalloproteinase inhibitors (MMPs) are a family of structurally related proteinases that have recently been identified as having important roles to play in several diseases, including cancer, neurodegenerative diseases and arthritis. More than 20 MMPs have been identified and the expression of several members of this family of enzymes (e.g. MMP-1, MMP-2, MMP-9) have been correlated with tumour progression and metastasis in several human and animal models.[115] Indeed, the number of different MMP family members expressed has been reported to increase with tumour progression and increasing levels of individual MMPs are observed with increasing tumour stage.[116] For example, an increased MMP-2 reactivity has been shown to correlate with poor prognosis, in terms of disease free survival, and metastasis in soft tissue sarcoma patients.[117] A key recent discovery in this area of research is that MMP-9 plays a crucial role in initiating the angiogenic switch, a process believed to be essential for the growth of malignant tumours.[118] These findings, in addition to the discovery that endogenous tissue inhibitors of MMPs (TIMPs) could interfere with tumour metastasis in experimental models, led to the hypothesis that the targeting of MMP activity may offer a novel approach to cancer treatment. Results from pre-clinical studies gave rise to significant optimism in this area and synthetic MMP inhibitors were rapidly developed, soon leading to clinical trials in cancer patients.[119]

The first MMP inhibitor studied extensively in various tumour models was batimastat (pictured), an inhibitor of MMP-1, 2, 3, 7 and 9. Pre-clinical studies showed a significant reduction in tumour growth when batimastat was administered shortly after tumour inoculation, although similar efficacy was not observed in more advanced tumour models.[120,121] In clinical studies, batimastat had poor oral bioavailability and could not be given intravenously; hence clinical studies were carried out using intraperitoneal or intrapleural administration. These studies led to the achievement of plasma levels that exceeded the IC_{50} concentrations of the drug determined for inhibition of MMPs in pre-clinical studies.[122] Further development of this agent was limited due to the absence of a suitable route for clinical administration. The first oral MMP inhibitor to enter clinical trials was marimastat (pictured), a potent inhibitor of several MMP enzymes. A phase I study with this agent in healthy volunteers showed it to be rapidly absorbed, achieving serum levels far in excess of the observed inhibitory concentration of 50% (IC_{50}) at doses that were well tolerated.[123] A number of phase II and phase III studies have been carried out with marimastat and other MMP inhibitors, and although results have indicated effects on serum tumour markers, used as surrogate markers of efficacy, there remains a lack of convincing data regarding efficacy as measured by response or survival rates. Recently published results from a phase II trial of marimastat in combination with temozolomide, for the treatment of recurrent and progressive glioblastoma multiforme, have suggested a significant increase in PFS as compared with previous results from the studies with temozolomide alone.[124] Although the use of marimastat in this drug combination study was associated with sometimes severe joint and tendon pain, leading to the removal of 11 per cent of patients from the study, results do suggest that MMP inhibitors may have a role to play in the treatment of this disease.

Batimastat

Marimastat

Despite the lack of clinical efficacy reported in phase II and III studies to date, there remains much interest in the development of MMP inhibitors in pre-clinical and clinical studies. Some non-peptide MMP inhibitors, such as BMS 275291, designed to improve the oral bioavailability and pharmaceutical properties of this class of drugs, are currently in phase III trials, although trials with other agents have been stopped. However, for significant gains to be made in this area of drug development, it is important to realize that these agents have multiple mechanisms of action in their inhibition of MMP. Currently, very little is known about the regulation of angiogenesis by MMP inhibitors, or whether this effect is more important than their actions in regulating apoptosis, invasion and metastasis.[125] With this information, a more rational approach to the design and use of MMP inhibitors may be possible.

Design of clinical trials for angiogenesis inhibitors

The hypothesis that the inhibition of tumour vasculature growth and development may provide a novel approach to anti-cancer therapy has been with us for many years. Indeed, it is now 10 years since the first angiogenic drug was first assessed in the clinic. Whilst some promising agents are advancing through to phase II and III trials, it has become apparent that the development of the angiogenesis inhibitors raises problems that were not encountered during clinical development of the cytotoxic chemotherapeutic agents.

In order to optimize the therapeutic use of antiangiogenic agents, it is important to identify both the specific molecular targets of the drugs and relevant surrogate markers for *in vivo* use. In particular, the use of positron emission tomography scanning and nuclear magnetic resonance imaging is likely to play an increasingly important role in quantification of the extent of angiogenesis inhibition in clinical trials, notably in phase I trials where MTD is of little significance in determining the optimal dose range of an antiangiogenic agent. It is certainly possible that many angiogenesis inhibitors that have recently been developed are not necessarily being used at optimal doses. Similarly, optimal dosing schedules for many of these drugs have not been defined, either when used alone or in combination therapy. Unexpected serious toxicity has recently been observed in combination studies of angiogenic inhibitors and chemotherapeutic agents, a phenomenon which may be related to an unnecessarily high dose of the antiangiogenic agent being used, as determined from phase I studies.[126] Once an optimum dose and schedule have been identified, another major hurdle presents itself in the form of the patient population to be studied in phase II trials. Whilst these antiangiogenic agents are most likely to be effective in an adjuvant setting, most phase II studies involve patients with advanced tumours resistant to conventional cytotoxic chemotherapy.

SUMMARY

Cancer chemotherapy is at a turning point such that, for the first time, it is possible to envisage treatments for individual patients that are targeted at the molecular and cellular pathology of their disease, and not simply at replicating cells. It is anticipated that therapies targeted at tumour-related molecular and cellular lesions will be both more active and less toxic than cytotoxic drugs and radiation. As described in this chapter, clinical results with, in particular, imatinib and trastuzumab for the treatment of CML, GIST and HER-2-overexpressing breast cancer are particularly encouraging, and a large number of other targeted therapies have been reviewed that hold considerable promise for many other tumour types. To date, the impact of targeted therapies has yet to be felt in paediatric oncology; however, trials in some diseases have been initiated, and as the use of non-cytotoxic therapies in adults increases, the pace of change in paediatric oncology will hopefully accelerate.

> ## KEY POINTS
>
> - There is now unequivocal evidence from studies in adults that targeted drugs designed to exploit the molecular and cellular pathology of cancer can have significant clinical activity.

- To date, only drugs designed to inhibit activated oncogenes have shown reproducible clinical activity. Although the development of agents to restore the function of tumour suppressor genes, or inhibit the products of immortality genes, is proving to be more challenging, a number of exciting approaches are being investigated.
- The inhibition of tumour-induced angiogenesis is an attractive target, and antiangiogenic therapies are being studied in a large number of clinical trials.
- Targeted agents have to date undergone only very limited evaluation in children, although many potential drug targets have been identified in paediatric cancers. Collaboration between pre-clinical drug developers and paediatric oncologists is urgently needed to identify targeted drugs for childhood malignancies.

REFERENCES

♦1. Rothenberg ML. Irintecan (CPT-11): recent developments and future direction – colorectal cancer and beyond. *Oncologist* 2001; **6**: 66–80.

♦2. Maroun JA. Capecitabine in the management of colorectal cancer. *Anticancer Ther* 2001; **1**: 327–33.

♦3. Agarwala SS, Kirkwood JM. Temozolomide, a novel alkylating agent with activity in the central nervous system, may improve the treatment of advanced metastatic melanoma. *Oncologist* 2000; **5**: 144–51.

♦4. Rodenhuis S. The status of high-dose chemotherapy in breast cancer. *Oncologist* 2000; **5**: 369–75.

♦5. Relling MV, Dervieux T. Pharmacogenetics and cancer therapy. *Nature* 2001; **1**: 99–108.

♦6. Danesi R, De Braud F, Fogli S et al. Pharmacogenetic determinants of anti-cancer drug activity and toxicity. *Trends Pharmacol Sci* 2001; **22**: 420–6.

♦7. Innocenti F, Ratain MJ. Update on pharmacogenetics in cancer chemotherapy. *Eur J Cancer* 2002; **38**: 639–44.

♦8. Shabbits JA, Krishna R, Mayer LD. Molecular and pharmacological strategies to overcome multidrug resistance. *Anticancer Ther* 2001; **1**: 585–94.

9. Fracasso PM, Brady MF, Moore DH et al. Phase II study of paclitaxel and valspodar (PSC 833) in refractory ovarian carcinoma: a gynecological oncology group study. *J Clin Oncol* 2001; **19**: 2975–82.

10. Toppmeyer D, Seidman AD, Pollak M et al. Safety and efficacy of the multidrug resistance inhibitor incel (biricodar; VX-710) in combination with paclitaxel for advanced breast cancer refractory to paclitaxel. *Clin Cancer Res* 2002; **8**: 670–8.

11. Piwnica-Worms D, Chiu M, Budding M et al. Functional imaging of multidrug-resistant p-glycoprotein with an organotechnetium complex. *Cancer Res* 1993; **53**: 977–84.

12. Quinn JA, Pluda J, Dolan ME et al. Phase II trial of carmustine plus O^6-benzylguanine for patients with nitrosourea-resistant recurrent or progressive malignant glioma. *J Clin Oncol* 2002; **20**: 2277–83.

♦13. Brown R, Strathdee G. Epigenomics and epigenetic therapy of cancer. *Trends Mol Med* 2002; **8**: S43-S48.

14. Slamon DJ, Clark GM, Wong SG et al. Human breast cancer – correlation of relapse and survival with amplification of the HER-2/neu oncogene. *Science* 1987; **235**: 177–82.

15. Slamon DJ, Clark GM. Amplification of c-erbB-2 and aggressive human breast tumours *Science* 1988; **240**: 1795–8.

16. Carter P, Presta L, Gorman CM et al. Humanization of an anti-P18HER2 antibody for human cancer therapy. *Proc Natl Acad Sci USA* 1992; **10**: 4285–9.

17. Webber SE, Bleckman TM, Attard J et al. Design of thymidylate synthase inhibitors using protein crystal structures: the synthesis and biological evaluation of a novel class of 5-substituted quinazolinoles. *J Med Chem* 1993; **36**: 733–46.

♦18. Hanahan D, Weinberg R. The hallmarks of cancer. *Cell* 2000; **100**: 57–70.

♦19. Blume-Jenson P, Hunter T. Oncogenic kinase signalling. *Nat Insight* 2001; **411**: 355–65.

20. Small EJ, Meyer M, Marshall ME et al. Suramin therapy for patients with symptomatic hormone-refractory prostate cancer: results of a randomised phase III trial comparing suramin plus hydrocortisone to placebo plus hydrocortisone. *J Clin Oncol* 2000; **18**: 1440–50.

21. Slamon DJ, Godolphin W, Jones LA et al. Studies of the HER-2/neu proto-oncogene in human breast and ovarian cancer. *Science* 1989; **244**: 707–12.

♦22. Baselga J. Targeting the epidermal growth factor receptor: a clinical reality. *J Clin Oncol* 2001; **19**: 41s-44s.

23. Cobleigh MA, Vogel CL, Tripathy D et al. Multinational study of the efficacy and safety of humanized anti-HER2 monoclonal antibody in women who have HER2-overexpressing metastatic breast cancer that has progressed after chemotherapy for metastatic disease. *J Clin Oncol* 1999; **17**: 2639–48.

●24. Slamon DJ, Leyland-Jones B, Shak S et al. Use of chemotherapy plus a monoclonal antibody against HER2 for metastatic breast cancer that overexpresses HER2. *N Engl J Med* 2001; **344**: 783–92.

25. Schneider JW, Chang AY, Rocco TP. Cardiotoxicity in signal transduction therapeutics: erbB2 antibodies and the heart. *Semin Oncol* 2001; **20**(Suppl. 16): 18–26.

♦26. de Bono JS, Rowinsky EK. The ErbB receptor family: a therapeutic target for cancer. *Trends Mol Med* 2002; **8**: S19–26.

27. Saltz L, Rubin M, Hochester H et al. Cetuximab (IMC-C225) plus irinotecan (CPT-11) is active in CPT-11-refractory colorectal cancer (CRC) that expresses epidermal growth factor receptor (EGFR) (abstract 7). *Proc Am Soc Clin Oncol* 2001; **20**: 3a.

28. Albanell J, Rojo F, Averbuch S et al. Pharmocodynamic studies of the epidermal growth factor receptor inhibitor ZD1839 in skin from cancer patients: histopathologic and molecular consequences of receptor inhibition. *J Clin Oncol* 2002; **20**: 110–24.

29. Baselga J. Targeting the epidermal growth factor receptor with tyrosine kinase inhibitors: Small molecules, big hopes. *J Clin Oncol* 2002; **20**: 2217–19.

30. Pietras RJ, Fendly BM, Chazin VR *et al.* Antibody to HER-2/*neu* receptor blocks DNA repair after cisplatin in human breast and ovarian cancer cells. *Oncogene* 1994; **9**: 1829–38.

♦31. Heinrich MC, Blanke CD, Druker BD, Corless CL. Inhibition of KIT tyrosine kinase activity: a novel molecular approach to the treatment of KIT-positive malignancies. *J Clin Oncol* 2002; **20**: 1692–703.

32. Eckhardt SG, Rizzo J, Sweeney KR *et al.* Phase I and pharmacologic study of the tyrosine kinase inhibitor SU101 in patients with advanced solid tumours. *J Clin Oncol* 1999; **17**: 1095–104.

♦33. Morin MJ. From oncogene to drug: development of small molecule tyrosine kinase inhibitors as anti-tumor and anti-angiogenic agents. *Oncogene* 2000; **19**: 6574–83.

♦34. Pollak MN, Schally AV. Mechanisms of antineoplastic action of somatostatin analogs. *Soc Exp Biol Med* 1998; **217**: 143–52.

♦35. Hejna M, Schmidinger M, Raderer M. The clinical role of somatostatin analogues as antineoplastic agents: much ado about nothing. *Ann Oncol* 2002; **13**: 653–68.

♦36. Adjei AA. Blocking oncogenic ras signalling for cancer therapy. *J Natl Cancer Inst* 2001; **93**: 1062–74.

♦37. Sebti SM, Hamilton AD. Farnesyltransferase and geranylgeranyltransferase I inhibitors and cancer therapy: lessons from mechanism and bench-to-bedside translational studies. *Oncogene* 2000; **19**: 6584–93.

38. Karp JE, Lancet JE, Kaufman SH *et al.* Clinical and biologic activity of the farnesyltransferase inhibitor R115777 in adults with refractory and relapsed acute leukemias: a phase I clinical-laboratory correlative trial. *Blood* 2001; **97**: 3361–9.

39. Britten CD, Rowinsky EK, Soignet S *et al.* A phase 1 pharmacological study of the farnesyl protein tranferase inhibitor L-778,123 in patients with solid malignancies. *Clin Cancer Res* 2001; **7**: 3894–903.

♦40. English JM, Cobb MH. Pharmacological inhibitors of MAPK pathways. *Trends Pharmacol Sci* 2002; **23**: 40–5.

♦41. Herrera R, Sebolt-Leopold JS. Unraveling the complexities of the Raf/MAP kinase pathway for pharmacological intervention. *Trends Mol Med* 2002; **8**: S27–31.

♦42. Lyons JF, Wilhelm S, Hibner B, Bollag G. Discovery of a novel Raf kinase inhibitor. *Endocr Relat Cancer* 2001; **8**: 219–25.

♦43. Mauro MJ, O'Dwyer M, Heinrich MC, Druker BJ. ST1571: a paradigm of new agents for cancer therapeutics. *J Clin Oncol* 2002; **20**: 325–34.

♦44. Šuša M, Missback M, Green G. Src inhibitors: drugs for the treatment of osteoporosis, cancer or both?. *Trends Pharmacol Sci* 2000; **21**: 489–95.

45. Basu A. The potential of protein-kinase-c as a target for anticancer treatment. *Pharmacol Ther* 1993; **59**: 257–80.

46. Propper DJ, McDonald AC, Man A *et al.* Phase I and pharmacokinetic study of PKC412, an inhibitor of protein kinase C. *J Clin Oncol* 2001; **19**: 1485–92.

♦47. Hurley LH. DNA and its associated processes as targets for cancer therapy. *Nature* 2002; **2**: 188–200.

♦48. Adams J. Proteasome inhibition: a novel approach to cancer therapy. *Trends Mol Med* 2002; **8**: S49–S54.

♦49. Szyf M. Towards a pharmacology of DNA methylation. *Trends Pharmacol Sci* 2001; **22**: 350–4.

♦50. Richon VM, O'Brien JP. Histone deacetylase inhibitors: a new class of potential therapeutic agents for cancer treatment. *Clin Cancer Res* 2002; **8**: 662–4.

♦51. Hupp TR, Lane DP, Ball KL. Strategies for manipulating the p53 pathway in the treatment of human cancer. *J Biochem* 2000; **352**: 1–17.

52. Foster BA, Coffey HA, Morin MJ, Rastinejad F. Pharmacological rescue of mutant P53 conformation and function. *Science* 1999; **286**; 2507–10.

53. Bykov VJN, Issaeva N, Shilov A *et al.* Restoration of the tumor suppressor function to mutant p53 by a low-molecular-weight compound. *Nat Med* 2002; **8**: 282–8.

♦54. Neckers L. Hsp90 inhibitors as novel cancer chemotherapeutic agents. *Trends Mol Med* 2002; **8**: S55–S61.

♦55. Sausville EA. Complexities in the development of cyclin-dependant kinase inhibitor drugs. *Trends Mol Med* 2002; **8**: S32–S37.

♦56. Senderowicz AM, Sausville EA. Preclinical and clinical development of cyclin-dependent kinase modulators. *J Natl Cancer Inst* 2000; **92**: 376–87.

57. Shay JW, Bacchetti S. A survey of telomerase activity in human cancer. *Eur J Cancer* 1997; **33**: 787–91.

♦58. Rhyu MS. Telomeres, telomerase and immortality. *J Natl Cancer Inst* 1995. **87**: 887–94.

59. Hiyama E, Hiyama K, Yokoyama T *et al.* Correlating telomerase activity levels with human neuroblastoma outcomes. *Nat Med* 1995; **1**: 249–55.

60. Dome JS, Chung S, Bergemann T *et al.* High telomerase reverse transcriptase (hTERT) and mRNA level correlates with disease recurrence in patients with favorable histology Wilms' tumor. *Cancer Res* 1999; **59**: 4301–7.

61. Tatematsu K, Nakayama J, Danbara M *et al.* A novel quantitative 'stretch PCR assay', that detects a dramatic increase in telomerase activity during the progression of myeloid lukemias. *Oncogene* 1996; **13**: 2265–74.

62. Engelhardt M, Ozkaynak MF, Drullinsky P *et al.* Telomerase activity and telomere length in pediatric patients with malignancies undergoing chemotherapy. *Leukemia* 1998; **12**: 13–24.

♦63. Bearss DJ, Hurley LH, Von Hoff DD. Telomere maintenance mechanisms as a target for drug development. *Oncogene* 2000; **19**: 6632–41.

♦64. De-Lange T, Jacks T. For better or for worse? Telomerase inhibition and cancer. *Cell* 1999; **98**: 273–5.

65. Sun DY, Thompson B, Cathers BE *et al.* Inhibition of human telomerase by a G-quadruplex-interative compound. *J Med Chem* 1997; **40**: 2113–16.

66. Perry PJ, Gowan SM, Reszka AP *et al.* 1.4 and 2.6-disubstituted amidoanthracene-9,10-dione derivatives as inhibitors of human telomerase. *J Med Chem* 1998; **41**: 3253–60.

67. Read M, Harrison RJ, Romagnoli B *et al.* Structure-based design of selective and patent G quadruplex-mediated telomerase inhibitors. *Proc Natl Acad Sci USA* 2001; **98**: 4844–9.

68. Damm K, Hammann U, Garin-Chesa P *et al.* A highly selective telomerase inhibitor limiting human cancer cell proliferation. *EMBO J* 2001; **20**: 6958–68.

♦69. Evans TRJ, Kaye SB. Retinoids: present role and future potential. *Br J Cancer* 1999; **80**: 1–8.

♦70. Chambon P. A decade of molecular biology of retinoic acid receptors. *FASEB J* 1996; **10**: 940–54.

71. Napoli JL. Retinoic acid biosynthesis and metabolism. *FASEB J* 1996; **10**: 993–1001.

72. Adamson PC, Widemann BC, Reaman GH *et al*. A phase 1 trial and pharmacokinetic study of 9-cis-retinoic acid (ALRT1057) in paediatric patients with refractory cancer: A joint Paediatric Oncology Branch, National Cancer Institute, and Children's Cancer Group Study. *Clin Cancer Res* 2001; **7**: 3034–9.

●73. Huang ME, Ye YC, Chen SR *et al*. Use of all-trans retinoic acid in the treatment of acute promyelocytic leukaemia. *Blood* 1988; **72**: 567–72.

74. Muindi J, Frankel SR, Miller WH *et al*. Continuous treatment with all-trans retinoic acid causes a progressive reduction in plasma drug concentrations – implications for relapse and retinoid resistance in patients with acute promyelocytic leukaemia. *Blood* 1992; **79**: 299–303.

●75. Matthay KK, Villablanca JG, Seeger RC *et al*. Treatment of high-risk neuroblastoma with intensive chemotherapy, radiotherapy, autologous bone marrow transplantation, and 13-cis-retinoic acid. *N Engl J Med* 1999; **341**: 1165–73.

76. Delia D, Aiello A, Lombardi L *et al*. N-(4-hydroxyphenyl)-retinamide induces apoptosis of malignant hematopoietic-cell lines including those unresponsive to retinoic acid. *Cancer Res* 1993; **53**: 6036–41.

77. Lovat PE, Ranalli M, Bernassola F *et al*. Synergistic induction of apoptosis of neuroblastoma by fenretinide or CD437 in combination with chemotherapeutic drugs. *Int J Cancer* 2000; **88**: 977–85.

♦78. Stein CA, Cohen JS. Oligodeoxynucleotides as inhibitors of gene-expression – a review. *Cancer Res* 1998; **48**: 2659–68.

♦79. Carter G, Lemoine NR. Antisense technology for cancer therapy – does it make sense? *Br J Cancer* 1993; **67**: 869–76.

♦80. Crooke ST. Progress toward oligonucleotide therapeutics – pharmacodynamic properties. *FASEB J* 1993; **7**: 533–9.

♦81. Curcio LD, Bouffard DY, Scanlon KJ. Oligonucleotides as modulators of cancer gene expression. *Pharmacol Ther* 1997; **74**: 317–32.

82. Rosolen A, Whitesell L, Ikegaki N *et al*. Antisense inhibition of single copy C-MYC protein in a neuroepithelioma cell-line. *Cancer Res* 1990; **50**: 6316–22.

83. Reed JC. A day in the life of the Bcl-2 protein: does the turnover rate of Bcl-2 serve as a biological clock for cellular lifespan regulation? *Leuk Res* 1996; **20**: 109–11.

84. Waters JS, Webb A, Cunningham D *et al*. Phase I clinical and pharmacokinetic study of Bcl-2 antisense oligonucleotide therapy in patients with non-Hodgkin's lymphoma. *J Clin Oncol* 2000; **18**: 1812–23.

85. Jansen B, Wacheck V, Heere-Ress E *et al*. BCL-2 antisense therapy for malignant melanoma: experiences from bench to bedside (abstract 59). *Clin Cancer Res* 2000; **6**: 4485.

86. Adesina AM, Dooley N, Yong VW, Nalbantoglu J. Differential role for protein kinase C-mediated signalling in the proliferation of medulloblastoma cell lines. *Int J Oncol* 1998; **45**: 759–68.

87. Dlugosz AA, Cheng C, Williams EK *et al*. Alterations in murine keratinocyte differentiation induced by activated ras(ha)

genes are mediated by protein-kinase C-alpha. *Cancer Res* 1994; **54**: 6413–20.

88. Nemunaitis J, Holmlund JT, Kraynak M *et al*. Phase I evaluation of ISIS 3521, an antisense oligodeoxynucleotide to protein kinase C-α, in patients with advanced cancer. *J Clin Oncol* 1999; **17**: 3586–95.

89. Yuen AR, Haldey J, Fisher GA *et al*. Phase I study of an antisense oligonucleotide to protein kinase C-alpha (ISIS 3521/CGP 64128A) in patients with cancer. *Clin Cancer Res* 1999; **5**: 3357–63.

90. Cunningham CC, Holmlund JT, Geary RS *et al*. A phase 1 trial of H-ras antisense oligonucleotide ISIS 2503 administered as a continuous intravenous infusion in patients with advanced carcinoma. *Cancer* 2001; **92**: 1265–71.

91. O'Dwyer PJ, Stevenson JP, Gallagher M *et al*. c-raf-1 depletion and tumor responses in patients treated with the c-raf-1 antisense oligodeoxynucleotide ISIS 5132 (CGP 69846A). *Clin Cancer Res* 1999; **5**: 3977–82.

92. Gewirtz AM. Developing oligonucleotide therapeutics for human leukaemia. *Anti-cancer Drug Design* 1997; **12**: 341–58.

93. Donehower R, Stewart D, Eisenhauer E *et al*. A phase I and pharmacokinetic (PK) study of MG98, a human DNA methyltransferase (Dnmt) mRNA inhibitor, given as a 2-hour twice weekly (BIW) infusion 3 out of every 4 weeks. *Clin Cancer Res* 2001; **7**(Suppl.): 133.

♦94. Carmeliet P, Jain RK. Angiogenesis in cancer and other diseases. *Nature* 2000; **407**: 249–57.

95. Folkman J. What is the evidence that tumors are angiogenesis dependent? *J Natl Cancer Inst* 1990; **82**: 4–6.

96. Hanahan D, Folkman J. Patterns and emerging mechanisms of the angiogenic switch during tumorigenesis. *Cell* 1996; **86**: 353–64.

♦97. Tosetti F, Ferrari N, De Flora S, Albini A. 'Angioprevention': angiogenesis is a common and key target for cancer chemopreventive agents. *FASEB J* 2002; **16**: 2–14.

98. Eggert A, Ikegaki N, Kwiatkowski J *et al*. High level expression of angiogenic factors is associated with advanced tumor stage in human neuroblastomas. *Clin Cancer Res* 2000; **6**: 1900–8.

99. Pavlakovic H, Von Schutz V, Rossler J *et al*. Quantification of angiogenesis stimulators in children with solid malignancies. *Int J Cancer* 2001; **72**: 756–60.

♦100. Kerbel RS. Clinical trials of antiangiogenic drugs: opportunities, problems, and assessment of initial results. *J Clin Oncol* 2001; **19**: 45s-51s.

101. O'Reilly MS, Holmgren L, Ching Y *et al*. Angiostatin – a novel angiogenesis inhibitor that mediates the suppression of metastases by a Lewis lung-carcinoma. *Cell* 1994; **79**: 315–28.

102. O'Reilly MS, Behm T, Shing Y *et al*. Endostatin: an endogenous inhibitor of angiogenesis and tumor growth. *Cell* 1997; **88**: 277–85.

103. Ezekowitz RAB, Mulliken JB, Folkman J. Interfon alfa-2A therapy for life-threatening hemangiomas of infancy. *N Engl J Med* 1992; **326**: 1456–63.

104. Tanaka T, Manome Y, Wen P *et al*. Viral vector-mediated transduction of a modified platelet factor 4 cDNA inhibits angiogenesis and tumor growth. *Nat Med* 1997; **3**: 437–42.

105. Ingber D, Fujita T, Kishimoto S *et al.* Synthetic analogs of fumagillin that inhibit angiogenesis and suppress tumor growth. *Nature* 1990; **348**: 555–7.

106. Yanase T, Tamura M, Fujita K *et al.* Inhibitory effect of angiogenesis inhibitor TNP-470 on tumor-growth and metastasis of human cell-lines in vitro and in vivo. *Cancer Res* 1993; **53**: 2566–70.

107. Shusterman S, Grupp SA, Barr R *et al.* The angiogenesis inhibitor TNP-470 effectively inhibits human neuroblastoma xenograft growth, especially in the the setting of subclinical disease. *Clin Cancer Res* 2001; **7**: 977–84.

108. Kudelka AP, Levy T, Verschraegen CF *et al.* A phase I study of TNP-470 administered to patients with advanced squamous cell cancer of the cervix. *Clin Cancer Res* 1997; **3**: 1501–5.

109. Bhargava P, Marshall JL, Rizvi N *et al.* A phase 1 and pharmacokinetic study of TNP-470 administered weekly to patients with advanced cancer. *Clin Cancer Res* 1999; **5**: 1989–95.

110. Fong TAT, Shawver LK, Sun L *et al.* SU5416 is a potent and selective inhibitor of the vascular endothelial growth factor receptor (Flk-1/KDR) that inhibits tyrosine kinase catalysis, tumor vascularization, and growth of multiple tumor types. *Cancer Res* 1999; **59**: 99–106.

111. Mendel DB, Laird AD, Smolich BD *et al.* Development of SU5416, a selective small molecule inhibitor of VEGF receptor tyrosine kinase activity, as an anti-angiogenesis agent. *Anticancer Drug Des* 2000; **15**: 29–41.

♦112. Ferrara N. Vascular endothelial growth factor. *Eur J Cancer* 1996; **32A**: 2413–22.

113. Rowe DH, Huang JZ, Kayton ML *et al.* Anti-VEGF antibody suppresses primary tumor growth and metastasis in an experimental model of Wilms' tumour. *J Pediatr Surg* 2000; **35**: 30–2.

♦114. Figg WD, Kruger EA, Price DK *et al.* Inhibition of angiogenesis: treatment options for patients with metastatic prostate cancer. *Invest New Drugs* 2002; **20**: 183–94.

♦115. Stetler-Stevenson WG, Yu AE. Proteases in invasion: matrix metalloproteinases. *Semin Cancer Biol* 2001; **11**: 143–52.

♦116. Nelson AR, Fingleton B, Rotherberg ML, Matrisian LM. Matrix metalloproteinases: biological activity and clinical implications. *J Clin Oncol* 2000; **18**: 1135–49.

117. Benassi MS, Gamberi G, Magagnoli G *et al.* Metalloproteinase expression and prognosis in soft tissue sarcomas. *Ann Oncol* 2001; **12**: 75–80.

118. Bergers G, Brekken R, McMahon G *et al.* Matrix metalloproteinase-9 triggers the angiogenic switch during carcinogenesis. *Nat Cell Biol* 2000; **2**: 737–44.

♦119. Hoekstra R, Eskens FALM, Verweij J. Matrix metalloproteinase inhibitors: current developments and future perspectives. *Oncologist* 2001; **6**: 415–27.

120. Davies B, Brown PD, East N *et al.* A synthetic matrix metalloproteinase inhibitor decreases tumor burden and prolongs survival of mice bearing human ovarian-carcinoma xenografts. *Cancer Res* 1993; **53**: 2087–91.

121. Chirivi RGS, Garofalo A, Crimmin MJ *et al.* Inhibition of the metastatic spread and growth of B16-BL6 murine melanoma by a synthetic matrix metalloproteinase inhibitor. *Int J Cancer* 1994; **58**: 460–4.

122. Beattie GJ, Smyth JF. Phase 1 study of intraperitoneal metalloproteinase inhibitor BB94 in patients with malignant ascites. *Clin Cancer Res* 1998; **4**: 1899–902.

♦123. Steward WP. Marimastat (BB2516): current status of development. *Cancer Chemother Pharmacol* 1999; **43**: 56S-60S.

124. Groves MD, Puduvalli VK, Hess KR *et al.* Phase II trial of temozolomide plus the matrix metalloproteinase inhibitor, marimastat, in recurrent and progressive glioblastoma multiforme. *J Clin Oncol* 2002; **20**: 1383–8.

♦125. Egeblad M, Werb Z. New functions for the matrix metalloproteinases in cancer progression. *Nat Rev* 2002; **2**: 161–74.

126. Marx GM, Steer CB, Harper P *et al.* Unexpected serious toxicity with chemotherapy and antiangiogenic combinations: time to take stock!. *J Clin Oncol* 2002; **20**: 1446–8.

29

Recent advances in radiotherapy

RUBIN SOOMAL & FRANK SARAN

INTRODUCTION

Radiotherapy as a treatment modality has undergone rapid changes in recent years with many more advances in development. The two major directions of research in paediatric radiotherapy over the last 10 years have been to conform the radiation to the target maximally and to enhance target definition with improved and new imaging modalities.

Machine hardware and the computing power of planning systems have begun to deliver the therapies first attempted over 40 years ago.[1] Recent technological progress has allowed clinicians to come closer to their goal of conforming the high doses of radiation to the target (conformal radiotherapy, CRT). Additionally, the latest imaging techniques can visualize normal tissues and tumours with improved anatomical definition as well as provide new functional and biological information to define that target in the first instance (multimodality imaging).[2]

Many of these developments have already been translated into clinical practice. In combination, these aim to deliver clinical benefits with a potential therapeutic gain from either improved tumour control or reduced toxicity, or both (i.e. improving the therapeutic ratio).

Progress has occurred in every component of the radiotherapy treatment pathway, from patient selection, immobilization and target definition to radiotherapy planning, verification and delivery. Furthermore, the use of twice-daily fractionation schedules (hyperfractionation) has the potential to improve patient outcome in selected rapidly proliferating tumours. The rationale for hyperfractionation is both to reduce the late effects of radiotherapy in children and prevent tumour repopulation, with the potential to improve tumour control. This is currently being explored in primitive neuroectodermal tumours (PNETs)[3-5] and in neuroblastoma[6] with some evidence of reduced late effects such as thyroid dysfunction.[7,8] Furthermore, the use of charged particles, e.g. protons instead of photons, offers further potential to spare normal tissues outside the high-dose radiotherapy volume compared with the best photon-based techniques.[9,10] At present, cost and availability limit the ability to access treatments using protons on a larger scale.

Some 'behind the scenes' technical advances cannot be discussed in depth here but are nonetheless important incremental steps in improving the overall quality of radiotherapy. The delivery of advanced radiotherapy is a complex multi-step process and the overall quality depends upon the 'weakest link', which may vary between departments.

The implementation of standardized protocols and central review by the large cooperative groups (SIOP and COG) has ensured minimum standards and improved outcome and has set an example for adult oncology. Online quality assurance of radiotherapy should allow a uniformity of practice and technique before the start of radiotherapy and will provide a prospectively gathered database of clinical data, pattern of failure and toxicity to guide future improvements. Incorporating the full three-dimensional (3D) dose–volume data may eventually allow detailed dose–response information for both normal tissues and tumours.[11,12] The USA has had a central database, QARC (Quality Assurance Review Centre), for many years with close involvement of the paediatric groups.[13]

In the paediatric setting, radiotherapy planning and treatment must be deliverable and acceptable to children of all ages, some of whom require treatment under a general anaesthetic (GA). Some new complex techniques may therefore not be practical for infants and small children, but others, such as radiotherapy using intensity-modulated radiotherapy (IMRT), may actually streamline the treatment process with an improved use of resources and reduced daily treatment time. IMRT is a technique of CRT that employs a non-uniform dose delivery and provides treatment possibilities in the form of critical organ avoidance and dose escalation not previously achievable. Yet IMRT utilizes novel planning and delivery techniques that require careful refinement, validation and evaluation, especially with regard to children, prior to widespread implementation.

The following paragraphs highlight some of the recent advances in external beam radiotherapy that are likely to affect paediatric oncology practice.

SET–UP AND PATIENT IMMOBILIZATION

Patient set-up, i.e. the position and immobilization of a patient for radiotherapy, is individually chosen for patient comfort as well as technical factors such as optimal access of treatment beams to target tissue. The degree of immobilization required varies according to tumour site and technique used. It needs to be both accurate and precise to provide reproducible positioning of the patient. Day-to-day variation should be measured in each department for different techniques to ensure adequate dose coverage and appropriate selection of safety margins around the gross tumour volume.[14] The most precise immobilization techniques are used in the field of neuro-oncology with methods of rigid immobilization, e.g. stereotactic radiosurgery (SRS) or stereotactic CRT (SCRT). This method has been employed for well-demarcated localized brain tumours such as craniopharyngiomas or low-grade gliomas.[15–18] Many technical solutions have been utilized for this problem, including a rigid relocatable frame with an individualized mouth-bite and head rest as well as frameless techniques (Figure 29.1).[14,19,20] These techniques can achieve a mean day-to-day reproducibility in the range 1–2 mm,[19,21] compared with the 4–5 mm variability associated with commercial thermoplastic masks. For children unable to use a frame-based system (e.g. those with inadequate dentition or requiring general anaesthetic), some centres have adapted the rigid frame using bony landmarks instead of a mouth-bite (i.e. nasal bridge or external

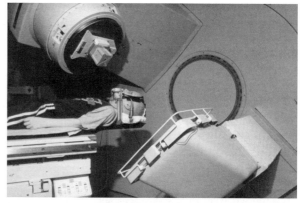

(a)

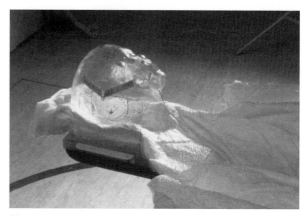

(b)

Figure 29.1 *Two methods of immobilization used for conformal radiotherapy. (a) A lightweight paediatric frame-based system with an individualized mouth-bite and a customized head rest. The rigid frame is fixed to the treatment couch of a linear accelerator and used for stereotactically guided conformal radiotherapy (SCRT). The mean day-to-day reproducibility using this type of system is approximately 1–1.5 mm. (b) A customized thermoplastic shell and moulded bag of polystyrene beads (VacFix). The VacFix bag is individually shaped and then hardened by vacuum to immobilize the head and upper body. The mean day-to-day reproducibility using such a system is approximately 1.5–2.5 mm.*

auditory canal) to aid fixation. The Royal Marsden and St Jude Children's Hospital have developed an alternative using a modified shell-based system with an individually shaped vacuum moulded bag of polystyrene beads, which has a reproducibility similar to a frame-based system.[14,19] If a single high-dose fraction of radiotherapy is delivered (SRS), a rigid frame is fitted via pins to the skull vault using local anaesthetic, eliminating any patient movement.

Stereotactic immobilization techniques have also been used for head and neck radiotherapy given the close proximity of many radiosensitive normal tissues.[22] The use of whole-body stereotactic frames for extracranial tumours is less well developed, but may have technical advantages for young children and targets close to the spinal cord.[23,24]

For thoracic tumours, control of patient breathing with the assistance of an active breathing control device is a further development entering clinical practice for selected tumours. This controls the delivery of radiation during a standardized breath-hold and minimizes the amount of lung and heart within the high-dose irradiation volume. As the use of such a device requires a degree of patient compliance, it may only be applicable for a subset of children, but has already been implemented for selected lung, breast and abdominal tumours in adults.[25]

RADIOTHERAPY VERIFICATION

Advances in verification include electronic portal imaging devices (EPIDs) fixed to the treatment machine. These allow an image of a treatment field on the linear accelerator to be taken and compared using bony landmarks to reference images from the planning computer or simulator. Enhanced imaging quality (e.g. amorphous silicon imagers) and computerized measurements have significantly enhanced the quality of treatment verification. Any new immobilization system is only validated as being superior if set-up is prospectively measured and analysed for a particular patient and group of patients treated with that system.[14]

Therapy machines are now being developed with an integrated orthovoltage source plus detector mounted on the linear accelerator at 90° to the treatment head and EPID. After the patient is set up for treatment, it rotates around the patient to produce a high-resolution soft tissue computed tomography (CT) scan. This allows a 3D check of the patient's internal and bony anatomy on a regular basis for image-guided or 'adaptive radiotherapy'.[26] This may allow on-line corrections to reduce even further the geometric uncertainties of daily treatment delivery during a fractionated course of radiotherapy.

IMAGING FOR RADIOTHERAPY PLANNING

Optimum visualization of the tumour volume and its surrounding anatomical structures is essential for any local cancer treatment. Soon after the introduction of CT scanners this modality was being adapted for radiotherapy planning to visualize internal structures and provide the required electron density data for planning computer systems for accurate dose calculation.[27] Even today this forms the basis of modern CT and planned 3D CRT.

Imaging defines the gross tumour volume (GTV). Depending on tumour type and biological behaviour, an individual margin is added to account for potential microscopic spread defining the clinical target volume (CTV). A further margin is then added to provide the planning target volume (PTV). This last margin incorporates internal organ movement and the uncertainties of daily repositioning and is the volume that should be encompassed by 95 per cent of the prescribed dose.[28,29] The rigid immobilization techniques that have been discussed in the previous section attempt to reduce this margin, thus exposing less normal tissue to high-dose irradiation.

Precise data to quantify the margin from GTV to CTV is lacking for many sites and is based on knowledge from pathological specimens, patterns of recurrence, past clinical trials and empirical experience. However, new functional imaging modalities and scan fusion technology may begin to change this in the future using biological information in conjunction with traditional anatomy.[2,30] Clinical positron emission tomography (PET) scanning has rapidly evolved over the last decade to provide functional tumour information. As part of initial staging procedures (over and above conventional methods such as chest radiography and CT scanning) it has altered patient selection for radiotherapy as well as aiding target definition, e.g. in Hodgkin's disease.[31,32] Clinicians have begun to integrate information from these new imaging tools into radiotherapy planning (multimodality imaging). Examples include fusion of a PET scan on to the planning CT scan for adult lung cancer to define the PTV and critical structures,[33,34] and PET fused with CT/MRI (magnetic resonance imaging) planning scans for head and neck cancer.[35] However, prospective trials to validate this technical advance with respect to patient-derived benefits are still outstanding.

The anatomical detail of helical CT is fused with the functional information of PET using commercially available software programs with a high degree of accuracy for sites such as the brain. However, this is relatively inaccurate for other anatomical regions due to changes in patient position and movement artefacts between scans. Some of these problems with regard to CT and PET have been solved with the introduction of combined or hybrid CT/PET scanners. These can perform both CT and PET scans with the patient in the same anatomical position during a single visit (Figure 29.2; see also Plate 30).

CT/MRI image fusion has been most successfully implemented for radiotherapy planning in neuro-oncology where there is minimal intracranial movement or distortion. Again this has been more difficult for other regions of the body, such as the pelvis and chest, which have problems of temporal and spatial correlation from MRI distortion and patient movement.[36,37] Some of these technical problems may be overcome using an open low-field MRI that reduces the distortion to only 1–2 mm for all regions of the body.[38]

Attempts have been made to utilize information from single photon emission computed tomography (SPECT),[39] PET[40] and magnetic resonance spectroscopy (MRS)[41,42]

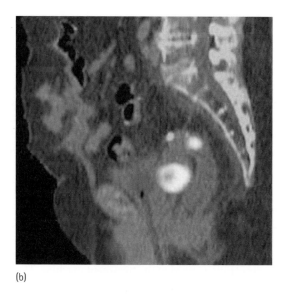

(a)   (b)

Figure 29.2 *Sagittal images from a combined or hybrid CT/PET scanner. (a) A PET scan showing marked [¹⁸F]-fluorodeoxyglucose uptake in a verified cervical tumour and a presacral focus consistent with a metastatic deposit. The concomitant CT scan did not demonstrate a pathologically enlarged lymph node in this location. (b) Fused CT/PET image that localizes the presacral uptake from the PET scan on to the CT scan, indicating metastatic spread to a regional lymph node. Such methods of combining anatomical details with biological tumour information are likely to improve staging accuracy and aid target definition for radiotherapy planning in the future. See also Plate 30. (Reproduced with the kind permission of CTI Molecular Imaging.)*

for gliomas to improve target definition. Results have shown a mismatch between anatomical and metabolic information for high-grade gliomas,[41] but also the possibility of reducing the clinical target volume for the irradiation of low-grade gliomas using MRS.[42] Lastly, mapping of the brain using functional MRI may allow selective avoidance of regions of the brain to reduce the risk of a specific functional impairment due to radiotherapy or surgery.[43,44]

All of these technologies increase the complexity of treatment and require prospective assessment and validation prior to routine implementation but have technical advantages suggestive of potential patient derived benefits.

RADIOTHERAPY PLANNING

Radiotherapy techniques continue to evolve and minimize the volume of normal tissue irradiated to a dose associated with a specified toxicity. The aim is to maintain adequate and homogeneous coverage of tumour PTV while minimizing dose to critical normal tissues in close proximity. It is particularly important in children to minimize all potential long-term radiation-induced sequelae, because they receive radiotherapy at a stage of growth and development. Late sequelae of radiation in children may include among others impaired cognitive development, altered physical appearance and organ dysfunction, with the subsequent impairment of quality of life. Second tumours and complications potentiated by

tumour damage as well as the other treatment modalities also contribute to late morbidity and mortality.[45–52]

Newer techniques of radiotherapy involve maximum conformation of high-dose radiation to the target with sparing of normal tissue. Figure 29.3 summarizes some of the particles, machines and delivery techniques currently in use or development. These techniques include 3D CRT using fixed beams, SCRT or SRS and IMRT. Radiotherapy is usually delivered with the machine gantry fixed, but techniques that move the gantry during treatment (arc therapy) have also been combined with other developments (intensity-modulated arc therapy, IMAT). All techniques have in common the issues of improved patient immobilization, target localization and treatment delivery with some variation in the method used. Using more complex radiation techniques aims to augment the conformity of the delivered dose to the PTV, but as well as increasing the complexity they may also increase the volume of normal tissue receiving low or very low doses of radiation. These lower doses have to be taken into account when comparing and assessing different plans and choosing the final treatment plan. The increase in tissues receiving even low doses compared with conventional 2D or 3D coplanar treatment techniques may be enough to increase the risk of a second malignant neoplasm, e.g. thyroid, salivary and skin cancers,[53–55] or impair growth.

Significant efforts have been devoted to the development of proton therapy for clinical use. Protons are particles that can deposit their energy at a set depth into tissue with virtually no exit of dose beyond the PTV. Compared

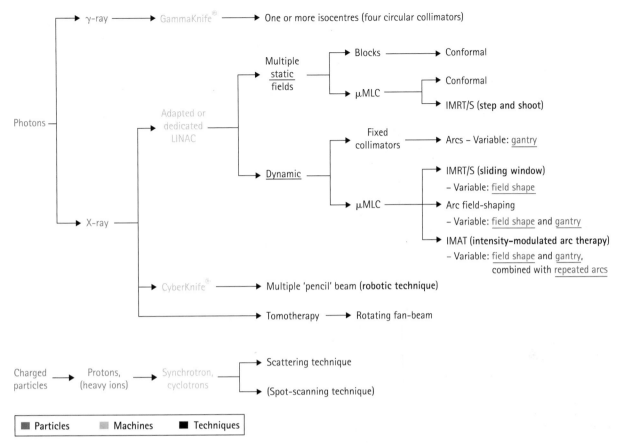

Figure 29.3 *Particles, machines and treatment techniques currently used or being developed for conformal radiotherapy, demonstrating the variety of options available for radiosurgery or stereotactic guided conformal radiotherapy. IMRT, intensity-modulated radiotherapy; MLC, multi-leaf collimator. (Reproduced with the kind permission of Stefano Gianolini, Royal Marsden Hospital, Sutton UK.)*

with conformal photon plans, this has clear technical advantages in terms of reducing the volume of normal tissue irradiated, which is particularly relevant for young children. Examples of tumours treated in this manner are low-grade optic pathway tumours, medulloblastoma and neuroblastoma (see Plate 31).[9,10,56,57] However, cost and limited availability currently prevent its widespread use, as a dedicated cyclotron is a mandatory requirement to produce the high-energy protons.

Rival plans from different techniques can be evaluated and compared in terms of the physical dose distribution within the target and relevant normal tissues for which a probability of tumour control (tumour control probability, TCP) and toxicity (normal tissue complication probability, NTCP) may be estimated. The level of tolerance to radiotherapy of a certain tissue is usually set at an agreed level for a given clinical setting. It is a complex function for a given tissue and depends on the volume irradiated, total dose delivered, dose per fraction, radiation energy and overall treatment time. The risk to experience a predefined toxicity is an overall probability and not predictive for any given patient. Development of a late toxicity can be difficult to estimate as it also depends on factors such as age, co-morbid disease, genetic susceptibility, tumour-related damage, surgery and chemotherapy. Newer radiation techniques may have clear technical advantages, but aim to improve current practice by impacting on this tolerance and reducing toxicity or allowing dose escalation with an equivalent toxicity.

Increased complexity of planning and delivery of radical radiotherapy are appropriate for some tumour sites to optimize the therapeutic ratio for radical treatments (the balance between treatment toxicity and clinical benefit). This is also appropriate in selected palliative settings. There has been a stepwise development in radiotherapy from a conventional parallel pair based on bony landmarks to multiple fields and 3D CRT using stereotaxy.

For 3D CRT, the planning CT scan is transmitted to a planning computer on which the target and relevant critical structures are contoured for each relevant CT slice. Use of the CT data improves visualization of the 3D relationships between target and critical normal structures. Different beam arrangements can be evaluated using the planning software before selecting a final plan providing

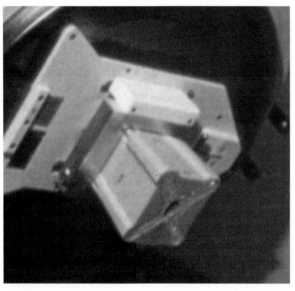

(a)

(b)

Figure 29.4 *Examples of field shaping methods for conformal radiotherapy (CRT). (a) Multi-leaf collimator (MLC) integrated into the head of a linear accelerator showing how the shape of a treatment field may be conformed by computer-controlled movement of each pair of leaves (i.e. conformed to the target volume or in this case a 'bear' shape). For 'dynamic' intensity-modulated radiotherapy (IMRT), the distance between each pair of leaves can be varied with the beam continuously switched on. (b) A customized conformal lead alloy block derived from the beam's eye view facility of a three-dimensional planning computer system. As each field of the treatment plan is treated in turn, the individualized customized block relating to it is attached to the treatment machine.*

the optimal physical dose distribution. This may involve beams entering the patient in a single plane (coplanar) or exploiting all three dimensions (non-coplanar). Unnecessary portions of each beam are shielded so that the shape of each beam conforms to the shape of the target in each 'beam's eye view' (BEV) direction. This is accomplished using a customized shielding block physically fitted on to the radiotherapy linear accelerator for each individual field or by using automated computer-controlled metal leaves (multi-leaf collimators, MLCs) that are incorporated into the head of the machine (Figure 29.4).

Radiotherapy planning studies have been used to demonstrate the physical benefits of 3D CRT (improved target definition, target coverage as well as avoidance of critical structures) for adult tumours[58] and paediatric tumours such as parameningeal rhabdomyosarcoma.[59] Clinical benefits are generally inferred from these planning studies and non-randomized clinical studies.[60,61] However, randomized evidence quantifying the clinical benefits of CRT does exist for prostate cancer. Studies have demonstrated reductions in acute and late toxicity[62,63] as well as improved biochemical local control[64,65] and have provided a proof of principle.

STEREOTACTIC RADIOTHERAPY

Stereotaxy (stereotactic radiotherapy) refers to the use of a fiducial system of relocation in 3D space originally developed for neurosurgery. This has been adapted for radiotherapy[66,67] to exploit the benefits of precise patient repositioning and improved immobilization, which are essential for the accurate delivery of radiotherapy (see 'Set-up and patient immobilization'). The largest experience with stereotactic radiotherapy has been gained in the fields of neuro-oncology and head and neck cancers. It can be used for fractionated radiotherapy using a relocatable frame (SCRT) or as a single fraction with a frame fixed by pins to the skull vault under local anaesthetic (SRS).

SCRT has been used in paediatric neuro-oncology for well-demarcated, slow-growing tumours such as low-grade gliomas and craniopharyngiomas.[15,16] The data from the planning CT scan is fused with a dedicated planning MRI sequence to provide improved visualization of the neuroanatomy to better differentiate tumour from normal tissue. The CT scan provides additional information such as details of the extent of the calcification associated with craniopharyngiomas or improved visualization of the bony extent of a meningioma not visible on MRI.[68] The fused CT and MRI scans are interpreted within the context of all previous imaging and in collaboration with the neuroradiologist and neurosurgeon in charge. The standard use of SCRT with reduced margins, compared with previous practice, still requires careful prospective monitoring. This should preferably be done in the context of a clinical trial to ensure local control is comparable to that achieved with previous techniques.

The ideal way of delivering homogeneous doses to non-spherical lesions with the optimum sparing of normal tissue is through multiple fixed fields conforming to the shape of the lesion.[69] This is achieved by shaped shielding with a multi-leaf collimator (MLC) or a mini-multi-leaf collimator (mMLC) using narrower leaves as well as through individually shaped lead-alloy shielding blocks.[70,71] Paediatric tumours suitable for SCRT are usually centrally located and well localized on imaging. For those measuring 3–6 cm in diameter, i.e. the majority, the optimum sparing of normal brain is achieved with four to six conformal non-coplanar fixed fields.[72] SCRT allows a high-precision localized treatment that minimizes the volume of normal brain receiving high doses of radiation while maintaining a homogeneous dose within the target volume and is feasible in younger children, even under general anaesthetic.[19,73]

Recent reports of SCRT in children with low-grade gliomas, intracranial germ cell tumours and craniopharyngiomas[16–18,74] are encouraging. There have been no cases of tumour recurrence directly adjacent to the high-dose regions suggestive of geographical misses and tumour control has been within historical experience. However, follow-up is still generally short and some relevant endpoints have not been reached, but there is a suggestion of reduced late toxicity.[75] The Boston group has reported their results of conservative surgery and SCRT for paediatric craniopharyngioma with a programme of prospective neurocognitive and memory assessments before and following the radiotherapy.[76] The St Jude experience also suggests reduced toxicity with this approach compared with initial aggressive surgery alone.[77] Prospective outcome data of this quality are essential to monitor the toxicity of a management policy of conservative surgery and SCRT as well as to compare it with other management policies.

SCRT and SRS have also been implemented for head and neck cancer, particularly for re-irradiation and for IMRT, e.g. of nasopharyngeal carcinoma.[78,79] The advantages are to minimize the volume of tissue re-irradiated and avoid critical structures in close proximity, such as major and minor salivary glands.

SRS is used to deliver a single ablative fraction of radiation akin to surgical ablation but without the damage and risks that surgical access may entail. A single fraction avoids the inconvenience of fractionated radiotherapy over many weeks but loses the benefit of fractionation to minimize late toxicity.

SRS can be delivered on a conventional linear accelerator using either an arc or a fixed-field technique or via a dedicated radiotherapy unit using 201 fixed cobalt (^{60}Co)

sources (GammaKnife®). The GammaKnife produces an equally rapid fall-off in dose away from the target compared with a linear accelerator.[80,81] Due to technical constraints, GammaKnife or linear accelerator SRS is usually restricted to tumour sizes of 3–3.5 cm at a 'safe' distance from known sensitive organs at risk, such as the optic chiasm, significantly limiting their use in children. Treating complex shapes or tumours larger than 3.5 cm using SRS leads to dose inhomogeneity and undesirable hotspots of up to twice the prescribed dose within the target and potentially the surrounding normal tissues.

SRS has a place in selected cases where standard fractionated radiotherapy has failed,[82,83] but its use in children should remain restricted to experienced centres. Radiosurgical ablation of intact nerve fibres, e.g. hypothalamus, mesial temporal lobes and limbic pathways, either within or in close proximity to the target, affects memory and neurocognitive outcomes[76] and thus SRS requires a high level of expertise or should be substituted by fractionated SCRT.

Benign conditions such as arteriovenous malformations (AVMs) have also been treated with SRS. The late effects of this ablative form of radiotherapy on the vasculature are specifically utilized to obliterate the malformation and this is used as a surrogate end-point of treatment success.[84,85] However, it is still controversial if this technique reduces the incidence of AVM-associated bleeding in the long term.

INTENSITY–MODULATED RADIOTHERAPY

Radiation beams usually have a uniform intensity or fluence across the field. In the past, simple methods of modifying radiation intensity have been used (e.g. wedges or compensating filters). IMRT involves the production of non-uniform beam intensity across a field (Figure 29.5) using advanced planning, verification and delivery techniques. The non-uniform intensity is summated in 3D for all the treatment fields and permits the creation of concavities into the high-dose distribution. IMRT can, therefore, produce more conformal dose distributions for irregular targets that contain concavities than was previously achievable. This spares critical structures lying within these concavities or in close proximity to the target (conformal avoidance). The benefits include adequate target coverage and the possibility of dose escalation whilst keeping critical structures within predetermined dose levels. IMRT also offers the ability to create inhomogeneous dose distributions that place a 'hotspot' in regions at higher risk of tumour recurrence, providing the ability to deliver a concomitant boost[86] as well as avoiding radiosensitive tissues (dose painting).

The complex planning peculiar to IMRT (inverse planning) involves stipulating desired dose and volume constraints for the target and critical structures. The planning computer then attempts to meet these by generating fluence profiles for predefined fields. These fluence profiles are then recalculated in an iterative manner until an 'optimized' solution is reached with the desired balance of target coverage and organ at risk avoidance. The optimum number of fields, their directions and planning objectives applicable to most tumours of a particular tumour site are termed the 'class' solution. Class solutions are under development for many tumour sites and in the future this optimization and search for the best solution may also be computer-automated.[87]

Currently there are several different methods of generating a field's fluence profile to deliver an optimized IMRT plan. This includes, for example, the manufacture of a physical 3D metal compensator or different ways of

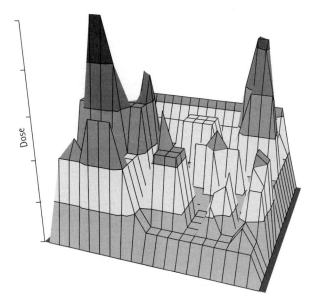

Figure 29.5 *An example of an intensity-modulated radiotherapy (IMRT) fluence profile for a single field, demonstrating the dose variation across the beam. Along the path of irradiation the peaks of higher radiation intensity correspond to tumour-containing areas, and troughs correspond to normal tissue or critical structures.*

using MLC leaves under computer control, e.g. step and shoot (Figure 29.6). For further details of how these are delivered and for which tumours, we refer readers to reviews of the different techniques in current use and development[88,89] and a consensus document from the IMRT Collaborative Working Group.[90]

At present, clinical data on outcome are sparse, but data showing the potential clinical gains are appearing for adult cancers.[91–93] Planning studies have shown clear physical advantages for spinal cord and parotid avoidance in head and neck cancers,[94] and the early clinical outcome studies regarding xerostomia have corroborated this.[92,93,95]

IMRT is in a period of rapid evolution as more reliable and efficient technologies are introduced and tested. The technology is becoming less work-intensive and expensive with 'off the shelf' hardware and software solutions now available. However, there are many quality assurance issues that still need to be solved and IMRT requires specific expertise. For some tumours, detailed knowledge regarding target definition is lacking, limiting the safe use of IMRT, but this may be improved by the integration of new imaging technologies into the planning process.

SUMMARY AND THE FUTURE

The major research directions have been related to CRT (including SCRT, SRS and IMRT) and multimodality imaging (MRI, MRS, PET, SPECT etc.) to improve target definition. Most recent technical advances in radiotherapy are not easily testable in the paediatric setting, as relevant clinical end-points are multifactorial and difficult to measure. Randomized evidence does exist for some advances, such as the value of 3D CRT to reduce acute and late toxicity and improve biochemical tumour control in prostate cancer. Although these results are not directly applicable to the paediatric setting, they represent an important proof of principle. Prospective vigorous academic testing has still to be pursued in this area to prove and quantify the benefits from modern radiotherapy

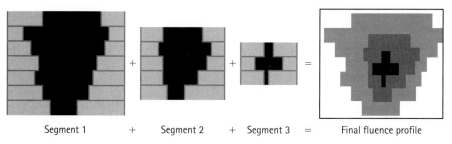

| Segment 1 | + | Segment 2 | + | Segment 3 | = | Final fluence profile |

Figure 29.6 *Step-and-shoot intensity-modulated radiotherapy (IMRT) delivery. For each segment, each leaf of the multi-leaf collimator (represented by the horizontal bars) is moved under computer control to shape the treatment aperture. Each segment is treated in turn with the sum, creating the final fluence profile for that field. The darker areas in the final fluence profile represent higher doses.*

planning and delivery techniques rather than relying on simplistic selected physical dose distributions or radiobiological models with their limitations.[96,97] Techniques such as IMRT have opened up new avenues of critical organ avoidance, dose escalation and concomitant boosts aiming at reducing toxicity and improving tumour control. However, it is not possible or it may not be appropriate to perform prospective, randomized controlled trials for every technical advance in radiotherapy or for each tumour site, due to small patient numbers and lack of appropriate measurement tools for specified end-points in growing children such as vision or quality of life. Only limited information can be derived from comparison with historical series, as significant changes have occurred in staging, imaging, surgery, pathology and chemotherapy over time, making these comparisons notoriously difficult and academically unsatisfactory. Progress in radiation oncology is not achieved by an improvement in a single step within the process but by continuous improvement of the whole pathway. Yet clinicians need to take care not to be enticed into implementing expensive new treatment technologies without clear evidence of patient-derived benefits.[98]

KEY POINTS

- The role of radiotherapy in the management of paediatric malignancies is constantly changing.
- Radiotherapy is increasingly individualized.
- The overall quality of advanced radiotherapy is a complex multi-step process and the 'weakest link' may vary between departments.
- Conformal 3D planned radiotherapy (CRT) maximally conforms the high doses of radiation to the target volume and aims to improve the therapeutic ratio.
- Intensity-modulated radiotherapy (IMRT) is a new method of CRT. This technique uses novel planning and delivery methods and, at present, is in a period of rapid evolution. Another method is the use of protons instead of photons, but limited availability and high costs prohibit widespread use.
- The incorporation of new imaging modalities (e.g. MRS, PET) into radiotherapy planning may improve anatomical and biological target volume definition (multimodality imaging).
- Radiotherapy as a treatment modality is able to rapidly implement new technology and techniques that demonstrate technical advantages over 'conventional' approaches.

- This is achieved at the expense of a significant increase in treatment complexity and must therefore demonstrate measurable patient-derived benefits.
- The evaluation of new treatment techniques should preferably be undertaken in the context of prospective national and international studies.

REFERENCES

1. Proimos BS. Beam-shapers oriented by gravity in rotational therapy. *Radiology* 1966; **87**(5): 928–32.
♦2. Ling CC, Humm J, Larson S *et al.* Towards multidimensional radiotherapy (MD-CRT): biological imaging and biological conformality. *Int J Radiat Oncol Biol Phys* 2000; **47**(3): 551–60.
3. Gandola L, Cefalo G, Massimino M *et al.* Hyperfractionated accelerated radiotherapy (HART) after intensive postoperative sequential chemotherapy for metastatic medulloblastoma. International Society of Paediatric Oncology SIOP XXXIV Annual Meeting. *Med Pediatr Oncol* 2002; **39**(4): 248.
4. Allen JC, Donahue B, DaRosso R, Nirenberg A. Hyperfractionated craniospinal radiotherapy and adjuvant chemotherapy for children with newly diagnosed medulloblastoma and other primitive neuroectodermal tumors. *Int J Radiat Oncol Biol Phys* 1996; **36**(5):1155–61.
5. Prados MD, Edwards MS, Chang SM *et al.* Hyperfractionated craniospinal radiation therapy for primitive neuroectodermal tumors: results of a phase II study. *Int J Radiat Oncol Biol Phys* 1999; **43**(2): 279–85.
6. Kushner BH, Wolden S, LaQuaglia MP *et al.* Hyperfractionated low-dose radiotherapy for high-risk neuroblastoma after intensive chemotherapy and surgery. *J Clin Oncol* 2001; **19**(11): 2821–8.
7. Ricardi U, Corrias A, Einaudi S *et al.* Thyroid dysfunction as a late effect in childhood medulloblastoma: a comparison of hyperfractionated versus conventionally fractionated craniospinal radiotherapy. *Int J Radiat Oncol Biol Phys* 2001; **50**(5): 1287–94.
8. Corrias A, Einaudi S, Ricardi U *et al.* Thyroid diseases in patients treated during pre-puberty for medulloblastoma with different radiotherapic protocols. *J Endocrinol Invest* 2001; **24**(6): 387–92.
9. Hug EB, Nevinny-Stickel M, Fuss M *et al.* Conformal proton radiation treatment for retroperitoneal neuroblastoma: introduction of a novel technique. *Med Pediatr Oncol* 2001; **37**(1): 36–41.
10. Lin R, Hug EB, Schaefer RA *et al.* Conformal proton radiation therapy of the posterior fossa: a study comparing protons with three-dimensional planned photons in limiting dose to auditory structures. *Int J Radiat Oncol Biol Phys* 2000; **48**(4): 1219–26.
11. Lee SW, Fraass BA, Marsh LH *et al.* Patterns of failure following high-dose 3-D conformal radiotherapy for high-grade astrocytomas: a quantitative dosimetric study. *Int J Radiat Oncol Biol Phys* 1999; **43**(1): 79–88.

12. Pai HH, Thornton A, Katznelson L et al. Hypothalamic/ pituitary function following high-dose conformal radiotherapy to the base of skull: demonstration of a dose-effect relationship using dose-volume histogram analysis. Int J Radiat Oncol Biol Phys 2001; **49**(4): 1079–92.

13. Halperin EC, Laurie F, Fitzgerald TJ. An evaluation of the relationship between the quality of prophylactic cranial radiotherapy in childhood acute leukemia and institutional experience: a Quality Assurance Review Center – Pediatric Oncology Group study. Int J Radiat Oncol Biol Phys 2002; **53**(4): 1001–4.

14. Zhu Y, Stovall J Jr, Butler L et al. Comparison of two immobilization techniques using portal film and digitally reconstructed radiographs for pediatric patients with brain tumors. Int J Radiat Oncol Biol Phys 2000; **48**(4): 1233–40.

15. Tarbell NJ, Barnes P, Scott RM et al. Advances in radiation therapy for craniopharyngiomas. Pediatr Neurosurg 1994; **21**(Suppl 1): 101–7.

16. Saran FH, Baumert BG, Khoo VS et al. Stereotactically guided conformal radiotherapy for progressive low-grade gliomas of childhood. Int J Radiat Oncol Biol Phys 2002; **53**(1): 43–51.

●17. Merchant TE, Zhu Y, Thompson SJ et al. Preliminary results from a phase II trial of conformal radiation therapy for pediatric patients with localised low-grade astrocytoma and ependymoma. Int J Radiat Oncol Biol Phys 2002; **52**(2): 325–32.

18. Debus J, Kocagoncu KO, Hoss A et al. Fractionated stereotactic radiotherapy (FSRT) for optic glioma. Int J Radiat Oncol Biol Phys 1999; **44**(2): 243–8.

19. Adams EJ, Suter BL, Warrington AP et al. Design and implementation of a system for treating paediatric patients with stereotactically-guided conformal radiotherapy. Radiother Oncol 2001; **60**(3): 289–97.

20. Ryken TC, Meeks SL, Pennington EC et al. Initial clinical experience with frameless stereotactic radiosurgery: analysis of accuracy and feasibility. Int J Radiat Oncol Biol Phys 2001; **51**(4): 1152–8.

21. Karger CP, Jakel O, Debus J et al. Three-dimensional accuracy and interfractional reproducibility of patient fixation and positioning using a stereotactic head mask system. Int J Radiat Oncol Biol Phys 2001; **49**(5): 1493–504.

22. Chou RH, Wilder RB, Wong MS, Forster KM. Recent advances in radiotherapy for head and neck cancers. Ear Nose Throat J 2001; **80**(10): 704–7, 711–14, 716.

23. Lohr F, Debus J, Frank C et al. Noninvasive patient fixation for extracranial stereotactic radiotherapy. Int J Radiat Oncol Biol Phys 1999; **45**(2): 521–7.

24. Wulf J, Hadinger U, Oppitz U et al. Stereotactic radiotherapy of extracranial targets: CT-simulation and accuracy of treatment in the stereotactic body frame. Radiother Oncol 2000; **57**(2): 225–36.

25. Wong JW, Sharpe MB, Jaffray DA et al. The use of active breathing control (ABC) to reduce margin for breathing motion. Int J Radiat Oncol Biol Phys 1999; **44**(4): 911–19.

26. Jaffray DA, Siewerdsen JH, Wong JW et al. Flat-panel cone-beam computed tomography for image-guided radiation therapy. Int J Radiat Oncol Biol Phys 2002; **53**(5): 1337–49.

27. Dobbs HJ, Parker RP, Hodson NJ et al. The use of CT in radiotherapy treatment planning. Radiother Oncol 1983; **1**(2): 133–41.

28. International Commission on Radiation Units and Measurements. ICRU Report 50. Prescribing, Recording and Reporting Photon Beam Therapy. Bethesda, MD: ICRU; 1993.

29. International Commission on Radiation Units and Measurements. ICRU Report 62. Prescribing, Recording and Reporting Photon Beam Therapy (supplement to ICRU Report 50). Bethesda, MD: ICRU; 1999.

30. Rosenman J. Incorporating functional imaging information into radiation treatment. Semin Radiat Oncol 2001; **11**(1): 83–92.

31. Partridge S, Timothy A, O'Doherty MJ et al. 2-Fluorine-18-fluoro-2-deoxy-D glucose positron emission tomography in the pretreatment staging of Hodgkin's disease: influence on patient management in a single institution. Ann Oncol 2000; **11**(10): 1273–9.

32. Spaepen K, Stroobants S, Dupont P et al. Can positron emission tomography with [(18)F]-fluorodeoxyglucose after first-line treatment distinguish Hodgkin's disease patients who need additional therapy from others in whom additional therapy would mean avoidable toxicity? Br J Haematol 2001; **115**(2): 272–8.

●33. Mah K, Caldwell CB, Ung YC et al. The impact of (18)FDG-PET on target and critical organs in CT-based treatment planning of patients with poorly defined non-small-cell lung carcinoma: a prospective study. Int J Radiat Oncol Biol Phys 2002; **52**(2): 339–50.

34. Erdi YE, Rosenzweig K, Erdi AK et al. Radiotherapy treatment planning for patients with non-small cell lung cancer using positron emission tomography (PET). Radiother Oncol 2002; **62**(1): 51–60.

35. Nishioka T, Shiga T, Shirato H et al. Image fusion between 18FDG-PET and MRI/CT for radiotherapy planning of oropharyngeal and nasopharyngeal carcinomas. Int J Radiat Oncol Biol Phys 2002; **53**(4): 1051–7.

♦36. Khoo VS, Dearnaley DP, Finnigan DJ et al. Magnetic resonance imaging (MRI): considerations and applications in radiotherapy treatment planning. Radiother Oncol 1997; **42**(1): 1–15.

37. Khoo VS. MRI – 'magic radiotherapy imaging' for treatment planning? Br J Radiol 2000; **73**(867): 229–33.

38. Krempien RC, Schubert K, Zierhut D et al. Open low-field magnetic resonance imaging in radiation therapy treatment planning. Int J Radiat Oncol Biol Phys 2002; **53**(5): 1350–60.

39. Grosu AL, Weber W, Feldmann HJ et al. First experience with I-123-alpha-methyl-tyrosine spect in the 3-D radiation treatment planning of brain gliomas. Int J Radiat Oncol Biol Phys 2000; **47**(2): 517–26.

40. Nuutinen J, Sonninen P, Lehikoinen P et al. Radiotherapy treatment planning and long-term follow-up with [(11)C]methionine PET in patients with low-grade astrocytoma. Int J Radiat Oncol Biol Phys 2000; **48**(1): 43–52.

41. Pirzkall A, McKnight TR, Graves EE et al. MR-spectroscopy guided target delineation for high-grade gliomas. Int J Radiat Oncol Biol Phys 2001; **50**(4): 915–28.

42. Pirzkall A, Nelson SJ, McKnight TR et al. Metabolic imaging of low-grade gliomas with three-dimensional magnetic resonance spectroscopy. Int J Radiat Oncol Biol Phys 2002; **53**(5): 1254–64.

43. Hamilton RJ, Sweeney PJ, Pelizzari CA *et al.* Functional imaging in treatment planning of brain lesions. *Int J Radiat Oncol Biol Phys* 1997; **37**(1): 181–8.

44. Fried I. Magnetic resonance imaging and epilepsy: neurosurgical decision making. *Magn Reson Imaging* 1995; **13**(8): 1163–70.

●45. Ris MD, Packer R, Goldwein J *et al.* Intellectual outcome after reduced-dose radiation therapy plus adjuvant chemotherapy for medulloblastoma: a Children's Cancer Group study. *J Clin Oncol* 2001; **19**(15): 3470–6.

●46. Mulhern RK, Kepner JL, Thomas PR *et al.* Neuropsychologic functioning of survivors of childhood medulloblastoma randomized to receive conventional or reduced-dose craniospinal irradiation: a Pediatric Oncology Group study. *J Clin Oncol* 1998; **16**(5): 1723–8.

47. Hogeboom CJ, Grosser SC, Guthrie KA *et al.* Stature loss following treatment for Wilms tumor. *Med Pediatr Oncol* 2001; **36**(2): 295–304.

48. Constine LS, Woolf PD, Cann D *et al.* Hypothalamic-pituitary dysfunction after radiation for brain tumors. *N Engl J Med* 1993; **328**(2): 87–94.

49. Eiser C, Jenney ME. Measuring symptomatic benefit and quality of life in paediatric oncology. *Br J Cancer* 1996; **73**(11): 1313–16.

50. Walter AW, Hancock ML, Pui CH *et al.* Secondary brain tumors in children treated for acute lymphoblastic leukemia at St Jude Children's Research Hospital. *J Clin Oncol* 1998; **16**(12): 3761–7.

●51. Neglia JP, Friedman DL, Yasui Y *et al.* Second malignant neoplasms in five-year survivors of childhood cancer: childhood cancer survivor study. *J Natl Cancer Inst* 2001; **93**(8): 618–29.

●52. Mertens AC, Yasui Y, Neglia JP *et al.* Late mortality experience in five-year survivors of childhood and adolescent cancer: the Childhood Cancer Survivor Study. *J Clin Oncol* 2001; **19**(13): 3163–72.

53. Ron E, Lubin JH, Shore RE *et al.* Thyroid cancer after exposure to external radiation: a pooled analysis of seven studies. *Radiat Res* 1995; **141**(3): 259–77.

54. Modan B, Chetrit A, Alfandary E *et al.* Increased risk of salivary gland tumors after low-dose irradiation. *Laryngoscope* 1998; **108**(7): 1095–7.

55. Shore RE, Moseson M, Xue X *et al.* Skin cancer after X-ray treatment for scalp ringworm. *Radiat Res* 2002; **157**(4): 410–18.

56. Fuss M, Hug EB, Schaefer RA *et al.* Proton radiation therapy (PRT) for pediatric optic pathway gliomas: comparison with 3D planned conventional photons and a standard photon technique. *Int J Radiat Oncol Biol Phys* 1999; **45**(5): 1117–26.

57. Miralbell R, Lomax A, Russo M. Potential role of proton therapy in the treatment of pediatric medulloblastoma/primitive neuro-ectodermal tumors: spinal theca irradiation. *Int J Radiat Oncol Biol Phys* 1997; **38**(4): 805–11.

58. Emami B, Purdy JA, Simpson JR *et al.* 3-D conformal radiotherapy in head and neck cancer. The Washington University experience. *Front Radiat Ther Oncol* 1996; **29**: 207–20.

59. Michalski JM, Sur RK, Harms WB, Purdy JA. Three dimensional conformal radiation therapy in pediatric parameningeal rhabdomyosarcomas. *Int J Radiat Oncol Biol Phys* 1995; **33**(5): 985–91.

60. Hazuka MB, Martel MK, Marsh L *et al.* Preservation of parotid function after external beam irradiation in head and neck cancer patients: a feasibility study using 3-dimensional treatment planning. *Int J Radiat Oncol Biol Phys* 1993; **27**(3): 731–7.

61. Sandler HM, McLaughlin PW, Ten Haken RK *et al.* Three dimensional conformal radiotherapy for the treatment of prostate cancer: low risk of chronic rectal morbidity observed in a large series of patients. *Int J Radiat Oncol Biol Phys* 1995; **33**(4): 797–801.

62. Koper PC, Stroom JC, van Putten WL *et al.* Acute morbidity reduction using 3DCRT for prostate carcinoma: a randomized study. *Int J Radiat Oncol Biol Phys* 1999; **43**(4): 727–34.

●63. Dearnaley DP, Khoo VS, Norman AR *et al.* Comparison of radiation side-effects of conformal and conventional radiotherapy in prostate cancer: a randomised trial. *Lancet* 1999; **353**(9149): 267–72.

64. Dearnaley DP, Hall E, Jackson C *et al.* Phase III trial of dose escalation using conformal radiotherapy in prostate cancer: side effects and PSA control. *Br J Cancer* 2001; **85**(Suppl 1): 15.

65. Dearnaley DP. Radiotherapy and combined modality approaches in localised prostate cancer. *Eur J Cancer* 2001; **37**(Suppl 7): S137–45.

66. Graham JD, Warrington AP, Gill SS, Brada M. A non-invasive, relocatable stereotactic frame for fractionated radiotherapy and multiple imaging. *Radiother Oncol* 1991; **21**(1): 60–2.

67. Schlegel W, Pastyr O, Bortfeld T *et al.* Stereotactically guided fractionated radiotherapy: technical aspects. *Radiother Oncol* 1993; **29**(2): 197–204.

68. Khoo VS, Adams EJ, Saran F *et al.* A Comparison of clinical target volumes determined by CT and MRI for the radiotherapy planning of base of skull meningiomas. *Int J Radiat Oncol Biol Phys* 2000; **46**(5): 1309–17.

69. Laing RW, Bentley RE, Nahum AE *et al.* Stereotactic radiotherapy of irregular targets: a comparison between static conformal beams and non-coplanar arcs. *Radiother Oncol* 1993; **28**(3): 241–6.

70. Shiu AS, Kooy HM, Ewton JR *et al.* Comparison of miniature multileaf collimation (MMLC) with circular collimation for stereotactic treatment. *Int J Radiat Oncol Biol Phys* 1997; **37**(3): 679–88.

71. Adams EJ, Cosgrove VP, Shepherd SF *et al.* Comparison of a multi-leaf collimator with conformal blocks for the delivery of stereotactically guided conformal radiotherapy. *Radiother Oncol* 1999; **51**(3): 205–9.

72. Perks JR, Jalali R, Cosgrove VP *et al.* Optimization of stereotactically-guided conformal treatment planning of sellar and parasellar tumors, based on normal brain dose volume histograms. *Int J Radiat Oncol Biol Phys* 1999; **45**(2): 507–13.

73. Jalali R, Brada M, Perks JR *et al.* Stereotactic conformal radiotherapy for pituitary adenomas: technique and preliminary experience. *Clin Endocrinol (Oxf)* 2000; **52**(6): 695–702.

74. Zissiadis Y, Dutton S, Kieran M *et al.* Stereotactic radiotherapy for pediatric intracranial germ cell tumors. *Int J Radiat Oncol Biol Phys* 2001; **51**(1): 108–12.

♦75. Loeffler JS, Kooy HM, Tarbell NJ. The emergence of conformal radiotherapy: special implications for pediatric neuro-oncology. *Int J Radiat Oncol Biol Phys* 1999; **44**(2): 237–8.

76. Carpentieri SC, Waber DP, Scott RM *et al.* Memory deficits among children with craniopharyngiomas. *Neurosurgery* 2001; **49**(5): 1053–7 (discussion 1057–8).

77. Merchant TE, Kiehna EN, Sanford RA *et al.* Craniopharyngioma: the St Jude Children's Research Hospital experience 1984–2001. *Int J Radiat Oncol Biol Phys* 2002; **53**(3): 533–42.

78. Pai PC, Chuang CC, Wei KC *et al.* Stereotactic radiosurgery for locally recurrent nasopharyngeal carcinoma. *Head Neck* 2002; **24**(8): 748–53.

79. Ahn YC, Kim DY, Huh SJ. Fractionated stereotactic radiation therapy for locally recurrent nasopharynx cancer: report of three cases. *Head Neck* 1999; **21**(4): 338–45.

80. Phillips MH, Stelzer KJ, Griffin TW *et al.* Stereotactic radiosurgery: a review and comparison of methods. *J Clin Oncol* 1994; **12**(5): 1085–99.

81. Verhey LJ, Smith V, Serago CF. Comparison of radiosurgery treatment modalities based on physical dose distributions. *Int J Radiat Oncol Biol Phys* 1998; **40**(2): 497–505.

82. Hodgson DC, Goumnerova LC, Loeffler JS *et al.* Radiosurgery in the management of pediatric brain tumors. *Int J Radiat Oncol Biol Phys* 2001; **50**(4): 929–35.

83. Chiou SM, Lunsford LD, Niranjan A *et al.* Stereotactic radiosurgery of residual or recurrent craniopharyngioma, after surgery, with or without radiation therapy. *Neuro-oncol* 2001; **3**(3): 159–66.

84. Smyth MD, Sneed PK, Ciricillo SF *et al.* Stereotactic radiosurgery for pediatric intracranial arteriovenous malformations: the University of California at San Francisco experience. *J Neurosurg* 2002; **97**(1): 48–55.

85. Levy EI, Niranjan A, Thompson TP *et al.* Radiosurgery for childhood intracranial arteriovenous malformations. *Neurosurgery* 2000; **47**(4): 834–41 (discussion 841–2).

86. Butler EB, Teh BS, Grant WH, 3rd *et al.* Smart (simultaneous modulated accelerated radiation therapy) boost: a new accelerated fractionation schedule for the treatment of head and neck cancer with intensity modulated radiotherapy. *Int J Radiat Oncol Biol Phys* 1999; **45**(1): 21–32.

87. Rowbottom CG, Nutting CM, Webb S. Beam-orientation optimization of intensity-modulated radiotherapy: clinical application to parotid gland tumours. *Radiother Oncol* 2001; **59**(2): 169–77.

♦88. Nutting C, Dearnaley DP, Webb S. Intensity modulated radiation therapy: a clinical review. *Br J Radiol* 2000; **73**(869): 459–69.

♦89. Webb S. Advances in three-dimensional conformal radiation therapy physics with intensity modulation. *Lancet Oncol* 2000; **1**(1): 30–6.

90. Intensity-modulated radiotherapy: current status and issues of interest. *Int J Radiat Oncol Biol Phys* 2001; **51**(4): 880–914.

91. Zelefsky MJ, Fuks Z, Hunt M *et al.* High-dose intensity modulated radiation therapy for prostate cancer: early toxicity and biochemical outcome in 772 patients. *Int J Radiat Oncol Biol Phys* 2002; **53**(5): 1111–16.

92. Eisbruch A, Kim HM, Terrell JE *et al.* Xerostomia and its predictors following parotid-sparing irradiation of head-and-neck cancer. *Int J Radiat Oncol Biol Phys* 2001; **50**(3): 695–704.

93. Eisbruch A. Intensity-modulated radiotherapy of head-and-neck cancer: encouraging early results. *Int J Radiat Oncol Biol Phys* 2002; **53**(1): 1–3.

94. Eisbruch A, Foote RL, O'Sullivan B *et al.* Intensity-modulated radiation therapy for head and neck cancer: emphasis on the selection and delineation of the targets. *Semin Radiat Oncol* 2002; **12**(3): 238–49.

95. Lee N, Xia P, Quivey JM *et al.* Intensity-modulated radiotherapy in the treatment of nasopharyngeal carcinoma: an update of the UCSF experience. *Int J Radiat Oncol Biol Phys* 2002; **53**(1): 12–22.

96. Amols HI, Ling CC. EUD but not QED. *Int J Radiat Oncol Biol Phys* 2002; **52**(1): 1–2.

97. Wu Q, Mohan R, Niemierko A, Schmidt-Ullrich R. Optimization of intensity-modulated radiotherapy plans based on the equivalent uniform dose. *Int J Radiat Oncol Biol Phys* 2002; **52**(1): 224–35.

98. Halperin EC. Overpriced technology in radiation oncology. *Int J Radiat Oncol Biol Phys* 2000; **48**(4): 917–18.

Late effects and supportive care

30

Acute complications

STEPHEN P. LOWIS, NICHOLAS GOULDEN & ANTHONY OAKHILL

Acute complications of therapy for malignant disease are common, reflecting the narrow therapeutic index of most anti-cancer drugs, and the variable patterns of organ involvement of paediatric malignancies. The importance of complications lies in the immediate danger to life, as with acute infection, and with the delays and reduction of subsequent therapy often caused; intensity of treatment is a determinant of therapeutic success for many tumours. Hence there is a possibility to improve treatment outcomes for patients by optimizing therapy and reducing complications.

The most frequently encountered complications are:

- nausea and vomiting
- bone marrow failure with its consequences of infection
- poor nutrition.

These will be dealt with separately below. Specific therapy-related acute complications that are discussed include tumour lysis syndrome, convulsions and other neurological problems.

Haematological problems are central to many emergencies in oncology. At presentation, and during conventional and high-dose chemotherapy, the consequences of bone marrow failure are diverse. Infection risk correlates with the depth and duration of neutropenia, and the risk of haemorrhage similarly correlates with thrombocytopenia. Hyperleucocytosis at presentation leads to many secondary effects. Inappropriate activation of the clotting system, diffuse intravascular coagulation and thrombotic thrombocytopenia have many causes, and have widespread and profound effects on the patient. The spectrum of trigger factors for these factors differs in oncology patients, since both the disease and the treatment may contribute. A thorough understanding of the processes involved and indications for intervention is essential for managing such patients, and a section relating to these is included in this chapter.

Many emergencies are iatrogenic, albeit unpredicted. Organ-specific toxicities are relatively common in oncology and many are well recognized. Bone marrow failure, mucositis and extravasation-related skin toxicity are such examples, but other toxicities, though relatively uncommon, also affect major organs. Such toxicities represent oncological emergencies which may be poorly recognized by inexperienced staff. Actinomycin-D-related veno-occlusive disease, cytarabine- or L-asparaginase-related pancreatitis and ifosfamide-related encephalopathy are examples of these, and prompt action reduces morbidity and mortality. The iatrogenic nature of many oncological emergencies offers hope for improvement. For example, better understanding of chemotherapeutic drugs allows safer treatment with more predictable effects. For some, as with the now well understood relationship between exposure to high levels of L-asparaginase and vascular thrombosis, particularly with other pro-coagulant risk factors, a pharmacological explanation has been found. For others, adverse side-effects remain unexplained.

For all of the complications described in this chapter, early recognition is an important part of appropriate management. Limitation of the extent of initial harm and prevention of secondary effects will lead to a greater chance of successful recovery.

Within the setting of bone marrow transplantation (BMT), complications are common and more difficult to overcome. Prolonged bone marrow failure, multiple drug therapy, repeated blood product transfusions, graft-versus-host disease and donor engraftment all contribute to overall greater difficulties, and are addressed separately in Chapter 25. Finally, the supportive care of children with incurable disease, particularly of pain control, is of major importance, and is discussed in greater detail in Chapter 34.

NAUSEA AND VOMITING

Background

Nausea and vomiting are of major significance in chemotherapy and radiotherapy, being both common and, at times, severe. The early and effective control of symptoms is of major importance both for determining the patient's ability to tolerate a given regimen and for their long-term nutritional state. Compliance with therapy, especially that of adolescent patients, may be affected by the nauseating effect of some therapeutic regimens. Early control is also important because the association of nausea and vomiting with administration of chemotherapy may lead to significant problems with anticipatory symptoms. Control of nausea and vomiting is more readily maintained by prevention than by increasing therapy once it has become established.

Emesis is controlled by the vomiting centre, located in the lateral reticular formation of the medulla, along with fibres of the VIII and X nuclei. In experimental animals, vomiting is provoked by electrical stimulation of the vomiting centre, whilst local destruction will prevent vomiting. In the normal individual, the vomiting centre receives inputs from:

- vestibular apparatus
- higher brainstem
- visceral afferents
- the chemoreceptor trigger zone (CTZ).

The CTZ is localized in the area postrema of the fourth ventricle, at which site the blood–brain barrier is relatively poorly developed. It receives afferent fibres from the vestibular nucleus and, in addition, many emetic agents appear to exert their effect directly upon the CTZ, which contains a high density of receptors for dopamine, serotonin, histamine and acetylcholine. Impulses are then transmitted to the vomiting centre, causing emesis.[1]

The integrity of the CTZ is necessary for the production of motion sickness, but is not an absolute requirement for vomiting; afferent impulses from the viscera via the vagus nerve or from the frontal cortex may still trigger vomiting where the CTZ has been experimentally ablated.

Antiemetic agents act by inhibition of one or more of the receptors in the CTZ, and in some cases by reducing visceral afferent impulses. Higher cortical afferent stimuli may have a great effect, and administration of chemotherapy in an environment appropriate to the needs of the child should always be the ideal; a quiet, calm ward is appropriate for young adults, whereas a busy, general paediatric ward is likely to be preferred by young children. The avoidance of strong cooking smells is to be recommended.

Antiemetic therapy

Control of nausea and vomiting may be achieved with a single drug, but more commonly two or more agents may be necessary, depending on the emesis-inducing potential of the chemotherapy agents and on the individual patient. Antiemetic agents may be grouped as given below. Their use according to an emetic control 'ladder', as reported by Foot and Hayes,[2] is recommended.

5HT₃ ANTAGONISTS

Type 3 receptors for serotonin are of major importance in chemotherapy-induced emesis, and $5HT_3$ receptors are abundant in both the gastrointestinal tract and the CTZ. Cisplatin administration has been shown to cause release of 5HT, presumably from intestinal mucosa,[3] which may explain the severe and often prolonged vomiting associated with this drug. Specific antagonists of $5HT_3$ receptors, the first of which was ondansetron, although granisetron and tropisetron are both now available, have improved control dramatically. Ondansetron has been shown to be significantly more effective than high-dose metoclopramide in cisplatin-induced emesis[4] and than metoclopramide-diphenhydramine in children receiving a variety of chemotherapy regimens.[5] For highly emetogenic regimens it is the drug of choice. Ondansetron[6] and granisetron[7] produce significantly better control of symptoms than tropisetron. Side-effects of therapy appear to be relatively minor, and include diarrhoea, dizziness, headaches, urticaria, rashes and transient elevation of liver enzymes. The major contraindication appears to be financial, and this is compounded by inappropriate prescription where less costly antiemetic regimens may prove equally successful. The administration of escalating doses, or more frequent doses, of ondansetron is less likely to be of benefit than coadministration of a second antiemetic agent such as a corticosteroid or an antidopaminergic agent.

ANTIDOPAMINERGIC AGENTS

Dopamine D2 receptors are abundant in the CTZ, and dopamine is excitatory to neurons in the area postrema of dogs. Antidopaminergic agents (e.g. domperidone) have antiemetic effects. The most widely used of these are the neuroleptic agents, phenothiazines and butyrophenones.

Phenothiazines (chlorpromazine, prochlorperazine) have antipsychotic effects attributable to their antidopaminergic action, and chlorpromazine in particular also has anticholinergic and antihistaminergic activity. Chlorpromazine has an antiemetic effect at doses which are generally less than those required for antipsychotic action, and the risk of extrapyramidal side-effects is correspondingly less. Chlorpromazine may induce hypotension, light-sensitive skin rashes and cholestatic jaundice.

Butyrophenones (haloperidol, droperidol, domperidone) have also been used, although less frequently than phenothiazines. High-dose haloperidol has been reported to be similar in efficacy to metoclopramide in cisplatin-induced emesis, although the risk of extrapyramidal side-effects remains. Butyrophenones are reported to cause less sedation and hypotension than phenothiazines. Domperidone, in particular, also acts by increasing gastric emptying, and thereby reducing afferent impulses from the viscera.

Metoclopramide is a substituted benzamide which was originally developed as a prokinetic agent. Part of its antiemetic action relates to enhancement of gastric emptying and increase of gastro-oesophageal tone, but it also has both antidopaminergic and antiserotonin activity centrally. The antidopaminergic activity is dose-limiting and extrapyramidal side-effects are common, particularly in younger patients.[8,9] Nevertheless, high-dose metoclopramide (2 mg/kg) was the best agent for cisplatin-induced emesis until the development of specific 5HT$_3$ antagonists.

The risk of precipitating an oculogyric crisis remains with all antidopaminergic agents, and the appropriate therapy should be readily available. The use of benzhexol, benztropine or orciprenaline is generally recommended, although intravenous diazepam may also be used with caution. A controlled intravenous dose, titrated to the patient's symptoms, is effective and has the theoretical benefit of inducing some retrograde amnesia. Extrapyramidal disorders of movement may prove more resistant to treatment, but may respond to low doses of phenytoin if anticholinergic agents are not effective.

CORTICOSTEROIDS

Corticosteroids have some antiemetic activity as single agents, and it has been suggested that this is related to changes in cell permeability or antiprostaglandin activity. Their use is more commonly confined to coadministration with other antiemetic agents. Corticosteroids have been shown to markedly increase the antiemetic activity of 5HT$_3$ antagonists[10] and metoclopramide,[11] and increases in the activity of phenothiazines (prochlorperazine, chlorpromazine), haloperidol, nabilone, and lorazepam have also been reported.

BENZODIAZEPINES

As single agents, benzodiazepines have little antiemetic effect, but act as anxiolytic, sedative and amnesia-inducing agents. Lorazepam, in particular, has been used in combination with other antiemetic agents in patients with significant anticipatory vomiting. The sedative effects of other agents such as phenothiazines and cannabinoids may also contribute to their antiemetic action in this way.

CANNABINOIDS

Anecdotal reports of reduced emesis in patients using marijuana led to formal studies of cannabinoids in moderately emetogenic chemotherapy. Tetrahydrocannabinol and nabilone have both been found to be effective, although side-effects including dysphoria, sedation and vertigo are relatively common.[12,13] Coadministration of prochlorperazine has been shown to reduce the incidence of dysphoria.[14]

ANTIHISTAMINIC AGENTS

Histamine H1 and muscarinic cholinergic receptors are present in high concentrations in the nuclei of the solitary tract (VIII and X), and the efficacy of antihistamines in the prevention of motion sickness has been known since the 1940s. The value of these in chemotherapy-induced emesis is limited, but they may be effective in overcoming the emetic effect of high doses of opiates.

ANTICHOLINERGIC AGENTS

Anticholinergic agents may reduce the risk of extrapyramidal side-effects seen with antidopaminergic drugs, but are of uncertain benefit for chemotherapy-induced emesis. In patients receiving palliative care, however, nausea associated with disseminated disease or with high doses of opiate analgesia is often improved by hyoscine. The reduction of secretions seen with anticholinergic agents is also often of benefit.

DELAYED VOMITING

Delayed vomiting is particularly associated with cisplatin, and may reflect gastrointestinal damage rather than drug-induced receptor stimulation. Delayed emesis may prove difficult to control, and benefit from anti-5HT$_3$ agents has not been shown. Kris et al.[15] reported reduced delayed vomiting in patients receiving oral dexamethasone and metoclopramide compared with placebo.

COMBINATION THERAPY

Given that it is often the least experienced members of the oncology team who are responsible for prescription of antiemetic medication, many units have developed 'in house' protocols for different anticipated degrees of emesis. An example of such a policy, in current use at the Royal Hospital for Sick Children, Bristol is given in Figure 30.1. The audited results of therapy according to this protocol have been published by Foot and Hayes.[2] A similar approach to antiemetic therapy was subsequently published by Hesketh et al.[16] Cytotoxic agents are categorized into four groups according to the severity of their emetic potential. In a series of 134 courses of chemotherapy in 60 children undergoing treatment for solid and haematological malignancies, including BMT, antiemetic control was achieved with this regimen in 82 per cent. Failure of antiemetic control was defined as two vomits or retches, or 4 hours of continued nausea in 24 hours. Overall, control was obtained on 89 per cent of days of chemotherapy.

TUMOUR LYSIS SYNDROME

The term tumour lysis syndrome (TLS) describes the metabolic effects produced by rapid death of tumour cells at the time of initial presentation. This may be spontaneous, but more commonly appears once therapy has begun. Cell breakdown releases large amounts of metabolites into the extracellular space, and these breakdown products are excreted principally by the kidneys. Potassium, phosphate, urate and other purine metabolites are of greatest importance, and accumulation of these may lead to renal impairment and life-threatening electrolyte imbalance.

Tumour lysis is most often associated with lymphoid malignancies with a high proliferative index, large tumour load and often high sensitivity to initial chemotherapy. B- and T-cell non-Hodgkin's lymphoma, and T-cell acute lymphoblastic leukaemia (ALL) are most commonly associated, but TLS may be seen with other tumours presenting with widespread or bulky disease if a rapid response to chemotherapy is seen. TLS has been reported to occur with induction therapy of acute myeloid leukaemia (AML), metastatic rhabdomyosarcoma, neuroblastoma, hepatoblastoma, hepatocellular carcinoma, and as a feature of haemophagocytic lymphohistiocytosis.[17–19]

Chemotherapy is the most common precipitant of TLS, although precipitants of cell death, including infection, anaesthesia and surgery, have been reported to act as trigger factors. Regardless of the cause, the management of TLS is the same, and aims to avoid fluid overload, protect renal function (by ensuring maximal diuresis and avoiding deposition of urate and phosphate), and identify and correct life-threatening hyperkalaemia.

Features of TLS

Rapid cell breakdown presents a large solute load to the systemic circulation. Urate, produced, in particular, from the breakdown of purines, is relatively insoluble, especially at low pH, and may precipitate in concentrated urine. Forced diuresis and correction of tissue hypoperfusion or acidosis form an essential part of prevention.

The most rapidly hazardous consequence of TLS is hyperkalaemia, although this can typically be managed medically unless there is concurrent renal impairment. Hyperkalaemia is treated as in any other setting, with diuresis if possible, correction of acidosis, oral or rectal resonium, salbutamol or glucose and insulin infusions. Peritoneal or haemodialysis may be necessary. The patient must be monitored closely with electrocardiography (ECG), and i.v. magnesium sulphate may be given to reduce the risk of dysrhythmia.

Hyperuricaemia is the most common finding in patients with TLS and acute renal failure, and its prevention has proven to be valuable in reducing the incidence of nephropathy. Historically, allopurinol, which inhibits xanthine oxidase, and hence production of urate, has been the drug most commonly used for this. More recently, urate oxidase has proven to be highly successful in patients at high risk of developing TLS. Recent publications have confirmed the safety and efficacy of recombinant urate oxidase, and its superiority to allopurinol in reducing plasma uric acid levels.[21–23] In time, this will undoubtedly become the drug of choice in newly diagnosed high-risk patients.

There is a theoretical risk that the efficacy of urate oxidase will be reduced if given after recent allopurinol: inhibition of xanthine oxidase will cause accumulation of hypoxanthine and xanthine with potential problems from these compounds. Effective inhibition removes the substrate for urate oxidase, and its action is therefore made less significant. If use of urate oxidase is anticipated, it is wise to start it before any dose of allopurinol is administered.

Acute renal failure may develop as a consequence of urate load, or because of deposition of calcium phosphate. Phosphate excretion rises rapidly with tumour breakdown, and the calcium–phosphate solubility product may be exceeded. Deposition of calcium phosphate crystals may occur in the microvasculature and renal tubules when the product of calcium and phosphate concentrations exceeds 60 mg/dL. Hyperphosphataemia is common in patients with non-Hodgkin's lymphoma and reported in virtually all of those with uraemia.

High plasma phosphate concentrations induce hypocalcaemia, which in turn leads to reduced urinary

Chemotherapy regimens

Antiemetics

A Age > 5 years

B Age ≤ 5 years

5 | As below with addition of lorazepam | As below with addition of promethazine + chlorpromazine

High

Carboplatin ▲
Cisplatin ▲
Cyclophosphamide (>1 g/m²) ▲
4
Cytosine (>500 mg/m²) ●
Ifosfamide
TBI

- Consider moving up to next different block if recent antiemetic failure
- Consider moving sideways B→A if borderline age
- If patient suffers from anticipatory nausea and vomiting, consider giving dose of lorazepam the night before chemotherapy

4 Before chemotherapy
* Ondansetron i.v.
and
■ Dexamethasone i.v.
Followed by
* Ondansetron i.v./p.o. 12 hours post
■ Dexamethasone i.v./p.o. 12-hourly ± metoclopramide

4 Before chemotherapy
* Ondansetron i.v.
and
■ Dexamethasone i.v.
Followed by
* Ondansetron i.v./p.o. 12 hours post
■ Dexamethasone i.v./p.o. 12-hourly ± prochlorperazine

Actinomycin D
Adriamycin
Busulphan
Cyclophosphamide (500 mg–1 g/m²) ▲
Cytosine (100–500 mg/m²)
Daunorubicin
Epirubicin
M-AMSA
Methotrexate (>3 g/m²)
Mitoxantrone
Procarbazine 1st dose only

3

* Give ondansetron on day(s) of most emetogenic treatments only
▲ Delayed emesis risk. Give extra dose of ondansetron at 24 hours post
■ Do NOT give dexamethasone if:
1) Chemotherapy includes steroids
2) Brain tumours – during chemotherapy
Discuss with consultant for use in delayed emesis

3 Before chemotherapy
* Ondansetron i.v.
Followed by
* Ondansetron i.v./p.o. 12 hours post ± metoclopramide

3 Before chemotherapy
* Ondansetron i.v.
Followed by
* Ondansetron i.v./p.o. 12 hours post ± prochlorperazine p.o./p.r.

Cyclophosphamide (<500 mg/m²)
Cytosine (<100 mg/m²)
Methotrexate (<3 g/m²)
Procarbazine – 2nd dose onwards
Triple IT
RADIOTHERAPY – Lower chest, abdomen, spine

2

2 Metoclopramide p.o./i.v. PRN

2 Prochlorperazine p.o./p.r. PRN or promethazine i.v. PRN

Asparaginase
Bleomycin
Methotrexate IT
Vinblastine
Vincristine
VP-16

1 Antiemetic failure =
4 hours of nausea
or
2 vomits in a 24-hour period

1 NO MEDICATION

1 NO MEDICATION

Low

ONDANSETRON
i.v. 5 mg/m² (maximum 8 mg)
Dilute in 20–50 mL of normal saline and give over 15 minutes
p.o. ≤ 1.2 m² 4 mg
> 1.2 m² 8 mg

DEXAMETHASONE
Before chemotherapy
8 mg/m² (maximum 8 mg) i.v.
Followed by
8 mg/m²/day i.v./p.o. in divided doses (maximum dose 1.2 mg)
Infuse over 15 minutes in normal saline

LORAZEPAM
p.o. Age ≤ 10 years 0.5 mg
Age >10 years 1 mg
up to t.d.s.
Not recommended <5 years

PROMETHAZINE + CHLORPROMAZINE
i.v. 0.5 mg/kg
may alternate every 2 hours PRN
Dilute in 20 mL normal saline and infuse over 15–20 minutes

METOCLOPRAMIDE
p.o./i.v. 0.5 mg/kg/day in three divided doses
Infuse slowly in normal saline

PROCHLORPERAZINE
p.o./p.r.
750 μg/kg/day in three divided doses

Figure 30.1 *The Royal Hospital for Sick Children, Bristol, Oncology and Haematology Unit: guidelines for use of antiemetics. IT, intrathecal; TBI, total body irradiation.*

phosphate reabsorption. Tubular deposition of calcium phosphate leads to nephrocalcinosis, and this may be made worse by attempts to correct low plasma calcium levels. Hypocalcaemia is rarely symptomatic and correction should not be attempted unless the patient does develop symptoms.

Management

Avoidance of TLS must be the goal for all patients. Recognition of those patients at significant risk – those with large tumour or leukaemia burden, lymphoid malignancy, or already showing metabolic signs of rapid tumour breakdown – must lead to early intervention with hyperhydration, avoidance of any potassium supplementation, diuresis and reduction of serum urate with either allopurinol or urate oxidase.

Despite such measures, TLS will develop in the occasional patient, and further management requires intensive monitoring. Hyperkalaemia is the immediate concern for such patients, and ECG monitoring is essential. Measures to reduce elevated potassium levels need to be taken promptly. Oral or rectal potassium binding resonium may be effective, but is not usually well tolerated in the young, unwell child. Nebulized salbutamol is effective, but usually only in the short term. Glucose and insulin infusions are similarly effective.

In the presence of established acute renal failure, early dialysis or haemofiltration is usually required. The patient must be catheterized, and administered fluids must be reduced to the previous hour's urine output plus insensible losses. The most common indications for dialysis are volume overload and hyperkalaemia not responding to medical management, but uraemia, hyperphosphataemia and symptomatic hypocalcaemia may also be causes. On occasions, the need to administer further chemotherapy may also require dialysis.

BONE MARROW FAILURE

Background

Expert management of bone marrow failure is the cornerstone of successful application of the intensive treatment protocols used in modern paediatric oncology. In the following section we will outline approaches to the treatment of anaemia, leucopenia and thrombocytopenia. In reality, isolated failure of one particular haemopoietic lineage is uncommon and varying degrees of pancytopenia are the rule. Moreover, common principles of management apply:

- Decisions to treat (particularly to transfuse blood products) should be based on symptoms and signs

and not numbers. The speed of development of cytopenia, its expected duration and other risks, such as the presence of mucositis or a residual intracranial mass, should all be taken into account. Failure to respond to therapy should lead to careful reappraisal and consideration of alternative strategies rather than slavish repetition.

- Staff, parents and patients must understand fully the risk of transfusion therapies. A local transfusion protocol should be in place and, in the UK, should conform to the guidelines set out by the British Committee for Standards in Haematology (BCSH).

- Quality assurance with regular audit of outcome is required. This is often overlooked when considering the outcome of clinical trials. In addition, regular training of all staff in the management of transfusions is vital.

- It should be recognized that this is a rapidly changing field and clinicians must be prepared to change their own policies and prejudices, which may have been built up over decades. Examples of recent change are the re-emergence of granulocyte infusions and the development of outpatient approaches to febrile neutropenia.

Transfusion of blood products

BASIC PRINCIPLES

Whilst the transfusion of blood, platelets and plasma is essential to the successful treatment of patients suffering from malignant disease, it is important to minimize the exposure of children to these products when possible. The indication for, and benefit from, their use must be clearly documented each time a patient receives a transfusion. Failure to do so is a serious omission and may lead to litigation.

Personnel who are unfamiliar with haematology and oncology are often confused as to the indications for irradiation, leucodepletion and the use of cytomegalovirus (CMV)-negative products. These are discussed below.

Irradiation

All blood products contain alloreactive lymphocytes and natural killer (NK) cells. Following transfusion these are killed by the immune system of the recipient and cause no clinical problem in immunocompetent patients. If the recipient is significantly immunosuppressed, however, the transfused white cells may engraft in the recipient and cause transfusion-associated graft-versus-host disease (TA-GvHD). TA-GvHD is almost always progressive and rapidly fatal. Irradiation of blood components prevents TA-GvHD and is performed by the Blood Service prior to issue. The indications for the use of irradiated blood products are shown in Table 30.1.

Table 30.1 *Specification of red cells and platelets for non-bone marrow transplant (BMT) patients (all products are leucodepleted at source)*

	Irradiation	CMV negative[b]
Suspected or known immunodeficiency (including Di-George)	Y	Y
Solid tumours		
High-dose therapy[a]	Y	N
Hodgkin's disease	Y	N
Fludarabine	Y	N
Other solid tumours	N	N
Aplastic anaemia	Y	N
Acute and chronic leukaemias		
ALL MRC 99/R2	N	N
AML XII	N	N
Fludarabine (FLAG)	Y	N
Hydroxyurea/anagrelide	N	N
Allogeneic blood transfused at the time of bone marrow/PBSC harvest	Y	N
HLA-matched platelets	Y	N
Post-BMT patients	Y	N
Granulocyte transfusions	Y	Y

CMV, cytomegalovirus; PBSC, peripheral blood stem cell.
[a] High-dose therapy is currently defined as any procedure requiring stem cell rescue. Irradiation should commence at the start of conditioning for allo-BMT and auto-BMT/PBSC patients and at the start of primary therapy prior to stem cell collection for autologous PBSC patients.
[b] All children under 1 year of age, regardless of diagnosis, should receive CMV-negative products.

It is also important to note that:

- all HLA-matched products should be irradiated regardless of recipient immune status
- all granulocyte transfusions should be irradiated, regardless of recipient immunity
- fresh frozen plasma (FFP) and cryoprecipitate do contain white cells but these are destroyed in the process of freeze and thaw and irradiation is therefore not required
- leucodepletion does **not** prevent TA-GvHD and must **not** be used as a substitute for irradiation.

It is our own practice to state that the requirement for irradiated blood products is lifelong, i.e. once a child is designated to receive irradiated blood, unirradiated blood products should never again be administered.

Leucodepletion (leucocyte depletion)
Transfused white cells may transmit infection, in particular CMV. This may lead to primary CMV disease in a seronegative recipient. An equal concern is that a patient infected with CMV by transfusion may then subsequently reactivate virus during a stem cell transplant (SCT). Reduction of the dose of transfused white cells to less than 5×10^6/L using a white cell filter has been shown to prevent transmission of CMV to the recipient. In order to achieve adequate quality control, leucodepletion is performed by the Blood Service prior to issue of the product. A further advantage of leucodepletion is the reduction in the generation of anti-white cell and antiplatelet antibodies. White cell antibodies can lead to transfusion reactions and also increase the likelihood of rejection of an allogeneic SCT. Antiplatelet antibodies are associated with refractoriness to platelet transfusion and an increased risk of bleeding. In 1998 the UK government recommended universal leucodepletion of blood products in response to concerns over transmission of variant Creutzfeld–Jakob disease (vCJD). For this reason, all red cells, platelets and FFP are now leucodepleted. Leucodepletion does not prevent TA-GvHD and must not be used as a substitute for irradiation.

CMV-negative blood products
In most children there is good evidence that leucodepletion prevents the transmission of CMV by transfusion. However, there are still only minimal data on the use of leucodepletion alone in infants and for this reason it is still recommended that all children under 1 year receive leucodepleted blood products from CMV-negative donors. Leucodepletion of granulocyte transfusions is clearly inappropriate and for this reason all granulocytes should be obtained from CMV-negative donors.

TRANSFUSION REACTIONS

An acute transfusion reaction should be suspected if the patient has a sudden rise in temperature of more than 1°C, develops a rash or a rigor, or becomes unwell in any way. A reaction may occur after the transfusion has finished or may be caused by a previous unit.

Major reactions which require immediate action
Acute intravascular haemolysis (IVH) is mostly caused by the transfusion of ABO-incompatible blood and often occurs during transfusion of the first few millilitres of blood. Infective shock is caused by bacterial contamination of the blood product, commonly with *Pseudomonas*, *Yersinia* or *Staphylococcus*. In the acute situation, both IVH and infective shock lead to circulatory collapse, disseminated intravascular coagulation (DIC) and acute renal failure. It is often not possible to differentiate between intravascular haemolysis and infective shock in the acute situation and either diagnosis should be suspected if one or more of the following are present:

- shortness of breath/hypoxia/chest pain
- back pain, flank or loin tenderness

- hypotension or poor perfusion
- haemoglobinuria.

Treatment involves immediate disconnection of the blood and institution of a crystalloid infusion to ensure volume expansion. All documentation relating to the transfusion should be checked and a senior medical laboratory scientific officer in the transfusion laboratory contacted. Further treatment includes standard management of renal failure and DIC and prompt administration of broad-spectrum antibiotics.

Anaphylaxis, characterized by bronchospasm, oedema and circulatory collapse, is rare and should lead to suspicion of IgA deficiency. If this is proven, further transfusion can normally be achieved with washed red cells and platelets and plasma from IgA-deficient donors. Transfusion-related acute lung injury is an acute pulmonary insult caused by transfusion of plasma containing antibodies. Although rare, it can easily be confused with pulmonary oedema through volume overload. Treatment involves cessation of transfusion and treatment as for adult respiratory distress syndrome.

Minor reactions where it may be possible to continue transfusion

Urticarial reaction occurs in 1–2 per cent of transfusions and is mediated by antibodies in the patient to infused plasma proteins or the infusion of allergens that bind to IgE antibodies in the patient. It is more likely to occur after transfusion of platelets or plasma. Treatment involves temporary discontinuation of transfusion and administration of an antihistamine.

Febrile non-haemolytic transfusion reactions may be due either to antileucocyte antibodies in the patient's serum, which react with white cells or platelets present in the transfusion, or to cytokines/interleukins that are released from white cells into red cells and platelets during storage. This is the commonest type of transfusion reaction and is especially frequent in multi-transfused patients. It is characterized by a sudden rise in temperature (>1°C), often with rigors, but in the absence of features suggestive of a major reaction (see above). Treatment involves temporary discontinuation of transfusion and administration of an antipyretic.

ANAEMIA

Anaemia, defined as the presence of a blood haemoglobin below the normal range for the patient's age, is very common in children receiving chemotherapy (possible causes are summarized in Box 30.1). By contrast, symptomatic anaemia is much less frequent. This reflects the fact that in most cases the low haemoglobin results from

---

Box 30.1 *Causes of anaemia in oncology patients*

Reduced production
- Anaemia of chronic disease
- Iron deficiency
- Folate deficiency
- Red cell aplasia (parvovirus infection)
- Chemotherapy
- Marrow infiltration
- Myelofibrosis

Post-transplant
- Graft failure (rejection, GvHD)
- Erythrophagocytosis

Haemolysis
Immune-mediated
- Transfusion related
  - intravascular (ABO)
  - extravascular (anti-Kidd, D, Kell or Duffy)
  - delayed (anti-Kidd, D, Kell or Duffy)
- Cold agglutinins (mycoplasma infection)
- Warm agglutinins (Hodgkin's disease)

Non-immune-mediated
- Sepsis
- Disseminated intravascular coagulation
- Thrombotic thrombocytopenic purpura
- Haemolytic-uraemic syndrome (post-BMT)
- Pre-existing abnormality
  - glucose-6-phosphatase (X-linked)
  - pyruvate kinase deficiency (autosomal recessive)
  - sickle cell disease, hereditary spherocytosis

Dilutional

Haemorrhage

---

reduced red cell production rather than rapid blood loss or haemolysis; the onset is slow. The life span of red cells in health is 120 days, and thus in pure red cell aplasia the haemoglobin will fall by 1 g/dL per week. Indeed, the marrow is often capable of some reticulocyte production in spite of chemotherapy. This is exemplified by consideration of children receiving maintenance therapy for ALL who are often anaemic but rarely symptomatic. It is important to note that chemotherapy-induced hypoplasia can be exacerbated by underlying congenital red cell disorders, haematinic deficiency, chronic blood loss and infection with parvovirus B19. The development of unexpectedly profound anaemia in a child receiving a low-intensity protocol should, therefore, prompt investigation.

Anaemia associated with rapid haemolysis or bleeding may be life-threatening and requires urgent diagnosis and management. Haemolysis may be immune (secondary to drugs, disease or infection) or mechanical [DIC, thrombotic thrombocytopenic purpura/haemolytic-uraemic syndrome (TTP/HUS) or haemangioma]. Acute blood loss is usually evident clinically and appropriate blood replacement is made. Occasionally, an acute bleed may remain occult (intracerebral, retroperitoneal).

In many cases, children with leukaemia are severely anaemic at diagnosis. Transfusion may be indicated for relief of symptoms. Moreover, many diagnostic procedures are undertaken under anaesthetic and there is often a perceived need to raise the haemoglobin prior to such procedures. If the presenting white cell count is high, particularly in AML where the blasts are large, there is a risk that transfusion may lead to an increase in whole blood viscosity and cerebral or pulmonary vascular compromise. In such cases, it is not appropriate to transfuse simply to facilitate anaesthesia.

Treatment

TRANSFUSION OF ALLOGENEIC RED CELLS

Products available for transfusion

In the UK, red cells are supplied as red cell concentrates suspended in optimal additive solution (OAS). The haematocrit of this product is usually around 65 per cent. This product has a shelf-life of up to 42 days if unirradiated. This long shelf-life has meant that it has been possible to subdivide units into small 'paedipacks' which may limit donor exposure in infants and neonates. It is no longer possible to obtain whole blood and, in rare cases where this is required (exchange transfusion and priming of cell separators in small children), coadministration of FFP or albumin is recommended.

When to transfuse

The introduction to the recent BCSH *Guidelines for the Clinical Use of Red Cell Transfusion* stated that there is no consensus as to the precise indications for red cell use. This is certainly true in paediatric oncology. Nevertheless, the guidelines provide a sound basis for clinical practice. In each case, it is important to recognize the inherent danger and expense of transfusion. The cause of anaemia should be defined and transfusions only administered where no effective alternatives exist (e.g. iron deficiency should be treated with iron, not allogeneic red cells). Moreover, it is important to recognize that there is no universal transfusion trigger (usually 7–8 g/dL) and assessment by an experienced clinician is the optimal approach. In acute blood loss, the effects of anaemia should be differentiated from those of hypovolaemia; crystalloid may be very effective treatment for loss of up to 30 per cent blood volume.

On the basis of the above, we believe the following are clear indications for red cell transfusion:

- symptomatic anaemia as determined by an experienced clinician
- a rapid and anticipated continuing fall in haemoglobin (e.g. associated with documented infection, consumptive coagulopathy)
- anaemia developing during intensive chemotherapy, where recovery will be delayed for many weeks
- anaemia developing before planned radiotherapy: optimal delivery of oxygen to involved fields is needed in order for the generation of free radicals, and it is common practice to ensure a haemoglobin above 10 g/dL.

ERYTHROPOIETIN

Recombinant human erythropoietin (rhEPO) has been shown to lead to a sustained increase in haemoglobin in adult patients receiving treatment for a wide variety of malignancies. Experience in children with cancer is limited, but the drug is widely used in paediatric nephrology and appears to be safe. A small number of case reports of the successful use of EPO in children who decline transfusion for religious reasons have been published and this should certainly be considered in such patients. It seems likely that concerns over the risk of allogeneic transfusion will drive an increased interest in the use of EPO in oncology.

AUTOLOGOUS TRANSFUSION AND INTRAOPERATIVE RED CELL SALVAGE

As with EPO, widespread use of these procedures has largely been restricted to adult medicine. We have personal experience of the use of acute isovolaemic dilution in children without malignancy weighing as little as 20 kg after EPO priming. Whilst this is unlikely to be appropriate in children who have already received very intensive chemotherapy there may be a role for those with less aggressive tumours.

THROMBOCYTOPENIA

As with anaemia, thrombocytopenia most commonly reflects suppression of marrow production by chemotherapy. In health, a platelet has a mean life span of approximately 8–11 days,[25] i.e. 10 per cent of the total platelet mass must be replaced each day. Thrombocytopenia therefore appears more rapidly than anaemia. In general, the degree of thrombocytopenia induced by a given protocol parallels the degree of anaemia and leucopenia, although for some agents, such as carboplatin, temozolamide and other alkylating agents, there may be a disproportionate and prolonged reduction in platelet production.

Box 30.2 *Causes of thrombocytopenia in cancer patients*

Reduced production
- Chemotherapy (esp. carboplatin)
- Infiltration
- Myelofibrosis

Post-transplant
- Graft failure (rejection, GvHD)
- Viral infection (CMV, HIV)

Increased consumption
Immune-mediated
- Drug related (co-trimoxazole, rifampicin, heparin, valproate)
- Hodgkin's disease (IgG)
- Anti-HLA antibodies
- Antiplatelet antibodies
- HIV infection

Non-immune
- Heparin
- Sepsis
- Disseminated intravascular coagulation

Post-transplant
- Thrombotic thrombocytopenic purpura
- Haemolytic-uraemic syndrome (post-BMT)

Sequestration
- Hypersplenism

Dilution
- Massive transfusion

Artefact
- Heparinized sample
- Clot

Thrombocytopenia may also arise as a result of other processes, and these must also be considered. The most common are sequestration in an enlarged spleen, consumption due to DIC or coadministration of amphotericin B and immunological destruction, including that induced by heparin (see Box 30.2).

Transfusion of allogeneic platelets

PRODUCTS AVAILABLE FOR TRANSFUSION

Traditionally, therapeutic doses of platelets were obtained by combining material from up to six separate donors. The last decade has seen a switch away from pooling to the use of single donor collections obtained by apheresis.

This limits donor exposure and also allows in-line leucodepletion. In the UK, platelets are currently supplied in two forms:

- an adult therapeutic dose equivalent (ATD) contains approximately 3.0×10^{11} platelets per pack in a volume of 150–350 mL
- a paediatric platelet product is a quarter of an ATD, and contains approximately 0.75×10^{11} platelets in a volume of 35–75 mL

WHEN TO TRANSFUSE

The major complication of thrombocytopenia is bleeding. Assessment of the risk of bleeding must take account of both platelet function and number. The former is impaired by uraemia, drugs and fever. The decision to transfuse a child with significant mucosal, retinal or internal bleeding is straightforward. It is important to note that platelets are generally ineffective in idiopathic thrombocytopenic purpura (ITP) and are relatively contraindicated in TTP or type II heparin-induced thrombocytopenia.

Most physicians agree that transfusion of an asymptomatic child to a platelet count of at least 50 is appropriate prior to invasive procedures such as insertion of central venous catheters and lumbar punctures. In the UK, prophylactic transfusion prior to the administration of intramuscular L-asparaginase is not recommended.

In contrast with the treatment of anaemia, most oncologists agree that there is a threshold for prophylactic administration of platelets in the absence of active bleeding. The 1987 Consensus Conference agreed that this was 20×10^9/L. More recently, studies in adult patients have concluded that this threshold may be lowered to 10×10^9/L, and this figure is applied in many paediatric units. Indeed, there is evidence that the risk of spontaneous intracranial haemorrhage is very low until the platelet count is less than 5×10^9/L in patients with no evidence of significant cutaneous mucosal or retinal bleeding.

ASSESSING EFFICACY – REFRACTORINESS TO PLATELET TRANSFUSION

Two measures are used to assess the efficacy of platelet transfusion. The most important is a clinical determination of whether bleeding has been controlled or prevented. A second measure is the effect on the platelet count. Whilst a number of relatively complex formulae exist for calculation of the platelet increment, a simple rule of thumb is that after a dose of 10 mL/kg of platelets one would expect that the platelet count would rise by 10–20×10^9/L 24 hours later.

Failure to achieve an increment at 24 hours or sooner in the persistently symptomatic child should alert the clinician to the fact that the child may be refractory to platelets. An increment at 1 and 24 hours should then be obtained after the next transfusion. Two broad mechanisms are responsible for refractoriness to platelet transfusion. Most common are non-immune causes such as splenomegaly, DIC, fever, sepsis and amphotericin B therapy. In some of these cases, administration of double or treble doses may generate an adequate increment. A less common but important mechanism is the development of alloantibodies in the recipient. These are usually HLA antibodies, and the transfusion of irradiated HLA-matched platelets can overcome the problem.

In general, patients with non-immune refractoriness show a more rapid fall in platelets after transfusion, but this crude method of assessment is not very specific. Therefore, we recommend that all children refractory to platelets should be discussed with the transfusion service. HLA matching should be performed early in treatment in order to allow rapid provision of HLA-matched platelets when required.

NEUTROPENIA

Background

Neutropenia may be strictly defined as an absolute neutrophil count of less than 1.5×10^9/L, although in practice a count of 1×10^9/L in a patient who has recently received chemotherapy is generally taken as the threshold. The neutropenic patient is susceptible to bacterial and fungal infection. The risk of infection is a function of the depth and duration of neutropenia as well as the integrity of mechanical barriers such as the skin and gut mucosa. Most studies indicate a relatively limited increased risk of infection until the neutrophil count falls below 0.5×10^9/L.

Management

PROPHYLACTIC ANTIBIOTICS AND ANTIFUNGALS

Neutropenia does not in itself require treatment, and where marrow recovery is anticipated in the near future, none would usually be given. The appropriate use of therapeutic antibiotics giving broad cover of both Gram-negative and Gram-positive organisms has contributed greatly to the marked fall in mortality due to infection over the past 20 years. In general oncology, the widespread use of prophylactic antimicrobials is to be discouraged as there is no proof of efficacy and genuine concern over the emergence of resistant organisms. By contrast, prophylactic antibiotics and, in particular, antifungals are justified after allogeneic BMT.

ADMINISTRATION OF GRANULOCYTE COLONY–STIMULATING FACTOR

Normal granulocyte development proceeds over a period of 6–10 days. A neutrophil remains in the peripheral circulation for a mean of 7 hours. Both maturation and margination of neutrophils are under the control of granulocyte-colony stimulating factor (G-CSF). Therapeutic use of G-CSF, particularly in non-myeloid malignancy, has been shown to shorten the time to recovery of neutrophil count after BMT. However, this was not associated with a reduction of in-patient stay. The value of G-CSF in patients receiving conventional chemotherapy is still unclear: whereas the use of G-CSF has been shown to shorten the duration of neutropenia, and improve adherence to chemotherapy schedules, there are no data about effect on outcome. Routine use of G-CSF is therefore not widely recommended.

In contrast, G-CSF is often used in patients in whom maximal antibiotic and antifungal therapy has failed to control infection. Although there is anecdotal evidence that administration of G-CSF in such patients may be effective, ethical considerations are such that proof of efficacy in controlled trials is impossible.

Perhaps the least controversial role of G-CSF is to mobilize stem cells. Peripheral blood stem cell (PBSC) harvesting performed with count recovery following a myelosuppressive course of chemotherapy, augmented by G-CSF, generally allows collection of sufficient stem cells to repopulate the bone marrow on two or more occasions, and dose escalation well beyond normal maximum tolerated doses is possible. The profound neutropenic phase following high-dose therapy may be (largely) eliminated, and bone marrow reconstitution following PBSC reinfusion is more rapid than following autologous BMT.

GRANULOCYTE TRANSFUSIONS

In the 1980s, there was a vogue for the widespread use of transfusion of allogeneic granulocytes derived from donor whole blood or buffy coat. Evidence that such transfusions were of value in the treatment or prophylaxis of infection was scant, and there were reports of pulmonary toxicity of white cells particularly when coadministered with amphotericin. Granulocyte transfusion was therefore abandoned by most physicians.

Interest in granulocyte transfusion has been rekindled by the discovery that apheresis of a healthy donor who has received a single dose of steroid and G-CSF can safely yield therapeutically effective doses of white cells. This approach is increasingly used in high-risk BMT patients and is likely to become more as the intensity of general oncology protocols increases. It is interesting to note that significant pulmonary toxicity of G-CSF-mobilized white cells has not been reported. This may reflect testing of recipients for antineutrophil antibodies as well as more considered use of amphotericin products.

DISORDERS OF COAGULATION

Normal coagulation

Damage to the endothelium of a blood vessel leads to a series of reactions, the final effect of which is to achieve haemostasis. The normal endothelium synthesizes prostacyclin (PGI_2) and von Willebrand factor. PGI_2 is a potent vasodilator, and damage leads to a loss of this production. This, in association with generation of other vasoactive hormones (vasoactive amines, 5HT, thromboxane A_2) associated with platelet activation, leads to local vasoconstriction. Systemic effects (sympathetic innervation, catecholamine release) potentiate this effect. von Willebrand factor adsorbs to exposed collagen and binds to the platelet glycoprotein membrane receptor, GP1b, allowing platelet adhesion.

Platelet adhesion leads to a change of shape from disc to rounded, with extension of pseudopods and release of ADP and 5HT (activation), leading to aggregation. In addition, granules release fibrinogen, which binds to platelet glycoprotein receptors IIb and IIIa, and potentiates aggregation. This loose primary platelet plug is held together by strands of cross-linked fibrin, which is in turn generated by the action of thrombin on fibrinogen. Thrombin is generated by activation of the clotting cascade. It is now known that this occurs primarily through direct activation of factor VII by 'tissue factor'. Amplification of the process is provided by factors VIII, IX and XI.

Abnormalities of coagulation

It is important to remember that children with malignant disease may also have an underlying congenital bleeding diathesis. For many patients, diagnosis and treatment of cancer represent their first major haemostatic challenge. Nevertheless, acquired coagulopathy is more common and causes are listed in Box 30.3.

DIC is characterized by inappropriate and excessive activation of coagulation, which may be acute or chronic. The patient usually has evidence of frank bleeding, although in chronic DIC, thromboembolic complications may occur. There is evidence of consumption of cellular blood products (haemolysis, thrombocytopenia), and of coagulation factors [prolonged thrombin clotting time (TCT), prothrombin time (PT), partial thromboplastin time (PTT)]. An underlying cause is always present and should be sought. In patients with

Box 30.3 *Causes of acquired coagulopathy*

Disseminated intravascular coagulation
- Infection
  - bacterial (Gram-negative sepsis, clostridia)
  - fungal
  - viral [CMV, varicella (purpura fulminans)]
  - parasitic (falciparum malaria)
  - rickettsial
- Malignant disease (leukaemia, metastatic solid tumours)
- Hepatic failure (actinomycin D)
- Incompatible transfusion
- Anaphylaxis
- Widespread tissue damage
  - haemorrhagic shock
  - trauma (surgery)
  - hypothermia
- Giant haemangioma (Kasabach–Merritt)

Liver disease

Vitamin K deficiency
- Malabsorption
- Vitamin K antagonists
- Biliary obstruction
- Bowel sterilization with reduced intake

Heparin therapy

Haemolytic–uraemic syndrome

L-asparaginase

Massive transfusion

Inhibitors of coagulation
- Factor VIII
- Lupus anticoagulant

Acquired deficiency of von Willebrand factor

---

bacterial sepsis in particular, DIC may be one of many coexistent problems associated with life-threatening illness. Diagnosis is made on the basis of a low platelet count, reduced fibrinogen, elevated levels of fibrinogen degradation products (commonly termed D-dimer, FDP or XDP) and prolongation of the TCT. In chronic DIC, increased synthesis of coagulation factors may compensate for increased utilization, and there may be no abnormality of PT or PTT. Nevertheless, DIC is associated with inappropriate consumption of coagulation factors, and this is not excluded by a single normal investigation.

DIC is commonly associated with myeloid leukaemia, in particular AML M3 and M5. In most cases, treatment of DIC is supportive with treatment of the underlying cause. In M3 AML the use of all-*trans*-retinoic acid (ATRA) as a differentiating agent has helped to reduce the numbers of patients who die because of DIC.

Management of coagulopathy

Coagulation factors should be replaced using FFP. It is important to note that FFP contains relatively little fibrinogen and the addition of cryoprecipitate may be of value in cases of aggressive fibrinogenolysis. Heparin is now rarely used in DIC.

Coagulopathy associated with asparaginase therapy is well documented, and may present with haemorrhagic or thromboembolic complications. Asparaginase causes reduced protein synthesis and, in particular, leads to low levels of factors IX, XI and fibrinogen, and of antithrombin III and plasminogen. In a series of 18 children treated for ALL who developed coagulopathy, five presented with cerebral infarction, four with haemorrhagic infarcts, five with cerebral haemorrhage and a further five had deep venous thrombosis.[26] The majority of patients presented between days 13 and 24 of treatment. Thrombosis associated with the central venous catheters is a particular concern during induction of ALL with asparginase and steroids.

The activity of factors II, VII, IX and X is dependent on post-translational gamma carboxylation. This reaction takes place in the liver and is dependent on vitamin K1 absorbed from the gut. Vitamin K deficiency may arise secondary to malnutrition or malabsorption. Liver disease may develop as a result of infection secondary to transfusion, or following chemotherapy. Acute severe derangement of liver function is described with actinomycin D therapy,[27] and an incidence of 3 per cent in patients with Wilms' tumour was reported in the UKW1 trial.[28] Although severe, the prognosis in these patients with appropriate care was very good, and no further hepatic impairment was seen when the patients were subsequently re-challenged. Administration in divided doses is common practice, although the incidence of hepatotoxicity appears to be dose-dependent.

Clinically significant acquired inhibitors of coagulation are uncommon in children. However, the association between Wilms' tumour and acquired von Willebrand's disease should always be considered prior to surgery.

INFECTION

Infection in the immunocompromised host presents a tremendous challenge in cancer care in terms of clinical assessment and treatment in a potentially life-threatening situation. The financial costs to our health services are enormous, particularly with the use of newer antibiotics and antifungals. It is important, therefore, that centres delivering this care should have protocols of investigation and management that are appropriate to that centre whilst ensuring a safe outcome for the patient.

The emphasis on an individual centre approach is important as patterns of infection and antibiotic resistance vary considerably. For example, the incidence of vancomycin-resistant enterococci (VRE) and methicillin-resistant *Staphylococcus aureus* (MRSA) may be totally different in units within the same geographical location.

Host defences are breached by a number of insults, including:

- the underlying disease, which may lead to neutropenia and immunodeficiency
- therapy, which in addition to the underlying disease may cause mucositis
- breaks in the integument, particularly by central venous catheters.

Bacterial infections

Neutropenia is the major factor for most patients and events. Bacteraemia in the neutropenic patient had a mortality of over 80 per cent before the use of empirical antibiotics,[29] with the frequency and severity of infection being universally correlated with the degree of neutropenia, the incidence of infection being greater (30–60 per cent) when the neutrophil count was as low as 0.1×10^9/L. It must be emphasized that life-threatening infection can occur when the patient has more than 1×10^9/L neutrophils, emphasizing the need for vigilance and careful clinical assessment.

Empirical broad-spectrum antibiotic therapy in patients with fever and neutropenia has reduced morbidity and mortality dramatically. This was first shown by Schimpff et al.[30] and confirmed by many later studies.[31] Before considering appropriate antibiotic regimens, it is important to review the changing pattern of pathogens seen over the past decades. In the early years, Gram-negative organisms predominated, particularly *Pseudomonas aeruginosa*. The use of empirical antibiotics, therefore, mandated the use of agents effective against these organisms.

The commonest Gram-positive organism was *Staphylococcus aureus*, but this was to change during the 1980s, with *S. epidermidis* becoming more frequent. More recently we have seen the advent of other Gram-positive organisms, particularly *Streptococcus viridans*.

The reasons for these changes are complex, but include the widespread use of indwelling central venous catheters and prophylactic antibiotics. The use of more intensive chemoradiotherapy has led to severe mucositis, accounting for the increase in viridans streptococci from the mouth and enterococci from the gut. The latter is particularly worrying with the development of vancomycin resistance. Bacteraemia in such patients has a high mortality rate.

The choice of empirical antibiotics is a difficult one. As stated above, it is dependent on centre experience of incidence of specific infection and patterns of resistance. During the 1970s, it was vital to provide anti-*Pseudomonas* cover, usually with a combination of an aminoglycoside and an appropriate penicillin. This approach is still valid today as, although infections with Gram-positive cocci are now more frequent, clinical deterioration (with the exception of streptococci and enterococci) is less acute than with Gram-negative organisms and there may be a rationale for awaiting results of culture.

During the 1980s and 1990s, third-generation cephalosporins and carbapenems were developed. These drugs are not only effective against Gram-negative bacilli but also have some potency against Gram-positive cocci. The concept of monotherapy was thus developed. This is still not accepted widely, despite being in the guidelines for the Infectious Disease Society of America. This may be due to the experience of clinicians who found that combination therapy improved the outcomes for patients with *Pseudomonas aeruginosa*.

Recently, new strategies of treatment have been developed based on risk assessment.[32] These risk groups have been defined in adults and it may be possible to evaluate them in the paediatric setting. Defining a patient as low risk (which may very well be the majority) would allow a more rational approach to empirical therapy. Monotherapy with drugs such as meropenem, imipenem or one of the latest generation of antibiotics may be more acceptable. For low-risk patients it may even be appropriate to consider oral therapy as an outpatient.[33]

Gram-positive organisms are now the commonest causes of bacteraemia. It could be argued that vancomycin or teicoplanin should be used in front-line empirical therapy. The consensus, however, is that this should only be the case in centres with a high incidence of *Streptococcus viridans* or where the patient is colonized with MRSA. Vancomycin and teicoplanin would therefore be reserved for resistant fever or positive cultures of sensitive organisms. One important reason for this in the case of vancomycin is the risk of renal impairment, particularly in a patient who has been exposed to multiple renal toxins.

There are two further complications in the management of febrile neutropenia, both dependent on the centre's 'microbiological soup' and the degree of risk for the individual patient. Firstly, what to do when a patient's fever has not responded to first-line empirical therapy and is culture-negative. Most centres will have a protocol for changing antibiotics which will include greater Gram-positive cover, but it should also be remembered that it is important to re-examine and re-culture the patient. It may be appropriate for X-ray and computed tomography (CT) examination to be performed. If there is no response after a further 48 hours, then, in patients at high risk, an antifungal should be prescribed.

The second complication is to decide how long patients whose temperature responds should be treated. The majority of patients are culture-negative and there are several potential avenues of treatment: continue antibiotics until the neutrophil count reaches 0.5×10^9/L and then stop; continue a full course (7–10 days); or stop and use an appropriate oral antibiotic. The decision, again, should be made on the risk status of the patient, i.e. supposed length of neutropenia and intensity of preceding chemotherapy.

If the cultures are positive then the appropriate antibiotic should be continued for 10–14 days, unless there is a deep-seated staphylococcal infection, in which case it should be longer.

Pneumonitis

The most important cause of interstitial pneumonitis in patients undergoing treatment for ALL was *Pneumocystis carinii* until the use of prophylactic co-trimoxazole. This is still the case in those who fail to take their medication (usually given on 2 days a week) or in whom it has been discontinued because of its bone marrow-suppressive effect. In the latter scenario, its replacement with inhaled pentamidine or oral dapsone should be considered.

With the prevention of *Pneumocystis carinii* pneumonitis, community-acquired infections have become the predominant cause of interstitial pneumonitis. *Mycoplasma pneumoniae*, respiratory syncytial virus and other organisms are now more common. Bronchoalveolar lavage, to confirm the diagnosis and allow appropriate therapy to be instituted, should be considered.

Viral infections

The normal child has at least four viral infections a year and we can therefore suppose that the child with cancer will have at least as many. Episodes of fever and neutropenia may have a viral aetiology. The importance of viral infections as pathogens depends on the degree of immunosuppression (i.e. treatment of stage I Wilms' tumour compared with haploidentical SCT) as well as the individual virus.

Recent controversies over immunization for mumps, measles and rubella (MMR) means that there is now an increasing risk of measles infection, which has a high morbidity with pneumonitis. The only action that can be taken when a susceptible patient comes into contact with an infected child is the use of immunoglobulin and the halting of chemotherapy, although how effective this will be in preventing giant cell pneumonia or later encephalitis is debatable.

Varicella zoster is a common viral infection in the community. Before the availability of acyclovir, the high morbidity rate was due to lung, liver and central nervous system (CNS) infection. The role of a varicella vaccine still remains controversial both for community use and for those at greatest risk (children with ALL). Immuno-suppressed patients who come into contact with varicella can be managed by passive immunization with zoster immunoglobulin, which needs to be given within 72 hours of contact. Many physicians would now choose to use acyclovir to prevent development of disease. This drug has a vital role in the management of proven zoster in the immunosuppressed child.

The greatest risk from viruses is within the setting of allogeneic SCT. This is particularly so with the increasing use of donors other than matched siblings, where immunosuppression is even greater and immune reconstitution takes much longer. Recently, there have been great advances made in detection, prevention and treatment of the important pathogens.

The use of prophylactic acyclovir is not only effective for herpes simplex (although, increasingly, resistance is occurring) and varicella zoster, but when used in high dose it is effective in preventing and delaying CMV disease. The latter has been a major cause of morbidity in allogeneic SCT, particularly in adults where donor and recipient are more likely to be positive. The increasing use of unrelated and adult haploidentical donors means that more paediatric patients are at risk. Strategies have therefore been developed to prevent CMV infection: firstly, the use of high-dose acyclovir as prophylaxis[34] and subsequently the advent of polymerase chain reaction (PCR) detection to enable very early diagnosis. Infection can then be treated with ganciclovir, preventing development of disease. The latter can be used as prophylaxis but unfortunately is associated with cytopenias. Death from CMV is now rare but risks from neutropenia due to ganciclovir cannot be underestimated.

The partial victory over CMV has seen the importance of other viruses increase, particularly adenovirus and respiratory syncitial virus. The latter is common in the community and all measures should be taken to prevent its occurrence on a SCT unit. Epidemics also happen and have a mortality of up to 10 per cent from pneumonia. The use of inhaled and/or intravenous ribavirin is controversial.

Recently, serious adenovirus infections have become a concern for the most susceptible patients. The disease often presents with gastroenteritis but may lead to pneumonitis and rapidly fatal hepatitis. Attempts at early detection by PCR in blood may offer an opportunity for therapy with cidofovir, although its effectiveness is yet to be proven.

Immunosuppressed patients cannot remain cocooned but precautions and prophylaxis against viruses should be considered for each individual.

Fungal infections

The incidence of fungal infections has increased for many reasons, including more intensive therapy and prolonged neutropenia (AML therapy and SCT), prolonged broad-spectrum antibiotic use, mucositis, corticosteroids and indwelling catheters (particularly leading to candidiasis). The most common infections are due to *Candida* species and invasive aspergillosis, although there are increasing reports of other organisms such as *Fusarium* species.

The most common presentation of candidal infection involves the gastrointestinal tract with oral, oesophageal and perineal thrush. Many patients are at risk but particularly those on induction therapy for ALL. Prophylaxis with nystatin and the use of fluconazole as either prophylaxis or treatment are effective in most patients, with the commonest species being *C. albicans*; others, *C. tropicalis*, *C. glabrata* and *C. krusei*, are also important pathogens and may have resistance to the favoured antifungals.

Invasive candidiasis leading to visceral involvement is a life-threatening complication. The CNS, liver and spleen, eye and lung are all important sites, but diagnosis may be difficult and is dependent on positive blood cultures and, in hepatosplenic infections, a classical appearance on computed tomography screening. Treatment involves prolonged courses with amphotericin B.

Invasive aspergillosis is perhaps the most difficult infection to diagnose as well as to treat. Serological and molecular testing are disappointing and radiological appearances typical of aspergillosis occur late in the course of the disease. CT signs and biopsy remain the gold standard for diagnosis.

The commonest organism seen is *A. fumigatus*, but *A. flavus* and *A. niger* also occur. Spores of these species occur naturally in the environment but are particularly common when building work is taking place. Attempts at prophylaxis in the most seriously at-risk patients (prolonged neutropenia and SCT) may be beneficial and many units have a policy of using low-dose amphotericin or itraconazole. Whether this will decrease the morbidity is yet to be seen.

Most patients with aspergillosis present with continuing fever despite the use of broad-spectrum antibiotics. Empirical use of amphotericin with the assumption of fungal infection has decreased the incidence of *Candida* and probably *Aspergillus*. Unfortunately, amphotericin is a toxic compound in terms of both acute toxicity with infusion and also longer-term problems with renal tubular damage. The likelihood of cure in many children with cancer means that, in order to prevent late effects on the kidney, lipid amphotericin products are used. These are tremendously costly but much better tolerated.[35]

Documented invasive aspergillosis has a very high mortality of around 80 per cent. The cornerstone of treatment remains amphotericin B, perhaps with the use of granulocyte/monocyte-colony stimulating factor (GM-CSF; to mobilize monocytes) and surgery in discrete pulmonary lesions. New compounds are being developed and trials are underway comparing them with lipid formulations of amphotericin. At present, the most interesting drugs are in the classes of triazoles and echinocandins. The triazoles, voriconazole and posaconazole, are derivations of fluconazole and itraconazole, respectively, and have good broad-spectrum antifungal activity. They appear to have low toxicity and, in a study by Walsh et al.,[36] compared favourably with liposomal amphotericin.

The echinocandins belong to a new class of antifungal medication and act on the fungal cell wall. Caspofungin is well tolerated and trials are taking place comparing this to amphotericin B.

The future should provide us with effective prophylaxis and treatment of invasive aspergillosis, perhaps with the newer drugs in combination where the sites of action are different and not in competition. At present, the costs in terms of morbidity and mortality of fungal infection as well as the financial implications of its prevention and treatment remain high.

NUTRITIONAL SUPPORT

Background

Poor nutrition, or rather the inability to maintain nutritional status, in children with cancer is common and relates to the malignant disease, acute and long-term effects of therapy, poor oral intake and intercurrent complications such as infection. It is a major cause of morbidity and mortality, leading to progressive wasting, weakness and debilitation. Compromised immune function, potential therapy intolerance and, ultimately, death may result.

Dietary intake may present a significant psychological problem for children and their carers. For many children, food refusal may represent the only way available to them to exercise control over their body. This may be made worse by learned patterns of behaviour because of previous experience of nausea or vomiting, and it may prove difficult to break a cycle of gradual starvation.

Protein-calorie malnutrition exists when the intake of macronutrients is inadequate to meet metabolic requirements. The incidence of protein energy malnutrition (PEM) is reported to be between 6 and 50 per cent, and is more common and more severe in patients with extensive, progressive or unresponsive disease.[37] PEM is also more common in patients receiving intensive chemotherapy, abdominal or pelvic irradiation, or abdominal surgery, or with psychiatric depression, and in patients with certain malignancies, such as Ewing's sarcoma, than with others.

The reasons for PEM are various, and stem from both tumour and host factors, although separation of the two components may not be possible. Cancer patients usually have an oral intake which is inadequate to maintain body mass. This arises from many causes, which are summarized in Box 30.4. Anorexia is the most common cause of decreased nutrient intake and is found in 15–25 per cent

of all cancer patients at the time of diagnosis; it is almost universal in patients with widely metastatic disease. Anorexia may arise because of biochemical disturbance, the patient's response to the tumour, or paraneoplastic effects of the tumour itself.[38,39]

Cachexia is a progressive and severe wasting, often seen in patients with advanced cancer. In part, this is produced by inadequate calorie intake, but cancer cachexia differs from simple starvation. The normal physiological response to moderate or severe starvation is to reduce resting metabolic requirements. Normal individuals adapt to starvation by decreasing their basal metabolic rate, whereas in cancer patients this ability is lost, and in fact an inverse correlation appears to be present.[40] The patient is anorexic and listless with marked muscle wasting, fat depletion and visceral atrophy. Biochemical abnormalities may be severe, with increased gluconeogenesis from protein, glucose intolerance, hypoglycaemia, hypoalbuminaemia, hyperlipidaemia and possibly lactic acidosis. All of these abnormalities may not be present in the child with malignancy, but hyperlipidaemia and increased turnover of free fatty acids have been identified even before weight loss has occurred.[41] Abnormalities of glucose and protein metabolism have been reported in non-cachectic adult patients with lung cancer[42] and sarcoma.[43]

Mediators of cancer cachexia

Although the exact mechanisms causing cancer cachexia are unknown, several theories regarding its pathogenesis

Box 30.4 *Causes of impaired oral intake*

- General malaise
- Anorexia
- Pain
    - mucositis
    - oesophagitis
    - gastritis
- Altered taste perceptions
    - chemotherapy
    - mineral deficiency (zinc especially)
    - increased awareness of urea in meat
- Unpalatable hospital food
- Inappropriate mealtimes
- Overuse of favourite foods
- Psychological
    - learned food aversion
    - depression, anxiety
    - control of self and family
- Nausea, vomiting and diarrhoea
- Ileus, gastrointestinal stasis, constipation
- Surgical complications

point to a complex mix of tumour, host and treatment variables.

There is evidence that cytokines, particularly tumour necrosis factor (TNF), interleukins (ILs) 1 and 6 and interferon, mediate some of the effects of cachexia. Levels of IL-6 have been shown to increase with increased tumour load in mice,[44] whilst exogenous administration of IL-1 causes weight loss and anorexia in rats.[45] In addition, some tumours may exert paraneoplastic effects with release, for example, of vasoactive peptides or anorexia-inducing metabolites.[46] Peptides, oligonucleotides and other metabolites that may cause anorexia and cachexia may alter the sense of taste or even have a direct effect on the hypothalamus. Early satiety or fullness is common in anorexic cancer patients.

The effects of chemotherapy, radiotherapy and inter-current infection contribute greatly to overall nutritional failure. Nausea and vomiting, mucositis, diarrhoea and constipation are commonly experienced by patients receiving chemotherapy. Abdominal radiotherapy, including scatter radiation in patients receiving craniospinal radiotherapy, may be associated in the short term with nausea and vomiting and significant mucositis, and in the long term may cause strictures and chronic radiation enteritis. Patients receiving radiotherapy to the oropharynx, head or neck may develop severe local symptoms which cause long-term nutritional difficulties. Acute mucositis, gingivitis and dysphagia may be replaced in the longer term by dry mouth, trismus, poor oral hygiene and dental caries, all of which may reduce oral intake.

Patients with neutropenic fever have markedly increased metabolic rate, and the increase in this is proportional to the magnitude of fever. Prolonged, marked neutropenia after chemotherapy is therefore more likely to be associated with nutritional problems than otherwise.

Psychological and social factors will affect a child's desire and willingness to eat. A child undergoing intensive therapy may become depressed or anxious and, depending on developmental age, may become negativistic towards parents or staff seeking to encourage eating. A feeling of loss of control or helplessness is common, and refusing to eat, or at least controlling food intake, may be the only way in which an older child may retain some control. Persistent nausea or vomiting may lead to learned food aversion or vomiting even without administered chemotherapy. Finally, the disruption to normal family life and the necessary time in hospital may make an adequate food intake impossible for an unwell child.

Recent studies have reported a positive impact of exercise (e.g. walking or mild aerobic) on the sense of well-being, nausea and vomiting, and nutritional intake. Patients forced to rely on artificial feeding methods (including forced oral feeding as well as enteral or parenteral feeding) can experience depression, body image changes and stress related to problems with feeding tubes and equipment.

Problems related to nutrition have been identified by cancer patients as the most important factor in affecting their sense of well-being, more important than sexuality and continued employment.

Nutritional assessment of the child with cancer

Nutritional assessment should be made at the time of diagnosis and frequently throughout the course of therapy in order to assess any immediate or subsequent need for intervention. It must be remembered that, for a child, lack of weight gain constitutes a deterioration in nutritional status. Assessment should include a detailed dietary history, calculation of energy and protein intake as well as the nutritional requirements, anthropometric measurement and consideration of biochemical indices.

DIETARY HISTORY

This is an individual's normal dietary intake for a typical day. Dietary history should be considered along with relevant medical problems, including food intolerance or allergy, likes and dislikes. All patients should have their height and weight, and in young children head circumference, recorded and plotted on centile charts along with any previously recorded measurements, and this should continue at regular intervals throughout treatment. As a general rule, a weight for height which is less than 80 per cent of the 50th centile value for the child's age is a reasonable indicator that nutritional intervention is required. Similarly, any recent loss of ≥5 per cent of body weight warrants investigation and possible intervention, and a dietary intake of <75 per cent of the required nutritional intake for 7 days is an indication for intervention.

ANTHROPOMETRIC ASSESSMENT

Measurement of mid-arm circumference (MAC) and skin fold thickness in triceps, biceps, subscapular and supra-iliac regions allows accurate estimation of body fat deposition. Anthropometry is valuable, particularly where a child has a large tumour which may contribute to overall body weight; any such measurement must always be done by a trained operator, and if possible the same operator on each occasion. Centile charts for values at each site are available. Parameters have been developed, such as the arm muscle area and the mid-arm muscle circumference, that attempt to estimate lean muscle mass, but these are less commonly used. At the Bristol Royal Hospital for Children, the parameters of most value are found to be dietary history, weight for height and age, documented or reported weight loss and documented caloric intake. MAC and nitrogen balance may

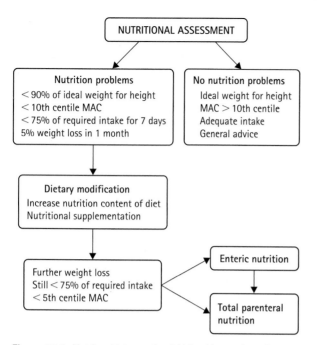

Figure 30.2 *Nutrional intervention. MAC, mid-arm circumference.*

also be of value. An algorithm for nutritional intervention is given in Figure 30.2.

Biochemical parameters used for nutritional assessment

All biochemical parameters will to some extent illustrate metabolic processes, but some are particularly useful in defining or monitoring patients requiring nutritional support.[47]

PROTEIN METABOLISM

Serum albumin

Albumin has a long half-life in the absence of significant protein loss (from renal or gastrointestinal tract) and is of value in long-term assessment of nutritional state, but may be normal in the presence of acute deterioration in nutritional state. False elevation may occur with dehydration, and a falsely low estimate of nutritional state may be made with coexistent renal or liver dysfunction and over-hydration. In evaluating the effect of total parenteral nutrition (TPN) in children with cancer, Rickard *et al.*[48] noted a fall in albumin when TPN was commenced, and a later normalization at 28 days. A poor correlation between serum albumin and weight for height centiles has been reported by van Eys.[49] Albumin probably reflects nutritional 'repletion' less well than other indicators.

Prealbumin

The half-life of prealbumin is approximately 2–3 days, and reduced production associated with poor nutrition will more rapidly cause a fall in prealbumin level.

Transferrin

The half-life of transferrin is short (4–10 days) and will allow assessment of nutritional status more acutely than serum albumin. Transferrin is, however, synthesized in response to iron deficiency and may be falsely low with coexistent renal dysfunction.

Retinol binding protein

Retinol binding protein (RBP) has a half-life of 12 hours and the total body pool is small. Rapid changes in levels of RBP may occur in response to changes in nutritional state, although levels are elevated in renal dysfunction, and decreased with liver dysfunction and deficiency of vitamin A and zinc.

Nitrogen balance

An accurate estimate of the daily protein nitrogen intake together with a measured urinary nitrogen level is a direct measurement of overall nitrogen balance, although this remains accurate only when renal function remains constant. Serum creatinine will also reflect total body muscle mass, although normal renal function is again required.

Protein breakdown products estimation

Histidine is found predominantly in actin and myosin, and estimation of 3-methylhistidine has been used to evaluate muscle protein breakdown. Levels may be falsely elevated in acute sepsis, and dietary protein may contribute to elevated levels. The assay is expensive and has not been widely adopted.

Altered amino acid patterns have been identified in non-stressed, malnourished patients, with alterations seen in the ratio of essential to non-essential amino acids. There is, however, only a poor correlation with degree of malnutrition, and a variety of disease states cause markedly varying patterns.

CARBOHYDRATE METABOLISM

Blood glucose concentration

Normoglycaemia in the non-stressed, normal but starved individual is associated with an elevated glucagon:insulin ratio. The response to a glucose load in such patients is exaggerated, as insulin levels rise and glucagon levels fall. In stressed patients, there is evidence of more marked gluconeogenesis, with elevated anaerobic metabolism to lactate. In the stressed patient, elevated catecholamine, corticosteroid and glucagon secretion may cause hyper-glycaemia, whereas in the severely cachectic patient, depletion of carbohydrate reserves may lead to varying hypoglycaemia.

LIPID METABOLISM

Triglyceride levels

Triglyceride levels are an indicator of lipid clearance after exogenous lipid administration, but not necessarily of lipid oxidation. In the stressed patient, triglyceride concentrations will be normal or slightly raised, as lipolysis occurs despite adequate glucose administration. With worsening sepsis, for example, decompensation may occur, and more marked elevation of triglycerides may occur. As peripheral clearance of triglyceride falls with worsening tissue perfusion, incomplete fatty acid oxidation will occur, and abnormal lipid deposition may occur. This may be due to, or enhanced by, the presence of increased insulin concentrations, reduced lipoprotein lipase concentration in skeletal muscle or carnitine deficiency.

Ketone body levels

Elevated levels of acetoacetate and β-hydroxybutyrate are seen in starvation, and under normal conditions there is free conversion between the two, a process which involves production of NADH with acetoacetate. In the stressed, starving patient, increased lactate production may be associated with depletion of NAD^+, and reduced generation of acetoacetate may follow. Increased production of β-hydroxybutyrate from long-chain acyl-CoA will also lead to an elevation of the β-hydroxybutyrate: acetoacetate ratio.

Effects of nutritional intervention

The implications of developing PEM in a child are potentially great. Well nourished children are better able to withstand the effects of chemotherapy and radiotherapy,[50] have a better immune response[51] and are better tempered and more able to play and participate in activities of their family. Most importantly, the loss of more than 10–15 per cent of body weight is itself associated with significant mortality, this being due to a combination of increased susceptibility to infection, metabolic disturbance and specific deficiencies. In one study of 286 children with malignant disease, nutritional status was directly correlated with freedom from relapse, either localized or distant.[52] The potential impact of nutritional intervention is great, therefore, both in the short term and in the development of late sequelae.

Nutritional intervention has been shown to be effective in the reversal of tumour-associated weight loss,[48,53] and there is considerable evidence that hyperalimentation allows administration of chemotherapy and radiotherapy on time and with fewer complications than with inadequate nutrition.[54] Hence, where effective therapy is available, nutritional intervention may be of value in improving therapy.

The question of whether nutritional support may enhance tumour growth is not fully answered. Tumour growth will normally continue at the expense of the host, but enhanced tumour growth has been reported in animals receiving supplementation. The selective chelation of iron by desferrioxamine is currently under investigation as a therapeutic modality in neuroblastoma, and enhanced growth of a neuroblastoma has been described in one patient receiving nutritional supplementation.[55] In a randomized trial of nutritional intervention in adult patients with cancer, a worse outcome was associated with those patients receiving TPN, and this has been confirmed in several series[56] (see van Eys[49] for a review). In patients with neuroblastoma, poor nutritional status has been reported to be of prognostic significance, but nutritional intervention is not associated with an effect on survival.

The beneficial effect of parenteral nutrition in patients undergoing BMT has been shown in several studies and a survival benefit has been reported in a series of 137 children and young adult patients for those patients receiving TPN rather than conventional nutrition.[57] In nine young patients receiving TPN to a target of 160 per cent of estimated basal energy expenditure, no significant change in weight, lean body mass or body fat was recorded, although a significant reduction in body cell mass and a negative nitrogen balance over the entire study period were seen.[58]

Methods of nutritional support

Guidelines for nutritional intervention in current use at the Bristol Royal Hospital for Children are given in Figure 30.2. All patients are reviewed by a dietician at diagnosis and throughout treatment. Those patients who have no nutritional problems are given both verbal and written dietary advice regarding potential problems that may occur. Initial nutritional support is with high-calorie normal foods, to which glucose polymers in solid or liquid form may be added. Complete nutritional supplements may also be added, although acceptance of these is variable. Patients with significant and continuing weight loss, those receiving highly intensive therapy and very young children, may require nasoenteric feeding. It is essential to prepare a child of any age for a procedure such as passing a nasogastric tube. The threat of a nasogastric tube is often made to a child with poor nutritional intake, which often makes the process difficult and unpleasant for the child should a tube be required. Successful enteral nutrition requires the cooperation of the child.

Flexible fine-bore and silk tubes are generally well tolerated and commercially produced sterile feeds are most appropriate. These are, in general, nutritionally complete, and formulations appropriate to young children are now available. Administration by a nasogastric tube is best accomplished as frequent small feeds, whereas nasojejunal feeds require a continuous infusion. The strength and volume of feed administered are best increased slowly over 4 days in order to avoid diarrhoea. Patients who have specific abnormalities of gastrointestinal function, such as short bowel syndromes or malabsorption, will require specifically designed formulae (such as hydrolysed protein, peptide or elemental feeds), which in general are unpalatable and require nasoenteric administration.

Energy requirements for children receiving chemotherapy or suffering side-effects from this are greater than for normal children and oral intake may be greatly reduced. Initial target oral intake should be 50–70 per cent of estimated average requirement for energy (EAR; 1991 Department of Health figures) for age. The majority of malnourished children will gain weight on this amount, but intake should be increased to 100 per cent of EAR, or more if necessary.

In patients with specific pharyngeal problems causing difficulties with oral administration of feeds (severe mucositis, oesophagitis, bulbar palsy, primary tumour involvement and radiotherapy to the oropharynx), gastrostomy or jejunostomy feeding may prove valuable. Endoscopic gastrostomy can be safely performed in most patients with minimal morbidity and may allow normal nutrition to be maintained in the presence of severe oropharyngeal disease. Where a gastrostomy is considered, the presence of significant gastro-oesophageal reflux must be excluded, and, if present, a surgical anti-reflux procedure considered.

Specialized feeds may be given if there are particular problems. A child with extensive gut mucosal toxicity may benefit from small volumes of hydrolysed feed. For some, temporary lactose intolerance may follow a period of mucositis, and withdrawal of milk based feeds may be of benefit.

GLUTAMINE SUPPLEMENTATION

Nutritional support in the presence of mucositis may be impossible without TPN. Glutamine is said to be the major energy source for intestinal epithelial cells,[59] and supplementation with glutamine has been used, aiming to reduce the duration of this period after chemotherapy. Effects upon T lymphocytes in adult patients have been described,[60] and have been associated with decreased severity of mucositis in patients receiving autologous (but not allogeneic) BMTs.[59] Van Zaanen et al.[61] reported a clinical benefit of glutamine (dipeptide)-supplemented TPN in patients receiving intensive chemotherapy, with greater weight gain in the supplemented patients, but no effect on toxicity was seen. Oral supplementation was not associated with any reduction in days receiving TPN, length of hospitalization, number of days or grade of mucositis compared with placebo when administered to patients undergoing high-dose chemotherapy.[62]

PARENTERAL NUTRITION

Parenteral nutrition (PN) may be indicated where weight loss continues despite enteral nutrition, or where gastrointestinal abnormalities prevent this route from being used. Most patients with these requirements will already have appropriate central venous access, although multiple concomitant medication may severely impair the ability to administer the required volumes. PN prescription is beyond the remit of a chapter such as this but general considerations are described below.

Fluids
Total fluid requirements, including inappropriate gastrointestinal, urinary and other losses, must be considered.

Carbohydrate
Glucose is the preferred carbohydrate source and may be administered at high concentration (20–25 per cent) via the central route. Approximately 50 per cent of energy requirements should be given as carbohydrate. Calculation of energy requirements in adults is made according to predicted basal metabolic rate (BMR), using reference tables, or the Harris–Benedict equation.

For children, no such equation exists, and nutritional requirements should be estimated according to age-specific tables. A diet providing the reference nutrient intake (defined as that level of intake that will provide adequate nutrients for 97.5 per cent of the healthy child population) should provide for adequately nourished children with cancer, and higher requirements are indicated in the presence of malnutrition.

Protein
Protein is normally administered as a balanced mixture of synthetic amino acids, together with adequate carbohydrate and lipid to prevent catabolism.

Fat
Fat is usually administered as an isotonic solution derived from soya bean oil, glycerol and egg yolk phospholipid. Approximately 30 per cent of calories should normally be administered as lipid, but this is contraindicated where there is evidence of sepsis or liver impairment.

Minerals and vitamins
These are supplemented using commercially available preparations, although it must be remembered that mineral requirements may be considerably greater in patients who receive chemotherapy. Renal tubular losses of sodium, potassium, calcium and magnesium may be markedly increased as a result of prior or concomitant therapy with cisplatin, ifosfamide and, in particular, amphotericin.

Parenteral nutrition requirements must always be adjusted according to the clinical situation and biochemical measurements.

Conclusions

Protein energy malnutrition in children receiving chemotherapy is common, may be severe and may continue for prolonged periods of time. Nutritional intervention will contribute to an improved feeling of well-being for patients and their families. The possibility that improved nutrition may adversely affect tumour responsiveness must be balanced against the improved ability of a well child to tolerate intensive chemotherapy and radiotherapy, and appropriate intervention should begin at diagnosis and continue throughout the course of treatment. The long-term effects of a period of PEM and of other nutritional deficiency must be considered with other sequelae of treatment.

MANAGEMENT OF ACUTE NEUROLOGICAL COMPLICATIONS

Alterations in the level of consciousness of a patient, confusion, disorientation and convulsions must always be regarded as serious events. Changes in neurological states are more common in patients with brain tumours, but may occur in any patient undergoing treatment for malignant disease. The process involved in managing such events is similar to that for any other patient, but important additional considerations must be made, reflecting a different spectrum of potential causes of such problems.

The approach to investigation of an acute change in neurological state should be the same as for any acutely unwell child, although the relative likelihood of particular causes differs. The assessment must include an immediate assessment of vital signs and appropriate resuscitation without delay. For a child suffering generalized seizures, these must be controlled and initial investigations undertaken whilst this is begun. It is important to establish the underlying malignant diagnosis, stage and sites affected by disease, since the possibility exists that these may directly cause symptoms. Recent therapy must be documented and the possibility that the patient may be thrombocytopenic assessed. Anaemia, infection and haemorrhage are all recognized causes of a changing neurological state. If intracranial haemorrhage in a thrombocytopenic patient is a likely diagnosis, platelets should be given without delay.

Initial assessment of the child requires quantification of the level of change of consciousness. The Glasgow Coma Scale is appropriate for all children, and is familiar to most medical and nursing staff. An adaptation of this, suitable for use with children below the age of 5 years, has been reported to be reproducible between observers and is given in Table 30.2.[63] A low score in a child of any age indicates a high risk of further deterioration, and urgent need for investigation and treatment.

Further assessment of the patient should exclude the possibility of raised intracranial pressure and look for signs of cerebral herniation. Initial herniation of one or both temporal lobes through the tentorium may be followed by complete recovery, but herniation of the pons or medulla through the foramen magnum may not. Mechanical damage to the brain, ischaemia and haemorrhage may lead to irrecoverable loss, and these may be incompatible with life. A rapid assessment of the patient

Table 30.2 *Modified Glasgow Coma Scale. Modified James Scale*[63]

	>5 years		<5 years
Eye opening			
4		Spontaneous	
3		To voice	
2		To pain	
1		None	
Verbal			
5	Orientated		Alert, babbles, coos, words or sentences: normal
4	Confused		Less than usual ability, irritable cry
3	Inappropriate words		Cries to pain
2	Incomprehensible sounds		Moans to pain
1	Nor response to pain		No response to pain
Motor			
6	Obeys commands		Normal spontaneous movements
5		Localizes to supraocular pain (>9 months)	
4		Withdraws from nailbed pressure	
3		Flexion to supraocular pain	
2		Extension to supraocular pain	
1		No response to supraocular pain	

Table 30.3 *Investigations of non-traumatic coma in children with malignant disease*

Investigation	Risk factors	Possible abnormality	Further investigation if abnormal	Possible diagnosis
Blood glucose	Nutrition	Hypoglycaemia	Insulin, blood ammonia, lactate, blood and urine amino acids, urine organic acids	Hypoglycaemia secondary to poor intake
	L-asparaginase			Pancreatitis, diabetic ketoacidosis
Sodium	Poor intake, vomiting, ifosfamide, cisplatin	Hypernatraemia	Urinary sodium, osmolality, tubular reabsorption of phosphate	Dehydration, possible renal tubular leak
	Pituitary region tumour, hyperhydration	Hyponatraemia	See specific protocol	Fluid overload, SIADH
Urea	Poor intake, vomiting, ifosfamide, cisplatin	Dehydration	Serum creatinine	Dehydration
LDH	BMT, cyclosporin	Raised		TTP
AST/ALT	BMT, cyclosporin	Raised		TTP
	Actinomycin D, 6-thioguanine, busulphan	Hepatic impairment		Veno-occlusive disease
	High-dose therapy	Hepatic impairment		Direct organ toxicity
FBC and film	Recent chemotherapy	Anaemia	CT/MRI brain	Intracranial haemorrhage
		Thrombocytopenia	CT/MRI brain	Intracranial haemorrhage
		Leucocytosis	Infection screen	Meningitis
	Infection, shocked, BMT	DIC/TTP	CT/MRI brain	Intracranial haemorrhage
PT, APTT, fibrinogen, D-dimers	Poor nutrition, malabsorption	Reduced vitamin K-dependent factor production	CT/MRI brain	Intracranial haemorrhage
	Infection, active disease	DIC (TTP)		
Blood culture			CT/MRI brain	Intracranial haemorrhage
Stool culture If clinically indicated		Bacteraemia, *Shigella*, enteroviruses		

Investigation	Predisposing factors	Finding	Further test	Interpretation
CT/MRI brain		Primary tumour, metastasis		Recurrent or progressive disease
	Prior radiotherapy	Mass lesion ± cavitation		Radionecrosis
	Leukaemia	Infiltration	FBC, BM aspiration	Leukaemic relapse
	L-asparaginase, dehydration, hyperleucocytosis, recent neurosurgery (intracranial germ cell tumour)	Infarct	MRI/angiography	Infarct
		Haemorrhage		
		Hydrocephalus		Tumour progression, shunt dysfunction
		Focal low density		
		Abscess		Abscess, herpes, tumour
		Diffuse oedema		
		Frontotemporal abnormality	CSF virology, PCR	Herpes virus encephalopathy
Lumbar puncture[a]				
Cytospin	Leukaemia, lymphoma	Blasts		Relapse
Culture				Meningitis (bacterial, viral, opportunistic)
PCR for TB				
PCR for viruses				
EEG		Epileptiform discharges		Status epilepticus

ALT, alanine aminotransaminase; APTT, activated partial thromboplastin time; AST, aspartate aminotransferase; BM, bone marrow; CSF, cerebrospinal fluid; DIC, disseminated intravascular coagulation; EEG, electroencephalogram; FBC, full blood count; IVIG, intravenous immunoglobulin; LDH, lactate dehydrogenase; PCR, polymerase chain reaction; PT, prothrombin time; SIADH, syndrome of inappropriate antidiuretic hormone; TTP, thrombotic thrombocytopenic purpura; WCC, white cell count.

[a] After CT/MRI, FBC, clotting.

Box 30.5 *Causes of impaired level of consciousness in oncology patients, additional to those affecting all children*

Metabolic
- Hypoglycaemia
- Hyperglycaemia (diabetic ketoacidosis)
- Hyponatraemia
- Hypernatraemia
- Uraemia

Drug related
- Steroid psychosis/depression
- Ifosfamide-related encephalopathy
- Melphalan, busulphan neurotoxicity
- Cyclosporin neurotoxicity
- L-asparaginase-induced thromboembolic disease
- Cytarabine encephalopathy
- Methotrexate leucoencephalopathy
- Sedative analgesia
- Opiates, benzodiazepines, phenothiazines, cannabinoids

Infection: meningitis, encephalitis
- Bacterial
- Viral
- Opportunistic, include fungal
- Neurosurgery-related (ventriculitis, shunt infection)

Haemorrhage, thrombosis
- Thrombocytopenia
- Disseminated intravascular coagulation
- Thrombotic thrombocytopenic purpura
- Coagulation factor hypoproduction (malnutrition, malabsorption, L-asparaginase-related)
- Dehydration
- Sepsis

Tumour–related
- Primary CNS tumour
- Metastatic tumour
- Paraneoplastic
- Post-neurosurgery complication
- Subdural/extradural collection, haematoma
- Infection – ventriculitis, meningitis
- Infarction, haemorrhage
- Posterior fossa syndrome
- Shunt dysfunction

possible secondary neurological damage to the patient. Box 30.5 summarizes causes that are particularly relevant to the child with malignant disease. An approach to the investigation of non-traumatic coma in children with known malignant disease is given in Table 30.3, which is an adaptation of that published by Kirkham[64] for children without known malignant disease.

Severe neurological impairment requires intensive care support and involvement of a paediatric neurologist. Where a transient change is seen, clearly associated with administration of a chemotherapeutic or other drug, the drug must be stopped immediately. Ifosfamide is well reported to be associated with such an encephalopathy;[65,66] risk factors for its development include oral administration, renal impairment, bulky abdominal disease and poor nutritional status. Discontinuation of the infusion is usually, but not always, associated with rapid recovery.[67,68] Methylene blue has been found to reverse the acute neurotoxic effects rapidly[69] and should be routinely available on the oncology ward. Busulphan is similarly associated with a risk of inducing fits, and prophylactic anticonvulsant medications are typically given in BMT conditioning regimens containing this drug.

KEY POINTS

- Early control of nausea and vomiting may reduce subsequent problems with anticipatory symptoms. Control of nausea and vomiting is more readily maintained by prevention than by increasing therapy once it has become established. The use of an emetic control 'ladder' is advisable.
- The place of the new class of antiemetic agents, the substance P/neurokinin 1 receptor inhibitors, is not yet clear. $5HT_3$ antagonists remain the most effective group of antiemetic agents for the majority of chemotherapy-related nausea and vomiting in children.
- Tumour lysis is associated with highly proliferative malignancies and large tumour load. Chemotherapy is the most common precipitant, but infection, anaesthesia and surgery may also lead to TLS.
- The safety and efficacy of recombinant urate oxidase, and its superiority to allopurinol in reducing plasma uric acid levels, seem clear, and its use in high-risk situations is advised.
- The use of blood product support in oncology is increasing, but decisions to transfuse blood products should be based on symptoms and signs and not numbers. Failure to respond to therapy should lead to careful reappraisal and

to assess intracranial pressure (ICP) is therefore mandatory, and immediate measures to reduce pressure instigated if required.

Impaired consciousness in all children should be systematically and rapidly investigated in order to minimize consideration of alternative strategies. The indication for, and benefit from, their use must be clearly documented each time a patient receives a transfusion. Wherever possible, use of blood products should be kept to a minimum.

- There is no consensus for the precise indications for red cell use, but sensible indications include symptomatic anaemia, rapid and anticipated continuing fall in haemoglobin, and anaemia developing during intensive chemotherapy or before planned radiotherapy. It seems likely that concerns over the risk of allogeneic transfusion will drive an increased interest in the use of erythropoeitin in oncology.
- The choice of empirical antibiotics for patients with fever and neutropenia should be based on local bacteriological sensitivities and on the risk presented by the patient. Outpatient monotherapy after initial stabilization is increasingly being investigated.
- Established fungal infection has a high mortality, and prophylactic antifungal medication is increasingly used. Novel antifungal agents – the triazoles (voriconazole and posaconazole) and echinocandins (caspofungin) – seem effective and well tolerated.
- Alterations in the level of consciousness of a patient, confusion, disorientation and convulsions must always be regarded as serious events. Initial assessment of the child requires quantification of the level of change of consciousness using the Glasgow Coma Scale. Assessment must assess the possibility of raised intracranial pressure and cerebral herniation, in order to avoid irreversible changes.

REFERENCES

1. Borison H, Wang SC. Physiology and pharmacology of vomiting. *Pharmacol Rev* 1953; **5**: 193.
2. Foot AB, Hayes C. Audit of guidelines for effective control of chemotherapy and radiotherapy induced emesis. *Arch Dis Child* 1994; **71**(5): 475–80.
3. Stables R, Andrews PL, Bailey HE *et al*. Antiemetic properties of the 5HT3-receptor antagonist, GR38032F. *Cancer Treat Rev* 1987; **14**: 333–6.
4. Marty M, Pouillart P, Scholl S *et al*. Comparison of the 5-hydroxytryptamine3 (serotonin) antagonist ondansetron (GR 38032F) with high-dose metoclopramide in the control of cisplatin-induced emesis. *N Engl J Med* 1990; **322**(12): 816–21.
5. Koseoglu V, Kurekci AE, Sarici U *et al*. Comparison of the efficacy and side-effects of ondansetron and metoclopramide-diphenhydramine administered to control nausea and vomiting in

children treated with antineoplastic chemotherapy: a prospective randomized study. *Eur J Pediatr* 1998; **157**(10): 806–10.
6. Stiakaki E, Savvas S, Lydaki E *et al*. Ondansetron and tropisetron in the control of nausea and vomiting in children receiving combined cancer chemotherapy. *Pediatr Hematol Oncol* 1999; **16**(2): 101–8.
7. Aksoylar S, Akman SA, Ozgenc F, Kansoy S. Comparison of tropisetron and granisetron in the control of nausea and vomiting in children receiving combined cancer chemotherapy. *Pediatr Hematol Oncol* 2001; **18**(6): 397–406.
8. Kris MG, Tyson LB, Gralla RJ *et al*. Extrapyramidal reactions with high-dose metoclopramide. *N Engl J Med* 1983; **309**(7): 433–4.
9. Allen JC, Gralla R, Reilly L *et al*. Metoclopramide: dose-related toxicity and preliminary antiemetic studies in children receiving cancer chemotherapy. *J Clin Oncol* 1985; **3**(8): 1136–41.
10. Smith DB, Newlands ES, Rustin GJ *et al*. Comparison of ondansetron and ondansetron plus dexamethasone as antiemetic prophylaxis during cisplatin-containing chemotherapy. *Lancet* 1991; **338**(8765): 487–90.
11. Allan SG, Cornbleet MA, Warrington PS *et al*. Dexamethasone and high dose metoclopramide: efficacy in controlling cisplatin induced nausea and vomiting. *Br Med J* (*Clin Res Ed*) 1984; **289**(6449): 878–9.
12. Sallan SE, Cronin C, Zelen M, Zinberg NE. Antiemetics in patients receiving chemotherapy for cancer: a randomized comparison of delta-9-tetrahydrocannabinol and prochlorperazine. *N Engl J Med* 1980; **302**(3): 135–8.
13. Abrahamov A, Mechoulam R. An efficient new cannabinoid antiemetic in pediatric oncology. *Life Sci* 1995; **56**(23-24): 2097–102.
14. Cunningham D, Forrest GJ, Soukop M *et al*. Nabilone and prochlorperazine: a useful combination for emesis induced by cytotoxic drugs. *Br Med J* (*Clin Res Ed*) 1985; **291**(6499): 864–5.
15. Kris MG, Gralla RJ, Clark RA *et al*. Incidence, course, and severity of delayed nausea and vomiting following the administration of high-dose cisplatin. *J Clin Oncol* 1985; **3**(10): 1379–84.
16. Hesketh PJ, Kris MG, Grunberg SM *et al*. Proposal for classifying the acute emetogenicity of cancer chemotherapy. *J Clin Oncol* 1997; **15**(1): 103–9.
17. Khan J, Broadbent VA. Tumor lysis syndrome complicating treatment of widespread metastatic abdominal rhabdomyosarcoma. *Pediatr Hematol Oncol* 1993; **10**(2): 151–5.
18. Hain RD, Rayner L, Weitzman S, Lorenzana A. Acute tumour lysis syndrome complicating treatment of stage IVS neuroblastoma in infants under six months old. *Med Pediatr Oncol* 1994; **23**(2): 136–9.
19. Lobe TE, Karkera MS, Custer MD *et al*. Fatal refractory hyperkalemia due to tumor lysis during primary resection for hepatoblastoma. *J Pediatr Surg* 1990; **25**(2): 249–50.
21. Pui CH. Urate oxidase in the prophylaxis or treatment of hyperuricemia: the United States experience. *Semin Hematol* 2001; **38**(4 Suppl 10): 13–21.

22. Patte C, Sakiroglu O, Sommelet D. European experience in the treatment of hyperuricemia. *Semin Hematol* 2001; **38**(4 Suppl 10): 9–12.

23. Goldman SC, Holcenberg JS, Finklestein JZ *et al.* A randomized comparison between rasburicase and allopurinol in children with lymphoma or leukemia at high risk for tumor lysis. *Blood* 2001; **97**(10): 2998–3003.

25. Stuart MJ, Murphy S, Oski FA. A simple nonradioisotopic technic for the determination of platelet life-span. *N Engl J Med* 1975; **292**: 1310–13.

26. Priest JR, Ramsay NKC, Stgeinherz PG *et al.* A syndrome of thrombosis and hemorrhage complicating L-asparaginase therapy for childhood acute lymphoblastic leukaemia. *J Pediatr* 1982; **100**: 984–9.

27. D'Angio GJ. Hepatotoxicity and actinomycin D. *Lancet* 1990; **1**: 1290.

28. Pritchard J, Imeson J, Barnes J *et al.* Results of the United Kingdom Children's Cancer Study Group first Wilms' tumor study. *J Clin Oncol* 1995; **13**: 124–33.

29. Bodey GP, Buckley M, Sathe YS, Freireich EJ. Quantitative relationships between circulating leukocytes and infection in patients with acute leukemia. *Ann Intern Med* 1966; **64**(2): 328–40.

30. Schimpff SC, Satterlee W, Young WM *et al.* Empiric therapy with carbenicillin and gentamicin for febrile patients with cancer and granulocytopenia. *N Engl J Med* 1971; **284**: 1061–5.

31. EORTC. International Antimicrobial Therapy Co-operative Group. Ceftazidime combined with a short or long course of amikacin for empirical therapy of gram-negative bacteraemia in cancer patients with granulocytopenia. *N Engl J Med* 1987; **317**: 1692–9.

32. Talcott JA, Siegel RD, Finberg R *et al.* Risk assessment in cancer patients with fever and neutropenia: a prospective, two center validation of a prediction rule. *J Clin Oncol* 1992; **10**: 316–22.

33. Freifeld A, Marchigiani D, Walsh T *et al.* A double-blind comparison of empirical oral and intravenous antibiotic therapy for low risk febrile patients with neutropenia during cancer chemotherapy. *N Engl J Med* 1999; **341**: 305–11.

34. Prentice HG, Gluckman E, Powles RL *et al.* Impact of long-term aciclovir on CMV infection and survival after allogeneic bone marrow transplantation. *Lancet* 1994; **343**(8900): 749–53.

35. Walsh TJ, Finberg RW, Arndt S *et al.* Liposomal amphotericin B for empirical therapy in patients with persistent fever and neutropenia. *N Engl J Med* 1999; **340**: 764–71.

36. Walsh TJ, Pappas P, Winston DJ *et al.* Voriconazole compared with liposomal amphotericin B for empirical antifungal therapy in patients with neutropenia and persistent fever. *N Engl J Med* 2002; **346**(4): 225–34.

37. Rickard KA, Baehner RL, Coates TD *et al.* Supportive nutritional intervention in pediatric cancer. *Cancer Res* 1982; **42**(2 Suppl): 766s–73s.

38. Theologides A. Anorexia-producing intermediary metabolites. *Am J Clin Nutr* 1976; **29**(5): 552–8.

39. Theologides A. Cancer cachexia. *Cancer* 1979; **43**(5 Suppl): 2004–12.

40. Young VR. Energy metabolism and requirements in the cancer patient. *Cancer Res* 1977; **37**(7 Pt 2): 2336–47.

41. Legaspi A, Jeevanandam M, Starnes HF, Jr. Brennan MF. Whole body lipid and energy metabolism in the cancer patient. *Metabolism* 1987; **36**(10): 958–63.

42. Heber D, Chlebowski RT, Ishibashi DE *et al.* Abnormalities in glucose and protein metabolism in noncachectic lung cancer patients. *Cancer Res* 1982; **42**(11): 4815–19.

43. Inculet RI, Stein TP, Peacock JL *et al.* Altered leucine metabolism in noncachectic sarcoma patients. *Cancer Res* 1987; **47**(17): 4746–9.

44. Jablons D, McIntosh J, Mule JJ *et al.* Induction of interferon-beta 2/interleukin-6 by cytokine administration and detection of circulating interleukin-6 in the tumor bearing state. *Ann NY Acad Sci* 1989; **557**: 157–60.

45. Hellerstein MK, Meydani SN, Meydani M *et al.* Interleukin-1-induced anorexia in the rat. Influence of prostaglandins. *J Clin Invest* 1989; **84**(1): 228–35.

46. McNamara M, Alexander R, Norton J. Cytokines and their rôle in the pathophysiology of cancer cachexia. *J Parenter Enteral Nutr* 1992; **16**: 50s–55s.

47. Mattox TW, Teasley-Strausburg KM. Overview of biochemical markers used for nutrition support. *DICP* 1991; **25**(3): 265–71.

48. Rickard KA, Grosfeld JL, Kirksey A *et al.* Reversal of protein-energy malnutrition in children during treatment of advanced neoplastic disease. *Ann Surg* 1979; **190**(6): 771–81.

49. van Eys J. Effect of nutritional status on responses to therapy. *Cancer Res* 1982; **42**(2 Suppl): 747s–53s.

50. Rickard KA, Coates TD, Grosfeld JL *et al.* The value of nutrition support in children with cancer. *Cancer* 1986; **58**(8 Suppl): 1904–10.

51. Neumann CG, Jelliffe DB, Zerfas AJ, Jelliffe EF. Nutritional assessment of the child with cancer. *Cancer Res* 1982; **42**(2 Suppl): 699s–712s.

52. Donaldson S, Jundt S, Riccour C *et al.* Radiation enteritis in children. A retrospective review, clinicopathologic correlation and dietary management. *Cancer* 1975; **35**: 1167–78.

53. Nixon DW. Hyperalimentation in the undernourished cancer patient. *Cancer Res* 1982; **42**(2 Suppl): 727s–8s.

54. Rickard KA, Loghmani ES, Grosfeld JL *et al.* Short- and long-term effectiveness of enteral and parenteral nutrition in reversing or preventing protein-energy malnutrition in advanced neuroblastoma. A prospective randomized study. *Cancer* 1985; **56**(12): 2881–97.

55. English W, Suskind R, Damrongsak D *et al.* Can growth of neuroblastoma be influenced by a child's nutritional state? *Clin Pediatr* 1975; **14**: 868.

56. Shamberger RC, Brennan MF, Goodgame JT Jr *et al.* A prospective, randomized study of adjuvant parenteral nutrition in the treatment of sarcomas: results of metabolic and survival studies. *Surgery* 1984; **96**(1): 1–13.

57. Weisdorf SA, Lysne J, Wind D *et al.* Positive effect of prophylactic total parenteral nutrition on long-term outcome of bone marrow transplantation. *Transplantation* 1987; **43**(6): 833–8.

58. Cheney CL, Abson KG, Aker SN *et al.* Body composition changes in marrow transplant recipients receiving total parenteral nutrition. *Cancer* 1987; **59**(8): 1515–19.

59. Anderson PM, Ramsay NK, Shu XO *et al.* Effect of low-dose oral glutamine on painful stomatitis during bone marrow transplantation. *Bone Marrow Transplant* 1998; **22**(4): 339–44.

60. O'Riordain MG, Fearon KC, Ross JA *et al.* Glutamine-supplemented total parenteral nutrition enhances T-lymphocyte response in surgical patients undergoing colorectal resection. *Ann Surg* 1994; **220**(2): 212–21.

61. van Zaanen HC, van der Lelie H, Timmer JG *et al.* Parenteral glutamine dipeptide supplementation does not ameliorate chemotherapy-induced toxicity. *Cancer* 1994; **74**(10): 2879–84.

62. Coghlin Dickson TM, Wong RM, Offrin RS *et al.* Effect of oral glutamine supplementation during bone marrow transplantation. *J Parenter Enteral Nutr* 2000; **24**(2): 61–6.

63. Tatman A, Warren A, Williams A *et al.* Development of a modified paediatric coma scale in intensive care clinical practice. *Arch Dis Child* 1997; **77**(6): 519–21.

64. Kirkham F. Non-traumatic coma in children. *Arch Dis Child* 2001; **85**: 303–12.

65. Cantwell BM, Carmichael J, Ghani S, Harris AL. A phase II study of ifosfamide/mesna with doxorubicin for adult soft tissue sarcoma. *Cancer Chemother Pharmacol* 1988; **21**(1): 49–52.

66. Lowis SP, Pearson AD, Reid MM, Craft AW. Prohibitive toxicity of a dose-intense regime for metastatic neuroblastoma containing ifosfamide, doxorubicin and cisplatin. *Cancer Chemother Pharmacol* 1993; **31**(5): 415–18.

67. Bruggers CS, Friedman HS, Tien R, Delong R. Cerebral atrophy in an infant following treatment with ifosfamide. *Med Pediatr Oncol* 1994; **23**(4): 380–3.

68. Shuper A, Stein J, Goshen J *et al.* Subacute central nervous system degeneration in a child: an unusual manifestation of ifosfamide intoxication. *J Child Neurol* 2000; **15**(7): 481–3.

69. Pelgrims J, De Vos F, Van den Brande J *et al.* Methylene blue in the treatment and prevention of ifosfamide-induced encephalopathy: report of 12 cases and a review of the literature. *Br J Cancer* 2000; **82**(2): 291–4.

31

Growth and endocrine late effects

W. HAMISH B. WALLACE, MARK F. H. BROUGHAM & HELEN A. SPOUDEAS

INTRODUCTION

Treatment of childhood cancer has markedly improved over the past few decades, such that around 80 per cent of children with cancer will be alive 5 years from diagnosis.[1] The number of long-term survivors is therefore increasing, and it has been estimated that by the year 2010, 1 in 250 young adults will have been treated for cancer in childhood.[2]

As a result there has been a change in emphasis from 'cure at any cost' to one in which quality of life during and after treatment has become important. Therefore, whilst still striving to improve survival, attention must be directed to minimizing adverse effects of treatment, in both the short and long term. Late sequelae are particularly important in the paediatric population due to their impact on normal growth and development.

Late effects of cancer treatment include:

- growth impairment
- disorders of the endocrine system, including infertility and hypothyroidism
- abnormalities of cardiac and pulmonary function
- renal and hepatic impairment
- second malignancies
- cognitive and psychosocial complications.

Collectively, endocrine disorders represent the commonest long-term complication, with one study suggesting

approximately 40 per cent of cancer patients as having at least one endocrine abnormality at follow-up.[3]

This chapter will focus on the consequences of cancer treatment on growth and endocrine function. In addition, the impact on puberty and fertility will be discussed. Long-term follow-up of these patients is essential in order that adverse effects are diagnosed early, and appropriate counselling and therapeutic intervention are instituted. Awareness of the aetiology and prevalence of late complications will allow treatment modifications that will improve the quality of life for long-term survivors of childhood cancer.

HYPOTHALAMIC–PITUITARY DYSFUNCTION

The hypothalamic–pituitary axis is central to the control of the endocrine system, and therefore disruption of this axis will have far-reaching consequences. Cranial irradiation is known to cause hypothalamic–pituitary dysfunction,[4] and the resultant hormone deficiency is dependent on the total dose of radiation received and the fractionation schedule.[5]

A tissue's radiosensitivity is directly proportional to its mitotic activity and inversely proportional to its cellular differentiation.[6] Therefore the effects of irradiation on slowly proliferating cell populations, such as the brain, are manifest only with time. Thus, depending upon radiation dose, hypothalamic–pituitary function may be progressively lost with increasing time since treatment.[7,8] This may not simply be due to delayed effects of radiotherapy on the axis as a whole, but may also reflect subsequent pituitary dysfunction secondary to earlier hypothalamic damage, as there is evidence that the hypothalamus is more radiosensitive than the pituitary.[9,10] This is suggested by suppression of insulin-mediated and spontaneous growth hormone (GH) secretion following irradiation,[11] yet the GH response to hypothalamic releasing factors is preserved.[12] However, the pituitary response to growth hormone-releasing hormone (GHRH) does decline with time,[12] and thus direct pituitary damage remains a late contributory factor.

This has implications with regard to follow-up and investigation of pituitary function. Pituitary function tests currently used rely on pharmacological provocation tests to detect deficiencies. However, there is evidence that radiation, or pre-existing brain injury, impairs normal central hormonal release mechanisms such that discrepancies between physiological secretion of pituitary hormones and peak responses to certain provocation tests occur.[11,13] The resulting neurosecretory dysfunction can have clinical significance, particularly during the pubertal growth spurt, when an increased GH secretion is required. Therefore the prevalence of hypopituitarism may be underestimated by standard provocation tests. Unfortunately, assessment of physiological secretion by overnight profile is difficult in practical terms, and currently remains a research tool. This emphasizes the importance of continued long-term follow-up and clinical vigilance for these patients.

Of further importance in differentiating between hypothalamic and pituitary disease are the implications with regard to therapeutic intervention. Treating endocrine deficits with hypothalamic-releasing factors requires intact pituitary function. Thus GHRH can be used following radiotherapy to improve growth, but this may be less effective than using recombinant GH in this situation.[14] This is, at least in part, because the response to GHRH additionally depends on intact hypothalamic somatostatin secretion, which is also disturbed by irradiation.[11,15]

An additional risk factor important in neuroendocrine late effects is the age of the child at the time of radiotherapy. There is evidence to suggest that younger children are more sensitive than older children and adults to radiation-induced damage of the hypothalamic–pituitary axis.[16]

Of the pituitary hormones, GH secretion is the most radiosensitive,[7] with doses as low as 18 Gy causing GH deficiency.[17] Subsequently, with increasing radiation dose and time from treatment, deficiencies are seen in gonadotrophin, corticotrophin and thyrotrophin secretion, commonly in that order.[7] Thus patients suffer an evolving post-irradiation endocrine deficit which is dose- and fractionation-dependent, and hierarchical in nature

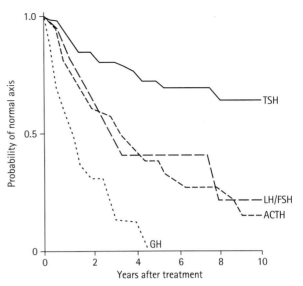

Figure 31.1 *Life-table analysis indicating probabilities of initially normal hypothalamic–pituitary target gland axes remaining normal after radiotherapy. ACTH, adrenocorticotrophic hormone; FSH, follicle-stimulating hormong; GH, growth hormone; LH, luteinizing hormone; TSH, thyroid-stimulating hormone.*

(Figure 31.1). A similar dose-dependent aetiology has been demonstrated in animal models,[18] but in the rat, thyroid-stimulating hormone (TSH) secretion is affected early, along with prolactin secretion, perhaps reflecting their common developmental origin,[19] whilst secretion of gonadotrophin and adrenocorticotrophic hormone (ACTH) secretion is relatively well preserved.[18]

Therefore, in summary, pituitary deficiencies are likely to be multiple, and manifest rapidly and completely in younger children, those receiving higher radiation doses and where tumours are centrally positioned. By comparison, deficits may be single, evolve more slowly or be qualitative rather than quantitative in nature after irradiation to more distant tumours or after lower cranial doses (Box 31.1). This will result in a cohort of survivors who may require hormone replacement therapy as adults, despite not requiring treatment as children.

GROWTH HORMONE DEFICIENCY

Growth hormone deficiency is the commonest endocrine abnormality following cranial irradiation. Short stature after cancer treatment has been well documented, particularly following cranial and craniospinal irradiation.[20] The effect on final height is more profound with treatment at a younger age.[21] The aetiology of short stature following treatment for childhood cancer is multifactorial and these issues will be discussed later, but GH deficiency has an important role.

Box 31.1 *Endocrine deficits following different doses of radiation to the hypothalamic–pituitary axis and recommendations for follow-up*

All patients

- Measure height at least 6-monthly until established normal pubertal growth spurt, then annually to final height
- Consider sitting height measurement
- Pubertal staging (including testicular volume in boys)

Dose of radiation to hypothalamic–pituitary axis
No radiotherapy
Monitor as above.

<24 Gy
At risk of:
- Early puberty
- Attenuated pubertal growth spurt

>24 Gy
At risk of:
- Growth hormone deficiency
- Early or delayed puberty
- Multiple pituitary hormone deficiency

Refer for endocrine assessment if:
- Height velocity <5 cm/year (i.e. falling off centiles)
- Suspicion of puberty at age <9 years
- Loss of harmony between growth and puberty
- Height <10th centile
- Dose to hypothalamic–pituitary axis >30 Gy
- Total body irradiation (at risk of skeletal dysplasia independent of GH status)

Risk factors
- Radiotherapy to CNS/spine (including total body irradiation)
- Brain tumours (even without radiotherapy)

As well as the effect on height, GH deficiency has also been implicated in causing a reduced lean body mass and increased fat mass,[22] metabolic abnormalities including an adverse lipid profile and glucose intolerance,[23] a reduction in bone mineral density[24] and impaired quality of life.[25]

Whilst other aspects of treatment and, indeed, the disease itself also play a role in the deleterious effects listed above, GH deficiency is important, and because of this, replacement with recombinant GH therapy has been advocated. This treatment has demonstrated an improved growth response in children with GH deficiency after cranial irradiation.[26]

In addition to the benefits observed in growth, replacement therapy has also been shown to reduce fat mass and increase muscle mass, reduce the cardiovascular risk factor profile, increase bone mineral density and improve quality of life[27–30] in adult survivors. However, it should perhaps be noted that many of the patients studied have had multiple, severe and long-term pituitary deficiencies.

It is now well accepted to treat documented GH deficiency in childhood with replacement doses of recombinant human GH. Unfortunately, the diagnosis of GH deficiency can be problematic, particularly in the early post-irradiation period.[11] Measurements of mean or peak GH secretion will miss deficits confined to qualitative, subtle disturbances in pulsatility and also those in which there is an inability to augment pubertal GH secretion adequately.[31,32] In addition, measurements of insulin-like growth factors and their binding proteins are unreliable indicators of GH secretion in this situation.[33] These difficulties make it imperative that all children are fully assessed following cranial irradiation and GH insufficiency considered.

Due to the evolving nature of GH insufficiency in these children, it is important that treatment with recombinant GH is commenced as early as possible in at-risk groups. Indeed, even if the cause of growth impairment is unclear, a trial of GH treatment may be appropriate.

Recombinant GH is usually given as a daily subcutaneous injection. Replacement therapy is normally discontinued once attainment of final height has been achieved. However, given the additional benefits of treatment discussed above, there is some evidence to suggest that replacement therapy, at a reduced dose, should be continued into adulthood.[34]

Growth hormone is, however, potentially mitogenic, and there have been concerns raised regarding its use in cancer survivors. There was concern that GH therapy could be associated with an increased risk of relapse of leukaemia and brain tumours.[35] In addition, a recent report has suggested an increased risk of colorectal cancer in adults treated with human pituitary GH prior to 1985.[36]

Lymphocyte natural killer activity is reduced in some patients with GH deficiency.[37] In addition, lymphocytes possess GH receptors, and therefore, if leukaemic transformation has occurred, GH therapy could potentially accelerate this process. However, much higher concentrations than those used therapeutically are required for this to occur.[38] Indeed, long-term studies of patients treated with physiological replacement doses of recombinant GH have failed to demonstrate any such increased risk,[39–41] although continued surveillance is essential. As discussed above, GH therapy should be commenced early to achieve a maximal response. However, in view of the concerns raised, most centres do not advocate introducing therapy within the first 2 years after cancer treatment, as this is the time of highest relapse rate.

HYPOTHALAMIC–PITUITARY–GONADAL AXIS

Gonadotrophin deficiency

With higher doses of cranial irradiation, damage to the hypothalamic–pituitary axis can also disrupt gonadotrophin secretion. Indeed, patients receiving radiation doses of 35–45 Gy have demonstrated subsequent deficiencies in follicle-stimulating hormone (FSH) and luteinizing hormone (LH) secretion.[5] In addition, as with growth hormone, the prevalence of gonadotrophin deficiency increases with time following irradiation.

The clinical sequelae of gonadotrophin deficiency exhibit a broad spectrum of severity, from subclinical abnormalities detectable only by gonadotrophin-releasing hormone (GnRH) testing, to a significant reduction in circulating sex hormone levels and delayed puberty.

As discussed earlier, the hypothalamus is more radiosensitive than the pituitary gland and therefore the aetiology of hypogonadism in the majority of patients after cranial irradiation is hypothalamic GnRH deficiency.[42] This opens up the possibility of using exogenous GnRH as replacement therapy with the aim of restoring gonadal function and fertility.

Early and precocious puberty

In contrast to the situation described above, it appears that, paradoxically, lower doses of cranial irradiation can cause premature activation of the hypothalamic–pituitary–gonadal axis, thus leading to early or precocious puberty. Precocious puberty is defined as the onset of puberty prior to the age of 8 years in girls and 9 years in boys, whereas early puberty is categorized as onset between 8 and 10 years in girls and 9 and 11 years in boys.

The precise aetiology of radiation-induced early puberty is thought to be via disinhibition of cortical influences on the hypothalamus. Before 1992 in the United Kingdom, all children with acute lymphoblastic leukaemia (ALL) received cranial irradiation as central nervous system (CNS) directed treatment, in order to prevent recurrent CNS disease. The dose used was 18–24 Gy, which is generally lower than that required to treat solid tumours of the CNS. Subsequently it has been noted that this treatment is associated with a higher incidence of early and precocious puberty, predominantly affecting girls.[43] Indeed, the incidence of early puberty in boys receiving cranial irradiation for ALL is no higher than in the normal population.[44] This is likely to reflect sex differences in the control of the onset of puberty. However, higher doses of cranial irradiation, such as that required for brain tumours, can lead to the early onset of puberty in both sexes.[45]

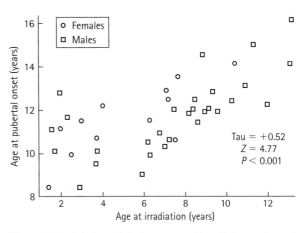

Figure 31.2 *Relationship between age at irradiation and age at pubertal onset in 41 children who received cranial/craniospinal irradiation for a brain tumour or irradiation for acute lymphoblastic leukaemia.*

Therefore early puberty as a consequence of cranial irradiation is dose-dependent, and the dose threshold of this effect is gender-specific. In addition, with higher doses of irradiation, a patient may enter puberty early but subsequently develop gonadotrophin deficiency, thus suggesting differential effects of radiotherapy with time. Treatments to delay puberty in this situation should therefore be used with caution.

The timing of pubertal onset is also related to the age of the child at the time of irradiation,[45] with treatment at a younger age resulting in more profound disturbances in the timing of puberty (Figure 31.2). The consequence of entering puberty early is a premature pubertal growth spurt followed by early epiphyseal fusion and a reduction in final adult height.

As discussed earlier, GH deficiency is common in patients who have received cranial irradiation. Although the duration of puberty is usually normal,[21,46] the combination of undiagnosed GH deficiency with early puberty further reduces final height potential by reducing peak height velocity.[46]

In addition to an overall reduction in height, growth in children after treatment is often disproportionate in that much of their height loss is due to a reduction in sitting height.[47] Spinal growth plays an important role during the latter part of the pubertal growth spurt, and early puberty coincident with undiagnosed GH deficiency clearly has a deleterious effect. In addition, irradiation involving the spine will further disrupt spinal growth, which will only partially respond to GH therapy. It has also been noted that the younger the child is at the time of irradiation, the greater the subsequent skeletal disproportion.[48]

As previously mentioned, GH replacement therapy is effective in improving final height. In view of the effects discussed above, if pubertal onset is early, it is also advantageous to suppress pubertal progression and delay skeletal fusion with GnRH analogues, in order to ensure height potential can be maximized. Indeed, combined treatment with GH and a GnRH analogue in this situation improves the height prognosis[49] and final adult height, although the height obtained remains lower than the target height.[50]

It is therefore essential that these patients are followed up indefinitely after treatment with regard to their growth and puberty. This involves 6-monthly clinical assessment of pubertal status and auxology measurements and, when indicated, biochemical assessment of GH and gonadotrophin secretion, and radiological assessment of their bone age.

FERTILITY

Whilst cranial irradiation can disrupt the onset of puberty or arrest its progress, the gonads themselves can be directly damaged by radiotherapy involving the spinal or pelvic area or by systemic chemotherapy. This damage may result in subfertility or infertility in both males and females.[51–54]

The effects of radiotherapy

The gonads are sensitive to radiotherapy, and the subsequent damage depends on the field of treatment, total dose and fractionation schedule.[54–57] Fractionation usually improves the therapeutic margin, but there is evidence to suggest that the gonads are an exception,[6,58] and that fractionation may be more harmful to gonadal function by reducing the time available for repair.

In males, doses as low as 0.1–1.2 Gy can have detectable effects on spermatogenesis,[55,56] with doses over 4 Gy causing a more permanent detrimental effect.[54,55] Somatic cells are more resistant to damage from radiotherapy than germ cells. Leydig cells, responsible for testosterone production in the male, are damaged at doses of around 20 Gy in prepubertal boys and up to 30 Gy in sexually mature males.[59,60] Therefore many patients will produce testosterone and develop normal secondary sexual characteristics, despite severe impairment of spermatogenesis.

In females, total body, abdominal or pelvic irradiation may cause ovarian and uterine damage and, as with males, the degree of impairment depends on the radiation dose, fractionation schedule and age at the time of treatment.[53,61–63] Depletion of primordial follicles is proportional to the oocyte pool, and therefore the younger the child at the time of radiotherapy, the larger the oocyte pool (Figure 31.3), and hence the later the onset of premature menopause, for a given dose of radiation. The human oocyte is highly sensitive to radiation, the LD_{50} having been estimated at less than 4 Gy.[61] Indeed, a recent study that provides a solution to the Faddy–Gosden

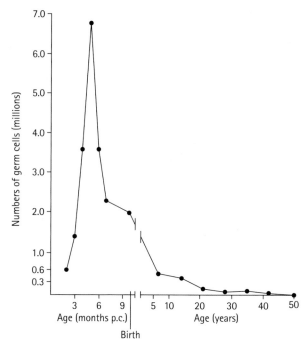

Figure 31.3 *The exponential decline of a fixed population of oocytes from the time of birth. p.c., post-conception.*

model of follicle decline in healthy women[64] estimates that the human oocyte is perhaps even more radiosensitive, with an LD_{50} of less than 2 Gy.[65] Premature menopause may be induced in women over the age of 40 years following treatment with 6 Gy, whilst significantly higher doses are required to destroy the oocyte pool completely and induce ovarian failure in younger women and children.[61]

Irradiation involving the uterus in childhood is associated with an increased incidence of nulliparity, spontaneous miscarriage and intrauterine growth retardation.[62,63,66] The mechanisms underlying these problems remain unclear, but reduced elasticity of the uterine musculature and uterine vascular damage has been suggested.[63,66] It is essential to counsel patients appropriately, and the obstetrician must be aware of the potential problems.

The effects of chemotherapy

Cytotoxic chemotherapy can damage the gonads, and the extent of this damage is dependent upon the agent administered, the age and sex of the patient, and the dose received.[52,67–70] A number of agents have been identified as being gonadotoxic, including procarbazine, cisplatin and the alkylating agents such as cyclophosphamide, melphalan and chlorambucil, although the relative contribution of each individual drug is often difficult to determine as most treatments are administered as multi-agent regimens (Box 31.2).

As with radiotherapy involving the testes, the germinal epithelium is more sensitive to the detrimental effects of chemotherapy than the somatic cells. Therefore, after receiving gonadotoxic chemotherapy, male patients may be rendered oligospermic or azoospermic, but testosterone production by the Leydig cells is unaffected and therefore secondary sexual characteristics develop normally.[71,72] Following higher doses of chemotherapy, Leydig cell dysfunction may also become apparent.[73]

Treatment of Hodgkin's disease has involved the use of procarbazine and alkylating agents such as chlorambucil and cyclophosphamide. Whilst this treatment leads to excellent survival rates, more than 90 per cent of male patients have subsequently developed permanent azoospermia.[67,71] Because of this, treatment of Hodgkin's disease has been modified in an attempt to reduce the gonadotoxicity.[74] Whilst procarbazine and alkylating agents are still used, cycles containing these drugs are alternated with cycles containing anthracycline agents, which, although potentially cardiotoxic, do not affect spermatogenesis. These 'hybrid' regimens result in significantly less gonadotoxicity.[75]

Although females are less susceptible to gonadotoxicity after chemotherapy, ovarian dysfunction is well recognized following treatment.[67]

Ovarian failure is seen in a significant number of females after treatment for Hodgkin's disease.[76,77] The causative agents again include procarbazine and the alkylating agents, and as with radiotherapy these effects are dose- and age-related.[67,76–79]

Long-term follow-up is essential for these patients as a significant number will enter the menopause early.[80] This has implications not only for fertility, but also for the additional medical complications of premature menopause, including osteoporosis.

Box 31.2 *Gonadotoxic chemotherapy agents*

Alkylating agents
Cyclophosphamide
Ifosfamide
Nitrosoureas e.g. carmustine, lamustine
Chlorambucil
Melphalan
Busulphan

Vinca-alkaloids
Vinblastine

Anti-metabolites
Cytarabine

Others
Cisplatin
Procarbazine

Potential for fertility after treatment

Due to the varied nature of the gonadal insult following chemotherapy or radiotherapy, it can often be very difficult to predict whether a child undergoing cancer treatment will subsequently have impaired fertility as an adult. The risk of subfertility can be categorized according to the type of malignancy and associated treatment (Box 31.3). However, this only represents an approximate guide and thus counselling children and their families with regard to future fertility can be very difficult. In addition, there are reports of patients having received sterilizing treatment who have subsequently demonstrated recovery of spermatogenesis or ovarian function,[81,82] which not only

Box 31.3 *Best assessment of risk[a] of subfertility following current treatment for childhood cancer by disease*

Low risk of subfertility
- Acute lymphoblastic leukaemia
- Wilms' tumour
- Soft tissue sarcoma – stage 1
- Germ cell tumours (with gonadal preservation and no radiotherapy)
- Retinoblastoma
- Brain tumour
  - surgery only
  - cranial irradiation <24 Gy

Medium risk of subfertility
- Acute myeloblastic leukaemia
- Hepatoblastoma
- Osteosarcoma
- Ewing's sarcoma
- Soft tissue sarcoma
- Neuroblastoma
- Non-Hodgkin's lymphoma
- Hodgkin's disease – 'hybrid therapy'
- Brain tumour
  - craniospinal radiotherapy
  - cranial irradiation >24 Gy

High risk of subfertility
- Total body irradiation
- Localized radiotherapy: pelvic/testicular
- Chemotherapy conditioning for bone marrow transplant
- Hodgkin's disease – alkylating agent-based therapy
- Soft tissue sarcoma – metastatic

---

[a]Low risk is assessed at <20 per cent, high risk as >80 per cent. Medium risk is difficult to quantify. Males are more susceptible to subfertility following chemotherapy than females, although females may be at risk of premature menopause.

---

has implications for counselling with regards to infertility, but also demonstrates the importance of discussing contraception with patients whose fertility status is uncertain. This also highlights the need for better long-term prospective studies of reproductive function in future childhood cancer trials.

Determining the impact of chemotherapy and radiotherapy on gonadal function currently involves regular clinical assessment of pubertal status, biochemical assessment of gonadotrophins and sex steroids, menstrual history in females and semen analysis in males. However, in prepubertal children, clinical assessment such as this is not possible and biochemical assessment is unreliable because the hypothalamic–pituitary–gonadal axis is relatively quiescent in this age group. Thus, it is currently not possible to detect gonadal damage early, due to the lack of a sensitive marker of gonadal function in prepubertal children.

There is currently much interest in inhibin B as a potential marker of gonadotoxicity in this age group. Inhibin B is secreted predominantly from Sertoli cells in males and developing antral follicles in females,[83,84] and plays an important role in spermatogenesis and folliculogenesis in adult males and females, respectively. There is evidence to suggest that gonadotoxic chemotherapy is associated with a reduction in inhibin B levels.[85] However, this relationship has not been clearly demonstrated in the prepubertal age group,[86] and it remains to be seen if inhibin B will become a useful tool in fertility assessment of these children in the future.

Offspring of childhood cancer survivors

Concerns have been raised that offspring of survivors of cancer may be more at risk of congenital abnormalities or even cancer. The mutagenic potential of cancer therapy could potentially cause problems in a fetus conceived with gametes produced after such treatment. A large epidemiological study has failed to demonstrate any such link,[87] except in those with familial malignancies. A recent study[72] investigated the integrity of spermatozoal DNA in men who had undergone treatment for childhood cancer. These sperm did not carry a greater burden of damaged DNA as compared with age-matched controls, which provides further reassurance, particularly with regard to the use of spermatozoa in assisted reproduction techniques following cancer therapy.

Fertility protection and preservation

Infertility after treatment for childhood cancer can have a huge detrimental impact as the patient enters adult life. Assisted reproductive therapy (ART) has developed extremely rapidly since 1978, when the first baby was born following such techniques, and there is now much interest in developing techniques to protect or preserve reproductive potential in the cancer patient.

As cytotoxic treatment acts predominantly on rapidly dividing cells, protection of male fertility has been attempted with hormonal manipulation, in an attempt to suppress the reproductive axis and induce testicular quiescence, thus protecting spermatogonia from the cytotoxic effects. Despite encouraging results in animal models,[88] application of this technique in human studies has thus far been disappointing.[89,90] Inter-species differences in spermatogenesis and optimal timing of hormonal intervention in relation to cytotoxic treatment may explain these disappointing results.

Preservation of fertility is obviously dictated by sexual maturity, and the only established options currently available are cryopreservation of spermatozoa in the male, oocytes in the female, or embryos in those with a partner. These techniques require time and can be problematic, particularly in the paediatric population. Sperm banking is not universally practised and there are few adequate 'adolescent-friendly' facilities. In addition, the specimens are often of poor quality, and this is further compromised by long-term cryopreservation. In postpubertal females, cryopreservation of oocytes is possible but inefficient, and storage of embryos is not applicable to the paediatric age group. In addition, both techniques require a stimulated cycle and a period of about 5–8 weeks.

Options in prepubertal children are limited and remain entirely experimental, but advances in assisted reproduction techniques have also focused attention on the possibility of preserving gonadal tissue for future use.[91–93]

In theory, testicular or ovarian tissue harvested and stored before sterilizing cancer therapy could be autotransplanted following cure, thus restoring natural fertility. Alternatively, stored tissue could be matured in vitro to produce gametes for fertilization with assisted reproduction techniques.

Procedures such as intracytoplasmic sperm injection (ICSI) now offer increased hope to men with severely reduced sperm counts and even 'azoospermia', provided the single sperm necessary can be obtained by testicular extraction.[94] Harvesting stem cells from testes before treatment, with subsequent autotransplantation on completion of therapy, has great potential, but much work needs to be done before clinical application of this technique.[92] Autotransplantation of cryopreserved ovarian cortical slices has yielded promising results in animal models, with restoration of ovarian function in sheep.[95]

Harvesting gonadal tissue for future use is an exciting prospect, but the technology raises a number of important ethical and legal issues. There are concerns regarding the protection of children's reproductive rights, and also about obtaining valid informed consent, both for storage and for future use of cryopreserved material. In addition, given the absence of proven therapeutic benefit and the potential risk associated with these procedures, together with the uncertainty of predicting infertility from new chemotherapeutic and reproductive strategies, it is questionable whether such experimentation is justified or ethical in children.[96] Of further concern with regard to autotransplantation in patients following treatment for cancer is the theoretical possibility of reintroducing malignant cells.

These issues must be addressed so that new techniques are adequately regulated.[97] This will ensure that children with cancer have a realistic and safe prospect for fertility in the future.[98]

THYROID DISORDERS

Thyroid disorders can occur following treatment for childhood cancer, either via disruption of the hypothalamic–pituitary–thyroid axis or following direct damage to the thyroid gland itself. The abnormalities can be of thyroid function, usually with hypothyroidism, or can manifest as thyroid nodules. In addition, there is a small risk of secondary thyroid cancer.[99]

Cranial irradiation can disrupt the hypothalamic–pituitary–thyroid axis, resulting in central hypothyroidism.[7] The incidence of radiation-induced TSH deficiency is dose-dependent[5] and this part of the axis appears to be the least vulnerable to radiation damage.[7,18] In children, disturbances of the hypothalamic–pituitary–thyroid axis are uncommon with doses lower than 40 Gy.[100]

The biochemical diagnosis of central hypothyroidism relies on levels of TSH and thyroid hormone (free T_4). However, there is some evidence to suggest that subtle abnormalities of thyrotrophin secretion, not detected in this manner, can be significant enough to have clinical implications. Thus TSH and free T_4 may fall within the normal range, yet more detailed investigation of TSH dynamics suggests clinically significant central hypothyroidism.[101] This damage may occur at lower doses of irradiation than that suggested above.

The implications of this may be important in deciding thresholds for intervention with thyroxine supplements, and this may be particularly important in the paediatric population as reduced thyroid function may affect growth[102] and physical and intellectual performance. Further work needs to be done in order to demonstrate the functional significance of these findings before the criteria for clinical intervention are modified. However, this again demonstrates the importance of follow-up and clinical vigilance in these children after treatment.

Thyroid abnormalities may also occur following direct damage to the thyroid gland itself. This is usually secondary to radiotherapy where the neck falls within the radiation field, including craniospinal irradiation, although chemotherapy can potentiate this radiation-induced damage.[103] Chemotherapy alone rarely affects thyroid function, although damage has been reported following intensive treatment with busulphan and cyclophosphamide,[104] as used for conditioning prior to bone marrow transplantation.

Hypothyroidism is the commonest abnormality following direct thyroid damage,[105] and this is usually initially in the form of compensated hypothyroidism with an elevated TSH and normal thyroxine. Despite this, thyroxine replacement may be justified in order to reduce the theoretical risk of thyroid cancer,[106] thought to be secondary to prolonged stimulation of the thyroid gland. Risk factors for developing hypothyroidism in this manner include higher doses of neck irradiation, female sex and older age at diagnosis. The greatest risk is during the first 5 years following treatment,[105] although other causes, such as autoimmunity, should also be excluded.

Hyperthyroidism is less common but can occur following neck irradiation, with those patients receiving higher doses being at greater risk.[105]

In addition to abnormalities in thyroid function, neoplasms of the thyroid gland, both benign and malignant, are more frequent following irradiation involving the neck.[99,107,108] The risk of developing thyroid neoplasia increases with higher doses of radiotherapy[109] and with younger age at the time of treatment.[110] In addition, females are at higher risk of developing thyroid cancer.[111]

Benign thyroid nodules include adenomas, focal hyperplasia and colloid nodules. Papillary carcinoma is the commonest thyroid cancer that develops secondary to irradiation,[111] which, if detected early, is associated with a high cure rate. Thus long-term follow-up of these children must include regular examination of the thyroid gland, and some advocate the use of ultrasound as a screening tool.[112]

HYPOTHALAMIC–PITUITARY–ADRENAL AXIS

The hypothalamic–pituitary–adrenal axis appears to be relatively radioresistant.[18] Abnormalities in ACTH or cortisol secretion are uncommon after low-dose cranial irradiation.[113] However, ACTH deficiency is potentially life-threatening, its symptoms are often subtle and it should be considered in patients receiving higher doses of irradiation, in excess of 50 Gy, and in those patients treated for pituitary or closely related tumours.[7] Lifelong replacement is necessary and is particularly problematic if posterior pituitary dysfunction is also present, such as after craniopharyngiomas.

As with the assessment of thyroid function, the incidence of abnormalities may be underestimated due to the diagnostic difficulty in evaluating the hypothalamic–pituitary–adrenal axis. In addition, clinical signs of cortisol deficiency can be non-specific and thus the diagnosis may be missed. The insulin tolerance test is regarded as the gold standard but can be problematic, particularly in the paediatric population, due to the consequences of severe hypoglycaemia, and must therefore be carried out according to rigorous protocols in units experienced in its use.

Excessive tiredness in a patient who has been treated with cranial irradiation should warrant testing of the hypothalamic–pituitary–adrenal axis. Hydrocortisone replacement is important, and increased doses are required for intercurrent illness and surgery.

Treatment of childhood leukaemia and lymphoma involves the use of corticosteroids as part of the chemotherapy regimen. The doses used are sufficient to cause suppression of the hypothalamic–pituitary–adrenal axis, although this is rarely associated with clinical manifestations of adrenal insufficiency.[114] However, if courses are inadvertently prolonged, consideration should be given to hydrocortisone substitution pending biochemical evidence of recovery being obtained.

OTHER PITUITARY HORMONES

Prolactin secretion is inhibited by dopamine from the hypothalamus. Cranial irradiation can disrupt this inhibitory control, resulting in hyperprolactinaemia. However, this is very unusual in children[115] and is unlikely to have any clinical significance.

Deficiency of antidiuretic hormone (ADH) secondary to cranial irradiation has not been described. However, central diabetes insipidus can be associated with childhood cancer, in particular with intracranial tumours involving the pituitary gland, or temporarily following cranial surgery in this region.[116] In addition, although a rare complication, diabetes insipidus has been described in association with acute leukaemia,[117] secondary to leukaemic infiltration of the pituitary gland. Despite treatment of the underlying malignancy, the hormone deficiency usually persists.

The syndrome of inappropriate ADH secretion (SIADH), with water retention and secondary hyponatraemia, has also been associated with malignancy, both from the disease itself and from aspects of its treatment,[118] although normally only in the short term and not as a long-term complication. The malignancies particularly associated with SIADH are more commonly seen in the adult population and include intrathoracic tumours, gastrointestinal cancers, breast and prostatic cancer and primary brain tumours. However, some treatments can cause SIADH in both children and adults, and this includes a number of cytotoxic drugs such as the vinca alkaloids, cisplatin, cyclophosphamide and melphalan. Other aspects of treatment, such as intrathoracic infection and artificial ventilation, have also been associated with SIADH.

Cerebral salt wasting, which can be severe in any child with a cranial insult, also causes hyponatraemia and a high urinary osmolality and can thus be confused with SIADH. However, unlike SIADH, it is associated with a large diuresis. Careful salt and fluid balance should be maintained in these patients and their cortisol reserve carefully assessed.

GROWTH AND BONE METABOLISM FOLLOWING TREATMENT OF CHILDHOOD CANCER

Impairment of growth is frequently seen following treatment for cancer in childhood.[20] Normal growth requires a complex interaction between the skeleton, the endocrine system and the overall health of the child, and thus the aetiology of poor growth following childhood cancer is usually multifactorial. Both the disease itself and the treatment, with chemotherapy, radiotherapy or surgery, can contribute to the deleterious effect observed.

Nutritional problems, reduced physical activity, disturbances in bone and mineral homeostasis, delayed or arrested puberty and psychosocial dysfunction all contribute to problems with growth and bone metabolism. As a consequence, children may fail to reach their height potential and are at risk of reduced bone mineral density, leading to osteopenia, osteoporosis and perhaps pathological fractures in later life.[20,119–121]

The effects of radiotherapy

We have discussed the impact radiotherapy can have on the endocrine system, and how the resultant disturbance can affect growth. However, radiotherapy can also exert a direct effect upon the skeletal system.

Spinal growth plays an important role in determining final height, and this may be compromised following radiotherapy involving the spine. This includes craniospinal irradiation,[48] total body irradiation,[122] and thoracic and abdominal irradiation.[123] Radiotherapy causes permanent disruption of the epiphyses, and the consequence of this on spinal growth results in skeletal disproportion, with a greater reduction in sitting height as compared with leg length. This effect is more pronounced the younger the child is at the time of treatment.[48] Cranial irradiation alone can also result in skeletal disproportion,[47] owing to the endocrine effects discussed earlier, although the consequences are less pronounced (Figure 31.4).

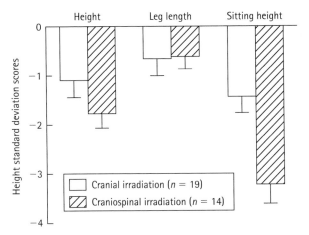

Figure 31.4 *Adult height without endocrine therapy of 33 patients irradiated in childhood for brain tumours.*

Scoliosis and kyphosis have long been recognized as complications of radiotherapy involving the spine.[124] However, with more modern techniques, in particular the use of megavoltage radiotherapy and symmetrical irradiation of the vertebral bodies, these complications are less frequent,[125] although they may still occur as radiotherapy can cause asymmetry of the paraspinal muscles. Thus radiotherapy can have a detrimental effect on spinal growth, and so sitting height and spinal curvature should be routinely examined as part of the follow-up for these patients.

In a similar manner, localized radiotherapy can disrupt the growth of a particular area of the body that falls within the radiation field.[126] This may result in skeletal hypoplasia and atrophy of overlying soft tissue, which can involve areas of the head and neck[126] or the extremities.[127] Whilst this may not affect overall growth, the problems encountered as a result can have a devastating impact upon the child.

The effects of chemotherapy

Chemotherapeutic agents generally target rapidly dividing cells. Because of this they may affect normal growth and bone activity.[119,128]

Growth has been extensively studied during and after treatment for ALL. ALL is the commonest childhood malignancy and, unlike many other cancers, is treated with ongoing chemotherapy of varying intensity over a prolonged period of time. With current UK protocols, treatment lasts for at least 2 years, extending up to 3 years in boys. Prior to 1992, cranial radiotherapy, to prevent CNS disease, was part of the management for all children with ALL. This is no longer used routinely and therefore the majority of patients will now receive chemotherapy alone.

Growth deceleration has been demonstrated during treatment for ALL, and this effect is most marked during the first year of treatment[129] and in younger children.[130] Different studies have reported growth decelerations of varying severity. Kirk *et al.*[131] reported significant growth retardation following treatment for ALL, with a mean standing height standard deviation score (SDS) of −1.37 at 6 years after diagnosis, compared with −0.44 observed by Clayton *et al.*[129] after the same time period. Varying intensities of chemotherapy protocols are likely to explain these differences, with patients from the former study having received treatment with the more intensive LSA_2L_2 protocol.

Obviously many of the longer-term studies, such as those discussed above, include children who received radiotherapy in addition to chemotherapy, and, as previously noted, this will have a detrimental effect on growth. However, studies investigating the role of chemotherapy alone have also demonstrated an impact on growth, although the magnitude of this effect is less marked.[132,133]

The impact of chemotherapy on the growth of long bones has been demonstrated by measurement of lower leg length during different phases of treatment for ALL.[134] In this study, growth of the lower leg was effectively stopped during periods of intensive chemotherapy. With less intensive 'maintenance' chemotherapy, the growth returned to a rate comparable to that of healthy children, and this was followed by a compensatory 'catch-up' period of accelerated growth velocity following cessation of treatment.

Thus catch-up growth does occur but only after chemotherapy is stopped, which may be up to 3 years after diagnosis. However, there is evidence to suggest that this catch-up growth tends to be complete in patients who receive chemotherapy alone, whereas those who have received radiotherapy still have a suboptimal final height in adulthood.[135,136]

Bone development is maximal during puberty, and peak bone mass is reached at around 20 years of age.[137] This can be disrupted by childhood cancer and its treatment. Indeed, a reduced bone mineral density (BMD), as measured by surrogate two-dimensional measures on dual-energy X-ray absorptiometry (DEXA) scans, has been demonstrated after treatment for childhood ALL[138] and other malignancies.[120] These surrogate measures need interpreting with care but any reduction in BMD is important. The aetiology of this is likely to be multifactorial and secondary to both the disease itself and its treatment. This can involve alterations in calcium absorption, vitamin D metabolism, insulin-like growth factors and their binding proteins, hypogonadism and GH deficiency.[139–143]

Various bone markers can be measured in order to assess the impact of chemotherapy on the dynamics of bone turnover and growth. In a prospective study of 22 children with ALL, markers of bone formation, bone resorption, soft tissue turnover and the GH axis were measured.[139] At diagnosis, bone turnover was low, probably secondary to GH resistance associated with the disease itself. During intensive phases of chemotherapy there was further suppression of the markers of bone and soft tissue turnover. However, these markers increased dramatically during periods of less intensive treatment.

Of the chemotherapeutic agents used, steroids and methotrexate have been particularly implicated in playing a pathological role in bone homeostasis.[139] Steroids cause retardation of bone growth, both directly (by decreasing osteoblast activity and turnover) and indirectly (by altering calcium homeostasis).[144,145] Decreased intestinal absorption and increased urinary excretion of calcium cause secondary hyperparathyroidism and, consequently, bone resorption. Methotrexate also inhibits bone growth, probably via inhibition of osteoblast proliferation and differentiation, secondary to folate deficiency.[146,147]

Other factors affecting growth and bone metabolism

As described earlier, the disease itself as well as its treatment can have a detrimental impact on growth and bone metabolism. In leukaemia, infiltration and expansion of the bone marrow spaces with leukaemic cells may destroy the spongiosa. In addition, the leukaemic cells themselves may secrete factors such as osteoblast-inhibiting factor and parathyroid hormone-related peptide, further contributing to the bone loss.[148]

In addition to the direct effects of the disease, other factors in these children are important. Poor nutrition, reduced physical activity and immobilization, prolonged hospitalization and psychosocial factors may all play a role in certain children, although the relative impact of each of these factors is difficult to ascertain.

Therapeutic intervention

Therapeutic intervention in endocrine dysfunction, e.g. with GH and GnRH analogues, may be essential in ensuring adequate growth after treatment for childhood cancer. However, of equal importance is the consideration of the factors discussed above, as these are all part of the long-term management of such children. Optimal nutrition, physical activity and psychosocial support are all vital for these children as they progress through treatment, if later morbidity is to be avoided.

Changes in bone homeostasis may predispose children to osteopenia, premature osteoporosis and possibly pathological fractures in later life. Assessment of calcium status and BMD at the end of treatment may enable early identification of these patients with impaired skeletal development and allow the institution of potential therapeutic interventions. Nutritional support, ensuring an adequate calcium intake, exercise to optimize body weight and physical fitness, and medical intervention with calcitonin, vitamin D and bisphosphonate treatment may all improve the BMD in these patients.[120,138]

OBESITY

Excessive weight gain is a recognized complication of certain childhood malignancies, in particular suprasellar tumours and ALL.

Obesity is frequently seen in patients with craniopharyngioma, with one recent study demonstrating severe obesity [defined as a body mass index (BMI) greater than three standard deviations above the mean] in 44 per cent of patients at follow-up.[149] The aetiology of this is likely to be multifactorial, although it appears to be associated with hypothalamic damage.[150] This results in hyperinsulinaemia secondary to disinhibition of vagal tone at the pancreatic beta cell, and may also result in insensitivity to endogenous leptin,[151] which normally inhibits appetite via hypothalamic receptors. In addition, increased bioavailability of insulin-like growth factor has been implicated.[152]

Obesity is well documented following treatment for ALL, and a number of risk factors have been postulated. Those children with ALL who received cranial irradiation as part of their treatment have an increased BMI as compared with their peers, and remain at significant risk of becoming overweight in adulthood.[153] GH deficiency is likely to play a role, but other important factors may include damage to areas of the brain that normally control appetite and body composition. Indeed, as with craniopharyngioma, higher leptin levels have been noted in these patients, which may reflect leptin insensitivity.[154]

Obesity after treatment for ALL has also been described in patients who have not received cranial irradiation,[155] although this has not been demonstrated in all studies.[153] The aetiology of excess weight gain in this patient group is likely to be multifactorial, and a number of risk factors have been suggested. Children with ALL are less active than their peers, both during[156] and after[157] treatment, and this appears to be one of the most important factors contributing to the excess weight gain observed.

Obesity in this patient group is also more pronounced in girls[158] and is more likely in those who are younger and thinner at diagnosis.[159] There may also be a familial contribution, with a significant number of obese patients having an obese mother.[160] In addition, pulsed steroids are used throughout ALL treatment regimens, causing a significant increase in energy intake, which further contributes to the prevalence of obesity in these children.[161]

Dietetic input is essential in these patient groups, in order to optimize nutrition and body composition. The importance of physical activity and a healthy lifestyle must also be emphasized.

CONCLUSIONS

The successful treatment of childhood cancer is associated with significant morbidity in later life. The major challenge faced by paediatric oncologists today is to sustain the excellent survival rates whilst striving to achieve optimal quality of life.

Endocrine dysfunction and complications of growth, development and bone metabolism form a significant part of this morbidity, and thus awareness of these complications with appropriate long-term follow-up and early intervention are essential in the management of these children. Involvement of all members of the multidisciplinary team, including oncologists, radiotherapists, endocrinologists, specialist nurses, dieticians and many others, is vital in the ongoing care of patients after childhood cancer treatment.

In the UK, strategies are being developed in order to define a comprehensive programme of follow-up,[162] together with the centralization of data to fully evaluate the late effects of childhood cancer therapy.[163] It is hoped that, in the future, treatment protocols may be further modified in order to reduce the impact of these late effects and subsequently improve the quality of life for these children as they progress into adulthood.

KEY POINTS

- As increasing numbers of children survive cancer, long-term side-effects of treatment are becoming increasingly important. Disorders of growth and the endocrine system are the commonest late effects observed in this patient group.
- Cranial irradiation can disrupt the hypothalamic–pituitary axis, causing widespread endocrine dysfunction. GH secretion is particularly radiosensitive, and thus deficiency of this hormone is the commonest abnormality following this treatment.
- Cranial irradiation can also affect normal pubertal progression. The combination of precocious puberty and GH deficiency can have a profound effect on the final height attained by these children and thus appropriate follow-up and treatment are essential.

- Fertility, in both males and females, can be affected by cancer treatment received prepubertally. This can be secondary to both radiotherapy and certain chemotherapeutic agents.
- The likelihood of reduced fertility in later life is very difficult to predict, although certain treatments, such as that for Hodgkin's disease and conditioning prior to bone marrow transplantation, are particularly gonadotoxic.
- Techniques that may protect or preserve fertility in these children are currently under investigation.
- Treatment for childhood cancer can also affect thyroid function, most commonly resulting in hypothyroidism. Secondary thyroid neoplasms have also been noted.
- Reduced bone density is described after treatment for childhood cancer. The aetiology of this is multifactorial and secondary to both treatment and the disease itself.
- Long-term follow-up in a multidisciplinary setting, clinical vigilance and awareness of the potential problems are of paramount importance in this patient group. We must aim to reduce the impact of late effects as these children enter adolescence and adult life.

REFERENCES

1. Mertens AC, Yasui Y, Neglia JP et al. Late mortality experience in five-year survivors of childhood and adolescent cancer: the Childhood Cancer Survivor Study. J Clin Oncol 2001; **19**: 3163–72.
2. Bleyer WA. The impact of childhood cancer on the United States and the world. CA Cancer J Clin 1990; **40**: 355–67.
3. Sklar CA. Overview of the effects of cancer therapies: the nature, scale and breadth of the problem. Acta Paediatr Suppl 1999; **88**: 1–4.
4. Constine LS, Woolf PD, Cann D et al. Hypothalamic-pituitary dysfunction after radiation for brain tumors. N Engl J Med 1993; **328**: 87–94.
5. Littley MD, Shalet SM, Beardwell CG et al. Radiation-induced hypopituitarism is dose-dependent. Clin Endocrinol (Oxf) 1989; **31**: 363–73.
6. Coggle JE. The effect of radiation at the tissue level. In: Biological Effects of Radiation. London: Taylor and Francis, 1983; 89–109.
7. Littley MD, Shalet SM, Beardwell CG et al. Hypopituitarism following external radiotherapy for pituitary tumours in adults. Q J Med 1989; **70**: 145–60.
8. Clayton PE, Shalet SM. Dose dependency of time of onset of radiation-induced growth hormone deficiency. J Pediatr 1991; **118**: 226–8.

9. Jorgensen EV, Schwartz ID, Hvizdala E *et al.* Neurotransmitter control of growth hormone secretion in children after cranial radiation therapy. *J Pediatr Endocrinol* 1993; **6**: 131–42.

10. Schmiegelow M, Lassen S, Poulsen HS *et al.* Growth hormone response to a growth hormone-releasing hormone stimulation test in a population-based study following cranial irradiation of childhood brain tumors. *Horm Res* 2000; **54**: 53–9.

11. Spoudeas HA, Hindmarsh PC, Matthews DR, Brook CG. Evolution of growth hormone neurosecretory disturbance after cranial irradiation for childhood brain tumours: a prospective study. *J Endocrinol* 1996; **150**: 329–42.

12. Lustig RH, Schriock EA, Kaplan SL, Grumbach MM. Effect of growth hormone-releasing factor on growth hormone release in children with radiation-induced growth hormone deficiency. *Pediatrics* 1985; **76**: 274–9.

13. Bercu BB, Diamond FB Jr. Growth hormone neurosecretory dysfunction. *Clin Endocrinol Metab* 1986; **15**: 537–90.

14. Ogilvy-Stuart AL, Stirling HF, Kelnar CJ *et al.* Treatment of radiation-induced growth hormone deficiency with growth hormone-releasing hormone. *Clin Endocrinol (Oxf)* 1997; **46**: 571–8.

15. Ogilvy-Stuart AL, Wallace WH, Shalet SM. Radiation and neuroregulatory control of growth hormone secretion. *Clin Endocrinol (Oxf)* 1994; **41**: 163–8.

16. Shalet SM, Beardwell CG, Pearson D, Jones PH. The effect of varying doses of cerebral irradiation on growth hormone production in childhood. *Clin Endocrinol (Oxf)* 1976; **5**: 287–90.

17. Brennan BM, Rahim A, Mackie EM *et al.* Growth hormone status in adults treated for acute lymphoblastic leukaemia in childhood. *Clin Endocrinol (Oxf)* 1998; **48**: 777–83.

18. Robinson IC, Fairhall KM, Hendry JH, Shalet SM. Differential radiosensitivity of hypothalamo-pituitary function in the young adult rat. *J Endocrinol* 2001; **169**: 519–26.

19. Dattani MT, Robinson IC. The molecular basis for developmental disorders of the pituitary gland in man. *Clin Genet* 2000; **57**: 337–46.

20. Muller HL, Klinkhammer-Schalke M, Kuhl J. Final height and weight of long-term survivors of childhood malignancies. *Exp Clin Endocrinol Diabetes* 1998; **106**: 135–9.

21. Ogilvy-Stuart AL, Shalet SM. Growth and puberty after growth hormone treatment after irradiation for brain tumours. *Arch Dis Child* 1995; **73**: 141–6.

22. de Boer H, Blok GJ, Van der Veen EA. Clinical aspects of growth hormone deficiency in adults. *Endocr Rev* 1995; **16**: 63–86.

23. Talvensaari K, Knip M. Childhood cancer and later development of the metabolic syndrome. *Ann Med* 1997; **29**: 353–5.

24. Kaufman JM, Taelman P, Vermeulen A, Vandeweghe M. Bone mineral status in growth hormone-deficient males with isolated and multiple pituitary deficiencies of childhood onset. *J Clin Endocrinol Metab* 1992; **74**: 118–23.

25. Stabler B. Impact of growth hormone (GH) therapy on quality of life along the lifespan of GH-treated patients. *Horm Res* 2001; **56**(Suppl. 1): 55–8.

26. Vassilopoulou-Sellin, Klein MJ, Moore BD III *et al.* Efficacy of growth hormone replacement therapy in children with organic growth hormone deficiency after cranial irradiation. *Horm Res* 1995; **43**: 188–93.

27. Murray RD, Darzy KH, Gleeson HK, Shalet SM. GH-deficient survivors of childhood cancer: GH replacement during adult life. *J Clin Endocrinol Metab* 2002; **87**: 129–35.

28. Pfeifer M, Verhovec R, Zizek B. Growth hormone (GH) and atherosclerosis: changes in morphology and function of major arteries during GH treatment. *Growth Horm IGF Res* 1999; **9**(Suppl. A): 25–30.

29. Longobardi S, Di Rella F, Pivonello R *et al.* Effects of two years of growth hormone (GH) replacement therapy on bone metabolism and mineral density in childhood and adulthood onset GH deficient patients. *J Endocrinol Invest* 1999; **22**: 333–9.

30. Lagrou K, Xhrouet-Heinrichs D, Massa G *et al.* Quality of life and retrospective perception of the effect of growth hormone treatment in adult patients with childhood growth hormone deficiency. *J Pediatr Endocrinol Metab* 2001; **14**(Suppl. 5): 1249–62.

31. Moell C, Garwicz S, Westgren U *et al.* Suppressed spontaneous secretion of growth hormone in girls after treatment for acute lymphoblastic leukaemia. *Arch Dis Child* 1989; **64**: 252–8.

32. Crowne EC, Moore C, Wallace WH *et al.* A novel variant of growth hormone (GH) insufficiency following low dose cranial irradiation. *Clin Endocrinol (Oxf)* 1992; **36**: 59–68.

33. Achermann JC, Hindmarsh PC, Brook CG. The relationship between the growth hormone and insulin-like growth factor axis in long-term survivors of childhood brain tumours. *Clin Endocrinol (Oxf)* 1998; **49**: 639–45.

34. Vahl N, Juul A, Jorgensen JO *et al.* Continuation of growth hormone (GH) replacement in GH-deficient patients during transition from childhood to adulthood: a two-year placebo-controlled study. *J Clin Endocrinol Metab* 2000; **85**: 1874–81.

35. Watanabe S, Tsunematsu Y, Fujimoto J, Komiyama A. Leukaemia in patients treated with growth hormone (letter). *Lancet* 1988; **1**: 1159–60.

36. Swerdlow AJ, Higgins CD, Adlard P, Preece MA. Risk of cancer in patients treated with human pituitary growth hormone in the UK, 1959–1985: a cohort study. *Lancet* 2002; **360**: 273–7.

37. Kiess W, Doerr H, Eisl E *et al.* Lymphocyte subsets and natural-killer activity in growth hormone deficiency (letter). *N Engl J Med* 1986; **314**: 321.

38. Zadik Z, Estrov Z, Karov Y *et al.* The effect of growth hormone and IGF-1 on clonogenic growth of hematopoietic cells in leukemic patients during active disease and during remission – a preliminary report. *J Pediatr Endocrinol* 1993; **6**: 79–83.

39. Ogilvy-Stuart AL, Ryder WD, Gattamaneni HR *et al.* Growth hormone and tumour recurrence. *Br Med J* 1992; **304**: 1601–5.

40. Swerdlow AJ, Reddingius RE, Higgins CD *et al.* Growth hormone treatment of children with brain tumors and risk of tumor recurrence. *J Clin Endocrinol Metab* 2000; **85**: 4444–9.

•41. Sklar CA, Mertens AC, Mitby P *et al.* Risk of disease recurrence and second neoplasms in survivors of childhood cancer treated with growth hormone: a report from the Childhood Cancer Survivor Study. *J Clin Endocrinol Metab* 2002; **87**: 3136–41.

42. Hall JE, Martin KA, Whitney HA *et al.* Potential for fertility with replacement of hypothalamic gonadotrophin-releasing hormone in long term female survivors of cranial tumors. *J Clin Endocrinol Metab* 1994; **79**: 1166–72.

43. Leiper AD, Stanhope R, Preece MA *et al.* Precocious or early puberty and growth failure in girls treated for acute lymphoblastic leukaemia. *Horm Res* 1988; **30**: 72–6.

44. Quigley C, Cowell C, Jimenez M *et al.* Normal or early development of puberty despite gonadal damage in children treated for acute lymphoblastic leukaemia. *N Engl J Med* 1989; **321**: 143–51.

45. Ogilvy-Stuart AL, Clayton PE, Shalet SM. Cranial irradiation and early puberty. *J Clin Endocrinol Metab* 1994; **78**: 1282–6.

46. Didcock E, Davies HA, Didi M *et al.* Pubertal growth in young adult survivors of childhood leukaemia. *J Clin Oncol* 1995; **13**: 2503–7.

47. Davies HA, Didcock E, Didi M *et al.* Disproportionate short stature after cranial irradiation and combination chemotherapy for leukaemia. *Arch Dis Child* 1994; **70**: 472–5.

48. Shalet SM, Gibson B, Swindell R, Pearson D. Effect of spinal irradiation on growth. *Arch Dis Child* 1987; **62**: 461–4.

49. Cara JF, Kreiter ML, Rosenfield RL. Height prognosis of children with true precocious puberty and growth hormone deficiency: effect of combination therapy with gonadotrophin releasing hormone agonist and growth hormone. *J Pediatr* 1992; **120**: 709–15.

50. Adan L, Souberbielle JC, Zucker JM *et al.* Adult height in 24 patients treated for growth hormone deficiency and early puberty. *J Clin Endocrinol Metab* 1997; **82**: 229–33.

51. Waring AB, Wallace WHB. Subfertility following treatment for childhood cancer. *Hosp Med* 2000; **61**: 550–7.

52. Whitehead E, Shalet SM, Jones PH *et al.* Gonadal function after combination chemotherapy for Hodgkin's disease in childhood. *Arch Dis Child* 1982; **57**: 287–91.

53. Wallace WH, Shalet SM, Crowne EC *et al.* Ovarian failure following abdominal irradiation in childhood: natural history and prognosis. *Clin Oncol (R Coll Radiol)* 1989; **1**: 75–9.

54. Speiser B, Rubin P, Casarett G. Aspermia following lower truncal irradiation in Hodgkin's disease. *Cancer* 1973; **32**: 692–8.

55. Centola GM, Keller JW, Henzler M, Rubin P. Effect of low-dose testicular irradiation on sperm count and fertility in patients with testicular seminoma. *J Androl* 1994; **15**: 608–13.

56. Clifton DK, Bremner WJ. The effect of testicular x-irradiation on spermatogenesis in man. A comparison with the mouse. *J Androl* 1983; **4**: 387–92.

57. Rowley MJ, Leach DR, Warner GA, Heller CG. Effect of graded doses of ionizing radiation on the human testis. *Radiat Res* 1974; **59**: 665–78.

58. Ash P. The influence of radiation on fertility in man. *Br J Radiol* 1980; **53**: 271–8.

59. Shalet SM, Tsatsoulis A, Whitehead E, Read G. Vulnerability of the human Leydig cell to radiation damage is dependent upon age. *J Endocrinol* 1989; **120**: 161–5.

60. Castillo LA, Craft AW, Kernahan J *et al.* Gonadal function after 12-Gy testicular irradiation in childhood acute lymphoblastic leukaemia. *Med Pediatr Oncol* 1990; **18**: 185–9.

61. Wallace WH, Shalet SM, Hendry JH *et al.* Ovarian failure following abdominal irradiation in childhood: the radiosensitivity of the human oocyte. *Br J Radiol* 1989; **62**: 995–8.

62. Sanders JE, Hawley J, Levy W *et al.* Pregnancies following high-dose cyclophosphamide with or without high-dose busulfan or total-body irradiation and bone marrow transplantation. *Blood* 1996; **87**: 3045–52.

63. Bath LE, Critchley HO, Chambers SE *et al.* Ovarian and uterine characteristics after total body irradiation in childhood and adolescence: response to sex steroid replacement. *Br J Obstet Gynaecol* 1999; **106**: 1265–72.

64. Faddy MJ, Gosden RG. A model conforming the decline in follicle numbers to the age of menopause in women. *Hum Reprod* 1996; **11**: 1484–6.

65. Wallace WHB, Thomson AB, Kelsey TW. The radiosensitivity of the human oocyte. *Hum Reprod* 2003; **18**: 117–21.

66. Critchley HO, Wallace WH, Shalet SM *et al.* Abdominal irradiation in childhood; the potential for pregnancy. *Br J Obstet Gynaecol* 1992; **99**: 392–4.

67. Mackie EJ, Radford M, Shalet SM. Gonadal function following chemotherapy for childhood Hodgkin's disease. *Med Pediatr Oncol* 1996; **27**: 74–8.

68. Wallace WH, Shalet SM, Lendon M, Morris-Jones PH. Male fertility in long-term survivors of childhood acute lymphoblastic leukaemia. *Int J Androl* 1991; **14**: 312–19.

69. Wallace WH, Shalet SM, Crowne EC *et al.* Gonadal dysfunction due to cis-platinum. *Med Pediatr Oncol* 1989; **17**: 409–13.

70. Watson AR, Rance CP, Bain J. Long term effects of cyclophosphamide on testicular function. *Br Med J (Clin Res Ed)* 1985; **291**: 1457–60.

71. Kreuser ED, Xiros N, Hetzel WD, Heimpel H. Reproductive and endocrine gonadal capacity in patients treated with COPP chemotherapy for Hodgkin's disease. *J Cancer Res Clin Oncol* 1987; **113**: 260–6.

72. Thomson AB, Campbell AJ, Irvine DS *et al.* Semen quality and spermatozoal DNA integrity in survivors of childhood cancer: a case-control study. *Lancet* 2002; **360**: 361–7.

73. Gerl A, Muhlbayer D, Hansmann G *et al.* The impact of chemotherapy on Leydig cell function in long term survivors of germ cell tumors. *Cancer* 2001; **91**: 1297–303.

♦74. Thomson AB, Wallace WH. Treatment of paediatric Hodgkin's disease: a balance of risks. *Eur J Cancer* 2002; **38**: 468–77.

75. Viviani S, Santoro A, Ragni G *et al.* Gonadal toxicity after combination chemotherapy for Hodgkin's disease. Comparative results of MOPP vs ABVD. *Eur J Cancer Clin Oncol* 1985; **21**: 601–5.

76. Waxman JH, Terry YA, Wrigley PF *et al.* Gonadal function in Hodgkin's disease: long-term follow-up of chemotherapy. *Br Med J (Clin Res Ed)* 1982; **285**: 1612–13.

77. Clark ST, Radford JA, Crowther D *et al.* Gonadal function following chemotherapy for Hodgkin's disease:

a comparative study of MVPP and a seven-drug hybrid regimen. *J Clin Oncol* 1995; **13**: 134–9.

78. Chiarelli AM, Marrett LD, Darlington G. Early menopause and infertility in females after treatment for childhood cancer diagnosed in 1964–1988 in Ontario, Canada. *Am J Epidemiol* 1999; **150**: 245–54.

79. Whitehead E, Shalet SM, Blackledge G *et al.* The effect of combination chemotherapy on ovarian function in women treated for Hodgkin's disease. *Cancer* 1983; **52**: 988–93.

80. Bryne J, Fears TR, Gail MH *et al.* Early menopause in long-term survivors of cancer during adolescence. *Am J Obstet Gynecol* 1992; **166**: 788–93.

81. Marmor D, Duyck F. Male reproductive potential after MOPP therapy for Hodgkin's disease: a long-term survey. *Andrologia* 1995; **27**: 99–106.

82. Nasir J, Walton C, Lindow SW, Masson EA. Spontaneous recovery of chemotherapy-induced primary ovarian failure: implications for management. *Clin Endocrinol (Oxf)* 1997; **46**: 217–19.

83. Anderson RA, Sharpe RM. Regulation of inhibin production in the human male and its clinical applications. *Int J Androl* 2000; **23**: 136–44.

84. Roberts VJ, Barth S, el-Roeiy A, Yen SS. Expression of inhibin/activin subunits and follistatin messenger ribonucleic acids and proteins in ovarian follicles and the corpus luteum during the human menstrual cycle. *J Clin Endocrinol Metab* 1993; **77**: 1402–10.

85. Wallace EM, Groome NP, Riley SC *et al.* Effects of chemotherapy-induced testicular damage on inhibin, gonadotrophin, and testosterone secretion: a prospective longitudinal study. *J Clin Endocrinol Metab* 1997; **82**: 3111–15.

86. Andersson AM, Muller J, Skakkebaek NE. Different roles of prepubertal and postpubertal germ cells and Sertoli cells in the regulation of serum inhibin B levels. *J Clin Endocrinol Metab* 1998; **83**: 4451–8.

87. Hawkins MM, Draper GJ, Smith RA. Cancer among 1,348 offspring of survivors of childhood cancer. *Int J Cancer* 1989; **43**: 975–8.

88. Meistrich ML, Kangasniemi M. Hormone treatment after irradiation stimulates recovery of rat spermatogenesis from surviving spermatogonia. *J Androl* 1997; **18**: 80–7.

89. Johnson DH, Linde R, Hainsworth JD *et al.* Effect of a luteinizing hormone releasing hormone agonist given during combination chemotherapy on post-therapy fertility in male patients with lymphoma: preliminary observations. *Blood* 1985; **65**: 832–6.

90. Thomson AB, Anderson RA, Irvine DS *et al.* Investigation of suppression of the hypothalamic-pituitary-gonadal axis to restore spermatogenesis in azoospermic men treated for childhood cancer. *Hum Reprod* 2002; **17**: 1715–23.

91. Brinster RL, Zimmermann JW. Spermatogenesis following male germ-cell transplantation. *Proc Natl Acad Sci USA* 1994; **91**: 11298–302.

92. Schlatt S, von Schonfeldt V, Schepers AG. Male germ cell transplantation: an experimental approach with a clinical perspective. *Br Med Bull* 2000; **56**: 824–36.

93. Newton H. The cryopreservation of ovarian tissue as a strategy for preserving the fertility of cancer patients. *Hum Reprod Update* 1998; **4**: 237–47.

94. Damani MN, Masters V, Meng MV *et al.* Post-chemotherapy ejaculatory azoospermia: fatherhood with sperm from testis tissue with intracytoplasmic sperm injection. *J Clin Oncol* 2002; **20**: 930–6.

95. Baird DT, Webb R, Campbell BK *et al.* Long-term ovarian function in sheep after ovariectomy and transplantation of autografts stored at –196°C. *Endocrinology* 1999; **140**: 462–71.

96. Spoudeas HA, Wallace WHB, Walker D. Is germ cell harvest and storage justified in minors treated for cancer? (letter) *Br Med J* 2000; **320**: 316.

♦97. Multidisciplinary Working Group convened by the British Fertility Society. A Strategy for Fertility Services for Survivors of Childhood Cancer. *Hum Fert* 2003; **6**: A1–A40.

98. Wallace WH, Walker DA. Conference consensus statement: ethical and research dilemmas for fertility preservation in children treated for cancer. *Hum Fertil (Camb)* 2001; **4**: 69–76.

99. Black P, Straaten A, Gutjahr P. Secondary thyroid carcinoma after treatment for childhood cancer. *Med Pediatr Oncol* 1998; **31**: 91–5.

100. Sklar CA, Constine LS. Chronic neuroendocrinological sequelae of radiation therapy. *Int J Radiat Oncol Biol Phys* 1995; **31**: 1113–21.

101. Rose SR, Lustig RH, Pitukcheewanont P *et al.* Diagnosis of hidden central hypothyroidism in survivors of childhood cancer. *J Clin Endocrinol Metab* 1999; **84**: 4472–9.

102. Rose SR. Isolated central hypothyroidism in short stature. *Pediatr Res* 1995; **38**: 967–73.

103. Livesey EA, Brook CG. Thyroid dysfunction after radiotherapy and chemotherapy of brain tumours. *Arch Dis Child* 1989; **64**: 593–5.

104. Michel G, Socie G, Gebhard F *et al.* Late effects of allogeneic bone marrow transplantation for children with acute myeloblastic leukaemia in first complete remission: the impact of conditioning regimen without total body irradiation – a report from the Societe Francaise de Greffe de Moelle. *J Clin Oncol* 1997; **15**: 2238–46.

●105. Sklar C, Whitton J, Mertens A *et al.* Abnormalities of the thyroid in survivors of Hodgkin's disease: data from the Childhood Cancer Survivor Study. *J Clin Endocrinol Metab* 2000; **85**: 3227–32.

106. Doniach I, Kingston JE, Plowman PN, Malpas JS. The association of post-radiation thyroid nodular disease with compensated hypothyroidism. *Br J Radiol* 1987; **60**: 1223–6.

107. Kaplan MM, Garnick MB, Gelber R *et al.* Risk factors for thyroid abnormalities after neck irradiation for childhood cancer. *Am J Med* 1983; **74**: 272–80.

108. Fleming ID, Black TL, Thompson EI *et al.* Thyroid dysfunction and neoplasia in children receiving neck irradiation for cancer. *Cancer* 1985; **55**: 1190–4.

109. de Vathaire F, Hardiman C, Shamsaldin A *et al.* Thyroid carcinomas after irradiation for a first cancer during childhood. *Arch Intern Med* 1999; **159**: 2713–19.

110. Ron E, Modan B, Preston D *et al.* Thyroid neoplasia following low-dose radiation in childhood. *Radiat Res* 1989; **120**: 516–31.

111. Inskip PD. Thyroid cancer after radiotherapy for childhood cancer. *Med Pediatr Oncol* 2001; **36**: 568–73.

112. Crom DB, Kaste SC, Tubergen DG *et al.* Ultrasonography for thyroid screening after head and neck irradiation in childhood cancer survivors. *Med Pediatr Oncol* 1997; **28**: 15–21.

113. Crowne EC, Wallace WH, Gibson S *et al.* Adrenocorticotrophin and cortisol secretion after low dose cranial irradiation. *Clin Endocrinol (Oxf)* 1993; **39**: 297–305.

114. Kuperman H, Damiani D, Chrousos GP *et al.* Evaluation of the hypothalamic-pituitary-adrenal axis in children with leukemia before and after 6 weeks of high-dose glucocorticoid therapy. *J Clin Endocrinol Metab* 2001; **86**: 2993–6.

115. Rappaport R, Brauner R, Czernichow P *et al.* Effect of hypothalamic and pituitary irradiation on pubertal development in children with cranial tumors. *J Clin Endocrinol Metab* 1982; **54**: 1164–8.

116. Wang LC, Cohen ME, Duffner PK. Etiologies of central diabetes insipidus in children. *Pediatr Neurol* 1994; **11**: 273–7.

117. Frangoul HA, Shaw DW, Hawkins D, Park J. Diabetes insipidus as a presenting symptom of acute myelogenous leukemia. *J Pediatr Hematol Oncol* 2000; **22**: 457–9.

118. Sorensen JB, Andersen MK, Hansen HH. Syndrome of inappropriate secretion of antidiuretic hormone (SIADH) in malignant disease. *J Intern Med* 1995; **238**: 97–110.

119. Ogilvy-Stuart AL, Shalet SM. Effect of chemotherapy on growth. *Acta Paediatr Suppl* 1995; **411**: 52–6.

120. Arikoski P, Komulainen J, Riikonen P *et al.* Reduced bone density at completion of chemotherapy for a malignancy. *Arch Dis Child* 1999; **80**: 143–8.

121. Haddy TB, Mosher RB, Reaman GH. Osteoporosis in survivors of acute lymphoblastic leukaemia. *Oncologist* 2001; **6**: 278–85.

122. Thomas BC, Stanhope R, Plowman PN, Leiper AD. Growth following single fraction and fractionated total body irradiation for bone marrow transplantation. *Eur J Pediatr* 1993; **152**: 888–92.

123. Wallace WH, Shalet SM, Morris-Jones PH *et al.* Effect of abdominal irradiation on growth in boys treated for a Wilms' tumor. *Med Pediatr Oncol* 1990; **18**: 441–6.

124. Riseborough EJ, Grabias SL, Burton RI, Jaffe N. Skeletal alterations following irradiation for Wilms' tumor: with particular reference to scoliosis and kyphosis. *J Bone Joint Surg Am* 1976; **58**: 526–36.

125. Rate WR, Butler MS, Robertson WW Jr, D'Angio GJ. Late orthopedic effects in children with Wilms' tumor treated with abdominal irradiation. *Med Pediatr Oncol* 1991; **19**: 265–8.

126. Larson DL, Kroll S, Jaffe N *et al.* Long-term effects of radiotherapy in childhood and adolescence. *Am J Surg* 1990; **160**: 348–51.

127. Gonzalez DG, Breur K. Clinical data from irradiated growing long bones in children. *Int J Radiat Oncol Biol Phys* 1983; **9**: 841–6.

128. van Leeuwen BL, Kamps WA, Jansen HW, Hoekstra HJ. The effect of chemotherapy on the growing skeleton. *Cancer Treat Rev* 2000; **26**: 363–76.

129. Clayton PE, Shalet SM, Morris-Jones PH, Price DA. Growth in children treated for acute lymphoblastic leukaemia. *Lancet* 1988; 1 (8583): 460–2.

130. Schriock EA, Schell MJ, Carter M *et al.* Abnormal growth patterns and adult short stature in 115 long-term survivors of childhood leukaemia. *J Clin Oncol* 1991; **9**: 400–5.

131. Kirk JA, Raghupathy P, Stevens MM *et al.* Growth failure and growth-hormone deficiency after treatment for acute lymphoblastic leukaemia. *Lancet* 1987; 1(8526): 190–3.

132. Sklar C, Mertens A, Walter A *et al.* Final height after treatment for childhood acute lymphoblastic leukaemia: comparison of no cranial irradiation with 1800 and 2400 centigrays of cranial irradiation. *J Pediatr* 1993; **123**: 59–64.

133. Ahmed SF, Wallace WH, Kelnar CJ. An anthropometric study of children during intensive chemotherapy for acute lymphoblastic leukaemia. *Horm Res* 1997; **48**: 178–83.

134. Ahmed SF, Wallace WH, Crofton PM *et al.* Short-term changes in lower leg length in children treated for acute lymphoblastic leukaemia. *J Pediatr Endocrinol Metab* 1999; **12**: 75–80.

135. Hokken-Koelega AC, van Doorn JW, Hahlen K *et al.* Long-term effects of treatment for acute lymphoblastic leukemia with and without cranial irradiation on growth and puberty: a comparative study. *Pediatr Res* 1993; **33**: 577–82.

136. Birkebaek NH, Clausen N. Height and weight patterns up to 20 years after treatment for acute lymphoblastic leukaemia. *Arch Dis Child* 1998; **79**: 161–4.

137. Kroger H, Kotaniemi A, Kroger L, Alhava E. Development of bone mass and bone density of the spine and femoral neck – a prospective study of 65 children and adolescents. *Bone Miner* 1993; **23**: 171–82.

138. Arikoski P, Komulainen J, Voutilainen R *et al.* Reduced bone mineral density in long-term survivors of childhood acute lymphoblastic leukemia. *J Pediatr Hematol Oncol* 1998; **20**: 234–40.

139. Crofton PM, Ahmed SF, Wade JC *et al.* Effects of intensive chemotherapy on bone and collagen turnover and the growth hormone axis in children with acute lymphoblastic leukaemia. *J Clin Endocrinol Metab* 1998; **83**: 3121–9.

140. Arikoski P, Komulainen J, Riikonen P *et al.* Alterations in bone turnover and impaired development of bone mineral density in newly diagnosed children with cancer: a 1-year prospective study. *J Clin Endocrinol Metab* 1999; **84**: 3174–81.

141. Halton JM, Atkinson SA, Fraher L *et al.* Altered mineral metabolism and bone mass in children during treatment for acute lymphoblastic leukaemia. *J Bone Miner Res* 1996; **11**: 1774–83.

142. Henderson RC, Madsen CD, Davis C, Gold SH. Bone density in survivors of childhood malignancies. *J Pediatr Hematol Oncol* 1996; **18**: 367–71.

143. Hoorweg-Nijman JJ, Kardos G, Roos JC *et al.* Bone mineral density and markers of bone turnover in young adult survivors of childhood lymphoblastic leukaemia. *Clin Endocrinol (Oxf)* 1999; **50**: 237–44.

144. Gaynon PS, Lustig RH. The use of glucocorticoids in acute lymphoblastic leukaemia of childhood. Molecular, cellular,

and clinical considerations. *J Pediatr Hematol Oncol* 1995; **17**: 1–12.

145. Atkinson SA, Halton JM, Bradley C *et al*. Bone and mineral abnormalities in childhood acute lymphoblastic leukaemia: influence of disease, drugs and nutrition. *Int J Cancer Suppl* 1998; **11**: 35–9.

146. Scheven BA, van der Veen MJ, Damen CA *et al*. Effects of methotrexate on human osteoblasts in vitro: modulation by 1,25-dihydroxyvitamin D3. *J Bone Miner Res* 1995; **10**: 874–80.

147. Uehara R, Suzuki Y, Ichikawa Y. Methotrexate (MTX) inhibits osteoblastic differentiation in vitro: possible mechanism of MTX osteopathy. *J Rheumatol* 2001; **28**: 251–6.

148. Halton JM, Atkinson SA, Fraher L *et al*. Mineral homeostasis and bone mass at diagnosis in children with acute lymphoblastic leukaemia. *J Pediatr* 1995; **126**: 557–64.

149. Muller HL, Bueb K, Bartels U *et al*. Obesity after childhood craniopharyngioma – German multi-center study on pre-operative risk factors and quality of life. *Klin Padiatr* 2001; **213**: 244–9.

150. de Vile CJ, Grant DB, Hayward RD *et al*. Obesity in childhood craniopharyngioma: relation to post-operative hypothalamic damage shown by magnetic resonance imaging. *J Clin Endocrinol Metab* 1996; **81**: 2734–7.

151. Roth C, Wilken B, Hanefeld F *et al*. Hyperphagia in children with craniopharyngioma is associated with hyperleptinaemia and a failure in the down-regulation of appetite. *Eur J Endocrinol* 1998; **138**: 89–91.

152. Tiulpakov AN, Mazerkina NA, Brook CG *et al*. Growth in children with craniopharyngioma following surgery. *Clin Endocrinol (Oxf)* 1998; **49**: 733–8.

153. Sklar CA, Mertens AC, Walter A *et al*. Changes in body mass index and prevalence of overweight in survivors of childhood acute lymphoblastic leukaemia: role of cranial irradiation. *Med Pediatr Oncol* 2000; **35**: 91–5.

154. Brennan BM, Rahim A, Blum WF *et al*. Hyperleptinaemia in young adults following cranial irradiation in childhood: growth hormone deficiency or leptin insensitivity? *Clin Endocrinol (Oxf)* 1999; **50**: 163–9.

155. Reilly JJ, Blacklock CJ, Dale E *et al*. Resting metabolic rate and obesity in childhood acute lymphoblastic leukaemia. *Int J Obes Relat Metab Disord* 1996; **20**: 1130–2.

156. Reilly JJ, Ventham JC, Ralston JM *et al*. Reduced energy expenditure in preobese children treated for acute lymphoblastic leukemia. *Pediatr Res* 1998; **44**: 557–62.

157. Warner JT, Bell W, Webb DK, Gregory JW. Daily energy expenditure and physical activity in survivors of childhood malignancy. *Pediatr Res* 1998; **43**: 607–13.

158. Odame I, Reilly JJ, Gibson BE, Donaldson MD. Patterns of obesity in boys and girls after treatment for acute lymphoblastic leukaemia. *Arch Dis Child* 1994; **71**: 147–9.

159. Reilly JJ, Ventham JC, Newell J *et al*. Risk factors for excess weight gain in children treated for acute lymphoblastic leukaemia. *Int J Obes Relat Metab Disord* 2000; **24**; 1537–41.

160. Shaw MP, Bath LE, Duff J *et al*. Obesity in leukemia survivors: the familial contribution. *Pediatr Hematol Oncol* 2000; **17**: 231–7.

161. Reilly JJ, Brougham M, Montgomery C *et al*. Effect of glucocorticoid therapy on energy intake in children treated for acute lymphoblastic leukaemia. *J Clin Endocrinol Metab* 2001; **86**: 3742–5.

♦162. Scottish Intercollegiate Guidelines Network. *Guideline 76: Long Term Follow-up of Survivors of Childhood Cancer*. A national clinical guideline. Edinburgh: SIGN, 2004.

163. Wallace WHB, Blacklay A, Eiser C *et al*. Developing strategies for long term follow up of survivors of childhood cancer. *Br Med J* 2001; **323**: 271–4.

32

Other organ sequelae

MICHAEL C. G. STEVENS & GABRIELE CALAMINUS

INTRODUCTION

The long-term consequences of successful treatment of malignant disease can be relevant to those of all ages but they are most important for those cured of cancer in childhood who will benefit most from life-years gained.[1] Reports of the frequency and severity of late effects of treatment vary widely, and accurate estimates of incidence and severity are difficult to define. Three key points need to be considered. First, although the definition of terms such as 'significant' and 'problem' as applied to the kind of issues which may emerge after successful treatment for cancer in childhood will vary according to the perspective of the person making the judgement, it is clear that this is not a trivial issue. Recent cohort studies have given estimates of the proportion of adult survivors experiencing problems of between 33 and 75 per cent.[2,3] The second issue is that the data available are influenced by the methods used to evaluate survivors. Systematic observations derived from large, representative populations are the ideal and the emergence of data from a large epidemiological study of cancer survivors in the United States (the Childhood Cancer Survivors Study)[4] will be enormously important in defining the scale of the problem more precisely. A similar study (the British Childhood Cancer Survivors Study) is now underway in the UK and has the added advantage that it is a population-based cohort study.[5] Thirdly, late effects of treatment may not only evolve with time from treatment for an individual survivor but they are likely to change with era of diagnosis as therapy has changed and survival improved.

Historically, early experience in paediatric oncology rarely concerned itself with the late sequelae of treatment: achieving survival was the primary challenge. As survival rates have improved, attention has been increasingly and appropriately directed towards a reduction in the consequences of the treatment itself. For example, in the treatment of Hodgkin's disease and Wilms' tumour, survival rates have been maintained despite a reduction in the overall intensity of treatment used for most patients. For many other diagnoses, however, survival rates have only recently been achieved at a level that justifies an approach which reflects this concern.[6]

Although detailed studies of defined groups of survivors are necessary to identify morbidity in relation to specific components of therapy, cause of death after apparent cure of the primary disease has been shown to be a useful proxy for important treatment-related late effects.[7] The number of deaths attributable to, for example, cardiotoxicity and second malignancy is a cause for concern and represents a target for reduction in the future. It is important to recognize that the greatest threat to survival beyond 5 years remains the inadequate treatment of the primary disease[8] and it would be difficult to argue other than that the principal efforts of the paediatric oncologist should still be directed towards the development and application of treatments to ensure cure. It is essential that the lessons learned from survivors of previous treatments are incorporated into the design of future strategies and it is inevitable that attention to the late sequelae of treatment will become an increasing responsibility for paediatric oncologists in the next decade.

Although many individual late effects are closely linked with specific forms of therapy, one of the challenges for the future will be to understand more about other factors that influence interindividual variation in the morbidity seen. For example, some of the variation in risk may be accounted for by individual biological or genetic susceptibility. This is best illustrated in studies of patients with second malignant tumours where some carry a predisposing germ-line mutation.[9]

A summary of known major sequelae of current therapies is given in Box 32.1.

Box 32.1 *Potential major non-endocrine long-term sequelae according to individual treatment risk factors*

All chemotherapy
- Dental caries
- Increased benign naevi

Actinomycin D
- Potentiates radiation damage

All alkylating agents
- Second malignancy
- Cyclophosphamide
  - Haemorrhagic cystitis/bladder fibrosis
  - Possible cardiotoxicity
  - Possible pulmonary toxicity
- Ifosfamide
  - Haemorrhagic cystitis/bladder fibrosis
  - Renal tubular and glomerular toxicity
- Nitrosoureas and busulphan
  - Pulmonary toxicity

All anthracyclines
- Cardiotoxicity
- Doxorubicin
  - Possible risk factor for second malignancy

Bleomycin
- Pulmonary toxicity

Carboplatin
- Ototoxicity (at high doses)
- Renal toxicity (at high doses)

Cisplatin
- Ototoxicity
- Renal toxicity

Epipodophyllotoxins
- Secondary leukaemia

Methotrexate
- Neuropsychological damage
- Liver dysfunction?

Steroids
- Cataract
- Osteoporosis

All radiotherapy
- Second malignancy

TBI
- Cataract
- Cardiotoxicity
- Pulmonary toxicity

Cranial
- Neuropsychological damage
- Leucoencephalopathy
- Incomplete hair regrowth
- Cataract

Head, neck and face
- Dental problems
- Cosmetic hypoplasia
- Cataract

Spinal
- Sitting height disproportion
- Scoliosis
- Pulmonary, cardiac or renal toxicity depending on field

Thoracic
- Cardiovascular disease
- Potentiates anthracycline cardiotoxicity
- Pulmonary toxicity
- Breast hypoplasia

Abdomen
- Liver, renal or bowel dysfunction depending on field
- Adverse pregnancy outcome

Pelvis
- Bladder fibrosis
- Adverse pregnancy outcome

Limbs
- Hypoplasia/asymmetry

Surgery
- Consequences are site- and procedure-dependent

SECOND MALIGNANCY

General risk and aetiological factors

Concern about the risk of second cancer ranks high in literature relating to the health of long-term survivors of cancer in childhood. It is only recently, however, that large populations of survivors have been followed up for long enough periods of time to allow the scale of the risk of subsequent cancer to be estimated with any certainty. It is still too early to identify the true lifetime risk and this will be likely to vary as changes in treatment exposure evolve with changes in clinical practice.[10] Recent estimates from the North American Childhood Cancer Survivors Study (CCSS) suggest a cumulative incidence of 3.2 per cent at 20 years from diagnosis of first cancer with an excess absolute risk of 1.9 per 1000 years of follow-up.[11] In a cohort of French and British survivors, cumulative risk of second cancer was estimated at 4.9 per cent at 25 years (although this excluded secondary leukaemia) and 7.7 per cent at 30 years.[12] The data suggest that, as time goes by, there is a decrease in risk for survivors relative to others of the same age in the general population (because background cancer risk increases with age); the actuarial risk increases with longer follow-up.

Risk of second malignancy relates both to the nature of treatment received and to possible genetic susceptibility. In the CCSS as well as in other paediatric cancer registries,[13] bone tumours and breast cancer represented the two most frequently encountered second cancer types and, after controlling for the impact of radiation exposure, the highest risk of developing any second cancer was linked to young age at diagnosis, primary diagnosis and exposure to anthracycline or epipodophyllotoxin chemotherapy. It is well recognized that risk relates, in part, to primary diagnosis. Survivors of Hodgkin's disease are at higher than average risk of second cancer,[14] as are survivors of bone and soft tissue sarcoma.[15,16] In contrast, survivors of childhood leukaemia are at relatively low risk if they have not received cranial radiation or significant exposure to alkylating agents or epipodophyllotoxins.[17]

Genetic risk associated with conditions such as hereditary retinoblastoma (in which, in particular, bone and soft tissue sarcomas occur with an increasing rate over time, especially in radiation fields) and neurofibromatosis type 1 is well described, representing the inactivation of tumour suppressor genes RB-1 and NF-1. Examples of other non-treatment-associated links between primary and secondary tumours which can be explained on this basis are those between sarcoma and breast cancer,[18] and between hepatoblastoma and colon cancer.[19] It is likely that other genetic polymorphisms will be identified in the future which may determine the relative risk of adverse sequelae following exposure to chemotherapy and radiation. These could interact with other environmental factors or lifestyle behaviours to create complex interrelationships governing the health of survivors, including their risk of a second cancer.

Radiotherapy

The role for radiotherapy in the treatment of many primary cancers is now considerably reduced, even for CNS-directed therapy in leukaemia, although there are many survivors who have received such treatment in the past. Nevertheless, radiation remains an important treatment for some patients who will remain at risk of second malignancy as a consequence. Variables include age at exposure, type of normal tissue in the radiation field, and total dose.

Doses from 12 to 60 Gy have been implicated in the induction of second cancer. Relatively low-dose exposure has been implicated in thyroid and CNS tumours whilst sarcomas are associated with doses greater than 30 Gy. A dose–response relationship appears to exist and one study suggested that exposure to a dose greater than 30 Gy conveyed a relative risk of secondary sarcoma 20–100 times that of the normal population.[20] Some alarming statistics have emerged in relation to risk in certain subgroups of patients. For example, data from studies of survivors of Hodgkin's disease have suggested that the actuarial risk of breast cancer in females who received radiation to the mediastinum may be as high as 33 per cent. Risks may be even higher in women who were exposed to radiotherapy during adolescence.[21] Interaction with chemotherapy, particularly alkylating agents and anthracycline drugs, has been implicated in the risk of secondary bone tumours associated with radiation.[22] Finally, second cancers induced by radiation are significantly more frequent in patients who have an established genetic predisposition to their first cancer – best illustrated by the known risk associated with hereditary retinoblastoma.[23]

Chemotherapy-induced malignancy

There are clear data to implicate alkylating agents and epipodophyllotoxins in the aetiology of secondary leukaemia.[24,25] There also appear to be characteristic clinical and biological differences which relate to the use of these two groups of drugs. These include a longer latent interval (median 4–7 years after exposure) and a demonstrable dose-effect relationship for leukaemia induced by alkylating agents, whilst leukaemia associated with epipodophyllotoxins occurs at a median of only 1–3 years and the risk is more likely to be affected by dose scheduling than by dose. Moreover, the finding of a chromosome abnormality involving 11q23 (the locus of the *MLL* gene) is frequent in leukaemia induced by epipodophyllotoxins, whilst leukaemia associated with exposure to alkylating agents may be characterized by deletions of chromosomes 5 and 7.[26]

Data relating to risk after exposure to other classes of chemotherapy are rare, but anthracyclines and anti-metabolites have been implicated. One study identified doxorubicin as a possible risk factor in secondary leukaemia,[27] and in a study of patients with secondary bone sarcoma, a history of exposure to anthracyclines appeared to reduce the latent interval of occurrence of the second tumour from the time of first diagnosis.[28] A recent study of secondary brain tumours suggested a possible synergistic role for anti-metabolite drugs.[29]

Surveillance

The mean latency for solid tumours after radiation is about 15 years and it is still too soon to know whether survival from childhood cancer predisposes to increased risk of some of the more common tumours in adult life. The implication is that there is a need for lifelong surveillance, creating important practical and emotional issues for the survivors and, in the case of those with known or suspected genetic risk, for the wider family. A balanced view needs to be provided from the follow-up clinic with opportunities for regular examination, screening tests and discussion of the risks. Healthy lifestyle advice, e.g. about smoking and diet, is sensible and worthwhile.

NEUROLOGICAL AND NEURO-PSYCHOLOGICAL SEQUELAE

There are now a considerable number of studies in the literature evaluating the neurological/neuropsychological sequelae of treatment for children with leukaemia and brain tumours. Particular areas of study have focused on the role of central nervous system (CNS) irradiation and the use of intrathecal (IT) methotrexate for CNS prophylaxis. More recently, attention has been extended to evaluate the impact of total body irradiation (TBI) given prior to bone marrow transplantation (BMT).

Experience from children treated for acute lymphoblastic leukaemia (ALL) has provided important insight into the risk of neuropsychological damage. Two groups of patients can be identified: patients treated with cranial irradiation with other forms of CNS prophylaxis (usually IT methotrexate) and the more recent experience of children who received CNS prophylaxis with chemotherapy (intravenous and/or IT methotrexate) without cranial radiotherapy.[30,31] Children treated with cranial

radiotherapy at doses between 18 and 24 Gy show a lower full IQ scale, verbal IQ and verbal comprehension, performance IQ and have impaired perceptual organization compared with patients receiving only IT methotrexate. These effects are most prominent in patients aged <3 years at the time of treatment.[32] Although young age at treatment is probably the most important risk factor at a given dose range,[33] dose itself is important, as indicated by the outcome for children receiving higher doses for treatment of brain tumours and for children who receive a second course of cranial radiation after CNS relapse.[34] The effect on neuropsychological performance of a reduction in prophylactic radiation dose from 24 to 18 Gy has not yet been adequately assessed and at least one early report concluded that the doses are equally neurotoxic.[35]

Most treatment strategies for leukaemia now avoid cranial radiotherapy for CNS protection and incorporate intravenous and/or IT methotrexate as the preferred form of CNS prophylaxis. So far, published data suggest that methotrexate alone does not cause significant cognitive impairment[36] but there is now possible concern from an observation that dexamethasone may play a role in the development of neurocognitive late effects in leukaemia patients.[37]

Children with brain tumours are disadvantaged by the direct effects of the tumour and by the consequences of surgical resection in addition to the use of radiotherapy and chemotherapy at high doses.[38] In one review, neurocognitive late effects were reported in 40–100 per cent of childhood brain tumour survivors.[39] Deficits are generally noted in the areas of intellectual ability, academic achievement, memory, attention, visual perceptual ability and language. Clinical experience suggests that brain tissue injury becomes increasingly apparent over the years after completion of therapy.[40] Tumour location plays an important role. Supratentorial tumours are associated with greater cognitive impairment than infratentorial tumours, even when whole-brain radiation was not used in the treatment.[41]

Most studies of neuropsychological functioning in paediatric brain tumour patients have focused on the sequelae of radiation therapy.[42] Overall IQ declines over a period of years after the end of treatment. One study of survivors of medulloblastoma who received radiation doses between 35 and 50 Gy showed that whilst 58 per cent had IQ scores above 80 at 5 years after radiation, only 15 per cent achieved this after 10 years of follow-up. Specific learning disabilities are also most common amongst children with brain tumours treated with irradiation.[43,44] For example, these children often struggle with mathematics, have attention and memory problems, and express difficulties with concentration and speed of thought.[45] Hemispheric tumours are possibly more likely to result in cognitive impairments and some have suggested that left-sided lesions are more likely to be associated with verbal or language-based deficits, whilst right-sided lesions are associated with visual perceptual deficits.[46]

A reduction of cranial irradiation doses below 24 Gy may reduce the incidence and severity of such sequelae,[47] but the challenge will be to establish whether this can be achieved without compromising tumour control. The severity of academic disadvantage experienced by children with brain tumours is clearly correlated with age at diagnosis.[48] It is also important to recognize that survivors of brain tumours may also experience important sensory and motor deficits or seizures that will contribute to their overall quality of life.[49]

Although chronic neurotoxicity from cranial radiation usually manifests as intellectual and educational difficulty, a small minority of patients develop leucoencephalopathy with severe intellectual, sensory and physical handicaps. The risk is greatest in those who have received more than one course of cranial radiotherapy, usually in combination with IT and systemic methotrexate.[50] Correlation of neurological outcome with structural abnormalities seen on computed tomography (CT) or magnetic resonance imaging (MRI) scans is notoriously difficult, although some studies report correlation between neurocognitive deficits and decreased normal white matter.[51] Leucoencephalopathy does not cause spinal cord symptoms but there is a risk of radiation myelopathy at particularly high doses (50 Gy) which may present with evidence of progressive cord damage.

Long-term neurological damage from chemotherapy other than methotrexate is very rare despite the recognition of various acute neurological effects. However, recent data suggest that a proportion of children treated for leukaemia have persisting fine or gross motor difficulties, possibly due to demyelinating lesions in peripheral nerves.[52]

Children who have undergone BMT may carry an additional risk of long-term neuropsychological toxicity, particularly following conditioning therapy involving TBI. Some studies have revealed a specific pattern of impairment in attention and memory,[53] and confirm the important adverse impact of young age at time of treatment.[54] More recently, reports have described a correlation with long-term cyclosporin medication. It is postulated that neurological abnormalities in long-term survivors of BMT can be associated with chronic graft-versus-host disease (GvHD) and the resulting immunosuppression.[55]

The major practical concern for the care of the child with any neurological/neuropsychological deficit is to maximize early rehabilitation by ensuring that appropriate assessments are undertaken and remedial help offered. It is particularly important to establish a close liaison with school staff and to ensure that educational expectations are not unrealistically diminished.

CARDIAC TOXICITY

Cardiac toxicity may arise as a consequence of exposure to radiotherapy or chemotherapy, or a combination of both. Overall, anthracycline drugs are the most frequent and important cause of cardiac toxicity in survivors of cancer in childhood.

Anthracycline cardiotoxicity

The cardiotoxic effects of anthracycline drugs have been recognized for some years, yet the natural history is still not clearly defined. Acute toxicity is rare but can occur during treatment or within months of completing treatment. It may present with heart failure or an abnormal rhythm state. These changes may either stabilize with treatment or evolve into chronic cardiomyopathy. The spectrum of long-term toxicity may range from subclinical dysfunction[56,57] to irreversible cardiac failure requiring cardiac transplantation.[58] The major concern in relation to the long-term surveillance of survivors is that late clinical cardiotoxicity can develop in apparently asymptomatic patients after an interval of up to 20 years.[59,60] One recent cohort study estimated a cumulative risk of clinical heart failure of 5 per cent within 15 years of starting anthracycline treatment.[61]

The mechanism of cardiac damage is probably multifactorial and not entirely understood, although free radical-mediated damage is probably the most significant element of the process.[62] The risk is clearly related to cumulative dose exposure. Whilst the anatomical damage (as revealed by endomyocardial biopsy) increases linearly with increasing dose, functional effects may be minimal for many patients although the risk increases sharply after dose exposure exceeds 500 mg/m^2.[63] Dose intensity, young age, female gender, pre-existing heart disease, cardiac radiation and length of follow-up are all important additional factors.[64] Additive exposure to cyclophosphamide has been implicated, particularly at higher doses,[65] although these data derive from relatively little experience. There is also weak indirect evidence to implicate the role of ifosfamide,[66] but this has not been confirmed.

The precise incidence of both clinical and subclinical myocardial damage is uncertain and critical review of the literature reveals considerable methodological criticisms in many of the studies published in this area.[67,68] The poor predictability of non-invasive monitoring techniques is of particular concern in children. Most experience relates to the utility of echocardiography. Other techniques to detect early evidence of myocardial damage have utilized cardiac treponin[69,70] and radionuclide scintigraphy,[71,72] but there is no clear consensus about their validity as predictors of late clinical toxicity.

Efforts to reduce the risk of cardiotoxicity include limitation of cumulative dose exposure and the use of alternative schedules of administration, anthracycline analogues and cardioprotective agents. Several studies have shown that reduced peak plasma levels, achieved by fractionating doses and utilizing continuous infusion schedules, can lower the risk of cardiotoxicity, although the long-term benefit of this approach has yet to be demonstrated.[73] Any attempt to modify the schedule by which anthracycline drugs are administered must also consider the potential for a reduction in treatment efficacy and the potentiation of other side-effects.[74] Most of the clinical experience in the published literature relates to treatment with doxorubicin and, to a lesser extent, daunorubicin. Epirubicin is the most frequently used of the other anthracycline analogues and, milligram for milligram, is probably less cardiotoxic.[75]

Serious interest in cardioprotective agents has mainly focused around the role of ICRF-187 (dexrazoxane). Data from adult studies support its cardioprotective properties. Paediatric experience is largely anecdotal although the data available support its value in reducing the risk of short-term subclinical cardiotoxicity.[76] No large randomized studies have yet shown definite proof of its value in paediatric practice[77] and additional studies with larger numbers of patients are needed to determine if any short-term cardioprotection will reduce the incidence of late cardiac complications in long-term survivors.

The most recent alternative approach to achieving a reduction in cardiotoxicity has been the evaluation of liposomal delivery systems for anthracycline (Dauno-Xome). Useful clinical studies of its efficacy in children are underway and its pharmacokinetic characteristics have been defined.[78]

The available data support the hypothesis that the administration of anthracyclines to children leads to a lifelong reduction in myocardial mass, the effect of which, with further growth, may result in reduced cardiac reserve. The implications of such effects are, first, the necessity to follow all survivors who have received anthracyclines with appropriate monitoring of cardiac function and, second, the need to offer advice about exercise and lifestyle. There may be an increased risk of cardiac decompensation when additional stress is imposed by factors as varied as growth hormone therapy, during the peak adolescent growth spurt, in pregnancy by hypervolaemic weight gain and the cardiovascular stress of vaginal delivery, or from certain types of exercise.

The optimal strategy for the long-term monitoring of patients who have received anthracyclines is debated. The cardiology committee of the Children' Cancer Study Group has published guidelines[79] that include advice about monitoring during therapy as well as the surveillance of survivors. These emphasize the importance of end-of-treatment echocardiography (performed within 3 months of the last anthracycline dose) in determining the frequency of subsequent surveillance. The recommendations include provision for an electrocardiogram (ECG) and echocardiogram every 2–3 years following therapy, and a radionuclide angiogram and 24-hour continuous ECG recording every 5 years. The latter investigation is included because of concern about dysrhythmia in addition to impairment of ventricular function. It is not clear that the risk is sufficient to justify this approach in all patients, particularly those who have a normal echocardiogram and who have not been exposed to high doses of anthracycline. In fact this guideline exceeds current practice in most centres in the UK, and possibly elsewhere. Standard ECG monitoring to detect prolonged QTc may offer a simpler screening method; this has been associated both with impending cardiomyopathy[80] and, in its congenital form, with sudden death from dysrhythmia. Ultimately, what is required is the development of an effective non-invasive method that can detect cardiac damage at the time of drug administration and will correlate with late outcome.

The best approach to the treatment of asymptomatic myocardial dysfunction is unclear but the use of angiotensin-converting enzyme (ACE) inhibitor drugs is now common practice in this setting, although long-term benefit remains uncertain. Treatment of established cardiac failure requires conventional management, but some patients have required cardiac transplantation for irreversible cardiomyopathy. Advice about lifestyle, smoking, obesity and diet should not be ignored.

Consequences of mediastinal radiation

Several reports suggest that mediastinal irradiation may not only potentiate anthracycline toxicity but can also predispose to premature coronary artery disease. One study reported the relative risk of death from heart disease to be 3.5 times greater after a dose of more than 30 Gy to the mediastinum.[81] In addition, radiation can cause constrictive pericarditis, although this is unusual at doses lower than 40 Gy, and at the highest doses, fibrous endocardial thickening affects heart valves. Overall risk appears to be dose-related but toxicity varies with fractionation and there may be a significantly lower threshold for single-fraction TBI and a higher dose tolerance when the cardiac field is incomplete. Damage probably occurs at a lower dose in children than in adults. In general, patients who have had doses to the mediastinum in excess of 30 Gy need to be advised about the risk of coronary artery disease, given appropriate lifestyle advice and encouraged to seek immediate advice if symptomatic. There are no established recommendations about ECG stress testing under these circumstances.

PULMONARY FUNCTION

Consequences of pulmonary radiotherapy

Pneumonitis followed by pulmonary fibrosis is a well recognized radiation response. The physiological changes noted in patients damaged by radiotherapy during adolescence or adult life are largely those of fibrosis, with loss of lung volume and reduced compliance. Functionally important late changes are more likely to occur in patients who have shown acute pulmonary toxicity. This rarely occurs at doses below 30 Gy when given by daily fractionation.[82] In contrast, the problems experienced by survivors of treatment given in childhood may also relate to restriction in the growth of the chest wall, as well as to the specific effects on the lung.[83] One early study of long-term follow-up of children treated for Wilms' tumour who received radiotherapy to the lungs showed that virtually all had evidence of restrictive lung disease,[84] but it is probable that children treated in more recent years not only received lower doses but were also treated with more favourable fractionation schedules.[85]

It is important to recognize that spinal radiotherapy fields may also deliver significant lung doses.[86] In the future, children surviving treatment with BMT and TBI may provide the most important group of survivors at risk of late pulmonary complications following radiotherapy, although other factors (GvHD, infection) also contribute.[87]

Chemotherapy-induced lung toxicity

A number of chemotherapy agents have been associated with pulmonary damage, of which bleomycin, the nitrosoureas and cyclophosphamide are likely to be of most concern.

The risk of acute bleomycin toxicity is typically associated with increasing cumulative dose, and may be potentiated by exposure to high levels of oxygen or coexistent infection. Such episodes may be fatal, but withdrawal of the drug may lead to reversal of the changes, although some patients will persist with X-ray and/or pulmonary function changes.[88] There has been little recent attention to this issue in the literature and no studies have linked acute bleomycin toxicity with late pulmonary toxicity.

Toxicity to BCNU is well recognized and dose-related. Evidence of fibrosis has been reported in over 50 per cent of patients receiving cumulative doses greater than 1500 mg/m^2.[89] Discontinuation of therapy may not prevent progressive deterioration. There are also reports of toxicity with other nitrosoureas and with cyclophosphamide, busulphan, melphalan and methotrexate.[90] Reports of reduced lung function in survivors of ALL suggest that multiple factors may be implicated.[91,92] Loss of lung volume from surgery for pulmonary metastatectomy may be an additional factor in some patients, particularly those surviving metastatic bone and soft tissue sarcoma.

There are no data addressing the potential additive role of environmental factors (smoking or occupational exposures) but it is logical to advise patients at risk to avoid such additional hazards.

GASTROINTESTINAL AND LIVER TOXICITY

Bowel toxicity

The overall incidence of late gastrointestinal toxicity is remarkably low given the frequency with which acute toxicity is experienced by patients during treatment. There is little or no evidence that chemotherapy causes important late gastrointestinal damage. Adhesions, strictures and malabsorption are all described consequences of radiation therapy. The risks appear to be dose-related but there is little in the literature relating specifically to children and, in general, experience of the consequences of radiation to the bowel must be extrapolated from data in adults. There is evidence to suggest that the risk of late sequelae is increased after the occurrence of acute bowel toxicity during treatment[93] and radiation may enhance the risk of obstruction from adhesions in children who have undergone laparotomy.[94] Overall, however, the incidence of problems in patients who receive radiation for Wilms' tumour is reassuringly low.[95] There may, however, be a small number of patients who survive after high-dose radiation to small fields, particularly in the pelvis, who have long-term complications including stricture and continence problems.

Resection of small bowel may theoretically raise concern about vitamin B$_{12}$ malabsorbtion, and diarrhoea may result from bile salt malabsorbtion. The risk relates to the extent of the resection and should be defined at the time of surgery.

Other causes of chronic bowel pathology include chronic GvHD following allogeneic BMT and the sequelae of serious infection (e.g. stricture after oesophageal candidiasis or typhlitis)

Liver toxicity

Chronic radiation damage to the liver is recognized and may result in fibrosis and portal hypertension.[96] The role of chemotherapy in the aetiology of long-term liver dysfunction seems fairly unimportant despite the frequency with which acute changes in liver function are encountered during treatment. Acute, severe and life-threatening hepatotoxicity (veno-occlusive disease) is encountered in a small number of children treated with actinomycin D and is being increasingly recognized in schedules incorporating high-dose chemotherapy with stem cell support.[97] The late complications of this have not yet been evaluated but earlier reports of this syndrome are reassuring.[98]

Hepatic fibrosis may arise from administration of methotrexate. The risk may be greatest in relation to chronic oral administration for prolonged periods and in this context the best evidence may derive from experience in non-malignant disease.[99] Despite histological changes, the risk of functional liver damage seems small. Earlier data suggest that the risk from weekly oral dose schedules or from high-dose intravenous methotrexate is also very low.[100]

In patients who have undergone BMT, chronic GvHD is the most likely cause of chronic liver disease. Symptomatic or subclinical liver damage may also be linked to transfusion-related infection (hepatitis B and C or cytomegalovirus). Long-term liver function is, of course, of particular concern in the small but increasing number of children who have undergone liver transplantation for hepatic tumours.

GENITOURINARY FUNCTION

Kidney

The consequences of unilateral nephrectomy (usually undertaken for Wilms' tumour) are rarely found to be important in clinical practice. Although a number of authors have documented an increased risk of hypertension, proteinuria and even mild reduction in glomerular filtration rate (GFR) in a minority of patients, the need for indefinite surveillance of renal function in this population is controversial, particularly when low-intensity chemotherapy has been used.[101] The requirement for very long-term follow-up of patients treated for Wilms' tumour will be influenced by the presence of other potential risk factors such as exposure to anthracycline drugs and the use of radiation.

Irradiation of the kidney is tolerated to doses of approximately 20 Gy (although tissue tolerance is less in very young children) and the risk of functional damage increases above this threshold. However, the use of higher doses to an abdominal field without shielding the kidney is unusual and important sequelae relating to renal function from radiotherapy alone are rarely encountered in practice. A more important issue is that radiation may be an additive risk factor for nephrotoxicity following certain kinds of chemotherapy (see below).

Cisplatin and ifosfamide are still the most important chemotherapy agents implicated in both acute and late renal damage. Published experience with very long-term

follow-up (i.e. greater than 20 years) is still limited for patients treated with these agents although there are ample data about acute effects.[102] Cisplatin causes both glomerular and tubular damage, the latter characteristically resulting in hypomagnesaemia. Partial recovery has been reported[103] and it is generally believed that, although the risk of damage is dose-related, it is not progressive once treatment has been discontinued.

There is a considerable body of work in the literature describing the acute toxicity of ifosfamide. Tubular damage (affecting both proximal and distal tubules) is the most frequent and clinically important element. This may result in severe renal loss of potassium, phosphate and bicarbonate and the full renal Fanconi's syndrome has been described. Bone mineralization can be affected and, in a very small number of patients, has been reported to progress to overt renal rickets.[104] Toxicity is dose-dependent although there is an element of individual susceptibility and the risks may be greater in young children and those who have been previously exposed to other risk factors such as cisplatin, renal radiotherapy or unilateral nephrectomy. The influence of administration schedule (short vs. continuous infusion) and mesna uroprotection are unknown, but the avoidance of cumulative doses above 60–80 g/m^2 is probably the most important way in which to limit risk.[105]

Other drugs, including carboplatin, high-dose cyclophosphamide and methotrexate, are also implicated in effects on renal function[58] and it is also important to remember that many drugs used in the supportive care of children receiving chemotherapy (e.g. aminoglycoside antibiotics and amphotericin) have an important renal toxicity profile which may be additive.

Bladder and urinary tract

Radiotherapy to the bladder can induce fibrosis with loss of bladder volume and disturbance of voluntary sphincter control. The effect is probably mediated via vascular damage to the bladder wall and depends on both the volume and dose of radiation. There is concern that this may also result in a risk of second malignancy. Radiation in early childhood may also interfere with the growth of the bladder, compounding the reduction in volume caused by fibrosis. Children with sarcoma arising from the bladder or other pelvic sites are amongst those most likely to require radiotherapy. The late functional consequences of their treatment may also reflect attempts at surgical resection. Problems with bladder capacity and continence are not uncommon.[106] Similar damage may affect the ureters and urethra, but radiation effects at these sites are likely only at very high doses. Patients who have received radiation to the bladder are not only at risk of bladder dysfunction but may have an increased risk of bladder malignancy, and cystoscopy should be considered whenever survivors experience haematuria.

Acute damage to the bladder from the effects of cyclophosphamide and ifosfamide is now largely abolished by the concurrent use of mesna, but there are many survivors of the pre-mesna era, some of whom may also have received pelvic radiotherapy. The consequences may be cumulative.[107]

Effects on other pelvic organs are less well described but fibrosis and growth impairment are characteristic of all radiation field injuries. Data from adults suggest that prostatic damage may have an effect on seminal ejaculate volume (and possibly function), and there is good evidence that uterine radiation has important long-term effects on pregnancy outcome.[108] Fibrosis and stricture of the vagina can occur after both surgery and radiotherapy and may require plastic surgical intervention.[109]

MUSCULOSKELETAL AND OTHER SOFT TISSUE DAMAGE

Damage to skeletal growth can follow even relatively low doses of radiation. The impact relates mainly to the total dose received but also reflects the size of the radiation field, dose per fraction and the age of the child at the time of treatment. Concomitant chemotherapy may accentuate the effect by enhancing the acute radiation reaction but rarely accounts for bone or soft tissue damage alone. Concern about bone mineral density and late osteoporosis is becoming more prominent,[110] particularly in survivors of ALL.[111,112] This is not restricted to those who received cranial radiation (who may therefore also be at risk of growth hormone insufficiency), and steroid therapy and reduced levels of physical activity are also implicated.[113,114] Recent reports of metabolic bone damage following ifosfamide-induced renal tubular toxicity represent another risk.

Limbs

Inclusion of epiphyses within the radiation treatment volume will have a major impact on limb growth and may predispose to the risk of slipped epiphysis. Osteonecrosis is rare and occurs only at particularly high radiation doses. Pathological fracture is unlikely except if there has been primary bone disease. Exostoses (osteocartilaginous outgrowths) are said to be relatively common within radiation fields but perhaps occur less frequently with megavoltage techniques and the risk of malignant degeneration is reported but rare. Lower limb length discrepancies, in particular, may require surgical intervention to prevent functional difficulties.

Spine

The risk of scoliosis from growth asymmetry is minimized by the practice of including the full width of the vertebral column in any radiation field including or adjacent to the spine, but unilateral hypoplasia or fibrosis of soft tissue may contribute to the development of a spinal curve. Regular inspection is required to detect and monitor the early occurrence of any spinal curvature and this is particularly important during the adolescent growth spurt. Disproportion in the sitting-to-standing height ratio arises when a significant length of vertebral column is irradiated, and the effects are maximal in children treated at a young age. It is estimated that a dose of 35–40 Gy to the whole spine before the age of 5 years may result in an average height loss of up to 16 cm.[115]

Craniofacial skeleton

Severe cosmetic damage can result from a radiation field directed to the face or orbit.[116] It is important to recognize that the consequent growth asymmetry will not be apparent to its maximal degree until pubertal growth is complete (see also 'Dental problems' and 'Visual problems' below).

Muscle and other soft tissue

Soft tissue hypoplasia after radiotherapy is difficult to quantitate and is usually associated with underlying skeletal damage. The overall effect is usually more cosmetic than functional, but fibrosis may restrict adjacent joint movement and cause pain. The developing breast may be damaged by relatively small doses of radiotherapy: 10 Gy will result in hypoplasia and failure of lactation, and over 20 Gy can ablate breast development entirely, requiring surgical augmentation in adult life.[117] Accelerated vascular degeneration is at least a theoretical concern when major arteries are included in radiation fields.[118]

Skin and hair

Alopecia induced by chemotherapy is almost always reversible but recovery after radiation therapy may be incomplete. Although this is unusual at the lower doses used for CNS prophylaxis in leukaemia (<24 Gy), it represents a problem for some patients treated for brain tumours to doses ⩾50 Gy. Skin pigmentation induced by chemotherapy and radiotherapy may persist but usually resolves slowly with time. Skin in radiation fields may appear thin and show increased telangiectatic markings. Both basal cell carcinoma and melanoma are reported as second malignancies following radiotherapy and sun exposure will recapitulate radiation damage and require appropriate precautions against sunburn. Children receiving chemotherapy are reported to develop increased numbers of benign naevi, the significance of which is uncertain.[119]

HAEMATOLOGICAL AND IMMUNOLOGICAL DYSFUNCTION

These are areas which have attracted little attention, given the importance of the changes in the bone marrow and immune function during therapy. The assumption is that these systems recover completely with time after treatment, but there is documentation of persistent subclinical bone marrow damage even after conventional chemotherapy[120] and similar changes are reported after radiotherapy.[121] These observations may be of relevance to the risk of treatment-induced secondary leukaemia.

Splenectomy during staging for Hodgkin's disease (now uncommon in clinical practice) is a long-term risk factor for sepsis although splenic damage from radiotherapy seems unlikely at doses below 20 Gy.[122] Reduction in both measures of humoral and cell-mediated immunity have also been reported after treatment for Hodgkin's disease, a risk which may be potentiated by total nodal irradiation. Prolonged immunosuppression is a major issue for survivors of BMT, especially those with chronic GvHD. Re-immunization is usually recommended, and revised guidelines for this have recently been issued in the UK.[123]

EYES, EARS AND TEETH

Hearing

Cisplatin is a well recognized cause of hearing loss and the effect may be potentiated by radiation, a particular risk in children receiving combined modality treatment for brain tumours,[124] although isolated radiation-induced hearing loss is rare. The long-term importance of cisplatin-induced deafness is likely to be more profound in children damaged in early life, before speech is fully developed, and in those whose loss extends below the high-frequency range. Augmentation with hearing aids may be helpful if there is significant loss below 4000 Hz. Carboplatin may have similar toxicity but only when used at particularly high dose. Some children experience problems with chronic otitis after radiation and middle ear drainage procedures may be required.

Visual problems

Chemotherapy is rarely, if ever, implicated in visual damage, except the well known association between steroid therapy and cataract formation. However, late radiation damage may affect all parts of the eye, the orbit and surrounding soft tissue. The most important consequences are cataract and dry eye.

Cataract formation depends on dose and fractionation but the lens is the most radiosensitive region of the eye and evidence of cataract may emerge within 2–3 years of treatment. In one report, 80 per cent of survivors of treatment involving TBI given at a dose of 10 Gy in a single fraction developed cataracts within 3 years, compared with less than 20 per cent of patients who were treated with 12–15 Gy in six to seven fractions.[125] Scatter from cranial radiation (e.g. for CNS prophylaxis in ALL or from the whole CNS field in medulloblastoma) may be sufficient to cause damage but direct doses for orbital sarcoma almost inevitably cause damage to the lens.[126] Careful radiotherapy planning and techniques to shield the lens, where feasible, are essential to minimize risk but cataracts do not always cause significant visual disturbance, their rate of progression is very variable and they can usually be treated surgically.

Dry eye is a consequence of damage both to tear production and to the cornea and conjunctiva. Trauma and infection must be managed aggressively and the use of artificial tear drops may maintain protection.

Dental problems

Direct irradiation to the mouth is damaging to developing teeth and to salivary glands and taste buds. As expected, effects are dose- and field size-related, but even patients receiving CNS-directed treatment may receive a significant dose to the parotid glands in addition to an 'exit' dose to the mouth from the spinal field. The combination of reduced salivary function, with dry mouth, and a direct dose to teeth may result in accelerated caries in addition to disrupted dental development. A generally deleterious effect of chemotherapy is recognized, including an increased risk of dental caries,[127] although this is not supported by all studies. Parents and patients should be instructed about the importance of good general dental care and oral hygiene. Children who receive high-dose fields direct to the mouth (e.g. those with head and neck sarcomas) should probably remain under surveillance in a specialist dental clinic.

PREGNANCY AND OFFSPRING

Despite reports of high fetal loss in some survivors, outcome of pregnancy is likely to be normal for all women except those who have received radiation to the abdomen.[128] One recent study reported an increased risk of low birth weight in babies born to women who had pelvic radiation.[129] These are likely to be women at high risk of infertility, in which case there is also concern that structural and vascular changes induced by radiation to the uterus could also limit potential for successful pregnancy after *in vitro* fertilization and embryo reimplantation.[130] There is no evidence that chemotherapy has long-lasting adverse effects on uterine function.

Current data are reassuring in relation to the risk of congenital abnormality or childhood malignancy in the offspring of children born to long-term survivors.[131,132] Detailed studies of offspring born to survivors using assisted reproduction are necessary in the future.[133]

PSYCHOSOCIAL ISSUES

Some studies which have examined adult survivors of childhood cancer indicate that the majority are in good health with a balanced psychological status, a normal social life and an adequate capacity to cope with daily life.[134,135] Nevertheless, several recent cohort studies have identified a significant incidence of measurable problems in adult survivors.[2,136,137] It is also clear that difficulties relating to less easily measured issues such as fatigue, social functioning, self-esteem and post-traumatic stress are identifiable,[138] even where the survivors have reported similar or significantly better levels of functioning in some areas than controls. It has been suggested that this might be a consequence of psychological mechanisms to compensate or even overcompensate for any objectively measurable consequences of surviving cancer in childhood.[139] The most important issue is that, although elements of the physical and neuropsychological impact of treatment can be measured in long-term survivors, there is relatively little information from survivors themselves about their perception of the impact of such problems on their lives.[140] Furthermore, the impact of the treatment experience itself and the way in which family and individual social functioning may have been changed as a result may have an impact on perceived quality of life, at both a subjective and an objective level. It is becoming more and more important to be able to measure the subjective impact of the illness and its treatment both in children with cancer and in survivors. However, the relatively low incidence of childhood cancer, the variety of types of cancer and of the treatment involved, and the wide age range at the time of treatment all contribute to the practical and methodological problems related to quality of life (QoL) assessment.[141,142]

Not all survivors carry the same burden. Survivors of brain tumours are seen to be particularly disadvantaged and QoL assessment in these patients also reflects the high frequency of neurocognitive dysfunction and motor and sensory neurological disability encountered in these patients. Another increasingly important group of patients are those surviving megatherapy and BMT. Potentially, they may have to carry the highest burden of late sequelae due to the cumulative toxicity of therapy received. These patients may also be affected by prolonged hospitalization and periods of isolation. Reassuringly, limited data suggest that QoL after megatherapy and autologous bone marrow rescue was judged to be good by a majority of survivors.[143] A recent large study of survivors of ALL and Wilms' tumour suggested no increase in psychiatric disorder when compared with a control group, but there was still evidence of poorer functioning in the area of relationships and friendships.[144]

It is important to recognize that surviving treatment for cancer in childhood is not necessarily an entirely negative experience at an individual level and that positive aspects of survival are well documented.[145] Nevertheless there is good evidence that some survivors experience practical difficulties in adult life, including problems with employment and insurability. In this respect there is an important advocacy role for health professionals in minimizing any discrimination that may be experienced by survivors. The importance of educational achievement on self-esteem, employability and earnings potential justifies considerable effort to ensure that schooling is supported at the time of treatment and thereafter. One of the major barriers to this has been the unnecessarily lowered expectations of teachers and the over-protectiveness of parents, but there are many examples of educational intervention programmes which seek to resolve this.

Empowering survivors to cope with real or perceived, actual or potential problems requires a clear strategy for their education about the treatment they received and its implications. Strategies include emphasis on 'exit' interviews at the end of treatment and during adolescence and the provision of written information containing details of the individual's disease and treatment history, including recommendations for follow-up.[146] For most patients this should form part of an ongoing contact with a long-term follow-up programme, the aim of which is to continue to support and inform survivors whilst collecting long-term data that will be important in influencing the design of future treatments and in advising later cohorts of survivors.

PROGRAMMES OF CARE FOR SURVIVORS

Given the range of potential complications that may emerge after successful treatment for cancer in childhood, it would be reasonable to assume that programmes should be available that undertake systematic surveillance of survivors and offer appropriate opportunities for education, screening and intervention. In fact, there are remarkably few published guidelines for follow-up and, where these exist, content is often somewhat empirical.[147,148] There are also few clear models for the optimal structure of follow-up programmes, particularly as there is uncertainty about the role of adult cancer services and a blurring of responsibility between paediatric and adult-based care.[149]

When determining a plan for the long-term follow-up of an individual patient, the surveillance strategy should be based on the treatment actually received (Figure 32.1). A record of cumulative drug and radiation exposures and details of significant surgical interventions should be compiled at the end of treatment and the follow-up plan matched to the risk factors thus identified.

Although it is common practice for most survivors to remain under long-term surveillance, it is not clear whether this policy is justified in all cases.[150] Nevertheless, it is important that sufficient data are collected to ensure that the true cost of cure can be defined and that systems evolve that provide appropriate transition for adult survivors from paediatric to adult health care settings. One of the key challenges to be met is to ensure that all survivors receive sufficient information to allow them to make choices about their future care. Evidence so far suggests that this needs to be improved.[151] There is

also valuable experience to highlight the important role that specialist nurses can contribute to the care and education of survivors.[152]

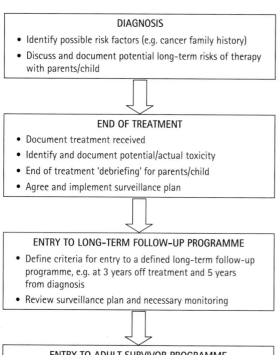

Figure 32.1 *Possible approach to the organization of long-term follow-up.*

KEY POINTS

- Surveillance strategies for survivors should be defined according to treatment actually received, and the presence of known predisposing risk factors. Better models of care are required to define the optimal structure of follow-up programmes for adult survivors.
- The ultimate impact of any late effect of treatment will depend, to a significant effect, on the perspective of the person making the judgement. More work is needed to develop tools to assess the quality of life of survivors.
- Data from earlier literature is frequently based on anecdotal clinical experience or derived from selected populations. There is a need to obtain more information from the systematic study of large-scale, preferably population-based, cohorts of survivors.
- Second malignancy remains one the most serious risks facing survivors of cancer in childhood. Risks are significantly higher relative to those of the same age in the general population and the cumulative incidence is probably between 3 and 5 per cent after 20 years' follow-up.
- Survivors of brain tumours are significantly more disadvantaged than those with other diagnoses. The reasons include the risk of neuropsychological sequelae from cranial radiation and the significant possibility of motor and sensory neurological disability experienced by these patients.
- Survivors of therapy including allogeneic BMT potentially carry the heaviest burden and are at risk of multi-organ damage.
- The precise incidence of subclinical and clinical cardiac toxicity following treatment with anthracycline drugs is uncertain. Effective, non-invasive techniques are needed to detect cardiac damage during treatment and to correlate this with late outcome.

REFERENCES

1. Donaldson SS. Lessons from our children. *Int J Radiat Oncol Biol Phys* 1993; **26**: 739–49.
2. Stevens MCG, Mahler H, Parkes S. The health status of adult survivors of childhood cancer. *Eur J Cancer* 1998; **34**: 694–8

3. Lackner H, Benesch M, Schagerl S et al. Prospective evaluation of late effects after childhood cancer therapy with a follow up of over 9 years. Eur J Pediatr 2000; **159**: 750–8.

4. Robison LL, Mertens AC, Boice JD et al. Study design and cohort characteristics of the Childhood Cancer Survivor Study: a multi institutional collaborative project. Med Pediatr Oncol 2002; **38**: 229–39.

◆5. Hawkins MM, Stevens MCG. The long term survivors. Br Med Bull 1996; **52**: 898–923.

6. Stiller CA. Population based survival rates for childhood cancer in Britain. 1980–91. Br Med J 1994; **309**: 1612–16.

7. Hawkins MM, Kingston JE, Kinnier Wilson LM. Late deaths after treatment for childhood cancer. Arch Dis Child 1990; **65**: 1356–63.

8. Robertson CM, Hawkins MM, Kingston JE. Late deaths and survival after childhood cancer. Br Med J 1994; **309**: 162–6.

9. Malkin D, Jolly KW, Barbier N et al. Germ line mutation of the p53 suppressor gene in children and young adults with second malignant neoplasms. N Engl J Med 1992; **326**: 1309–15.

◆10. Meadows AT. Second tumours. Eur J Cancer 2001; **37**: 2074–81.

11. Neglia JP, Friedman DL, Yasuy Y et al. Second malignant neoplasms in five year survivors of childhood cancer: a report from the Childhood Cancer Survivors Study. J Natl Cancer Inst 2001; **93**: 618–29.

12. De Vathaire F, Hawkins M, Campbell S et al. Second malignant neoplasms after a first cancer in childhood: temporal pattern of risk according to type of treatment. B J Cancer 1999; **79**: 1884–93.

13. Kaatsch P, Haaf G, Michaelis J. Childhood malignancies in Germany – methods and results of a nationwide registry. Eur J Cancer 1995; **31A**: 993–9.

14. Sankila R, Garwicz S, Olsen JH et al. Risk of subsequent malignant neoplasms among 1,641 Hodgkin's disease patients diagnosed in childhood and adolescence: a population based study in the five Nordic countries. Association of Nordic Cancer registries and the Nordic Society of Pediatric Hematology and Oncology. J Clin Oncol 1996; **14**: 1442–6.

15. Tucker MA, D'Angio GJ, Boice JD et al. Bone sarcomas linked to radiotherapy and chemotherapy in children. N Engl J Med 1991; **317**: 588–93.

16. Heyn R, Haeberlen V, Newton WA et al. Second malignant neoplasms in children treated for rhabdomyosarcoma. J Clin Oncol 1993; **11**: 262–70.

17. Loning L, Zimmermann M, Reiter A et al. Secondary neoplasms subsequent to Berlin-Frankfurt-Munster therapy of acute lymphoblastic leukemia in childhood: significantly lower risk without cranial radiotherapy. Blood 2000; **95**: 2770–5.

18. Varley KM, McGowan G, Thorncroft M et al. Germline mutations of TP53 in Li-Fraumeni families: an extended study of 39 families. Cancer Res 1997; **57**: 3245–52.

19. Garber JE, Li FG, Kingston JE et al. Hepatoblastoma and familial adenomatous polyposis. J Natl Cancer Inst 1988; **80**: 1626–8.

20. Paulussen M, Ahrens S, Lehnert M et al. Second malignancies after Ewing tumor treatment in 690 patients from a cooperative German/Austrian/Dutch study. Ann Oncol 2001; **12**: 1619–30

21. Bhatia S, Robison LL, Oberlin O et al. Breast cancer and other second neoplasms following childhood Hodgkin's disease: a report from the Late Effects Study Group. N Engl J Med 1996; **33**: 745–51.

22. Hawkins MM, Kinnier Wilson LM, Burton HS et al. Radiotherapy, alkylating agents and the risk of bone cancer after childhood cancer. J Natl Cancer Inst 1996; **88**: 270–8.

23. Wong FL, Boice JD, Abramson DH. Cancer incidence after retinoblastoma: radiation dose and sarcoma risk. J Am Med Assoc 1997; **278**: 1262–7.

24. Hawkins MM, Kinnear-Wilson M, Stovall MA et al. Epipodophylollotoxins, alkylating agents and radiation and risk of secondary leukaemia after childhood cancer. Br Med J 1992; **304**: 951–8.

25. Pui CH, Ribiero RC, Hancock ML et al. Acute myeloid leukemia in children treated with epipodophyllotoxins for acute lymphoblastic leukaemia. N Engl J Med 1991; **325**: 1682–7.

26. Bhatia S, Davies SM, Robison LL. Leukemia. In: Neugut AI, Meadows AT, Robinson E, eds. Multiple Primary Cancers. Philadelphia: Lippincott Williams and Wilkins, 1999; 257–75.

27. Tucker MA, Meadows AT, Boice JD. Leukemia after therapy with alkylating agents for childhood cancer. J Natl Cancer Inst 1987; **78**: 459–64.

28. Newton WA, Meadows AT, Shimada H et al. Bone sarcomas as second malignant neoplasms following childhood cancer. Cancer 1991; **67**: 193–201

29. Relling RV, Rubnitz JE, Rivera GK et al. High incidence of secondary brain tumours after radiotherapy and antimetabolites. Lancet 1999; **354**: 34–9.

30. Langer T, Martus P, Ottensmeier H et al. CNS late-effects after ALL therapy in childhood. Part III: neuropsychological performance in long-term survivors of childhood ALL: impairments of concentration, attention, and memory. Med Pediatr Oncol 2002; **38**: 320–8.

31. Hill JM, Kornblith AB, Jones D et al. A comparative study of the long term psychosocial functioning of childhood acute lymphoblastic leukemia survivors treated by intrathecal methotrexate with or without cranial radiation. Cancer 1998; **82**: 208–18.

32. Waber DP, Shapiro BL, Carpentieri SC et al. Excellent therapeutic efficacy and minimal late neurotoxicity in children treated with 18 grays of cranial radiation therapy for high-risk acute lymphoblastic leukemia: a 7-year follow-up study of the Dana-Farber Cancer Institute Consortium Protocol 87–01. Cancer 2001; **92**: 15–22.

33. Jannoun L. Are cognitive and educational development affected by age at which prophylactic therapy is given in acute lymphoblastic leukaemia? Arch Dis Child 1983; **58**: 953–8.

34. Longeway K, Mulhern R, Crisco J et al. Treatment of meningeal relapse in childhood acute lymphoblastic leukemia: II. A prospective study of intellectual loss specific to CNS relapse and therapy. Am J Pediatr Hematol Oncol 1990; **12**: 45–50.

35. Tamaroff M, Miller DR, Murphy ML et al. Immediate and long-term posttherapy neuropsychologic performance in children with acute lymphoblastic leukemia treated without central nervous system radiation. J Pediatr 1982; **101**: 524–9.

36. Kingma A, Van Dommelen RI, Mooyaart EL *et al.* No major cognitive impairment in young children with acute lymphoblastic leukemia using chemotherapy only: a prospective longitudinal study. *J Pediatr Hematol Oncol* 2002; **24**:106–14.

37. Waber DP, Carpentieri SC, Klar N *et al.* Cognitive sequelae in children treated for acute lymphoblastic leukemia with dexamethasone or prednisone. *J Pediatr Hematol Oncol* 2000; **22**: 206–13.

◆38. Anderson DM, Rennie KM, Ziegler JP *et al.* Medical and neurocognitive late effects among survivors of childhood central nervous system tumors. *Cancer* 2001; **92**: 2709–19.

39. Glauser TA, Packer RJ. Cognitive deficits in long term survivors of childhood brain tumors. *Childs Nerv Syst* 1991; **7**: 2–12.

40. Hoppe-Hirsch E, Renier D, Lellouch-Tubiana A *et al.* Medulloblastoma in childhood: progressive intellectual deterioration. *Childs Nerv Syst* 1990; **6**: 60–5.

41. Levisohn L, Cronin-Golomb A, Schmahmann JD. Neuropsychological consequences of cerebellar tumour resection in children: cerebellar cognitive affective syndrome in a paediatric population. *Brain* 2000; **123**: 1041–50.

42. Roman DD, Sperduto PW. Neuropsychological effects of cranial radiation: current knowledge and future directions. *Int J Radiat Oncol Biol Phys* 1995; **31**: 983–98.

43. Johnson DL, McCabe MA, Nicholson HS *et al.* Quality of long term survival in young children with medulloblastoma. *J Neurosurg* 1994; **80**: 1004–110.

44. Radcliffe J, Bunin GR, Sutton LN *et al.* Cognitive deficits in long-term survivors of childhood medulloblastoma and other noncortical tumors: age dependent effects of whole brain radiation. *Int J Dev Neurosci* 1994; **12**: 327–34.

45. Deutsch M, Thomas PR, Krischer J *et al.* Results of a prospective randomized trial comparing standard dose neuraxis irradiation (3,600 cGy/20) with reduced neuraxis irradiation (2,340 cGy/13) in patients with low-stage medulloblastoma. A Combined Children's Cancer Group-Pediatric Oncology Group Study. *Pediatr Neurosurg* 1996; **24**: 167–76.

46. Ellenberg L, McComb JG, Siegel SE, Stowe S. factors affecting intellectual outcome in pediatric brain tumor patients. *Neurosurgery* 1987; **21**: 638–44.

47. Mulhern RK, Kepner JL, Thomas PR *et al.* Neuropsychologic functioning of survivors of childhood medulloblastoma randomized to receive conventional or reduced-dose craniospinal irradiation: a Pediatric Oncology Group study. *J Clin Oncol* 1998; **16**: 1723–8.

48. Radcliffe J, Packer RJ, Atkins TE *et al.* Three and four year cognitive outcome in children with non cortical brain tumors treated with whole brain radiotherapy. *Ann Neurol* 1992; **32**: 551–5.

49. Mostow EN, Byrne J, Connelly RR, Mulvihill JJ. Quality of life in long term survivors of CNS tumors of childhood and adolescence. *J Clin Oncol* 1991; **9**: 592–9.

50. Pizzo P, Poplack DG, Bleyer WA. Neurotoxicities of current leukemia therapy. *J Pediatr Hematol Oncol* 1979; **1**: 127–38.

51. Mulhern RK, Reddick WE, Palmer SL *et al.* Neurocognitive deficits in medulloblastoma survivors and white matter loss. *Ann Neurol* 1999; **46**: 834–41.

52. Harila-Saari AH, Vainionpaa LK, Kovala TT *et al.* Nerve lesions after therapy for childhood acute lymphoblastic leukemia. *Cancer* 1998; **82**: 200–7.

53. Arvidson J, Kihlgren M, Hall C, Lonnerholm G. Neuropsychological functioning after treatment for hematological malignancies in childhood, including autologous bone marrow transplantation. *Pediatr Hematol Oncol* 1999; **16**: 9–21

54. Smedler AC, Bolme P. Neuropsychological deficits in very young bone marrow transplant recipients. *Acta Paediatr* 1995; **84**: 429–33.

55. Padovan CS, Yousry TA, Schleuning M *et al.* Neurological and neuroradiological findings in long-term survivors of allogeneic bone marrow transplantation. *Ann Neurol* 1998; **43**: 627–33.

56. Lipshultz SE, Colan SD, Gelber RD *et al.* Late cardiac effects of doxorubicin therapy for children with acute lymphoblastic leukaemia in childhood. *N Engl J Med* 1991; **324**: 808–15.

57. Sorensen K, Levitt G, Sebag-Montefiore D *et al.* Cardiac function in Wilms' tumor survivors. *J Clin Oncol* 1995; **13**: 1546–56.

58. Levitt G, Bunch K, Rogers CA *et al.* Cardiac transplantation in childhood cancer survivors. *Eur J Cancer* 1996; **32A**: 826–30.

59. Steinherz LJ, Steinherz PG, Tan TC *et al.* Cardiac toxicity 4 to 20 years after completing anthracycline therapy. *J Am Med Assoc* 1991; **266**: 1672–7.

60. Goorin AM, Chauvenet AR, Perez-Atayde AR *et al.* Initial congestive heart failure six to ten years after doxorubicin chemotherapy for childhood cancer. *J Pediatr* 1990; **116**: 144–7.

61. Kremer LCM, van Dalen EC, Offringa M *et al.* Anthracycline induced clinical heart failure in a cohort of 607 children: long term follow up study. *J Clin Oncol* 2001; **19**: 191–6.

62. Boucek RJ. Mechanism for anthracycline induced cardiomyopathy: clinical and laboratory correlations. *Prog Pediatr Cardiol* 1998; **8**: 59–70

63. Von Hoff DD, Rozeneweig M, Layard M *et al.* Daunomycin induced cardiotoxicity in children and adults. *Am J Med* 1977; **62**: 200–8.

◆64. Levitt G. Cardioprotection. *Br J Haematol* 1999; **106**: 860–9.

65. Steinherz LJ, Steinherz PG, Mangiacasale D *et al.* Cardiac changes with cyclophosphamide. *Med Pediatr Oncol* 1981; **9**: 417–22.

66. Oberlin O, Habrand JL, Zucker JM *et al.* No benefit from ifosfamide in Ewing's sarcoma: a non randomised study of the French Society of Pediatric Oncology. *J Clin Oncol* 1992; **10**: 1407–12

◆67. Kremer LC, Van Dalen EC, Offringa M, Voute PA. Frequency and risk factors of anthracycline induced clinical heart failure in children: a systematic review. *Ann Oncol* 2002; **13**: 503–12.

◆68. Kremer LC, Van Der Pal HJ, Offringa M *et al.* Frequency and risk factors of subclinical cardiotoxicity after anthracycline therapy in children: a systematic review. *Ann Oncol* 2002; **13**: 819–29.

69. Lipshultz SE, Rifai N, Sallan SE *et al.* Predictive value of cardiac troponin T in pediatric patients at risk for myocardial injury. *Circulation* 1997; **96**: 2496–7.

70. Kremer LC, Bastiaansen BA, Offringa M *et al.* Treponin T in the first 24 hours after administration of chemotherapy and the detection of myocardial damage in children. *Eur J Cancer* 2002; **38**: 686–9.

71. Maini CL, Sciuto R, Ferraironi A *et al*. Clinical relevance of radionuclide angiography and anti myosin immunoscintigraphy for risk assessment in epirubicin cardiotoxicity. *J Nucl Cardiol* 1997; **4**: 502–8.

72. Kremer LC, Tiel-van Buul MM, Ubbink MC *et al*. Indium-111-antimyosin scintigraphy in the early detection of heart damage after anthracycline therapy in children. *J Clin Oncol* 1999; **17**: 1208.

73. Nysom K, Colan SD, Lipschultz SE. Late cardiotoxicity following anthracyclinen therapy for childhood cancer. *Prog Pediatr Cardiol* 1998; **8**: 121–38.

74. Bielack SS, Ertmann R, Kempf-Bielack B, Winkler K. Impact of scheduling on toxicity and clinical efficacy of doxorubicin: what do we know in the mid nineties? *Eur J Cancer* 1996; **32A**: 1652–60.

75. de Valeriola D. Dose optimization of anthracyclines. *Anticancer Res* 1994; **14**: 2307–14.

76. Bu'Lock FA, Gabriel HM, Oakhill A *et al*. Cardioprotection by ICRF 187 against high dose anthracycline toxicity in children with malignant disease. *Br Heart J* 1993; **70**: 185–8.

77. Lipshultz SE. Dexrazoxone for protection against cardiotoxic effects of anthracyclines in children. *J Clin Oncol* 1996; **14**: 328–30.

78. Bellott R, Auvrignon A, Leblanc T *et al*. Pharmacokinetics of liposomal daunorubicin (DaunoXome) during a phase I-II study in children with relapsed acute lymphoblastic leukaemia. *Cancer Chemother Pharmacol* 2001; **47**: 15–21.

79. Steinherz LJ, Graham T, Hurwitz R *et al*. Guidelines for monitoring of children during and after anthracycline therapy: report of the cardiology committee of the Children's Cancer Study Group. *Pediatrics* 1992; **89**: 942–9.

80. Bender KS, Shematek JP, Leventhal BG *et al*. QT prolongation associated with anthracycline cardiotoxicity. *J Pediatr* 1984; **105**: 442–4.

81. Hancock SL, Tucker MA, Hoppe RT. Factors affecting late mortality from heart disease after treatment for Hodgkin's disease. *J Am Med Assoc* 1993; **270**: 1949–55.

82. Gross NJ. Pulmonary effects of radiation therapy. *Ann Intern Med* 1977; **86**: 81–92.

83. Miller RW, Fusner JE, Fink RJ *et al*. Pulmonary function abnormalities in long term survivors of childhood cancer. *Med Pediatr Oncol* 1986; **14**: 202–7.

84. Benoist MR, Lemerle J, Jean R *et al*. Effects on pulmonary function of whole lung irradiation for Wilms' tumour in children. *Thorax* 1982; **37**: 175–80.

85. Paulino AC, Wen BC, Brown CK *et al*. Late effects of children treated with radiation therapy for Wilms' tumour. *Int J Radiat Oncol Biol Phys* 2000; **46**: 1239–46.

86. Jacacki RI, Schramm CM, Donahue BR *et al*. Restrictive lung disease following treatment for malignant brain tumors: a potential late effect of craniospinal irradiation. *J Clin Oncol* 1995; **13**: 1478–85.

87. Cerveri I, Zoia MC, Fulgoni P *et al*. Late pulmonary sequelae after childhood bone marrow transplantation. *Thorax* 1999; **54**: 131–5.

88. Eigen H, Wyszomierski D. Bleomycin lung injury in children. Pathophysiology and guidelines for management. *Am J Pediatr Hematol Oncol* 1985; **7**: 71–8.

89. O'Driscoll BR, Hasleton PS, Taylor PM *et al*. Active lung fibrosis up to 17 years after chemotherapy with carmustine (BCNU) in childhood. *N Engl J Med* 1990; **323**: 378–82.

90. Makipernaa A, Heino A, Laitinen LA *et al*. Lung function following treatment of malignant tumours with surgery, radiotherapy or cyclophosphamide in childhood. *Cancer* 1989; **63**: 625–30.

91. Shaw NA, Tweeddale PM, Eden OB. Pulmonary function in childhood leukaemia survivors. *Med Pediatr Oncol* 1989; **17**: 149–54.

92. Jenney ME, Faragher EB, Jones PH, Woodcock A. Lung function and exercise capacity in survivors of childhood leukaemia. *Med Pediatr Oncol* 1995; **24**: 222–30.

93. Donaldson SS, Jundt S, Ricour C *et al*. Radiation enteritis in children – a retrospective review, clinicopathologic correlation and dietary management. *Cancer* 1975; **35**: 1167–78.

94. Hays DM, Turnberg JL, Chen TT *et al*. Complications relating to 234 staging laparotomies performed in the Intergroup Hodgkin's Disease in Childhood Study. *Surgery* 1984; **96**: 471–8.

95. Taylor RE. Morbidity from abdominal radiotherapy in the first United Kingdom Children's cancer Study Group Wilms' Tumour Study. *Clin Oncol* 1997; **9**: 381–4.

96. Barnard JA, Marshall GS, Neblett WW *et al*. Non cirrhotic portal fibrosis after Wilms' tumour therapy. *Gastroenterology* 1986; **90**: 1054–6.

◆97. Ribaud P, Gluckman E. Hepatic veno-occlusive disease. *Pediatr Transplant* 1999; **3**: 41–4.

98. Raine J, Bowman A, Wallendszus K, Pritchard J. Hepatopathy-thrombocytopenia syndrome – a complication of dactinomycin therapy for Wilms' tumour: a report form the United Kingdom Children's Cancer Study Group. *J Clin Oncol* 1991; **9**: 268–73.

99. Hashkes PJ, Balistreri WF, Bove KE *et al*. The long term effect of methotrexate function on the liver in patients with juvenile rheumatoid arthritis. *Arthritis Rheum* 1997; **40**: 2226–34.

100. McIntosh S, Davidson DI, O'Brien Rt *et al*. Methotrexate hepatopathy in children with leukemia. *J Pediatr* 1977; **90**: 1019–21.

101. Raney RB, Heyn R, Cassady R *et al*. Late effects of cancer therapy on the genitourinary tract in children. In: Schwartz CL, Hobbie WL, Constine LS, Ruccione KS, eds. *Survivors of Childhood Cancer: Assessment and Management*. St Louis: Mosby, 1994: 132–43.

◆102. Skinner R, Pearson ADJ, Coulthard MG *et al*. Assessment of chemotherapy associated nephrotoxicity in children with cancer. *Cancer Chemother Pharmacol* 1991; **28**: 81–92.

103. Brock PR, Koliouskas DE, Barrett TM *et al*. Partial reversibility of cisplatin nephrotoxicity in children. *J Pediatr* 1991; **118**: 531–4.

104. Skinner R, Sharkey IM, Pearson ADJ. Ifosfamide, mesna and nephrotoxicity in children. *J Clin Oncol* 1993; **11**: 173–90.

105. Skinner R, Cotterill SJ, Stevens MCG. Risk factors for nephrotoxicity after ifosfamide treatment in children: a UKCCSG Late Effects Group Study. *Br J Cancer* 2000; **82**: 1636–45.

106. Raney RB, Heyn R, Hays D et al. Sequelae of treatment in 109 patients followed for five to fifteen years after diagnosis of sarcoma of the bladder and prostate: a report from the Intergroup Rhabdomyosarcoma Committee. Cancer 1993; 71: 2387–94

107. Levine LA, Ritchie JP. Urological complications of ifosfamide. J Urol 1989; 141: 1063–9.

108. Critchley HO, Wallace WH, Shalet SM et al. Abdominal irradiation in childhhod: the potential for pregnancy. Br J Obstet Gynaecol 1993; 99: 392–4.

109. Flamant F, Gerbaulet A, Nihoul-Fekete C et al. Long term sequelae of conservative treatment by surgery, brachytherapy and chemotherapy for vulval and vaginal rhabdomyosarcoma in children. J Clin Oncol 1990; 8: 1847–53.

110. Aisenberg J, Hsieh K, Kalaitzoglou G et al. Bone mineral density in young adult survivors of childhood cancer. J Pediatr Hematol Oncol 1998; 20: 241–5.

111. Ariskoski P, Komulainen J, Voutilainen R et al. Reduced bone mineral density in long term survivors of childhood acute lymphoblastic leukemia. J Pediatr Hematol Oncol 1998; 20: 234–40

◆112. Gleeson HK, Darzy K, Shalet SM. Late endocrine, metabolic and skeletal sequelae following treatment of childhood cancer. Best Pract Clin Endocrinol Metab 2002; 16: 335–48.

113. Strauss AJ, Su JT, Kimball Dalton VM et al. Bony morbidity in children treated for acute lymphoblastic leukemia. J Clin Oncol 2001; 19: 3066–72.

114. Warner JT, Evans WD, Webb DKH et al. Relative osteopenia after treatment for acute lymphoblastic leukemia. Pediatr Res 1998; 45: 544–51

115. Silber JH, Littman PS, Meadows AT. Stature loss following skeletal irradiation for childhood cancer. J Clin Oncol 1990; 8: 304–12.

116. Raney RB, Asmar L, Vassilopoulou-Sellin R et al. Late complications of therapy in 213 children with localized, nonorbital soft-tissue sarcoma of the head and neck: a descriptive report from the Intergroup Rhabdomyosarcoma Studies (IRS)-II and – III. IRS Group of the Children's Cancer Group and the Pediatric Oncology Group. Med Pediatr Oncol 1999; 33: 362–71.

117. Rosenfield NS, Haller JO, Berson WE et al. Failure of development of the growing breast after radiotherapy. Pediatr Radiol 1989; 19: 124–7.

118. Nylander G, Pettersson F, Swedenborg J. Localized arterial occlusions in patients treated with pelvic field radiation for cancer. Cancer 1978; 41: 2158–61.

119. Hughes BR, Cinliffe WJ, Bailey CC. Excess benign melanocytic naevi after chemotherapy for malignant disease in childhood. Br Med J 1989; 299: 88–91.

120. Testa NG, Bhavnani M, Will A et al. Long term bone marrow damage following treatment for acute lymphoblastic leukaemia. Haematology 1988; 8: 279–87.

121. Vogel JM, Kimball JR, Foley HT et al. Effect of extensive radiotherapy on the marrow granulocyte reserves of patients with Hodgkin's disease. Cancer 1986; 21: 798–804.

122. Stevens MCG, Brown E, Zipursky A. The effect of abdominal radiation on spleen function: a study in children with Wilms' tumor. Pediatric Hematol Oncol 1986; 3: 69–72.

123. Royal College of Paediatrics and Child Health. Immunisation of the Immunocompromised Child: Best Practice Statement. (http://www.rcpch.ac.uk/publications/recent_publications/Immunocomp.pdf) London: Royal College of Paediatrics and Child Health, 2002.

124. Schell M, McHaney V, Green AA. Hearing loss in children and young adults receiving cisplatin with or without prior cranial irradiation. J Clin Oncol 1989; 7: 754–60.

125. Deeg HJ, Flournoy N, Sullivan KM et al. Cataracts after total body irradiation and marrow transplantation: a sparing effect of dose fractionation. Int J Radiat Oncol Biol Phys 1984; 10: 957–64.

126. Raney RB, Anderson JR, Kollath J et al. Late effects of therapy in 94 patients with localized rhabdomyosarcoma of the orbit: Report from the Intergroup Rhabdomyosarcoma Study (IRS)-III, 1984-1991. Med Pediatr Oncol 2000; 34: 413–20

127. Purdell Lewis DJ, Stalman MS, Leeuw JA et al. Long term results of chemotherapy and the developing dentition: caries risk and developmental aspects. Community Dent Oral Epidemiol 1988; 16: 68–71.

◆128. Green DM. Fertility and pregnancy outcome after treatment for cancer in childhood or adolescence. Oncologist 1997; 2: 171–9.

129. Green DM, Whitton JA, Stovall M et al. Pregnancy outcome of female survivors of childhood cancer: A report from the Childhood Cancer Survivor Study. Am J Obstet Gynecol 2002; 187: 1070–80

130. Critchley HOD, Wallace WHB, Shalet SM et al. Abdominal radiation in childhood; the potential for fertility. Br J Obstet Gynaecol 1992; 99: 392–4.

131. Li FP, Fine W, Jaffe N et al. Offspring of patients treated for cancer in childhood. J Natl Cancer Inst 1979; 62: 1193–7.

132. Hawkins MM, Draper GJ, Smith RA. Cancer among 1348 survivors of childhood cancer. Int J Cancer 1989; 43: 975–8.

◆133. Thomson AB, Critchley HOD, Wallace WHB. Fertility and progeny. Eur J Cancer 2002; 38: 1634–44.

134. Makipernaa A. Long-term quality of life and psychosocial coping after treatment of solid tumours in childhood. A population-based study of 94 patients 11-28 years after their diagnosis. Acta Paediatr Scand 1989; 78: 728–35.

135. Apajasalo M, Sintonen H, Siimes MA et al. Health-related quality of life of adults surviving malignancies in childhood. Eur J Cancer 1996; 32A: 1354–8.

136. Lackner H, Benesch M, Schargerl S et al. Prospective evaluation of late effects after childhood cancer therapy with a follow up over 9 years. Eur J Pediatr 2000; 159: 750–8.

137. Humpl T, Fritsche M, Bartels U, Gutjahr P. Survivors of childhood cancer for more than twenty years. Acta Oncol 2001; 40: 44–9.

138. Hobbie WL, Stuber M, Meeske K et al. Symptoms of posttraumatic stress in young adult survivors of childhood cancer. J Clin Oncol 2000; 18: 4060–6.

139. Elkin TD, Phipps S, Mulhern RK, Fairclough D. Psychological functioning of adolescent and young adult survivors of pediatric malignancy. Med Pediatr Oncol 1997; 29: 582–8.

◆140. Jenney MEM, Levitt GA. The quality of survival after childhood cancer. Eur J Cancer 2002; 38: 1241–50.

141. Bradlyn AS, Ritchey Ak, Harris CV *et al*. Quality of life research in pediatric oncology. *Cancer* 1996; **78**: 1333–9

142. Eiser C, Jenney MEM. Measuring symptomatic benefit and quality of life in paediatric oncology. *Br J Cancer* 1996; **73**: 1313–16.

143. Kanabar DJ, Attard-Montalto S, Saha V *et al*. Quality of life in survivors of childhood cancer after megatherapy with autologous bone marrow rescue. *Pediatr Hematol Oncol* 1995; **12**: 29–36.

144. Mackie E, Hill J, Kondryn H, McNally R. Adult psychosocial outcomes in long term survivors of acute lymphoblastic leukaemia and Wilms' tumour: a controlled study. *Lancet* 2000; **355**: 1310–14.

145. Greenberg HS, Kazak AE, Meadows AT. Psychological functioning in cancer survivors. *J Pediatr* 1989; **114**: 488–93.

146. Ruccione KS. Issues in survivorship. In: Schwartz CL, Hobbie WL, Constine LS, Ruccione KS, eds. *Survivors of Childhood Cancer: Assessment and Management*. St Louis: Mosby, 1994.

147. Kissen GDN, Wallace WHB. *Long Term Follow Up Therapy Based Guidelines*. Leicester: United Kingdom Children's Cancer Study Group, 1995.

148. Masera G, Chesler M, Jancovic M *et al*. SIOP working committee on psychosocial issues in pediatric oncology: guidelines for care of long term survivors. *Med Pediatr Oncol* 1966; **27**: 1–2.

149. Rosen DS. Transition to adult health care for adolescents and young adults with cancer. *Cancer* 1992; **71**: 3411–14.

150. Wallace WHB, Blacklay A, Eiser C *et al*. Developing strategies for long term follow up of survivors of childhood cancer. *Br Med J* 2001; **323**: 271–4.

151. Kadan-Lottick NS, Robison LL, Gurney JG *et al*. Childhood cancer survivors' knowledge about their past diagnosis and treatment. *J Am Med Assoc* 2002; **287**: 1832–9.

152. Gibson F, Soanes L. Long term follow up following childhood cancer: maximising the contribution from nursing. *Eur J Cancer* 2001; **37**: 1859–68.

33

Palliative care in paediatric oncology

RICHARD D. W. HAIN & JANET HARDY

As adults and as parents, we naturally expect that children will outlive us. Thankfully, only a relatively small proportion of parents whose children develop cancer have to face the unthinkable: the death of their son or daughter during childhood. Nevertheless, and despite the continuing improvement in prognosis, cancer remains a principal cause of death in childhood outside infancy, and good palliative care remains an integral part of management of the child with cancer.

CHANGING TO PALLIATIVE TREATMENT

Pallium is the Latin for cloak. Palliation covers up and hides from view the effects of cancer, rather than dealing with the cancer itself. To palliate is to relieve without curing.

The senses of 'palliative' and 'curative' are therefore, in some ways, antithetical and it is tempting to imagine that practical palliative care and curative care are similarly mutually exclusive. In reality, palliative and curative approaches are very far from being opposed, and indeed should be seen as complementary. They share a common principle: that of the balance of burden and benefit. The aim of all medical intervention is ultimately to improve the quality of the child's life. A clinician is faced with a series of judgements about the benefit of the intervention to the patient relative to the burden it imposes. Complete cure of an underlying disease is a good way to improve the quality of life and may justify considerable burden (such as intensive chemotherapy) in the short and even in the long term.

Cure is not, however, the only way to improve the quality of a child's life. For example, from a child's point of view, the impact of leukaemia may be the pain it causes, rather than leukaemia itself. If leukaemia cannot be abolished, the medical team can, and should, put themselves in a position to offer relief from pain.

So, palliative and curative phases are underpinned by the same approach to treatment. That is, diagnostic and therapeutic interventions are considered appropriate only when the potential benefit to the patient is considered to outweigh the potential burden. With this in mind, the oncology team should feel confident that even when cure is no longer possible, they can have a valuable role in helping children to enjoy the rest of their life.

One practical application of this common approach is that good symptom control should not be reserved for the final few weeks of a child's life. Traditionally, professionals caring for children have often been reluctant to prescribe some medications, particularly opioids, on the grounds that they are powerful drugs that should be reserved until the child is close to death. Even during potentially curative therapy, however, good symptom control offers improved quality of life with little burden to the patient. There is probably no point during treatment when the benefits of good symptom management, in all its dimensions, should not be available.

The same cannot always be said of antineoplastic therapy, which usually includes toxic medications that have a significant negative impact on a child's well-being. The use of cytotoxics is, of course, mandatory at presentation of most children's cancers, but becomes optional for many after relapse, and may well be contraindicated once there is no longer any prospect of cure. This gives the paediatric oncologist the unenviable task of explaining that antineoplastic treatment is to stop. For many families it is a shattering blow. However unpleasant children find chemotherapy, it may have been a feature of their life for many months or years and represents for most their only defence against a deadly disease. Withdrawal in the absence of a cure can mean only one thing: that treatment has failed.

Communications at this point in the course of a child's disease have therefore to be very sensitively handled. The key points are summarized in Box 33.1. The news must

Box 33.1 *Key points in news-giving*

1. **Set the scene**
   Private place
   Uninterrupted (give bleep to someone else)
   Invite relevant others – child, ward staff etc.
   Ensure eye contact on same level (ideally all sit)
   Speak in an unhurried way
   Never look at clock or watch

2. **Alignment**
   What does family already know?
   What does family understand?
   What are they expecting from you in this interview?

3. **Exchanging information**
   Acknowledge what is already known and understood
   Use it as basis for giving new information – use family's vocabulary
   Prioritize: what are most important and/or immediate concerns?
   Repeat and summarize as often as necessary

4. **Checking back**
   What has family understood ?
   Did they receive the message you intended to give?
   Have you answered what they needed to hear?
   Go back to step 3 as often as necessary

5. **Closing**
   Reassure family members that they are not expected to remember everything
   Invite further questions (go back to step 3 if necessary)
   'Permit' further questions in the future – of you, ward staff, junior doctors etc.
   Make arrangement to meet again
   Summarize once again

be given clearly and in a way that allows it to be received without ambiguity, but at the same time in a way that respects the coping strategies of the family. This is considered further in the section on 'Talking with families'.

WHERE TO LOOK AFTER THE CHILD

At the time they receive the news that cure is no longer possible, the family members of a child with cancer are often ambivalent about continuing their involvement with the hospital unit. On the one hand, the paediatric oncology centre and/or shared care centre have been a major part of their lives for many weeks, months or even years, while on the other, everything about the environment may serve to remind them of repeated unpleasant interventions and investigations which have ultimately proven fruitless. Many families choose to avoid attending hospital as far as possible. The challenge for the paediatric oncology team is then to ensure quality palliative care is provided in the child's home or a children's hospice.

Home is the environment favoured by most families, and there is evidence that parental adaptation after death is better if it can be supported at home.[1] This is most commonly achieved through a team of paediatric oncology outreach nurses, backed up medically by the consultant in paediatric oncology and/or palliative medicine as well as by the family's GP. Typically, the outreach team has been involved with the family from diagnosis, providing a link between oncology centre, shared care centre and primary care team in the home. The place of the outreach team becomes particularly important in the palliative phase. Their role is to liaise with and coordinate the various professionals who are needed in the care of the child. The exact composition of the wider 'team' that emerges in this way is different for each individual child. For many, the paediatric oncologist will remain the key medical professional. For others, the GP will be the key, with the paediatric oncologist simply providing support, while for others, again, it will be a community paediatric nurse or a paediatrician who takes this role. Some children will require input from psychologists, pain specialists, play therapists or chaplains, while for others these may not be necessary. The paediatric oncology outreach nurse team potentially provides a flexible and effective means of delivering palliative care to a child in the home. Where one is available, the support of a specialist in paediatric or adult palliative medicine can be invaluable.

This 'outreach model' is well established in paediatric oncology and is very effective. Perhaps for this reason, it remains relatively unusual for paediatric oncology patients to be admitted to a children's hospice.[2] Children with cancer typically account for less than 10 per cent of admissions to most children's hospices. Nevertheless, a children's hospice potentially provides a valuable resource for the families of children dying from cancer. Hospices provide a home-like environment in which there is nevertheless access to 24-hour nursing care. Most provide facilities for families to stay with the child, which may allow parents, in particular, to have a break without having to sacrifice precious time with their child. Medical support for children's hospices is usually provided by GPs. Some children's hospice doctors have developed considerable expertise in symptom control, while others will prefer to have more support from the referring consultant. Although there is sometimes the potential for duplication or, worse, conflict of approaches between the paediatric oncology team and the children's hospice, this can usually be resolved by discussion. The children's hospice movement provides paediatric oncologists with a third alternative, between home and hospital.

Management of the palliative phase on an acute paediatric oncology unit is usually less than ideal.[3] The needs of the child and the family during this period are often for working through spiritual and psychological issues, and for building up a store of memories against the time when the child will no longer be there. These things take time, a resource in short supply on any acute unit. Nevertheless, a small minority of families prefer the child to die in hospital. This can be for a variety of reasons, but is often because they cannot bear the thought of having to live where their child has died, or because of fears that complex symptoms may be difficult to manage there. Exploring these issues can often be reassuring, and avoid the need for prolonged admission.

Where hospital admission is unavoidable, the aim should be to create, as far as possible, a home-like environment. This can most easily be done by setting aside a single room and allowing the family to bring in such soft furnishing, toys etc. as they see fit. It is tempting for the ward team to avoid intruding on the family's grief, partly because of a worry that the encounter will take too long during a busy ward round. Paradoxically, it is in fact possible for a family to feel more isolated on an acute ward surrounded by professionals than at home where contact is limited to a visit every day or two. It is important that a member of the ward team makes time to sit and talk to the family each day. Generally, this does not take as long as one expects and a great deal of discussion can take place in a 5- or 10-minute encounter.

SYMPTOM MANAGEMENT

Pain

One rational and common-sense approach to pain in a child has been summarized in the letters QUEST,[4]

i.e. **q**uestion the child, **u**se pain rating tools, **e**valuate behaviour, **s**ensitize parents and **t**ake action (or **t**reat).

ASSESSMENT

The purpose of pain assessment is twofold:

* to assess the severity of pain
* to assess the nature of pain, with a view to making a diagnosis of its cause.

A useful mnemonic 'PQRST' has been devised to help summarize the aspects of pain that should be recorded:

* *Precipitating (or relieving) factors.* Pain on movement of a limb may be the result of a pathological fracture. Pain relieved by defaecation suggests that constipation is the cause. This part of the assessment should include attention to the medications that have been effective. Most pain is at least partially opioid-responsive.
* *Quality.* Children are sometimes surprisingly clear in their descriptions of what pain feels like. Descriptors that imply a change of sensation, such as numbness, paraesthesia, hyperaesthesia or burning, are suggestive of a neuropathic type pain. One child explained that: 'It felt as though petrol has been poured all over my leg and set on fire.' Other descriptors that suggest a deep, intense but well localized pain are suggestive of bone pain, most commonly due to metastases to the bone cortex. A common description is 'like toothache in my arm'.
* *Radiation.* Neuropathic pain is typically distributed in a recognizably dermatomal pattern and this is often indicated by the child with a sweeping gesture of the hand. In contrast, bone pain is typically well circumscribed and is often indicated by pointing with one finger. Sympathetic mediated nerve pain is rather unusual in children with cancer and is distributed in a vascular rather than a dermatomal pattern.
* *Severity.* A variety of scales have been developed to assess the severity of pain in children.[5,6] Most are variations on the simple visual analogue scale[7,8] and are effective for children old enough to use them.[9–11] The best validated among these[12–19] use facial expression as an index for the severity of pain. Whilst this is very appropriate for the measurement of acute pain, it is much less relevant to the assessment of cancer-related pain, which typically persists for many hours or days. Furthermore, a child may be able to avoid pain, but only by remaining very still.[20] Such a child might not express pain but would certainly be in need of analgesia. The DEGR scale[21,22] recognizes these difficulties, and was developed specifically for use in paediatric oncology. Unfortunately, to date it has only been validated in a small French study but it

warrants further attention. For younger children, there may be no alternative but to make assumptions about the child's experience of pain based on observations by those who know the child best. Nurses and, even more, parents are the most likely to recognize a behaviour pattern in the child that indicates pain. Attenuation of such behaviour in response to relatively pure analgesics such as opioids is diagnostic of pain, but the absence of a response may be due to under-treatment. If there is some doubt, pain should usually be assumed and a therapeutic trial of adequate analgesia instituted.

- *Timing*. Neuropathic and bone pains are both usually constant in nature. Pain may be intermittent for a variety of reasons. The cause itself may be intermittent (e.g. a pathological fracture may be painful only when moved), the pain may be of an episodic nature itself (e.g. intestinal colic due to lactulose, stimulant laxatives or constipation), or the dose of regular medication may be too small, which results in intermittent breakthrough pain. The distinction between these three is clearly important as the management will be rather different for each.

In order to address all five aspects of pain assessment, a thorough history (Box 33.2) and examination are needed. Where appropriate, it may also be necessary to consider further investigations. Once it is clear that cure is no longer possible, however, investigations should be ordered only after careful consideration. Most require attendance at hospital and many an injection or blood test. It can even be argued, for example, that it is unnecessary to order a bone scan to demonstrate bony metastases, since in the context of known metastatic disease, asymptomatic metastases need no treatment and symptomatic ones can be treated empirically using radiotherapy or analgesic medications.

Box 33.2 *Pain – key points in history and examination*

Diagnosis
- Precipitating or relieving factors
- Quality of pain
- Radiation
- Severity
- Timing

Assessment 'QUEST'[4]
- Question the child
- Use measurement scales
- Evaluate behaviour
- Sensitize parents to possibility of pain
- Take action (treat) appropriately

This rational and systematic approach to diagnosis and assessment of pain illustrate once again that the palliative phase can be marked by the same rigorous attention to principle that should characterize the curative phase. This is also true of management.

APPROACHES TO PAIN MANAGEMENT

Pain management, like other aspects of palliative management of a child, requires an analytical and systematic approach, with careful attention to the principles and evidence base that underpin our understanding of the pathophysiology of symptoms. At the same time, the approach has to be pragmatic. Where there is no evidence, it may be necessary to fall back on what has been effective in other individual children, or what has worked in the particular child in question.

The World Health Organization has proposed a standardized approach to pain management in children.[23–25] There are three steps, as follows:

1. simple analgesia (effectively just paracetamol since aspirin is not widely used in paediatrics)
2. 'minor' opioids for mild-to-moderate pain (codeine, dihydrocodeine)
3. 'major' opioids for moderate-to-severe pain (morphine, fentanyl, diamorphine).

Medications at the next step should be introduced as soon as those at the step before have become ineffective, usually through disease progression. An important corollary is that there should be no rotation within a step. Once codeine is ineffective, there is no advantage in changing to other minor opioids. This is least true at step 3 (major opioids), where the characteristics of individual major opioids may make one preferable over another.

It can be argued that in children there is little need for the middle step (minor opioids). Children are more resilient than adults to the effects of opioids. A small dose of a major opioid is, in any case, pharmacologically identical with a large dose of minor opioid. Nevertheless, for some parents (and indeed some professionals) there is some comfort in the availability of an intermediate step.

At each stage, appropriate adjuvants should be introduced. The selection of an appropriate adjuvant depends on an accurate diagnosis of the likely nature of the pain. It is important to recognize that even the most effective adjuvant is less likely to be of benefit than an opioid, but that the two are complementary, not alternative.

There are essentially three phases in the management of pain in a child with cancer.

1. *Selection of a starting dose.* A starting dose can be chosen from a paediatric formulary,[26] or else converted from a dose of opioids a child is already receiving. The regular dose should in the first instance be prescribed as immediate-acting

morphine 4-hourly regularly (not 'as needed'). At the same time a breakthrough dose equivalent to this 4-hourly dose should also be prescribed.

2. *Titration of the dose upwards to establish the child's analgesic needs.* The regular dose should be reviewed regularly. Where the child has needed one or more breakthrough doses during any two consecutive 24-hour periods, the extra doses should be totalled and added to the regular dose. The breakthrough dose should be increased accordingly.

3. *Maintenance of analgesia.* It is usually possible to find a steady dose for a period of days or even weeks, despite disease progression and the theoretical development of tolerance. In this phase, it is usually convenient to change the immediate-release morphine to an alternative preparation such as MST or MXL. Fentanyl transdermally is increasingly a popular alternative (see below). Even during this phase, it is important to keep the dose under review. The child's requirements for opioid will usually (although by no means always) increase as the child approaches death.

INCIDENT PAIN

Intermittent pain can be very difficult to treat,[27–29] particularly when severe, such as abdominal colic. A dose of analgesia that is adequate for the pain at its worst may be unmanageably toxic at other times. Management of the acute episodes of pain may be made difficult by the duration of onset of the medication, so that the peak analgesic effect occurs some time after the pain has remitted spontaneously.

ANALGESICS

Simple analgesics

Paracetamol is an extremely effective analgesic in children and carries very little toxicity. It is rarely enough

alone to treat cancer pain but is an often helpful additional drug at all steps. Paracetamol is antipyretic but not anti-inflammatory and, in contrast with aspirin, has no effect on platelet aggregation.

Minor opioids

There are many minor opioids. Codeine is the most widely known and used in children in the UK. Minor opioids are simply weak opioids. They are nevertheless powerfully constipating and most children receiving them should also start prophylactic laxatives. There is little to be gained from switching from one minor opioid to another. If minor opioids become ineffective, the appropriate manoeuvre is to move to the next step (major opioids). Children who have been receiving minor opioids will already have developed some tolerance to some of the adverse effects of major opioids and can often start at a higher dose, which can be calculated by conversion on the basis of relative potencies (Table 33.1).

There are a number of opioids that are intermediate in potency between minor and major. These include tramadol and pethidine (meperidine). Neither has established a role in the management of cancer pain in children. The active metabolites of pethidine accumulate and can cause seizures.[30,31]

Major opioids

Generally speaking, morphine is the major opioid of choice for the management of cancer pain in children. It is familiar and generally well tolerated. Immediate-release formulations are ideal for breakthrough pain, but for maintenance analgesia they need to be given six times a day, which is inconvenient. Contrary to what was once believed, there is little evidence that outside infancy children are more sensitive to opioids than adults. Indeed, the reverse may be nearer the truth.[32–38]

Slow-release formulations are available that can be given twice or even once daily. However, the pharmacokinetics of these in children seems to be erratic,[39] such

Table 33.1 *Relative potency of common opioids, and their potential advantages over morphine*

Opioid	Advantage over morphine	Relative potency compared with oral morphine (approx.)
Diamorphine (s.c. or i.v.)	More soluble	1.5
Fentanyl (patch)	Patch formulation	100
	Less constipation[45]	
	?Less itch	
	?Less retention	
Methadone (p.o.)	Anti-neuropathic activity[47,48]	Variable
Hydromorphone (p.o.)	None	5
Pethidine	None	0.125
Tramadol	None	0.25
Oxycodone	None	1

i.v., intravenous; p.o., per os; s.c., subcutaneous.

that they often need to be given more frequently and this can limit their usefulness in individual patients.

There are few good data regarding the occurrence of adverse effects of opioids in children, and much of what follows is anecdotal. Constipation is almost universal with children requiring major opioids. Significant respiratory depression is unusual in the presence of pain, and nausea and vomiting appear to be less common than in adults (while laxatives should always be prescribed when commencing major opioid therapy in children, it is not usually necessary routinely to add an antiemetic). In contrast, pruritus and urinary retention may be more common. The former may respond to ondansetron[40–42] or even naloxone.[43]

Fentanyl is a powerful major opioid which potentially offers some patients a number of benefits over morphine.[44–46] It is available in a transdermal formulation so that there is no need for needles or syringe drivers, and it may cause less constipation.[45] Fentanyl is a useful second-line major opioid for children unable to tolerate morphine, because of either its formulation or its adverse effects.

Diamorphine is believed to be metabolized to morphine immediately on entering the bloodstream and therefore has the same benefits and disadvantages. Its big advantage over morphine is that it is very much more soluble. This means large doses can be dissolved in relatively small volumes, making it particularly suitable for use in syringe drivers. It is relatively unusual in paediatric practice to need doses of morphine that are so high they could not be dissolved in a practical volume. Nevertheless it is common practice for diamorphine to be employed effectively as a parenteral form of morphine, when and if one becomes necessary. Diamorphine parenterally is about three times the potency of the same dose of morphine by mouth.

Hydromorphone is another major opioid,[34] five to 10 times as potent but otherwise little different from morphine. Its main role is as a parenteral opioid in countries where diamorphine is not yet available. Methadone is unique among opioid analgesics in possessing antagonist activity against the NMDA receptor,[47,48] which is responsible for mediating neuropathic pain.[49,50] It has been used in children,[51,52] but its role remains unclear.

There are a number of routes available to give medication in children. Where possible, the oral route is preferred. The intravenous route is often easily available, as many children will retain some form of central venous access following chemotherapy. There is anecdotal evidence that tolerance to opioids develops more rapidly by this route, though this is difficult to explain.

The subcutaneous route is widely used in adult palliative medicine and is gaining acceptability in the paediatric speciality. Most major opioids, and indeed many other medications for symptom relief, can be given subcutaneously. Intermittent boluses, e.g. of breakthrough opioid, can be given through indwelling subcutaneous cannulas. Continuous 24-hour infusions containing one or even several compatible medications can also be given by this route. Diamorphine is compatible with a wide range of other drugs, including most antiemetics and several anxiolytics and sedatives.[53–55] Nebulized opioids have been studied in adults.[56] There is no evidence for their effectiveness in relieving dyspnoea, but they do provide patient and family with an acute intervention that need not wait for the arrival of a doctor or nurse.

Transdermal formulations, particularly of fentanyl and hyoscine, are often useful in paediatric palliative care as they can avoid the need for needles. There have been paediatric studies of fentanyl in a lozenge delivery system[57] with encouraging results.

Some medications lend themselves to topical administration. Topical opioids have been used admixed with wound dressings in the management of pain associated with pressure sores.[58–62] Individual patients report relief but there is little published evidence.

Novel routes have also been used in children. Medications have been given intranasally (e.g. midazolam), rectally (e.g. diazepam) and via the buccal route (e.g. lorazepam). Some of these have their own drawbacks; intranasal or buccal medications can taste unpleasant, and some children find the rectal route unacceptably undignified and invasive. Nevertheless, for many they may provide useful alternatives to needles.

NON-STEROIDAL ANTI-INFLAMMATORY DRUGS (NSAIDs)

There are a number of NSAIDs available. They are used as adjuvants in the management of cancer-related bone pain[63–67] and, indeed, other forms of cancer pain. Although minor adverse effects such as gastric irritation are relatively common, NSAIDs are generally well tolerated.[68] Where adverse effects persist, NSAIDs can be made more tolerable by the concurrent prescription of antacids[69–71] (particularly omeprazole), gastric mucosal protectants (misoprostol) or the use of Cox-2 selective drugs[72–74] such as rofecoxib. NSAIDs should be used with some caution in patients also receiving steroids,[75] or with lymphoproliferative disorders such as leukaemia, since NSAIDs inhibit platelet aggregation and can increase the likelihood of bleeding in the presence of low platelets.

ADJUVANTS FOR NEUROPATHIC PAIN

There is now good evidence[76,77] that antidepressants and anticonvulsants are useful adjuvants in the management of neuropathic pain. There is little evidence to support a preference for one as first-line medication over the other, but carbamazepine has the advantage of a long track record in paediatrics. The adjuvant effect of amitriptyline can be manifest at doses well below those needed for antidepression. Newer anticonvulsants and antidepressants, such as vigabatrin, fluoxetine and especially gabapentin,[78–84] are probably effective, although to date there is little evidence for their use in children. Ketamine is widely used in adults,[27,48,85,86] and increasingly in children[87,88] with neuropathic pain. There is little evidence to support the use of oral ketamine even in adults.

STEROIDS

Their protean pharmacological effects make steroids very useful in the palliative management of children with cancer. However, their propensity for causing side-effects means that in most cases it is only a relatively short time before the benefits of their use are outweighed by the threat to a child's quality of life. Even where long-term adrenal suppression is not a concern, the development of a cushingoid facies has a profound impact on a child's self-image and the way he or she is treated by other children. This can mean the difference between attending school or not.

Generally speaking, steroids should be prescribed in the palliative phase only for limited courses of 3 or 5 days each. Dexamethasone is typically preferred in the palliative phase but may cause more profound changes in personality and more sleep disturbance.

Where steroids are co-prescribed with NSAIDs, it is prudent to prescribe a prophylactic gastric protectant such as omeprazole and/or misoprostol.

Indications for steroids in palliative management of children with cancer include:

- nausea and vomiting, particularly prescribed alongside high-dose metoclopramide or ondansetron, or when raised intracranial pressure is the cause
- neuropathic pain caused by tumour compression, if prescribed within 48 hours of the onset of pain
- pain and nausea caused by liver infiltration by metastatic disease (e.g. neuroblastoma or sarcoma)
- other situations where reducing the oedema around a tumour can help alleviate symptoms (such as dyspnoea due to pulmonary metastases)
- superior vena cava obstruction (although rare in paediatric patients it can complicate lymphomas and other tumours of the mediastinum) or in any condition that causes thrombus to occlude the collecting systems of the upper thorax. By reducing oedema, steroids can improve facial swelling and symptoms of headache, flushing and uncomfortable fullness of the face
- stimulation of appetite – although eating is often a major concern to the family of a child, it is usually

more appropriate to explore their expectations and establish realistic goals than to prescribe steroids.

PALLIATIVE CHEMOTHERAPY

The main value of chemotherapy to patients is when it offers the possibility of a cure. Once this is no longer likely, the toxicity of chemotherapy means it is usually inappropriate. However, there are exceptions, e.g. chemotherapy agents that are relatively well tolerated, and that are effective in reducing, though not abolishing, the burden of malignant cells, with some symptom benefit. Vincristine has an acceptable side-effect profile, and combined with short courses of steroids can be a very effective adjunct in the management of bone pain caused by marrow infiltration by advanced leukaemia. Oral etoposide has been widely used in the palliative phase for a variety of malignancies.[89–92] However, the dose requires careful ongoing review, since it can cause hair loss and neutropenia, which may precipitate hospital admission for sepsis. Once again, a clinical judgement must be made about the balance of burden and benefit to the patient.

Families will often ask about new or experimental agents. This raises difficult ethical questions. On the one hand, the drugs are by definition of no proven benefit and may – indeed probably will – cause unpleasant side-effects. On the other hand, for some older children, experimental chemotherapy offers them the valuable opportunity to feel they have been able to help others. There is no reason in principle why experimental chemotherapy should not be offered. However, the paediatric oncologist should understand that most families who request it believe that it may do some good. It is important to ensure families understand that the chance of an improvement in the cancer is very limited, and that the expected benefit from participation in phase I or II studies is to other people. This needs to be made explicit by the clinician if families are to give truly informed consent.

RADIOTHERAPY

Radiotherapy is a powerful tool in palliation of symptoms.[93] It is highly effective in improving symptoms, even where they are caused by relatively resistant tumour such as osteosarcoma. A relatively small reduction in tumour mass can often have a disproportionate effect on symptoms.

Where bone metastases can be diagnosed clinically, a single dose of localized radiation can often be directed at the lesion without need for further imaging. Radiotherapy to chest tumours or pulmonary metastases can often relieve dyspnoea and/or haemoptysis. Where neuropathic pain is caused by compression by tumour, prompt radiotherapy can greatly enhance the effectiveness of systemic medications and may render them unnecessary.

In general, wherever symptoms are directly caused by the presence of tumour, it is worth seeking the advice of a radiotherapist as to whether it will be a helpful modality.

ANAESTHETIC BLOCKS

Procedures that require needles should, on the whole, be used only with caution in children requiring palliative care. However, there are times when the benefit outweighs the burden to the child. Epidural infusions of opioid and local anaesthetic can be highly effective. More specific blocks using local anaesthetic are done only infrequently in children, but offer effective alternatives in the management of opioid-resistant pains. Intra-abdominal tumours such as Wilms' or neuroblastoma may impinge on the coeliac plexus, causing intractable neuropathic pain which can be moderated using a coeliac plexus block. Blocks require the skilled input of an appropriately experienced anaesthetist.

Epidural infusions can be managed in the community by the liaison team. It is important to ensure that all those involved with the care of the child recognize that the infusion is into the epidural space, since the pumps and the medications may be the same but the doses are usually 10 times lower.

PSYCHOLOGICAL HELP FOR PAIN

In considering a rational approach to management, it has so far been necessary to consider the experience of pain in a systematic fashion. This has meant breaking it down firstly into its physical component and then further into various causal subtypes. This risks presenting pain as one or more unidimensional phenomena happening in parallel. In reality, pain, like all human experience, occurs simultaneously in all of the physical, psychosocial and existential (spiritual) dimensions. Having anatomized pain for the purpose of learning the principles, a process of reintegration is now necessary when applying them to the care of real patients.

The term 'total pain' is often used to describe a syndrome in which the physical component is a relatively minor part. Probably all pain should be considered 'total pain' but it is certainly true that for some children it becomes clear that no amount of physical intervention will be sufficient to manage their pain. Fear, anger, guilt, grieving, sadness and lack of understanding are all part of the experience of pain, but they do not respond well to analgesics.

If possible, a child's understanding of the pain and its causes should be explored. This can often be done effectively by the nurse or doctor, but where they are available the services of a child psychologist or play therapist should be enlisted. For many children, pain is made worse by a lack of understanding or, more commonly,

by the awareness[94] that something serious is happening about which they are being kept in the dark. For others, there are existential issues of guilt and anger to consider.

For some patients there may be coexistent psychiatric illness, particularly anxiety or depression. These are probably under-diagnosed in children. Whilst it is clear that uncontrolled pain can cause depression, it should also be borne in mind that untreated depression can make the experience of pain intolerable. Depression has been described as 'learned helplessness' and is an understandable but treatable response to terminal cancer and intractable pain. Paediatric oncologists should be prepared to offer counselling and, if necessary, medications in managing pathological depression in children.

Gastrointestinal problems

The pattern of symptoms experienced by children with cancer is probably little different from those of adults.[95,96] After pain, the commonest single symptom is nausea and vomiting. The pathophysiology of vomiting is complex, involving numerous chemotransmitters at receptors in the gut wall, in the liver, at the chemoreceptor trigger zone and in the vomiting centre itself. Superimposed on this basic system are higher cortical influences such as anxiety. Whatever the afferent arm, the efferent is mediated through acetylcholine in the vagus nerve.

In order to treat nausea and vomiting effectively, it is first necessary once again to have a systematic approach to diagnosis of the cause. This is the basis for rational prescribing of an antiemetic. For example, where damage to the gastrointestinal mucosa is thought to be the major cause, $5HT_3$ antagonists[97–101] such as ondansetron and high-dose metoclopramide are appropriate choices. On the other hand, where a central cause is suspected, cyclizine (anticholinergic and antihistamine) is a good first choice. It is worth remembering that irrespective of the cause, an anticholinergic is likely to be at least partially effective, through its effect on the vagus nerve.

In practice, nausea and vomiting are often multifactorial or else the cause cannot easily be identified. If the first-line antiemetic fails, a suitable second line[102] is levomepromazine (methotrimeprazine). This drug belongs to the phenothiazine group and acts at most of the major receptors involved in nausea and vomiting. It can therefore be seen as a 'broad spectrum' antiemetic. The mechanisms of nausea and vomiting, together with an approach to management in palliative medicine, have been thoroughly reviewed.[103]

Constipation is common among children with cancer. Many require opioids, and may be both relatively dehydrated and immobile. Opioid-induced constipation requires a stimulant and a softening laxative. Senna and magnesium hydroxide are a traditional combination and are very effective. More conveniently, co-danthrusate combines both functions in a single preparation. Lactulose, though often prescribed in paediatrics, has only a doubtful place in the management of opioid-induced constipation. It is primarily an osmotic laxative, whose metabolites cause flatulence and colic but have very little useful impact on increasing peristalsis. Novel approaches, such as the use of oral naloxone for opioid-induced constipation[104–106] and erythromycin to stimulate motilin receptors,[107] have not been widely used in children and are not yet well supported by evidence but carry little in the way of adverse effects.

Rarer symptoms associated with the gastrointestinal tract include diarrhoea, hiccoughs and pruritus caused by jaundice. There are therapeutic strategies available for all of these and it is worth consulting a local specialist consultant in paediatric or adult palliative medicine.

Respiratory problems

Dyspnoea is a sensation that breathing has become subjectively unpleasant. It may occur in as many as 40 per cent of children with cancer.[95,108] In considering how best to treat it, it is important to distinguish between breathing that has become unpleasant due to pain (for which the appropriate treatment is analgesia) and that due to other causes.[109,110] The lower respiratory tract is equipped with receptors sensitive to stretch, fluid and hypoxia. The sensations are coordinated in the respiratory centre in the medulla. Higher cortical centres processing anxiety and fear, and the respiratory centre are mutually influential.

Opioids given orally or parenterally relieve dyspnoea at a number of different levels.[109,110] The dose required to relieve dyspnoea is approximately half that required to relieve pain, but the two frequently coexist. Benzodiazepines (particularly midazolam) help to reduce anxiety but also act directly on the respiratory centre to reduce the sensation of dyspnoea. Face mask oxygen appears only to be effective in relieving the dyspnoea of hypoxia. Anecdotal reports of relief in other situations may reflect the influence of oxygen blowing on the face, an effect which can be reproduced using a fan, or opening a window. Similarly, nebulized opioids have been the subject of considerable research, which does not support their routine use.[56,110]

A common pattern of dyspnoea, particularly among teenagers, is the sudden panic attack. The main essential in managing such attacks is to give the patient or family the means to intervene rapidly at the moment breathlessness develops, in order to avoid a spiral of breathlessness and panic. Sublingual benzodiazepines such as lorazepam, or parenteral midazolam may have a valuable role here, as may face mask oxygen.

Where the cause of dyspnoea is pneumothorax or pleural effusion, there is sometimes a possibility of surgical intervention to relieve the problem. In practice, the need for admission to hospital and general anaesthetic makes these unsuitable for most children, and in any case the problems often recur. If they are necessary, concurrent pleurodesis should be considered to reduce the risk of recurrence.

Other symptoms

The child with terminal cancer has to die from something. The aim of a palliative approach is to prevent, as far as is possible, the symptoms that are distressing and unpleasant while allowing the disease itself to take its course. To this end it is usually a good idea to anticipate with the family what symptoms are likely to supervene, and to arrange for measures to control them to be available at short notice. Pain crises, feelings of suffocation and choking, severe agitation, catastrophic haemorrhage and convulsions are five of the commonest 'emergencies' to consider. Pain and choking have been dealt with elsewhere in this chapter.

AGITATION

Agitation can be exacerbated by the profusion of medications received by many of these children. The management is to rationalize medications, combined, if necessary, with haloperidol and midazolam for acute symptom control. There is some evidence that adequate hydration in adults can reduce the risk of agitation,[111,112] perhaps by improving the renal excretion of toxic metabolites.

CATASTROPHIC HAEMORRHAGE

Though rare, this is very frightening for the family and, if conscious, the child. Midazolam and other major anxiolytics have their place here, too, but a practical support is to have green surgical towels on hand. The sight even of a small haemorrhage on light-coloured bedclothes is frightening and the use of surgical towels can reduce this.

CONVULSIONS

Without treatment, convulsions commonly complicate the terminal phase of children with brain tumours, or those who suffer intercerebral haemorrhage as a result of thrombocytopenia. Where convulsions are thought likely, prophylactic anticonvulsants may be indicated early in the palliative management. Acute interventions include phenobarbitone infusion subcutaneously. This has the additional advantage of offering excellent sedation.

Rectal diazepam offers the family the opportunity to intervene to curtail a seizure.

Summary

Although children are very different from adults, particularly in the psychosocial, emotional and spiritual dimensions, many of the techniques of symptom control that have been developed in adults can have an application to paediatric patients, and particularly in those with cancer. When faced with difficult symptomatology, it is always worth seeking advice from a specialist paediatric or adult palliative medicine physician.

BLOOD AND PLATELET TRANSFUSIONS

Suppression of red cell and platelet production is common in the advanced stages of many malignancies, particularly lymphoproliferative disorders such as leukaemia. No-where is the potential conflict between an 'interventionist' approach and a 'palliative' one more clearly demonstrated than in the decision as to whether or not to offer transfusions of blood or platelets. Offering such a transfusion usually involves the child in visits to the hospital, which may be unwelcome. Routinely maintaining an 'adequate' haemoglobin or platelet count risks sending out very mixed messages about prognosis.

On the other hand, even relatively invasive procedures may be justified if the benefit outweighs the burden to the individual patient. Transfusions of both blood and platelets can sometimes offer significant improvement in the quality of a child's life. Symptoms of anaemia can include fatigue, dyspnoea and drowsiness. Thrombocytopenia can lead to the appearance of unsightly and worrying bruises as well as haemorrhages, particularly from the nasal and oral mucosae. Catastrophic haemorrhage is, in reality, rather uncommon, but the mere possibility can cause great anxiety to both patient and family in the presence of more minor bleeding.

As with all palliative manoeuvres, the decision to offer a full blood count and then a transfusion of blood or platelets should be made on the basis of the balance of burden and benefit in that individual patient. Where appropriate and practical, transfusions should ideally be offered in the child's home. For some patients, however, a visit to the oncology unit for transfusion can offer a welcome reminder that the unit is still available for support, even though cure is no longer possible.

Other factors that should be taken into account when deciding the balance of burden and benefit include the presence or otherwise of an indwelling central venous catheter and therefore the need for a needle, and the risk – usually small – of a distressing transfusion-related reaction.

PSYCHOLOGICAL SUPPORT

Talking with families

In breaking bad news, the job of the paediatric oncologist is to create the opportunity for the family to receive the message. Actually giving the information is only a small part of giving bad news.[113–115]

The main purpose of the interview for the physician is perhaps not simply to give information to the family. Rather, it should be a process of information exchange between oncologist and family. The oncologist has information about the disease; the family members have information about their prior understanding, their expectations, hopes and fears. In an ideal world, at the end of the interview, everyone involved would share all the relevant information. In reality, this is hampered by a number of barriers. Families rarely hear or understand all that is said to them, even after many repetitions. It is difficult for families to formulate the questions they want to ask, and, having done it, even more difficult for them to articulate these in the context of an emotional interview carried out in a hospital, often without good facilities for such discussions. It is important to remember that in exchanging information in this way, the playing field is not level; the family is at a natural disadvantage.

The first step is to find out what family members already understand ('alignment') by asking them. This serves a number of purposes simultaneously. Allowing people to talk, rather than simply speaking at them, gives them a chance to begin to be more relaxed, which will make it easier to hear what the oncologist has to say. Allowing family members to explain what they already understand also allows the oncologist to assess their factual knowledge and (perhaps more importantly) their understanding of it. The message given is rarely the message that is received. So, for example, it is not uncommon for families to know that multiple metastases have developed, but not to recognize that this makes cure impossible. Quite apart from its value in information exchange, this process of discovering what people already know before telling them what you want to say is simply a matter of courtesy. If it is not done, the impression received will be one of arrogance and an uncaring attitude.

Very often, the process of alignment reveals that family members know and understand much of what the paediatric oncologist wished to break to them. Indeed, commonly it becomes clear that they were expecting news that was even worse. Many parents expect their child to experience relentlessly increasing levels of pain, perhaps culminating in a catastrophic haemorrhage in the middle of the night at home when there is no one to support them. This scenario is, in reality, rather unlikely, and allowing the family to set the agenda at the beginning of the discussion can have the effect of transforming a discussion about bad news into an opportunity to reassure and comfort.

It is essential that decisions are made clearly and unambiguously. It is common for family members to misinterpret or misremember what is said. This is not because the consultant has failed to speak clearly, but because they find it hard to take in. The only solution to this is to be clear in the first place, and then to check that it has been understood by asking.

It is not always easy for families to ask the questions they wish to of a consultant, and questions should be actively solicited. The question 'Do you want to ask me anything about what I have just said?' may seem clumsy but can provide a valuable invitation for family members to explore further what the oncologist has said in a way that is accommodated by their own agenda.

Professionals as well as parents are generally reluctant to involve children in these difficult discussions, despite evidence that children have quite a sophisticated understanding of death and dying from an early age.[94,116,117] The risk is that, without access to the truth, children will construct an alternative explanation for the sadness and tension they observe among the rest of the family. They may consider that they must, in some way, have been responsible, and feel guilty, or simply be fearful of some vague but intense horror. Such ill-defined terrors are typically far worse than fear of what is actually likely.

Using a combination of verbal and symbolic approaches, often through play,[118] it is frequently possible to understand children's perspective enough to explore their understanding and interpretation of what is going on. This requires a sensitive, confident and skilled approach, often in collaboration with a child psychologist or other trained professional.

Generally speaking, the more open communication can be within a family, the better,[119-121] but families' own communication styles vary in their capacity for open discussions. Some families will never get to a point where they feel comfortable about their child knowing the truth.

Bereavement

Paediatric oncology, like other paediatric subspecialities, encompasses to some extent all three tiers of health care. During the years a child receives potentially curative treatment, the paediatric oncology team becomes the first port of call for most health care issues.

An appropriate extension of this family-centred, 'primary care' role is to offer families support after the child has died. The paediatric oncology team is then faced with a dilemma very familiar to those working in primary care: how proactive to be. On the one hand, the family needs support. On the other, they do not always welcome endless reminders of their involvement with the hospital.

Many families value the chance to meet the paediatric oncologist after the child's death. For some, this may simply be a question of an opportunity to say thank-yous and goodbyes to members of the team. For some, other issues may need to be addressed. However careful the team is to keep a family informed, there are often misunderstandings, and for some families these can assume particular importance after the child has died. Concerns may centre on a particular incident, perhaps unrelated to the actual circumstances of the child's death. The chance to go through their child's notes with the consultant or another member of the team can be very much appreciated. It offers the opportunity to have questions answered at the moment they occur, and emphasizes that there is no desire for secrecy.

Memorial services and organized opportunities for bereaved families in the unit to meet can also be supportive.

Longer-term support is often more appropriately provided by the clinical nurse specialist or social workers on the team. This has to proceed in a way and at a rate that is appropriate for the individual family. This can be hard for the carers; it can be difficult to avoid a feeling of rejection if a family chooses not to continue to engage with the team.

The range of grieving that is 'normal' is extremely wide. It is important to distinguish between helpful coping mechanisms and complicated grief. Factors that can make the grieving process more difficult include social and emotional isolation, difficulty in expressing grief (either due to inherent reluctance to discuss issues or to a lack of opportunity to do so), and pre-existing psychological or psychiatric vulnerability such as depression. None of these makes complicated grief inevitable, and their absence does not necessarily protect.

The role of the paediatric oncology team is usually to support normal grief and to recognize complicated grief among the bereaved family.[122] Where the latter is suspected, it is important to seek the involvement of appropriate specialists in mental health, such as psychologists or psychiatrists. Ongoing support can be offered through appropriate literature, telephone helplines[123] and group support.

Simply by being children, siblings are at risk of complicated grief. Children need special provision in order to express normal grief. There are very few such facilities currently and this is an area that needs considerable investment. In the meantime, there is much to be gained by encouraging families to be open with other children in the family. Where they feel able, siblings should be encouraged to attend funerals and address questions directly to the paediatric oncology team. Children's questions can often be disconcertingly blunt. It is important that members of the team deal with questions in a confident and open manner. Well meant deceits are usually counterproductive. Children are, on the whole, able to cope with loss and death, but they find untruths from adults much more difficult.

Support for staff

In our modern medical system, it has usually been assumed that professional carers are there to look after other people, rather than requiring support themselves. The reality is that paediatric oncology, despite the ever brightening prospects for cure, remains a speciality with high emotional casualties. For some staff, the effects may be very obvious, but for others they may manifest more subtly; they may have difficulty talking to patients or develop tactics to distance themselves from difficult emotional situations.[124] The effectiveness of the team in supporting the family of a child dying from cancer can therefore be imperilled.[115]

The development of such counterproductive tactics can be minimized by the provision of support for the team, particularly during the palliative phase. This can be done through regular input from skilled 'supervisors', and also simply through helping team members feel confident in their own skills. Such confidence comes from adequate education in aspects of listening, communicating effectively and symptom control. Considerable support is now available from specialists in palliative medicine, especially from the adult speciality, but increasingly from specialists in paediatric palliative care.

Summary

In summary, it is understandable that as paediatric oncologists, trained to diagnose and to try to cure cancer in childhood, we find it more uncomfortable to manage a child whose treatment has failed. However, palliative medicine in children can be a very active alternative to curative treatment. Like paediatric oncology, palliative care in children with cancer is characterized by a rational and systematic approach, a pragmatic mix of evidence basis and empiricism, and continual re-evaluation of the balance between burden and benefit.

PALLIATIVE MEDICINE IN CHILDREN: WHAT CAN BE LEARNED FROM THE ADULT SPECIALITY?

Increasing numbers of paediatricians are specializing in palliative medicine, and the opportunities for paediatricians to gain training in symptom control are expanding. Nevertheless, it will be many years before there are enough consultants to ensure that all children with cancer who need it can have access to specialist paediatric palliative medicine. In the meantime, it is essential that paediatric oncology teams recognize the value of input from adult specialists. This section considers some of the advances in adult palliative medicine that may impact on the paediatric speciality.

WHO ANALGESIC LADDER

In 1986, the WHO developed a set of guidelines for the treatment of pain following the recognition that pain control was a neglected public health issue.[125] The WHO three-step analgesic ladder aimed to give health care workers worldwide a simple scheme for controlling pain, using a relatively small number of drugs to be delivered regularly by mouth according to the individual needs of each patient (Figure 33.1). The principles of the scheme are equally applicable to the treatment of pain in children as they are in adults, apart from minor changes, e.g. the avoidance of aspirin and drugs that cannot be delivered as an elixir. A paediatric version of the ladder was published in 1998.[25]

The ladder has been criticised over recent years. Despite its widespread dissemination, pain is still poorly managed throughout the world.[126] This is generally assumed to be because of inadequate provision of analgesia, but in recent times, the ladder itself has been questioned. There is very little hard evidence to support the use of the ladder. Trials

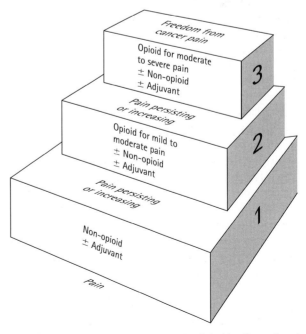

Figure 33.1 *The WHO three-step analgesic ladder. (Reproduced with kind permission from the World Health Organization.[25])*

claiming an efficacy of 70–95 per cent with respect to successful pain management in adults have been shown to be flawed, primarily because of poor methodology. There have been no randomized controlled trials, and many of the studies were retrospective and had short or variable follow-up. There were high withdrawal rates and insufficient detail with respect to outcome measures.[126,127] Furthermore, many of the step 1 drugs have been shown to be more efficacious than those traditionally used at step 2.[128]

The WHO ladder for adults has subsequently been revised to take some of these concerns into account, as follows:

- The NSAIDs are now classed as step 1 drugs rather than as adjuvants (and acknowledged to bridge steps 1 and 2).
- The use of an opioid as well as a non-opioid at step 2 is based on the principle that the mid-range opioids (codeine and dextropropoxyphene) should not be used alone but should be used in combination as in co-proxamol (paracetamol plus dextropropoxyphene) or co-codamol (paracetamol plus codeine).
- The terms 'weak' and 'strong' opioids have been replaced by 'opioids for mild to moderate pain' and 'opioids for moderate to severe pain' to reflect the fact that there is no clear distinction between different opioids.
- The list of recommended drugs has been increased to take account of new agents now available.

It has been argued that step 2 should be removed altogether and that it makes sense to progress from step 1 straight to low-dose morphine. Others have proposed a mechanistic approach to pain management based on the clinically perceived anatomical and pathophysiological mechanisms of pain generation, e.g. somatic versus visceral or neurogenic pain.[129]

Despite these criticisms, it must be stressed that the WHO ladder is established globally as a simple, user-friendly guide that can be employed in a large number of different countries, across all age groups and in different clinical environments. It is supported by considerable clinical experience and expert opinion and should not be discarded simply because of the lack of supporting evidence. Many paediatricians would argue that at the present time, the emphasis should be to ensure that the basic principles of pain management are adhered to, and that drugs are given regularly by mouth and according to the needs of the individual child.

ALTERNATIVE OPIOIDS

Morphine is the WHO opioid of choice for moderate-to-strong pain.[125] This premise is supported in the guidelines of the European Association of Palliative Care (EAPC)[130] and is rarely questioned.

It is well recognized in clinical practice, however, that between 10 and 30 per cent of adult patients do not benefit from morphine because of inadequate analgesia or intolerable side-effects.[131] Therefore, many patients are 'rotated' or 'switched' to an alternative opioid in an attempt to both improve pain control and lessen toxicity. There are several uncontrolled studies claiming benefit from such a manoeuvre[131,132] and many postulated mechanisms as to why there should be a benefit, including incomplete cross-tolerance and differential binding at receptor sites.[133] It is difficult to explain, however, how one opioid can be vastly different from another if they are acting at the same basic receptor.[134] It has been suggested that because of the uncertainty regarding equianalgesic opioid doses,[135] a rotation to an alternative opioid may simply equate with a dose reduction and therefore less toxicity.

Differences in toxicity and tolerability may be secondary to different pathways of metabolism. Morphine, for instance, undergoes glucuronidation to the metabolites, morphine-3-glucuronide (M3G) and morphine-6-glucuronide (M6G). M3G is the major toxic metabolite and is inactive as far as analgesia is concerned, while M6G is a rather minor metabolite which is powerfully analgesic. Both M3G and M6G can accumulate in renal failure, as of course does morphine itself. Both glucuronides are produced by the liver and therefore appear in reduced concentrations in anhepatic patients. The impact of hepatic failure on morphine metabolism is thus complex, since the body cannot convert mor-phine into either its minor analgesic or its major toxic metabolite.

Several alternative opioids have 'niche' or special indications. Fentanyl, delivered by a transdermal patch system, is ideal for patients unable to take drugs by mouth.[46] Young children dislike the process of patch removal, however, which can be likened to taking off a sticking plaster. Methadone is a cheap drug that has been around for many years and is thought to have some activity in neuropathic pain.[136] The process of titration is very different from that of morphine, however, and toxic metabolites can accumulate with prolonged use. Oxycodone is increasingly being used as the alternative opioid of choice in adult practice. It has greater bioavailability, fewer active metabolites and a more predictable pharmacokinetic profile compared with morphine. It produces equivalent analgesia to morphine with fewer reported incidences of nausea, pruritus and hallucinations when compared with morphine in controlled trials.[137] Its pharmacokinetics have been studied in adults[137–139] but nothing has been published on children other than occasional reports in non-cancer-related pain.[140–142] Hydromorphone is unlikely to be sufficiently different from morphine to justify its use as an alternative opioid. Diamorphine remains the parenteral opioid of choice. Those children who develop intolerable side-effects, e.g. nightmares, hallucinations or respiratory depression at a dose necessary for satisfactory pain relief, may benefit from a rotation to fentanyl or the related synthetic opioid alfentanil, especially in those patients with renal impairment.[143]

There are a large number of alternative opioids on the market, many of which have claimed superiority over morphine.[45,136] EAPC guidance states that there is insufficient evidence to date to suggest that any drug other than morphine should be the 'strong opioid' of choice.[130]

THE USE OF DRUGS BEYOND LICENCE

Recent audits in both palliative care and paediatric clinical practice have found that many licensed drugs are used in clinical situations that fall outside the remit of the licence, i.e. 'off-label'. This applies to drugs used for different age groups, different indications, doses or route of administration. A survey of drug use in paediatric wards in Europe and the UK found that almost half of all prescriptions were either unlicensed or off-label.[144] This is even more common in specialist palliative care units where such prescriptions may affect two-thirds of in-patients.[145] Examples include the use of carbamazepine or amitriptyline for neuropathic pain, levomepromazine for nausea and most of the drugs commonly delivered subcutaneously in palliative care, e.g. midazolam, cyclizine and hyoscine butylbromide. Many alternative opioids (hydromorphone, methadone and oxycodone) are not recommended for use in children.[146] Moreover, it is unlikely that a licence for most drugs used off-label will ever be obtained. The use of drugs for unlicensed indications is often supported by expert opinion and many years of clinical experience and there is often no financial incentive on the part of pharmaceutical companies to extend licences.

This has led to some concern in recent years from a clinical governance perspective and because of the possibility of accusations of clinical negligence when using drugs in this way. Patient information leaflets distributed when a drug is dispensed may well state that 'the medicine is not recommended for children'. In order to help communication with parents and children and to avoid misunderstanding, a generic patient information leaflet has been produced by the Royal College of Paediatricians and Child Health (RCPCH) to be included in all paediatric prescriptions. Peer approval for the use of many drugs beyond licence is documented in such publications as *Medicines for Children*[26] and the *Palliative Care Formulary*.[147] Position statements for the use of drugs beyond licence have been issued by both the Association of Palliative Medicine[148] and the RCPCH.[149]

It is acknowledged that the use of drugs beyond licence in palliative care is both necessary and common. There remains a need for the formulation of national frameworks, guidelines and standards for the use of drugs in this manner.

EVIDENCE BASE

Palliative medicine is hampered as a speciality by the paucity of evidence on which to base clinical practice. For example, in 2001, an expert working group of the EAPC published a set of guidelines on the use of opioids for the management of cancer pain.[130] The 20 key recommendations could only be supported by randomized controlled trial evidence in six cases. In over 50 per cent of cases, the recommendation is based on expert opinion alone.

This situation is not just limited to the use of opioids for pain control, but applies to the management of many other symptoms. For example, there are multiple randomized controlled trials in the use of antiemetics for the control of chemotherapy- or radiotherapy-induced nausea and vomiting,[150,151] but very few for the management of nausea and vomiting related to other factors, e.g. opioid-induced. Although there are a growing number of systematic reviews in the area of symptom control, these usually rely heavily on case reports, anecdotal data and expert opinion. Trials in paediatric palliative care are even more sparse, with much of the practice adopted from adult palliative care and non-cancer paediatric experience.

It is well recognized that clinical trials in palliative care are very difficult to undertake.[152] The patients are often of poor performance status and the study dropout rate is high. Although about 80 per cent of children with cancer are entered into UK Children's Cancer Study Group phase III studies, less than 10 per cent are ever entered into phase II studies. It has been shown, however, that patients are usually more than willing to participate if asked. It is the failure of health care professionals to approach adult patients about the possibility of entering a trial that is often the limiting factor.[153] Children's understanding of research is affected by their age and developmental maturity, by how much information they are provided with and by what opportunity they have been given to ask questions.[154] Research participation in children with cancer has been shown to be positively correlated with a sense of control over illness.[155]

Many of the common practices in palliative care have become firmly established on the basis of little more than physician preference and anecdote. To be taken seriously as a speciality in its own right, palliative care must be seen to justify what it does.[156]

WHAT IS THE ROLE OF AN ADULT PALLIATIVE CARE TEAM IN CARING FOR CHILDREN WITH ADVANCED CANCER?

Whilst palliative care in the UK is a highly developed speciality in its own right, palliative care in paediatrics is still in its infancy.[157] There are very few paediatricians specifically trained in the area. The work has largely been done by those with an interest in palliative care, or by those whose expertise overlaps or encompasses palliative care (e.g. paediatric oncologists caring for children with brain tumours or chest physicians with an interest in cystic fibrosis). In the absence of a well-developed paediatric palliative care service, should children with advanced disease be cared for by paediatric oncologists or by adult palliative care physicians?

There are practical issues that make it difficult for adult teams to provide palliative care to small children. Many adult palliative carers will have had very little exposure to, or experience in, paediatric palliative care. Young children are not 'little adults' and the diseases and symptomatology are different. Furthermore, according to the United Nations' *Convention on the Rights of the Child*,[158] it is not permissible for a physician treating adults to have sole medical responsibility for a child without the collaboration of a paediatrician.

Although community teams should enable most children to be cared for at home, in-patient admission is sometimes necessary to optimize symptom control. Adult in-patient units will not have suitable facilities and are rarely appropriate for children.[159] Adult services are unlikely to have the range of social work/psychological support available in most paediatric units. Families may be reluctant to lose strong attachments they have built up with a paediatric team and paediatricians may not want to lose contact with their patients.

On the other hand, palliative care is a highly developed speciality in adult practice and many of the approaches used in adults can be carried over into paediatrics. The holistic principles of palliative care, emphasizing physical, social and spiritual care of patients and families, apply to all age groups. Some experience in paediatric palliative care is now an essential requisite for the training of speciality registrars in palliative care and most communities are well served by highly skilled clinical nurse specialists. There are very few drugs and procedures used for the palliation of symptoms in adults that cannot be used in children. In many areas, there will be little expertise in pain and symptom control outside adult palliative care units and genuine concern by community paediatric teams regarding their ability to care for a dying child. The expertise of an adult palliative care service can be a very valuable resource and collaboration can greatly enhance the palliative care offered to a child.

A multidisciplinary and multiprofessional approach, with input if necessary from both adult teams and paediatricians, seems the most ideal. A model that allows for patient/parent choice regarding the focus and preferred place of care has been developed in some centres.[160,161] This is particularly important for adolescents whose care so often falls between adult and paediatric services.[162]

KEY POINTS

- Palliative care is an active and total approach to care, embracing physical, emotional, social and spiritual elements. It focuses on enhancement of quality of life for the child and support for the family and includes management of distressing symptoms, provision of respite, and care through death and bereavement.
- Palliative management should always be rational and take into account the balance between burden and benefit to the child.
- A rational approach may be evidence-based at some times and empirical at other times.
- Use of medications for off-label and unlicensed indications is a necessary and common practice both in paediatrics and in palliative medicine.
- Palliative care should ideally be provided in the home. Other resources, especially children's hospices, can provide valuable respite as well as an alternative for families who do not wish a death to take place at home.
- Palliative care cannot be delivered by one discipline or profession alone. Good team-working between doctors and nurses, primary, secondary and tertiary care, and sometimes between paediatric and adult services, requires very good communication and professional sensitivity.
- There is a right and a wrong way to prescribe medications, even in the palliative phase.
- Good symptom control requires specialist expertise and anticipation of likely problems. This is particularly true in the immediate terminal phase.
- The paediatric oncology team has a unique role in supporting a family before, during and after the palliative phase. However, the responsibility of the team is often to recognize the need for the expertise of others. This may include psychologists, bereavement counsellors and chaplains as well as specialists in paediatric palliative care (if available), GPs, children's hospices and adult palliative medicine teams.
- Expression of normal grief can be difficult in today's culture, particularly for children. Many resources can help, including the telephone 'help lines'.

REFERENCES

●1. Lauer ME, Mulhern RK, Wallskog JM, Camitta BM. A comparison study of parental adaptation following a child's death at home or in the hospital. *Pediatrics* 1983; **71**(1): 107–12.

2. Burne SR, Dominica F, Baum JD. Helen House – a hospice for children: analysis of the first year. *Br Med J (Clin Res Ed)* 1984; **289**(6459): 1665–8.

3. Goldman A, Beardsmore S, Hunt J. Palliative care for children with cancer – home, hospital, or hospice? *Arch Dis Child* 1990; **65**(6): 641–3.

4. Baker CM, Wong DL. QUEST: a process of pain assessment in children. *Orthop Nurs* 1987; **6**(1): 11–21.

♦5. Franck LS, Greenberg CS, Stevens B. Pain assessment in infants and children. *Pediatr Clin North Am* 2000; **47**(3): 487–512.

♦6. Hain RDW. Pain scales in children: a review. *Palliat Med* 1997; **11**(5): 341–50.

7. Huskisson EC. Visual analogue scales. In: Melzack R, ed. *Pain Management and Assessment.* New York: Raven Press, 1983; 33–7.

8. Price DD, McGrath PA, Rafii A, Buckingham B. The validation of visual analogue scales as ratio scale measures for chronic and experimental pain. *Pain* 1983; **17**: 45–56.

9. Hester NKO, Foster R, Kristensen K. Measurement of pain in children: generalizability and validity of the pain ladder and the poker chip tool. In: Tyler DC, Krane EJ, eds. *Advances in Pain Research and Therapy.* New York: Raven Press, 1990; **15**: 79–84.

10. Kuttner L, LePage T. Face scales for the assessment of pediatric pain: a critical review. *Can J Behav Sci/Rev Can Sci Comp* 1989; **21**(2): 198–209.

11. Bieri D, Reeve RA, Champion GD *et al.* The faces pain scale for the self-assessment of the severity of pain experienced by children: development, initial validation, and preliminary investigation for ratio scale properties. *Pain* 1990; **41**: 139–50.

12. Beyer JE, Wells N. The assessment of pain in children. *Pediatr Clin North Am* 1989; **36**(4): 837–54.

13. Beyer A. Content validity of an instrument to measure young children's perception of the intensity of their pain. *J Pediatr Nurs* 1986; **1**(6): 386–95.

14. Beyer JE, Villarruel AM, Denyes M. *The Oucher: The New User's Manual and Technical Report.* Denver, CO: University of Colorado Health Sciences Center, 1988.

15. Beyer A. Convergent and discriminant validity of a self-report measure of pain intensity for children. *Children's Health Care* 1988; **16**(4): 274–82.

16. Jordan-Marsh M, Yoder L, Hall D, Watson R. Alternate Oucher form testing: gender, ethnicity, and age variations. *Res Nurs Health* 1994; **17**(2): 111–18.

17. Knott C, Beyer J, Villarruel A *et al.* Using the Oucher developmental approach to pain assessment in children. *MCN Am J Matern Child Nurs* 1994; **19**(6): 314–20.

18. Beyer JE, Denyes MJ, Villarruel AM. The creation, validation, and continuing development of the Oucher: a measure of pain intensity in children. *J Pediatr Nurs* 1992; **7**(5): 335–46.

19. Beyer JE, Knott CB. Construct validity estimation for the African-American and Hispanic versions of the Oucher Scale. *J Pediatr Nurs* 1998; **13**(1): 20–31.

20. Gauvain-Piquard A, Rodary C, Lemerle J. L'atonie psychomotrice: signe majeur de douleur chez l'enfant de moins de 6 ans. *J Paris Pediatrie* 1988: 249–52.

●21. Gauvain-Piquard A, Rodary C, Rezvani A, Serbouti S. The development of the DEGR(R): A scale to assess pain in young children with cancer. *Eur J Pain* 1999; **3**(2): 165–76.

22. Gauvain-Piquard A, Rodary C, Francois P *et al.* Validity assessment of DEGR scale for observational rating of 2–6 year old child pain. *J Pain Symptom Manage* 1991; **6**(3): 171.

23. Ventafridda V, Tamburini M, Caraceni C *et al.* A validation study of the WHO method for cancer pain relief. *Cancer* 1987; **59**: 850–6.

♦24. World Health Organization. *Cancer as a Global Problem.* Geneva: WHO, 1984.

♦25. World Health Organization. Guidelines for analgesic drug therapy. In: *Cancer Pain Relief and Palliative Care in Children.* Geneva: WHO/IASP, 1998; 24–8.

26. Hull D, Burns A, Stephenson T *et al. Medicines for Children,* 1st edn. London: Royal College of Paediatrics and Child Health; 1999.

27. Pal SK, Cortiella J, Herndon D. Adjunctive methods of pain control in burns. *Burns* 1997; **23**(5): 404–12.

28. Michaud L, Gottrand F, Ganga-Zandzou PS *et al.* Nitrous oxide sedation in pediatric patients undergoing gastrointestinal endoscopy. *J Pediatr Gastroenterol Nutr* 1999; **28**(3): 310–14.

29. Martin JP, Sexton BF, Saunders BP, Atkin WS. Inhaled patient-administered nitrous oxide/oxygen mixture does not impair driving ability when used as analgesia during screening flexible sigmoidoscopy. *Gastrointest Endosc* 2000; **51**(6): 701–3.

30. Kussman BD, Sethna NF. Pethidine-associated seizure in a healthy adolescent receiving pethidine for postoperative pain control. *Paediatr Anaesth* 1998; **8**(4): 349–52.

31. Pryle BJ, Grech H, Stoddart PA *et al.* Toxicity of norpethidine in sickle cell crisis. *Br Med J* 1992; **304**(6840): 1478–9.

32. Esmail Z, Montgomery C, Courtrn C *et al.* Efficacy and complications of morphine infusions in postoperative paediatric patients. *Paediatr Anaesth* 1999; **9**(4): 321–7.

33. McRorie TI, Lynn AM, Nespeca MK *et al.* The maturation of morphine clearance and metabolism. *Am J Dis Child* 1992; **146**(8): 972–6.

●34. Collins JJ, Geake J, Grier HE *et al.* Patient-controlled analgesia for mucositis pain in children: a three-period crossover study comparing morphine and hydromorphone. *J Pediatr* 1996; **129**(5): 722–8.

35. Hunt A, Joel S, Dick G, Goldman A. Population pharmacokinetics of oral morphine and its glucuronides in children receiving morphine as immediate-release liquid or sustained-release tablets for cancer pain. *J Pediatr* 1999; **135**(1): 47–55.

36. Hain RD, Hardcastle A, Pinkerton CR, Aherne GW. Morphine and morphine-6-glucuronide in the plasma and cerebrospinal fluid of children. *Br J Clin Pharmacol* 1999; **48**(1): 37–42.

37. Lynn A, Nespeca MK, Bratton SL *et al.* Clearance of morphine in postoperative infants during intravenous infusion: the influence of age and surgery. *Anesth Analg* 1998; **86**(5): 958–63.

38. Hartley R, Green M, Quinn M, Levene MI. Pharmacokinetics of morphine infusion in premature neonates. *Arch Dis Child* 1993; **69**: 55–8.

39. Hunt TL, Kaiko RF. Comparison of the pharmacokinetic profiles of two oral controlled-release morphine formulations in healthy young adults. *Clin Ther* 1991; **13**(4): 482–8.

40. Arai L. The use of ondansetron to treat pruritis associated with intrathecal morphine in two paediatric patients. *Paediatr Anaesth* 1996; **6**(4): 337–9.

41. Sanger GJ, Twycross R. Making sense of emesis, pruritus 5HT- & 5HT$_3$-receptor antagonists. *Prog Palliat Care* 1996; **4**: 7–8.

42. Kyriakides K, Hussain SK, Hobbs GJ. Management of opioid-induced pruritus: a role for 5HT$_3$ antagonists? *Br J Anaesth* 1999; **83**(3): 439–41.

43. Nelson TW, Lilly JK 3rd, Baker JD 3rd, Ackerly JA. Treatment of pruritus secondary to epidural morphine. Prophylactic v. PRN naloxone. *W V Med J* 1988; **84**(5): 183–5.

●44. Hunt AM, Goldman A, Devine T, Phillips M. Transdermal fentanyl for pain relief in a paediatric palliaitve care population. *Palliat Med* 2001; **15**: 405–12.

●45. Ahmedzai S, Brooks D. Transdermal fentanyl versus sustained-release oral morphine in cancer pain: preference, efficacy, and quality of life. The TTS-Fentanyl Comparative Trial Group. *J Pain Symptom Manage* 1997; **13**(5): 254–61.

●46. Collins JJ, Dunkel IJ, Gupta SK *et al.* Transdermal fentanyl in children with cancer pain: feasibility, tolerability, and pharmacokinetic correlates. *J Pediatr* 1999; **134**: 319–23.

47. Stringer M, Makin MK, Miles J, Morley JS. D-morphine, but not l-morphine, has low micromolar affinity for the non-competitive N-methyl-D-aspartate site in rat forebrain. Possible clinical implications for the management of neuropathic pain. *Neurosci Lett* 2000; **295**(1–2): 21–4.

48. Sang CN. NMDA-receptor antagonists in neuropathic pain: experimental methods to clinical trials. *J Pain Symptom Manage* 2000; **19**(suppl. 1): S21–5.

49. Ripamonti C, De Conno F, Groff L *et al.* Equianalgesic dose/ratio between methadone and other agonists in cancer pain: comparison of two clinical experiences. *Ann Oncol* 1998; **9**(1): 79–83.

50. Carpenter KJ, Chapman V, Dickenson AH. Neuronal inhibitory effects of methadone are predominantly opioid receptor mediated in the rat spinal cord *in vivo*. *Eur J Pain* 2000; **4**: 19–26.

●51. Shir Y, Shenkman Z, Shavelson V *et al.* Oral methadone for the treatment of severe pain in hospitalized children: a report of five cases. *Clin J Pain* 1998; **14**(4): 350–3.

52. Miser AW, Chayt KJ, Sandlund JT *et al.* Narcotic withdrawal syndrome in young adults after the therapeutic use of opiates. *Am J Dis Child* 1986; **140**(6): 603–4.

53. Grassby PF, Hutchings L. Drug combinations in syringe drivers: the compatibility and stability of diamorphine with cyclizine and haloperidol. *Palliat Med* 1997; **11**(3): 217–24.

54. Vermeire A, Remon JP. Compatibility and stability of ternary admixtures of morphine with haloperidol or midazolam and dexamethasone or methylprednisolone. *Int J Pharm* 1999; **177**(1): 53–67.

55. Schrijvers DEA. Determination of compatibility and stability of drugs used in palliative care. *J Clin Pharm Ther* 1998; **23**(4): 311–14.

56. Zeppetella G. Nebulized morphine in the palliation of dyspnoea. *Palliat Med* 1997; **11**: 267–75.

57. Sharar SR, Bratton SL, Carrougher GJ *et al.* A comparison of oral transmucosal fentanyl citrate and oral hydromorphone for inpatient pediatric burn wound care analgesia. *J Burn Care Rehabil* 1998; **19**(6): 516–21.

58. Back IN, Finlay I. Analgesic effect of topical opioids on painful skin ulcers. *J Pain Symptom Manage* 1995; **10**(7): 493.

59. Flock P, Gibbs L, Sykes N. Diamorphine-metronidazole gel effective for treatment of painful infected leg ulcers. *J Pain Symptom Manage* 2000; **20**(6): 396–7.

60. Krajnik M, Zylicz Z, Finlay I *et al.* Potential uses of topical opioids in palliative care – report of 6 cases. *Pain* 1999; **80**(1–2): 121–5.

61. Ramesh PR, Santhosh AR, Kumar KS. Topical morphine in Ayurveda. *Palliat Med* 1998; **12**(1): 64.

62. Twillman RK, Long TD, Cathers TA, Mueller DW. Treatment of painful skin ulcers with topical opioids. *J Pain Symptom Manage* 1999; **17**(4): 288–92.

63. Thomsen CB, Crawford ME, Sjogren P. Malignant bone pain. *Ugeskr Laeger* 1997; **159**(16): 2364–9.

64. Johnson JR, Miller AJ. The efficacy of choline magnesium trisalicylate (CMT) in the management of metastatic bone pain: a pilot study. *Palliat Med* 1994; **8**(2): 129–35.

65. Portenoy RK. Cancer pain management [review]. *Semin Oncol* 1993; **20**(2 suppl. 1): 19–35.

66. Portenoy RK. Pharmacologic management of cancer pain [review]. *Semin Oncol* 1995; **22**(2 suppl. 3): 112–20.

67. Payne R. Mechanisms and management of bone pain. *Cancer* 1997; **80**(8 Suppl.): 1608–13.

68. Levick S, Jacobs C, Loukas DF *et al.* Naproxen sodium in treatment of bone pain due to metastatic cancer. *Pain* 1988; **35**(3): 253–8.

●69. Yeomans ND, Tulassay Z, Juhasz L *et al.* A comparison of omeprazole with ranitidine for ulcers associated with nonsteroidal antiinflammatory drugs. Acid Suppression Trial: Ranitidine versus Omeprazole for NSAID-associated Ulcer Treatment (ASTRONAUT) Study Group. *N Engl J Med* 1998; **338**(11): 719–26.

●70. Hawkey CJ, Karrasch JA, Szczepanski L *et al.* Omeprazole compared with misoprostol for ulcers associated with nonsteroidal antiinflammatory drugs. Omeprazole versus Misoprostol for NSAID-induced Ulcer Management (OMNIUM) Study Group. *N Engl J Med* 1998; **338**(11): 727–34.

71. Yeomans ND. New data on healing of nonsteroidal anti-inflammatory drug-associated ulcers and erosions. Omeprazole NSAID Steering Committee. *Am J Med* 1998; **104**(3A): 56S–61S (discussion 79S–80S).

72. Shah AA, Thjodleifsson B, Murray FE *et al.* Selective inhibition of COX-2 in humans is associated with less gastrointestinal injury: a comparison of nimesulide and naproxen. *Gut* 2001; **48**(3): 339–46.

73. Mandell BF. COX 2-selective NSAIDs: biology, promises, and concerns. *Cleve Clin J Med* 1999; **66**(5): 285–92.

74. Miyamoto H, Saura R, Harada T et al. The role of cyclooxygenase-2 and inflammatory cytokines in pain induction of herniated lumbar intervertebral disc. Kobe J Med Sci 2000; **46**(1–2): 13–28.

75. Piper JM, Ray WA, Daugherty JR, Griffin MR. Corticosteroid use and peptic ulcer disease: role of nonsteroidal anti-inflammatory drugs. Ann Intern Med 1991; **114**(9): 735–40.

♦●76. McQuay HJ, Tramer M, Nye BA et al. A systematic review of antidepressants in neuropathic pain. Pain 1996; **68**: 217–27.

♦●77. McQuay HJ, Carroll D, Jadad AR et al. Anticonvulsant drugs for management of pain: a systematic review. Br Med J 1995; **311**: 1047–52.

78. Backonja M, Beydoun A, Edwards KR et al. Gabapentin for the symptomatic treatment of painful neuropathy in patients with diabetes mellitus: a randomized controlled trial. J Am Med Assoc 1998; **280**(21): 1831–6.

79. Caraceni A, Zecca E, Martini C, De Conno F. Gabapentin as an adjuvant to opioid analgesia for neuropathic cancer pain. J Pain Symptom Manage 1999; **17**(6): 441–5.

80. Chandler A, Williams JE. Gabapentin, an adjuvant treatment for neuropathic pain in a cancer hospital. J Pain Symptom Manage 2000; **20**(2): 82–6.

81. Dallocchio C, Buffa C, Mazzarello P, Chiroli S. Gabapentin vs. amitriptyline in painful diabetic neuropathy: an open-label pilot study. J Pain Symptom Manage 2000; **20**(4): 280–5.

82. Morello CM, Leckband SG, Stoner CP et al. Randomized double-blind study comparing the efficacy of gabapentin with amitriptyline on diabetic peripheral neuropathy pain. Arch Intern Med 1999; **159**(16): 1931–7.

83. Rowbotham M, Harden N, Stacey B et al. Gabapentin for the treatment of postherpetic neuralgia: a randomized controlled trial. J Am Med Assoc 1998; **280**(21): 1837–42.

84. Rusy LM, Troshynski TJ, Weisman SJ. Gabapentin in phantom limb pain management in children and young adults: report of seven cases. J Pain Symptom Manage 2001; **21**(1): 78–82.

85. McDonnell FJ, Sloan JW, Hamann SR. Advances in cancer pain management. Curr Pain Headache Rep 2001; **5**(3): 265–71.

86. Lloyd-Williams M. Ketamine for cancer pain. J Pain Symptom Manage 2000; **19**(2): 79–80.

87. Takahashi H, Miyazaki M, Nanbu T et al. The NMDA-receptor antagonist ketamine abolishes neuropathic pain after epidural administration in a clinical case. Pain 1998; **75**(2–3): 391–4.

88. Persson J, Axelsson G, Hallin RG, Gustafsson LL. Beneficial effects of ketamine in a chronic pain state with allodynia, possibly due to central sensitization. Pain 1995; **60**(2): 217–22.

●89. Davidson A, Gowing R, Lowis S et al. Phase II study of 21 day schedule oral etoposide in children. New Agents Group of the United Kingdom Children's Cancer Study Group (UKCCSG). Eur J Cancer 1997; **33**(11): 1816–22.

90. Haim N, Ben-Shahar M, Epelbaum R. Prolonged daily administration of oral etoposide in lymphoma following prior therapy with adriamycin, an ifosfamide-containing salvage combination, and intravenous etoposide. Cancer Chemother Pharmacol 1995; **36**(4): 352–5.

91. Ng A, Taylor GM, Eden OB. Secondary leukemia in a child with neuroblastoma while on oral etoposide: what is the cause? Pediatr Hematol Oncol 2000; **17**(3): 273–9.

●92. Schiavetti A, Varrasso G, Maurizi P et al. Ten-day schedule oral etoposide therapy in advanced childhood malignancies. J Pediatr Hematol Oncol 2000; **22**(2): 119–24.

93. Crellin AM, Marks A, Maher EJ. Why don't British radiotherapists give single fractions of radiotherapy for bone metastases? Clin Oncol 1989; **1**: 63–6.

94. Bluebond-Langner M. The Private Worlds of Dying Children. Princeton, NJ: Princeton University Press; 1978.

95. Wolfe J, Grier HE, Klar N et al. Symptoms and suffering at the end of life in children with cancer. N Engl J Med 2000; **342**(5): 326–33.

96. Hain RDW, Hughes E. Children referred for specialist palliative care: First 25 patients. Arch Dis Child 2001; **84**(Suppl. 1): A56–7.

97. DeMulder HM, Seynaeve S, Vermorken JB et al. Ondansetron compared with high-dose metaclopramide in prophylaxis of acute and delayed cisplatin-induced nausea and vomiting. Ann Intern Med 1990; **113**: 834–40.

98. White L, Daly SA, Zhestkova N et al. A comparison of oral ondansetron syrup or intravenous ondansetron loading dose regimens given in combination with dexamethasone for the prevention of nausea and emesis in pediatric and adolescent patients receiving moderately/highly emetogenic chemotherapy. Pediatr Hematol Oncol 2000; **17**: 445–55.

●99. Pinkerton CR, Williams D, Wootton C et al. 5HT3 antagonist ondansetron – an effective outpatient antiemetic in cancer treatment. Arch Dis Child 1990; **65**: 822–5.

100. Currow DC, Coughlan M, Fardell B, Cooney NJ. Use of ondansetron in palliative medicine. J Pain Symptom Manage 1997; **13**: 301–7.

101. Tramer M, Moore RA, Reynolds DJM, McQuay HJ. A quantitative systematic review of ondansetron in treatment of established post-operative nausea and vomiting. Br Med J 1997; **314**: 1088–92.

102. Twycross RG, Barkby GD, Hallwood PM. The use of low dose levomepromazine (methotrimeprazine) in the management of nausea and vomiting. Prog Palliat Care 1997; **5**(2): 49–53.

♦103. Twycross R, Back I. Nausea and vomiting in advanced cancer. Eur J Palliat Care 1998; **5**(2): 39–45.

104. Kreek M-J, Schaefer RA, Hahn EF, Fishman J. Naloxone, a specific opioid antagonist, reverses chronic idiopathic constipation. Lancet 1983; **1**: 261–2.

105. Meissner W, Schmidt U, Hartmann M et al. Oral naloxone reverses opioid-induced constipation. Pain 2000; **84**: 105–9.

106. Sykes NP. An investigation of the ability of oral naloxone to correct opioid-related constipation in patients with advanced cancer. Palliat Med 1996; **10**: 135–44.

107. Peeters TL. Erythromycin and other macrolides as prokinetic agents. Gastroenterology 1993; **105**: 1886–99.

108. Hain RDW, Patel N, Crabtree S, Pinkerton CR. Respiratory symptoms in children dying from malignant disease. Palliat Med 1995; **9**: 201–6.

109. Ripamonti C, Bruera E. Dyspnea: pathophysiology and assessment. J Pain Symptom Manage 1997; **13**(4): 220–32.

♦110. Davis CL. The therapeutics of dyspnoea. *Cancer Surv Palliat Med* 1994; **21**: 85–98.

●111. Bruera E, Franco JJ, Maltoni M *et al.* Changing pattern of agitated impaired mental status in patients with advanced cancer: association with cognitive monitoring, hydration and opioid rotation. *J Pain Symptom Manag* 1995; **10**(4): 287–91.

●112. Lawlor PG, Gagnon B, Mancini IL *et al.* Occurrence, causes, and outcome of delirium in patients with advanced cancer: a prospective study. *Arch Intern Med* 2000; **160**(6): 786–94.

♦113. Ptacek JT, Eberhardt TL. Breaking bad news. A review of the literature. *J Am Med Assoc* 1996; **276**(6): 496–502.

114. Franks A. Breaking bad news and the challenge of communication. *Eur J Palliat Care* 1997; **4**(2): 61–5.

♦115. Buckman R. Breaking bad news: why is it still so difficult? *Br Med J* 1984; **288**: 1597–9.

116. Lansdown R, Benjamin G. The development of the concept of death in children aged 5–9 years. *Child Care Health Dev* 1985; **11**(1): 13–20.

117. Kane B. Children's concepts of death. *J Gen Psychol* 1979; **134**: 141–53.

118. Goldman A, Christie D. Children with cancer talk about their own death with their families. *Pediatr Hematol Oncol* 1993; **10**: 223–31.

♦●119. Mulhern RK, Lauer ME, Hoffman RG. Death of a child at home or in the hospital: subsequent psychological adjustment of the family. *Pediatrics* 1983; **71**: 743–7.

120. Spinetta JJ. Impact of cancer on the family. *Front Radiat Ther Oncol* 1981; **16**: 167–76.

121. Spinetta JJ, Swarner JA, Sheposh JP. Effective parental coping following the death of a child from cancer. *J Pediatr Psychol* 1981; **6**(3): 251–63.

122. Worden JW. *Grief Counselling and Grief Therapy*, 2nd edn. London: Tavistock/Routledge, 1991.

123. Child Death Helpline. +44(0)800 282986. Operates 7–10pm every evening and 10am–1pm Wednesday.

♦124. Maguire P. Barriers to psychological care of the dying. *Br Med J (Clin Res Ed)* 1985; **291**(6510): 1711–13.

125. World Health Organization (WHO). *Cancer Pain Relief: a Guide to Opioid Availability*, 2nd edn. Geneva: WHO, 1996.

♦126. Jadad AR, Browman GP. The WHO analgesic ladder for cancer pain management. *J Am Med Assoc* 1995; **274**(23): 1870–3.

127. Mercadante S. Pain treatment and outcomes for patients with advanced cancer who receive follow-up care at home. *Cancer* 1999; **85**: 1849–58.

♦128. McQuay H, Moore A. *An Evidence-based Resource for Pain Relief. Acute Pain: Conclusion.* Oxford: Oxford University Press, 1998; 187–92.

129. Ashby MA, Fleming BG, Brooksbank M *et al.* Description of a mechanistic approach to pain management in advanced cancer. Preliminary report. *Pain* 1992; **51**: 153–61.

♦130. European Association for Palliative care (EAPC) Expert Working Group of the Research Network. Morphine and alternative opioids in cancer pain: the EAPC recommendations. *Br J Cancer* 2001; **84**(5): 587–93.

131. De Stoutz ND, Bruera E, Suarez-Almazoe M. Opioid rotation for toxicity reduction in terminal cancer patients. *J Pain Symptom Manage* 1995; **10**(5): 378–84.

132. Ashby MA, Martin P, Jackson KA. Opioid substitution to reduce adverse effects in cancer pain management. *Med J Aust* 1999; **170**: 68–71.

133. Fallon M. Opioid rotation: does it have a role? *Palliat Med* 1997; **11**: 177–8.

134. McQuay H. Opioids in pain management. *Lancet* 1999; **353**: 2229–32.

♦135. Pereira J, Lawlor P, Vigano A *et al.* Equianalgesic dose ratios for opioids: a critical review and proposals for long-term dosing. *J Pain Symptom Manage* 2001; **22**: 672–87.

136. Collins JJ, Berde CB. Management of cancer pain in children. In: Pizzo PA, Poplack DG, eds. *Principles and Practice of Pediatric Oncology*, 3rd edn. Philadelphia: Lippincott-Raven, 1997.

♦137. Shah S, Hardy J. Oxycodone: a review of the literature. *Eur J Palliat Care* 2001; **8**(3): 93–6.

138. Davis MP, Homsi J. The importance of cytochrome P450 monooxygenase CYP2D6 in palliative medicine. *Support Care Cancer* 2001; **9**: 442–51.

139. Tallgren M, Olkkola KT, Seppala T *et al.* Pharmacokinetics and ventilatory effects of oxycodone before and after liver transplantation. *Clinical Pharmacol Ther* 1997; **61**(6): 655–61.

140. Atchinson NE, Osgood PF, Carr DB *et al.* Pain during burn dressing change in children: relationship to burn area, depth and analgesic regimens. *Pain*: 1991; **47**(1): 41–5.

141. Kalso E. Pharmacokinetics and ventilatory effects of intravenous oxycodone in postoperative children. *Br J Clin Pharmacol* 1995; **39**(20): 214–15.

142. Sharar SR, Carrougher GJ, Selzer K *et al.* A comparison of oral transmucosal fentanyl citrate and oral oxycodone for pediatric outpatient wound care. *J Burn Care Rehabil* 2002; **23**(1): 27–31.

♦143. Davies G, Kingswood C, Street M. Pharmacokinetics of opioids in renal dysfunction. *Clin Pharmacokinet* 1996; **31**(6): 410–22.

144. Conroy S, Choonara I, Impicciatore P *et al.* Survey of unlicensed and off label drug use in paediatric wards in European countries. *Br Med J* 2000; **320**: 79–82.

145. Pavis H, Wilcock A. Prescribing of drugs for use outside their licence in palliative care: survey of specialists in the United Kingdom. *Br Med J* 2001; **323**: 484–5.

146. BMA/RPSGB. *British National Formulary (BNF)*. London: British Medical Association and Royal Pharmaceutical Society of Great Britain, 2002.

147. Twycross R, Wilcocks A, Thorp S. *Palliative Care Formulary*. Abingdon: Radcliffe Medical Press, 1998.

148. Association for Palliative Medicine (APM) and the Pain Society. *The Use of Drugs Beyond Licence in Palliative Care and Pain Management. A Position Statement Prepared on Behalf of the APM and the Pain Society*. London: APM/Pain Society, 2002.

149. Royal College of Paediatrics and Child Health. *Position Statement on the Use of Licensed and Unlicensed Medicines*. London: RCPCH, 2000.

●150. Dick GS, Meller ST, Pinkerton CR. Randomised comparison of ondansetron with metochlorpramide and dexamethasone for chemotherapy-induced emesis. *Arch Dis Child* 1995; **73**: 243–5.

♦151. Fauser AA, Fellhauer M, Hoffman M *et al.* Guidelines for anti-emetic therapy: acute emesis. *Eur J Cancer* 1999; **35**(3): 361–70.

152. Grande GE, Todd CJ. Issues in research: why are trials in palliative care so difficult? *Palliat Med* 2000; **14**(1): 69–74.

153. Ling J, Rees E, Hardy J. What influences participation in clinical trials in palliative care in a cancer centre? *Eur J Cancer* 2000; **36**: 621–6.

154. Devine T. Presenting a case for involving children with a terminal illness in clinical trials. *Int J Palliat Nurs* 2001; **7**(10): 482–4.

155. Dorn LD, Susman EJ, Fletcher JC. Informed consent in children and adolescents: age, maturation and psychological state. *J Adolesc Health* 1995; **16**(3): 185–90.

156. Hardy JR. Placebo-controlled trials in palliative care: the argument for. *Palliat Med* 1997; **11**: 415–18.

157. Hain R. The view from a bridge. *Eur J Palliat Care* 2002; **9**(2): 75–7.

158. United Nations. *Convention on the Rights of the Child.* London: HMSO, 1991.

159. Association for Children with Life-Limiting and Threatening Illnesses and their Families (ACT). *Children in Adult Hospices.* Bristol: ACT, 1996.

160. McQuillan R, Finlay I. Facilitating the care of terminally ill children. *J Pain Symptom Manage* 1996; **12**: 320–4.

161. Edwards J. A model of palliative care for the adolescent with cancer. *Int J Palliat Nurs* 2001; **7**(10): 485–8.

162. Thornes R, for Joint Working Party on Palliative Care for Adolescents and Young Adults. *Palliative Care for Young People Aged 13–24.* Bristol: Association for Children with Life-threatening or Terminal Conditions and their Families (ACT), National Council for Hospice and Specialist Palliative Care Services, Scottish Partnership Agency for Palliative and Cancer Care (SPAPCC), 2001.

34

Caring for the child with cancer within a model of shared care

JACKIE EDWARDS & LOUISE HOOKER

INTRODUCTION

The improved outcomes for children and teenagers with cancer are related to developments in treatment, supportive care and service provision, to the extent that in many cases survival is expected although never certain. There is evidence that centralized paediatric oncology care is associated with improved survival.[1] As increased numbers of patients have been referred to paediatric oncology treatment centres, these centres have developed specialist services and facilities and significant expertise in clinical management.[2] Centralized care is not without its drawbacks, and attempts have been made to understand the problems that families experience. These may include increased travelling, disruption to family life, financial costs, social isolation and additional stress.[3–5]

The development of intensive treatment for poor-risk groups, requiring high-dependency in-patient care has been paralleled by expansion in the range of drug regimens designed to be administered in outpatient settings, or even in the home. These developments have an impact on the delivery of both treatment and care, as existing systems of care are adapted and new systems devised to respond to the physical and psychosocial needs of children, teenagers and their families in both the short and long term. One such response is the increased use of systems of shared care, in an attempt to combine the survival advantage of specialist treatment with the benefits of locally available services, and to ensure appropriate utilization of high-cost specialist services. Although it

was once unusual for paediatric patients to receive cancer treatment within primary or secondary services, in some areas shared care involving these providers is now well established, and local care provision is now a guiding principle informing the organization of cancer services. 'Wherever possible effective and appropriate cancer services should be provided within a patient's home or as close to their home as is feasible.'[6]

For the purposes of this chapter, shared care is defined as a planned arrangement for clinical management whereby specialist paediatric oncology centres and local children's services jointly participate in the provision of childhood cancer care. Within the UK National Health Service, shared care arrangements in paediatric oncology are based on a 'hub and spoke' model[7] involving a paediatric oncology centre (POC), paediatric oncology shared care units (POSCUs) in district general hospitals, and community and/or primary care teams (Figure 34.1).

There is a lack of evidence related to the outcomes of shared medical management of childhood cancer. A single study of children with acute lymphoblastic leukaemia (ALL) reported that prognosis was not affected by a policy of shared care with paediatricians working in district general hospitals.[8] A small number of papers describe strategies that may support shared care practice, including clinical management guidelines, information packs for general practitioners,[9] parent-held records,[10] joint outreach clinics and educational programmes.[11] The role of the paediatric oncology outreach nurse specialist (POONS) has been cited as one that potentially supports

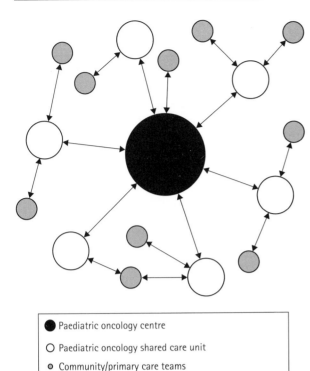

● Paediatric oncology centre

○ Paediatric oncology shared care unit

◉ Community/primary care teams

↕ Two-way movement of patients between care providers

Figure 34.1 *Hub and spoke model of shared care.*

developments in all these areas, and some evaluation of these roles has been undertaken.[12–14]

A number of potential problems related to shared care have been reported; continuity of care, conflicting advice, and differences in procedures have been cited as examples,[15] and it has been suggested that ineffective shared care can leave families feeling isolated, insecure and vulnerable.[14] A factor in determining success has been postulated to be whether a 'critical mass' (related to workload) of oncology experience is maintained at shared care units.[16] However, much of the evidence is anecdotal and represents the opinions of individual practitioners or centres.

In the absence of published evaluation of shared care in paediatric oncology, it is worth identifying where lessons may be learnt from other areas. The most extensive body of evidence relates to integrated primary and secondary level care in the management of chronic physical conditions such as asthma, diabetes and hypertension in adults. The main findings of these studies are summarized below. However, evaluation of the impact of different organizational models on disease outcomes is difficult,[17] and in studies designed to compare treatment outcomes, the contribution made by the method of care delivery is usually disregarded.

- If treatment is shared in an ad hoc or unstructured fashion, patient outcomes may be adversely affected in comparison to specialist-only care,[18,19] but well coordinated shared care can offer equally good, and

sometimes improved, outcomes compared with traditional methods.[20,21]

- Patients may initially have reservations about the involvement of non-specialists, but many evaluate shared care programmes positively once they have experienced them, notably in terms of convenience, ease of access to medical advice and relationships with local service providers.[20,21]
- Shared care systems can offer potential cost savings for both health services and patients, but these depend upon the organizational arrangements of individual providers.[19,21]

Teenagers with cancer – a particular challenge for shared care

The needs of teenagers with cancer present further challenges for service provision through shared care. For many teenagers and young adults, the care provided in paediatric or adult cancer settings is largely unsuitable, and there are proposals for dedicated teenage units[22,23] and for community staff to have specific training in their care needs.[24] Yet this group represents a small minority of cancer patients, and to date there are only a few professionals who specialize in adolescent health care, and limited training opportunities. In addition, the 'cut-off' age for many paediatric hospital and community services is 16 years, and over this age, involvement of adult primary and secondary care services will be required. These services may have different pressures, priorities and working practices from children's teams, and, as many adult cancer units will not be familiar with paediatric treatment protocols due to the infrequency of their involvement, abandoning shared care in favour of treatment in the paediatric or adolescent oncology centre may appear the only option. Opportunities exist for motivated paediatric and adult cancer teams to share the management of these patients, and patient-specific care packages that identify key-worker and consultative roles of paediatric and adult, generalist, cancer and palliative care practitioners are perhaps the best way forward.[24]

PROFESSIONAL ROLES WITHIN THE SHARED CARE MODEL

The challenges of managing the patient pathway within the matrix of service provision should not be underestimated. Coordination of care is essential to delivering a seamless service, and this requires effective collaboration between the many health care professionals involved, with clear lines of communication. Clarifying responsibility and accountability for aspects of patient and family care is vital to ensure that patient safety and standards of care are maintained. This requires effort to understand and address negative perceptions that may exist within and across institutional boundaries and the health care disciplines.

The paediatric oncology centre

Investigation, diagnosis and staging, cancer, the delivery of complex cancer treatment, including radiotherapy, monitoring of treatment response and cancer research will be undertaken within the paediatric oncology centre. In addition, this is the appropriate setting for high-risk, high-dependency, complex supportive care and management of the critically ill child. Provision of information about diagnosis and treatment, and patient or parent teaching, e.g. about managing central venous access devices, monitoring blood counts and care of the child at home, are usually the remit of specialist nursing staff at the centre, although it should be remembered that learning continues throughout treatment and local teams may be required to continue or reinforce teaching or clarify misconceptions. For these reasons, local teams need access to copies of information booklets and explicit information about details of diagnosis and prognosis that have been given to families.

Establishing psychosocial support for children, teenagers and their families provided by specialist allied health professionals is a particularly valuable role for the paediatric oncology centre specialist team, especially around the time of diagnosis or recurrence. This provides the foundations of psychosocial care upon which the family can rely throughout treatment and beyond, although they may also be able to access local support services that will work in tandem with the specialist teams. The clinical psychologist, social worker, play therapist, schoolteacher and hospital chaplain will be able to describe their roles in relation to children and families receiving shared care. Often they will have links with their local counterparts and be able to explain how they communicate and cooperate with each other. Similarly, in well functioning shared care networks, the dietician, physiotherapist and other allied health professionals will have established working practices with local services to appropriately support recipients of shared care, and these should be explained to families.

It is important that the specialist team describes the operation of shared care to families at the start of treatment, giving practical examples about what aspects of care will be undertaken in which setting. This relies upon the POC team having a genuine understanding of, and demonstrating confidence in, the teams who provide local care. The provision of information about local services and contact details provides families with some security as they prepare for discharge. Family members may have initial misgivings about returning to the shared care unit, and this is often based on the fact that at diagnosis they were referred to the centre, interpreting this as evidence of the local team's inability to care for children with cancer. The consultant paediatric oncologist should clearly explain that they retain overall responsibility for the child's cancer treatment, and that this is not affected by the fact that some care may be given locally. Families often find it a challenge to transfer their trust from specialist to local teams, and any steps that can be taken to provide information and give evidence of teamwork between shared care partners will demonstrate both acknowledgement of families' concerns and support of local colleagues. Families need to have realistic expectations of local services, so that differences in routines and practices are not misinterpreted as a failure in local care. Families should be encouraged to voice their concerns, and any reported difficult experiences explored with shared care colleagues at an early stage, to enable parents to develop confidence in the system.

The role of the paediatric oncology outreach nurse (POON) is to work alongside hospital and community health and social care practitioners. In relation to shared care, the aim is to provide families with ongoing support from the point of diagnosis, throughout treatment and beyond, to coordinate transitions between care settings and to support the integration of specialist cancer care at the tertiary centre with secondary and primary care. For the child who requires palliative care when the child and family wish to remain at home, the POON can assist in facilitating community and primary health care to attain this outcome. A primary role within the delivery of care for the POON is to 'empower' primary and community professionals with the knowledge and skills required in caring for the child in the community.[14] This is described below with reference to specific community and primary care team members.

There is role diversity in the functions of the POON in differing parts of the UK. Hunt,[14,35] in a study of the working practices of the POON, found that while some provided a 'hands-on' approach (carrying out specialist care in the community), others provide a 'hands off' approach (facilitating specialist care, carried out by others). The latter model of care has been greatly facilitated by the increased number and expertise of children's community nursing (CCN) teams.

The paediatric oncology shared care unit

The principle of integrating aspects of a patient's cancer treatment near to a patient's home with units that are equipped with the necessary knowledge and skills in the delivery of supportive care was stressed by the Expert Advisory Group on Cancer.[6] From the family's perspective, evidence of integration between the shared care unit and the oncology centre begins at initial referral. It is important that the child and family are informed of the potential

Box 34.1 *Policy on chickenpox contact and use of VZIG (varicella zoster immunoglobulin)*

Definition of significant exposure to varicella zoster		
Index case	Timing of exposure	Duration of exposure
Clinical chicken pox and disseminated zoster (incubation period 14–21 days from contact; infectious period 48 hours before rash and until all vesicles are dry)	48 hours before rash until all lesions have crusted	Contact in same room for 15 minutes Face to face contact
Shingles or localized zoster	Day of onset of rash until all lesions have crusted	Contact in same room for 15 minutes Face to face contact

Who gets VZIG?

- All immunocompromised persons without a history of chickenpox are known to be VZV IgG-negative or equivocal
- Immunocompromised children known to be VZV IgG-positive should have their VZV IgG re-tested as close to the date of exposure as possible (no later than 7 days from contact). If this is negative or equivocal, VZIG IgG should be given
- Patients undergoing transplantation who have received many transfusions or immunoglobulin may have acquired VZ antibody passively; these patients do not need VZIG if antibody is detected at the time of exposure
- Patients with bleeding disorders who cannot receive an intramuscular injection should be given intravenous normal immunoglobulin
- Patients who have received VZIG should be isolated for up to 28 days after exposure, to protect susceptible patients and staff
- Acyclovir prophylaxis should start at day 10 of contact for 4 weeks for patients who are particularly high-risk, e.g. conditioning for bone marrow transplant or surgery within 4 weeks
- The child and family should be informed that VZIG will not prevent acquiring chickenpox but should reduce the morbidity and provide a degree of protection for up to 3 weeks

diagnosis (using the term cancer or tumour, to prevent misunderstanding) and what will occur as part of the diagnostic procedures prior to attendance at the cancer centre.

In general, where shared care operates, supportive care, such as management of febrile neutropenic episodes, thrombocytopenia and anaemia, occurs within secondary services, together with any other aspect of physical supportive care requiring in-patient admission. Many shared care units are able to administer simple outpatient chemotherapy to children who are established on treatment regimens, particularly continuing therapy for ALL.[25] A smaller number have the resources to offer more complex day-case or in-patient chemotherapy care, with the explicit agreement of the oncology centre. Timely, accurate and comprehensive communication is required between shared care units and oncology centres, specifically relating to adjustments to doses, disease control and toxicity. Return of clinical trials data is a particular responsibility where aspects of children's cancer treatment are shared.

The role of supportive care in reducing treatment-related mortality is now recognized as a vital component of care.[26,27] This includes the prevention and management of infections following the administration of chemotherapy. Infectious diseases were once a relatively common problem for the patient during cancer treatment, particularly chickenpox and measles.[28] Treatment-related deaths from infectious diseases such as

Pneumocystis carinii and measles decreased from 6 per cent in 1980 to 1 per cent in 1997 for children treated for ALL within MRC UKALL trials.[29] Chickenpox (varicella) and shingles (herpes zoster) carry significant mortality for patients during treatment and up to 6–12 months following completion of treatment. Close contact with siblings in the home and children at school means these sites can be the sources of the highest level of exposure to chickenpox and measles.

A universal policy on chickenpox contact and VZIG (varicella zoster immunoglobulin) has been provided by the Royal College of Paediatrics and Child Health (2000) (see Box 34.1).[30]

Shared care in the community

The benefits of community care for children and teenagers with malignancy are numerous (Box 34.2). One potential drawback is that health care professionals within the community may be less familiar with the specific needs, assessment and management required for children and teenagers receiving cancer treatments, creating a sense of insecurity and vulnerability for families.[12] Where shared care is in operation, it is imperative that efforts are made to ensure that non-specialists in the community can acquire the necessary knowledge and

Box 34.2 *The benefits of community care*

- The psychological trauma that is associated with repeated and prolonged periods of hospitalization for children is minimized[31]
- A reduced risk of infection with resistant hospital microbiological flora[32]
- The potential for disruption to family life is reduced. For example, children are able to return to school during treatment and the parents can return to work[33]
- Home care enhances a family's sense of normality, which, in turn, is conducive to the child's well-being[34]

expertise, and that everyone understands the unique, equally important roles of the generalist and the specialist team members, as well as the relationship between the key players.

Continuing care such as blood sampling to monitor full blood count, assessment of nutritional status and surveillance of general health and education, and meeting palliative care needs occur within the community delivered by primary and community staff.

The primary health care team

In the UK, primary health teams are composed of the general practitioner (GP), district nurse (DN), practice nurse and health visitor (HV), based in a local health centre. Primary care services are usually the first contact with health services for families of children with cancer and therefore form the basis of their experience at a uniquely vulnerable time. Prompt referral for investigation that will provide a diagnosis of childhood cancer and access to treatment is therefore important both to ensure optimum care and to maintain the family's confidence in their GP, and the health care system as a whole.

An individual GP may encounter perhaps one child or teenager with cancer throughout their career. The GP's knowledge of the variety and specificity of presentations of malignant disease at this stage may understandably be limited, particularly as these symptoms may be, at first, indistinguishable from more common and less significant childhood ailments. Many children with cancer present to the GP with subtle symptoms.[36] Such symptoms, e.g. lethargy, fatigue, easy bruising, loss of appetite and viral type illnesses, can lead to patients and families being referred to the cancer centre with lengthy histories of repeated visits to the GP. Parents frequently seek medical advice from a GP only after first exploring over-the-counter medications or non-pharmaceutical

strategies.[37] Therefore, for parents/carers to take their child to a GP is of significance. Many parents report disputes with their GP due to a perceived delay in obtaining a diagnosis. To reduce this, it is recommended that medical practitioners within primary or secondary services should do the following if faced with repeated concern:[38]

- If no abnormality is found after examination of the child, explain this to the parents, but also stress and be prepared to examine the child again if the symptom persists.
- Always take seriously parents who state that, although they do not know what is wrong, they know their child is 'not right'.
- Beware of categorically telling parents nothing is wrong with their child.
- Note how often the child has been seen. If after a few visits nothing can be found, consider asking a colleague or paediatrician to see the child.

Following a cancer diagnosis, the role of the GP during the child's treatment can often appear somewhat insignificant, yet in supporting parents, siblings and extended family, primary care can play an important role. Faulkner *et al.*[39] explored the challenges facing family members during a child's diagnosis and treatment, and found that a diversity of meanings exist, shaped by past experience of cancer, culture and knowledge. Thus, it is pivotal that the paediatric oncologist informs the GP of the patient's diagnosis promptly, and keeps him or her updated throughout treatment about the child's progress and significant events. In the UK, responsibility for in-depth liaison with the GP lies with the POON, and should occur as soon as the diagnosis has been confirmed. Establishing a good relationship between the GP, the family and the POON will become particularly crucial if the child eventually requires terminal care.

The GP, with ongoing responsibility for the health care of the whole family, has a role in supporting informed consent in relation to uptake of immunizations. High uptake from 1988 for the combined vaccination against measles, mumps and rubella (MMR)[40] reduced the cases of measles within the community, with reported knock-on effects in terms of cases and mortality in children with cancer. Yet with a reduction in uptake rates of MMR since 1997,[41] there is concern that a rise in confirmed cases may occur. It is essential that families be advised to immunize the child's siblings as per the immunization schedule and for primary health care staff to continue health education programmes to maintain and support herd immunity within communities. Guidelines for immunization during and following standard treatment and for children following intensive chemotherapy regimens (allogeneic haemopoietic stem cell transplant/ rescue) have been provided by the Royal College of Paediatrics and Child Health.[30] These are being followed by the regional children's cancer centres within the UK for all immunocompromised children during treatment and following cessation of treatment (see Box 34.3 for outline of practice).

The health visitor

The role of health visitors in the UK was once to focus predominantly on preventative care and health education especially for families where there were children under 5 years of age.[42] Now, as well as supporting the

Box 34.3 *Guidelines for immunizations in children following cancer treatment*

Immunizations during and until 6 months after completion of standard treatment
- All children who are immunocompromised must not receive live vaccines during cancer treatment and for the following 6 months after cessation of treatment. This will include MMR, oral polio vaccine (OPV), Bacille Calmette–Guérin (BCG), oral typhoid and yellow fever. Inactivated polio vaccine (IPV) can be administered in place of OPV.
- Influenza vaccine is recommended annually in the autumn for all patients receiving chemotherapy, and for those still within 6 months of completion of chemotherapy.

Immunizations 6 months and later after completing treatment
- At 6 months following completion of treatment, administer an additional booster of diphtheria, tetanus, acellular pertussis, IPV, Hib, MeningoC and MMR. Subsequent routine booster doses (e.g. pre-school) will not be necessary if they are scheduled to be given within 1 year of this additional dose.
- If the patient has previously had BCG and is considered to be in a high-risk group for tuberculosis, check tuberculin test and, if negative, revaccinate. If patient has not previously had BCG, immunize according to local policy. Ensure that the primary health care team is informed.
- Varicella zoster is not routinely administered within the UK.

HLA-identical sibling donor allogeneic or syngeneic haemopoietic stem cell transplantation (HSCT)
- At 12 months post-HSCT, administer:
  - diphtheria, tetanus, acellular pertussis: three doses at monthly intervals
  - IPV: three doses at monthly intervals
  - Hib: three doses at monthly intervals
  - MeningoC: three doses at monthly intervals
- At 15 months post-HSCT, administer:
  - pneumococcal vaccine: give conjugate vaccine initially, followed by polysaccharide vaccine once the child is 24 months post-HSCT
  - if the child is under 24 months of age, give three doses of conjugate vaccine at monthly intervals (NB. polysaccharide vaccine to follow later)
- At 18 months and 24 months post-HSCT, administer:
  - MMR (providing that they have been off all immunosuppressive treatment for at least 12 months)
  - these two doses should usually be given with a minimum 6-month interval, but the second dose can be given 4 weeks after the first in the event of a measles outbreak
- At 24 months post-HSCT, administer:
  - polysaccharide pneumococcal vaccine: one dose
- Every autumn, administer:
  - influenza vaccine (for as long as the patient remains clinically immunocompromised or is considered to be at increased risk from influenza virus infection)

Any other allogeneic HSCT
- Re-immunization schedule as above, but starting and continuing 6 months later (i.e. starting at 18 months post-HSCT)

Re-immunization of autologous HSCT recipients
- Re-immunization programme should commence 1 year after an autologous HSCT; the schedule is identical to that for HLA-identical sibling donor allogeneic or syngeneic HSCT (see above)

child and family with cancer, their important function involves health promotion and health education in collaboration with fellow members of the primary health care team.[43] It is the role of the POON to make contact with a family's HV to inform them of the diagnosis and planned treatment strategies. The HV will play a key role for children who experience developmental difficulties due to the diagnosis and/or side-effects of the cancer treatment, facilitating early referral to appropriate agencies, such as Portage training and the community paediatrician. In addition, HVs can help to support families in the home by organizing practical support such as voluntary babysitters, home help or family aid through social services, or by providing psychological support.

The community team

The multidisciplinary teams in the community setting have important roles in children's cancer care. In the UK, a community children's team may comprise personnel from health and social care, educational services and the voluntary sector, and include children's community nurses (CCNs), a community paediatrician, school nurse, schoolteachers, allied health professionals and lay carers. The availability of multidisciplinary team members and the constitution of teams demonstrate marked geographical variation. Community teams may provide home care for all groups of children, although teams also exist that have a specific remit for the care of children with life-limiting or life-threatening conditions, and may be organizationally related to hospice services. Coordinating the input from members of these teams, to provide the best possible package of appropriate, knowledgeable and skilled care for individual children with cancer and their families, is a particular responsibility of the POON.

In the UK, the care of the sick child in the home environment has only been made possible because of the increase in CCNs.[44] CCNs are educated firstly to become children's nurses and then undertake specialist children's community nurse training.[45] The proliferation of POONs and the development of CCN roles have significantly influenced decisions about the provision of children's cancer care in the UK. The existence of experienced children's nurses in the community has made possible the safe early discharge of children, e.g. during the early phase of induction treatment. It is now not unusual for a child with a diagnosis of ALL to be discharged home as early as 5–7 days after treatment has begun. Teamwork between all the shared care partners is required if these families are to receive optimum emotional and informational support out of hospital, as well as assuring the child's safety and welfare.

The existence of the POON and CCN has also enabled certain technical aspects of cancer treatments to be given in the child's home, by either a POON or a CCN with appropriate knowledge and skills. Additionally, parental involvement in some aspects of their child's care has become common practice. It has now become routine in some areas for children with established central venous access to undergo blood sampling,[46] and receive intravenous antibiotics, antiemetics and chemotherapy in the home when it is safe, acceptable and feasible to do so.[47–49] Parents can receive training to manage their child's central venous access device, insert nasogastric tubes and set up enteral feeds, administer oral chemotherapy, intravenous chemotherapy and intravenous antibiotics. Despite this increased responsibility, a study by Hooker and Kohler of parents who undertook training and provided intravenous therapy to their child at home reported benefits to family life.[47] Carefully coordinated input from the POON, and community and primary health care teams in providing emotional and nursing support at home may ensure that children are cared for safely in the home, and that parents are not pressurized to undertake complex home care, nor overburdened by their decision to do so.

It is predominantly the responsibility of the POON to initiate a referral to the CCN, although this may be done by other professionals, depending on local service configuration and practice. Joint home visits by the POON and CCN following the child's diagnosis can assist in planning individualized family-centred care and provide an opportunity for education and training in relation to the child's condition, treatment and expected progress, and about specific nursing interventions required. These activities will enhance clarification of roles for both the professionals and the family, facilitate team-working and provide explicit evidence of collaboration to all parties involved in the child's care.

Physical disability related to some cancers, such as brain and spinal tumours and osteosarcomas, may require assessment and advice regarding adjustment of living arrangements and school establishments by the physiotherapist and occupational therapist. Practical aids such as wheelchairs, toilet and bathing equipment can be provided. The psychological trauma of living with a life-threatening condition may require interventions from the child psychologist, psychiatrist and social support provided by social workers. Respite care offered by voluntary organizations can reduce family stress and anxiety and assist with household chores, and a befriending service may be available. In many communities, youth workers and spiritual leaders can be a valuable source of support. Referral to a member of the team can occur through a POON, the children's community nursing service, members of the multidisciplinary team at the cancer centre or through the primary health care team, depending upon the specific resources available in each child's community. To avoid duplications, it is important to establish which key professional will make referrals in partnership with the child and family members.

EDUCATIONAL ISSUES FOR THE CHILD WITH CANCER

Education plays a vital role throughout a child's formative years. For those children who miss significant periods of schooling due to repeated or prolonged hospital admissions, the role of the hospital-based teacher is vital. Some children may require home tuition during and following cancer treatment, e.g. those who have undergone bone marrow transplantation procedures in whom prolonged profound immune suppression will delay the return to school. Early school re-integration wherever possible is widely accepted to be the best option in relation to both education and social outcomes, but this can present something of a challenge to achieve. A child may develop changes in self-image because of the impact of the disease and the physical consequences of treatment. This may lead to the child opting out of the educational system, which can be traumatic in the short term and have detrimental consequences throughout that child's life. Schoolteachers may also be diffident in accepting children with cancer back into the classroom and may not have appropriately high expectations in terms of their survival or educational achievement. The POON or CCN can assist in reducing the anxiety associated with a child's return to school, by liaising with the school and (with the parent's consent) sharing information regarding the diagnosis, treatment and the possible physical, psychological and social side-effects that the child may experience. It is the role of the POON and/or the CCN to assist families in informing the child's nursery, playgroup, school or college of the precautions related to chickenpox or measles exposure, if needed. Referral by the POON/CCN to the school nursing service is important. Health surveillance and health education for the pupil while in the educational system[50] can play an important role in advising the teaching team, and supporting the child with cancer to return to, and maintain attendance at, school.

Neutropenia is not, in itself, universally considered to be a reason for children to stay away from school as long as they are physically well, their teachers know to respond if they become unwell, and a parent can be contacted to collect their child from school in a timely manner. Treatment-related fatigue is to be expected, and this may be a limiting factor to children attending full time.

Some children will have particularly significant challenges in maintaining their education and fulfilling their potential. For the child with a brain tumour who has received radiotherapy and surgery, the associated morbidity of physical disability and cognitive developmental delay will mean that specialized teaching input may be required.[51] In the UK, such children may need to have a formal assessment of special educational needs, in order to receive the additional educational support they require. Referral to the community paediatrician will be required to assist in this process and to monitor the child's 'special' needs during the school years.

ORGANIZATIONAL ISSUES

In order for shared care systems to deliver continuity and consistency in approach and clinical care across organizational and team boundaries, a number of organizational strategies and structures are required. Families' negative experiences of shared care are often related to inconsistencies they notice between care providers, in terms of specialist knowledge, facilities and the details of clinical procedures. All professional partners collaborating in shared care arrangements have a responsibility to take steps to minimize these differences. It is proposed here that the POC, with overall responsibility for the quality of care,[52] should take a lead in determining the expectations of shared care arrangements, and take active steps to support local teams in the development of expertise and services. Local teams who undertake shared care are accountable for the care they provide and, as such, for ensuring that staff have the necessary knowledge and clinical expertise, and securing resources and management recognition and support to provide safe, appropriate oncology care to the agreed level.

Communication

During a child's treatment, the centre must provide shared care units with clear treatment plans and accurate, up-to-date information, most crucially about any alterations to the planned treatment, such as dose reductions or other clinical management problems. Use of e-mail, fax and patient-held records[10] can provide a useful supplement to telephone contact and written correspondence. The centre team has a responsibility to provide 24-hour specialist telephone advice and support to shared care colleagues and families, and this should be reflected in a centre's staffing levels and on-call arrangements. Staff in shared care units should be encouraged to ask for advice and, in particular, discuss any sick children at an early stage, to ensure appropriate management and to expedite timely admission to the centre if their clinical condition requires specialist care. It is helpful to identify communication routes and people to contact regarding specific aspects of care, and the interaction between teams should be characterized by willingness to collaborate, a shared concern for patients and genuine two-way communication.

Education and training

There is an obvious need for the providers of the different components of shared care to have the expertise to enable the delivery of high-quality care. Continuing professional development activities for medical, nursing and allied health professionals should be relevant to the roles and responsibilities that they are undertaking. There is a need for training programmes in general paediatric oncology care, and for specific skills such as:

- management of central venous access devices
- cytotoxic chemotherapy administration
- supportive and palliative care.

It can be argued that provision of training for shared care practice should be the responsibility of the specialist team, and it may well be that the resources to do so cost-effectively can only exist within the paediatric oncology centre. It is clearly the responsibility of the oncology centre team to ensure that shared care colleagues have an opportunity to update their knowledge and skills, particularly in relation to changes in practice and new treatment regimens.

Clinical management guidelines

The development of clinical management guidelines can support the practice and decision-making of non-specialists. A comprehensive guide containing sound clinical advice, based on robust evidence where available, provided to all practitioners and updated annually to ensure currency is a prerequisite to the specialists' extended sphere of clinical accountability that is obligatory in shared care. Additionally, practical information regarding organizational and administrative issues can aid clear, appropriate communication between shared care partners. Guidelines should stress the importance of timely, appropriate clinical intervention, communication and discussion of clinical progress with the paediatric oncology centre team, and reinforce the 24-hour availability of specialist advice and retrieval of a sick child back to the specialist centre should this be necessary. Content may include:

- initial management of the child with suspected cancer, prior to referral to the specialist centre
- administration of chemotherapy to agreed protocols, as agreed with the specialist centre, including

prevention and management of chemotherapy-related side-effects such as nausea and vomiting
- supportive care related to the disease or treatment – monitoring of bone marrow suppression, blood product support, management of neutropenic fever and infections such as chickenpox and measles contact, *Pneumocystis carinii* pneumonia, fluid and electrolyte imbalance and nutritional support
- guidance related to pain management and other palliative care issues – this may also be included, to encourage consistency of approaches when children receive treatment in different care settings.

The oncology handbook may usefully contain outlines of procedural practice, in order to encourage consistency between care providers, e.g.:

- management of central venous access devices, blood sampling and exit-site care
- administration of cytotoxic chemotherapy, including home chemotherapy
- use of syringe-drivers in palliative care.

Organizational guidelines

In addition to clinical management guidelines, shared care partner organizations could usefully develop agreed practices for the operational management of care across each group of care providers that constitute a clinical network for paediatric oncology services, e.g.:

- defined roles and responsibilities of paediatric oncology centre and shared care units
- criteria for selecting patients for whom shared care is appropriate – these may be clinical, psychosocial or organizational and may include a child's age, diagnosis, treatment regimen, family circumstances or geographical location
- agreements regarding levels of care to be undertaken, or expected of specific providers, appropriate to the requirements of different patient groups and the available resources[16]
- communication routes and expected standards and practices.

On a larger scale, development of national service standards, in line with those available for adult cancer services in the UK, could provide a framework to guide clinicians and managers to develop high-quality integrated care, and a sound basis upon which to make decisions about resource allocation and service configuration. However, the credibility of such organizational standards for systems of shared care will be dependent on obtaining evidence about its clinical and cost-effectiveness, which is negligible at present. Models of shared care delivery should reflect the needs, priorities and responsibilities of all those involved – health and social care professionals, health care purchasers and providers, and, crucially, the service users: children and teenagers with cancer and their families.

KEY POINTS

- Centralized, specialist care has played a significant role in the dramatically improved outcomes for children with cancer, but can have negative psychosocial consequences for families and is expensive for service providers.
- Systems of shared care have been developed in an attempt to combine the survival gains of centralized treatment with the practical and social advantages of local care and best use of health care resources.
- Successful shared care requires clinical, organizational and professional motivation, and significant effort by all parties involved, to deliver high-quality family-focused services across organizational boundaries.
- There is a pressing need for high-quality research to evaluate the outcomes of shared care in paediatric oncology.
- Ultimately, the success of any system of shared care depends on professionals' willingness and commitment to the venture, which can be gained by reinforcing the value of all partners' contributions, and agreement on organization, development and information-sharing.[53]

REFERENCES

1. Stiller C. Centralisation of treatment and survival rates for cancer. *Arch Dis Child* 1988; **63**: 23–30.
2. Hollis R. Childhood cancer into the 21st century. *Paediatr Nurs* 1997; **9**: 12–15.
3. Bodkin CM, Pigott TJ, Mann JR. Financial burden of childhood cancer. *Br Med J* 1982; **284**: 1542–4.
4. Lansky S, Cairns N, Clark G, Lowman J *et al.* Childhood cancer: non-medical cost of the illness. *Cancer* 1979; **43**: 403–8.
5. Bignold S, Cribb A, Ball S. *Nursing Families of Children with Cancer: the Work of the Paediatric Oncology Outreach Nurse Specialists.* A report to Cancer Relief Macmillan Fund and the Department of Health. London: Kings College, 1994.
6. Expert Advisory Group on Cancer. *A Policy Framework for Commissioning Cancer Services.* London: Department of Health, 1995.
7. Ham C, Smith J, Temple J. *Hubs, Spokes and Policy Cycles.* London: King's Fund, 1998.
8. Muir K, Parkes S, Boon R *et al.* Shared care in paediatric oncology. *J Cancer Care* 1992; **1**: 15–17.
9. James JA, Harris DJ, Mott MG, Oakhill A. Paediatric oncology information pack for General Practitioners. *Br Med J* 1988; **296**: 97–8.
10. Hooker L, Williams J. Parent-held shared care records: bridging the communication gaps. *Br J Nurs* 1996; **5**: 738–41.
11. Hooker L, Milburn M. Taking practice forward in paediatric oncology: the impact of a newly-developed education programme for nurses working in shared care hospitals. *Eur J Oncol Nurs* 200; **4**: 48–52.
12. Bignold S, Cribb A, Ball S. Creating a 'seamless web of care' – the work of paediatric oncology outreach nurse specialist. In: Richardson A, Wilson-Barnett J, eds. *Nursing Research in Cancer Care.* London: Scutari Press, 1995; 67–79.
13. Evans M, Kelly P. Bringing support home for families of children with cancer. *Br J Nurs* 1995; **4**: 395–8.
14. Hunt JA. Empowering health care professionals: a relationship between primary health care teams and paediatric oncology outreach nurse specialists. *Eur J Oncol Nurs* 1998; **2**: 27–33.
15. Gibson F, Williams J. Network of care for children and teenagers with cancer: an overview for adult cancer nurses. *J Cancer Nurs* 1997; **1**: 200–7.
16. Patel N, Sepion B, Williams J. Development of a shared care programme for children with cancer. *J Cancer Nurs* 1997; **1**: 147–50.
17. Eastwood AJ, Sheldon TA. Organisation of asthma care: what difference does it make? A systematic review of the literature. *Qual Health Care* 1996; **5**: 134–43.
18. Hayes TM, Harries J. Randomised controlled trial of routine clinical care versus routine general practice care for type 2 diabetes. *Br Med J* 1984; **289**: 728–30.
19. Day JL, Humphreys H, Alban-Davies H. Problems of comprehensive shared diabetes care. *Br Med J* 1987; **294**: 1590–2.
20. Grampian Asthma Study of Integrated Care (GRASSIC). Integrated care for asthma: a clinical, social and economic evaluation. *Br Med J* 1994; **308**: 559–64.
21. DICET (Diabetes Integrated Care Evaluation Team). Integrated care for diabetes: clinical, psychosocial and economic evaluation. *Br Med J* 1994; **308**: 1208–12.
22. Barrett A. Where should patients be treated? In: Selby P, Bailey C, eds. *Cancer and the Adolescent.* London: BMJ Publishing Group, 1996; 242–50.
23. Souhami RL, Whelan J, McCarthy JF, Kilby A. Benefits and problems of an adolescent unit. In: Selby P, Bailey C, eds. *Cancer and the Adolescent.* London: BMJ Publishing Group, 1996; 276–83.
24. Edwards J. A model of care for the adolescent with cancer. *Int J Palliat Care.* 2001; **7**: 485–8.
25. Chessels JM. Maintenance treatment and shared care in lymphoblastic leukaemia. *Arch Dis Child* 1993; **73**: 368–73.
26. Lampert F, Henze G. Acute lymphoblastic leukaemia. In: Pinkerton CR, Plowman PN, eds. *Paediatric Oncology. Clinical Practice & Controversies.* London: Chapman & Hall Medical, 1997; 258–77.
27. Chessells J. Recent advances in management of acute leukaemia. *Arch Dis Child* 2000; **82**: 438–42.

28. Lowis SP, Oakhill A. Management of acute complications of therapy. In: Pinkerton CR, Plowman PN, eds. *Paediatric Oncology. Clinical Practice & Controversies:* London: Chapman & Hall Medical, 1997; 677–705.

29. Hargrave DR, Hann IM, Richards SM *et al.* Progressive reduction in treatment-related deaths in medical research council childhood lymphoblastic leukaemia trials from 1980 to 1997 (UKALL VIII, X and XI). *Br J Haematol* 2001; **112**: 293–9.

30. Royal College of Paediatrics and Child Health. *Immunisation of the Immunocompromised Child: Best Practice Statement.* London: RCPCH, 2002.

31. Muller DJ, Harris PJ, Wattley L. *Nursing Children: Psychology Research and Practice.* London: Harper and Row Publishers, 1986.

32. Campbell S, Glasper EA. *Children's Nursing.* London: Mosby, 1995.

33. Hooker L, Palmer S. Administration of chemotherapy. In Gibson F, Evans M, eds. *Paediatric Oncology. Acute Nursing Care.* London: Whurr, 1999: 22–58.

34. While AE. An evaluation of a paediatric home care scheme. *J Adv Nurs* 1991; **16**: 1413-21.

35. Hunt JA. The paediatric community nurse specialist: the influence of employment location and funders on models of practice. *J Adv Nurs* 1995; **22**: 126–33.

36. Holland M. Paediatric cancer: does primary care help or hinder? *Cancer Services Insight* (www.totalhealthcaremedia.com), 2001.

37. Neill S. Acute childhood illness at home: the parent's perspective. *J Adv Nurs* 2000; **31**: 821–32.

38. Dixon-Woods M, Findlay M, Young B *et al.* Parents' account of obtaining a diagnosis of childhood cancer. *Lancet* 2001; **357**: 670–4.

39. Faulkner A, Peace G, O'Keeffe C. *When a Child Has Cancer.* London: Chapman and Hall, 1995.

40. Salisbury D, Begg N. *Immunisation against Infectious Diseases.* London: The Stationery Office, 1996.

41. Lunts E, Cowper D. Parents refusing MMR: do GPs and health visitors understand why? *Community Pract* 2002; **75**: 94–6.

42. Robertson C. *Health Visiting in Practice.* London: Churchill Livingstone, 1998.

43. Hall D. Change, continuity and function of the community health visitor. *Community Pract* 2000; **73**: 870–2.

44. Whiting M. 1888–1988: 100 years of community children's nursing. In: Muir J, Sidley A, eds. *Textbook of Community Children's Nursing.* London: Baillière Tindall, 2000: 15–31.

45. Livesey P. Setting the agenda for education. In: Muir J, Sidley A, eds. *Textbook of Community Children's Nursing.* London: Baillière Tindall, 2000: 85–99.

46. Bravery K. Paediatric intravenous therapy in practice. In: Dougherty L, Lamb J, eds. *Intravenous Therapy in Nursing Practice.* London: Churchill Livingstone, 1999; 401–45.

47. Hooker L, Kohler J. Safety, efficacy, and acceptability of home intravenous therapy administered by parents of pediatric oncology patients. *Med Pediatr Oncol* 1999; **32**: 421–6.

48. RCN. *Administering Intravenous Therapy to Children in the Community Setting.* London: Royal College of Nursing, 2001.

49. Edwards J, Breen M. Administration of intravenous chemotherapy for children & teenagers with cancer in the home. *Cancer Nurs Pract* 2002; **1**(5): 26–9.

50. Farrow S. The role of the school nurse in promoting health. In: Scriven A, Orme J, eds. *Health Promotion: Professional Perspectives.* London: Open University Press, 1996; 144–56.

51. Zucchinelli V, Bouffett E. Academic future of children treated for brain tumours. Single-center study of 27 children. *Arch Pediatr* 2000; **7**: 933–41.

52. United Kingdom Children's Cancer Study Group. *The Resources and Requirements of a UKCCSG Treatment Centre.* Leicester: UKCCSG, 1997.

53. Van Damme R, Drummond N, Beattie J, Douglass G. Integrated care for patients with asthma: views of general practitioners. *Br J Gen Pract* 1994; **44**: 9–13.

Index